DIABETO-CARDIOLOGY

A Companion to **BRAUNWALD'S**

HEART DISEASE

CARDIOLOGY

A Companion to BRAUNWALD'S
HEART DISEASE

EDITION
2

DARREN K. McGUIRE, MD, MHSc, FAHA, FESC

Professor of Internal Medicine-Cardiology
University of Texas Southwestern Medical Center
Parkland Health System
Dallas, Texas

NIKOLAUS MARX, MD, FESC, FAHA

Professor of Medicine/Cardiology
Head of the Department of Internal Medicine I
University Hospital Aachen
Aachen, Germany

ELSEVIER

Elsevier
1600 John F. Kennedy Blvd.
Ste 1800
Philadelphia, PA 19103-2899

DIABETO-CARDIOLOGY: A COMPANION TO BRAUNWALD'S HEART DISEASE, SECOND EDITION ISBN: 978-0-323-87862-3

Senior Content Strategist: Melanie Tucker
Senior Content Development Specialist: Vasowati Shome
Publishing Services Manager: Deepthi Unni
Project Manager: Nayagi Anandan
Design Direction: Renee Duenow

Printed in India

Last digit is the print number: 9 8 7 6 5 4 3 2 1

To my family, trainees, colleagues, collaborators,
and in honor of the patients we treat.
Best, Darren

To my family.
Best, Niko

Contributors

Aaron W. Aday, MD, MSc
Assistant Professor
Division of Cardiovascular Medicine, Department of Medicine
Vanderbilt University Medical Center
Nashville, Tennessee

David Aguilar, MD, MSc
Professor
Department of Internal Medicine, Division of Cardiovascular Medicine
University of Texas Southwestern Medical Center
Dallas, Texas

Clare Arnott, MBBS (Hons), PhD, FRACP
Associate Professor, Program Director
Cardiovascular
The George Institute for Global Health
Syndey, New South Wales, Australia
Staff Specialist
Cardiology
Royal Prince Alfred Hospital
Newtown, New South Wales, Australia

Joshua A. Beckman, MD, MS
Chief
Division of Vascular Medicine
Department of Medicine
UT Southwestern Medical Center
Dallas, Texas

David D. Berg, MD, MPH
Assistant Professor
Department of Medicine
Brigham and Women's Hospital, Harvard Medical School
Boston, Massachusetts

Deepak L. Bhatt, MD, MPH, MBA
Director of Mount Sinai Fuster Heart Hospital
Mount Sinai Fuster Heart Hospital
Icahn School of Medicine at Mount Sinai
New York, Massachusetts
Dr. Valentin Fuster Professor of Cardiovascular Medicine (with Tenure)
Icahn School of Medicine at Mount Sinai
New York, Massachusetts

Petter Bjornstad, MD
Professor
Medicine
University of Washington
Seattle, Washington

Julia Brandts, MD, Dr
Physician
Department of Internal Medicine I
University Hospital Aachen
Aachen, Germany
Honorary Research Associate
School of Public Health
Imperial College London
London, United Kingdom

Michael R. Brennan, MS, DO, FACP, FACE
Head of Endocrinology, Corwellhealth East
Section Head, Assistant Program Director Endocrinology Fellowship
Endocrinology
Corwellhealth William Beaumont University Hospital
Assistant Professor
Oakland University
Assistant Professor
Michigan State University

Juliana C.N. Chan, MBChB, MD, FRCP
Professor of Medicine and Therapeutics
Department of Medicine and Therapeutics
The Chinese University of Hong Kong
Shatin, Hong Kong

Melanie J. Davies, CBE, MBChB, MD, FRCP, FRCGP, FMedSci
Professor of Diabetes Medicine
Diabetes Research Unit
University of Leicester
Leicester, United Kingdom

Pierre Henri Ducluzeau, MD, PhD
Service d'Endocrinologie Diabétologie et Nutrition
Centre Hospitalier Universitaire et Faculté de Médecine
Université de Tours
Tours, France

Leonard E. Egede, MD, MS
Professor & Chair
Department of Medicine
University at Buffalo
Buffalo, New York

Frank Joachim Erbguth, MD, PhD
Professor
Department of Neurology
Paracelsus Medical University-Nuremberg General Hospital
Nuremberg, Germany

Brendan M. Everett, MD, MPH
Associate Professor
Department of Medicine, Division of Cardiovascular Medicine
Brigham and Women's Hospital and Harvard Medical School
Boston, Massachusetts

Wenjun Fan, PhD
Assistant Professor
Epidemiology & Biostatistics
University of California, Irvine
Irvine, California

Laurent Fauchier, MD
Professor of Cardiology
Cardiologie
Centre Hospitalier Universitaire Trousseau, Faculté de Médecine, Université François Rabelais
Tours, France

Barry A. Franklin, PhD
Director (Emeritus), Preventive Cardiology and Cardiac Rehabilitation
Corewell Health, William Beaumont, University Hospital
Michigan
Professor, Internal Medicine
Oakland University William Beaumont School of Medicine
Michigan

Baptist Gallwitz, MD, Prof, Dr
Former Deputy Head of Department
Department of Medicine IV (Diabetology, Endocrinology, Nephrology)
Eberhard Karls University Tübingen
Tübingen, Germany
Media Speaker
German Diabetes Association (DDG)
Berlin, Germany

Baris Gencer, MD, MPH
Associate Professor
Service of Cardiology
CHUV
Lausanne, Switzerland

Revital L. Gorodeski-Baskin, MD
Clinical Associate Professor
Department of Endocrinology
University Hospitals of Cleveland
Cleveland, Ohio

Colin James Greaves, PhD, C Psychol
Professor
School for Sport, Exercise and Rehabilitation Sciences
University of Birmingham
Birmingham, United Kingdom

Jennifer B. Green, MD
Professor of Medicine
Department of Medicine, Division of Endocrinology
Duke University School of Medicine
Durham, North Carolina

Richard Haynes, DM, FRCP
Professor
Clinical Trial Service Unit, Nuffield Department of Population Health
University of Oxford
Oxford, United Kingdom
Honorary Consultant Nephrologist
Oxford Kidney Unit
Oxford University Hospitals NHS Foundation Trust
Oxford, United Kingdom

Joseph Henson, PhD
Associate Professor
Diabetes Research Centre
University of Leicester
Leicester, United Kingdom

Adrian F. Hernandez, MD, MHS
Executive Director of Duke Clinical Research Institute
Medicine
Duke University School of Medicine
Durham, North Carolina
Vice Dean
Cardiology
Duke University School of Medicine
Durham, North Carolina
Professor of Medicine
Duke Clinical Research Institute
Durham, North Carolina

William Guy Herrington, MA MBBS MD FRCP FERA
Professor of Clinical Trials and Epidemiology of Kidney Disease
Nuffield Department of Population Health
University of Oxford
Oxford, United Kingdom
Honorary Consultant Nephrologist
Oxford Kidney Unit
Churchill Hospital
Oxford, United Kingdom

Hans-Ulrich Häring, MD
German Center for Diabetes Research (DZD)
Neuherberg, Germany

Juan F. Iglesias, MD
Interventional Cardiologist
Cardiology
Geneva University Hospitals
Geneva, Switzerland

Silvio E. Inzucchi, MD
Professor
Internal Medicine (Endocrinology)
Yale University School of Medicine
New Haven, Connecticut
Clinical Chief
Endocrinology
Yale-New Haven Hospital
New Haven, Connecticut
Director
Yale Diabetes Center
Yale-New Haven Hospital
New Haven, Connecticut

Calvin Ke, MD, PhD, FRCPC
Assistant Professor
Department of Medicine and Institute of Health Policy, Management and Evaluation
University of Toronto
Toronto, Ontario, Canada
Clinician Scientist and Staff Endocrinologist
Department of Medicine
University Health Network
Toronto, Ontario, Canada

Kamlesh Khunti, FRCGP, FRCP, MD, PhD, FMedSci
Diabetes Research Centre
University of Leicester
Leicester, United Kingdom

Mikhail Kosiborod, MD, FACC, FAHA
Professor of Medicine
CV Research
Saint Luke's Mid America Heart Institute
Kansas City, Missouri

Lee-Ling Lim, MBBS, PhD, FRCP
Associate Professor
Department of Medicine
Universiti Malaya
Kuala Lumpur, Malaysia
Clinical Associate Professor (Honorary)
Department of Medicine and Therapeutics
The Chinese University of Hong Kong
Hong Kong SAR, China

Kasia J. Lipska, MD, MHS
Associate Professor
Internal Medicine (Endocrinology)
Yale School of Medicine
New Haven, Connecticut

Cecilia C. Low Wang, MD
Professor
Department of Medicine, Division of Endocrinology, Metabolism and Diabetes
University of Colorado Anschutz Medical Campus
Aurora, Colorado

Katharina Marx-Schütt, MD, FESC
Senior Consultant
Department of Internal Medicine I
University Hospital RWTH Aachen
Aachen, Germany

Wendy M. Miller, MD, FACP, DABOM
Section Head
Nutrition and Preventive Medicine
Corewell Health-East
Royal Oak, Michigan
Professor
Internal Medicine
Oakland University William Beaumont School of Medicine
Rochester, Michigan
Medical Director
Weight Control Centers
Corewell Health East
Royal Oak, Michigan

Ian J. Neeland, MD, FAHA, FACC
Director, UH Center for Cardiovascular Prevention
University Hospitals Harrington Heart and Vascular Institute
University Hospitals Cleveland Medical Center
Cleveland, Ohio
Associate Professor
Department of Medicine
Case Western Reserve University School of Medicine
Cleveland, Ohio

Michelle L. O'Donoghue, MD, MPH
McGillycuddy Logue Endowed Chair of Cardiovascular Medicine
Cardiovascular Division
Brigham and Women's Hospital
Boston, Massachusetts
Senior Investigator
TIMI Study Group
Associate Professor of Medicine
Harvard Medical School

Neha Pagidipati, MD, MPH
Medicine
Duke Clinical Research Institute
Durham, North Carolina

Ambarish Pandey, MD, MSCS
Associate Professor
Internal Medicine
UT Southwestern Medical Center
Dallas, Texas

Anushka A. Patel, MBBS, PhD, FRACP
Chief Executive Officer
The George Institute for Global Health, UNSW
Sydney, New South Wales, Australia

Jorge Plutzky, MD
Director, Preventive Cardiology
Cardiovascular Medicine
Brigham and Women's Hospital Harvard Medical School
Boston, Massachusetts
Faculty
Harvard Medical School
Boston, Massachusetts

Kausik K. Ray, BSc, MBChB, FRCP, MD, MPhil, FACC, FESC, FAHA, FMedSci
Professor of Public Health
Primary Care and Public Health
Imperial College London
London, United Kingdom
Honorary Consultant Cardilogist
Cardiology
Imperial College NHS Trust
London, United Kingdom

Marco Roffi, MD
Director
Interventional Cardiology Unit
Cardiology Division University Hospital
Geneva, Switzerland
Associate Professor
Interventional Cardiology Unit
Cardiology Division University Hospital
Geneva, Switzerland

Naveed Amjid Sattar, MBChB, PhD, FMedSci
Professor of Metabolic Medicine
School of Cardiovascular and Metabolic Health
University of Glasgow
Glasgow, United Kingdom

Ann Marie Schmidt, MD
Dr. Iven Young Professor of Endocrinology,
Department of Medicine
Professor
Department of Biochemistry and Molecular Pharmacology
Professor
Department of Pathology
NYU Grossman School of Medicine
New York, New York

Kalie L. Tommerdahl, MD, MS
Associate Professor
Pediatric Endocrinology
University of Washington School of Medicine
Seattle, Washington

Renu Virmani, MD
President Emeritus and Founder
Department of Pathology
CVPath Institute, Inc.
Gaithersburg, Maryland

Rebekah J. Walker, PhD
Associate Professor
Department of Medicine
University at Buffalo
Buffalo, New York
Chief
Division of Population Health
Department of Medicine
University at Buffalo
Buffalo, New York

Joni S. Williams, MD, MPH
Associate Professor
Medicine
Medical College of Wisconsin
Milwaukee, Wisconsin

Nathan D. Wong, PhD, FACC, FAHA
Professor and Director, Heart Disease Prevention Program
Mary and Steve Wen Cardiovascular Division
University of California, Irvine School of Medicine
California

Thomas Yates, PhD
Professor
Diabetes Research Centre
University of Leicester
Leicester, United Kingdom

Foreword

It is well established that cardiovascular disorders (CVD) remain the leading causes of death worldwide and that atherosclerosis and its complications lead the list of CVDs. Important risk factors for atherogenesis—hypertension, dyslipidemia, and smoking—are trending downwards (albeit too slowly), while type 2 diabetes mellitus (T2DM), also a cardinal risk factor for the development of atherosclerotic disease of coronary, carotid, and other systemic arteries, has grown rapidly to affect more than 400 million persons globally. Therefore cardiologists and other health care deliverers and their trainees must learn how to prevent, assess, and manage T2DM as they have become accustomed to managing the traditional risk factors. Similarly, diabetologists (or endocrinologists) must learn how to prevent and recognize atherosclerotic heart disease and heart failure, complications that are responsible for the most frequent causes of death of patients with T2DM. As a consequence, these two specialties—cardiology and diabetology—are now "joined at the hip."

We are pleased to welcome the second edition of *Diabeto-cardiology* as an important companion to *Braunwald's Heart Disease*. This book has succeeded in placing into a single text much of what is known about the effects of T2DM on CVD. Fortunately, two classes of antihyperglycemic drugs—incretin mimetics including glucagon-like peptide receptor agonists (GLP-1RAs) and sodium-glucose cotransporters (SGLT)-2 inhibitors—are now widely used for the treatment of persons with T2DM. Both classes are also beneficial on cardiac and kidney function, with the former reducing body weight substantially. This Companion provides useful information on these agents as well.

This book is eminently readable, thorough but not encyclopedic. The authors, ably led by the talented editors, Drs. McGuire and Marx, are international authorities who have provided excellent and up-to-date information in this rapidly expanding field which is positioned at the intersection of cardiology and diabetology. The optimal care of patients with T2DM requires a team approach involving both diabetologists and cardiologists. It is likely that as the incidence of the combination of T2DM and CVD continues to rise, it will become necessary to create a new subspecialty—*Diabetocardiology*, and this book would be an excellent text to prepare health care professionals for this important field.

Eugene Braunwald
Boston, Massachusetts

Robert O. Bonow
Chicago, Illinois

Douglas L. Mann
St. Louis, Missouri

Gordon F. Tomaselli
Baltimore, Maryland

Deepak L. Bhatt
New York, New York

Scott D. Solomon
Boston Massachusetts

Peter Libby
Boston, Massachusetts

Preface

Over the past several decades, overweight/obesity and diabetes mellitus have become an increasing problem that constitutes a global epidemic, representing one of the most important chronic disease conditions in the world with critically important public health implications. Persons with diabetes exhibit an increased propensity to develop myriad cardiovascular diseases; its key sequelae are myocardial infarction, heart failure, stroke, peripheral arterial disease, atrial fibrillation, and cardiovascular death. Over this same time period, the cardiology community has increasingly recognized the adverse cardiovascular prognosis of persons with diabetes, with increasing understanding of the heterogeneity of efficacy of available medical and interventional strategies by diabetes status and a notable unmet clinical need to mitigate the incremental "residual" cardiovascular risk associated with diabetes. Based on these observations and resultant evolution of regulatory requirements for type 2 diabetes drug development around the world, it is only within the past few years that the cardiovascular effects and safety of antihyperglycemic therapies have begun to undergo rigorous assessment in large-scale randomized cardiovascular outcome trials focusing specifically on persons with diabetes. Thus the field of cardiovascular disease in diabetes has gained momentum over the past years, resulting in joint activities and guidelines from cardiology and professional recommendations from diabetes associations around the world, requiring and fostering a truly interdisciplinary collaborative research and clinical partnership among cardiologists, endocrinologists, primary care clinicians, nutritionists, exercise physiologists, pharmacists, and diabetes educators—reflected in the diverse authorship of chapters in this textbook.

The first edition of *Diabetes in Cardiovascular Disease: A Companion to Braunwald's Heart Disease* included 31 chapters that addressed the spectrum of topics relevant to the nexus of diabetes and cardiovascular disease. In this second edition renamed *Diabeto-Cardiology*, we present 27 chapters covering this spectrum of clinical care. These chapters cover the epidemiology, pathophysiologic and genetic underpinnings, clinical presentation and consequences, and diagnostic and therapeutic approaches for prevention and treatment of persons with diabetes at elevated risk for cardiovascular and kidney disease complications, and review systems approaches to apply such interventions. Each of the chapters is written by international leaders in their respective fields, and for us it has been a true pleasure and great honor to work with such a fabulous group of experts. They are our colleagues, collaborators, and friends and represent the remarkable interdisciplinary collaborative spirit bridging our specialties and advancing the field of science and health care for the betterment of our patients. We believe that this book will be an invaluable resource for cardiologists, diabetologists, nephrologists, primary care clinicians, and all other health care personnel taking care of patients with diabetes and with or at high risk for cardiovascular disease.

We thank our many friends, our colleagues, and the experts around the world who contributed to this book. Without their expertise and contribution, the textbook could not have been completed.

Darren K. McGuire

Nikolaus Marx

Acknowledgments

We offer our heartfelt gratitude to those who have supported the development of this textbook. First, to Professors Braunwald and Libby, who had the confidence to allow us to edit an addition to the family of texts with the internationally revered imprimatur of *Braunwald's Heart Disease*. Second, to our colleagues and friends around the world who accepted our invitation to author chapters and delivered such excellent content that most commonly exceeded our highest expectations. Finally, to the editorial staff at Elsevier who so ably assisted and facilitated the development of this book at every step of the way: Melanie Tucker, Vasowati Shome, Tarana Parveen, and Nayagi Anandan. To each of you, thank you.

Darren K. McGuire

Nikolaus Marx

Contents

Braunwald's Heart Disease Family of Books

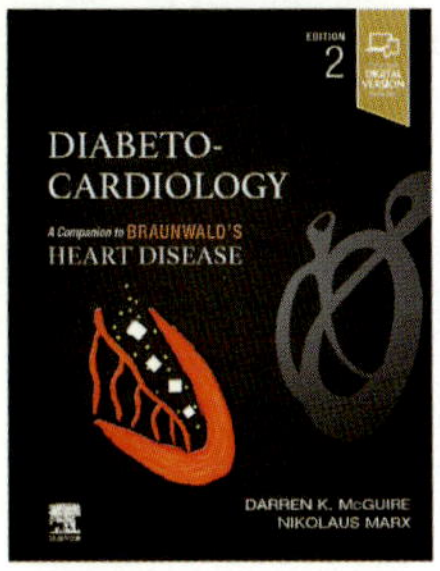

McGUIRE AND MARX
DIABETO-CARDIOLOGY

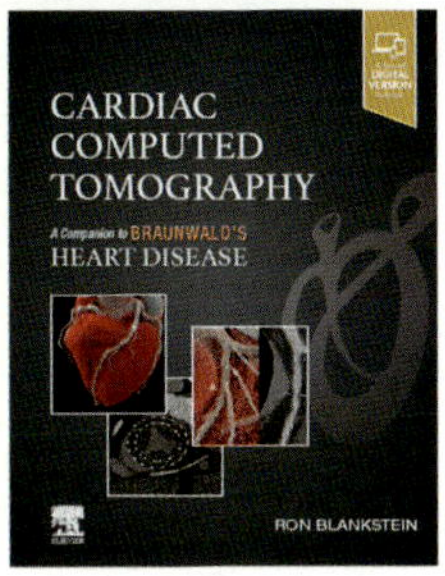

BLANKSTEIN
Computed Cardiac Tomography

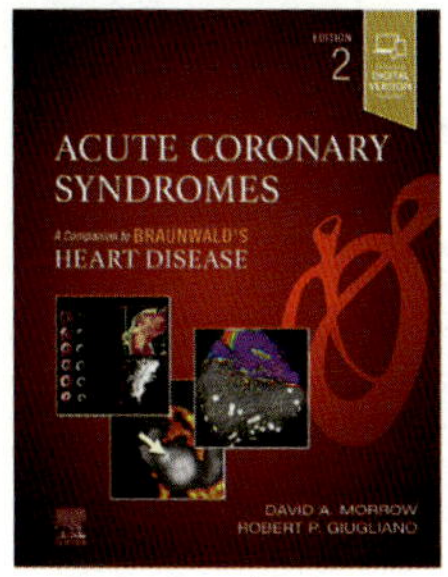

MORROW
Acute Coronary Syndromes

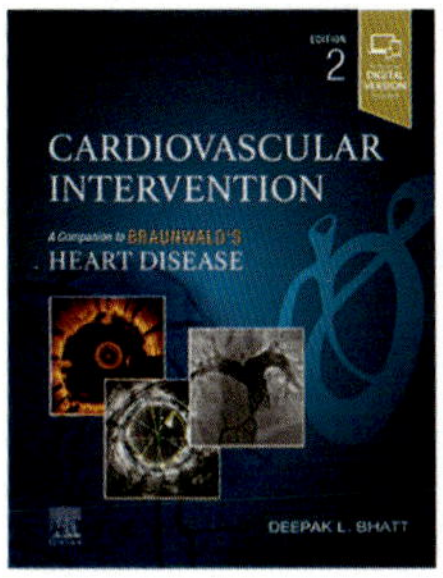

BHATT
Cardiovascular Intervention

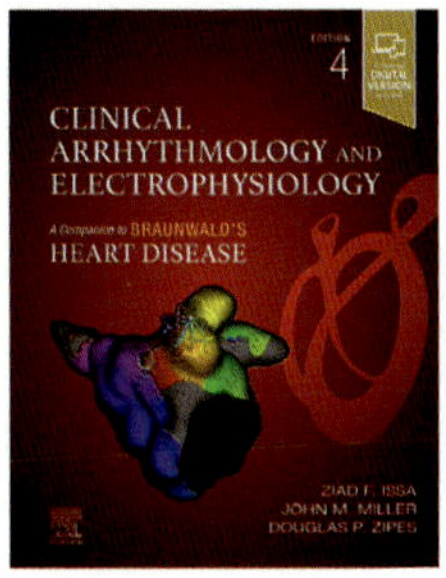

ISSA, MILLER, ZIPES
Clinical Arrhythmology and Electrophysiology

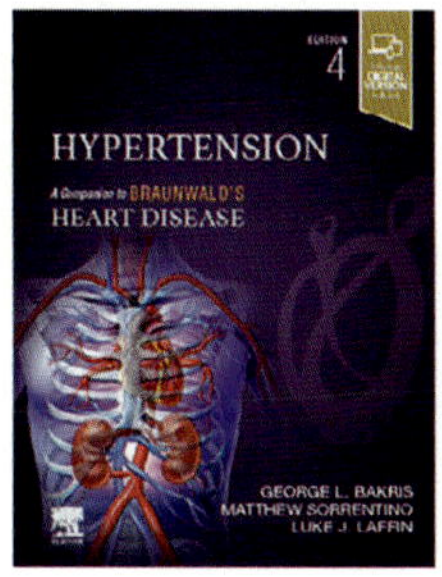

BAKRIS, SORRENTINO, AND LAFFIN
Hypertension

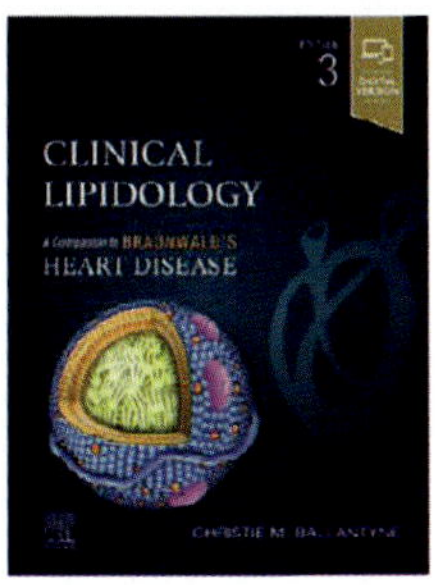

BALLANTYNE
Clinical Lipidology

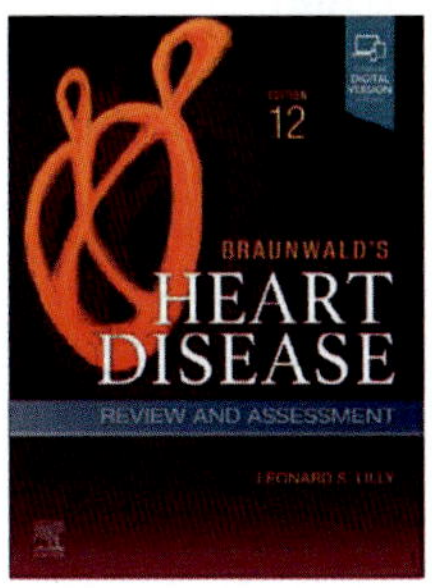

LILLY
Braunwald's Heart Disease Review and Assessment

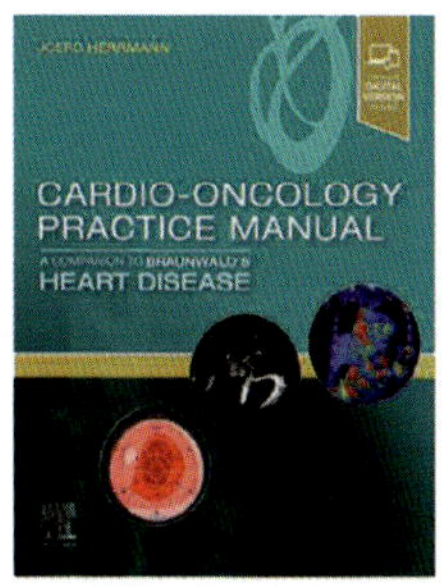

HERRMANN
Cardio-Oncology Practice Manual

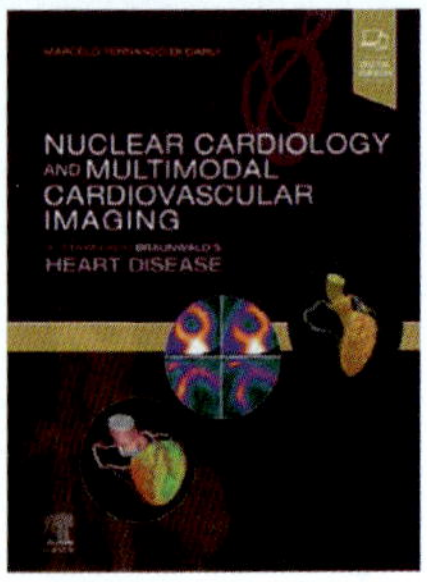

DI CARLI
Nuclear Cardiology and Multimodal Cardiovascular Imaging

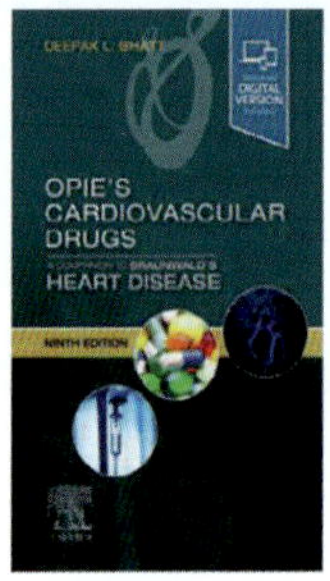

BHATT
Opie's Cardiovascular Drugs

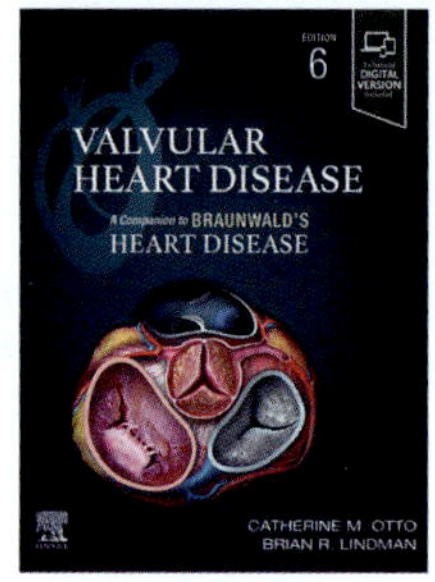

OTTO AND BONOW
Valvular Heart Disease

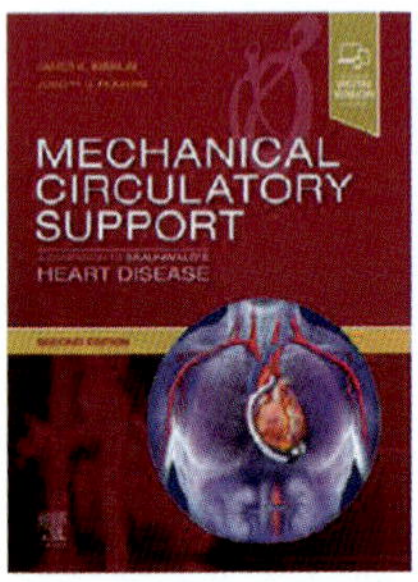

KIRKLIN AND ROGERS
Mechanical Circulatory Support

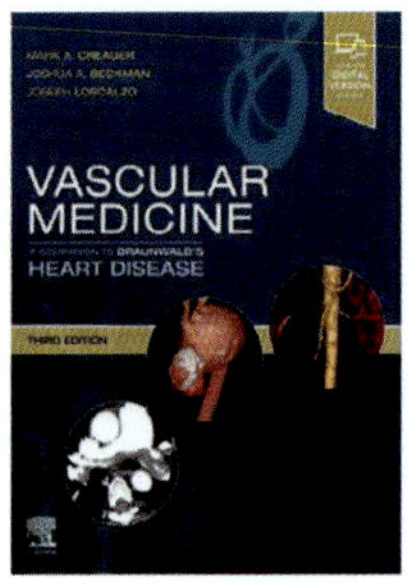

CREAGER
Vascular Medicine

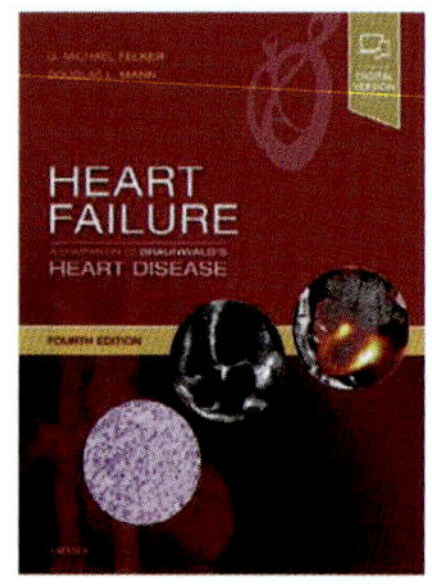

FELKER AND MANN
Heart Failure

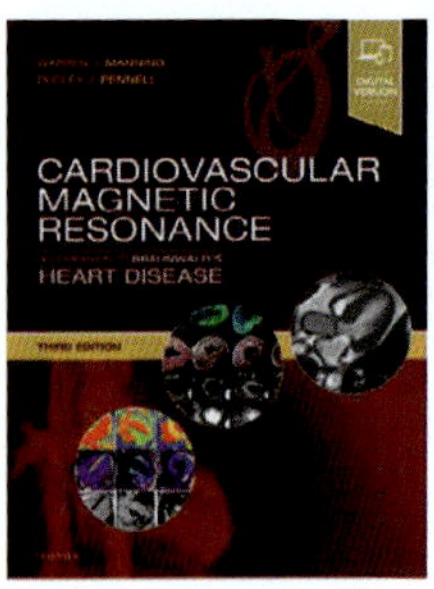

MANNING AND PENNELL
Cardiovascular Magnetic Resonance

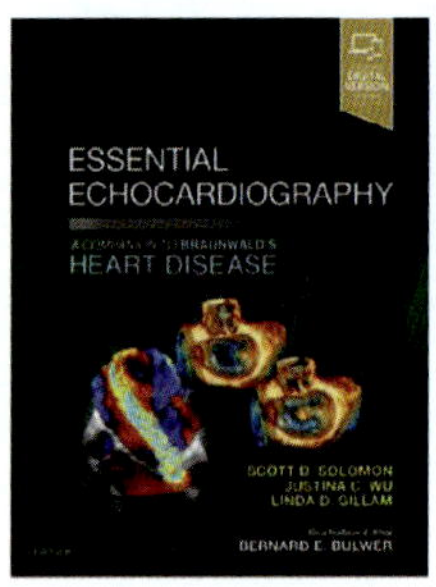

SOLOMON, WU, AND GILLAM
Essential Echocardiography

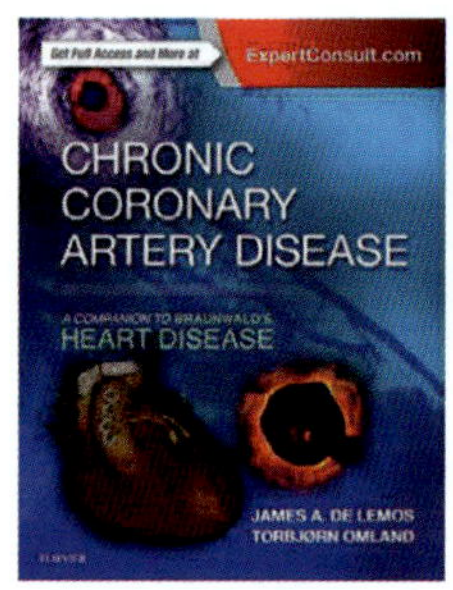

DE LEMOS AND OMLAND
Chronic Coronary Artery Disease

1 Definition and Epidemiology of Type 2 Diabetes Mellitus

CALVIN KE, JULIANA C.N. CHAN, AND LEE-LING LIM

Diabetes mellitus has reached epidemic proportions, costing an estimated US$1.015 trillion in direct health expenditures worldwide (12% of global health expenditure).[1] Although diabetes mellitus has a variety of forms with differing etiologies (e.g., autoimmune type 1 diabetes mellitus, type 2 diabetes mellitus, gestational diabetes mellitus, monogenic diabetes, drug-induced diabetes, diabetes due to pancreatic diseases or endocrinopathy[2]), most cases of diabetes mellitus—approximately 90% to 95%—are type 2 diabetes mellitus (hereafter referred to simply as *diabetes*). Diabetes affects multiple systems of the body and can result in serious and debilitating complications. In this chapter, we provide an overview of diabetes and its complications, describe the global burden of diabetes, discuss the causal underpinnings of diabetes, and conclude by reviewing strategies to prevent and manage diabetes.

TYPE 2 DIABETES MELLITUS: DEFINITIONS AND OVERVIEW

The maintenance of glucose homeostasis requires appropriate levels of insulin secretion. Diabetes is characterized by a "progressive loss of adequate [pancreatic] β-cell insulin secretion frequently on the background of insulin resistance."[3] Impaired glucose tolerance and impaired fasting glucose are together termed *prediabetes*, a precursor to and a risk factor for diabetes. The diagnostic criteria for prediabetes and diabetes are shown in Table 1.1. The fasting plasma glucose test, 2-h 75-g oral glucose tolerance test, and glycosylated hemoglobin A_{1c} (HbA_{1c}) test are used to screen for diabetes. In the absence of typical symptoms (e.g., polyuria, polydipsia, weight loss), diabetes is diagnosed by two abnormal results from these screening tests.

Diabetes is a heterogeneous condition that can manifest as a diversity of phenotypes.[5] Individual differences in factors such as islet biology and autoimmunity, incretin activity, insulin resistance (IR), and adipose tissue distribution may contribute, to varying degrees, to the development of diabetes. There is growing interest in using a "precision medicine" approach to individualize diabetes management according to phenotypic characteristics. Some experts have proposed that diabetes may be subclassified into discrete subgroups (severe insulin-deficient diabetes [SIDD], severe insulin-resistant diabetes [SIRD], mild obesity-related diabetes, and mild age-related diabetes) based on age at diagnosis, body mass index (BMI), glutamic acid decarboxylase antibodies, β-cell function, and IR. The latter two are often expressed as Homeostasis Model of Assessment-β (HOMA-β) and Homeostasis Model of Assessment insulin resistance (HOMA-IR), which are measures estimated from fasting plasma glucose and C-peptide (residual fraction of proinsulin after its cleavage into insulin).[6] These subgroups are associated with different prognoses (e.g., people with SIRD are more likely to develop kidney disease, while people with SIDD often require early insulin treatment and are at the risk of retinopathy) and highlight the heterogeneity of diabetes. Other epidemiological studies have indicated that HOMA-IR and HOMA-β are independently and additively associated with early onset of diabetes and early insulin requirement.[7]

Long-term hyperglycemia and its fluctuations, especially in the presence of other cardiometabolic risk factors, notably obesity, hypertension, and dyslipidemia, can lead to microvascular and macrovascular changes affecting multiple body systems, resulting in fatal and nonfatal complications. The most recognized complications of diabetes include myocardial infarction, stroke, heart failure, peripheral arterial disease, atrial fibrillation, chronic kidney disease, retinopathy including visual loss, and diabetic neuropathy.[8–10] Diabetes is also associated with other hitherto underappreciated complications, namely, infections (e.g., tuberculosis), liver diseases, mental illness, cancers, and cognitive impairment.[10,11] For a more thorough discussion of these complications, see Chapters 6 through 10, 12, 13, 15, 22, and 24 through 27.

TABLE 1.1 American Diabetes Association Diagnostic Criteria for Diabetes and Prediabetes[3]

		DIAGNOSTIC TEST		
		FASTING PLASMA GLUCOSE	OGTT[a]	HBA_{1C}
Type 2 diabetes[b]		≥126 mg/dL (7.0 mmol/L)	≥200 mg/dL (11.1 mmol/L)	≥6.5% (48 mmol/mol)
Prediabetes	Impaired fasting glucose[c]	100–125 mg/dL (5.6–6.9 mmol/L)		5.7–6.4% (39–47 mmol/mol)
	Impaired glucose tolerance		140–199 mg/dL (7.8–11.0 mmol/L)	

[a]Two-hour, 75-g oral glucose tolerance test.
[b]Two abnormal tests are required (either the same or different diagnostic test), unless the patient has classic symptoms of hyperglycemia and random plasma glucose ≥200 mg/dL (11.1 mmol/L).
[c]The World Health Organization defines impaired fasting glucose with a narrower range: 110 to 125 mg/dL (6.1–6.9 mmol/L), does not use HbA_{1c} (glycosylated hemoglobin A_{1c}) to diagnose prediabetes, and prefers the term "intermediate hyperglycemia" rather than prediabetes.[4]
OGTT, Oral glucose tolerance test.
Data from American Diabetes Association Professional Practice Committee. 2. Diagnosis and Classification of Diabetes: Standards of Care in Diabetes—2024. *Diabetes Care.* 2023;47(suppl 1):S20–S42.

In particular, diabetes is a risk factor for severe COVID-19 and associated mortality.[12] The relationship between diabetes and COVID-19 may be mediated by hyperglycemia, inflammation, altered immune status, and renin-angiotensin-aldosterone system activation. In the Emerging Risk Factor Collaboration study of 820,900 people in 97 prospective cohorts, individuals with diabetes had a 1.3- to 3-fold increased risk of death from conditions ranging from cardiovascular diseases and kidney failure to infections, mental disorders, and liver disease. Due to their propensity for developing these life-threatening conditions, people with diabetes die earlier than those without. For example, a person diagnosed with diabetes at the age of 50 years might lose around 6 years of life, although the prognosis can be improved by managing multiple risk factors.[11]

Although a loss of β-cell secretion to maintain normoglycemia is inherent to diabetes in general, people diagnosed with diabetes at a young age have an especially accelerated rate of β-cell function loss. *Young-onset diabetes* is often defined as diabetes diagnosed before the age of 40 years.[13] People with young-onset diabetes have a more aggressive course and longer duration of disease, thus resulting in a greater risk of cardiovascular-kidney and other complications of diabetes than people diagnosed with diabetes later in life.[14,15] The risk of complications is also greater than similarly aged people with type 1 diabetes, often due to concomitant cardiometabolic risk factors with delayed or suboptimal intervention. The incidence and prevalence rates of young-onset diabetes are particularly high among Asian, Black, and Indigenous populations in many countries, including the United States and Canada.[1,13]

There is strong evidence that treatment of multiple risk factors simultaneously in patients with diabetes improves outcomes.[12,16] Meta-analyses suggest that reducing HbA_{1c} by 0.9%, systolic blood pressure by 10 mm Hg, and low-density lipoprotein (LDL) cholesterol by 1 mmol/L might reduce the risk of cardiovascular disease and all-cause mortality by 10% to 20%.[15] In the Swedish National Diabetes Registry, having a higher number of risk factors within target ranges (HbA_{1c} < 7%, systolic BP < 140 mm Hg, LDL < 2.5 mmol/L, high physical activity, no smoking) was associated with marked reduction in risk of mortality, myocardial infarction, and stroke in a graded manner.[17] Clinical practice guidelines recommend that patients with diabetes undergo regular examination to detect silent complications (e.g., foot and eye examinations) and assess management of modifiable risk factors including lifestyle (e.g., physical activity, diet, smoking, sleep, emotional wellness) and cardiometabolic risk factors (e.g., blood glucose, HbA_{1c}, blood pressure, LDL cholesterol, triglycerides, body weight, kidney function including urinary albumin) and early use of organ-protective drugs (e.g., angiotensin-converting enzyme inhibitor or angiotensin receptor blocker, statins).[18] The achievement of these goals may be optimized by integrating assessment, education, and care services in a structured, team-based setting.[15,18,19] Furthermore, people at high risk of cardiovascular disease and those with established atherosclerotic cardiovascular disease (ASCVD), chronic kidney disease, or heart failure should be treated with a sodium-glucose cotransporter-2 inhibitor (if heart failure or chronic kidney disease predominates) or glucagon-like peptide-1 receptor agonist (if ASCVD predominates and especially in obese patients). Both of these drugs have been proven to prevent the onset or reduce the progression of these adverse outcomes.[18–20]

GLOBAL BURDEN OF DIABETES

Prevalence and Incidence

The number of people with diabetes has sharply increased from 151 million (2000) to 58,937 million (2024) worldwide (age 20–79 years; Table 1.2).[1] On current trends, the number of people with diabetes will rise to around 853 million by 2050. This increase is attributable to population growth and aging, as well as a rising burden of obesity. The *prevalence* rate of diabetes is defined as the proportion of a population with diabetes at a point in time. Globally, the prevalence rate of diabetes is 11.1% (age 20–79 years), and this figure is projected to rise to 13% by 2050. In the United States, there are around 38.5 million people with diabetes, and the prevalence rate is 15.7% (age 20–79 years). Over 80% of people with diabetes live in low- and middle-income countries (LMICs), such as China, India, and Pakistan (Table 1.3). The standardized prevalence of diabetes (which uses statistical adjustment to account for differences in age distribution across populations) is highest in Pakistan (31.4%), Marshall Islands (25.7%), Kuwait (25.6%), and Samoa (25.4%). Globally, around two-thirds of people with diabetes reside in urban areas, which have a higher prevalence (12.7%) of diabetes than rural areas (8.8%).[1] This urban-rural disparity is in part due to the rapid changes in environment and behaviors associated with urbanization and economic development.[1]

A substantial proportion of people with diabetes are undiagnosed. This proportion ranges from around 28.9% in high-income countries to 45.5% to 58.7% in LMICs.[1] Barriers to diagnosing diabetes include poor awareness among the public and healthcare providers, insufficient health system infrastructure, and lack of capacity or processes to detect diabetes. Delayed diagnosis increases the risk of presenting with advanced diabetes and severe complications.

The increasing prevalence of diabetes is an urgent public health issue with both societal and personal implications, calling for a multipronged strategy to reduce its burden. The *prevalence* rate is the proportion of people with diabetes among survivors at any one time. Thus in an aging society with a declining death rate, prevalence may continue to rise despite a falling number of new (incident) cases. Thus incidence rates are a preferred indicator to evaluate the impact of prevention strategies for controlling the epidemic of diabetes. The *incidence* rate of diabetes is defined as the number of new cases of diabetes divided by the person-time at risk over a particular period. An analysis of 23 high- and middle-income countries suggested that from 2010 to 2018, the incidence of diabetes had a declining trend in 19 of these countries (−1.1% to −10.8% per year), with an increasing trend in four of these countries (0.9%–5.6% per year).[21] Incidence trends in LMICs have not been similarly studied due to insufficient data. Together with the declining trends of death rates among people with diabetes in high-income countries,[22] these figures strongly demonstrate the preventable nature of diabetes and its complications.

TABLE 1.2 **Numbers of People With Diabetes (in Millions), 2024 and 2050 (20–79 Years), Globally[1]**

REGION	2024	2050
Middle East and North Africa	84.7	162.6
North America and Caribbean	56.2	68.1
Western Pacific	215.4	253.8
Southeast Asia	106.9	184.5
South and Central America	35.4	51.5
Europe	65.6	72.4
Sub-Saharan Africa	24.6	59.5
World	588.7	852.5

Data from IDF Diabetes Atlas, 10th Edition Committee. *IDF Diabetes Atlas*. 10th ed. International Diabetes Federation; 2021.

TABLE 1.3 **Countries With the Highest Number of People With Diabetes (20–79 Years), 2024 and 2050[1]**

COUNTRY	2021 (MILLIONS)	COUNTRY	2045 (MILLIONS)
China	148.0	China	168.3
India	89.8	India	156.7
United States	38.5	Pakistan	70.2
Pakistan	34.5	United States	43.0
Indonesia	20.4	Indonesia	28.6
Brazil	16.6	Egypt	24.7
Bangladesh	13.9	Brazil	24.0
Mexico	13.6	Bangladesh	23.1
Egypt	13.2	Mexico	19.9
Japan	10.8	Turkey	14.1

Data from IDF Diabetes Atlas, 11th Edition Committee. *IDF Diabetes Atlas*. 11th ed. International Diabetes Federation; 2025.

Management

There are substantial gaps in the management of cardiometabolic risk factors in people with diabetes.[23] In the United States, initial improvements in diabetes control observed from 1999 to 2010 have now stalled or partially reversed. The rate of achieving an HbA_{1c} <7% declined from 57.4% (2007–10) to 50.5% (2015–18), while the rate of attaining all glycemic, blood pressure, and LDL cholesterol targets has plateaued at 22.2% (2015–18).[24] Young adults and people without health insurance were less likely to meet treatment targets. A study of 28 LMICs showed that out of all people with diabetes, only 44% were aware of their diagnosis, 28% were treated, and 23% had an HbA_{1c} <8%—a pattern known as the care cascade.[25] In a study of 49 countries across Africa, the Middle East, South Asia, South and Central America, Asia, and Eastern Europe, the rate of achieving an HbA_{1c} <7% declined from 36.0% (2005) to 30.1% (2017).[26] Barriers to attaining treatment targets include insufficient investment and capacity in health systems and suboptimal organization of diabetes care for implementing risk assessment and management programs to allow for early intervention. Other reasons include socioeconomic factors, high medication costs, complex treatment regimens, and inadequate patient empowerment with suboptimal self-management and poor medication adherence.[15] In Hong Kong, a cosmopolitan city in South China with 7 million people, the introduction of a territory-wide diabetes risk assessment and management program in 2000 focusing on early intervention and patient empowerment was accompanied by progressive improvement in glycemic control against a backdrop of 50% to 70% decline in death and major cardiovascular event rates in 0.8 million people with diabetes in 2000 to 2016.[27–29]

Outcomes

Data from high-income countries suggest that the incidence of cardiovascular-kidney complications and mortality in people with diabetes has fallen since 1990.[10] In the United States, the incidence of myocardial infarction and stroke have each dropped by around two-thirds and one-half, respectively, from 1990 to 2010.[30] However, the greatest declines were limited to people aged 75 years or older. Similar overall declines have been reported in other high-income countries, such as Australia, Canada, and Sweden. The incidence of end-stage kidney disease among people with diabetes has declined by around 28% in the United States (1990–2010) and by 6% per year in China (2000–12). Nevertheless, in recent years, the number of people with end-stage kidney disease has grown by 11% in the United States and by 40% to 700% in other regions, including Russia, the Philippines, Malaysia, Korea, Australia, Taiwan, and Scotland. This increase may be in part due to increasing survival among people with diabetes. In a study of 16 high-income countries from 1995 to 2016, all-cause mortality dropped in most countries by 0.5% to 4.2% per year, with the largest decreases in East Asian regions such as Hong Kong, South Korea, Taiwan, and Singapore.[22]

In LMICs, there are limited data on the incidence of diabetes outcomes. It is estimated that the incidence of cardiovascular complications and premature mortality among people with diabetes is around two to three times higher than in high-income countries.[15] In the 10 LMICs with the highest number of people with diabetes (China, India, Brazil, Mexico, Indonesia, Egypt, Pakistan, Bangladesh, Turkey, Thailand), diabetes may cause over 3 million premature deaths every year between the ages of 30 and 69 years. Nearly half of these deaths are attributable to cardiovascular causes.[15]

CAUSAL UNDERPINNINGS OF TYPE 2 DIABETES

IR, often due to obesity, and impaired insulin secretion due to pancreatic β-cell dysfunction are crucial factors and occur early in the pathogenesis of diabetes.[15] Under physiological conditions, IR leads to compensatory hyperplasia of pancreatic β-cells to promote insulin secretion for maintaining glucose homeostasis and preventing the progression from normal glucose tolerance to prediabetes and overt diabetes.[31] Obesity and associated inflammation can induce IR, increase hepatic glucose production, and decrease peripheral glucose uptake in skeletal muscle and adipose tissue, leading to hyperglycemia.[32,33]

In people with poor β-cell reserves due to factors such as genetic predisposition, this abnormal milieu of glucolipotoxicity and low-grade inflammation can impair pancreatic β-cell function and decrease insulin secretion, leading to hyperglycemia and eventually overt diabetes. Of note, β-cell mass in people with prediabetes and diabetes is approximately 60% and 40%, respectively, compared to people without prediabetes or diabetes.[15] Persistent hyperglycemia in at-risk populations with prediabetes can further decrease β-cell mass and its functional capacity, thus making it harder for the body to maintain glucose homeostasis.[15] In the past two decades, advances in diabetes research have confirmed that the pathogenesis of diabetes involves a complex interaction of genetic, epigenetic, and environmental factors.[15,32]

GENETIC, EPIGENETIC, AND GENE-ENVIRONMENTAL INTERACTIONS

Although the natural history of diabetes has been traditionally described as a process of increasing age-related IR followed by declining β-cell function and impaired insulin secretion, it has been postulated that people at risk for diabetes may have a primary genetic defect in β-cell function.[34] In accordance with this hypothesis, family history is a strong and independent risk factor for diabetes that can interact with other lifestyle factors to bring about earlier development of diabetes at ages <40 years.[35] Family history as a risk factor not only reflects genetic inheritance but also shares environment and health-related behaviors within families and their effects on previous generations (Fig. 1.1).[36] Nutritional or metabolic factors can lead to temporal changes in the expression of genetic factors (so-called metabolic imprinting), which can persist throughout life. The "thrifty phenotype hypothesis" describes how maternal undernutrition (as occurs during famine or in less severe food shortages) changes the intrauterine environment, leading to fetal adaptations that can affect the child throughout life.[37] For the same mother, siblings born before and after the mother developed gestational diabetes had very different risks for glucose intolerance, despite sharing similar genetic profiles.[38] In a similar vein, self-reported ethnicity or race is sometimes interpreted as a proxy for genetic ancestry. However, interethnic differences in culture and socioeconomic determinants may interact with other environmental, psychological, and behavioral factors to influence the risk of diabetes.[39] This complexity is supported by the poor transferability of polygenic risk scores developed in European populations to other ethnic groups living in countries at different stages of economic development.[40]

With the advent of single- and multiancestry genome-wide association studies (GWAS), exome sequencing, and targeted array genotyping, a total of 237 genetic loci with 338 distinct association signals known to influence quantitative glycemic traits (including glucose, insulin, HbA_{1c} levels) and β-cell mass or function have been identified since 2005.[41] These results indicate that diabetes is a polygenic disease and that the patterns of genetic variation may inform risk stratification and prognostication for implementing personalized medicine in the prevention and treatment for diabetes.[42] Of note, known risk variants are generally common variants with a minor allele frequency of >0.05 with modest effect sizes. By combining these risk variants into a polygenic risk score, statistical power can be maximized to capture information on novel mechanistic insights into disease pathophysiology, clinical heterogeneity of disease predisposition and progression, and responses to targeted interventions.[43] A polygenic risk score based on the findings of a large-scale GWAS estimated a 20% heritability for the risk of diabetes among Europeans,[44] albeit with poor transferability to other ethnic groups with considerably lower explained variance.[40] Thus there remain unresolved questions over the generalizability of such data to non-European populations and the extent to which genetic data adds to disease prediction apart from family history, clinical data, and sociodemographic information.[43]

Even within the same family or same ethnic group, individuals exhibit variable susceptibility to diabetogenic environmental factors with varying outcomes depending on the individual genetic predisposition. This relationship

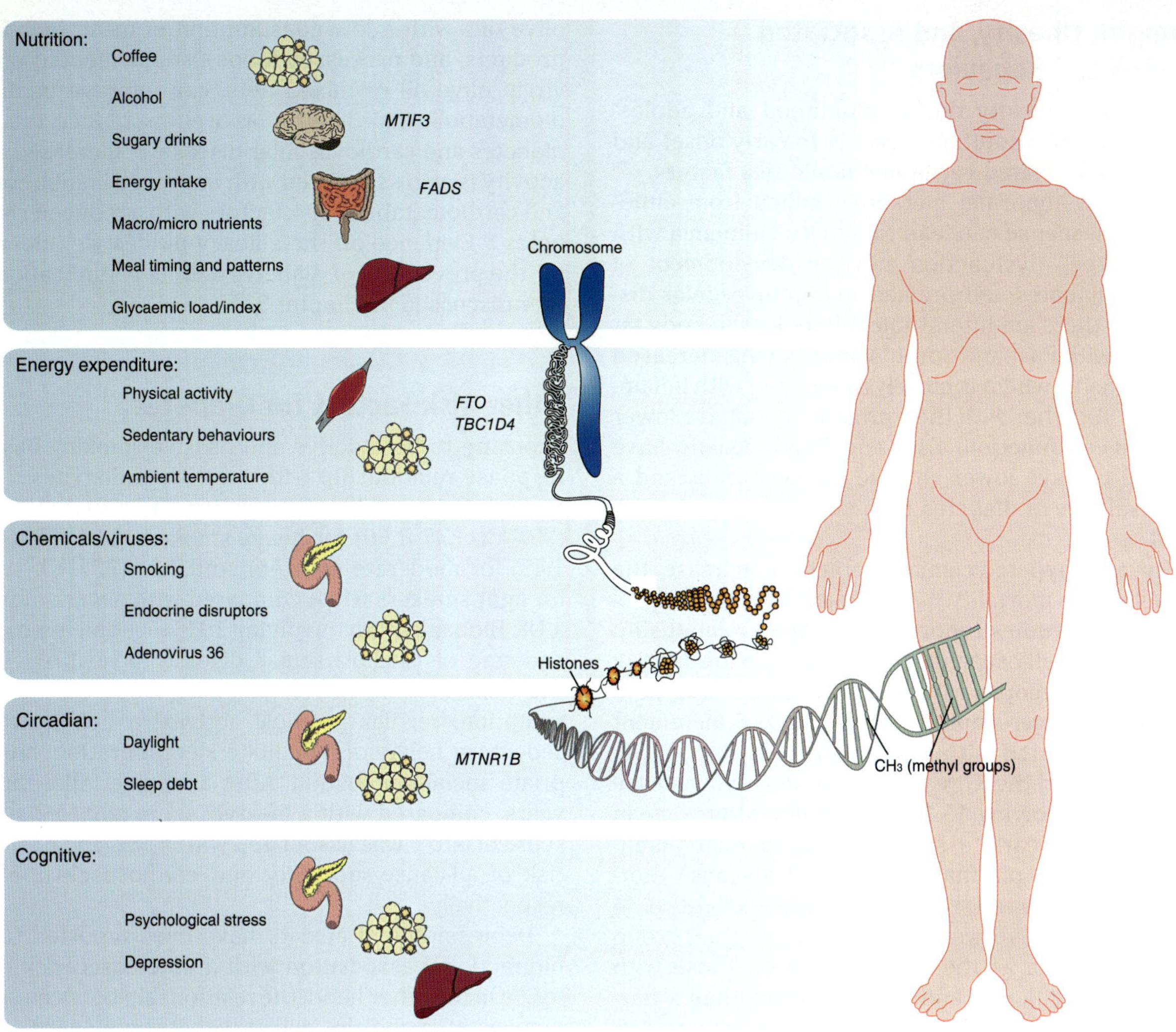

FIG. 1.1 Complex gene-environment interactions in the pathogenesis of type 2 diabetes mellitus (T2DM). In the presence of genetic predisposition, environmental factors such as nutrition, physical activity, chemicals, viruses, and sleep dysregulation can affect the transcriptional and regulatory processes (via methylation, chromatin modeling, or histone modifications), leading to the development and progression of T2DM. Several key environmental and health-related behaviors factors, candidate loci with evidence of gene-lifestyle interactions (such as *MTIF3*, *FADS*, *FTO*, *TBC1D4*, and *MTNR1B*), and target organs that can affect glycemia and adipose tissue regulation are shown here. From Franks, P.W., Poveda, A. Lifestyle and precision diabetes medicine: will genomics help optimise the prediction, prevention and treatment of type 2 diabetes through lifestyle therapy?. Diabetologia 60, 784–792 (2017). https://doi.org/10.1007/s00125-017-4207-5.

is referred to as the "gene × environment (G×E) interaction."[45] The G×E interaction occurs throughout life and is well illustrated by considering the Pima Indians, a Native American population living in the Southwestern United States and Mexico. Compared with Pima Indians living in the United States, Pima Indians living in Mexico are more physically active (mean physical activity of 27.4 vs. 7.6 hours/week) and less obese (prevalence of obesity, 13.2% vs. 69.3%).[46] Although both populations share a similar genetic predisposition for diabetes from an ethnic perspective, compared with Pima Indians living in the United States, Pima Indians living in Mexico have a lower prevalence of diabetes (8.0% vs. 37.5%). In the United Kingdom (UK) Biobank study, compared with those with low genetic risk and healthy behaviors, people with high genetic risk and healthy behaviors had a hazard ratio of 1.94 (95% confidence interval [CI], 1.30–2.90) for the risk of diabetes.[47] The independent and additive effects of health-related behaviors and genetic factors are further evidenced by the progressive increase in hazard ratio to 6.27 (95% CI, 4.53–8.68) in people with high genetic risk and intermediate lifestyle and 15.46 (95% CI, 10.82–22.08) among those with high genetic risk and poor lifestyle.

The frequent clustering of multiple risk factors in people with or at risk of developing diabetes can have additive effects on one another on impairing multiple organ function. Since genetic factors cannot be modified, there is a need to monitor modifiable clinical markers (e.g., blood glucose, HbA_{1c}, blood pressure, lipid profile, BMI, waist circumference, kidney function including albuminuria, and estimated glomerular filtration rate) and health-related behaviors (e.g., diet, physical activity, sleep, mood, alcohol use, tobacco use) to delay the onset of diabetes and prevent complications. Together with other emerging risk factors such as pathway-specific biomarkers, the microbiome, and psychosocial factors, it may be possible to build a unique profile of each individual, describing the potential causes, trajectory, and consequences of diabetes to increase the precision of prediction, prevention, prognostication, and treatment of this condition.[45,48]

Overweight, Obesity, and Associated Health-Related Behaviors

Overweight and obesity during childhood and adolescence can track into adult life, leading to early onset and worsening of associated cardiometabolic risk factors.[15,36] Exposure to an abnormal metabolic milieu from childhood and adolescence can lead to hyperinsulinemia with progressive β-cell dysfunction and the development of young-onset diabetes and premature cardiovascular disease. Of note, there are interethnic differences in body fat distribution, with East and South Asians having increased visceral adiposity, which is closely associated with inflammation.[34,49,50] Together with their propensity to have lower pancreatic β-cell function, East and South Asians have been shown to have lower glucose disposal rates and a higher prevalence of diabetes than non-Asians, given the same BMI.[34]

Obesity and hyperglycemia interact to increase the risk of premature mortality.[51] A meta-analysis of 230 prospective cohort studies reported a J-shaped relationship between BMI and all-cause mortality with the lowest risk observed among people with a BMI of 20 to 22 kg/m^2.[52] Among healthy never-smokers, every 5 kg/m^2 increment in BMI was associated with a 21% increased risk for all-cause mortality.[52] In the Korean National Health Insurance Service cohort involving 15,149,275 adults, after a mean follow-up of 13.7 years, a similar J-shaped relationship among BMI, fasting plasma glucose, and all-cause mortality was also observed.[51] Among people aged 18 to 44 years and using the overweight (BMI 25–27.4 kg/m^2) group with normoglycemia as the reference group, those with the lowest BMI <20 kg/m^2 and normoglycemia had a hazard ratio of 1.29 (95% CI, 1.25–1.33) for all-cause mortality. Using the same reference group, people with diabetes and overweight (BMI 25–27.4 kg/m^2) had a hazard ratio of 2.59 (95% CI, 2.39–2.82), and the leanest group (BMI < 20 kg/m^2) had a hazard ratio of 11.18 (95% CI, 10.20–12.25). The increased hazard ratio associated with low BMI might be confounded by other unmeasured factors, such as malnutrition or poor health, although BMI has been shown to be closely correlated with β-cell function, while central obesity is often considered a surrogate of visceral obesity with IR.[53,54]

Excessive caloric intake and poor diet quality, such as low intake of dietary fiber and high intake of foods with high glycemic index, notably sugar-sweetened beverages and foods with high content of saturated and trans fats, increase the risk of obesity, diabetes, and associated cardiometabolic diseases.[55] Consumption of a healthy diet with balanced nutrition has been shown to improve insulin action, reduce hepatic glucose production, and counteract the effect of obesity on the metabolic milieu.[15] A high-quality diet, especially maintained over the long term, is associated with a 26% reduced risk for diabetes. This efficacy is augmented when combined with high levels of leisure-time exercise and is associated with a 45% risk reduction for diabetes.[56] Both the DASH (Dietary Approaches to Stop Hypertension, a low-fat, high-fiber diet rich in vegetables, fruit, and low-fat dairy products) and Mediterranean-style diet (high intake of vegetables, beans, fruits, nuts, fish, and olive oils with a low consumption of meat, high-fat dairy products, and processed foods), supplemented with extra virgin olive oil or mixed nuts, can improve multiple cardiometabolic risk factors, as well as reduce the risk for diabetes and cardiovascular diseases.[57] Increased physical activity is also associated with improved insulin sensitivity and cardiometabolic risk factors with a reduced risk of diabetes.[58] Evidence on the efficacy of lifestyle interventions for the prevention of diabetes and its complications is further discussed in Chapter 3.

Other Risk Factors for Diabetes

Exposure to both active and passive smoking has a dose-response relationship with the risk of diabetes.[58] A meta-analysis reported that the relative risk of diabetes was 1.57 (95% CI, 1.47–1.66) for heavy smokers, 1.34 (95% CI, 1.27–1.41) for moderate smokers, and 1.21 (95% CI, 1.10–1.33) for light smokers when compared with never-smokers.[59] In a UK Biobank study involving 13,366 people with diabetes and free of cardiovascular disease, a healthy "lifestyle" was defined as no current smoking, moderate alcohol consumption, regular physical activity, a healthy diet, less sedentary behavior, adequate sleep duration, and appropriate social connection. After a median follow-up of 11.7 years, compared with a lifestyle score of 0 to 2, a lifestyle score of 6 to 7 was associated with a 58% and 65% reduced risk of all-cause mortality and cardiovascular mortality, respectively.

Depression and anxiety have been reported to have a bidirectional association with an increased risk of diabetes.[15] On the other hand, the relationship between socioeconomic status and the risk of diabetes may vary according to the national economic development.[60] In high-income countries, diabetes and obesity are more common among low socioeconomic status groups, while in LMICs, diabetes and obesity are more common among those with the highest socioeconomic status.[60,61] As an economy undergoes transition, these risks would also vary depending on levels of acculturation, inherent predisposition, and access to healthcare.

Epidemiological studies have reported that suboptimal sleep duration and quality are associated with an increased risk of diabetes and obesity.[62] Unhealthy sleep habits and patterns may perturb the neuroendocrine and autonomic nervous systems with increased hormones, such as leptin and ghrelin. These changes in the internal milieu can alter eating behaviors, leading to ectopic fat accumulation, worsening IR, and impaired glucose tolerance.[62]

Other emerging risk factors include long-term exposure to air pollutants, such as particulate matter $(PM)_1$, $PM_{2.5}$, and PM_{10}, which are associated with a 13% to 20% higher prevalence of diabetes, especially in people aged <50 years or with overweight or obesity (BMI > 25 kg/m^2).[63] There is also growing evidence suggesting that different patterns of gut microbiota may alter the metabolic and inflammatory milieu of the host to increase the risk of prediabetes and overt diabetes.[64] These host-microbiota interactions might be further modified by health-related behaviors and medications.

APPROACHES TO TRANSFORMING DIABETES PREVENTION AND CARE

To prevent diabetes and reduce the occurrence of its cardiovascular-kidney and other complications, a multilevel approach is required to target the society, community, and individual[15] (see also Chapters 3 and 4). Elements of this approach are summarized in Fig. 1.2. At the individual level, integrated assessment, education, and care services in a structured, team-based setting have been shown to improve clinical outcomes of diabetes. In a meta-analysis of 181 randomized controlled trials, quality improvement initiatives targeted at healthcare providers through team changes (e.g., delegating tasks to, or expanding the roles of, nonphysician personnel; using interprofessional teams to provide shared care); at patients through education and support to promote self-management; and at processes such as using tools (e.g., electronic diabetes registers) or people (e.g., trained healthcare assistants or peers) to relay information and enhance patient-provider communication had the greatest benefits in reducing HbA_{1c}, blood pressure, and LDL cholesterol.[65] Given the silent and progressive nature of diabetes, establishing diabetes registers can help organize routinely collected patient data and provide personalized information for risk stratification, empowerment of self-management, and individualized treatment.[15] These data can be leveraged to analyze population trends and develop outcome models to inform health policy and decision-making.

SUMMARY

Diabetes is a major public health problem associated with escalating healthcare costs. On a personal basis, diabetes can cause debilitating complications, leading to the loss of societal productivity and human suffering. The global burden of diabetes is large and growing, affecting populations in every region of the world. The largest burden of diabetes occurs in LMICs, where prevention is of utmost importance to reducing the costs and complications of this condition. Diabetes is caused by a confluence of factors including, but not limited to, health-related behaviors and genetic and environmental factors. Health-related behaviors, particularly physical inactivity; consumption of high-calorie, low-fiber diets; and poor sleep, can lead to adiposity with worsening insulin sensitivity and β-cell function, resulting in the progression from normal glucose tolerance to prediabetes and diabetes in at-risk individuals. To address this epidemic, a multilevel approach is needed to reduce the burden of diabetes on the society, community, and individual by creating a health-enabling environment and transforming care delivery aimed at promoting early detection, prevention, and treatment through empowerment and personalized care.

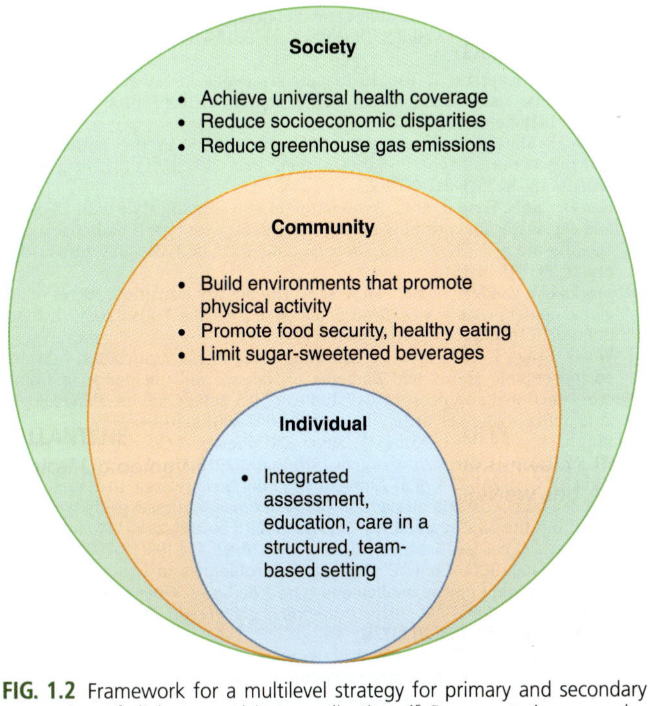

FIG. 1.2 Framework for a multilevel strategy for primary and secondary prevention of diabetes and its complications.[15] Representative examples for each category are indicated in the figure. From Chan JCN, Lim LL, Wareham NJ, et al. The Lancet Commission on diabetes: using data to transform diabetes care and patient lives. *Lancet*. 2020;396(10267):2019–2082. https://doi.org/10.1016/S0140-6736(20)32374-6.

REFERENCES

1. IDF Diabetes Atlas, 11th Edition Committee. *IDF Diabetes Atlas*. 11th ed. International Diabetes Federation; 2025.
2. Kong APS, Chow EYK, Chan JCN. *Other disorders with type 1 phenotype. Textbook of Diabetes*. John Wiley & Sons, Ltd; 2017:154–160. https://doi.org/10.1002/9781118924853.ch11.
3. American Diabetes Association Professional Practice Committee. 2. Diagnosis and classification of diabetes: standards of care in diabetes—2024. *Diabetes Care*. 2023;47(suppl 1):S20–S42. https://doi.org/10.2337/dc24-S002.
4. World Health Organization, International Diabetes Federation. *Definition and diagnosis of diabetes mellitus and intermediate hyperglycaemia: report of a WHO/IDF Consultation*; 2006. http://www.who.int/diabetes/publications/diagnosis_diabetes2006/en/.
5. McCarthy MI. Painting a new picture of personalised medicine for diabetes. *Diabetologia*. 2017;60(5):793–799. https://doi.org/10.1007/s00125-017-4210-x.
6. Ahlqvist E, Storm P, Käräjämäki A, et al. Novel subgroups of adult-onset diabetes and their association with outcomes: a data-driven cluster analysis of six variables. *Lancet Diabetes Endocrinol*. 2018;6(5):361–369. https://doi.org/10.1016/S2213-8587(18)30051-2.
7. Fan B, Wu H, Shi M, et al. Associations of the HOMA2-%B and HOMA2-IR with progression to diabetes and glycaemic deterioration in young and middle-aged Chinese. *Diabetes Metab Res Rev*. 2022;38(5):e3525. https://doi.org/10.1002/dmrr.3525.
8. UK Prospective Diabetes Study 6. Complications in newly diagnosed type 2 diabetic patients and their association with different clinical and biochemical risk factors. *Diabetes Res*. 1990;13(1):1–11.
9. Adler AI, Stratton IM, Neil HAW, et al. Association of systolic blood pressure with macrovascular and microvascular complications of type 2 diabetes (UKPDS 36): prospective observational study. *BMJ*. 2000;321(7258):412–419. https://doi.org/10.1136/bmj.321.7258.412.
10. Harding JL, Pavkov ME, Magliano DJ, Shaw JE, Gregg EW. Global trends in diabetes complications: a review of current evidence. *Diabetologia*. 2019;62(1):3–16. https://doi.org/10.1007/s00125-018-4711-2.
11. The Emerging Risk Factors Collaboration. Diabetes mellitus, fasting glucose, and risk of cause-specific death. *N Engl J Med*. 2011;364(9):829–841. https://doi.org/10.1056/NEJMoa1008862.
12. Lim S, Bae JH, Kwon HS, Nauck MA. COVID-19 and diabetes mellitus: from pathophysiology to clinical management. *Nat Rev Endocrinol*. 2021;17(1):11–30. https://doi.org/10.1038/s41574-020-00435-4.
13. Magliano DJ, Sacre JW, Harding JL, Gregg EW, Zimmet PZ, Shaw JE. Young-onset type 2 diabetes mellitus—implications for morbidity and mortality. *Nat Rev Endocrinol*. 2020;16(6):321–331. https://doi.org/10.1038/s41574-020-0334-z.
14. Nanayakkara N, Curtis AJ, Heritier S, et al. Impact of age at type 2 diabetes mellitus diagnosis on mortality and vascular complications: systematic review and meta-analyses. *Diabetologia*. 2021;64(2):275–287. https://doi.org/10.1007/s00125-020-05319-w.
15. Chan JCN, Lim LL, Wareham NJ, et al. The Lancet Commission on diabetes: using data to transform diabetes care and patient lives. *Lancet*. 2020;396(10267):2019–2082. https://doi.org/10.1016/S0140-6736(20)32374-6.
16. Gæde P, Vedel P, Larsen N, Jensen GV, Parving HH, Pedersen O. Multifactorial intervention and cardiovascular disease in patients with type 2 diabetes. *N Engl J Med*. 2003;348(5):383–393.
17. Rawshani A, Rawshani A, Franzén S, et al. Risk factors, mortality, and cardiovascular outcomes in patients with type 2 diabetes. *N Engl J Med*. 2018;379(7):633–644. https://doi.org/10.1056/NEJMoa1800256.

18. Marx N, Federici M, Schütt K, et al. 2023 ESC guidelines for the management of cardiovascular disease in patients with diabetes: developed by the task force on the management of cardiovascular disease in patients with diabetes of the European Society of Cardiology (ESC). *Eur Heart J*. 2023;44(39):4043–4140. https://doi.org/10.1093/eurheartj/ehad192.
19. American Diabetes Association Professional Practice Committee. 4. Comprehensive medical evaluation and assessment of comorbidities: standards of care in diabetes—2024. *Diabetes Care*. 2023;47(suppl 1):S52–S76. https://doi.org/10.2337/dc24-S004.
20. Buse JB, Wexler DJ, Tsapas A, et al. 2019 Update to: Management of hyperglycemia in type 2 diabetes, 2018. A consensus report by the American Diabetes Association (ADA) and the European Association for the Study of Diabetes (EASD). *Diabetes Care*. 2020;43(2):487–493. https://doi.org/10.2337/dci19-0066.
21. Magliano DJ, Chen L, Islam RM, et al. Trends in the incidence of diagnosed diabetes: a multicountry analysis of aggregate data from 22 million diagnoses in high-income and middle-income settings. *Lancet Diabetes Endocrinol*. 2021;9(4):203–211. https://doi.org/10.1016/S2213-8587(20)30402-2.
22. Magliano DJ, Chen L, Carstensen B, et al. Trends in all-cause mortality among people with diagnosed diabetes in high-income settings: a multicountry analysis of aggregate data. *Lancet Diabetes Endocrinol*. 2022;10(2):112–119. https://doi.org/10.1016/S2213-8587(21)00327-2.
23. Zhou B, Rayner AW, Gregg EW, Sheffer KE, Carrillo-Larco RM, Bennett JE, et al. Worldwide trends in diabetes prevalence and treatment from 1990 to 2022: a pooled analysis of 1108 population representative studies with 141 million participants. *Lancet*. 2024;404(10467):2077–2093.
24. Fang M, Wang D, Coresh J, Selvin E. Trends in diabetes treatment and control in U.S. adults, 1999–2018. *N Engl J Med*. 2021;384(23):2219–2228. https://doi.org/10.1056/NEJMsa2032271.
25. Manne-Goehler J, Geldsetzer P, Agoudavi K, et al. Health system performance for people with diabetes in 28 low- and middle-income countries: a cross-sectional study of nationally representative surveys. *PLoS Med*. 2019;16(3):e1002751. https://doi.org/10.1371/journal.pmed.1002751.
26. Aschner P, Gagliardino JJ, Ilkova H, et al. Persistent poor glycaemic control in individuals with type 2 diabetes in developing countries: 12 years of real-world evidence of the International Diabetes Management Practices Study (IDMPS). *Diabetologia*. 2020;63:711–721. https://doi.org/10.1007/s00125-019-05078-3.
27. Wu H, Lau ESH, Ma RCW, et al. Secular trends in all-cause and cause-specific mortality rates in people with diabetes in Hong Kong, 2001–2016: a retrospective cohort study. *Diabetologia*. 2020;63(4):757–766. https://doi.org/10.1007/s00125-019-05074-7.
28. Yang A, Wu H, Lau ESH, et al. Trends in glucose-lowering drug use, glycemic control, and severe hypoglycemia in adults with diabetes in Hong Kong, 2002–2016. *Diabetes Care*. 2020;43(12):2967–2974. https://doi.org/10.2337/dc20-0260.
29. Chan JCN, Lim LL, Luk AOY, et al. From Hong Kong diabetes register to JADE program to RAMP-DM for data-driven actions. *Diabetes Care*. 2019;42(11):2022–2031. https://doi.org/10.2337/dci19-0003.
30. Gregg EW, Li Y, Wang J, et al. Changes in diabetes-related complications in the United States, 1990–2010. *N Engl J Med*. 2014;370(16):1514–1523. https://doi.org/10.1056/NEJMoa1310799.
31. Kahn SE, Hull RL, Utzschneider KM. Mechanisms linking obesity to insulin resistance and type 2 diabetes. *Nature*. 2006;444(7121):840–846. https://doi.org/10.1038/nature05482.
32. Zheng Y, Ley SH, Hu FB. Global aetiology and epidemiology of type 2 diabetes mellitus and its complications. *Nat Rev Endocrinol*. 2018;14(2):88–98. https://doi.org/10.1038/nrendo.2017.151.
33. DeFronzo RA. From the triumvirate to the ominous octet: a new paradigm for the treatment of type 2 diabetes mellitus. *Diabetes*. 2009;58(4):773–795. https://doi.org/10.2337/db09-9028.
34. Ke C, Narayan KMV, Chan JCN, Jha P, Shah BR. Pathophysiology, phenotypes and management of type 2 diabetes mellitus in Indian and Chinese populations. *Nat Rev Endocrinol*. 2022;18:413–432. https://doi.org/10.1038/s41574-022-00669-4.
35. Cheung J, Lau E, Tsui C, et al. Combined associations of family history and self-management with age at diagnosis and cardiometabolic risk in 86,931 patients with type 2 diabetes: Joint Asia Diabetes Evaluation (JADE) Register from 11 countries. *BMC Med*. 2022 Jul 14;20(1):249. https://doi.org/10.1186/s12916-022-02424-y.
36. Kong AP, Luk AO, Chan JC. Detecting people at high risk of type 2 diabetes- How do we find them and who should be treated? *Best Pract Res, Clin Endocrinol Metab*. 2016;30(3):345–355. https://doi.org/10.1016/j.beem.2016.06.003.
37. Hales CN, Barker DJP. Type 2 (non-insulin-dependent) diabetes mellitus: the thrifty phenotype hypothesis. *Diabetologia*. 1992;35(7):595–601. https://doi.org/10.1007/BF00400248.
38. Pettitt DJ, Lawrence JM, Beyer J, et al. Association between maternal diabetes in utero and age at offspring's diagnosis of type 2 diabetes. *Diabetes Care*. 2008;31(11):2126–2130. https://doi.org/10.2337/dc08-0769.
39. Batai K, Hooker S, Kittles RA. Leveraging genetic ancestry to study health disparities. *Am J Phys Anthropol*. 2021;175(2):363–375. https://doi.org/10.1002/ajpa.24144.
40. Kamiza AB, Toure SM, Vujkovic M, et al. Transferability of genetic risk scores in African populations. *Nat Med*. 2022;28(6):1163–1166. https://doi.org/10.1038/s41591-022-01835-x.
41. Mahajan A, Spracklen CN, Zhang W, et al. Multi-ancestry genetic study of type 2 diabetes highlights the power of diverse populations for discovery and translation. *Nat Genet*. 2022;54(5):560–572. https://doi.org/10.1038/s41588-022-01058-3.
42. McCarthy MI, Mahajan A. The value of genetic risk scores in precision medicine for diabetes. *Expert Rev Precis Med Drug Dev*. 2018;3(5):279–281. https://doi.org/10.1080/23808993.2018.1510732.
43. Udler MS, McCarthy MI, Florez JC, Mahajan A. Genetic risk scores for diabetes diagnosis and precision medicine. *Endocr Rev*. 2019;40(6):1500–1520. https://doi.org/10.1210/er.2019-00088.
44. Mahajan A, Taliun D, Thurner M, et al. Fine-mapping type 2 diabetes loci to single-variant resolution using high-density imputation and islet-specific epigenome maps. *Nat Genet*. 2018;50(11):1505–1513. https://doi.org/10.1038/s41588-018-0241-6.
45. Franks PW, Merino J. Gene-lifestyle interplay in type 2 diabetes. *Curr Opin Genet Dev*. 2018;50:35–40. https://doi.org/10.1016/j.gde.2018.02.001.
46. Schulz LO, Bennett PH, Ravussin E, et al. Effects of traditional and western environments on prevalence of type 2 diabetes in Pima Indians in Mexico and the U.S. *Diabetes Care*. 2006;29(8):1866–1871. https://doi.org/10.2337/dc06-0138.
47. Said MA, Verweij N, van der Harst P. Associations of combined genetic and lifestyle risks with incident cardiovascular disease and diabetes in the UK Biobank Study. *JAMA Cardiol*. 2018;3(8):693–702. https://doi.org/10.1001/jamacardio.2018.1717.
48. Chung WK, Erion K, Florez JC, et al. Precision medicine in diabetes: a consensus report from the American Diabetes Association (ADA) and the European Association for the Study of Diabetes (EASD). *Diabetes Care*. 2020;43(7):1617–1635. https://doi.org/10.2337/dci20-0022.
49. Chan JCN, Malik V, Jia W, et al. Diabetes in Asia: epidemiology, risk factors, and pathophysiology. *JAMA*. 2009;301(20):2129–2140. https://doi.org/10.1001/jama.2009.726.
50. Ma RCW, Chan JCN. Type 2 diabetes in East Asians: similarities and differences with populations in Europe and the United States. *Ann NY Acad Sci*. 2013;1281(1):64–91. https://doi.org/10.1111/nyas.12098.
51. Jung MH, Yi SW, An SJ, Balkau B, Yi JJ, Kim H. Complex interaction of fasting glucose, body mass index, age and sex on all-cause mortality: a cohort study in 15 million Korean adults. *Diabetologia*. 2020;63(8):1616–1625. https://doi.org/10.1007/s00125-020-05160-1.
52. Aune D, Sen A, Prasad M, et al. BMI and all cause mortality: systematic review and non-linear dose-response meta-analysis of 230 cohort studies with 3.74 million deaths among 30.3 million participants. *BMJ*. 2016;353:i2156. https://doi.org/10.1136/bmj.i2156.
53. Yoon KH, Ko SH, Cho JH, et al. Selective β-cell loss and α-cell expansion in patients with type 2 diabetes mellitus in Korea. *J Clin Endocrinol Metab*. 2003;88(5):2300–2308. https://doi.org/10.1210/jc.2002-020735.
54. Després JP, Lemieux I. Abdominal obesity and metabolic syndrome. *Nature*. 2006;444(7121):881–887. https://doi.org/10.1038/nature05488.
55. Ludwig DS, Hu FB, Tappy L, Brand-Miller J. Dietary carbohydrates: role of quality and quantity in chronic disease. *BMJ*. 2018;361:k2340. https://doi.org/10.1136/bmj.k2340.
56. Yu D, Zheng W, Cai H, et al. Long-term diet quality and risk of type 2 diabetes among urban Chinese adults. *Diabetes Care*. 2018;41(4):723–730. https://doi.org/10.2337/dc17-1626.
57. Sikand G, Severson T. Top 10 dietary strategies for atherosclerotic cardiovascular risk reduction. *Am J Prev Cardiol*. 2020;4:100106. https://doi.org/10.1016/j.ajpc.2020.100106.
58. Kolb H, Martin S. Environmental/lifestyle factors in the pathogenesis and prevention of type 2 diabetes. *BMC Med*. 2017;15(1):131. https://doi.org/10.1186/s12916-017-0901-x.
59. Han H, Cao Y, Feng C, et al. Association of a healthy lifestyle with all-cause and cause-specific mortality among individuals with type 2 diabetes: a prospective study in UK biobank. *Diabetes Care*. 2022;45(2):319–329. https://doi.org/10.2337/dc21-1512.
60. Jaacks LM, Vandevijvere S, Pan A, et al. The obesity transition: stages of the global epidemic. *Lancet Diabetes Endocrinol*. 2019 Mar;7(3):231–240. https://doi.org/10.1016/S2213-8587(19)30026-9.
61. Wu H, Bragg F, Yang L, et al. Sex differences in the association between socioeconomic status and diabetes prevalence and incidence in China: cross-sectional and prospective studies of 0.5 million adults. *Diabetologia*. 2019;62(8):1420–1429. https://doi.org/10.1007/s00125-019-4896-z.
62. Ding C, Lim LL, Xu L, Kong AP. Sleep and obesity. *J Obes & Metab Syndr*. 2018;27(1):4–24. https://doi.org/10.7570/jomes.2018.27.1.4.
63. Yang BY, Qian ZM, Li S, et al. Ambient air pollution in relation to diabetes and glucose-homoeostasis markers in China: a cross-sectional study with findings from the 33 Communities Chinese Health Study. *Lancet Planet Health*. 2018 Feb;2(2):e64–e73. https://doi.org/10.1016/S2542-5196(18)30001-9.
64. Chu N, Chan JCN, Chow E. Pharmacomicrobiomics in western medicine and traditional Chinese medicine in type 2 diabetes. *Front Endocrinol (Lausanne)*. 2022;13:857090. https://doi.org/10.3389/fendo.2022.857090. PMID: 35600606; PMCID: PMC9114736.
65. Lim LL, Lau ESH, Kong APS, et al. Aspects of multicomponent integrated care promote sustained improvement in surrogate clinical outcomes: a systematic review and meta-analysis. *Diabetes Care*. 2018;41(6):1312–1320. https://doi.org/10.2337/dc17-2010.

2 Insulin Resistance: Pathophysiology, Molecular Mechanisms, and Genetic Insights

HANS-ULRICH HÄRING AND BAPTIST GALLWITZ

Type 2 diabetes mellitus (T2DM) is a chronic disturbance of glucose metabolism without the absolute insulin deficiency that is typical for type 1 diabetes. Rather, T2DM is characterized by a reduced efficacy of insulin action in different peripheral tissues (insulin resistance) as well as a disturbance in beta-cell function. These two important pathophysiologic characteristics in T2DM result in an imbalance of insulin availability and insulin demand. The clinical manifestation of the disease occurs mostly in the fourth to fifth decade of life, although alarming recent data show an increase in obesity and T2DM even in adolescents.

GENETIC FACTORS

T2DM is a polygenetic disease with heterogeneous phenotypes and different gene-environment interactions. A high genetic predisposition for T2DM has been shown in population studies (e.g., the Pima Indians) and in family studies. First-degree relatives of patients with T2DM have a significantly higher risk for T2DM than people without a hereditary or genetic risk.[1] Twin studies revealed a much higher diabetes concordance in homozygous twins compared to heterozygous twins. Although the existence of these genetic factors has been known for a considerable time, it was difficult to identify specific T2DM genes until recently, when genome-wide analyses and the human genome project led to progress in this field.[2–4]

The greatest success in T2DM genetics arose from the development and use of high-density single-nucleotide polymorphism (SNP) arrays in large case-control cohorts. Most of the gene variants could be confirmed in many ethnicities, whereas others, probably because of divergent risk allele frequencies, may have higher relevance for certain ethnic groups.[4]

Recent studies also provided evidence that SNPs associated with diabetes risk act in an additive manner to increase the diabetes risk.[4–6] Although significantly contributing to the T2DM risk, these gene-gene interactions do not yet allow a substantially better disease prediction than clinical risk factors (e.g., body mass index [BMI], age, sex, family history of diabetes, fasting glucose level, blood pressure [BP], and plasma triglycerides),[4,7–9] nor do they explain the heritability of T2DM.[4,5]

Beyond that, some of the diabetes-relevant genes are susceptible to persistent and partly inheritable epigenetic regulation—that is, DNA methylation and histone modifications—so gene-environment interactions are additional important factors that contribute to the complexity of T2DM genetics.[4,10–12]

Genome-wide association studies identified a series of T2DM risk loci that are mostly associated with impaired pancreatic beta-cell function.[3,13–37]

Although the underlying mechanisms by which common genetic variations within these loci affect beta-cell function are not completely understood, risk variants may alter glucose-stimulated insulin secretion,[3,14,16–18,30–34] proinsulin conversion,[3,38,39] and incretin secretion or incretin action.[3,40] Table 2.1 summarizes the most important diabetes genes and their functional roles.[4]

It has further become evident in recent studies that genetic variants in several diabetes risk genes may predict the treatment outcome of glucose-lowering drugs. Response to thiazolidinedione therapy has been associated with peroxisome proliferator–activated receptor gamma variations[3,41] in some, but not all, studies.[3,42,43] The genetic variants of the transcription factor 7-like 2 (TCF7L2, a transcription factor involved in the Wnt-signaling pathway and the most important genetic marker associated with T2DM) have been reported to influence

TABLE 2.1 Effects of Single-Nucleotide Polymorphisms (SNPs) in Confirmed T2DM Genes on Prediabetic Traits

GENE	LOCATION ON CHROMOSOME	TISSUE EXPRESSION (REPRODUCTIVE SYSTEM NOT INCLUDED)	VARIANTS (APPROXIMATE RISK ALLELE FREQUENCY IN EUROPEANS)	RISK ALLELE EFFECTS
ADAMTS9	3	Skeletal muscle, breast, thymus, kidney, prostate, pancreas, heart, lung, spinal cord, brain, all fetal tissues	rs4607103 (80%)	Unknown
CAPN10	2	Thymus, colon, bladder, brain, spleen, prostate, skeletal muscle, pancreas, heart, lymph node, lung, kidney	rs3792267 (70%), rs3842570 (40%), rs5030952 (90%)	Glucose-stimulated insulin secretion ↓; proinsulin conversion ↓; whole-body insulin sensitivity ↓
CDC123 \CAMK1D	10	Bone marrow, smooth muscle, kidney, prostate, colon, bladder, spleen, lung, lymph node, skin, breast, brain, liver, thymus and skin, retina, spleen, skeletal muscle, lung	rs12779790 (20%)	Insulin secretion ↓
CDKAL1	6	Bone marrow, breast, liver, spleen, prostate, retina, brain, lung, kidney, thymus, pancreas, skeletal muscle	rs7754840 (30%)	Glucose-stimulated insulin secretion ↓; proinsulin conversion ↓
CDKN2A /CDKN2B	9	Ubiquitous; bladder, colon, lung, spleen, skin, liver, breast, skeletal muscle, prostate, kidney, brain, pancreas, adipose tissue	rs10811661 (80%)	Glucose-stimulated insulin secretion ↓
ENPP1	6	Thyroid gland, kidney, skeletal muscle, breast, liver, skin, thymus, salivary gland, brain capillaries	rs1044498/K121Q (10%)	Whole-body insulin sensitivity ↓; insulin secretion ↓
FTO	16	Brain, pancreas, skeletal muscle, prostate, retina, heart, skin, breast, lung, kidney, liver, thymus, fetal brain, fetal kidney, fetal liver	rs8050136 (40%), rs9939609 (40%)	Overall fat mass ↑; energy intake ↑; cerebrocortical insulin sensitivity ↓
HHEX	10	Thyroid gland, brain, lymph node, spleen, liver, lung, kidney, breast, pancreas, thymus, skin, prostate, fetal pancreas	rs7923837 (60%)	Glucose-stimulated insulin secretion ↓
HNF1B	17	Colon, kidney, liver, thymus, retina, pancreas, prostate, lung	rs757210 (40%)	Unknown
IGF2BP2	3	Smooth muscle, colon, lung, retina, skeletal muscle, skin, kidney, thymus, fetal liver, fetal brain, pancreas	rs4402960 (30%)	Glucose-stimulated insulin secretion ↓
JAZF1	7	Lymph node, retina, pancreas, thymus, brain, skin, liver, skeletal muscle, lung, spleen, prostate	rs864745 (50%)	Insulin secretion ↓
KCNJ11	11	Pancreas, heart, pituitary gland, skeletal muscle, brain, smooth muscle	rs5219/E23K (50%)	Insulin secretion ↓; glucose dependent; suppression of glucagon secretion ↓
KCNQ1	11	Thyroid gland, bone marrow, prostate, heart, pancreas, lung, thymus, skin, liver, kidney	rs2237892 (90%), rs151290 (80%)	Insulin secretion ↓; incretin secretion ↓
MTNR1B	11	Retina, brain, pancreas	rs10830963 (30%), rs10830962 (40%), rs4753426 (50%)	Glucose-stimulated insulin secretion ↓
NOTCH2	1	Lung, skin, thyroid gland, skeletal muscle, smooth muscle, kidney, bladder, lymph node, breast, colon, prostate, spleen, brain, thymus, heart, liver, pancreas	rs10923931 (10%)	Unknown
PPARG	3	Adipose tissue, colon, lung, kidney, breast, spleen, skin, prostate, bone marrow, brain, skeletal muscle, liver	rs1801282/P12A (80%)	Whole-body insulin sensitivity ↓; adipose tissue insulin sensitivity ↓; insulin clearance ↓
SLC30A8	8	Pancreas, kidney, lung, breast, amygdala	rs13266634/R325W (70%)	Glucose-stimulated insulin secretion ↓; proinsulin conversion ↓
TCF7L2	10	Brain, lung, bone marrow, thyroid gland, colon, pancreas, skin, breast, kidney, liver, thymus, prostate	rs7903146 (30%), rs12255372 (30%), rs7901695 (30%)	Incretin-stimulated insulin secretion ↓; proinsulin conversion ↓; whole-body insulin sensitivity ↓; hepatic insulin sensitivity ↓
THADA	2	Ubiquitous	rs7578597/T1187A (90%)	Unknown
TSPAN8/ LGR5	12	Spinal cord, colon, skeletal muscle, prostate, liver, lung, pancreas, kidney, skeletal muscle, skin, brain, spinal cord	rs7961581 (30%)	Insulin secretion ↓
WFS1	4	Ubiquitous	rs10010131 (60%)	Incretin-stimulated insulin secretion ↓

Data from Staiger H, Machicao F, Fritsche A, Häring HU. Pathomechanisms of type 2 diabetes genes. *Endocr Rev.* 2009;30:557.

disease severity and therapeutic control,[3,44] including lifestyle intervention,[3,45] and the response to sulfonylureas and possibly incretin-based therapies.[3,46]

INSULIN RESISTANCE

T2DM, according to our present understanding, is a multifactorial disease characterized by insulin resistance of various degrees in different organs.[47] Insulin resistance is in most patients further accompanied by central obesity, arterial hypertension, dyslipidemia, and other risk factors for cardiovascular disease. The joint presence of these risk factors with or without manifest T2DM is summarized by the term "metabolic syndrome." The metabolic syndrome is a multifactorial metabolic disorder with a twofold to fourfold increased risk for cardiovascular disease (see Chapter 4).

The hormone insulin has a number of cellular effects and regulates not only glucose metabolism but also lipid and protein metabolism, as well as DNA synthesis and lipolysis (Fig. 2.1).[47] Any defect of these different cellular effects of insulin action can be seen as insulin resistance. In experimental medicine, the gold standard for measuring and quantifying insulin resistance is the euglycemic glucose clamp technique. This technique is too complicated and time and personnel consuming for everyday clinical practice; therefore a number of simpler tests for determining insulin resistance were developed. These are basically based on the assumption that a curvilinear relationship between insulin sensitivity and insulin secretion exists. In healthy patients it is possible to calculate the insulin sensitivity from the fasting plasma glucose concentration with a special formula for a hyperbolic relationship. However, this formula is not applicable for patients with a disturbance of glucose tolerance and diabetes because they show a disturbance in insulin secretion of varying degrees in addition to being insulin resistant. The presently available simple tests to determine insulin resistance in patients with diabetes are based on the measurements of the fasting plasma glucose and insulin concentrations (homeostatic model assessment [HOMA])[48] or on the completion of an oral glucose tolerance test (OGTT) with measurements of plasma glucose and insulin concentrations (e.g., HOMA-IR [HOMA model for insulin resistance], insulin sensitivity index [ISI][0,120], Matsuda index, and the Stumvoll index).[49–51] Whereas the glucose clamp technique is a reliable method for the quantification of insulin resistance, the previously mentioned simple tests do not allow an exact quantification for a single individual. Therefore the determination of insulin resistance with these tests in an individual clinical setting is feasible only in special situations. Frequent sources of error include, for example, the incorrect performance of the OGTT that will eventually lead to wrong conclusions in determining insulin resistance. In everyday clinical practice, insulin resistance can be more easily detected with symptoms such as central obesity or other factors of the metabolic syndrome. Therapeutic decisions are mainly based on these clinically visible characteristics and will lead to recommendations of lifestyle changes, body weight reduction, and pharmacologic interventions with oral glucose-lowering drugs such as metformin. It should be mentioned that insulin resistance may vary considerably depending on the patient's

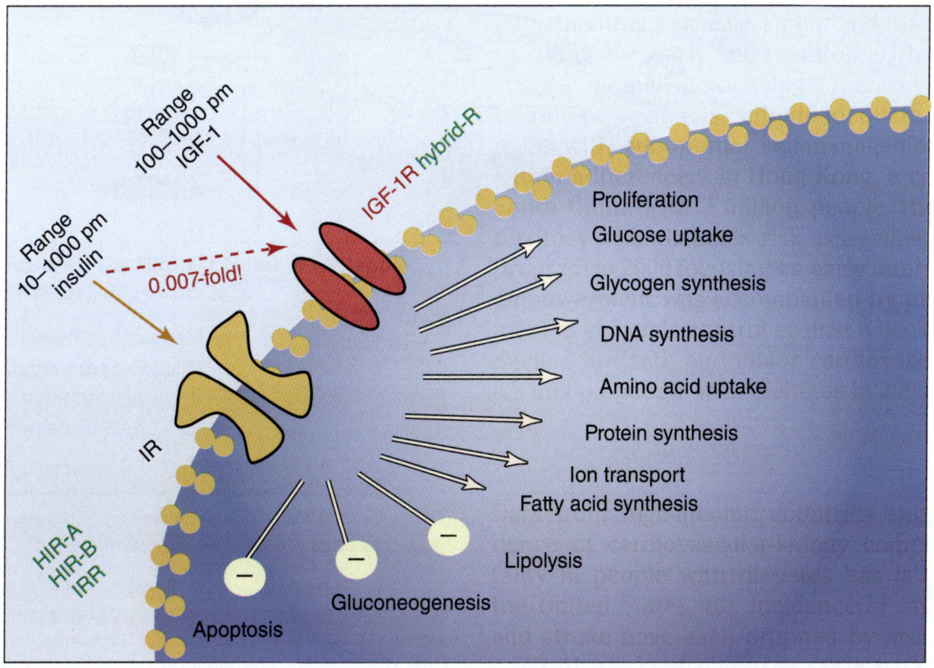

FIG. 2.1 Insulin receptor (*IR*)–mediated effects. The binding of a ligand to its receptor triggers the activation of signaling pathways through effector proteins that transduce signals to several intracellular second-messenger systems, which eventually lead to biologic actions. The figure shows the *IR* with three different isoforms (IRR, HIR-A, and HIR-B) as well as the structurally and functionally similar receptor for insulin-like growth factor (*IGF-1*). The biologic actions triggered by ligand binding of insulin are depicted in a schematic manner.

level of physical fitness and activity, body weight, and overall health (e.g., acute and chronic infections, tumors). Insulin resistance is a common and important risk factor for the development of T2DM and cardiovascular disease.[52–60] However, insulin resistance does not always lead to diabetes even though obesity is the most important risk factor. Only patients with a disturbance in insulin secretion or other risk factors will develop diabetes.

Insulin Signaling and Cellular Mechanisms of Insulin Resistance

Insulin effects are transmitted by insulin binding to a specific transmembrane insulin receptor. The receptor belongs to the family of tyrosine kinase receptors, like the receptors for many growth factors.[61] The active receptor is a dimer of two combined subunits. Insulin effects in the intact organism are mediated almost exclusively through the insulin receptor but can also be mediated by hybrid receptors that are formed by one subunit of the insulin receptor and another subunit of the receptor for insulin-like growth factor (IGF-1). Insulin binds with high affinity to its own receptor and with a 100 to 150 times lower affinity to the IGF-1 receptor. Therefore insulin binding to the IGF-1 receptor does not play a notable role at physiologic insulin plasma concentrations compared with IGF-1 effects at its own receptor.[62] The affinity toward insulin-IGF-1 hybrid receptors lies between that for the insulin receptor and that for the IGF-1 receptor. The binding of insulin to its receptor leads to a cascade of cellular signals that are mostly phosphorylation and dephosphorylation events. The docking proteins IRS-1 to IRS-4 (insulin receptor substrates) have been detected as primary intracellular substrates for postreceptor signaling. These transmit the insulin signal downstream into different cellular compartments after phosphorylation by the activated insulin receptor.[63,64] There are two distinctly different pathways in the intracellular insulin signal transmission. One pathway conveys the metabolic effects of insulin via the signaling molecules AKT/protein kinase B (PKB), and the other pathway transmits the mitogenic effects of insulin via the signaling proteins Ras/Raf/MAP kinase (Fig. 2.2).[47,62,64] Insulin resistance can, therefore, lead to a reduction of metabolic and mitogenic effects. Because redundancies and compensation mechanisms are present throughout the entire system of the intracellular signal transduction of the insulin signal, a disturbance of a single transmission element does not necessarily result in insulin resistance. Depending on the defects of the insulin signal transduction, metabolic and mitogenic effects of insulin may be affected to varying degrees.[65,66]

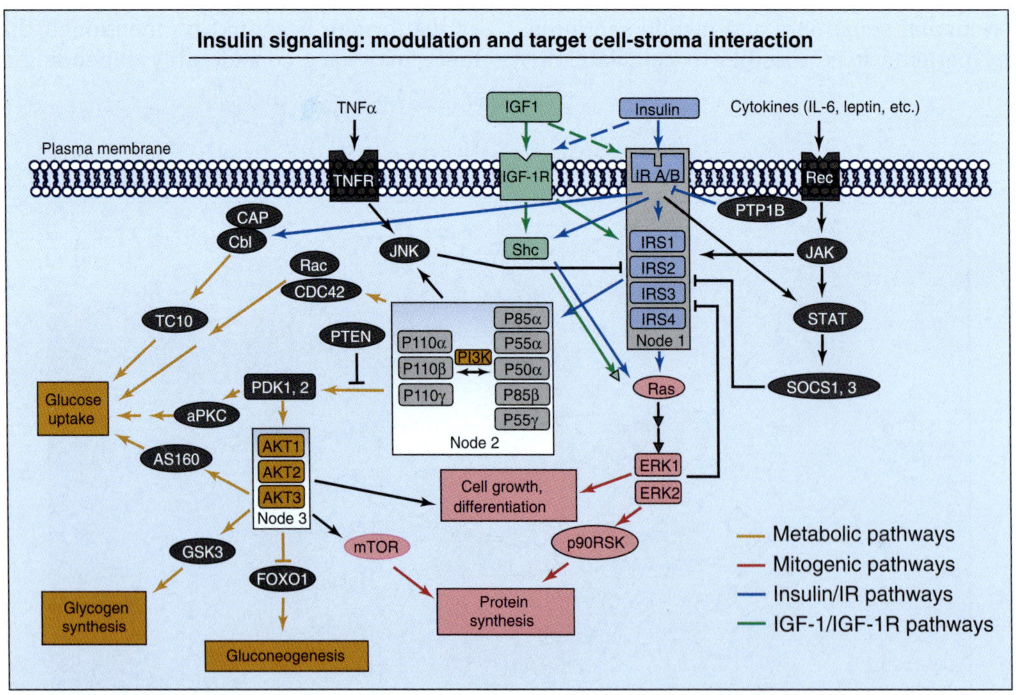

FIG. 2.2 Insulin signaling: modulation and target cell-stroma interaction. Critical nodes form an important part of the signaling network that functions downstream of the insulin receptor (*IR*) and the insulin-like growth factor 1 (*IGF-1*) receptor (*IGF-1R*). The important metabolic and mitogenic pathways are shown. Three important nodes in the insulin pathway are the IR and the IR substrates (*IRS*) 1 to 4 (node 1), the phosphatidylinositol 3-kinase (*PI3K*) with its several regulatory and catalytic subunits (node 2), and the three AKT/protein kinase B (PKB) isoforms (node 3). Downstream or intermediate effectors, as well as modulators, of these critical nodes include atypical protein kinase C (*aPKC*), AKT substrate of 160 kDa (*AS160*), Cas-Br-M (murine) ecotropic retroviral transforming sequence homologue (*Cbl*), Cbl-associated protein (*CAP*), cell-division cycle 42 (*CDC42*), extracellular signal-regulated kinase 1 and 2 (*ERK1* and *ERK2*), forkhead box O1 (*FOXO1*), glycogen synthase kinase 3 (*GSK3*), Janus kinase (*JAK*), c-Jun-*N*-terminal kinase (*JNK*), mammalian target of rapamycin (*mTOR*), p90 ribosomal protein S6 kinase (p90RSK), phosphoinositide-dependent kinase 1 and 2 (*PDK1, 2*), phosphatase and tensin homologue (*PTEN*), protein tyrosine phosphatase-1B (*PTP1B*), Ras, Rac, Src-homology-2-containing protein (*Shc*), suppressor of cytokine signaling (*SOCS*), signal transducer and activator of transcription (*STAT*), and Ras homologue gene family, member Q (ARHQ; also called TC10). *IL*, Interleukin; *TNFα* tumor necrosis factor α; *TNFR*, TNF-α receptor. (Modified from Taniguchi CM, Emanuelli B, Kahn CR. Critical nodes in signalling pathways: insights into insulin action. *Nat Rev Mol Cell Biol.* 2006;7:85–95.)

Insulin Receptor, Insulin Receptor Substrates, and PKB/AKT Proteins

Numerous investigations have been carried out to investigate possible mutations in the gene for the insulin receptor in T2DM. Only very few mutations have been found that are associated with the development of insulin resistance or T2DM.[67–69] Furthermore, most studies have not shown a significant reduction in insulin receptor molecules in peripheral target tissues and organs for insulin action.[70–73] Therefore quantitative changes in insulin receptor expression and insulin receptor mutations are not responsible for the development of insulin resistance in T2DM. It is interesting to note that a reduction in insulin receptor autophosphorylation was detected in vitro in tissues from patients with T2DM in numerous former investigations.[74] It is hypothesized that the reduced autophosphorylation of the insulin receptor is responsible for disturbed insulin signal transduction and consequently the development of insulin resistance. The reduction in autophosphorylation and autoactivation of the insulin receptor is partially caused by modifications in the receptor molecule by an increased phosphorylation of serine residues.[75,76] The changes in insulin receptor activity are most likely secondary phenomena resulting from the metabolic changes in T2DM (e.g., hyperglycemia, dyslipidemia). Studies demonstrating normalization of the insulin receptor activity after lifestyle interventions support this hypothesis.[77–80] Only in rare patients with severe insulin resistance syndromes have insulin receptor mutations been detected that are associated with a reduced binding affinity of insulin to the insulin receptor or to a diminished autophosphorylation and autoactivation of the insulin receptor. These severe insulin resistance syndromes, also referred to as *type A insulin resistance*, most often lead to glucose metabolism disorders during adolescence and are often associated with acanthosis nigricans and hyperandrogenism in females.[67,75] Other very rare insulin receptor mutations involving a complete loss of function lead to severe diseases such as leprechaunism.[81]

Functional studies on the activation of the IRSs and the phosphatidylinositol 3-kinase (PI 3-kinase) that binds to the IRS were performed predominantly in muscle cells and adipocytes of patients with T2DM. These in vitro studies revealed reduced activation of IRS-1 and IRS-2 as well as reduced PI 3-kinase/PKB activity in T2DM.[65,69,82,83] Defects in the insulin signaling cascade are therefore already present in the first steps of the signal transmission in insulin resistance and T2DM. Apart from these findings, genetic polymorphisms in the genes for the IRS proteins and the PI 3-kinase/PKB/AKT complex were found in T2DM—for example, Gly972Arg for IRS-1 and Met326Iso for PI 3-kinase.[84–87] The incidence and the functional relevance of these polymorphisms are very heterogeneous in different populations. These studies suggest that the diminished activation of IRS-1, IRS-2, and PI 3-kinase/AKT in muscle cells, hepatocytes, and adipocytes may be secondary to regulatory signal changes in metabolic disturbances. It is interesting to note that a disturbance of the metabolic signal pathway via IRS/PI 3-kinase/AKT is present in insulin resistance in T2DM, whereas the mitogenic pathway of the insulin signal via MAP kinase is not affected. In summary, in insulin resistance, a reduced cellular action of insulin is found concerning the metabolic but not the mitogenic effects of insulin.[65]

GLUCOSE TRANSPORT

The activation of the insulin signal transduction cascade leads to glucose transport into the cell. The insulin effect on the glucose transport system is mediated by a translocation of glucose transporters from the intracellular pools to the plasma membrane on the one hand and by the activation of the transporters in the plasma membrane on the other.[61,62] There are at least 12 different glucose transporter proteins in different tissues.[88] The insulin-dependent glucose transporter type 4 (GLUT-4) is the most widely expressed glucose transporter and is responsible for the largest proportion of glucose transport in muscle and adipose tissue. In addition to that, glucose-dependent glucose transporters such as GLUT-1 in the brain, GLUT-2 in the liver, and sodium-dependent transporters such as GLUT-3 in the gastrointestinal tract are also known. Investigations in muscle cells and adipocytes have been performed to elucidate whether a defect in the insulin-dependent glucose transporter GLUT-4 is responsible for the development of insulin resistance in T2DM. The results from these experiments were relatively heterogeneous and revealed a reduced expression of GLUT-4 in some studies, a defect in the translocation and activation of GLUT-4 in others, as well as an unchanged GLUT-4 expression in T2DM.[82,89,90] It is interesting to note that in studies of patients with T2DM, a reduced translocation of glucose transport vesicles to the plasma membrane was found, whereas GLUT-4 expression was unchanged.[91,92] In studies investigating possible mutations of GLUT-4 in T2DM, no functionally relevant defects were found.[93] In summary, in T2DM, a reduced capacity of insulin-dependent translocation of GLUT-4 vesicles to the plasma membrane is observed as a consequence of insulin resistance (Fig. 2.3).[94]

ROLE OF THE ADIPOCYTE AND OBESITY IN TYPE 2 DIABETES

Obesity is one of the most important predisposing factors for the development of insulin resistance and T2DM. In the past two decades, we have learned to discriminate which fat compartments contribute substantially to this development. Patients with an increased visceral (mesenteric and omental) fat mass, as well as people with increased liver fat mass, have an increased risk for insulin resistance and T2DM.[53] This explains why measuring the waist circumference and the waist-to-hip ratio predicts diabetes incidence more reliably than measuring the BMI. Increased subcutaneous fat depots in the hip, thigh, or gluteal region do not increase the risk for insulin resistance as long as there is no accompanying increase in visceral fat.[56] An increased subcutaneous fat accumulation around the hip and thigh is often observed in females and is termed *gynoid fat distribution*, whereas central obesity is more common in males and is termed *android fat distribution*. The causes of predominantly subcutaneous or visceral fat storage are genetic and also dependent on sex hormone concentrations and additional endocrine influences. The understanding of genetic causes for central obesity is just being unraveled, but hormones such as cortisol and androgens have already been identified as being important for the development of central obesity. Visceral fat cells express a higher number of cortisol receptors and are, therefore, more sensitive to react to increased plasma cortisol concentrations.[95] One hypothesis is that insulin resistance–induced obesity is caused by an overactivity of the neuroendocrine hormonal axes as well as by genetic predisposition.[95] One rare example of an extreme cause of central obesity and in this case a secondary cause of diabetes development is Cushing syndrome. Furthermore, hyperandrogenism in females predisposes them to central obesity.[96] These females frequently have polycystic ovary syndrome and an increased risk for the development of T2DM during middle age and later.

Visceral adipose tissue is now seen as an endocrine organ with respect to special functions concerning activation and secretion of numerous hormones and cytokines that mediate insulin resistance and chronic inflammation (Fig. 2.4).[97,98] Not only omental adipose tissue but also an increased fat content in hepatocytes, muscle cells, and even intrapancreatic fat play an important role in the development of insulin resistance and even in a decrease in insulin secretion (caused by intrapancreatic fat).[4,47,55,98–100] Free fatty acids are important mediators in central obesity. Elevated free fatty acid concentrations in plasma are found in insulin resistance and T2DM. These free fatty acids are most likely liberated by an increased lipolytic activity of the central and visceral fat depots and facilitate insulin resistance through an increased rate of fatty acid oxidation of the involved organs. Insulin and the sympathetic nervous system are important regulators of lipolysis. In central obesity, the increased sympathetic activity and reduced insulin action mediate the rate of lipolysis, which results in an increase of free fatty acids.[47,54,55]

In addition to free fatty acids, numerous other factors play a role in the development of insulin resistance. In patients with insulin resistance, the insulin-sensitizing hormone adiponectin has gained much attention in the past few years, not only because circulating levels of this adipokine are markers of T2DM and an elevated risk for cardiovascular disease but also because adiponectin is involved in the progression of these diseases.[47,101–104] Adiponectin is a protein that is synthesized and secreted by fat cells. In obese individuals, significantly reduced adiponectin plasma concentrations are observed compared with lean people. Adiponectin is present in serum in relatively high concentrations, and the serum concentrations show a negative correlation with BMI and a positive correlation with insulin resistance and even with the incidence of cardiovascular diseases.[101,102] The exogenous application of adiponectin under experimental conditions leads to an improvement in insulin sensitivity, a reduction in plasma glucose concentrations because of the activation of

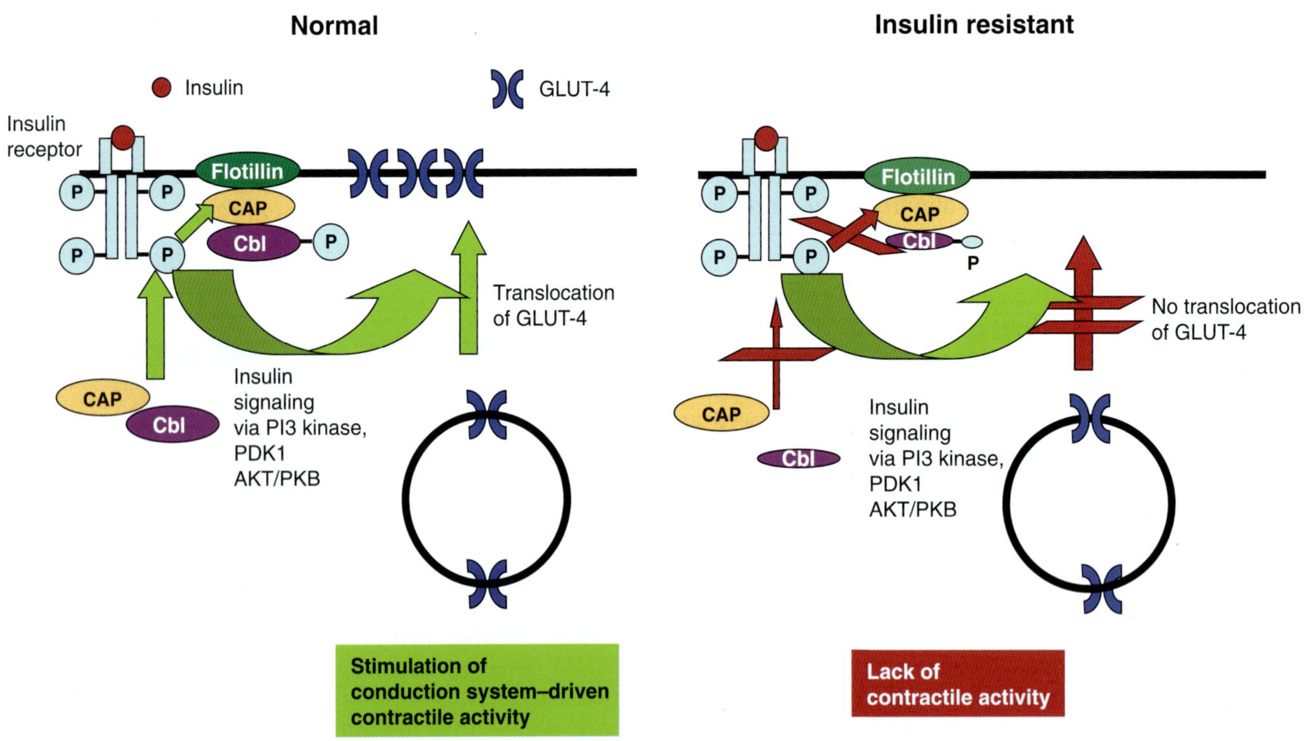

FIG. 2.3 Differences in the regulation of GLUT-4 translocation in cardiac myocytes under normal conditions and in insulin resistance. Under normal conditions in fully differentiated cardiac myocytes (*left*), insulin stimulates the activation of the PI3-K/PDK1/AKT signal transduction. Insulin further stimulates the phosphorylation of the protooncogene Cbl (Cas-Br-M [murine] ecotropic retroviral transforming sequence homologue) and its increased recruitment to a lipid raft-located complex containing flotillin and CAP (Cbl-associated protein). The joint activity of both pathways is a prerequisite for the translocation of the glucose transporter GLUT-4. In the insulin-resistant state in dedifferentiated cardiac myocytes (*right*), the stimulation of the PI3-K/PDK1/AKT signal transduction is unchanged. Cbl, on the other hand, is reduced, and furthermore Cbl phosphorylation is impaired. As a consequence, the translocation of GLUT-4 is inhibited and the pool of available GLUT-4 is also diminished. *PDK1*, Phosphoinositide-dependent kinase 1; *PKB*, protein kinase B; *PI3K*; phosphatidylinositol 3-kinase.

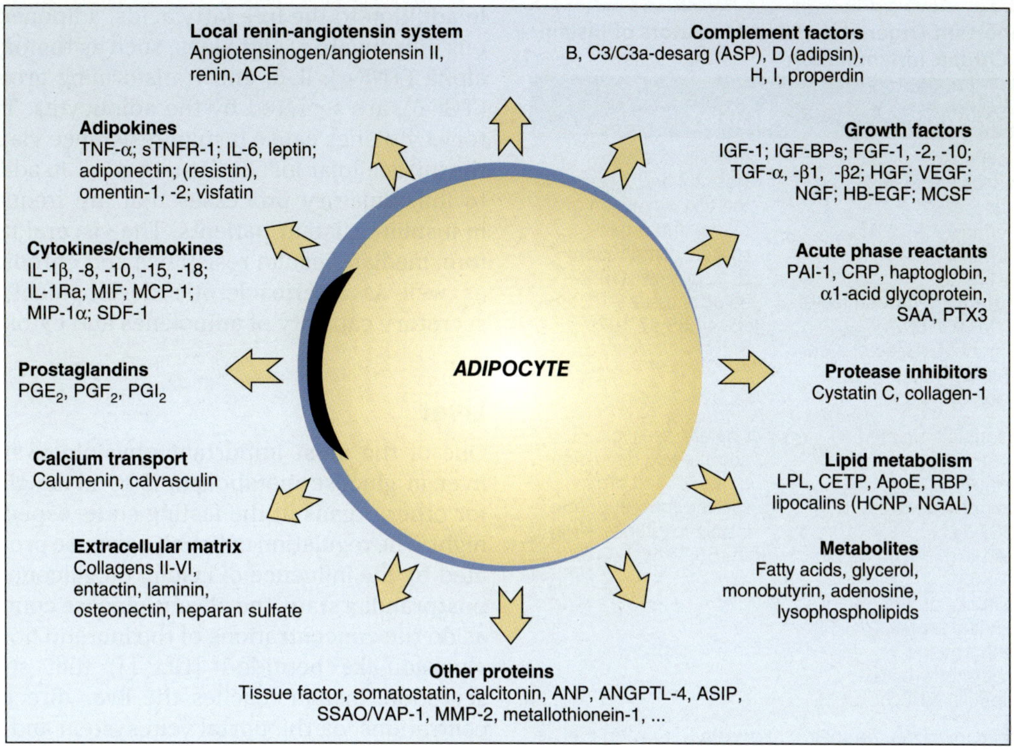

FIG. 2.4 **The adipocyte as endocrine organ.** The figure shows the different hormones, cytokines, inflammatory markers, growth factors, and other transmitter molecules that are secreted by the adipocyte. These substances are involved in inflammatory processes, insulin resistance, and vascular changes. *FGF*, Fetal growth factor; *IGF-1*, insulin-like growth factor 1; *IL*, interleukin; *TGF*, transforming growth factor; *TNF-α*, tumor necrosis factor alpha; *TNFR*, TNF-α receptor; *ACE*, Angiotensin converting enzyme; *CRP*, C reactive protein; *NGF*, Neural growth factor; *LPL*, Lipoprotein lipase; *PAI-1*, Plasminogen activator inhibitor; *PG*, Prostaglandin. (Modified from Staiger H, Häring HU. Adipocytokines: fat-derived humoral mediators of metabolic homeostasis. *Exp Clin Endocrinol Diabetes.* 2005;113:67.)

5′-AMP-kinase (adenosine monophosphate) and antiinflammatory effects.[103–105] These effects may also be responsible for the antidiabetic and antiarteriosclerotic properties of adiponectin. Adiponectin is, therefore, thought to be a protective protein that is not sufficiently synthesized and secreted by adipocytes in insulin-resistant patients and patients with type 2 diabetes. Other known adipokines (e.g., leptin, resistin, retinol-binding protein, glypican-4) are currently being evaluated to determine whether they might serve as important targets for preventing and treating T2DM and cardiovascular disease.[53,102,106]

Adipokines presently are the best-known "organokines," although several other classes of organokines have been identified (including myokines, lipokines, and hepatokines). Organokines are proteins exclusively or predominantly produced by and secreted from a specific tissue, but they are not simply markers of the function of their source tissue. All organokines have paracrine or endocrine actions or both (Table 2.2).[53,106,122]

TISSUE- AND ORGAN-SPECIFIC CONTRIBUTION TO INSULIN RESISTANCE

Muscle

Skeletal muscle plays an important role in glucose uptake. Approximately 80% of the glucose is transported into the skeletal muscle in an insulin-dependent manner. In this respect, the skeletal muscle is an important organ involved in the development of insulin resistance. This was demonstrated in glucose clamp experiments and positron emission tomography (PET) scan investigations that showed that in insulin resistance and T2DM, insulin-dependent glucose uptake into the skeletal muscle is significantly reduced.[90,91] Ectopic fat deposition also seems to be highly important for the development of insulin resistance of skeletal muscle. Increased intramyocellular fat depositions are found in insulin resistance and T2DM.[119,123,124] The ectopic fat deposition creates an altered metabolic atmosphere with increased free fatty acid concentrations and increased adipokines that lead to enhanced lipid oxidation and an increase in chronic inflammation, resulting in the development of insulin resistance and diminished glucose uptake into the skeletal muscle.[119] The cause of increased intramyocellular fat deposition in insulin resistance and T2DM is most likely a genetic disposition. The triglyceride accumulation in skeletal muscle in obesity derives from a reduced capacity for fat oxidation. An inflexibility in regulating fat oxidation, rather than a defect in fatty acid uptake, is related to insulin resistance and T2DM.[120] On the other hand, elevated circulating free fatty serum concentrations may secondarily lead to an increase in intramyocellular triglyceride accumulation.[121,125]

The humoral cross talk between skeletal muscle and liver seems to be of interest and importance; in animal studies, an acute increase in physical activity quickly and strongly regulates the expression of a large number of genes in the liver.[53,126,127]

In humans, aerobic fitness specifically regulates liver fat content but not total or visceral obesity.[53,108] Whether myokines are involved in this important cross talk between

TABLE 2.2 Important Organokines and Mediators of Insulin Resistance and Chronic Inflammation

ORGAN	IMPORTANT ORGANOKINES	REMARKS
Adipose tissue (visceral)	Adiponectin Interleukin-6 (IL-6) Leptin Omentin-1 Omentin-2 Resistin Transforming growth factor beta (TGF-β) Tumor necrosis factor alpha (TNF-α) Visfatin	For details, see also Figs. 2.4 and 2.5 and the text discussion of tissue- and organ-specific contribution to insulin resistance—adipose tissue (Refs. 47,55,97,107)
Liver	Angiopoietin-related protein 6 Fetuin-A Fetal growth factor 21 (FGF-21) Insulin-like growth factors (IGFs) Insulin-like growth factor–binding proteins (IGFBP) Selenoprotein P Sex hormone–binding globulin (SHBG)	For details, see Fig. 2.5, and the text discussion of tissue- and organ-specific contribution to insulin resistance—liver (Refs. 55,58,108–118)
Muscle	Brain-derived neurotrophic factor Erythropoietin (EPO) Interleukin-6 (IL-6) Interleukin-15 (IL-15) Interleukin-1β (IL-1β) Tumor necrosis factor alpha (TNF-α)	For details, see also the text discussion of tissue- and organ-specific contribution to insulin resistance—muscle (Refs. 85,91,119–121)

skeletal muscle and liver in humans needs to be further investigated and characterized.[53]

In addition to insulin-dependent glucose uptake, the transport of glucose into the skeletal muscle can also be mediated by physical activity in an insulin-independent manner. This insulin-independent glucose uptake is mainly mediated by an increase in the 5′-AMP-kinase concentration with the consecutive activation of the 5′-AMP-activated protein kinase (AMPK). Most data indicate that this pathway, activated by physical activity, is not altered in insulin resistance and in T2DM, in contrast to perturbations of insulin-dependent glucose transport.[90]

In this respect, interleukin-6 (IL-6) produced in the working muscle during physical activity could act as an energy sensor by activating AMP-activated kinase and enhancing glucose disposal, lipolysis, and fat oxidation.[123,124] In addition to the numerous positive effects of physical activity on all aspects of the metabolic syndrome and beyond, physical fitness and training improve glucose uptake into the skeletal muscle via the AMPK pathway.

Adipose Tissue

The role of central and visceral obesity in the development of insulin resistance was described previously. On a molecular level, the mediators secreted by the adipocytes in dependence of fat mass and fat distribution play an important role in the development of insulin resistance. In addition to the free fatty acids, adiponectin and numerous inflammatory cytokines, such as tumor necrosis factor alpha (TNF-α), IL-6, and transforming growth factor beta (TGF-β), are secreted by the adipocytes. These inflammatory cytokines cause insulin resistance via an inhibition of the intracellular insulin signaling.[47,107] In addition, they lead to inflammatory processes that are frequently observed in insulin-resistant patients. The visceral fat stores, therefore, mediate insulin resistance and chronic inflammation, as well as arteriosclerotic development, through their secretory capacity of adipokines and cytokines.[53,101,102]

Liver

One of the most important physiologic functions of the liver in glucose metabolism is to make glucose available for other organs in the fasting state, especially during the night. The regulation of hepatic glucose production is mediated by the influence of insulin on gluconeogenesis. In the postprandial state, the plasma glucose concentration rises, as do the concentrations of the incretin hormones (mainly glucagon-like peptide-1 [GLP-1]) that stimulate insulin secretion. Insulin reaches the liver directly in high concentrations via the portal vein system and physiologically suppresses hepatic glucose production, which would be counterproductive in the postprandial state, when plasma glucose is elevated already.[109] Only during the fasting state with low glucose and insulin concentrations do low insulin concentrations disinhibit hepatic gluconeogenesis, leading to sufficiently high glucose concentrations in the circulation in the fasting state. In insulin resistance and T2DM, an increased hepatic glucose production is observed that is caused by a diminished hepatocyte response to insulin failing to suppress gluconeogenesis.[110] Insulin resistance of the liver is typically detected in the clinical setting through elevated fasting glucose concentration, which is caused by the increased hepatic glucose production. Different mechanisms that lead to an increased hepatic gluconeogenesis are discussed: the insensitivity of the liver toward insulin itself on the one hand, but also elevated free fatty acid concentrations, as well as hyperglucagonemia, and increased activity of phosphoenolpyruvate-carboxykinase, a key enzyme of gluconeogenesis.[110,111] One important trigger for insulin resistance of the liver is the fat accumulation in this organ. Different studies have shown a correlation between triglyceride content in hepatocytes and insulin resistance within the liver.[53,58] Patients with T2DM frequently also have nonalcoholic steatohepatosis (MASH) or nonalcoholic fatty liver disease (MASLD), which are tightly correlated with insulin resistance.[53,58–60,112] Successful implementation of a lifestyle intervention may reduce liver fat mass and may improve insulin resistance.[53,58,108] The insulin-sensitizing effect of metformin and glitazones is partially explained by the reduction of the triglyceride content in the liver.[113,114] MASLD is the most common liver disease, and along with the worldwide increase in the prevalence of general and abdominal obesity, MASLD has become a prevalent general health problem in many industrialized countries. MASLD represents a continuum of liver disease from simple steatosis to MASH and cirrhosis. Up to 20% of patients with simple steatosis will develop MASH, and in a subgroup of these patients, MASH can progress further to MASH with fibrosis and cirrhosis.[53,112,115] Cirrhosis is the main risk factor for the development of hepatocellular carcinoma.[53,116] In addition, MASLD was identified as a strong and independent predictor of T2DM and cardiovascular disease.[53,117] Thus much effort is currently focused worldwide on precisely quantifying liver fat content in humans for predictive and therapeutic purposes.[53,117] However, this endeavor might not be sufficient to completely understand the pathophysiology of MASLD.

During conditions of a positive energy balance, subcutaneous and visceral adipose tissues expand in a manner that is predominantly genetically determined. Subcutaneous obesity is not strongly associated with metabolic diseases, whereas visceral obesity is a strong predictor of these diseases. Increased availability of fatty acids (resulting from increased lipolysis), increased subclinical inflammation, and dysregulation of adipokine production and release are thought to promote insulin resistance, atherosclerosis, and beta-cell dysfunction. Accumulation of lipids in the liver is also largely genetically determined, and two distinct phenotypes have been identified. When hepatic detoxification processes are active, storage of lipids in the liver is not associated with metabolic diseases. By contrast, when lipotoxicity is present, hepatic glucose production increases, and lipids are released with an atherogenic profile. Dysregulated hepatokine production also contributes to the development of metabolic diseases. The important heptokines are listed in Table 2.3, and Fig. 2.5 shows a schematic diagram of the putative roles of liver and adipose tissue in the development of metabolic diseases.[53]

The glycoprotein fetuin-A is an important hepatokine. It is a natural inhibitor of the insulin-stimulated insulin receptor tyrosine kinase and induces insulin resistance in rodents. In humans, circulating fetuin-A levels are positively associated with fat accumulation in the liver, insulin resistance, metabolic syndrome, and type 2 diabetes mellitus. In addition to inducing insulin resistance, fetuin-A is involved in subclinical inflammation and correlates positively with high-sensitive C-reactive protein levels in humans. It also induces cytokine expression in human monocytes and reduces the expression of the atheroprotective adipokine adiponectin in animals. Taken together, fetuin-A may represent a pathway linking fatty liver with cardiovascular events by inducing insulin resistance and inflammation. Indeed, an investigation in the cohort of the EPIC study (European Prospective Investigation into Cancer and Nutrition; EPIC-Potsdam) revealed a link between high plasma fetuin-A levels and an increased risk of myocardial infarction (MI) and ischemic stroke. High fetuin-A plasma concentrations led to a threefold to fourfold increased risk for MI and ischemic stroke.[118]

TABLE 2.3 Function of Important Hepatokines In Vitro and In Vivo

HEPATOKINE	EFFECTS: IN VITRO OR ANIMAL STUDIES	EFFECTS: IN HUMANS
Angiopoietin-related protein 6	Energy expenditure ↑ Obesity ↓ NAFLD ↓ Insulin resistance ↓	Insulin resistance ↑
Fetuin-A	Obesity ↔/↑ Insulin resistance ↑ Subclinical inflammation ↑	Obesity ↔ NAFLD ↑ Insulin resistance ↑ Subclinical inflammation ↑ T2DM ↑ CVD ↑
FGF-21	Energy expenditure ↑ Insulin resistance ↓ Beta-cell survival ↑	Obesity ↑ NAFLD ↑ Insulin resistance ↑
IGFs and IGFBPs	Insulin resistance ↔/↑/↓	Insulin resistance ↑/↓
Selenoprotein P	Insulin resistance ↑	Insulin resistance ↑ Subclinical inflammation ↑
Sex hormone–binding globulin	Sex hormone bioavailability ↑ Sex hormone signaling ↑	Obesity ↓ NAFLD ↓ Insulin resistance ↓ Subclinical inflammation ↓ T2DM ↓ Cardiovascular disease ↓

CVD, Cardiovascular disease; *FGF-21*, fetal growth factor 21; *IGF*, insulin-like growth factor; *IGFBs*, insulin-like growth factor–binding proteins; *T2DM*, type 2 diabetes mellitus.
Data from Stefan N, Häring HU. The role of hepatokines in metabolism. *Nat Rev Endocrinol.* 2013;9:144.

Brain

During the past years, an increasingly important role of the brain in the development of insulin resistance and obesity has been found. The brain is not only an important organ for glucose disposal but has recently also been recognized as an insulin-sensitive organ. IRs are expressed in brain tissue.[128] A high degree of insulin sensitivity of the human brain facilitates the loss of body weight and body fat during a lifestyle intervention.[129]

Furthermore, insulin has important functions in regulating satiety signals and energy expenditure within the central nervous system and therefore has an influence on the development of obesity.[130,131] Intracerebroventricular application of insulin promotes satiety in experimental models in animals and human studies.[131–133] Neutralizing insulin effects in the brain in animal experiments leads to hyperphagia and obesity[132] and a reduced peripheral action of insulin in the liver.[133] The results of these experiments point to insulin effects in the brain that most likely lead to a neurotransmitter response that has an influence on hepatic glucose production. The brain is therefore an important central regulator for peripheral insulin action in the liver.[54,57,130] Brain insulin resistance in humans has been associated with longterm adiposity and an unfavorable adipose tissue distribution, thus implicating it in the pathogenesis of subgroups of obesity and (pre)diabetes that are characterized by distinct patterns of body fat distribution. Encouragingly, emerging evidence suggests that brain insulin resistance could represent a treatable entity, thereby opening up novel therapeutic avenues to improve systemic metabolism and enhance brain functions, including cognition.[130]

Regarding interventions, two clinical trials showed that brain insulin resistance appears to be treatable. A nonpharmacological intervention with 8 weeks of exercise in

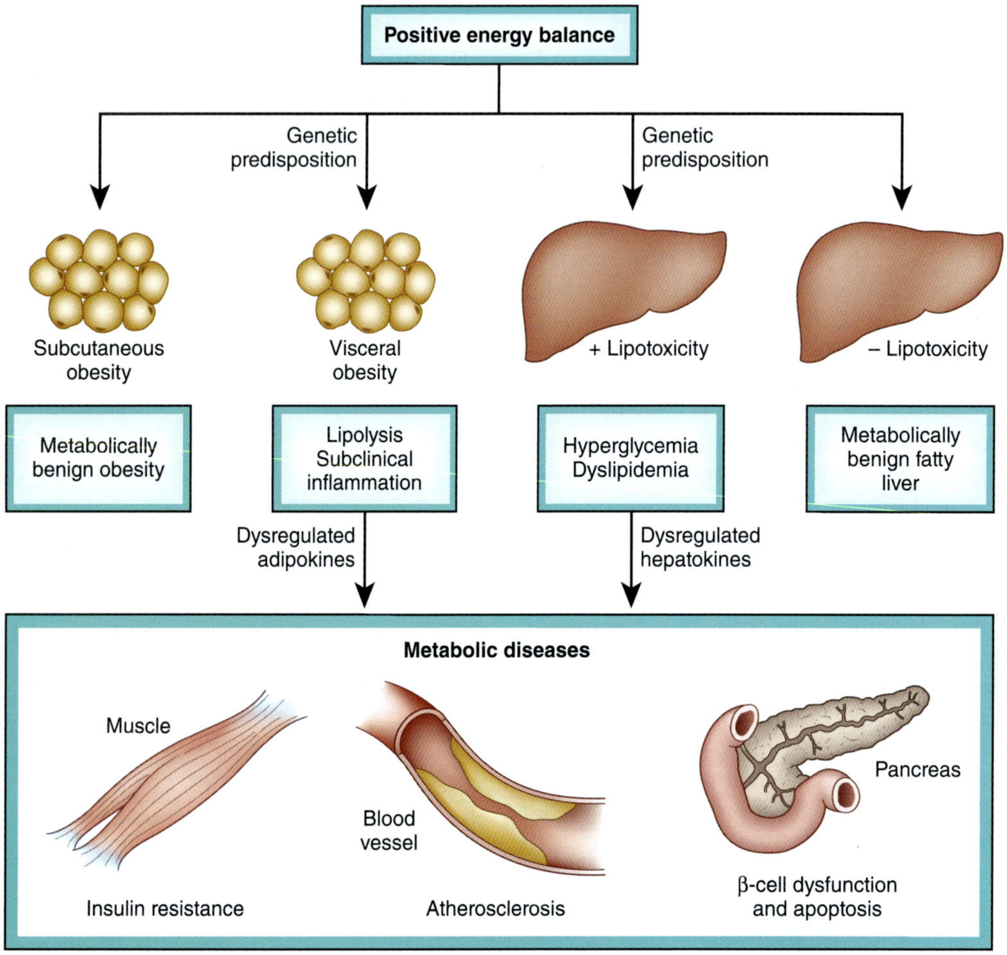

FIG. 2.5 Novel roles of liver and adipose tissue in the development of metabolic diseases. During conditions of a positive energy balance, subcutaneous and visceral adipose tissues expand in a manner that is predominantly genetically determined. Subcutaneous obesity is not strongly associated with metabolic diseases, whereas visceral obesity is a strong predictor of these diseases. Increased availability of fatty acids (resulting from increased lipolysis), increased subclinical inflammation, and dysregulation of adipokine production and release are thought to promote insulin resistance, atherosclerosis, and beta-cell dysfunction. Accumulation of lipids in the liver is also largely genetically determined, and two distinct phenotypes have been identified. When hepatic detoxification processes are active, storage of lipids in the liver is not associated with metabolic diseases. By contrast, when lipotoxicity is present, hepatic glucose production increases and lipids are released with an atherogenic profile. Dysregulated hepatokine production also contributes to the development of metabolic diseases. (Modified from Stefan N, Häring HU. The role of hepatokines in metabolism. *Nat Rev Endocrinol.* 2013;9:144.)

obese subjects improved insulin responsiveness in the dorsal striatum (putamen) to a level similar to that seen in lean individuals.[134] Another study evaluated pharmacological treatment with the sodium-glucose cotransporter 2 (SGLT2) inhibitor empagliflozin in subjects with prediabetes and overweight or obesity.[135] Empagliflozin over 8 weeks restored hypothalamic insulin sensitivity independently of body weight loss. Further analyses indicated that this improvement in hypothalamic insulin responsiveness seems to trigger the reduction of liver fat content and enhancement of fasting blood glucose levels that were also achieved with the SGLT2 inhibitor intervention.[135]

Improving and developing therapeutic methods for brain insulin resistance could potentially lead to novel preventative or therapeutic options for obesity and metabolic disorders on the one hand and perhaps also for related neurological and psychiatric conditions. Progress in this central and important promising area requires a multidisciplinary effort to translate research findings into clinical practice and improvement of therapeutic options.[131]

BETA-CELL DYSFUNCTION IN T2DM

Role of Insulin Secretion and Beta Cells in T2DM

Disturbed beta-cell function and a loss of beta-cell mass of the pancreatic islets play important pathogenetic roles in the development and progression of T2DM. Regarding the beta cell, a loss of insulin secretion and defects in the early phase of insulin secretion are important in the pathogenesis of T2DM. As diabetes progresses, a loss of beta-cell mass is also observed. In addition, a disturbance in glucagon secretion from the pancreatic alpha cells in the islet with hyperglucagonemia also contributes to the disorder of glucose metabolism. Although insulin resistance is relatively stable in the course of T2DM, the defects in beta-cell function and the loss of beta-cell mass are responsible for the progressive nature of the disease.

Pulsatility

Insulin secretion is regulated through a complex interplay of glucose, hormones, incretins, amino acids, and neuronal signals, among other factors. Physiologic insulin secretion follows a pulsatile pattern; in healthy individuals, every 5 to 10 minutes insulin is secreted in a pulse.[136,137] These short-lasting insulin pulses add up to an insulin secretion profile that is repeated every 80 to 150 minutes. The pulsatile secretion of insulin is significantly more effective in lowering plasma glucose concentrations than continuous secretion. Patients with T2DM already show defective pulsatile insulin secretion even before the clinical manifestation of their diabetes. This defect is characterized by a reduction in pulse frequency as well as lower amplitudes of the insulin pulses. These disturbances can be observed in glucose-dependent as well as glucose-independent fashion.[138,139] Insulin secreted from the beta cells reaches the liver via the portal system in the described pulsatile manner. It is degraded by approximately 60% in the liver and not distributed in the same pulsatile fashion into the systemic circulation. As a consequence of the defective pulsatile insulin secretion, hepatic glucose production is elevated.[140,141]

Glucose-Dependent Insulin Secretion

The insulin secretion response after glucose administration in healthy individuals has a typical biphasic pattern, with an immediate insulin secretion peak approximately 3 to 5 minutes after an intravenous glucose bolus and approximately 20 minutes after oral glucose administration, which lasts for around 10 minutes. This acute or first phase of insulin secretion is followed by a second phase with a slower and more sustained elevation of plasma insulin concentrations. The duration of the second phase of insulin secretion is dependent on the elevation of plasma glucose. The first phase of insulin secretion results from the liberation of insulin from the fast recruitable secretory vesicles that are close to the plasma membrane of the beta cell. The second phase of insulin secretion is recruited from a less readily recruitable reserve pool of insulin vesicles. This reserve pool comprises newly synthesized insulin vesicles and so-called storage vesicles and is located further away from the outside cell membrane of the beta cell.[142–145] In T2DM as well as in the prediabetic state of impaired glucose tolerance (Table 2.4 for classification),[146] a significantly reduced or even absent first phase of insulin secretion is observed after a glucose stimulus.[147,148] This defect in the first phase of insulin secretion especially has an impact on the postprandial glucose concentrations.[149] Several mechanisms have been reported to cause the defect in the first phase of insulin secretion: chronic hyperglycemia, elevated free fatty acid plasma concentrations, and a reduction in beta-cell mass. Some studies indicate that the first phase of insulin secretion can be restored by normalizing glucose metabolism. In addition to the described changes in the first phase of insulin secretion, the second phase is also changed in T2DM. Because of persistent hyperglycemia, the second phase of insulin secretion is often prolonged and more pronounced compared with the second phase in healthy individuals.[143–145,149] There is a reciprocal nonlinear hyperbolic relationship between insulin secretion and insulin resistance. Insulin secretion can therefore be evaluated only with respect to the amount of peripheral insulin resistance. In insulin-resistant patients with T2DM, elevated plasma insulin concentrations may be observed compared with healthy controls, but these may be inappropriately low in relation to the degree of insulin resistance or to the elevation of plasma glucose concentrations during chronic hyperglycemia and may not be sufficient to normalize the plasma glucose. The insulin secretion in T2DM is, therefore, insufficient and often inadequate to cover the actual demand for glucose normalization. In addition to the disturbed insulin secretion, a defect in glucagon secretion is found in T2DM. Usually an inappropriately high glucagon secretion is observed that mediates increased hepatic glucose production.[150] This hyperglucagonemia is partially caused by the lack of the tonic inhibition of glucagon secretion by insulin and beta-cell activity.[140,141,151]

Proinsulin-to-Insulin Ratio

In addition to the described defects in insulin secretion kinetics, in T2DM a change in the proinsulin-to-insulin ratio is observed that is characterized by a higher proinsulin secretion.[152] Insulin and C peptide are formed by the enzymatic cleavage of proinsulin in the secretory granules of the beta cells. In healthy individuals, approximately 2.5% of immunoreactive insulin originates from proinsulin or intermediate split products of proinsulin; in patients with T2DM, this proportion is much higher and amounts to approximately 8%. This finding indicates a defective or incomplete processing of proinsulin in T2DM.[152,153] It is interesting to note that in healthy individuals the proinsulin-to-insulin ratio is also dependent on the degree

TABLE 2.4 Classification and Detection of T2DM and Prediabetic States With a Standardized Oral Glucose Tolerance Test (OGTT, 75 g Glucose)

TIME POINT OF GLUCOSE MEASUREMENT	NORMOGLYCEMIA	IMPAIRED FASTING GLUCOSE (IFG)	IMPAIRED GLUCOSE TOLERANCE (IGT)	T2DM
Fasting (0 min)	<100 mg/dL<5.6 mmol/L	100–125 mg/dL 5.6–6.9 mmol/L		≥126 mg/dL ≥7.0 mmol/L
2-Hour postglucose	<140 mg/dL<7.8 mmol/L		140–199 mg/dL 7.8–11.0 mmol/L	≥200 mg/dL ≥11.1 mmol/L

Glucose is measured from venous plasma.
Data from American Diabetes Association. Diagnosis and classification of diabetes mellitus. *Diabetes Care*. 2013;36(suppl 1):S67.

of peripheral insulin resistance and the fasting plasma glucose concentration. The proinsulin proportions vary from a minimum of 8% under normoglycemic conditions to approximately 30% under overt hyperglycemia with glucose concentrations of 15 mmol/L.[154] It is hypothesized that chronic hyperglycemia is a continuous stimulatory impulse for insulin granules. Because of this chronic hypersecretion, matured insulin granules are depleted and immature insulin granules with a higher proportion of proinsulin prevail.[155] In addition, other mechanisms of defects in insulin biosynthesis that are not primarily dependent on hyperglycemia are discussed as being responsible for the increased proinsulin secretion in T2DM. Because proinsulin has only a very low insulin-like biologic activity, a further reduction of insulin action for insulin-sensitive organs results from the change in the proinsulin-to-insulin ratio. The increased proinsulin secretion is further seen as a marker for beta-cell stress and as a predictor for diabetes development.[152,153,156]

Incretin Hormones and T2DM

The so-called incretin effect describes the phenomenon by which orally ingested glucose elicits a significantly more pronounced insulin response than an intravenous glucose infusion with identical changes in plasma glucose concentrations. The incretin effect is mediated by the gastrointestinal hormones glucose-dependent insulinotropic peptide (GIP) and GLP-1, which are physiologically secreted after a meal, especially after carbohydrate consumption.[157] In healthy individuals the incretin effect is responsible for 50% to 70% of the postprandial insulin secretion.[158] In T2DM, the incretin effect is diminished, mostly because GIP has lost its insulinotropic activity as a result of chronic hyperglycemia.[159,160] Supraphysiologic concentrations of GLP-1 can restore glucose-dependent insulin secretion and normalize plasma glucose in T2DM, as long as sufficient beta-cell mass is still present. It is interesting to note that GLP-1 also inhibits glucagon secretion in a glucose-dependent manner. This effect also contributes to the glucose normalization observed under supraphysiologic GLP-1 plasma concentrations.[161] During the last decade, additional physiologic effects of GLP-1 were discovered that may help to normalize metabolism in T2DM.[157] GLP-1 also slows gastric emptying and thereby retards the resorption of carbohydrates; in rodent models, it increases beta-cell function and beta-cell mass. Like other gastrointestinal hormones, GLP-1 is also found as a neurotransmitter in the brain. GLP-1–containing neurons in the hypothalamus are involved in mediating satiety.[157,162] Novel data also describe cardiovascular effects of GLP-1 that seem to be favorable in T2DM or in patients with metabolic syndrome (e.g., improvement of left ventricular function in myocardial infarct models, reduction of BP).[163] Fig. 2.6 summarizes the pancreatic and extrapancreatic effects of GLP-1. The incretin-based therapies for T2DM with GLP-1 receptor agonists or with dipeptidyl peptidase (DPP-4) inhibitors that elevate endogenous GLP-1 plasma concentrations use these GLP-1 effects.[157,164] The most recent developments are: (1) the introduction of the combined GLP-1/GIP dual agonist tirzepatide for the therapy of type 2 diabetes and (2) the development of further dual- or triple-GLP-1/GIP/glucagon agonists for the treatment of T2DM and obesity.[165–168] The discovery and development of so-called gut hormone co-agonists as a new class of drugs for the treatment of diabetes and obesity is considered a transformative breakthrough in the field. Combining action profiles of multiple gastrointestinal hormones within a single molecule, these novel therapeutics achieve synergistic metabolic benefits.[169] The success of these agents in preclinical models and clinical trials suggests a promising future for multi-agonists in the treatment of metabolic diseases, with the most recent glucose-dependent insulinotropic peptide receptor:glucagon-like peptide-1 receptor:glucagon receptor (GIPR:GLP-1R:GCGR) triagonists rivaling the efficacy of bariatric surgery. However, further research is needed to fully understand how these therapies exert their effect on body weight.[169–171]

Beta-Cell Mass

Several studies have shown that at the time of T2DM diagnosis, beta-cell mass has already decreased to around 50% of the original beta-cell mass and that this amount of beta-cell reduction is critical.[172–174] With this reduction in beta-cell mass, for many middle-aged or older people,

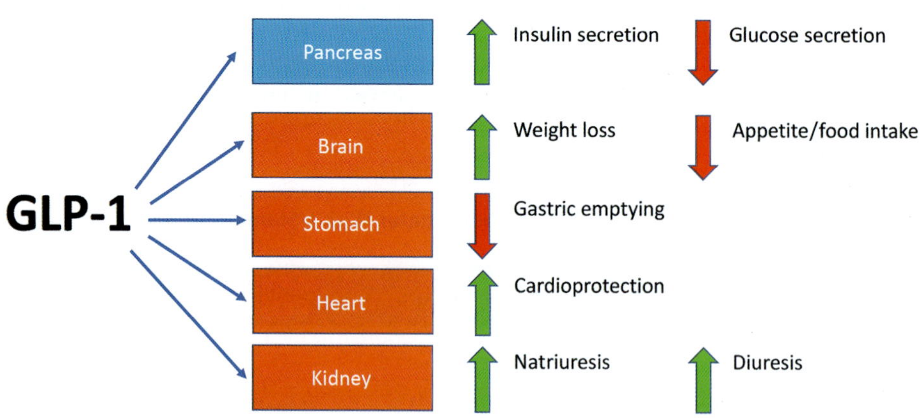

FIG. 2.6 Pancreatic and extrapancreatic effects of glucagon-like peptide-1 (*GLP-1*). The figure shows different direct pancreatic effects of GLP-1 on insulin and glucagon secretion as well as extrapancreatic effects with metabolic consequences in type 2 diabetes and obesity. (Modified from Baggio LL, Drucker D. Glucagon-like peptide-1 receptor co-agonists for treating metabolic disease. *Mol Metab.* 2021;46:101090.)

normal glucose metabolism is no longer possible. In people with marked insulin resistance, moderate loss of beta-cell mass may already lead to a manifestation of diabetes. Most patients with T2DM show a 40% to 50% reduction in beta-cell mass compared with a nondiabetic age-matched control group.[175,176] The loss of beta cells in comparison with the loss of other cell types within the pancreatic islet is relatively selective for the beta cells; the loss of the glucagon-secreting alpha cells or the somatostatin-producing delta cells is not observed in a comparable quantity in T2DM. Even though the exact causes for the reduced beta-cell mass in T2DM are not completely elucidated, programmed cell death (apoptosis) seems to play a key pathogenetic role. Secondary factors such as elevated free fatty acid plasma concentrations, oxidative stress, and chronic hyperglycemia (see the later discussion of glucose toxicity) lead to an increased rate of beta-cell apoptosis. Other possibilities, such as a reduced rate of beta-cell proliferation or beta-cell neogenesis, play most likely only a minor role in the reduction of beta-cell mass in T2DM.[177]

Glucose Toxicity

Chronic hyperglycemia leads to a desensitization of the beta cell toward a glucose stimulus. This effect is also described as glucose toxicity of the beta cell. Glucose toxicity does not seem to be a substantial pathogenetic factor for the development of T2DM or in early stages of the disease. In later stages of diabetes with overt chronic hyperglycemia, it may lead to an additional dysfunction of the beta cell contributing to a further decline of metabolic control.[178] It is interesting to note that the results from the United Kingdom Prospective Diabetes Study showed comparably progressive beta-cell dysfunction in the intensively treated patients as well as in the control group.[174] This finding indicates that plasma glucose concentrations may have less influence on the progressive beta-cell dysfunction.

Lipotoxicity

Free fatty acids from alimentary sources or endogenous pools are also involved in mediating beta-cell dysfunction. Elevated free fatty acid concentrations lead to a diminished glucose-dependent insulin secretion.[179,180] Investigations in vitro in beta-cell lines showed an increase of programmed cell death (apoptosis) of the cultured cells under the influence of elevated concentrations of free fatty acids. This effect is observed with saturated fatty acids but not with unsaturated fatty acids. An approximately 20-fold increased apoptosis rate of beta cells was induced by the fatty acids palmitate and stearate, which are predominantly found in fats from animal sources. Fatty acids from plant sources that are monounsaturated or polyunsaturated, such as oleate, palmitoleate, and linoleate, did not show the apoptotic effect. Saturated fatty acids most likely transmit apoptotic signals in beta cells via protein kinase C.[98,181] In epidemiologic studies, an association between the nutritional fat composition and beta-cell function has been suggested. A correlation between the intake of saturated fatty acids and the incidence of T2DM has been shown.[182,183]

SUMMARY

This chapter gives insight into the pathophysiology and mechanisms involved in insulin resistance, a paramount characteristic of T2DM.

On the genetic level, SNPs in genes associated with diabetes risk contribute to altered insulin signaling, insulin secretion, organ function, or organ cross-talk (e.g., among the intestine, the endocrine pancreas, the liver, the brain, and the adipose tissue).

The mechanisms involved in insulin resistance mainly occur after insulin binding to the insulin receptor, with insulin normally mediating metabolic effects via the signaling molecules AKT/PKB, as well as mitogenic effects via the signaling proteins Ras/Raf/MAP kinase. In insulin resistance, reduced cellular insulin action is found with respect to metabolic but not mitogenic effects of insulin. Defects in the insulin signaling cascade are already present in the first steps of the signal transmission in insulin resistance and T2DM.

The activation of the insulin signal transduction cascade leads to glucose transport into the cell. The insulin effect on the glucose transport system is mediated by a translocation of glucose transporters from the intracellular pools to the plasma membrane and activation of these transporters in the plasma membrane. The glucose transporter GLUT-4 plays a major role. A reduced capacity of insulin-dependent translocation of GLUT-4 to the plasma membrane is observed as a consequence of insulin resistance.

Concerning the cross-talk between various tissues, the adipose tissue and adipocytes contribute to the development of insulin resistance by producing and secreting mediators such as adipokines and cytokines that act on the muscle and other target tissues of insulin action. The visceral adipose tissue is now seen as an endocrine organ with respect to special functions concerning the activation and secretion of numerous hormones and cytokines that mediate insulin resistance and chronic inflammation. Chronic inflammation is associated with an increased risk for macrovascular complications in T2DM and the metabolic syndrome.

Insulin resistance also leads to lipid accumulation in the muscle and liver, aggravating the metabolic disturbances. In MASLD and MASH, hepatokines such as fetuin-A contribute to insulin resistance and most likely to the increased cardiovascular risk associated with this condition.

The brain has only recently been recognized as an important organ regulating insulin sensitivity. It contributes to energy expenditure and body weight regulation. Neutralizing insulin effects in the brain in animal experiments leads to hyperphagia and obesity and to a reduced peripheral action of insulin in the liver, indicating an important organ interaction between the brain and the liver.

In addition, defects in insulin secretion and pancreatic islet function contribute to the pathophysiology of T2DM. Multiple defects involving insulin secretion have been characterized in T2DM. These include a diminished or absent fast insulin response after a sharp rise in glucose concentration (the so-called first phase of insulin secretion), an increase in the secretion of proinsulin, a defect in the insulinotropic action of incretin hormones (i.e., a defect in the cross-talk between the small intestine and the endocrine pancreas), and a defect in the interdependent pulsatile secretions of insulin and glucagon. In addition to genetic backgrounds for these pathophysiologic findings (SNPs in diabetes candidate genes), glucotoxicity, lipotoxicity, and the effects of inflammatory cytokines (predominantly secreted by adipocytes) contribute to the defects in pancreatic beta-cell function and also the loss of beta-cell mass in T2DM.

REFERENCES

1. DeForest N, Majithia AR. Genetics of type 2 diabetes: implications from large-scale studies. Curr Diab Rep. 2022;22:227.
2. Hansen L. Candidate genes and late-onset type 2 diabetes mellitus. Susceptibility genes or common polymorphisms? Dan Med Bull. 2003;50:320.
3. Müssig K, Staiger H, Machicao F, et al. Genetic variants affecting incretin sensitivity and incretin secretion. Diabetologia. 2010;53:2289.
4. Staiger H, Machicao F, Fritsche A, et al. Pathomechanisms of type 2 diabetes genes. Endocr Rev. 2009;30:557.
5. Lango H, Palmer CN, Morris AD, et al. Assessing the combined impact of 18 common genetic variants of modest effect sizes on type 2 diabetes risk. Diabetes. 2008;57:3129.
6. Wagner R, Staiger H, Ullrich S, et al. Untangling the interplay of genetic and metabolic influences on beta-cell function: examples of potential therapeutic implications involving TCF7L2 and FFAR1. Mol Metab. 2014;3:261.
7. Lyssenko V, Jonsson A, Almgren P, et al. Clinical risk factors, DNA variants, and the development of type 2 diabetes. N Engl J Med. 2008;359:2220.
8. Meigs JB, Shrader P, Sullivan LM, et al. Genotype score in addition to common risk factors for prediction of type 2 diabetes. *N Engl J Med.* 2008;359:2208.
9. Vaxillaire M, Yengo L, Lobbens S, et al. Type 2 diabetes-related genetic risk scores associated with variations in fasting plasma glucose and development of impaired glucose homeostasis in the prospective DESIR study. *Diabetologia.* 2014;57:1601.
10. Ling C, Del Guerra S, Lupi R, et al. Epigenetic regulation of PPARGC1A in human type 2 diabetic islets and effect on insulin secretion. *Diabetologia.* 2008;51:615–622.
11. Ling C, Rönn T. Epigenetics in human obesity and type 2 diabetes. *Cell Metab.* 2019;29:1028.
12. Kleinert M, Clemmensen C, Hofmann SM, et al. Animal models of obesity and diabetes mellitus. *Nat Rev Endocrinol.* 2018;14:140.
13. Kirchhoff K, Machicao F, Haupt A, et al. Polymorphisms in the TCF7L2, CDKAL1 and SLC30A8 genes are associated with impaired proinsulin conversion. *Diabetologia.* 2008;51:597.
14. Lyssenko V, Nagorny CL, Erdos MR, et al. Common variant in MTNR1B associated with increased risk of type 2 diabetes and impaired early insulin secretion. *Nat Genet.* 2009;41:82.
15. Hughes AE, Hattersley AT, Flanagan SE, et al. Two decades since the fetal insulin hypothesis: what have we learned from genetics? *Diabetologia.* 2021;64:717.
16. Krentz NAJ, Gloyn AL. Insights into pancreatic islet cell dysfunction from type 2 diabetes mellitus genetics. *Nat Rev Endocrinol.* 2020;16:202.
17. Mattis KK, Gloyn AL. From genetic association to molecular mechanisms for islet-cell dysfunction in type 2 diabetes. *J Mol Biol.* 2020;432:1551.
18. Bernstein D, Golson ML, Kaestner KH. Epigenetic control of β-cell function and failure. *Diabetes Res Clin Pract.* 2017;123:24.
19. Rutter GA. Dorothy Hodgkin Lecture 2014. Understanding genes identified by genome-wide association studies for type 2 diabetes. *Diabet Med.* 2014;31:1480.
20. Pullen TJ, Rutter GA. Roles of lncRNAs in pancreatic beta cell identity and diabetes susceptibility. *Front Genet.* 2014;5:193.
21. Dimas AS, Lagou V, Barker A, et al. Impact of type 2 diabetes susceptibility variants on quantitative glycemic traits reveals mechanistic heterogeneity. *Diabetes.* 2014;63:2158.
22. Prokopenko I, Langenberg C, Florez JC, et al. Variants in MTNR1B influence fasting glucose levels. *Nat Genet.* 2009;41:77.
23. Rong R, Hanson RL, Ortiz D, et al. Association analysis of variation in/near FTO, CDKAL1, SLC30A8, HHEX, EXT2, IGF2BP2, LOC387761, and CDKN2B with type 2 diabetes and related quantitative traits in Pima Indians. *Diabetes.* 2009;58:478.
24. Sandhu MS, Weedon MN, Fawcett KA, et al. Common variants in WFS1 confer risk of type 2 diabetes. *Nat Genet.* 2007;39:951.
25. Saxena R, Gianniny L, Burtt NP, et al. Common single nucleotide polymorphisms in TCF7L2 are reproducibly associated with type 2 diabetes and reduce the insulin response to glucose in nondiabetic individuals. *Diabetes.* 2006;55:2890.
26. Saxena R, Voight BF, Lyssenko V, et al. Genome-wide association analysis identifies loci for type 2 diabetes and triglyceride levels. *Science.* 2007;316:1331.
27. Scott LJ, Mohlke KL, Bonnycastle LL, et al. A genomewide association study of type 2 diabetes in Finns detects multiple susceptibility variants. *Science.* 2007;316:1341.
28. Sladek R, Rocheleau G, Rung J, et al. A genome-wide association study identifies novel risk loci for type 2 diabetes. *Nature.* 2007;445:881.
29. Sparsø T, Andersen G, Albrechtsen A, et al. Impact of polymorphisms in WFS1 on prediabetic phenotypes in a population-based sample of middle-aged people with normal and abnormal glucose regulation. *Diabetologia.* 2008;51:1646.
30. Staiger H, Machicao F, Kantartzis K, et al. Novel meta-analysis-derived type 2 diabetes risk loci do not determine prediabetic phenotypes. *PLoS One.* 2008;3:e3019.
31. Staiger H, Machicao F, Schäfer SA, et al. Polymorphisms within the novel type 2 diabetes risk locus MTNR1B determine beta-cell function. *PLoS One.* 2008;3:e3962.
32. Staiger H, Machicao F, Stefan N, et al. Polymorphisms within novel risk loci for type 2 diabetes determine beta-cell function. *PLoS One.* 2007;2:e832.
33. Staiger H, StancÆkovÆ A, Zilinskaite J, et al. A candidate type 2 diabetes polymorphism near the HHEX locus affects acute glucose-stimulated insulin release in European populations: results from the EUGENE2 study. *Diabetes.* 2008;57:514.
34. Steinthorsdottir V, Thorleifsson G, Reynisdottir I, et al. A variant in CDKAL1 influences insulin response and risk of type 2 diabetes. *Nat Genet.* 2007;39:770.
35. Unoki H, Takahashi A, Kawaguchi T, et al. SNPs in KCNQ1 are associated with susceptibility to type 2 diabetes in East Asian and European populations. *Nat Genet.* 2008;40:1098.
36. Yasuda K, Miyake K, Horikawa Y, et al. Variants in KCNQ1 are associated with susceptibility to type 2 diabetes mellitus. *Nat Genet.* 2008;40:1092.
37. Zeggini E, Weedon MN, Lindgren CM, et al. Replication of genome-wide association signals in UK samples reveals risk loci for type 2 diabetes. *Science.* 2007;316:1336.
38. Loos RJ, Franks PW, Francis RW, et al. TCF7L2 polymorphisms modulate proinsulin levels and beta-cell function in a British Europid population. *Diabetes.* 2007;56:1943.
39. Stolerman ES, Manning AK, McAteer JB, et al. TCF7L2 variants are associated with increased proinsulin/insulin ratios but not obesity traits in the Framingham Heart Study. *Diabetologia.* 2009;52:614.
40. Del Bosque-Plata L, Martínez-Martínez E, Espinoza-Camacho MÁ, et al. The role of *TCF7L2* in type 2 diabetes. *Diabetes.* 2021;70:1220.
41. Kang ES, Park SY, Kim HJ, et al. Effects of Pro12Ala polymorphism of peroxisome proliferator-activated receptor gamma2 gene on rosiglitazone response in type 2 diabetes. *Clin Pharmacol Ther.* 2005;78:202.
42. Blüher M, Lubben G, Paschke R. Analysis of the relationship between the Pro12Ala variant in the PPAR gamma2 gene and the response rate to therapy with pioglitazone in patients with type 2 diabetes. *Diabetes Care.* 2003;26:825.
43. Florez JC, Jablonski KA, Sun MW, et al. Effects of the type 2 diabetes-associated PPARG P12A polymorphism on progression to diabetes and response to troglitazone. *J Clin Endocrinol Metab.* 2007;92:1502.
44. Kimber CH, Doney AS, Pearson ER, et al. TCF7L2 in the Go-DARTS study: evidence for a gene dose effect on both diabetes susceptibility and control of glucose levels. *Diabetologia.* 2007;50:1186.
45. Florez JC, Jablonski KA, Bayley N, et al. TCF7L2 polymorphisms and progression to diabetes in the diabetes prevention program. *N Engl J Med.* 2006;355:241.
46. Pearson ER, Donnelly LA, Kimber C, et al. Variation in TCF7L2 influences therapeutic response to sulfonylureas: a GoDARTs study. *Diabetes.* 2007;56:2178.
47. Matthaei S, Stumvoll M, Kellerer M, et al. Pathophysiology and pharmacological treatment of insulin resistance. *Endocr Rev.* 2000;21:585.
48. Bonora E, Targher G, Alberiche M, et al. Homeostasis model assessment closely mirrors the glucose clamp technique in the assessment of insulin sensitivity: studies in subjects with various degrees of glucose tolerance and insulin sensitivity. *Diabetes Care.* 2000;23:57.
49. Gutt M, Davis CL, Spitzer SB, et al. Validation of the insulin sensitivity index (ISI(0,120)): comparison with other measures. *Diabetes Res Clin Pract.* 2000;47:177.
50. Matsuda M, DeFronzo RA. Insulin sensitivity indices obtained from oral glucose tolerance testing: comparison with the euglycemic insulin clamp. *Diabetes Care.* 1999;22:1462.
51. Stumvoll M, Mitrakou A, Pimenta W, et al. Use of the oral glucose tolerance test to assess insulin release and insulin sensitivity. *Diabetes Care.* 2000;23:295.
52. Saltiel AR, Kahn CR. Insulin signalling and the regulation of glucose and lipid metabolism. *Nature.* 2001;414:799.
53. Stefan N, Häring HU. The role of hepatokines in metabolism. *Nat Rev Endocrinol.* 2013;9:144.
54. Heni M, Kullmann S, Preissl H, et al. Impaired insulin action in the human brain: causes and metabolic consequences. *Nat Rev Endocrinol.* 2015;11:701.
55. Siegel-Axel DI, Häring HU. Perivascular adipose tissue: An unique fat compartment relevant for the cardiometabolic syndrome. *Rev Endocr Metab Disord.* 2016;17:51.
56. Stefan N, Fritsche A, Schick F, et al. Phenotypes of prediabetes and stratification of cardiometabolic risk. *Lancet Diabetes Endocrinol.* 2016;4:789.
57. Kullmann S, Heni M, Hallschmid M, et al. Brain insulin resistance at the crossroads of metabolic and cognitive disorders in humans. *Physiol Rev.* 2016;96:1169.

58. Stefan N, Häring HU, Cusi K. Non-alcoholic fatty liver disease: causes, diagnosis, cardiometabolic consequences, and treatment strategies. *Lancet Diabetes Endocrinol.* 2019;7:313.
59. Gastaldelli A, Stefan N, Häring HU. Liver-targeting drugs and their effect on blood glucose and hepatic lipids. *Diabetologia.* 2021;64:1461.
60. Wagner R, Eckstein SS, Yamazaki H, et al. Metabolic implications of pancreatic fat accumulation. *Nat Rev Endocrinol.* 2022;18:43.
61. Häring HU. The insulin receptor: signalling mechanism and contribution to the pathogenesis of insulin resistance. *Diabetologia.* 1991;34:848.
62. Kellerer M, Lammers R, Häring HU. Insulin signal transduction: possible mechanisms for insulin resistance. *Exp Clin Endocrinol Diabetes.* 1999;107:97.
63. Lee YH, White MF. Insulin receptor substrate proteins and diabetes. *Arch Pharm Res.* 2004;27:361.
64. Taniguchi CM, Emanuelli B, Kahn CR. Critical nodes in signalling pathways: insights into insulin action. *Nat Rev Mol Cell Biol.* 2006;7:85.
65. Cusi K, Maezono K, Osman A, et al. Insulin resistance differentially affects the PI 3-kinase- and MAP kinase-mediated signaling in human muscle. *J Clin Invest.* 2000;105:311.
66. Pollak M. The insulin and insulin-like growth factor receptor family in neoplasia: an update. *Nat Rev Cancer.* 2012;12:159.
67. Moller DE, Yokota A, Flier JS. Normal insulin-receptor cDNA sequence in Pima Indians with NIDDM. *Diabetes.* 1989;38:1496.
68. O'Rahilly S, Choi WH, Patel P, et al. Detection of mutations in insulin-receptor gene in NIDDM patients by analysis of single-stranded conformation polymorphisms. *Diabetes.* 1991;40:777.
69. Strack V, Bossenmaier B, Stoyanov B, et al. A 973 valine to methionine mutation of the human insulin receptor: interaction with insulin-receptor substrate-1 and Shc in HEK 293 cells. *Diabetologia.* 1997;40:1135.
70. Caro JF, Ittoop O, Pories WJ, et al. Studies on the mechanism of insulin resistance in the liver from humans with noninsulin-dependent diabetes. Insulin action and binding in isolated hepatocytes, insulin receptor structure, and kinase activity. *J Clin Invest.* 1986;78:249.
71. Kellerer M, Sesti G, Seffer E, et al. Altered pattern of insulin receptor isotypes in skeletal muscle membranes of type 2 (non-insulin-dependent) diabetic subjects. *Diabetologia.* 1993;36:628.
72. Klein HH, Vestergaard H, Kotzke G, et al. Elevation of serum insulin concentration during euglycemic hyperinsulinemic clamp studies leads to similar activation of insulin receptor kinase in skeletal muscle of subjects with and without NIDDM. *Diabetes 344.* 1995:1310.
73. Farese RV, Sajan MP, Standaert ML. Insulin-sensitive protein kinases (atypical protein kinase C and protein kinase B/Akt): actions and defects in obesity and type II diabetes. *Exp Biol Med (Maywood).* 2005;230:593.
74. Obermaier-Kusser B, White MF, Pongratz DE, et al. A defective intramolecular autoactivation cascade may cause the reduced kinase activity of the skeletal muscle insulin receptor from patients with non-insulin-dependent diabetes mellitus. *J Biol Chem.* 1989;264:9497.
75. Dunaif A. Insulin resistance and the polycystic ovary syndrome: mechanism and implications for pathogenesis. *Endocr Rev.* 1997;18:774.
76. Kellerer M, Coghlan M, Capp E, et al. Mechanism of insulin receptor kinase inhibition in non-insulin-dependent diabetes mellitus patients. Phosphorylation of serine 1327 or threonine 1348 is unaltered. *J Clin Invest.* 1995;96:6.
77. Chibalin AV, Yu M, Ryder JW, et al. Exercise-induced changes in expression and activity of proteins involved in insulin signal transduction in skeletal muscle: differential effects on insulin-receptor substrates 1 and 2. *Proc Natl Acad Sci U S A.* 2000;97:38.
78. Freidenberg GR, Reichart D, Olefsky JM, et al. Reversibility of defective adipocyte insulin receptor kinase activity in non-insulin-dependent diabetes mellitus. Effect of weight loss. *J Clin Invest.* 1988;82:1398.
79. Zierath JR, Krook A, Wallberg-Henriksson H. Insulin action in skeletal muscle from patients with NIDDM. *Mol Cell Biochem.* 1998;182:153.
80. Clerk A, Sugden PH. The insulin receptor family in the heart: new light on old insights. *Biosci Rep.* 2022;42 BSR20221212.
81. Longo N, Wang Y, Smith SA, et al. Genotype-phenotype correlation in inherited severe insulin resistance. *Hum Mol Genet.* 2002;11:1465.
82. Krook A, Bjornholm M, Galuska D, et al. Characterization of signal transduction and glucose transport in skeletal muscle from type 2 diabetic patients. *Diabetes.* 2000;49:284.
83. Pratipanawatr W, Pratipanawatr T, Cusi K, et al. Skeletal muscle insulin resistance in normoglycemic subjects with a strong family history of type 2 diabetes is associated with decreased insulin-stimulated insulin receptor substrate-1 tyrosine phosphorylation. *Diabetes.* 2001;50:2572.
84. Marchetti P, Lupi R, Federici M, et al. Insulin secretory function is impaired in isolated human islets carrying the Gly (972)–>Arg IRS-1 polymorphism. *Diabetes.* 2002;51:1419.
85. Pedersen O. Genetics of insulin resistance. *Exp Clin Endocrinol Diabetes.* 1999;107:113.
86. Stumvoll M, Stefan N, Fritsche A, et al. Interaction effect between common polymorphisms in PPAR gamma2 (Pro12Ala) and insulin receptor substrate 1 (Gly972Arg) on insulin sensitivity. *J Mol Med.* 2002;80:33.
87. 'T Hart LM, Nijpels G, Dekker JM, et al. Variations in insulin secretion in carriers of gene variants in IRS-1 and -2. *Diabetes.* 2002;51:884.
88. Joost HG, Bell GI, Best JD, et al. Nomenclature of the GLUT/SLC2A family of sugar/polyol transport facilitators. *Am J Physiol.* 2002;282:E974.
89. Shepherd PR, Kahn BB. Glucose transporters and insulin action–implications for insulin resistance and diabetes mellitus. *N Engl J Med.* 1999;341:248.
90. Kakoti BB, Alom S, Deka K, et al. AMPK pathway: an emerging target to control diabetes mellitus and its related complications. *J Diabetes Metab Disord.* 2024;23:441.
91. Cline GW, Petersen KF, Krssak M, et al. Impaired glucose transport as a cause of decreased insulin-stimulated muscle glycogen synthesis in type 2 diabetes. *N Engl J Med.* 1999;341:240.
92. Williams KV, Price JC, Kelley DE. Interactions of impaired glucose transport and phosphorylation in skeletal muscle insulin resistance. A dose-response assessment using positron emission tomography. *Diabetes.* 2001;50:2069.
93. Kusari J, Verma US, Buse JB, et al. Analysis of the gene sequences of the insulin receptor and the insulin-sensitive glucose transporter (GLUT-4) in patients with common-type non-insulin-dependent diabetes mellitus. *J Clin Invest.* 1991;88:1323.
94. Rosenblatt-Velin N, Lerch R, Papageorgiou I, et al. Insulin resistance in adult cardiomyocytes undergoing dedifferentiation: role of GLUT4 expression and translocation. *FASEB J.* 2004;18:872.
95. Björntorp P, Rosmond R. Neuroendocrine abnormalities in visceral obesity. *Int J Obes Relat Metab Disord.* 2000;24(suppl 2):S80–S85.
96. Hirschberg AL. Hyperandrogenism and cardiometabolic risk in pre- and postmenopausal women-what is the evidence? *J Clin Endocrinol Metab.* 2024;109:1202.
97. Staiger H, Häring HU. Adipocytokines: fat-derived humoral mediators of metabolic homeostasis. *Exp Clin Endocrinol Diabetes.* 2005;113:67.
98. Gerst F, Wagner R, Oquendo MB, et al. What role do fat cells play in pancreatic tissue? *Mol Metab.* 2019;25:1.
99. Heni M, Machann J, Staiger H, et al. Pancreatic fat is negatively associated with insulin secretion in individuals with impaired fasting glucose and/or impaired glucose tolerance: a nuclear magnetic resonance study. *Diabetes Metab Res Rev.* 2010;26:200.
100. Machann J, Häring H, Schick F, et al. Intramyocellular lipid and insulin resistance. *Diabetes Obes Metab.* 2004;6:239.
101. Gilani A, Stoll L, Homan EA, et al. Adipose signals regulating distal organ health and disease. *Diabetes.* 2024;73:169.
102. Hafiane A. Adiponectin-mediated regulation of the adiponectin cascade in cardiovascular disease: updates. *Biochem Biophys Res Commun.* 2024;694:149406.
103. Ouchi N, Parker JL, Lugus JJ, et al. Adipokines in inflammation and metabolic disease. *Nat Rev Immunol.* 2011;11:85.
104. Turer AT, Scherer PE. Adiponectin: mechanistic insights and clinical implications. *Diabetologia.* 2012;55:2319.
105. Yamauchi T, Kamon J, Minokoshi Y, et al. Adiponectin stimulates glucose utilization and fatty-acid oxidation by activating AMP-activated protein kinase. *Nat Med.* 2002;8:1288.
106. Mitchell F. Obesity: glypican-4: role in insulin signalling. *Nat Rev Endocrinol.* 2012;8:505.
107. Hoene M, Weigert C. The role of interleukin-6 in insulin resistance, body fat distribution and energy balance. *Obes Rev.* 2008;9:20.
108. Kantartzis K, Thamer C, Peter A, et al. High cardiorespiratory fitness is an independent predictor of the reduction in liver fat during a lifestyle intervention in non-alcoholic fatty liver disease. *Gut.* 2009;58:1281.
109. Unger RH, Cherrington AD. Glucagonocentric restructuring of diabetes: a pathophysiologic and therapeutic makeover. *J Clin Invest.* 2012;122:4.
110. Kajani S, Laker RC, Ratkova E, et al. Hepatic glucagon action: beyond glucose mobilization. *Physiol Rev.* 2024;104:1021.
111. Wewer Albrechtsen NJ, Holst JJ, Cherrington AD, et al. 100 years of glucagon and 100 more. *Diabetologia.* 2023;66:1378.
112. Portincasa P, Baffy G. Metabolic dysfunction-associated steatotic liver disease: evolution of the final terminology. *Eur J Intern Med.* 2024;124:35.
113. Colca JR, Scherer PE. The metabolic syndrome, thiazolidinediones, and implications for intersection of chronic and inflammatory disease. *Mol Metab.* 2022;55:101409.
114. Lamos EM, Kristan M, Siamashvili M, et al. Effects of anti-diabetic treatments in type 2 diabetes and fatty liver disease. *Expert Rev Clin Pharmacol.* 2021;14:837.
115. European Association for the Study of the Liver; European Association for the Study of Diabetes; European Association for the Study of Obesity; Clinical Practice Guideline Panel. EASL-EASD-EASO Clinical Practice Guidelines on the management of metabolic dysfunction-associated steatotic liver disease (MASLD). *Diabetologia.* 2024;67:2375–2392. https://doi.org/10.1007/s00125-024-06196-3. Epub ahead of print. PMID: 38869512.
116. Bader H, Yamin S, Alshahwan H, et al. Association between metabolic-dysfunction-associated steatotic liver disease and hepatic cancer: current concepts and future challenges. *J Clin Med.* 2024;13:3132.
117. Cohen JC, Horton JD, Hobbs HH. Human fatty liver disease: old questions and new insights. *Science.* 2011;332:1519.
118. Weikert C, Stefan N, Schulze MB, et al. Plasma fetuin-a levels and the risk of myocardial infarction and ischemic stroke. *Circulation.* 2008;118:2555.
119. Petersen KF, Shulman GI. Pathogenesis of skeletal muscle insulin resistance in type 2 diabetes mellitus. *Am J Cardiol.* 2002;90:11G.
120. Kelley DE, Goodpaster B, Wing RR, et al. Skeletal muscle fatty acid metabolism in association with insulin resistance, obesity, and weight loss. *Am J Physiol.* 1999;277:E1130.
121. Lewis GF, Carpentier A, Adeli K, et al. Disordered fat storage and mobilization in the pathogenesis of insulin resistance and type 2 diabetes. *Endocr Rev.* 2002;23:201.
122. Pedersen BK, Febbraio MA. Muscles, exercise and obesity: skeletal muscle as a secretory organ. *Nat Rev Endocrinol.* 2012;8:457.

123. Böhm A, Weigert C, Staiger H, et al. Exercise and diabetes: relevance and causes for response variability. *Endocrine*. 2016;51:390.
124. Hoffmann C, Weigert C. Skeletal muscle as an endocrine organ: the role of Myokines in exercise adaptations. *Cold Spring Harb Perspect Med*. 2017;7:a029793.
125. Staiger H, Tschritter O, Machann J, et al. Relationship of serum adiponectin and leptin concentrations with body fat distribution in humans. *Obes Res*. 2003;11:368.
126. Weigert C, Hoene M, Plomgaard P. Hepatokines-a novel group of exercise factors. *Pflugers Arch*. 2019;471:383.
127. Hoene M, Weigert C. The stress response of the liver to physical exercise. *Exerc Immunol Rev*. 2010;16:163.
128. Havrankova J, Roth J, Brownstein M. Insulin receptors are widely distributed in the central nervous system of the rat. *Nature*. 1978;272:827.
129. Tschritter O, Preissl H, Hennige AM, et al. High cerebral insulin sensitivity is associated with loss of body fat during lifestyle intervention. *Diabetologia*. 2012;55:175.
130. Porte D, Jr, Seeley RJ, Woods SC, et al. Obesity, diabetes and the central nervous system. *Diabetologia*. 1998;41:863.
131. Heni M. The insulin resistant brain: impact on whole-body metabolism and body fat distribution. *Diabetologia*. 2024;67:1181.
132. Obici S, Feng Z, Karkanias G, et al. Decreasing hypothalamic insulin receptors causes hyperphagia and insulin resistance in rats. *Nat Neurosci*. 2002;5:566.
133. Obici S, Zhang BB, Karkanias G, et al. Hypothalamic insulin signaling is required for inhibition of glucose production. *Nat Med*. 2002;8:1376.
134. Kullmann S, Goj T, Veit R, et al. Exercise restores brain insulin sensitivity in sedentary adults who are overweight and obese. *JCI Insight*. 2022;7:e161498.
135. Kullmann S, Hummel J, Wagner R, et al. Empagliflozin improves insulin sensitivity of the hypothalamus in humans with prediabetes: a randomized, double-blind, placebo-controlled, phase 2 trial. *Diabetes Care*. 2022;45:398.
136. Goodner CJ, Walike BC, Koerker DJ, et al. Insulin, glucagon, and glucose exhibit synchronous, sustained oscillations in fasting monkeys. *Science*. 1977;195:177.
137. Laurenti MC, Matveyenko A, Vella A. Measurement of pulsatile insulin secretion: rationale and methodology. *Metabolites*. 2021;11:409.
138. O'Rahilly S, Turner RC, Matthews DR. Impaired pulsatile secretion of insulin in relatives of patients with non-insulin- dependent diabetes. *N Engl J Med*. 1988;318:1225.
139. Polonsky KS, Given BD, Hirsch LJ, et al. Abnormal patterns of insulin secretion in non-insulin-dependent diabetes mellitus. *N Engl J Med*. 1988;318:1231.
140. Meier JJ, Pennartz C, Schenker N, et al. Hyperglycaemia is associated with impaired pulsatile insulin secretion: effect of basal insulin therapy. *Diabetes Obes Metab*. 2013;15:258.
141. Menge BA, Grüber L, Jørgensen SM, et al. Loss of inverse relationship between pulsatile insulin and glucagon secretion in patients with type 2 diabetes. *Diabetes*. 2011;60:2160.
142. Porte Jr D, Pupo AA. Insulin responses to glucose: evidence for a two pool system in man. *J Clin Invest*. 1969;48:2309.
143. Bisht S, Singh MF. The triggering pathway, the metabolic amplifying pathway, and cellular transduction in regulation of glucose-dependent biphasic insulin secretion. *Arch Physiol Biochem*. 2024;9:1.
144. Henquin JC. The dual control of insulin secretion by glucose involves triggering and amplifying pathways in β-cells. *Diabetes Res Clin Pract*. 2011;93(suppl 1):S27.
145. Rorsman P, Renström E. Insulin granule dynamics in pancreatic beta cells. *Diabetologia*. 2003;46:1029.
146. American Diabetes Association Professional Practice Committee. 2. Diagnosis and classification of diabetes: standards of care in diabetes-2024. *Diabetes Care*. 2024;47(suppl 1):S20.
147. Stumvoll M, Fritsche A, Häring HU. Clinical characterization of insulin secretion as the basis for genetic analyses. *Diabetes*. 2002;51(suppl 1):S122.
148. Stumvoll M, Fritsche A, Stefan N, et al. A 60 minute hyperglycemic clamp is sufficient to assess both phases of insulin secretion. *Horm Metab Res*. 2000;32:230.
149. Gerich JE. Is reduced first-phase insulin release the earliest detectable abnormality in individuals destined to develop type 2 diabetes? *Diabetes*. 2002;51(suppl 1):S117.
150. Mitrakou A, Kelley D, Veneman T, et al. Contribution of abnormal muscle and liver glucose metabolism to postprandial hyperglycemia in NIDDM. *Diabetes*. 1990;39:1381.
151. Meier JJ, Kjems LL, Veldhuis JD, et al. Postprandial suppression of glucagon secretion depends on intact pulsatile insulin secretion: further evidence for the intraislet insulin hypothesis. *Diabetes*. 2006;55:1051.
152. Ramzy A, Kieffer TJ. Altered islet prohormone processing: a cause or consequence of diabetes? *Physiol Rev*. 2022;102:155.
153. Kahn SE, Halban PA. Release of incompletely processed proinsulin is the cause of the disproportionate proinsulinemia of NIDDM. *Diabetes*. 1997;46:1725.
154. Saad MF, Kahn SE, Nelson RG, et al. Disproportionately elevated proinsulin in Pima Indians with noninsulin-dependent diabetes mellitus. *J Clin Endocrinol Metab*. 1990;70:1247.
155. Rhodes CJ, Alarcón C. What beta-cell defect could lead to hyperproinsulinemia in NIDDM? Some clues from recent advances made in understanding the proinsulin-processing mechanism. *Diabetes*. 1994;43:511.
156. Chen YC, Taylor AJ, Verchere CB. Islet prohormone processing in health and disease. *Diabetes Obes Metab*. 2018;20(suppl 2):64.
157. Drucker DJ, Holst JJ. The expanding incretin universe: from basic biology to clinical translation. *Diabetologia*. 2023;66:1765.
158. Nauck MA, Homberger E, Siegel EG, et al. Incretin effects of increasing glucose loads in man calculated from venous insulin and C-peptide responses. *J Clin Endocrinol Metab*. 1986;63:492.
159. Nauck MA, Heimesaat MM, Orskov C, et al. Preserved incretin activity of glucagon-like peptide 1 [7-36 amide] but not of synthetic human gastric inhibitory polypeptide in patients with type-2 diabetes mellitus. *J Clin Invest*. 1993;91:301.
160. Nauck M, Stöckmann F, Ebert R, et al. Reduced incretin effect in type 2 (non-insulin-dependent) diabetes. *Diabetologia*. 1986;29:46.
161. Nauck MA, Kleine N, Orskov C, et al. Normalization of fasting hyperglycaemia by exogenous glucagon-like peptide 1 (7-36 amide) in type 2 (non-insulin-dependent) diabetic patients. *Diabetologia*. 1993;36:741.
162. Krieger JP. Intestinal glucagon-like peptide-1 effects on food intake: Physiological relevance and emerging mechanisms. *Peptides*. 2020;131:170342.
163. Ussher JR, Drucker DJ. Glucagon-like peptide 1 receptor agonists: cardiovascular benefits and mechanisms of action. *Nat Rev Cardiol*. 2023;20:463.
164. Holst JJ. Treatment of type 2 diabetes and obesity on the basis of the incretin system: The 2021 Banting Medal for Scientific Achievement Award Lecture. *Diabetes*. 2021;70:2468.
165. Gallwitz B. Clinical perspectives on the use of the GIP/GLP-1 receptor agonist tirzepatide for the treatment of type-2 diabetes and obesity. *Front Endocrinol (Lausanne)*. 2022;13 https://doi.org/10.3389/fendo.2022.1004044.
166. El K, Douros JD, Willard FS, et al. The incretin co-agonist tirzepatide requires GIPR for hormone secretion from human islets. *Nat Metab*. 2023;5:945.
167. Del Prato S, Gallwitz B, Holst JJ, et al. The incretin/glucagon system as a target for pharmacotherapy of obesity. *Obes Rev*. 2022;23:e13372. https://doi.org/10.1111/obr.13372.
168. Rosenstock J, Frias J, Jastreboff AM, et al. Retatrutide, a GIP, GLP-1 and glucagon receptor agonist, for people with type 2 diabetes: a randomised, double-blind, placebo and active-controlled, parallel-group, phase 2 trial conducted in the USA. *Lancet*. 2023;402:529.
169. Nogueiras R, Nauck MA, Tschöp MH. Gut hormone co-agonists for the treatment of obesity: from bench to bedside. *Nat Metab*. 2023;5:93.
170. Gutgesell RM, Nogueiras R, Tschöp MH, et al. Dual and triple incretin-based co-agonists: novel therapeutics for obesity and diabetes. *Diabetes Ther*. 2024;15:1069.
171. Nauck MA, Müller TD. Incretin hormones and type 2 diabetes. *Diabetologia*. 2023;266:1780.
172. Kumar AF, Gruessner RW, Seaquist ER. Risk of glucose intolerance and diabetes in hemipancreatectomized donors selected for normal preoperative glucose metabolism. *Diabetes Care*. 2008;31:1639.
173. Menge BA, Tannapfel A, Belyaev O, et al. Partial pancreatectomy in adult humans does not provoke beta-cell regeneration. *Diabetes*. 2008;57:142.
174. UK Prospective Diabetes Study (UKPDS) Group. Intensive blood-glucose control with sulphonylureas or insulin compared with conventional treatment and risk of complications in patients with type 2 diabetes. UK Prospective Diabetes Study (UKPDS) Group. *Lancet*. 1998;352:837.
175. Meier JJ, Menge BA, Breuer TG, et al. Functional assessment of pancreatic beta-cell area in humans. *Diabetes*. 2009;58:1595.
176. Butler PC, Meier JJ, Butler AE, et al. The replication of beta cells in normal physiology, in disease and for therapy. *Nat Clin Pract Endocrinol Metab*. 2007;3:75.
177. Hill TG, Hill DJ. The importance of intra-islet communication in the function and plasticity of the islets of Langerhans during health and diabetes. *Int J Mol Sci*. 2024;25:4070.
178. Yki-Järvinen H, Esko N, Eero H, et al. Clinical benefits and mechanisms of a sustained response to intermittent insulin therapy in type 2 diabetic patients with secondary drug failure. *Am J Med*. 1988;84:185.
179. Vilas-Boas EA, Almeida DC, Roma LP, et al. Lipotoxicity and β-cell failure in type 2 diabetes: oxidative stress linked to NADPH oxidase and ER stress. *Cells*. 2021;10:3328.
180. Unger RH. Lipotoxic diseases. *Annu Rev Med*. 2002;53:319.
181. Eitel K, Staiger H, Rieger J, et al. Protein kinase C delta activation and translocation to the nucleus are required for fatty acid-induced apoptosis of insulin-secreting cells. *Diabetes*. 2003;52:991.
182. Risi R, Vidal-Puig A, Bidault G. An adipocentric perspective of pancreatic lipotoxicity in diabetes pathogenesis. *J Endocrinol*. 2024;262:e230313.
183. Brayner B, Kaur G, Keske MA, et al. Novel approach to investigate the association between type 2 diabetes risk and dietary fats in a dietary pattern context: a scoping review. *Front Nutr*. 2023;10:1071855.

3 Lifestyle Interventions for the Prevention of Type 2 Diabetes Mellitus

JOSEPH HENSON, MELANIE J. DAVIES, COLIN JAMES GREAVES, KAMLESH KHUNTI, AND THOMAS YATES

INTRODUCTION

This chapter will principally focus on the evidence base for the prevention of type 2 diabetes mellitus (T2DM), which has developed exponentially over the last two decades, from efficacy trials through to real-world translational studies. In the first instance, an overview of the prevalence, terminology, and effectiveness of diabetes prevention strategies will be explored. Consideration will also be given to the epidemiological and experimental data pertaining to weight loss, diet, physical activity, and sedentary behavior in T2DM prevention. Finally, the challenge of implementing the evidence into the real world and the underlying role of behavior change will be discussed.

OVERVIEW OF PREVALENCE, ECONOMIC BURDEN, AND GLOBAL HEALTHCARE SYSTEMS

In 2021 the global prevalence of T2DM was estimated to be over half a billion (536.6 million), representing 10.5% of the total adult population aged 20 to 79 years.[1] This figure has increased by 16% compared with 2019 and 255% since 2000.[1,2] If this seemingly persistent trend continues, the prevalence of T2DM is likely to rise to 783 million by 2045.[1,2] Despite variation between and within countries, the rising figures can be partly attributed to earlier diagnosis, better management (leading to greater life expectancy), increased urbanization, and obesogenic "westernized" environments (partly driven by an inadequate diet, physical inactivity, and sedentary behavior).[3] That said, the projections are still likely to be conservative as they only consider demographic changes in populations relating to aging and urbanization and not changes in risk factor prevalence.

There is therefore an urgent need to develop and implement coordinated and multisectoral strategies to reduce the incidence of T2DM as it is one of the top 10 causes of death globally.[4] Indeed, together with cardiovascular disease, cancer, and respiratory disease, these conditions account for over 80% of all worldwide premature noncommunicable disease (NCD) deaths.[5] In response, the World Health Organization (WHO), the United Nations, and the Berlin Declaration (in collaboration with the International Diabetes Federation) have set global targets to encourage action to improve care and reinforce healthcare systems.[6–9] These actions include reducing premature death from NCDs, including diabetes, by 30% by 2030, while establishing national diabetes plans (see below sections) and achieving universal health coverage.[6,10] Similarly, the Lancet Commission on Diabetes provided a blueprint for reducing gaps in diabetes prevention, ongoing care, and professional knowledge. In particular, the use of data-driven modeling could avert up to 800,000 premature deaths in the top 10 low-to-middle-income countries with the highest populations of people with T2DM.[11]

Due to its adverse effect on people's health, T2DM also imposes a substantial economic burden. In the United Kingdom, for instance, the most comprehensive analysis to date (2010/2011) concluded that the direct cost of T2DM to the National Health Service (NHS) in the United Kingdom was £8.8 billion (£9.8 billion including all types of diabetes; corresponding to ~US$10.8 and 12 billion, respectively).[12] Around 80% is spent on complications, with treatment and intervention costs dominated by primary care and prescriptions. Of these, end-stage renal disease is associated with the largest increase in annual hospital costs, closely followed by lower limb amputation.[13] If the costs of treating a patient with T2DM remain consistent, the overall costs are set to account for 17% of the entire NHS budget over the next 20 years.[12] From a global perspective, assuming past trends continue, the economic burden of T2DM in 2030 will exceed 2015 levels by 88%.[14] Importantly, even if countries meet the sustainable development goals of decreasing mortality from T2DM by one-third,[6] the economic burden in 2030 will still be 61% higher than in 2015.[14]

IDENTIFICATION OF HIGH-RISK STATUS AND REFERRAL FOR DIABETES PREVENTION

Identifying those at high risk of T2DM allows elevated blood glucose levels to be recognized early, thus limiting potential overexposure to hyperglycemia and allowing the deployment of appropriate preventative strategies. T2DM resides at one end of a continuous glucose control spectrum, with normal glucose levels at the other. In between, there exists a "high-risk" condition called persons with nondiabetic hyperglycemia (NDH), historically defined as a composite of impaired fasting glucose (IFG) and/or impaired glucose tolerance (IGT). Over the last decade, guidelines have evolved to include HbA_{1c} in the diagnosis of NDH or T2DM. Various diagnostic thresholds exist for T2DM, alongside a second lower inclusion threshold to define those with NDH/high risk[15–17] (Table 3.1). Although there is ongoing debate about the advantages and disadvantages of the different diagnostic tests, NDH serves as an important marker for those who are at the greatest risk of developing T2DM.

In clinical practice, epidemiological, clinical, and laboratory risk factor information is often assimilated into a two-step process. For example, the National Institute for Health and Care Excellence (NICE) recommends involving the use of a risk assessment tool, validated in UK populations, followed by a venous blood test (fasting plasma glucose or HbA_{1c}) if deemed necessary.[19] This is also consistent with the ADA guidelines, where a diabetes risk test can be used to determine the appropriateness of clinical/laboratory testing for prediabetes in asymptomatic adults (diabetes.org/socrisktest). The risk score includes age, gender, history of gestational diabetes mellitus, family history of diabetes, high blood pressure, physical activity, and BMI, with those individuals scoring ≥5 considered to be at high risk of diabetes.

TABLE 3.1 ADA, WHO, NICE, and IDF Definitions for NDH/High Risk

	FASTING PLASMA GLUCOSE (mmol/L)	2-HOUR OGTT (mmol/L)	HbA_{1c} (mmol/mol)
ADA[16]	5.6–6.9	<7.8	39–46 (5.7%–6.4%)
WHO[17]	6.1–6.9	<7.8	42–46 (6.0%–6.4%)
NICE[15]	5.5–6.9	—	42–46 (6.0%–6.4%)
IDF[18]	6.1–6.9	<7.8	—

ADA, American Diabetes Association; *IDF*, International Diabetes Federation; *NDH*, Nondiabetic hyperglycemia; *NICE*, National Institute for Health and Care Excellence; *OGTT*, oral glucose tolerance test; *WHO*, World Health Organization.

In 2021 the US Preventive Services Task Force recommended prediabetes screening for asymptomatic individuals aged 35 to 70 years in those living with overweight/obesity (previously the lower cut-off age was 40 years).[20] The latest recommendations also suggest screening at a lower BMI (≥23 kg/m² if Asian American) and even younger ages in certain racial and ethnic minority groups (e.g., American Indian, Asian, Hispanic, and Black), which is likely associated with higher sensitivity (albeit with lower specificity).[21] These guidelines are also similar to those stipulated by NICE (outlined in Fig. 3.1), where the following groups are encouraged to have a risk assessment: those aged >40 (except pregnant females); those aged between 25 and 39 and of South Asian, Chinese, African-Caribbean, or Black African descent, or adults with preexisting conditions that increase the risk of T2DM (e.g., cardiovascular disease, hypertension, obesity, stroke, polycystic ovary syndrome, and a history of gestational diabetes).[19] The Leicester Diabetes Risk Score (http://riskscore.diabetes.org.uk) is one of several scores recommended by NICE for health practitioners and takes into account age, gender, BMI, ethnicity, family history of diabetes, and antihypertensive medication.[22] A score of 0 to 6 on the Leicester Diabetes Risk Score is deemed low risk, 7 to 15 is increased risk, 16 to 24 is moderate risk, and >25 is high risk. Other commonly used diabetes risk-prediction scores are the online Diabetes Risk Score and Finnish Diabetes Risk Score (FINDRISC).[19] It is expected that if a computer-based risk assessment tool is not available, the healthcare professional should provide a validated self-assessment questionnaire (e.g., the Cambridge diabetes risk score, the QDiabetes risk calculator, or the Leicester Practice Risk Score[19]) or provide information on how to access specific validated online self-assessment tools. This service has recently expanded (due to COVID-19), where a self-referral route via an online risk tool is available, meaning access is no longer restricted to a referral-only route (from general practice).[23]

Individuals with a high-risk score should be offered a venous blood test to identify possible T2DM. This may be fasting plasma glucose, an oral glucose tolerance test (OGTT), and/or HbA_{1c}. Individuals with a fasting plasma glucose (FPG) 99.0 to 124.2 mg/dL (5.5–6.9 mmol/L) or HbA_{1c} 42 to 47 mmol/mol (6.0%–6.4%) should be offered a referral to a local, evidence-based intensive lifestyle-change program with repeat blood, weight, and BMI measurements performed at least once a year. If the availability to deliver intensive lifestyle-change programs places is limited, those with FPG of 117.0 to 124.2 mg/dl (6.5–6.9 mmol/L) or HbA_{1c} of 44 to 47 mmol/mol (6.2%–6.4%) should be prioritized.

In contrast, for those individuals deemed to be at low/moderate risk of T2DM (FPG <5.5 mmol/L or HbA_{1c} <42 mmol/mol [6.0%]), guidance recommends that a brief consultation include communication of current low-risk status and risk-reduction advice with a reassessment at least every 5 years.

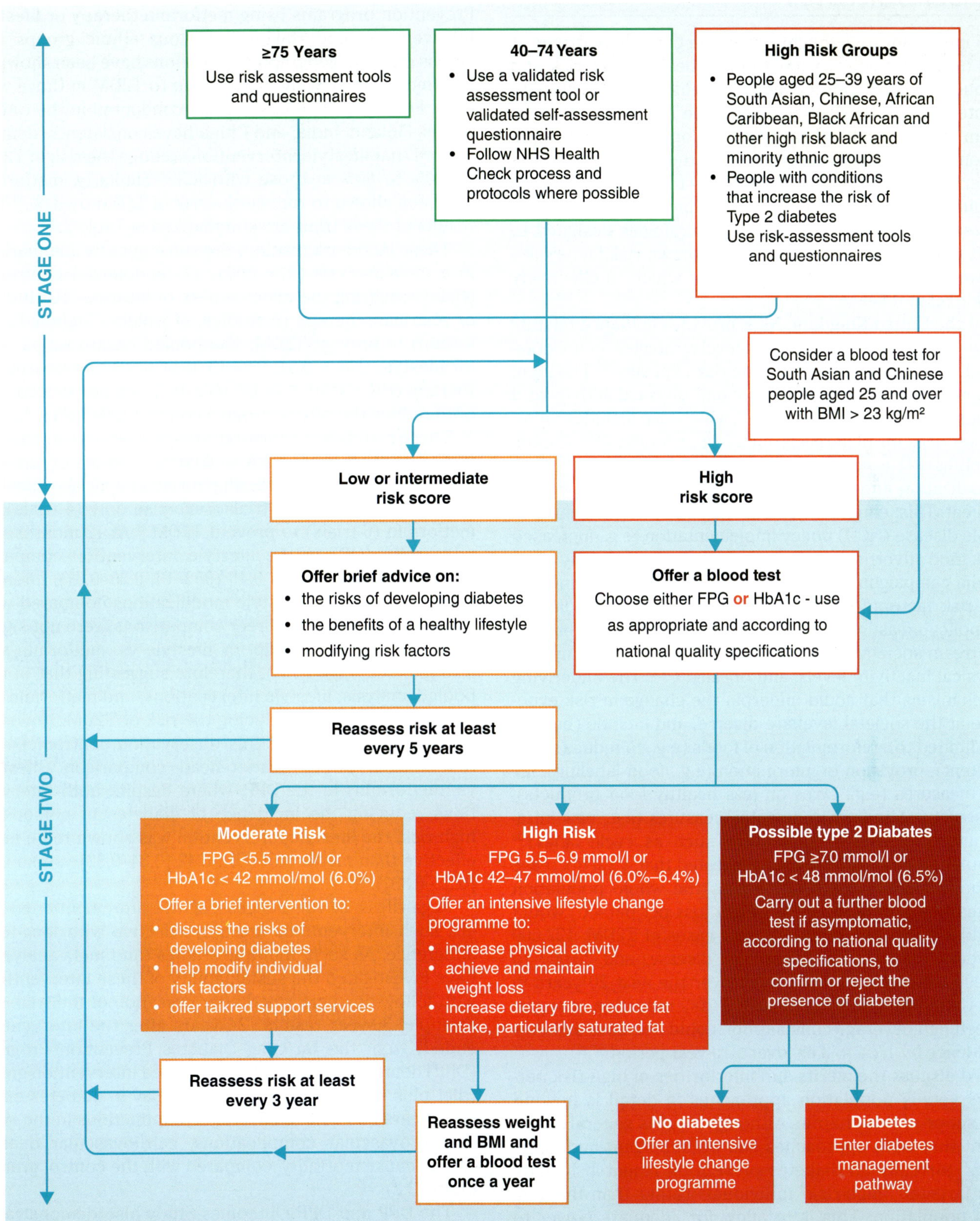

FIG. 3.1 NICE guidelines for the detection of individuals at high risk of type 2 diabetes mellitus (*T2DM*). Adapted from: National Institute for Clinical Excellence (2012) Preventing T2DM - risk identification and interventions for individuals at high risk (PH38). London: NICE.

HIGH-RISK VERSUS POPULATION-LEVEL APPROACHES TO THE PREVENTION OF TYPE 2 DIABETES MELLITUS

It is important to highlight one of the core conundrums at the heart of medical versus public health—high-risk and population-level approaches to prevention. The "high-risk" strategy seeks to identify susceptible individuals to offer them some individual protection. Conversely, the population-level strategy aims to reduce the mean level of the determinants of disease, and thereby the incidence, in the population as a whole. This "prevention paradox" was publicized by Geoffrey Rose, in which strategies designed to shift the population distribution of known risk factors are viewed as the only viable method in which to effectively tackle mass disease.[24]

In the United Kingdom, NICE provides guidance relating to the integration of population-level strategies on noncommunicable disease to reduce the risk exposure.[25] The main aim is to promote a healthy diet and physical activity at a community and population level, which also includes tailoring services for high-risk groups (e.g., minority ethnic communities). At a population level, modern-day society (i.e., globalization and urbanization) has changed how we live and eat. This, coupled with the stagnation of noncommunicable disease (NCD) policy implementation (e.g., increased junk food advertising and decreased physical activity mass media campaigns), has led to greater exposure to individual risk factors.[26] Population approaches are predicated by policy measures that have the potential to address the upstream societal drivers of unhealthy food consumption, physical inactivity levels, and obesity.[25,27,28] The underlying mechanisms that could underpin the change in risk exposure at the societal level are diverse, and include (but are not limited to): reformulation of foods (e.g., to reduce sugar content), provision of information (e.g., food labeling), fiscal measures (e.g., taxes on less healthy food products), or structural and environmental measures (e.g., new infrastructure for active commuting, such as cycle lanes).[28] Simulation models have also suggested that a 1% decrease in body mass index (BMI) across the whole population (roughly equating to 1 kg of weight loss per person) would avoid 179,000 to 202,000 incident cases of T2DM, 122,000 incident cases of cardiovascular disease, and 32,000 to 33,000 incident cases of cancer over the next 20 years in the United Kingdom.[29] Similarly, a 10% reduction in sugar-sweetened beverage consumption could decrease diabetes incidence by 1.7% to 3.6% over a 10-year period.[30]

To discuss the merits and inferiorities of high-risk persons versus population approaches in detail is beyond the scope of this chapter. Although there is general agreement that both approaches can be important and effective,[31] virtually all diabetes prevention research to date has targeted "high-risk" individuals rather than the general population. This is to allow for adequate power to test interventions with sample sizes and follow-up times that are affordable, practical, and feasible. The focus hereafter will be on approaches to T2DM prevention for high-risk individuals.

EFFECTIVENESS OF PREVENTION PROGRAMS AND LEGACY EFFECTS

Prevention programs using metformin therapy or lifestyle interventions undertaken in various ethnic groups and across different geographical locations have been shown to be effective at slowing progression to T2DM in those with NDH. For instance, efficacy trials conducted in the United States, Finland, India, and China have consistently demonstrated that lifestyle interventions reduce the risk of T2DM by 30% to 60% in those with IGT.[32] Similarly, metformin has been shown to reduce the risk of T2DM by 31%.[33] The results of these trials are summarized in Table 3.2.

These landmark results were subsequently summarized in a meta-analysis (n = 8084, 17 randomized controlled trials) assessing the effectiveness of lifestyle (10 studies) or pharmacotherapy (9 studies, of which 3 included metformin) to prevent T2DM. The pooled hazard ratios (HR) for lifestyle (HR = 0.51; 95% CI, 0.44–0.60) and pharmacotherapy (HR = 0.70; 95% CI, 0.62–0.79) demonstrated that both reduce the rate of progression to T2DM[32] (Fig. 3.2).

These results were corroborated in a network meta-analysis (n = 20,113) that encapsulated the results of randomized controlled trials assessing the effectiveness of lifestyle (20 trials), diet only (4 trials), exercise only (4 trials), or metformin (6 trials) to prevent T2DM.[41] At 12 months, the odds ratio (OR) in the lifestyle intervention compared with standard care was 0.46 (95% CI, 0.33–0.61). Interestingly, the effects of lifestyle modifications compared with other treatments by indirect comparisons were not significant (i.e., the odds ratio for lifestyle vs. metformin was 0.96 [95% CI, 0.58–1.73]), therefore suggesting that in this pooled analysis, lifestyle interventions, and metformin are similarly effective in reducing the risk of T2DM. However, it should be noted that this observation contradicts the randomized, direct head-to-head comparison (lifestyle vs. metformin) in the DPP, where despite both interventions reducing the incidence of diabetes in persons at high risk, the lifestyle intervention was shown to be more effective than metformin (OR: 0.42 [0.34–0.52] vsersu 0.69 [0.57–0.83]).[33]

Regardless of the success of the aforementioned trials, such interventions are only effective with long-term adherence. As such, multiple studies (and meta-analyses) have investigated the sustainability of these interventions with follow-ups performed after cessation of the trial. For example, 30-year results (24 years after the intervention ended) from the Da Qing Diabetes Prevention Program (DPP) demonstrated that the combined intervention group (diet plus exercise) had a median delay in diabetes onset of ~4 years and 26% to 35% relative reductions in the risks of microvascular complications, cardiovascular deaths, and all-cause mortality, compared with the control group[40] (Table 3.2).

The DPP and DPP Outcomes Study also demonstrated clinically meaningful levels of diabetes prevention at two decades after the cessation of the initial randomized treatment (lifestyle or metformin).[42] All participants who were receiving metformin in the randomized phase were offered

TABLE 3.2 A Summary of Major Diabetes Prevention Programs and Their Legacies

TRIAL NAME, LOCATION, PUBLICATION DATE & DURATION	POPULATION	INTERVENTION		OUTCOME	LEGACY
		CONTROL	INTERVENTION (S)	RELATIVE RISK (*I* VS. *C* 95% CIs)	
Diabetes Prevention Study (*DPS*), Finland (2003) 3 years[34]	*n* = 522, overweight with impaired glucose tolerance, 67% females	Limited advice on diet and exercise	Tailored, detailed advice on diet, weight reduction, and exercise	0.42 (0.3–0.7)	13-year follow-up showed that the corresponding HR during the postintervention follow-up was 0.67 (0.48, 0.95)[35] Among individuals who lost weight 2.5%–4.9% and 5% or more during the first year, the HR for the incidence of drug-treated diabetes was 0.63 (0.49, 0.81), and 0.71 (0.56–0.90) during a 7.4-year median follow-up[36]
Diabetes Prevention Program (*DPP*), United States (2002) Average = 2.8 years[33]	*n* = 3234 with impaired glucose tolerance, aged ≥25. Minimum BMI 24 (22 in Asians), 32% females, 54.7% White	Standard lifestyle recommendations	Intensive program of lifestyle modification or metformin therapy	Lifestyle = 0.42 (0.34–0.52) Metformin = 0.69 (0.57–0.83)	During a 22-year follow-up, diabetes incidence in the lifestyle group was reduced by 25% and 18% in the metformin group vs. placebo.
Indian Diabetes Prevention Program (*IDDP*), India (2006) 3 years[37]	*n* = 531 native Asian Indians with impaired glucose tolerance, aged 35–55, 21% females	Routine advice	Advice on a healthy diet and regular physical activity or metformin or both	Lifestyle = 0.71 (0.63–0.81) Metformin = 0.74 (0.65–0.81) Both = 0.72 (0.63– 0.80)	To be confirmed
The Diabetes Community Lifestyle Improvement Program (*D-CLIP*), India (2012) 3 years[38]	*n* = 578 overweight/ obese Asian Indians with IFG, IGT, or both, aged 20–65, 36.8% females	Routine care, which included: a single day with one-on-one visits with a physician, a dietitian, and a fitness trainer, and one group class on diabetes prevention	A group based and culturally appropriate lifestyle curriculum based on the DPP, plus metformin when needed	0.68 (0.50–0.93)	To be confirmed
Da Qing Study, China (1997) 6 years[39]	*n* = 530 Chinese with impaired glucose tolerance. All >25 years, 47% females	Routine advice	Diet group = individual and group counseling.[40] Exercise group = increase daily exercise.[40] Diet and exercise group = both interventions[40]	Exercise: 0.54 (0.2–0.9) Diet and exercise: 0.58 (0.4–0.9)	30-year follow-up showed that those in the combined lifestyle intervention groups had a 39% lower incidence (0.61 [0.45–0.83] of T2DM vs. control. The combined intervention group also had a median delay in diabetes onset of ~4 years[41]

CI, Confidence interval; *IFG*, impaired fasting glucose; *IGT*, impaired glucose tolerance; *T2DM*, type 2 diabetes mellitus.

continued treatment and all participants (regardless of randomization) received group-based lifestyle intervention. When compared with the placebo group, the reduction in diabetes incidence in the metformin group was –18% and –25% for the lifestyle intervention group[43] (Table 3.2).

A systematic review and meta-analysis (n = 5224) also demonstrated that those with NDH who received a lifestyle intervention had a 54% (95% CI, 34%–68%) and 36% (95% CI, 23%–47%) lower risk of progression to T2DM after 1 (16 trials) and 3 (11 trials) years, respectively.[44] Results from a 2017 meta-analysis also showed that participants receiving medication had a 29% lower diabetes risk at the end of the active intervention (RR = 0.71; 95% CI, 0.55–0.92) and that long-term follow-up of lifestyle interventions (mean follow-up, 7.2 years) yielded a 28% (95% CI, 14%–40%) reduced relative risk of developing T2DM.[45]

That said, despite a continued reduction in the risk of T2DM at 21 years of follow-up, recent results from the DPP Outcomes study demonstrate no significant differences in the incidence of major cardiovascular events (heart attacks, stroke, or cardiovascular death) in either the metformin or lifestyle group.[46] The disparity may be driven

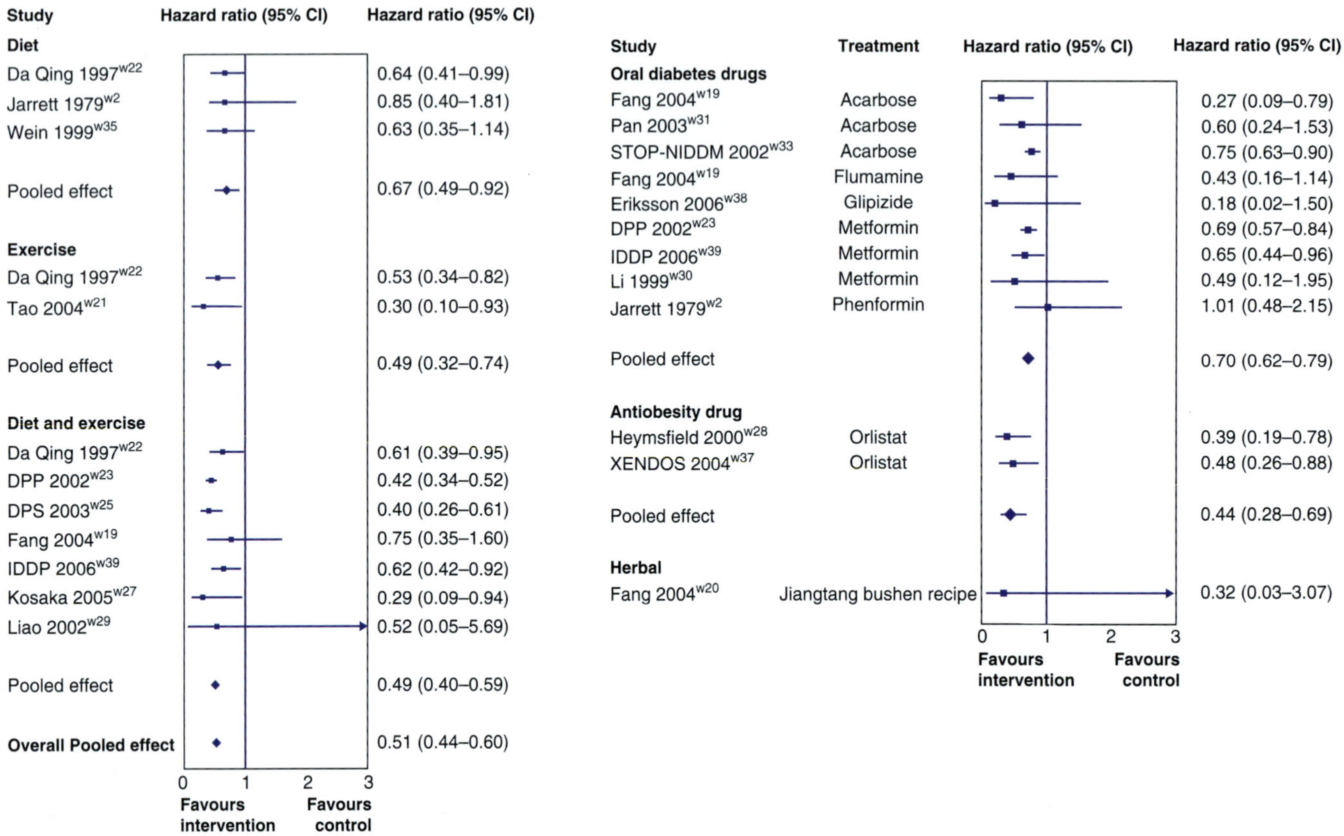

FIG. 3.2 Meta-analyses of effect of pharmacological, lifestyle, and herbal interventions on risk of developing type 2 diabetes. *CI*, Confidence interval.

by the reduced intensity of the lifestyle intervention and gradual decline in the adherence to metformin following the initial phase of the study. It should also be noted that in comparison to the Da Qing cohort, these participants were relatively low risk (in terms of cardiovascular disease [CVD] events). For example, the Da Qing cohort included a greater proportion of smokers, a higher prevalence of hypertension, and a higher overall CVD event rate. The participants from the DPP Outcomes study were also well controlled at follow-up, with 68% to 74% and 53% to 62% receiving antihypertensive and statin medications, respectively (compared to 16% and 4% at baseline).[46]

With obesity presenting an increasing challenge to public health, interest in novel pharmacological therapies (as outlined below) as an adjunct to lifestyle interventions may change the potency of future diabetes prevention programs.

ELEMENTS OF PREVENTION

Diet

It is well established that an inadequate diet is considered a major contributor to the incidence of T2DM.[47] More recently the evidence has converged from both prospective observational studies and randomized controlled trials to further highlight the importance of individual nutrients, foods, and dietary patterns in the prevention of T2DM. This is timely, as diet plays a pivotal role in the incidence of obesity.[48] As such, the importance of body weight (and subsequent reduction) in those with NDH places an emphasis on the cumulative energy deficit and the induction of a negative energy balance. Although physical activity is the most effective way of increasing our daily energy expenditure, the imbalance in the levels of energy intake (calorie excess) cannot be tackled by increasing activity alone.

CURRENT RECOMMENDATIONS

A large body of evidence (predominantly largely derived from long-term prospective studies, with limited evidence from randomized controlled trials) is available, examining the associations between certain food groups, dietary composition, and incidence of T2DM. Indeed, the evidence appears to support a common set of dietary approaches for the prevention of T2DM and chronic disease(s),[49] largely underpinned by evidence-based guidance to limit the daily consumption of highly processed foods and carbohydrates, particularly those consisting of rapidly digestible starches and sugars.[10,50,51]

These overarching messages were also outlined in an ADA consensus report that stated that macronutrient distribution should be based on individualized assessment of current eating patterns, preferences, and metabolic goals[52] (Fig. 3.3). This may be facilitated through a referral to an intensive lifestyle intervention program. As such, no ideal percentage of calories from carbohydrates, protein, and fat for all people with NDH was promulgated.

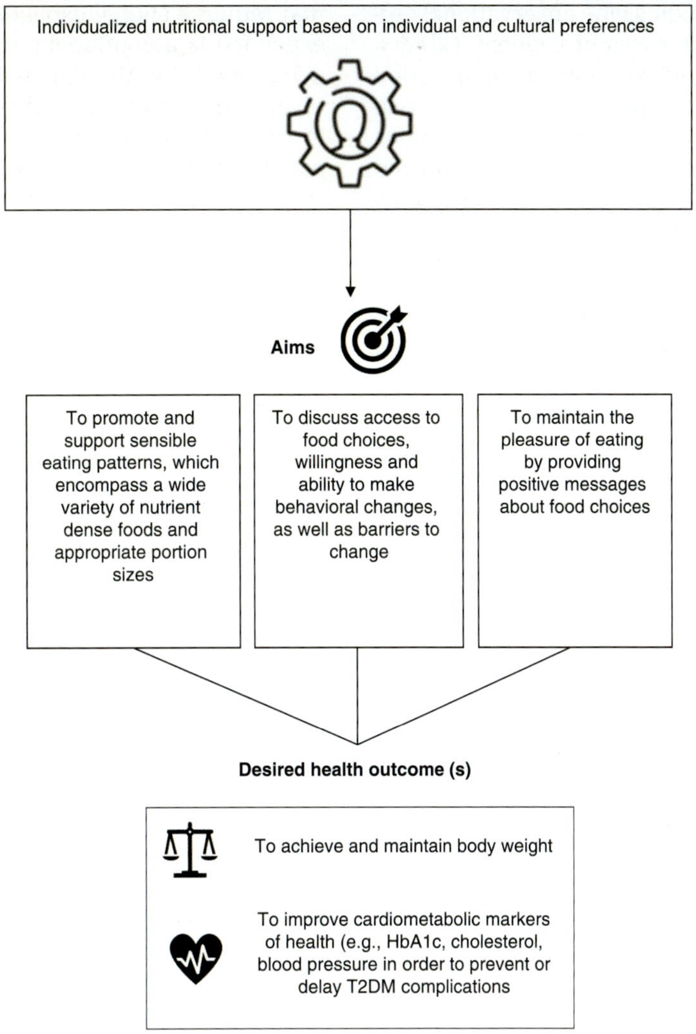

FIG. 3.3 Goals of nutrition therapy in the prevention of type 2 diabetes mellitus (*T2DM*). Adapted from Evert AB, Dennison M, Gardner CD, Garvey WT, Lau KHK, MacLeod J, et al. Nutrition Therapy for Adults With Diabetes or Prediabetes: A Consensus Report. *Diabetes Care* 2019;42(5):731–754.

EPIDEMIOLOGICAL EVIDENCE

The overarching recommendations were recently summarized by the Diabetes and Nutrition Study Group (DNSG) of the European Association for the Study of Diabetes (EASD).[51] These recommendations were preceded by a 2014 narrative review including results of meta-analyses of prospective cohort studies demonstrating that processed and unprocessed red meat, white rice, and sugar-sweetened beverages having a consistent, positive relation with T2DM. Conversely, green leafy vegetables, whole grains, and coffee were inversely associated with T2DM.[53]

More recently, a 2019 umbrella review of systemic reviews and meta-analyses (53 studies; 153 adjusted summary HRs) explored the associations between the incidence of T2DM and dietary behaviors or diet quality indices, food groups, beverages (including alcohol), macronutrients, and micronutrients.[47] Inverse associations were reported for whole grains (adjusted HR per additional 30 g/day = 0.87 [95% CI, 0.82–0.93]), cereal fiber (adjusted HR per additional 10 g/day = 0.75 [95% CI, 0.65–0.86]), and moderate alcohol intake (vs. no alcohol) (adjusted HR per 12–24 g = 0.75 [95% CI, 0.67–0.83]).[47] Conversely, red meat (adjusted HR per additional 100 g/day = 1.17 [95% CI, 1.08–1.26]), processed meat (adjusted HR per additional 50 g/day = 1.37 [95% CI, 1.22–1.54]), and sugar-sweetened beverages (adjusted HR per one serving/day = 1.26 [95% CI, 1.11–1.43]) were associated with a higher incidence of T2DM.[47]

Although the aforementioned findings are consistent with existing guidelines, diet involves a complex combination of foods and nutrients that act synergistically. As such, examining dietary patterns (e.g., Nordic,[54] Mediterranean[55]) may be more predictive of disease risk than investigations of single foods or nutrients. For instance, a Western diet (typically high in sugar-sweetened soft drinks, refined grains, and processed meat) was associated with a relative risk for T2DM of 1.49 (95% CI, 1.26–1.76) in 69,554 females (aged 38–63 years), when comparing the highest with lowest quintiles.[56]

The potential of plant-based dietary patterns to be used in the prevention of management of chronic disease (including T2DM) has also gained considerable traction over recent years. This dietary pattern places a greater emphasis on foods derived from plants (e.g., nuts, seeds, fruits and vegetables, whole grains) and includes lower consumption of or exclusion of animal products. A systematic review and meta-analysis including nine observational prospective studies (n = 307,099, cases of incident T2DM = 23,544) demonstrated a significant inverse association between higher adherence to a plant-based dietary pattern and risk of T2DM (RR = 0.77; 95% CI, 0.71–0.84) versus poorer adherence.[57] These associations were strengthened when fruits, vegetables, whole grains, legumes, and nuts were encapsulated within the definition of a plant-based dietary pattern (RR = 0.70; 95% CI, 0.62–0.79).[57] Similarly, a cohort study (n = 145,299 postmenopausal females, with a mean follow-up of 16 years) demonstrated that adherence to a Portfolio Diet, assessed with a score based on six components (high in plant protein [soy and pulses], nuts, viscous fiber, plant sterols, and monounsaturated fat and low in saturated fat and cholesterol) was prospectively associated with a lower risk of T2DM (HR = 0.77; 95% CI, 0.72–0.82).[58] Interestingly, the level of risk reduction was comparable to that of a Mediterranean diet (HR = 0.78; 95% CI, 0.74–0.83).[58]

EXPERIMENTAL EVIDENCE

Although these dietary approaches show some promise regarding the prevention of T2DM, weight loss is clearly the dominant determinant of the reduced risk of T2DM. Evidence suggests that dietary factors are unlikely to lead to any additional reductions in diabetes risk after accounting for weight loss. This was epitomized by findings from the DPP, where there was no independent effects of decreased percent fat on T2DM risk after adjustment for weight change.[59] Similarly, the effects of replacing saturated fatty acids with monounsaturated fatty acids or high glycemic index foods with low glycemic foods over 24 weeks had little effect on insulin sensitivity when body weight remained stable.[60] Even when weight loss is achieved through dietary manipulation, the methods appear to have similar effects upon insulin resistance. For example, an 8-week comparison between two weight loss diets (low-fat [20% fat, 60% carbohydrate] and low-carbohydrate diets [60% fat, 20% carbohydrate]) in 24 overweight/obese adults resulted in comparable effects on body weight (7.6% and 7.1% reduction in low carb and low fat, respectively) and insulin resistance, independent of macronutrient composition.[61]

These findings question the relative merits of different dietary approaches independent of weight loss. Arguably, the ideal diet is the one that is best adhered to by individuals so that they can stay on the diet as long as possible (i.e., a personalized approach). This recommendation was typified by results from a meta-analysis including 48 randomized controlled trials, showing that both low-carbohydrate and low-fat diets were elicited similar weight loss at 6 (~ –8 kg) and 12 months (~ –6 kg) when compared with no dietary intervention.[62] Although statistical differences existed among several well-publicized diets, the differences were minimal and unlikely to be important in those seeking to lose weight.

Physical Activity

Regular physical activity is a fundamental therapeutic aid in the prevention of T2DM. In its most rudimentary form, it is defined as any movement produced by skeletal muscles that requires energy expenditure.[63] The amount of energy expended is a continuous variable that is predominantly determined by the intensity, duration, and frequency of muscular movement. Its importance is promulgated in international guidelines, consensus documents, and patient decision aids.[64–69] Irrespective of mode, it provides an economically viable, nonpharmacological method for eliciting beneficial adaptations on glycemic control and a plethora of other health outcomes, some of which are highlighted and discussed below.

CURRENT RECOMMENDATIONS

Regular physical activity is recommended for all individuals, unless otherwise contraindicated, with national (The UK Chief Medical Officers [CMO], NICE) and international (ADA, WHO, American College of Sports Medicine [ACSM]) guidelines produced that apply to all age groups.[19,64–69] To discuss in detail is beyond the scope of this chapter; therefore we provide an abridged version here within and a summary in Table 3.3.

Those at a high risk of T2DM are encouraged to undertake a minimum of 150 minutes per week of moderate-intensity physical activity, which is congruent with the general population. Vigorous intensity can be substituted in for moderate in those who are already physically active with a minimum of 75 minutes per week suggested. This should be supplemented with two to three resistance, flexibility, and/or balance training sessions/week. Sedentary behaviors should also be limited (discussed in more detail below).[64] Regardless of subtle differences in their recommendations, each set of physical activity guidelines promulgates the use of a personalized, patient-centered approach to promotion, while considering personal limitations and preferences.

Although individuals are encouraged to work toward the aforementioned recommendations, the absolute targets are to a certain degree, arbitrary, as physiological and psychological benefits can be achieved at levels below and above these thresholds. It should be emphasized that although a higher intensity and duration of activity will elicit a greater range and magnitude of physiological adaptations, any form of increased movement has beneficial effects on overall health. For example, all intensities of physical activity are associated with a substantially lower risk of mortality in a graded association (up to a plateau of ~150 minutes per week of moderate-to-vigorous intensity and ~300 minutes per week for light-intensity physical activity).[70] Importantly, the graded relationship between physical activity achieved and health outcomes is curvilinear, suggesting that the gains of increased physical activity could be especially significant for those currently doing the lowest levels of activity (fewer than 30 minutes per week), as the associations with improvements in health per additional minute of physical activity will be proportionately greater.[69]

EPIDEMIOLOGICAL EVIDENCE

A meta-analysis summarized the epidemiological evidence examining the independent association of physical activity (after additionally adjusting for body weight) and T2DM

TABLE 3.3 A Summary of Sedentary Behavior and Physical Activity Guidelines

	SEDENTARY BEHAVIOR	PHYSICAL ACTIVITY LIGHT/MODERATE/ VIGOROUS INTENSITY)	RESISTANCE ACTIVITIES
American College of Sports Medicine (*ACSM*)[66,67]			
Adults	Adults should move more and sit less throughout the day. Some physical activity is better than none. Adults who sit less and do any amount of moderate-to-vigorous physical activity gain some health benefits.	150–300 minutes per week of moderate intensity; OR 75–150 minutes a week of vigorous-intensity aerobic physical activity; OR an equivalent combination of moderate- and vigorous-intensity aerobic activity.	Muscle-strengthening activities of moderate intensity that involve all major muscle groups on ≥2 days a week.
	As above	≥150 minutes a week to 300 minutes a week of moderate intensity; OR 75–150 minutes a week of vigorous-intensity aerobic physical activity; OR an equivalent combination of moderate- and vigorous-intensity aerobic activity. When adults with chronic conditions or disabilities are not able to meet the above key guidelines, they should engage in regular physical activity according to their abilities and should avoid inactivity.	As above
American Diabetes Association (*ADA*)[64]			
Adults with T2DM	All patients should reduce their daily levels of sedentary behavior. In particular, prolonged sitting should be interrupted at least every 30 minute with either light or moderate activity.	≥150 minutes of moderate-to-vigorous intensity activity weekly, spread over at least 3 days/week, with no more than two consecutive days without activity. Shorter durations (minimum 75 minutes/week) of vigorous-intensity or interval training may be sufficient for younger and more physically fit individuals. Increase total daily incidental (nonexercise) physical activity to gain additional health benefits. Encouraged as part of a whole-day approach.	2–3 sessions/week of resistance exercise on nonconsecutive days.
UK Chief Medical Officers guidelines[69]			
Adults	Adults should aim to minimize the amount of time spent being sedentary	Aim to be physically active every day ≥150 minutes per week of moderate-intensity activity (such as brisk walking or cycling); OR 75 minutes of vigorous-intensity activity (such as running); OR even shorter durations of very vigorous-intensity activity (such as sprinting or stair climbing); OR a combination of moderate- and vigorous-intensity activity.	≥2 days/week muscle-strengthening activities at moderate or greater intensity involving all major muscle groups (upper and lower).
World Health Organization (*WHO*)[65]			
Adults	Limit the amount of time spent being sedentary. In parallel, all adults should also aim for the recommended levels of moderate-to vigorous-intensity physical activity	≥150–300 minutes of moderate-intensity aerobic physical activity per week; OR at least 75–150 minutes of vigorous-intensity aerobic physical activity; OR an equivalent combination of moderate- and vigorous-intensity activity throughout the week.	≥2 days/week muscle-strengthening activities at moderate or greater intensity involving all major muscle groups.

incidence. In total, three studies (n = 261,618 participants and 19,417 events) were included.[71] To aid interpretation and in comparison to the aforementioned binary outcome, the authors derived a single, continuous physical activity metric. Overall, the results demonstrated an RR of 0.74 (95% CI, 0.72–0.77) for T2DM after adjustment for body weight and a similar level of risk when not adjusted for body weight (RR = 0.73; 95% CI, 0.68–0.79). Interestingly, the dose-response curve demonstrated a similar benefit when moving from inactive (0 METs) to 6 METs (RR = 0.77; 95% CI, 0.74–0.80), compared with moving from inactive to the MET h/week synonymous with current physical activity guidelines (11.25 MET h/week) (RR = 0.70; 95% CI, 0.54–0.90).[71] The inverse association between physical activity and T2DM incidence also exists after adjusting for genetic risk. For example, a recent prospective cohort analysis using the UK Biobank demonstrated that when compared to the least-active individuals, a dose-response association was observed for moderate-to-vigorous intensity physical activity (corresponding daily minutes (HRs and

95% CIs): 5.3 to 25.9 minutes/day (0.63 [0.53–0.75]), 26.0 to 68.4 minutes/day (0.41 [0.34–0.51]) and >68.4 minutes/day (0.26 [0.18–0.38]).[72] Interestingly, there was an interaction between moderate to vigorous physical activity (MVPA) and genetic risk score, suggesting larger absolute risk differences amongst those with a higher genetic risk.[72] Inverse associations have also been shown between various physical activity modalities and T2DM incidence. For instance, a meta-analysis including 81 studies reported that the RR for high versus low activity was 0.65 (95% CI, 0.59–0.71).[73] Similar results were also seen across the physical activity continuum with low (RR = 0.68; 95% CI, 0.52–0.90), moderate (RR = 0.66; 95% CI, 0.47–0.94), and vigorous activity (RR = 0.74; 95% CI, 0.70–0.79) all yielding significant inverse associations. More specifically, an RR of 0.85 (95% CI, 0.79–0.91) was also observed for walking. Although the strongest inverse association was seen for cardiorespiratory fitness (RR = 0.45; 95% CI, 0.29–0.70), the favorable associations also extended beyond aerobic activities, with resistance exercise displaying an RR of 0.72 (95% CI, 0.57–0.91) for high versus low resistance exercise.[74]

Experimental Evidence

GLYCEMIC CONTROL

Several reviews, consensus documents, and meta-analyses have summarized the health benefits of exercise training in T2DM-related outcomes (see Chapter XX), with favorable associations evident across the whole glucose spectrum and encompassing the continuum of human movement (from light activity through to high-intensity interval training [HIIT]).[67,75–78] For example, a meta-analysis including both those with normal glucose tolerance and NDH (25 studies [*n* = 870]) demonstrated that HIIT effectively reduced postprandial glucose (−0.37; 95% CI, −0.60 to −0.13) and insulin (−0.36; 95% CI, −0.68 to −0.04) levels when compared with a control group.[79] Subanalysis further showed that the results for glucose were only significant in those individuals identified as having NDH at a baseline (5 intervention arms).

Similarly, results from a meta-analysis (15 studies), not including those with T2DM, demonstrated that physical activity interventions were associated with significantly lower HbA_{1c} (effect size = 0.32; 95% CI, 0.01–0.62) versus control.[80] Interestingly, supervised physical activity programs (effect size = 0.33; 95% CI, 0.14–0.52) had greater magnitude of associations than physical activity counseling (effect size = 0.03; 95% CI, −0.13 to 0.20) and interventions <12 weeks and >150 minutes per week yielded the largest associations with improved glycemic control. This is similar to interventions in those living with T2DM, where a pooled analysis of 23 randomized controlled trials, ranging from 12 to 52 weeks of aerobic, resistance, or combined (aerobic plus resistance) exercise training elicited significant reductions in HbA_{1c} compared with nonexercise control participants (mean difference −0.73%, −0.57%, and −0.51%, respectively).[76] Interestingly, total duration greater than 150 minutes per week had the greatest effect on average reduction of HbA_{1c} (−0.89%), but even those below this threshold exhibited on average significant reductions in HbA_{1c} (−0.36%).[76] These results suggest that any form of sustained physical activity is likely to be beneficial for patients at a high risk of T2DM.

WHOLE-BODY BENEFITS

Aerobic exercise interventions are repeatedly found to induce clinically significant benefits on cardiorespiratory fitness (mean improvement in peak oxygen uptake [$\dot{V}O_2$ peak] ~12%) and glycemic control.[75,77,81,82] The evidence is also clear on a dose-response relationship, whereby activity of greater intensity, duration, or frequency will likely result in greater benefits.[83,84] Some of these short-term benefits include (but are not limited to): improvements in sleep quality, anxiety/stress management, blood pressure, and insulin sensitivity.[64–69] Chronic adaptions to sustained physical activity include the lowering of whole-body and ectopic lipid stores, improvements in endothelial function, improvements in cognitive function, reduction of systolic and diastolic blood pressure, promotion of a more favorable circulating lipid profile, reduced risk of cardiovascular morbidity, and all-cause mortality and improvements in glycemic control.[64,85–90]

THE IMPORTANCE OF STEPS AND MONITORING OF PHYSICAL ACTIVITY

The proliferation and popularity of newly developed wearable devices have streamlined the measurement, quantification, and prescription of habitual physical activity. Daily step counts provide an easy-to-understand metric of ambulation that are common to most (if not all) wearable devices. Moreover, steps can be categorized as light, moderate, or vigorous, providing a range of exertion choice in the context of physical activity monitoring and prescription. This is exemplified by analyses demonstrating that a 5- to 6-minute brisk intensity walk per day (~500 steps in 5 minutes) equates to ~4-year greater life expectancy.[73,91–93]

Previous studies have also shown that an increase of as little as 500 steps per day is associated with a 2% to 9% lower risk of cardiovascular morbidity and all-cause mortality, including those with NDH.[92,94–97] Ponsonby et al. also estimated that for any average daily step count, an additional 2000 steps was associated with a 25% lower incidence of NDH over 5 years.[98] Concurrent with the findings from the NAVIGATOR studies, the relationship between daily step count and health outcome appears linear.[94,99] For instance, Kraus et al. analyzed the relationship between baseline steps and the incidence of T2DM in 7118 participants (where 35% subsequently developed T2DM).[99] Results showed that each 2000-step increment in the average number of daily steps up to 10,000 was associated with >6% lower risk of progression toward T2DM.[100] In addition, recent results from the UK Biobank (median follow-up of 7.4 years, *n* = 162,155, of which 4442 participants developed T2DM), demonstrate that compared with self-reported slow walkers, self-reported brisk walkers have the same diabetes incidence rate 18.6 (females) and 16.0 (males) years later.[101] Moreover, the prospective associations between walking pace and the incidence of T2DM have been observed independent of adiposity, highlighting the potential benefits of combining brisk walking and weight management strategies in the prevention of T2DM.[102]

Physical activity trackers, particularly those that count steps, are effective in supporting physical activity behavior change through enabling goal setting and feedback. For example, results from a meta-analysis of 34 randomized controlled trials (n = 3793) showed a significant association of wearable tracker use (i.e., pedometers, accelerometers, or fitness trackers) with increased physical activity levels, which is amplified further when combined with health professional consultations.[103]

THE UNIQUE ROLE OF PHYSICAL ACTIVITY IN WEIGHT LOSS

Despite the impressive results of medication and/or surgery, existing therapeutic approaches (i.e., physical activity) still have a pivotal role to play. For instance, although the dual effects of weight loss and improved glycemic control associated with GLP-1RAs are appealing, a recent review examining the effect of GLP-1RA on changes in body composition demonstrated that the proportion of lean body mass reduction ranged between 20% and 50%, which is consistent with diet-induced weight loss and bariatric surgery.[104,105] Therefore multimodal (both aerobic and resistance) exercise can be used to help preserve lean mass during weight loss, while acting to increase cardiorespiratory fitness and improve physical function.[105–109] Muscle mass is critical to maintaining healthy human physiology, fundamentally providing the dynamic biomechanical device needed for locomotion, physical function, and the completion of essential daily activities.[110] It also plays a fundamental role in maintaining cellular homeostasis through contributing to a wide range of physiological processes, including regulating glucose, inflammation, hormonal, and energy balance.[111–113] Given that T2DM also represents a state of accelerated metabolic aging, some of the additional frailty risk (up to 5 times) may be underpinned by an increased loss of lean body mass and function.[114–116]

Sedentary Behavior

The term "sedentary behavior" (from the Latin word sedere, "to sit") is defined as "any waking behavior characterized by an energy expenditure ≤1.5 METs (multiples of the resting metabolic rate) while in a sitting or reclining posture".[117] One MET is the energy cost of resting quietly, often defined in terms of oxygen uptake as 3.5 mL/kg/min.[118] Given the fact that it is often impractical to measure energy expenditure, sedentary behavior should be operationally defined as any sitting or lying behavior conducted outside of structured exercise.

CURRENT RECOMMENDATIONS

Sedentary behavior has recently become more prominent in current physical activity guidelines (see above and Table 3.3). This important step forward is epitomized by the incorporation of new evidence-based recommendations on sedentary behavior within the 2020 WHO guidelines.[65] That said, given the relative infancy of the research, the overarching message for the general population and those at risk of chronic disease remains generic ("sit less").[65,69] In comparison, the ADA guidelines stipulate breaking sitting time at least every 30 minutes with light or moderate activity in those with T2DM[64] (see also Chapter XX).

EPIDEMIOLOGICAL EVIDENCE

Multiple meta-analyses have helped to highlight the importance of sedentary behavior by estimating the independent associations on the incidence of chronic disease(s) and markers of health, including those associated with T2DM.[119–122] Importantly, the strongest and most consistent associations are seen for risk of T2DM (when compared with the increased risk for all-cause and cardiovascular disease [CVD] mortality).[120] For instance, results from a meta-analysis including 11 prospective studies (n = 1,331,468), demonstrated a graded association between higher levels of TV viewing time with the incidence of T2DM.[123] TV viewing was estimated to be related to 29% (95% CI, 26%–32%) of T2DM incidence (vs. 5% for CVD mortality) with the largest associations with higher risk for T2DM seen <4 hours per day of TV viewing (1.12; 95 CI, 1.08–1.15) versus (1.02; 95% CI, 0.99–1.04) for CVD mortality.[123] A similarly sized graded association meta-analysis (n = 1,071,967; 13 cohort, 10 cross sectional), demonstrated that the risk of T2DM was 5% higher (total sedentary time) and 8% (TV viewing) for each 1-hour per day higher sedentary time.[124] When examining sitting time only (as opposed to TV viewing), results from a 2019 systematic review and meta-analysis (5 studies, n = 223,871) demonstrated higher risk for CVD (HR = 1.14; 95% CI, 1.04–1.23) and higher risk for incident diabetes (HR = 1.11; 95% CI, 1.01–1.19), independent of physical activity.[125]

EXPERIMENTAL EVIDENCE

Experimental research has complemented these epidemiological findings by examining the postprandial effects of breaking up bouts of prolonged sitting with standing or light-intensity activity. Multiple studies have demonstrated benefits on markers of metabolic health in those at high risk of T2DM.[126–130] Importantly, this also includes some alternative strategies that do not necessarily involve changes in posture. For example, seated arm ergometry (5 minutes every 30 minutes) has been shown to acutely lower postprandial glucose and insulin levels by 57% and 20%, respectively, when compared with prolonged sitting.[127] This mode of activity offers a viable alternative for those with weight-bearing difficulties or those who are wheelchair bound.

The acute effects of breaking up prolonged sitting on cardiometabolic outcomes in a largely overweight/obese cohort were summarized in a recent meta-analysis (number of randomized crossover trials = 7). The results showed that prolonged sitting punctuated with standing significantly reduced postprandial glucose (mean effect size = 0.31; 95% CI, 0.03–0.60). Similarly, light-intensity walking was also shown to attenuate the postprandial glucose (mean effect size = 0.72; 95% CI, 0.41–1,03) and insulin (mean effect size = 0.83; 95% CI, 0.48–1.18) response when compared with prolonged sitting.[131]

Results from another meta-analysis that included 20 experimental studies demonstrated that when compared with prolonged sitting, short, frequent bouts of light-intensity activity reduced postprandial glucose by 17.5% (95% CI, 8.4–31.7) and insulin levels by 25.1% (95% CI; −18.3 to −31.76).[132] Importantly, the effects on glucose were more pronounced in metabolically impaired individuals (−28.7%; 95% CI, −18.3 to −31.8) versus −20.1; 95% CI, −3.0 to −37.2).

The potential interindividual variability in the response to breaking up prolonged sitting has also been highlighted in a systematic review and meta-analysis, which included 42 studies.[133] Although breaking prolonged sitting with physical activity attenuated the postprandial glucose and insulin response, the greater magnitude of difference in glycemic measures was observed in people with a higher BMI.[134] These findings also corroborate a pooled analysis of four acute, randomized, experimental trials (n = 129, persons with NDH = 27.1%) examining the postprandial response (glucose and insulin) to three treatment conditions: prolonged sitting (6.5 hours) or prolonged sitting broken up with either standing or light-intensity physical activity (5 minutes every 30 minutes).[134] Reductions in postprandial insulin were modified by ethnicity, gender, and BMI. For instance, the response was more pronounced in South Asians versus White Europeans (–23.5% vs. –9.3%), females versus males (–21.2% vs. –17.6%), or those with a BMI ≥27.2 kg/m^2 (–22.9% vs. –18.2%). Glucose responses were also more pronounced in females (–6.8% vs. –1.7%) and those with a BMI ≥27.2 kg/m^2 (–6.7% vs. –3.4%).

Exploratory, post-hoc analysis of the *Stand and Move at Work* intervention, a multilevel intervention targeting reduction in sedentary time, also showed differences in the effect size, determined by glycemic status.[135] Although the intervention yielded reductions in sitting time at 12 months for the whole cohort (n = 487), the reductions in glucose, HbA_{1c}, body weight, and body fat were considerably larger and clinically meaningful in those with NDH or T2DM (n = 95).[135]

Therefore the current evidence suggests that breaking or reducing sedentary behavior is likely to be particularly important in those with NDH or associated risk factors. A reasonable goal may be to first break up sitting time with informal/light-intensity physical activity, which may also be more culturally acceptable to high-risk groups (e.g., South Asian females),[136] before progressing onto higher-intensity activities.

Weight Loss

Weight loss, whether achieved through lifestyle modification (i.e., diet and/or physical activity) and/or pharmacotherapy and/or surgery is known to enhance insulin sensitivity, reduce the workload on β-cells, and improve glucose tolerance in those with NDH. As such, given the inextricable association between T2DM and obesity, weight loss is a core aim of lifestyle prevention programs.[137,138] A 5% reduction in body weight (vs. baseline) is deemed a realistic and meaningful target, which equates to a ~30% improvement in whole-body insulin sensitivity[139] and decreases the conversion rate of NDH to T2DM by 56%.[33] Although it is true that for most outcomes a 5% weight loss is associated with benefits (and is often referred to as "clinically significant"), those who undertake and sustain physical activity combined with a healthy diet can still yield benefits below this threshold (weight loss ranging from no change to ~3%).[140] This is evidenced by the DPP, where those who achieved ~150 minutes per week of moderate-to-vigorous physical activity, but did not achieve "clinically significant weight loss," reduced their diabetes incidence by 44%.[59] Such observations are also consistent with the findings of the Finnish Diabetes Prevention Study.[141]

For those unable to attain adequate weight loss through lifestyle interventions, guidelines pertaining to obesity control also recommend pharmacological and/or surgical intervention. A number of pharmacological and surgical therapies have been shown to induce significant weight loss for persons with overweight or obesity. A few of these interventions have data supporting efficacy for prevention or delaying incident T2DM. Within this section, we discuss some of the key findings from clinical trials involving traditional (i.e., metformin) and novel (i.e., GLP-1RA and dual agonists) glucose-lowering therapies, with a particular focus on those with or at high risk of NDH.

METFORMIN

Metformin may be pivotal in diabetes prevention, as indicated by NICE prevention guidelines,[19] where benefits appear to be the strongest in adults at a higher risk of incident T2DM. For example, metformin has been shown to be more effective in younger (<60 years), obese individuals (BMI >35 kg/m^2) and in females with a history of gestational diabetes.[142,143] Metformin may also have favorable effects beyond its ability to improve insulin sensitivity (i.e., weight loss/maintenance).[144,145] The largest study to show the weight benefits of metformin in those with NDH is the DPP. As previously discussed, the metformin arm of the DPP reduced the incidence of diabetes by 31% in a 3-year period, but participants also experienced a mean weight loss of 2.1 kg.[33] Unsurprisingly, the degree of weight loss was strongly associated with adherence, where those participants displaying high levels of adherence over 2 years of follow-up demonstrated an average 3.5% reduction in body mass, compared with weight neural status in the low adherence group. Importantly, this weight loss persisted in the extended follow-up period over 10 years for the highly adherent group.[43]

The addition of metformin to a dietary intervention has also been shown to result in the maintenance of diet-induced weight loss in overweight and obese females with normoglycemia and hyperinsulinemia.[146] Results from a meta-analysis of randomized controlled trials also demonstrated that metformin does not increase body weight and may prevent weight gain from other glucose-lowering medications or induce small amounts of weight loss (−1.1 kg).[147]

However, due to the modest effects of weight loss (particularly when compared with other pharmacological options mentioned below), metformin is not approved as a weight loss agent. That said, it is frequently utilized in patients at high risk for metabolic complications and who do not tolerate other interventions. Furthermore, it can be combined with other glucose-lowering medications, including GLP-1RAs and dual agonists that may result in additional weight loss or weight maintenance.

GLP-1RA

In addition to increasing insulin secretion and synthesis, GLP-1RAs suppress glucagon secretion, slow gastric emptying, promote β-cell proliferation, and reduce food intake via the reduction of appetite and enhancement of satiety.[148] Liraglutide, a GLP-1RA, was initially approved as an adjunct therapy to diet and exercise for management of hyperglycemia of T2DM. Subsequently, its influence upon body weight has been investigated in multiple phase III and IV clinical trials. With particular relevance to diabetes prevention, The Satiety and Clinical Adiposity—Liraglutide Evidence (SCALE) Obesity and Prediabetes trial assessed the efficacy and safety of daily liraglutide injections (3mg) versus placebo injections.[149] After 56 weeks, the obesity and prediabetes cohort (n = 2487 participants; 61.2% with NDH) demonstrated 8% weight loss (vs. 2.6% in the placebo arm). Of these, 63.2% reached the clinically significant threshold for weight loss (≥5%) and 33.1% achieved ≥10%. The combination of weight loss and improved glycemic control (HbA_{1c} [−0.30%±0.28]) also likely contributed to the observed reductions in the prevalence of prediabetes (OR for NDH at 56 weeks = 0.30; 95% CI, 0.21–0.42) and the lower odds for incident T2DM (OR = 0.12; 95% CI, 0.04–0.38).[149] These promising results persisted at 3 years, where the time to onset of T2DM over 160 weeks was 2·7 times longer with liraglutide than with the placebo, yielding a HR of 0.21 (95% CI, 0.13–0.34). Liraglutide also induced greater weight loss at 160 weeks (vs. placebo) (–6.1% vs. –1.9%).[150]

Semaglutide is another example of a GLP-1RA used in the management of hyperglycemia of T2DM (1.0 or 2mg per week, via subcutaneous injection), with the capability of inducing significant weight loss, particularly when considered in the context of other available weight loss medications. For example, orlistat and the aforementioned liraglutide each induce ~4% to 8% weight reductions on average when compared with the placebo.[151] However, semaglutide more than doubles this weight loss. Indeed, findings from the Semaglutide Treatment Effect in People With Obesity (STEP) 8 trial, an open-label randomized controlled trial conducted in 338 participants, showed that after 68 weeks, those adults living with obesity achieved –15.8% weight loss with semaglutide (2.4mg, n = 126) versus 6.4% with liraglutide (3.0mg, n = 127).[152] The STEP 1 trial, a double-blind randomized controlled trial in 1961 in overweight/obese individuals, also demonstrated specific benefits in those with NDH. In those randomized to once-weekly subcutaneous semaglutide (2.4mg), 84.1% of those with NDH at baseline returned to normoglycemia after 68 weeks (vs. 47.8% in the placebo, plus lifestyle intervention arm).[153] This offers great potential for clinical improvement for those living with obesity and NDH. Table 3.4 describes the weight loss observed with semaglutide in the related phase III trials in more detail.

The benefits may also extend beyond weight loss, where the ability of 2.4mg weekly doses of semaglutide to reduce the risk of cardiovascular events in overweight/obesity (BMI = ≥27kg/m²) has recently been demonstrated in the SELECT trial. Indeed, alongside 10.2% weight loss at a 4-year follow-up (208 weeks),[157] semaglutide was also shown to be superior to placebo in reducing the incidence of death from cardiovascular causes, nonfatal myocardial infarction, or nonfatal stroke (HR: 0.80; 95% CI, 0.72–0.90) with a mean follow-up of 39.8 months.[158]

It is important to note that high-dose GLP-1RAs are only one of several promising new drug classes in development for obesity, and the results to date merely represent the start of a promising future. For instance, although

TABLE 3.4 Summary of the Semaglutide (2.4mg) Phase III Clinical Trials Applicable to NDH

TRIAL	POPULATION	CONCOMITANT LIFESTYLE THERAPY	WEIGHT LOSS AT 68 WEEKS (UNLESS OTHERWISE STATED)		PROPORTION ACHIEVING 5% WEIGHT LOSS	
			SEMAGLUTIDE (2.4mg)	PLACEBO	SEMAGLUTIDE (2.4mg)	PLACEBO
STEP 1[153]	1961 adults with BMI >30kg/m² or >27kg/m² with >1 weight-related comorbidity	Lifestyle intervention	−14.9%	−2.4%	86.4%	31.5%
STEP 3[154]	611 adults with BMI >30kg/m² or >27kg/m² with >1 weight-related comorbidity	Both groups received a low-calorie diet for 8 weeks, including behavioral therapy	−16.0%	−5.7%	86.6%	47.6%
STEP 4[155]	902 adults with BMI >30kg/m² or >27kg/m² with >1 weight-related comorbidity entered 20-week run-in Of these, 806 reached 2.4mg dose and were subsequently randomized	Lifestyle intervention	−17.4% −7.9% (from week 20)	−5.9% +6.9% (from week 20)	88.7%	47.6%
STEP 5[156]	304 adults with BMI >30kg/m² or >27kg/m² with >1 weight-related comorbidity	Both groups received a low-calorie diet and increased physical activity	−15.2% *at 104 weeks*	−2.6% *at 104 weeks*	77.1%	34.4%
STEP 8[152]	Once-weekly subcutaneous semaglutide, 2.4mg (16-week escalation; n=126), or matching placebo, or once-daily subcutaneous liraglutide, 3.0mg (4-week escalation; n=127), or matching placebo	Lifestyle intervention	Semaglutide = −15.8% Liraglutide = −6.4%	−1.9%.	Semaglutide = 87.2% Liraglutide = 58.1%	29.5%

NDH, Nondiabetic hyperglycemia.

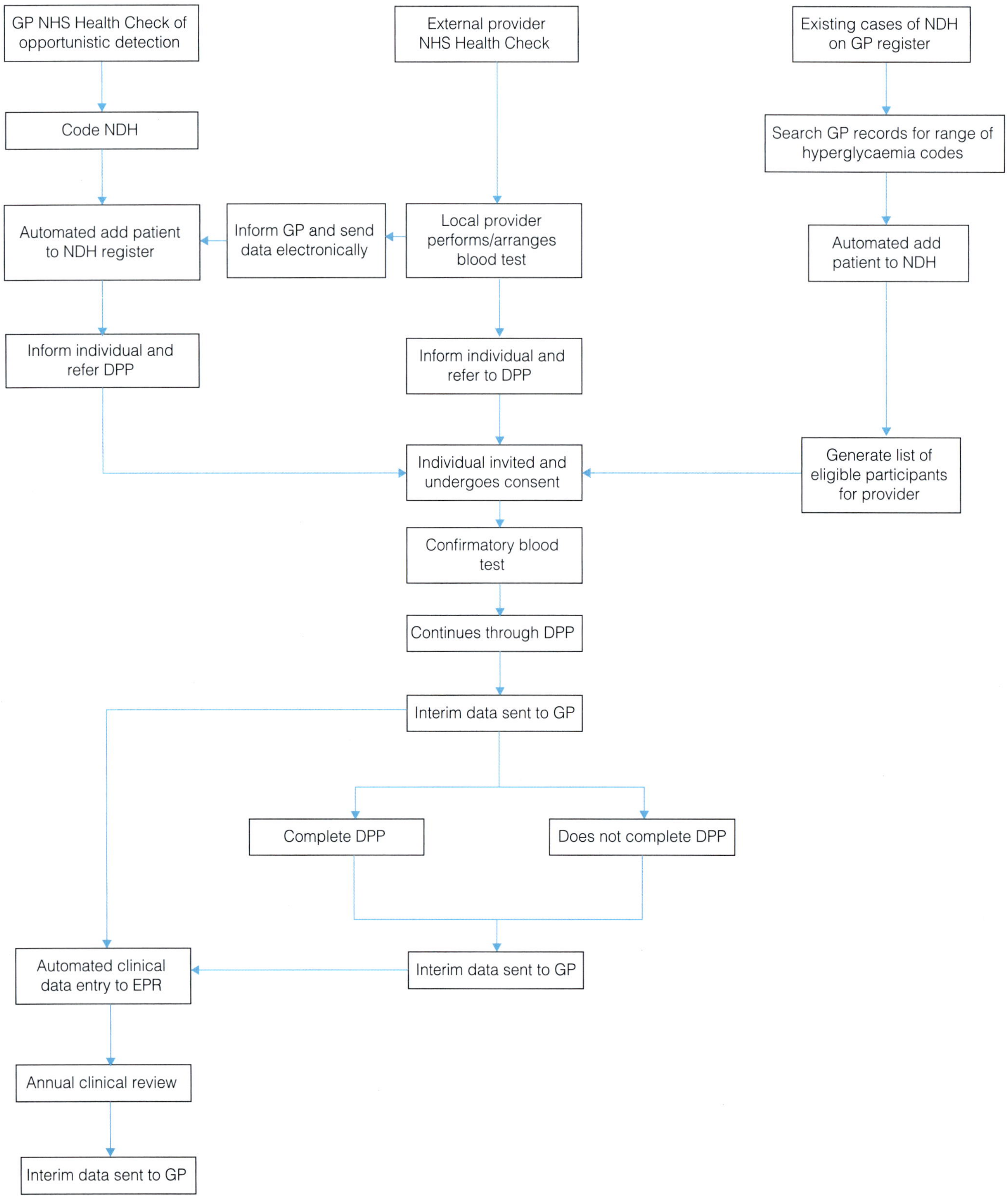

FIG. 3.4 NHS DPP referral pathway. *DPP*, Diabetes prevention program; *EPR*, electronic patient record; *NDH*, nondiabetic hyperglycemia; *NHS*, National Health Service. Adapted from NHS DPP: Primary Care Toolkit to support local implementation of the NHS DPP. https://www.england.nhs.uk/wp-content/uploads/2016/07/dpp-pc-toolkit.pdf

half again will adhere, leaving the majority and potentially those with the greatest risk of diabetes progression without meaningful benefit.

Although lifestyle interventions work for those who engage with them, they are unlikely to form a viable long-term solution to diabetes prevention by themselves. Individuals with NDH from different backgrounds and cultures may be responsive to a number of different strategies that modify the cognitive, social, and emotional processes that underpin their lifestyle behaviors. There are also a number of possible modes of intervention beyond persuasive face-to-face interaction (as mentioned previously), including modification of the physical environment and changes in food pricing or regulation and taxation. Hence, there may be considerable opportunities to further increase the efficiency and cost-effectiveness of programs to support lifestyle behavior change.

There is also a need for developing tailored diabetes prevention pathways that combine lifestyle intervention with other evidence-based therapies, such as metformin. The American Diabetes Association, the International Diabetes Federation, and the UK NICE guidelines already recommend some degree of tailoring whereby metformin can be combined with lifestyle modification if risk remains elevated or when other risk factors are present.[183,219,220] A stepwise approach to diabetes prevention was tested in the Diabetes Community and Lifestyle Improvement Program (D-CLIP), a randomized controlled trial of 578 Asian Indian adults with overweight or obesity at high risk of diabetes (defined as IFG, IGT, or both).[38] Patients in the intervention arm received a 6-month culturally tailored diabetes prevention lifestyle intervention with the stepwise addition of metformin twice daily at 4 months for those participants who were considered to still be at high risk. At 3 years, the intervention group had a relative risk reduction of 32%. The majority of the intervention participants (72%) required metformin in addition to lifestyle intervention. The intervention was found to be cost-effective.[221] The tailored combination of lifestyle therapy with metformin has yet to be integrated into national-level prevention programs.

CONCLUSION

Targeting T2DM prevention through reductions in our overall consumption of food and increased levels of physical activity (with interventions at both population level and those targeted to high-risk individuals) are currently the most viable and evidence-based methods for diabetes prevention. Indeed, a combination of low-risk behaviors (which includes a healthy diet and regular physical activity) is prospectively associated with an 80% lower risk of T2DM.[222] However, solely relying on an individual's adherence to diet and physical activity recommendations may not be enough to delay progression for a large proportion of the at-risk population. Thus, going forward, attention must also be given to pharmacological therapy or bariatric surgery to yield long-term societal benefits. The subsequent introduction of novel glucose-lowering medications (especially those with the potential for weight loss) and the national diabetes prevention programs herald an exciting time for diabetes prevention, and although real-world translation and finding ways to maximize maintenance of effects remain huge hurdles, it arguably also represents the best opportunity to stem the tide of the global T2DM pandemic.

REFERENCES

1. Sun H, Saeedi P, Karuranga S, Pinkepank M, Ogurtsova K, Duncan BB, et al. IDF Diabetes Atlas: global, regional and country-level diabetes prevalence estimates for 2021 and projections for 2045. Diabetes Res Clin Pract. 2022;183:109119.
2. International Diabetes Federation. Diabetes Atlas, 9th ed. 2019; Available from: http://www.idf.org/diabetesatlas.
3. Gassasse Z, Smith D, Finer S, Gallo V. Association between urbanisation and type 2 diabetes: an ecological study. BMJ Glob Health. 2017;2(4): e000473-000473. eCollection 2017.
4. Lin X, Xu Y, Pan X, Xu J, Ding Y, Sun X, et al. Global, regional, and national burden and trend of diabetes in 195 countries and territories: an analysis from 1990 to 2025. Sci Rep. 2020;10(1):14790. 9.
5. Collaborators G2RF. Global, regional, and national comparative risk assessment of 84 behavioural, environmental and occupational, and metabolic risks or clusters of risks for 195 countries and territories, 1990-2017: a systematic analysis for the Global Burden of Disease Study 2017. Lancet. 2018;392(10159):1923–1994.
6. United Nations. Transforming our world: the 2030 Agenda for Sustainable Development. 2021. Available from: https://sdgs.un.org/2030agenda.
7. World Health Organisation. Global action plan on physical activity 2018–2030: more active people for a healthier world. 2018. Available from: https://www.who.int/publications/i/item/9789241514187.
8. Ceriello A, Gavin 3rd JR, Boulton AJM, Blickstead R, McGill M, Raz I, et al. The Berlin Declaration: a call to action to improve early actions related to type 2 diabetes. How can specialist care help? *Diabetes Res Clin Pract.* 2018;139:392–399.
9. Khunti K, Gavin 3rd JR, Boulton AJM, Blickstead R, McGill M, Ceriello A, et al. The Berlin Declaration: a call to improve early actions related to type 2 diabetes. Why is primary care important? Primary Care Diabetes. 2018;12(5):383–392.
10. World Health Organisation. Global action plan for the prevention and control of noncommunicable diseases 2013-2020. 2013. Available from: https://apps.who.int/iris/handle/10665/94384.
11. Chan JCN, Lim LL, Wareham NJ, Shaw JE, Orchard TJ, Zhang P, et al. The Lancet Commission on Diabetes: using data to transform diabetes care and patient lives. *Lancet.* 2021;396(10267):2019–2082.
12. Hex N, Bartlett C, Wright D, Taylor M, Varley D. Estimating the current and future costs of type 1 and type 2 diabetes in the UK, including direct health costs and indirect societal and productivity costs. *Diabet Med.* 2012;29(7):855–862.
13. Keng MJ, Leal J, Bowman L, Armitage J, Mihaylova B, ASCEND Study Collaborative Group. Hospital costs associated with adverse events in people with diabetes in the UK. *Diabetes Obes Metab.* 2022;24(11):2108–2117.
14. Bommer C, Sagalova V, Heesemann E, Manne-Goehler J, Atun R, Barnighausen T, et al. Global economic burden of diabetes in adults: projections from 2015 to 2030. *Diabetes Care.* 2018;41(5):963–970.
15. Chatterton H, Younger T, Fischer A, Khunti K, Programme Development Group. Risk identification and interventions to prevent type 2 diabetes in adults at high risk: summary of NICE guidance. *BMJ.* 2012;345:e4624.
16. American Diabetes Association. Classification and diagnosis of diabetes: Standards of Medical Care in Diabetes-2021. *Diabetes Care.* 2021;44(Suppl 1): S15–S33.
17. World Health Organization. Use of glycated haemoglobin (HbA1c) in the diagnosis of diabetes mellitus. 2011. Available from: http://www.who.int/diabetes/publications/report-hba1c_2011.pdf.
18. International Diabetes Federation. Definition and diagnosis of diabetes mellitus and intermediate hyperglycaemia. 2006. Available from: https://www.idf.org/webdata/docs/WHO_IDF_definition_diagnosis_of_diabetes.pdf.
19. National Institute for Health and Care Excellence. Tpye 2 diabetes: prevention in people at high risk. 2017. Available from: https://www.nice.org.uk/guidance/ph38, 2022.
20. Davidson KW, Barry MJ, Mangione CM, Cabana M, Caughey AB, Davis EM, et al. Screening for prediabetes and type 2 diabetes: US Preventive Services Task Force recommendation statement. *JAMA.* 2021;326(8):736–743.
21. O'Brien MJ, Zhang Y, Bailey SC, Khan SS, Ackermann RT, Ali MK, et al. Screening for prediabetes and diabetes: clinical performance and implications for health equity. *Am J Prev Med.* 2023;64(6):814–823.
22. Gray LJ, Taub NA, Khunti K, Gardiner E, Hiles S, Webb DR, et al. The Leicester Risk Assessment score for detecting undiagnosed type 2 diabetes and impaired glucose regulation for use in a multiethnic UK setting. *Diabetic Med.* 2010;27(8):887–895.
23. National Health Service. Healthier You: Diabetes Prevention Programme. 2022. Available from: https://preventing-diabetes.co.uk/, 2022.
24. Rose G. Strategy of prevention: lessons from cardiovascular disease. *Br Med J (Clin Res Ed.* 1981;282(6279):1847–1851.
25. National Institute for Health and Care Excellence. Type 2 diabetes prevention: population and community-level interventions public health guideline [PH35]. 2011. Available from: https://www.nice.org.uk/guidance/ph35, 2022.

26. Allen LN, Wigley S, Holmer H, Barlow P. Non-communicable disease policy implementation from 2014 to 2021: a repeated cross-sectional analysis of global policy data for 194 countries. *Lancet Global Health*. 2023;11(4):e525–e533.
27. McGill R, Anwar E, Orton L, Bromley H, Lloyd-Williams F, O'Flaherty M, et al. Are interventions to promote healthy eating equally effective for all? Systematic review of socioeconomic inequalities in impact. *BMC Public Health*. 2015;15:457-457.
28. Mayne SL, Auchincloss AH, Michael YL. Impact of policy and built environment changes on obesity-related outcomes: a systematic review of naturally occurring experiments. *Obes Rev*. 2015;16(5):362–375.
29. Wang YC, McPherson K, Marsh T, Gortmaker SL, Brown M. Health and economic burden of the projected obesity trends in the USA and the UK. *Lancet*. 2011;378(9793):815–825.
30. Salgado MV, Penko J, Fernandez A, Konfino J, Coxson PG, Bibbins-Domingo K, et al. Projected impact of a reduction in sugar-sweetened beverage consumption on diabetes and cardiovascular disease in Argentina: a modeling study. *PLoS Med*. 2020;17(7):e1003224.
31. Fagg J, Valabhji J. How do we identify people at high risk of type 2 diabetes and help prevent the condition from developing? *Diabet Med*. 2019;36(3):316–325.
32. Gillies CL, Abrams KR, Lambert PC, Cooper NJ, Sutton AJ, Hsu RT, et al. Pharmacological and lifestyle interventions to prevent or delay type 2 diabetes in people with impaired glucose tolerance: systematic review and meta-analysis. *BMJ*. 2007;334(7588):299.
33. Knowler WC, Barrett-Connor E, Fowler SE, Hamman RF, Lachin JM, Walker EA, et al. Reduction in the incidence of type 2 diabetes with lifestyle intervention or metformin. *N Engl J Med*. 2002;346(6):393–403.
34. Lindstrom J, Louheranta A, Mannelin M, Rastas M, Salminen V, Eriksson J, et al. The Finnish Diabetes Prevention Study (DPS): lifestyle intervention and 3-year results on diet and physical activity. *Diabetes Care*. 2003;26(12):3230–3236.
35. Lindstrom J, Peltonen M, Eriksson JG, Ilanne-Parikka P, Aunola S, Keinanen-Kiukaanniemi S, et al. Improved lifestyle and decreased diabetes risk over 13 years: long-term follow-up of the randomised Finnish Diabetes Prevention Study (DPS). *Diabetologia*. 2013;56(2):284–293.
36. Rintamäki R, Rautio N, Peltonen M, Jokelainen J, Keinänen-Kiukaanniemi S, Oksa H, et al. Long-term outcomes of lifestyle intervention to prevent type 2 diabetes in people at high risk in primary health care. *Prim Care Diabetes*. 2021;15(3):444–450.
37. Ramachandran A, Snehalatha C, Mary S, Mukesh B, Bhaskar AD, Vijay V, et al. The Indian Diabetes Prevention Programme shows that lifestyle modification and metformin prevent type 2 diabetes in Asian Indian subjects with impaired glucose tolerance (IDPP-1). *Diabetologia*. 2006;49(2):289–297.
38. Weber MB, Ranjani H, Staimez LR, Anjana RM, Ali MK, Narayan KM, et al. The stepwise approach to diabetes prevention: results from the D-CLIP randomized controlled trial. *Diabetes Care*. 2016;39(10):1760–1767.
39. Pan XR, Li GW, Hu YH, Wang JX, Yang WY, An ZX, et al. Effects of diet and exercise in preventing NIDDM in people with impaired glucose tolerance. The Da Qing IGT and Diabetes Study. *Diabetes Care*. 1997;20(4):537–544.
40. Temprosa M. Diabetes Prevention Program Outcomes Study (DPPOS) (Version 6) [Dataset] NIDDK Central Repository. 2024, https://doi.org/10.58020/66x5-8y21.
41. Gong Q, Zhang P, Wang J, Ma J, An Y, Chen Y, et al. Morbidity and mortality after lifestyle intervention for people with impaired glucose tolerance: 30-year results of the Da Qing Diabetes Prevention Outcome Study. *Lancet Diabetes Endocrinol*. 2019;7(6):452–461.
42. Yamaoka K, Nemoto A, Tango T. Comparison of the effectiveness of lifestyle modification with other treatments on the incidence of type 2 diabetes in people at high risk: a network meta-analysis. *Nutrients*. 2019;11(6):1373. https://doi.org/10.3390/nu11061373.
43. Group DPPR. Long-term effects of metformin on diabetes prevention: identification of subgroups that benefited most in the Diabetes Prevention Program and Diabetes Prevention Program Outcomes Study. *Diabetes Care*. 2019;42(4):601–608.
44. Glechner A, Keuchel L, Affengruber L, Titscher V, Sommer I, Matyas N, et al. Effects of lifestyle changes on adults with prediabetes: a systematic review and meta-analysis. *Prim Care Diabetes*. 2018;12(5):393–408.
45. Haw JS, Galaviz KI, Straus AN, Kowalski AJ, Magee MJ, Weber MB, et al. Long-term sustainability of diabetes prevention approaches: a systematic review and meta-analysis of randomized clinical trials. *JAMA Intern Med*. 2017;177(12):1808–1817.
46. Goldberg RB, Orchard TJ, Crandall JP, Boyko EJ, Budoff M, Dabelea D, et al. Effects of long-term metformin and lifestyle interventions on cardiovascular events in the Diabetes Prevention Program and Its Outcome Study. *Circulation*. 2022;145(22):1632–1641.
47. Neuenschwander M, Ballon A, Weber KS, Norat T, Aune D, Schwingshackl L, et al. Role of diet in type 2 diabetes incidence: umbrella review of meta-analyses of prospective observational studies. *BMJ*. 2019;366:l2368.
48. Kopp W. How western diet and lifestyle drive the pandemic of obesity and civilization diseases. *Diabetes Metab Syndr Obes*. 2019;12:2221–2236.
49. Forouhi NG, Misra A, Mohan V, Taylor R, Yancy W. Dietary and nutritional approaches for prevention and management of type 2 diabetes. *BMJ*. 2018;361:k2234.
50. World Health Organisation. Guideline: sugars intake for adults and children. 2015.
51. Diabetes and Nutrition Study Group (DNSG) of the European Association for the Study of Diabetes (EASD). Evidence-based European recommendations for the dietary management of diabetes. *Diabetologia*. 2023;66(6): 965–985.
52. Evert AB, Dennison M, Gardner CD, Garvey WT, Lau KHK, MacLeod J, et al. Nutrition therapy for adults with diabetes or prediabetes: a consensus report. *Diabetes Care*. 2019;42(5):731–754.
53. Ley SH, Hamdy O, Mohan V, Hu FB. Prevention and management of type 2 diabetes: dietary components and nutritional strategies. *Lancet*. 2014;383(9933):1999–2007.
54. Chiavaroli L, Viguiliouk E, Nishi SK, Blanco Mejia S, Rahelić D, Kahleová H, et al. DASH dietary pattern and cardiometabolic outcomes: an umbrella review of systematic reviews and meta-analyses. *Nutrients*. 2019;11(2):338. 10.3390/nu11020338.
55. Uusitupa M, Khan TA, Viguiliouk E, Kahleova H, Rivellese AA, Hermansen K, et al. Prevention of type 2 diabetes by lifestyle changes: a systematic review and meta-analysis. *Nutrients*. 2019;11(11):2611. 10.3390/nu11112611.
56. Fung TT, Schulze M, Manson JE, Willett WC, Hu FB. Dietary patterns, meat intake, and the risk of type 2 diabetes in women. *Arch Intern Med*. 2004;164(20):2235–2240.
57. Qian F, Liu G, Hu FB, Bhupathiraju SN, Sun Q. Association between plant-based dietary patterns and risk of type 2 diabetes: a systematic review and meta-analysis. *JAMA Intern Med*. 2019;179(10):1335–1344.
58. Glenn AJ, Li J, Lo K, Jenkins DJA, Boucher BA, Hanley AJ, et al. The Portfolio diet and incident type 2 diabetes: findings from the Women's Health Initiative Prospective Cohort Study. *Diabetes Care*. 2023;46(1):28–37.
59. Hamman RF, Wing RR, Edelstein SL, Lachin JM, Bray GA, Delahanty L, et al. Effect of weight loss with lifestyle intervention on risk of diabetes. *Diabetes Care*. 2006;29(9):2102–2107.
60. Jebb SA, Lovegrove JA, Griffin BA, Frost GS, Moore CS, Chatfield MD, et al. Effect of changing the amount and type of fat and carbohydrate on insulin sensitivity and cardiovascular risk: the RISCK (Reading, Imperial, Surrey, Cambridge, and Kings) trial. *Am J Clin Nutr*. 2010;92(4):748–758.
61. Bradley U, Spence M, Courtney CH, McKinley MC, Ennis CN, McCance DR, et al. Low-fat versus low-carbohydrate weight reduction diets: effects on weight loss, insulin resistance, and cardiovascular risk: a randomized control trial. *Randomized Controlled Trial*. 2009;58(12):2741–2748.
62. Johnston BC, Kanters S, Bandayrel K, Wu P, Naji F, Siemieniuk RA, et al. Comparison of weight loss among named diet programs in overweight and obese adults: a meta-analysis. *JAMA*. 2014;312(9):923–933.
63. Caspersen CJ, Powell KE, Christenson GM. Physical activity, exercise, and physical fitness: definitions and distinctions for health-related research. *Public Health Rep*. 1985;100(2):126–131.
64. Colberg SR, Sigal RJ, Yardley JE, Riddell MC, Dunstan DW, Dempsey PC, et al. Physical activity/exercise and diabetes: a position statement of the American Diabetes Association. *Diabetes Care*. 2016;39(11):2065–2079.
65. Bull FC, Al-Ansari SS, Biddle S, Borodulin K, Buman MP, Cardon G, et al. World Health Organization 2020 guidelines on physical activity and sedentary behaviour. *Br J Sports Med*. 2020;54(24):1451–1462.
66. Garber AJ, Handelsman Y, Grunberger G, Einhorn D, Abrahamson MJ, Barzilay JI, et al. Consensus statement by the American Association of Clinical Endocrinologists and American College of Endocrinology on the comprehensive type 2 diabetes management algorithm: 2020 executive summary. *Endocr Pract*. 2020;26(1):107–139.
67. Kanaley JA, Colberg SR, Corcoran MH, Malin SK, Rodriguez NR, Crespo CJ, et al. Exercise/Physical activity in individuals with type 2 diabetes: a consensus statement from the American College of Sports Medicine. *Med Sci Sports Exerc*. 2022;54(2):353–368.
68. Davies MJ, Aroda VR, Collins BS, Gabbay RA, Green J, Maruthur NM, et al. Management of hyperglycemia in type 2 diabetes, 2022. A consensus report by the American Diabetes Association (ADA) and the European Association for the Study of Diabetes (EASD). *Diabetes Care*. 2022;45(11): 2753–2786.
69. Department of Health & Social Care. *UK Chief Medical Officers' Physical Activity Guidelines*. 2019. Available from: https://assets.publishing.service.gov.uk/government/uploads/system/uploads/attachment_data/file/832868/uk-chief-medical-officers-physical-activity-guidelines.pdf.
70. Ekelund U, Tarp J, Steene-Johannessen J, Hansen BH, Jefferis B, Fagerland MW, et al. Dose-response associations between accelerometry measured physical activity and sedentary time and all cause mortality: systematic review and harmonised meta-analysis. *BMJ*. 2019;366:l4570.
71. Wahid A, Manek N, Nichols M, Kelly P, Foster C, Webster P, et al. Quantifying the association between physical activity and cardiovascular disease and diabetes: a systematic review and meta-analysis. *J Am Heart Assoc*. 2016;5(9):e002495. https://doi.org/10.1161/JAHA.115.002495.
72. Luo M, Yu C, Del Pozo Cruz B, Chen L, Ding D. Accelerometer-measured intensity-specific physical activity, genetic risk and incident type 2 diabetes: a prospective cohort study. *Br J Sports Med*. 2023;57(19):1257–1264.
73. Rowlands AV, Edwardson CL, Davies MJ, Khunti K, Harrington DM, Yates T. Beyond cut points: accelerometer metrics that capture the physical activity profile. *Med.Sci.Sports Exerc*. 2018;50(6):1323–1332.
74. Aune D, Norat T, Leitzmann M, Tonstad S, Vatten LJ. Physical activity and the risk of type 2 diabetes: a systematic review and dose-response meta-analysis. *Eur J Epidemiol*. 2015;30(7):529–542.
75. Boule NG, Kenny GP, Haddad E, Wells GA, Sigal RJ. Meta-analysis of the effect of structured exercise training on cardiorespiratory fitness in type 2 diabetes mellitus. *Diabetologia*. 2003;46(8):1071–1081.
76. Umpierre D, Ribeiro PA, Kramer CK, Leitao CB, Zucatti AT, Azevedo MJ, et al. Physical activity advice only or structured exercise training and

association with HbA1c levels in type 2 diabetes: a systematic review and meta-analysis. *JAMA*. 2011;305(17):1790–1799.

77. Najafipour F, Mobasseri M, Yavari A, Nadrian H, Aliasgarzadeh A, Mashinchi Abbasi N, et al. Effect of regular exercise training on changes in HbA1c, BMI and VO_2max among patients with type 2 diabetes mellitus: an 8-year trial. *BMJ Open Diabetes Res Care*. 2017;5(1):e000414.
78. Hawley JA. Exercise as a therapeutic intervention for the prevention and treatment of insulin resistance. *Diabetes Metab Res Rev*. 2004;20(5): 383–393.
79. Khalafi M, Ravasi AA, Malandish A, Rosenkranz SK. The impact of high-intensity interval training on postprandial glucose and insulin: a systematic review and meta-analysis. *Diabetes Res Clin Pract*. 2022;186:109815.
80. Cavero-Redondo I, Peleteiro B, Álvarez-Bueno C, Artero EG, Garrido-Miguel M, Martinez-Vizcaíno V. The effect of physical activity interventions on glycosylated haemoglobin (HbA(1c)) in non-diabetic populations: a systematic review and meta-analysis. *Sports Med*. 2018;48(5):1151–1164.
81. Boule NG, Haddad E, Kenny GP, Wells GA, Sigal RJ. Effects of exercise on glycemic control and body mass in type 2 diabetes mellitus: a meta-analysis of controlled clinical trials. *JAMA*. 2001;286(10):1218–1227.
82. Pan B, Ge L, Xun YQ, Chen YJ, Gao CY, Han X, et al. Exercise training modalities in patients with type 2 diabetes mellitus: a systematic review and network meta-analysis. *Int J Behav Nutr Phys Act*. 2018;15(1):72–73.
83. Jelleyman C, Yates T, O'Donovan G, Gray LJ, King JA, Khunti K, et al. The effects of high-intensity interval training on glucose regulation and insulin resistance: a meta-analysis. *Obes Rev*. 2015;16(11):942–961.
84. Liubaoerjijin Y, Terada T, Fletcher K, Boule NG. Effect of aerobic exercise intensity on glycemic control in type 2 diabetes: a meta-analysis of head-to-head randomized trials. *Acta Diabetol*. 2016;53(5):769–781.
85. Garber CE, Blissmer B, Deschenes MR, Franklin BA, Lamonte MJ, Lee IM, et al. American College of Sports Medicine position stand. Quantity and quality of exercise for developing and maintaining cardiorespiratory, musculoskeletal, and neuromotor fitness in apparently healthy adults: guidance for prescribing exercise. *Med Sci Sports Exerc*. 2011;43(7):1334–1359.
86. Chudyk A, Petrella RJ. Effects of exercise on cardiovascular risk factors in type 2 diabetes: a meta-analysis. *Diabetes Care*. 2011;34(5):1228–1237.
87. Kraus WE, Powell KE, Haskell WL, Janz KF, Campbell WW, Jakicic JM, et al. Physical activity, all-cause and cardiovascular mortality, and cardiovascular disease. *Med Sci Sports Exerc*. 2019;51(6):1270–1281.
88. Yates T, Haffner SM, Schulte PJ, Thomas L, Huffman KM, Bales CW, et al. Association between change in daily ambulatory activity and cardiovascular events in people with impaired glucose tolerance (NAVIGATOR trial): a cohort analysis. *Lancet*. 2014;383(9922):1059–1066.
89. Kodama S, Tanaka S, Heianza Y, Fujihara K, Horikawa C, Shimano H, et al. Association between physical activity and risk of all-cause mortality and cardiovascular disease in patients with diabetes: a meta-analysis. *Diabetes Care*. 2013;36(2):471–479.
90. Sluik D, Buijsse B, Muckelbauer R, Kaaks R, Teucher B, Johnsen NF, et al. Physical activity and mortality in individuals with diabetes mellitus: a prospective study and meta-analysis. *Arch Intern Med*. 2012;172(17):1285–1295.
91. Piercy KL, Troiano RP, Ballard RM, Carlson SA, Fulton JE, Galuska DA, et al. The physical activity guidelines for Americans. *JAMA*. 2018;320(19):2020–2028.
92. Rowlands A, Davies M, Dempsey P, Edwardson C, Razieh C, Yates T. Wrist-worn accelerometers: recommending ~1.0 mg as the minimum clinically important difference (MCID) in daily average acceleration for inactive adults. *Br J Sports Med*. 2021;55(14):814–815.
93. Chudasama YV, Khunti KK, Zaccardi F, Rowlands AV, Yates T, Gillies CL, et al. Physical activity, multimorbidity, and life expectancy: a UK Biobank longitudinal study. *BMC Med*. 2019;17(1): 108-0.
94. Yates T, Haffner SM, Schulte PJ, Thomas L, Huffman KM, Bales CW, et al. Association between change in daily ambulatory activity and cardiovascular events in people with impaired glucose tolerance (NAVIGATOR trial): a cohort analysis. *Lancet*. 2014;383(9922):1059–1066.
95. Saint-Maurice PF, Troiano RP, Bassett DR, Jr, Graubard BI, Carlson SA, Shiroma EJ, et al. Association of daily step count and step intensity with mortality among US adults. *JAMA*. 2020;323(12):1151–1160.
96. Lee IM, Shiroma EJ, Kamada M, Bassett DR, Matthews CE, Buring JE. Association of step volume and intensity with all-cause mortality in older women. *JAMA Intern Med*. 2019;179(8):1105–1112.
97. Sheng M, Yang J, Bao M, Chen T, Cai R, Zhang N, et al. The relationships between step count and all-cause mortality and cardiovascular events: a dose-response meta-analysis. *J Sport Health Sci*. 2021;10(6):620–628.
98. Ponsonby AL, Sun C, Ukoumunne OC, Pezic A, Venn A, Shaw JE, et al. Objectively measured physical activity and the subsequent risk of incident dysglycemia: the Australian Diabetes, Obesity and Lifestyle Study (AusDiab). *Diabetes Care*. 2011;34(7):1497–1502.
99. Huffman KM, Sun JL, Thomas L, Bales CW, Califf RM, Yates T, et al. Impact of baseline physical activity and diet behavior on metabolic syndrome in a pharmaceutical trial: results from NAVIGATOR. *Metabolism*. 2014;63(4):554–561.
100. Kraus WE, Yates T, Tuomilehto J, Sun JL, Thomas L, McMurray JJV, et al. Relationship between baseline physical activity assessed by pedometer count and new-onset diabetes in the NAVIGATOR trial. *BMJ Open Diabetes Res Care*. 2018;6(1):e000523.
101. Boonpor J, Ho FK, Gray SR, Celis-Morales CA. Association of self-reported walking pace with type 2 diabetes incidence in the UK Biobank Prospective Cohort Study. *Mayo Clin Proc*. 2022;97(9):1631–1640.
102. Boonpor J, Parra-Soto S, Gore J, Talebi A, Lynskey N, Raisi A, et al. Association between walking pace and incident type 2 diabetes by adiposity level: A prospective cohort study from the UK Biobank. *Diabetes Obes Metab*. 2023;25(7):1900–1910.
103. Hodkinson A, Kontopantelis E, Adeniji C, van Marwijk H, McMillian B, Bower P, et al. Interventions using wearable physical activity trackers among adults with cardiometabolic conditions: a systematic review and meta-analysis. *JAMA Netw Open*. 2021;4(7):e2116382.
104. Magkos F, Fraterrigo G, Yoshino J, Luecking C, Kirbach K, Kelly SC, et al. Effects of moderate and subsequent progressive weight loss on metabolic function and adipose tissue biology in humans with obesity. *Cell Metab*. 2016;23(4):591–601.
105. Villareal DT, Chode S, Parimi N, Sinacore DR, Hilton T, Armamento-Villareal R, et al. Weight loss, exercise, or both and physical function in obese older adults. *N Engl J Med*. 2011;364(13):1218–1229.
106. Villareal DT, Aguirre L, Gurney AB, Waters DL, Sinacore DR, Colombo E, et al. Aerobic or resistance exercise, or both, in dieting obese older adults. *N Engl J Med*. 2017;376(20):1943–1955.
107. Weiss EP, Racette SB, Villareal DT, Fontana L, Steger-May K, Schechtman KB, et al. Lower extremity muscle size and strength and aerobic capacity decrease with caloric restriction but not with exercise-induced weight loss. *J Appl Physiol*. 2007;102(2):634–640.
108. Frimel TN, Sinacore DR, Villareal DT. Exercise attenuates the weight-loss-induced reduction in muscle mass in frail obese older adults. *Med Sci Sports Exerc*. 2008;40(7):1213–1219.
109. Yates T, Henson J, Sargeant J, King J, Ahmad E, Zaccardi F, et al. Exercise, pharmaceutical therapies and type 2 diabetes: looking beyond glycemic control to whole body health and function. *Transl Med Exerc Prescr*. 2021;1(1):33–42.
110. Reid KF, Fielding RA. Skeletal muscle power: a critical determinant of physical functioning in older adults. *Exerc Sport Sci Rev*. 2012;40(1):4–12.
111. Lundell LS, Massart J, Altintas A, Krook A, Zierath JR. Regulation of glucose uptake and inflammation markers by FOXO1 and FOXO3 in skeletal muscle. *Mol Metab*. 2019;20:79–88.
112. Sharma B, Dabur R. Role of pro-inflammatory cytokines in regulation of skeletal muscle metabolism: a systematic review. *Curr Med Chem*. 2020;27(13):2161–2188.
113. Wu H, Ballantyne CM. Skeletal muscle inflammation and insulin resistance in obesity. *J Clin Invest*. 2017;127(1):43–54.
114. Sayer AA, Dennison EM, Syddall HE, Gilbody HJ, Phillips DI, Cooper C. Type 2 diabetes, muscle strength, and impaired physical function: the tip of the iceberg? *Diabetes Care*. 2005;28(10):2541–2542.
115. Delmonico MJ, Harris TB, Visser M, Park SW, Conroy MB, Velasquez-Mieyer P, et al. Longitudinal study of muscle strength, quality, and adipose tissue infiltration. *Am J Clin Nutr*. 2009;90(6):1579–1585.
116. Park SW, Goodpaster BH, Strotmeyer ES, de Rekeneire N, Harris TB, Schwartz AV, et al. Decreased muscle strength and quality in older adults with type 2 diabetes the health, aging, and body composition study. *Diabetes*. 2006;55(6):1813–1818.
117. Tremblay MS, Aubert S, Barnes JD, Saunders TJ, Carson V, Latimer-Cheung AE, et al. Sedentary Behavior Research Network (SBRN) - Terminology Consensus Project process and outcome. *Int J Behav Nutr Phys Act*. 2017;14(1):75–78.
118. Ainsworth BE, Haskell WL, Whitt MC, Irwin ML, Swartz AM, Strath SJ, et al. Compendium of physical activities: an update of activity codes and MET intensities. *Med Sci Sports Exerc*. 2000;32(9 Suppl):498.
119. Edwardson CL, Gorely T, Davies MJ, Gray LJ, Khunti K, Wilmot EG, et al. Association of sedentary behaviour with metabolic syndrome: a meta-analysis. *PLoS One*. 2012;7(4):e34916.
120. Wilmot EG, Edwardson CL, Achana FA, Davies MJ, Gorely T, Gray LJ, et al. Sedentary time in adults and the association with diabetes, cardiovascular disease and death: systematic review and meta-analysis. *Diabetologia*. 2012;55(11):2895–2905.
121. Biswas A, Oh PI, Faulkner GE, Bajaj RR, Silver MA, Mitchell MS, et al. Sedentary time and its association with risk for disease incidence, mortality, and hospitalization in adults: a systematic review and meta-analysis. *Ann Intern Med*. 2015;162(2):123–132.
122. Grontved A, Hu FB. Television viewing and risk of type 2 diabetes, cardiovascular disease, and all-cause mortality: a meta-analysis. *JAMA*. 2011;305(23):2448–2455.
123. Patterson, et al.McNamara R, Tainio E, de Sa M, Smith TH, Sharp SJ AD, et al. Sedentary behaviour and risk of all-cause, cardiovascular and cancer mortality, and incident type 2 diabetes: a systematic review and dose response meta-analysis. *Eur J Epidemiol*. 2018;33(9):811–829.
124. Guo C, Zhou Q, Zhang D, Qin P, Li Q, Tian G, et al. Association of total sedentary behaviour and television viewing with risk of overweight/obesity, type 2 diabetes and hypertension: a dose-response meta-analysis. *Diabetes Obes Metab*. 2020;22(1):79–90.
125. Bailey DP, Hewson DJ, Champion RB, Sayegh SM. Sitting time and risk of cardiovascular disease and diabetes: a systematic review and meta-analysis. *Am J Prev Med*. 2019;57(3):408–416.
126. Henson J, Davies MJ, Bodicoat DH, Edwardson CL, Gill JM, Stensel DJ, et al. Breaking up prolonged sitting with standing or walking attenuates the postprandial metabolic response in postmenopausal women: a randomized acute study. *Diabetes Care*. 2016;39(1):130–138.
127. McCarthy M, Edwardson CL, Davies MJ, Henson J, Rowlands A, King J, et al. Breaking up sedentary time with seated upper body activity can regulate metabolic health in obese high risk adults: a randomised crossover trial. *Diabetes Obes Metab*. 2017;19(12):1732–1739.
128. Yates T, Edwardson CL, Celis-Morales C, Biddle SJH, Bodicoat D, Davies MJ, et al. Metabolic effects of breaking prolonged sitting with standing or light

walking in older South Asians and White Europeans: a randomized acute study. *J Gerontol A Biol Sci Med Sci*. 2018;75(1):139–146.

129. Dempsey PC, Larsen RN, Sethi P, Sacre JW, Straznicky NE, Cohen ND, et al. Benefits for type 2 diabetes of interrupting prolonged sitting with brief bouts of light walking or simple resistance activities. *Diabetes Care*. 2016;39(6):964–972.
130. Dunstan DW, Kingwell BA, Larsen R, Healy GN, Cerin E, Hamilton MT, et al. Breaking up prolonged sitting reduces postprandial glucose and insulin responses. *Diabetes Care*. 2012;35(5):976–983.
131. Buffey AJ, Herring MP, Langley CK, Donnelly AE, Carson BP. The acute effects of interrupting prolonged sitting time in adults with standing and light-intensity walking on biomarkers of cardiometabolic health in adults: a systematic review and meta-analysis. *Sports Med*. 2022;52(8):1765–1778.
132. Chastin SFM, De Craemer M, De Cocker K, Powell L, Van Cauwenberg J, Dall P, et al. How does light-intensity physical activity associate with adult cardiometabolic health and mortality? Systematic review with meta-analysis of experimental and observational studies. *Br J Sports Med*. 2018;53(6):370–376.
133. Loh R, Stamatakis E, Folkerts D, Allgrove JE, Moir HJ. Effects of interrupting prolonged sitting with physical activity breaks on blood glucose, insulin and triacylglycerol measures: a systematic review and meta-analysis. *Sports Med*. 2020;50(2):295–330.
134. Henson J, Edwardson CL, Celis-Morales CA, Davies MJ, Dunstan DW, Esliger DW, et al. Predictors of the acute postprandial response to breaking up prolonged sitting. *Med Sci Sports Exerc*. 2020;52(6):1385–1393.
135. Pereira MA, Mullane SL, Toledo MJL, Larouche ML, Rydell SA, Vuong B, et al. Efficacy of the 'stand and move at work' multicomponent workplace intervention to reduce sedentary time and improve cardiometabolic risk: a group randomized clinical trial. *Int J Behav Nutr Phys Act*. 2020;17(1):133.
136. Lucas A, Murray E, Kinra S. Heath beliefs of UK South Asians related to lifestyle diseases: a review of qualitative literature. *J Obes*. 2013;2013:827674.
137. McCarthy MI. Genomics, type 2 diabetes, and obesity. *N Engl J Med*. 2010;363(24):2339–2350.
138. Smyth S, Heron A. Diabetes and obesity: the twin epidemics. *Nat Med*. 2006;12(1):75–80.
139. Kitabchi AE, Temprosa M, Knowler WC, Kahn SE, Fowler SE, Haffner SM, et al. Role of insulin secretion and sensitivity in the evolution of type 2 diabetes in the diabetes prevention program. Effects of lifestyle intervention and metformin. *Diabetes*. 2005;54(8):2404–2414.
140. Ross R, Bradshaw AJ. The future of obesity reduction: beyond weight loss. *Nat Rev Endocrinol*. 2009;5(6):319–325.
141. Laaksonen DE, Lindstrom J, Lakka TA, Eriksson JG, Niskanen L, Wikstrom K, et al. Physical activity in the prevention of type 2 diabetes: the Finnish diabetes prevention study. *Diabetes*. 2005;54(1):158–165.
142. Aroda VR, Knowler WC, Crandall JP, Perreault L, Edelstein SL, Jeffries SL, et al. Metformin for diabetes prevention: insights gained from the Diabetes Prevention Program/Diabetes Prevention Program Outcomes Study. *Diabetologia*. 2017;60(9):1601–1611.
143. American Diabetes Association 9. Pharmacologic approaches to glycemic treatment: Standards of Medical Care in Diabetes-2021. *Diabetes Care*. 2021;44(Suppl 1):S111–S124.
144. Golay A. Metformin and body weight. *Int J Obes*. 2008;32(1):61–72.
145. Yerevanian A, Soukas AA. Metformin: mechanisms in human obesity and weight loss. *Curr Obes Rep*. 2019;8(2):156–164.
146. Mogul H, Freeman R, Nguyen K. Metformin-sustained weight loss and reduced android fat tissue at 12 months in EMPOWIR (enhance the metabolic profile of women with insulin resistance): a double blind, placebo-controlled, randomized trial of normoglycemic women with midlife weight gain. *Endocr Pract*. 2016;22(5):575–586.
147. Domecq JP, Prutsky G, Leppin A, Sonbol MB, Altayar O, Undavalli C, et al. Clinical review: drugs commonly associated with weight change: a systematic review and meta-analysis. *J Clin Endocrinol Metab*. 2015;100(2): 363–370.
148. Drucker DJ. Mechanisms of action and therapeutic application of glucagon-like peptide-1. *Cell Metab*. 2018;27(4):740–756.
149. Pi-Sunyer X, Astrup A, Fujioka K, Greenway F, Halpern A, Krempf M, et al. A randomized, controlled trial of 3.0 mg of liraglutide in weight management. *N Engl J Med*. 2015 Jul 2;373(1):11–22.
150. le Roux CW, Astrup A, Fujioka K, Greenway F, Lau DC, Van Gaal L, et al. 3 years of liraglutide versus placebo for type 2 diabetes risk reduction and weight management in individuals with prediabetes: a randomised, double-blind trial. *Lancet*. 2017;389(10007):1399–1409.
151. Pilitsi E, Farr OM, Polyzos SA, Perakakis N, Nolen-Doerr E, Papathanasiou AE, et al. Pharmacotherapy of obesity: available medications and drugs under investigation. 2019;92:170–192.
152. Rubino DM, Greenway FL, Khalid U, O'Neil PM, Rosenstock J, Sørrig R, et al. Effect of weekly subcutaneous semaglutide vs daily liraglutide on body weight in adults with overweight or obesity without diabetes: the step 8 randomized clinical trial. *JAMA*. 2022;327(2):138–150.
153. Wilding JPH, Batterham RL, Calanna S, Davies M, Gaal LFV, Lingvay I, et al. Once-weekly semaglutide in adults with overweight or obesity. *N Engl J Med*. 2021;384(11):989–1002.
154. Wadden TA, Bailey TS, Billings LK, Davies M, Frias JP, Koroleva A, et al. Effect of subcutaneous semaglutide vs placebo as an adjunct to intensive behavioral therapy on body weight in adults with overweight or obesity: the step 3 randomized clinical trial. *JAMA*. 2021;325(14):1403–1413.
155. Rubino D, Abrahamsson N, Davies M, Hesse D, Greenway FL, Jensen C, et al. Effect of continued weekly subcutaneous semaglutide vs placebo on weight loss maintenance in adults with overweight or obesity: the step 4 randomized clinical trial. *JAMA*. 2021;325(14):1414–1425.
156. Garvey WT, Batterham R, Bhatta M, Buscemi S, Christensen L, Frias J, et al. Two-year effect of semaglutide 2.4 mg vs Placebo in adults with overweight or obesity. STEP 5. *Canadian J Diabetes*. 2021;29:43.
157. Ryan DH, Lingvay I, Deanfield J, Kahn SE, Barros E, Burguera B, et al. Long-term weight loss effects of semaglutide in obesity without diabetes in the SELECT trial. *Nat Med*. 2024;30(7):2049–2057.
158. Lincoff AM, Brown-Frandsen K, Colhoun HM, Deanfield J, Emerson SS, Esbjerg S, et al. Semaglutide and cardiovascular outcomes in obesity without diabetes. *N Engl J Med*. 2023;389(24):2221–2232.
159. Jastreboff AM, Aronne LJ, Ahmad NN, Wharton S, Connery L, Alves B, et al. Tirzepatide once weekly for the treatment of obesity. *N Engl J Med*. 2022; 387(3):205–216.
160. Wilson JM, Nikooienejad A, Robins DA, Roell WC, Riesmeyer JS, Haupt A, et al. The dual glucose-dependent insulinotropic peptide and glucagon-like peptide-1 receptor agonist, tirzepatide, improves lipoprotein biomarkers associated with insulin resistance and cardiovascular risk in patients with type 2 diabetes. *Diabetes Obes Metab*. 2020;22(12):2451–2459.
161. Melson E, Ashraf U, Papamargaritis D, Davies MJ. What is the pipeline for future medications for obesity? *Int J Obes*. 2024;49(3):433–451.
162. Jastreboff AM, Kaplan LM, Frías JP, Wu Q, Du Y, Gurbuz S, et al. Triple-hormone-receptor agonist retatrutide for obesity: a phase 2 trial. *N Engl J Med*. 2023;389(6):514–526.
163. Carlsson LM, Peltonen M, Ahlin S, Anveden A, Bouchard C, Carlsson B, et al. Bariatric surgery and prevention of type 2 diabetes in Swedish obese subjects. *N Engl J Med*. 2012;367(8):695–704.
164. Pontiroli AE, Zakaria AS, Fanchini M, Osio C, Tagliabue E, Micheletto G, et al. A 23-year study of mortality and development of co-morbidities in patients with obesity undergoing bariatric surgery (laparoscopic gastric banding) in comparison with medical treatment of obesity. *Cardiovasc Diabetol*. 2018;17(1):161.
165. Bradley D, Magkos F, Klein S. Effects of bariatric surgery on glucose homeostasis and type 2 diabetes. *Gastroenterology*. 2012;143(4):897–912.
166. Venditti EM, Kramer MK. Diabetes Prevention Program community outreach: perspectives on lifestyle training and translation. *Am J Prev Med*. 2013;44(4 Suppl 4):339.
167. Davies MJ, Gray LJ, Troughton J, Gray A, Tuomilehto J, Farooqi A, et al. A community based primary prevention programme for type 2 diabetes integrating identification and lifestyle intervention for prevention: the let's prevent diabetes cluster randomised controlled trial. *Prev Med*. 2016;84:48–56.
168. Albright AL, Gregg EW. Preventing type 2 diabetes in communities across the U.S.: the National Diabetes Prevention Program. *Am J Prev Med*. 2013;44(4):346.
169. DiBenedetto JC, Blum NM, O'Brian CA, Kolb LE, Lipman RD. Achievement of weight loss and other requirements of the Diabetes Prevention and Recognition Program: a National Diabetes Prevention Program Network Based on Nationally Certified Diabetes Self-management Education Programs. *Diabetes Educ*. 2016 Dec;42(6):678–685.
170. Hawkes RE, Cameron E, Bower P, French DP. Does the design of the NHS Diabetes Prevention Programme intervention have fidelity to the programme specification? A document analysis. *Diabet Med*. 2020;37(8):1357–1366.
171. Diabetes Prevention Program (DPP) Research Group. The Diabetes Prevention Program (DPP): description of lifestyle intervention. *Diabetes Care*. 2002;25(12):2165–2171.
172. Uusitupa M, Louheranta A, Lindström J, Valle T, Sundvall J, Eriksson J, et al. The Finnish Diabetes Prevention Study. *Br J Nutr*. 2000;83(Suppl 1):137.
173. Aziz Z, Absetz P, Oldroyd J, Pronk NP, Oldenburg B. A systematic review of real-world diabetes prevention programs: learnings from the last 15 years. *Implement Sci*. 2015;10:172–176.
174. Johnson M, Jones R, Freeman C, Woods HB, Gillett M, Goyder E, et al. Can diabetes prevention programmes be translated effectively into real-world settings and still deliver improved outcomes? *A synthesis of evidence*. 2013;30(1):3–15.
175. Khunti K, Griffin S, Brennan A, Dallosso H, Davies MJ, Eborall HC, et al. Promoting physical activity in a multi-ethnic population at high risk of diabetes: the 48-month PROPELS randomised controlled trial. *BMC Med*. 2021;19(1):130–134.
176. Toro-Ramos T, Michaelides A, Anton M, Karim Z, Kang-Oh L, Argyrou C, et al. Mobile Delivery of the Diabetes Prevention Program in people with prediabetes: randomized controlled trial. *JMIR Mhealth Uhealth*. 2020;8(7):e17842.
177. Valabhji J, Barron E, Bradley D, Bakhai C, Khunti K, Jebb S. Effect of the COVID-19 pandemic on body weight in people at high risk of type 2 diabetes referred to the English NHS Diabetes Prevention Programme. *Lancet Diabetes Endocrinol*. 2021;9(10):649–651.
178. Baskerville R, Ricci-Cabello I, Roberts N, Farmer A. Impact of accelerometer and pedometer use on physical activity and glycaemic control in people with Type 2 diabetes: a systematic review and meta-analysis. *Diabet Med*. 2017;34(5):612–620.
179. Hodkinson A, Kontopantelis E, Adeniji C, Marwijk HV, McMillian B, Bower P, et al. Interventions using wearable physical activity trackers among adults with cardiometabolic conditions: a systematic review and meta-analysis. *JAMA Netw Open*. 2021 1;4(7):e2116382.
180. Hawkes RE, Cameron E, Miles LM, French DP. The fidelity of training in behaviour change techniques to intervention design in a National Diabetes Prevention Programme. *Int J Behav Med*. 2021;28(6):671–682.

181. Schwarz PEH, Timpel P, Harst L, Greaves CJ, Ali MK, Lambert J, et al. Blood sugar regulation for cardiovascular health promotion and disease prevention: JACC Health Promotion Series. *J Am Coll Cardiol*. 2018;72(15): 1829–1844.
182. Greaves CJ, Sheppard KE, Abraham C, Hardeman W, Roden M, Evans PH, et al. Systematic review of reviews of intervention components associated with increased effectiveness in dietary and physical activity interventions. *BMC Public Health*. 2011;11:119-119.
183. National Institute for Health and Care Excellence. Preventing type 2 diabetes: risk identification and interventions for individuals at high risk. 2012. Available from: https://www.nice.org.uk/guidance/ph38.
184. The National Institute for Health and Care Excellence (NICE). Type 2 diabetes prevention: population and community-level interventions. Public Health Guideline [PH35]. 2011. Available from: https://www.nice.org.uk/guidance/ph35/chapter/1-Recommendations
185. Valabhji J, Barron E, Bradley D, Bakhai C, Fagg J, O'Neill S, et al. Early outcomes from the English National Health Service Diabetes Prevention Programme. *Diabetes Care*. 2020;43(1):152–160.
186. Ely EK, Gruss SM, Luman ET, Gregg EW, Ali MK, Nhim K, et al. A national effort to prevent type 2 diabetes: participant-level evaluation of CDC's National Diabetes Prevention Program. *Diabetes Care*. 2017;40(10):1331–1341.
187. Dunkley AJ, Bodicoat DH, Greaves CJ, Russell C, Yates T, Davies MJ, et al. Diabetes prevention in the real world: effectiveness of pragmatic lifestyle interventions for the prevention of type 2 diabetes and of the impact of adherence to guideline recommendations: a systematic review and meta-analysis. *Diabetes Care*. 2014;37(4):922–933.
188. Galaviz KI, Weber MB, Straus A, Haw JS, Narayan KMV, Ali MK. Global Diabetes prevention interventions: a systematic review and network meta-analysis of the real-world impact on incidence, weight, and glucose. *Diabetes Care*. 2018;41(7):1526–1534.
189. Public Health England. A systematic review and meta-analysis assessing the effectiveness of pragmatic lifestyle interventions for the prevention of type 2 diabetes mellitus in routine practice. 2015. Available from: https://assets.publishing.service.gov.uk/media/5b6c484ae5274a2967e4cfc0/PHE_Evidence_Review_of_diabetes_prevention_programmes-_FINAL.pdf.
190. Shirinzadeh M, Afshin-Pour B, Angeles R, Gaber J, Agarwal G. The effect of community-based programs on diabetes prevention in low- and middle-income countries: a systematic review and meta-analysis. *Global Health*. 2019;15(1):10–14.
191. Staite E, Bayley A, Al-Ozairi E, Stewart K, Hopkins D, Rundle J, et al. A wearable technology delivering a Web-Based Diabetes Prevention Program to people at high risk of type 2 diabetes: randomized controlled trial. *JMIR Mhealth Uhealth*. 2020;8(7):e15448.
192. Sampson M, Clark A, Bachmann M, Garner N, Irvine L, Howe A, et al. Effects of the Norfolk diabetes prevention lifestyle intervention (NDPS) on glycaemic control in screen-detected type 2 diabetes: a randomised controlled trial. *BMC Med*. 2021;19(1):183.
193. Yates T, Edwardson CL, Henson J, Gray LJ, Ashra NB, Troughton J, et al. Walking Away from Type 2 diabetes: a cluster randomized controlled trial. *Diabet Med*. 2017;34(5):698–707.
194. Carraça E, Encantado J, Battista F, Beaulieu K, Blundell J, Busetto L, et al. Effective behavior change techniques to promote physical activity in adults with overweight or obesity: a systematic review and meta-analysis. *Obes Rev*. 2021;22(Suppl 4):e13258.
195. Gray LJ, Yates T, Troughton J, Khunti K, Davies MJ. Team LPD. Engagement, Retention, and Progression to Type 2 Diabetes: A Retrospective Analysis of the Cluster-Randomised Let's. *Prevent Diabetes Trial*. 2016 Jul 12;13(7):e1002078.
196. Greaves C, Poltawski L, Garside R, Briscoe S. Understanding the challenge of weight loss maintenance: a systematic review and synthesis of qualitative research on weight loss maintenance. *Health.Psychol.Rev*. 2017;11(2):145–163.
197. Gokal K, Amos-Hirst R, Moakes CA, Sanders JP, Esliger DW, Sherar LB, et al. Views of the public about Snacktivity™: a small changes approach to promoting physical activity and reducing sedentary behaviour. *BMC Public Health*. 2022;22(1):618.
198. Hartmann-Boyce J, Theodoulou A, Oke JL, Butler AR, Scarborough P, Bastounis A, et al. Association between characteristics of behavioural weight loss programmes and weight change after programme end: systematic review and meta-analysis. *BMJ*. 2021;374:n1840.
199. Sampson M, Clark A, Bachmann M, Garner N, Irvine L, Howe A, et al. Lifestyle intervention with or without lay volunteers to prevent type 2 diabetes in people with impaired fasting glucose and/or nondiabetic hyperglycemia: a randomized clinical trial. *JAMA Intern Med*. 2021;181(2):168–178.
200. Roberts S, Craig D, Adler A, McPherson K, Greenhalgh T. Economic evaluation of type 2 diabetes prevention programmes: Markov model of low- and high-intensity lifestyle programmes and metformin in participants with different categories of intermediate hyperglycaemia. *BMC Med*. 2018;16(1):16–14.
201. Gillies CL, Lambert PC, Abrams KR, Sutton AJ, Cooper NJ, Hsu RT, et al. Different strategies for screening and prevention of type 2 diabetes in adults: cost effectiveness analysis. *BMJ*. 2008;336(7654):1180–1185.
202. Leal J, Ahrabian D, Davies MJ, Gray LJ, Khunti K, Yates T, et al. Cost-effectiveness of a pragmatic structured education intervention for the prevention of type 2 diabetes: economic evaluation of data from the Let's Prevent Diabetes cluster-randomised controlled trial. *BMJ Open*. 2017;7(1):13592.
203. Zhuo X, Zhang P, Barker L, Albright A, Thompson TJ, Gregg E. The lifetime cost of diabetes and its implications for diabetes prevention. *Diabetes Care*. 2014;37(9):2557–2564.
204. Alva ML, Gray A, Mihaylova B, Leal J, Holman RR. The impact of diabetes-related complications on healthcare costs: new results from the UKPDS (UKPDS 84). *Diabet.Med*. 2015;32(4):459–466.
205. Jönsson B, Board CA. Revealing the cost of type II diabetes in Europe. *Diabetologia*. 2002; 45(7):5.
206. NHS England. NHS Diabetes Prevention Programme (NHS DPP). 2020. Available from: https://www.england.nhs.uk/diabetes/diabetes-prevention/, 2021.
207. NHS England. National Diabetes Audit: Non-Diabetic Hyperglycaemia, Diabetes Prevention Programme. 2023. Available from: https://digital.nhs.uk/data-and-information/publications/statistical/national-diabetes-audit-ndh-dpp/ndh-dpp-2021-22-detailed-analysis/diabetes-prevention-programme#chapter-index.
208. Ravindrarajah R, Sutton M, Reeves D, Cotterill S, Mcmanus E, Meacock R, et al. Referral to the NHS Diabetes Prevention Programme and conversion from nondiabetic hyperglycaemia to type 2 diabetes mellitus in England: A matched cohort analysis. *PLoS Med*. 2023;20(2):e1004177.
209. Centers for Disease Control and Prevention. National Diabetes Prevention Program. 2021. Available from: https://www.cdc.gov/diabetes/prevention/index.html.
210. Ross LW, Bana F, Blacher RJ, McDivitt J, Petty J, Beckner J, et al. Continuous stakeholder engagement: expanding the role of pharmacists in prevention of type 2 diabetes through the national diabetes prevention program. *Prev Chronic Dis*. 2020;17:E41.
211. Cannon MJ, Ng BP, Lloyd K, Reynolds J, Ely EK. Delivering the National Diabetes Prevention Program: Assessment of Enrollment in In-Person and Virtual Organizations. *J Diabetes Res*. 2022;2022:2942918.
212. Moin T, Damschroder LJ, AuYoung M, Maciejewski ML, Havens K, Ertl K, et al. Results from a trial of an online Diabetes Prevention Program Intervention. *Am J Prev Med*. 2018;55(5):583–591.
213. Van Rhoon L, Byrne M, Morrissey E, Murphy J, McSharry J. A systematic review of the behaviour change techniques and digital features in technology-driven type 2 diabetes prevention interventions. *Digit Health*. 2020;6:2055207620914427.
214. Bower P, Soiland-Reyes C, Heller S, Wilson P, Cotterill S, French D, et al. Diabetes prevention at scale: narrative review of findings and lessons from the DIPLOMA evaluation of the NHS Diabetes Prevention Programme in England. *Diabet.Med*. 2023;40(11):e15209.
215. Dunbar JA, Jayawardena A, Johnson G, Roger K, Timoshanko A, Versace VL, et al. Scaling up diabetes prevention in Victoria, Australia: policy development, implementation, and evaluation. *Diabetes Care*. 2014;37(4): 934–942.
216. Hardcastle SJ, Fortier M, Blake N, Hagger MS. Identifying content-based and relational techniques to change behaviour in motivational interviewing. *Health Psychol Rev*. 2017;11(1):1–16.
217. Ogden J. Celebrating variability and a call to limit systematisation: the example of the behaviour change technique taxonomy and the behaviour change wheel. *Health Psychol Rev*. 2016;10(3):245–250.
218. Devereux-Fitzgerald A, Powell R, Dewhurst A, French DP. The acceptability of physical activity interventions to older adults: a systematic review and meta-synthesis. *Soc Sci Med*. 2016;158:14–23.
219. Alberti KG, Zimmet P, Shaw J. International Diabetes Federation: a consensus on Type 2 diabetes prevention. *Diabet Med*. 2007;24(5):451–463.
220. Association AD. 5. Prevention or delay of type 2 diabetes. *Diabetes Care*. 2017;40(Suppl 1):S44–S47.
221. Islek D, Weber MB, Ranjit Mohan A, Mohan V, Staimez LR, Harish R, et al. Cost-effectiveness of a stepwise approach vs standard care for diabetes prevention in India. *JAMA Netw Open*. 2020;3(7):e207539.
222. Khan TA, Field D, Chen V, Ahmad S, Mejia SB, Kahleová H, et al. Combination of multiple low-risk lifestyle behaviors and incident type 2 diabetes: a systematic review and dose-response meta-analysis of prospective cohort studies. *Diabetes Care*. 2023;46(3):643–656.

4 Pharmacological and Surgical Interventions That Prevent or Remit Type 2 Diabetes

IAN J. NEELAND AND REVITAL L. GORODESKI-BASKIN

INTRODUCTION

Type 2 diabetes (T2D) is a multisystem disorder characterized by systemic insulin resistance and inadequate insulin secretion by pancreatic β-cells, leading to fasting and postprandial hyperglycemia. In turn, metabolic disarray activates the sympathetic nervous and renin-angiotensin-aldosterone systems leading to vascular complications in both the micro- and macrovascular beds. T2D is caused by impaired insulin secretion, impaired insulin action, and visceral obesity; alone or in combination, and all of these components are usually defective in patients with T2D. Furthermore, these components frequently interact. For example, reducing visceral obesity improves insulin sensitivity; improved insulin action leads to less demand for insulin secretion. Any intervention that improves glycemia also tends to normalize insulin secretion by reducing glucotoxicity impairing β-cell function. Strategies to prevent and/or remit T2D have therefore primarily focused on interventions that address one or more of these physiological drivers of T2D (Fig. 4.1).

Many randomized controlled clinical trials (RCTs) have tested interventions in persons without T2D but with impaired glucose tolerance (IGT; "prediabetes") or other T2D risk factors with the goal of preventing or delaying the onset of T2D. Most RCTs for prevention included only persons with prediabetes, with or without obesity or impaired fasting glucose (IFG). Therefore the effectiveness of medical and surgical interventions in persons who do not have prediabetes has not been well studied.

Remission of T2D is a diagnosis that is difficult to achieve and maintain. Improvement of glucose levels into the normal range can occur in some people living with diabetes, either spontaneously or after medical interventions, and in some cases can persist after withdrawal of glucose-lowering pharmacotherapy. Such sustained improvement may now be occurring more often due to newer forms of treatment. However, terminology for describing this process and objective measures for defining it are not well established, and the long-term risks versus benefits of its attainment are not well understood. An American Diabetes Association (ADA) group of international experts recently proposed the definition of remission of diabetes to be an achievement of a glycosylated hemoglobin (HbA_{1c}) of less than 6.5% (48 mmol/mol) for a minimum of 3 months following cessation of glucose-lowering pharmacotherapy (Table 4.1).[1]

RCTs testing lifestyle interventions that prevent or remit T2D, such as the Diabetes Prevention Program, in which a lifestyle intervention resulted in a 58% reduction in the incidence rate of T2D,[2] are important in patient care but are not discussed here (see Chapter 3). Furthermore, before pharmacological and/or surgical intervention can be applied in addition to lifestyle intervention, it is important to define what characteristics identify people most likely to benefit from these interventions. All the RCTs differed to some degree in eligibility criteria, but all included patients with some definition of prediabetes and most required patients to be living with overweight or obesity. In the US Diabetes Prevention Program, effects on T2D prevention varied with entry characteristics. In general, those with highest levels of T2D risk factors had the greatest reductions in T2D incidence, especially when expressed on an absolute, rather than risk ratio, scale.[3] In the future, selection of treatment candidates for drugs or surgery may also vary according to genotype.

Nonlifestyle interventions that prevent or remit T2D can be categorized into pharmacological (Table 4.2) and surgical methods (Table 4.3). Pharmacological interventions can then be subdivided by whether their primary effects target insulin secretion, insulin action, or visceral obesity. Surgical interventions are mostly focused on visceral obesity, although certain procedures can impact glucose and insulin metabolism very rapidly (within hours to days), long before substantial weight loss occurs. In the chapter that follows, the pharmacological and surgical methods shown to prevent or remit T2D will be discussed including the most contemporary evidence available.

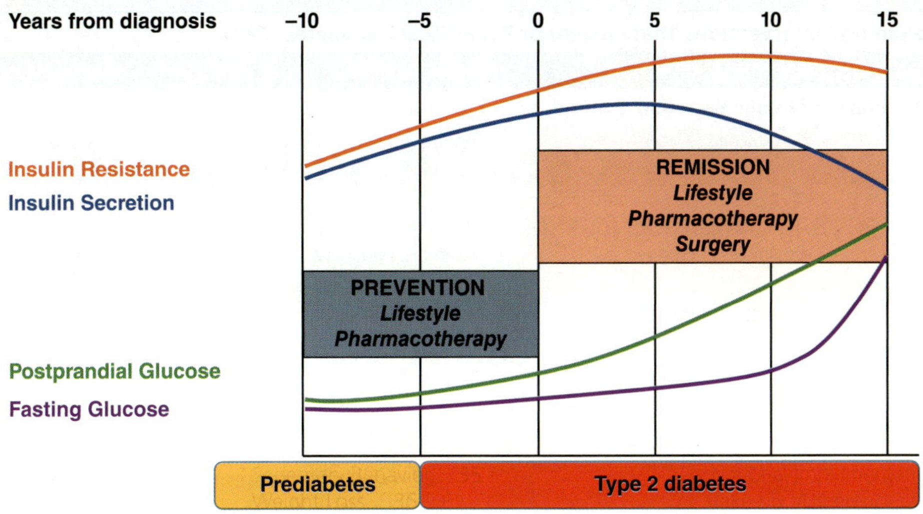

FIG. 4.1 Natural history and timing of interventions to prevent or remit type 2 diabetes. Insulin resistance and altered insulin secretion occur years before the onset of type 2 diabetes and result in ongoing β-cell stress. Concomitantly, postprandial and fasting glucose begin to increase over time until the threshold for diabetes diagnosis is reached. During this phase, interventions that prevent diabetes, such as lifestyle and pharmacotherapy, are key to halt the pathophysiology of β-cell dysfunction and loss. Once type 2 diabetes is diagnosed, interventions should focus on remission and include lifestyle, pharmacotherapy, and surgery.

TABLE 4.1 Remission of Type 2 Diabetes as Defined by the American Diabetes Association (*ADA*) International Expert Group

REMISSION OF TYPE 2 DIABETES DEFINED BY ADA EXPERT CONSENSUS[1]
Primary criteria: Return of glycosylated hemoglobin to <6.5% (<48 mmol/mol) that occurs spontaneously or following an intervention for a period of at least 3 months[a]
Alternative criteria: Fasting plasma glucose <126 mg/dl (<7.0 mmol/L) Glucose management indicator <6.5% calculated from a continuous glucose monitoring device

[a]Note: For surgical interventions, glycosylated hemoglobin to <6.5% (<48 mmol/mol) is required for at least 3 months after the procedure and 3 months after cessation of any pharmacotherapy.

PHARMACOLOGICAL INTERVENTIONS THAT PREVENT OR REMIT TYPE 2 DIABETES

Impaired Insulin Secretion

INSULIN

T2D develops slowly over years with the development of both insulin secretion impairment and insulin resistance (see Fig. 4.1). Acute glucotoxicity is a state of extreme hyperglycemia that is thought to be a driver of β-cell functional decline. Studies have initiated insulin at the early onset of T2D with the hope of restoring the early-phase insulin secretion and reaching remission.[4,5] It has been suggested that the administration of intense insulin can lead to a "β-cell rest," lowering the demand for insulin secretion.[4] The ORIGIN trial randomized 12,537 participants with IGT, IFG, or early T2D with cardiovascular (CV) risk factors to receive insulin glargine (target fasting blood glucose of <95 mg per deciliter) or standard care, plus n-3 fatty acids or placebo over a follow-up of 6.2 years. Although the CV outcomes rates were similar in both groups, the incidence of new-onset T2D was reduced by 28% in those with prediabetes in the insulin arm.[6,7] There were, however, higher rates of hypoglycemia and weight gain in the insulin glargine group. A significant legacy effect was noted with a 2-year passive follow-up as well.[8]

A study from Taiwan evaluated the effect of insulin administration to patients with newly diagnosed T2D with severe hyperglycemia. Patients were initially treated with intensive insulin administration over 10 to 14 days, then were randomized (50/50) for a span of 6 months of either oral antidiabetic drugs (OADs) or insulin (basal insulin twice per day).[5] Following the initial 6 months, the insulin group discontinued their insulin and were transitioned to OADs. Patients were then managed per national guidelines for the following 5 years. At the end of the 5 years, the HbA1c was lower in the initial insulin group, as was the rate of remission: 27.3% in the insulin group compared with 5.9% in the OAD group ($P = .048$).[5]

A meta-analysis of seven studies (n = 839 participants) looked at newly diagnosed T2D patients who were administered a short-term intensive insulin treatment for 14 to 21 days either through multiple daily injections or continuous subcutaneous insulin infusion. Four of these trials evaluated the long-term remission rates following the short-term intervention. In these studies, the drug-free remission after 3 months of follow-up was 66.2% (292 of 441 patients), after 6 months 58.9% (222 of 377 patients), after 12 months 46.3% (229 or 495), and after 24 months 42.1% (53 of 126 patients).[9] As evident in this data, the remission after short-term intensive insulin did diminish over time.[9]

SULFONYLUREAS AND NATEGLINIDE

Insulin secretion can be stimulated by sulfonylureas and nateglinide. The now-unavailable sulfonylurea, tolbutamide, was tested for diabetes prevention in the 1960s. These studies preceded current definitions of prediabetes and T2D, so the terms used to describe these trials have slightly different definitions than those used today. The Bedford (UK) trial of tolbutamide evaluated 241 adults with IGT randomized to tolbutamide or placebo and to

TABLE 4.2 Pharmacological Interventions That Prevent or Remit Type 2 Diabetes (*T2D*)

PHARMACOLOGIC INTERVENTION	MECHANISM OF ACTION	EFFECT ON T2D	MAIN ADVERSE EFFECTS
Medications That Target Impaired Insulin Secretion			
Insulin glargine	Basal insulin	28% Reduction in T2D incidence 21%–66% rate of T2D remission	Hypoglycemia Weight gain Diarrhea Infection
Nateglinide	Insulin secretagogue	No reduction in T2D incidence	Hypoglycemia Weight gain
Medications That Target Impaired Insulin Action			
Metformin	Improves insulin sensitivity, decreases intestinal and hepatic glucose production	18%–31% Reduction in T2D incidence	Gastrointestinal (nausea, vomiting, flatulence, diarrhea, bloating)
Thiazolidinediones	Improves target cell responsiveness to insulin and preserves insulin secretion	62%–72% Reduction in T2D incidence	Edema Weight gain Hypertension
Medications That Target Visceral Obesity			
Liraglutide	GLP-1 agonist Slows gastric emptying Central decrease in appetite	80% Reduction in risk of T2D incidence	Hypoglycemia Gastrointestinal (nausea, vomiting, decreased appetite, abdominal pain)
Tirzepatide	GIP and GLP-1 agonist Slows gastric emptying Central decrease in appetite	81%–86% Remission of T2D 31%–52% remission to normoglycemia	Gastrointestinal (nausea, vomiting, decreased appetite, abdominal pain) Sinus tachycardia
Dapagliflozin	SGLT2-Inhibitor Reduces reabsorption of filtered glucose Lowers renal threshold for glucose	33% Reduction in T2D incidence	Genitourinary infections Acute kidney injury Volume depletion Euglycemic diabetic ketoacidosis
Orlistat	Gastric and pancreatic lipase reversible inhibitor Decreases absorption of dietary fat	37% Reduction T2D incidence	Abdominal pain Flatulence GU injections
Medications With Alternative Mechanisms			
Acarbose	Competitive inhibitor of pancreatic alpha-amylase and intestinal alpha-glucosidase	25%–61% Reduction in T2D incidence	Flatulence Diarrhea Abdominal pain
Vitamin D	Improves B-cell function	11% Reduction in T2D incidence (not statistically significant)	None
Zinc	Decreases B-cell destruction and oxidative stress	Reduction in fasting glucose by 10.9 mg/dL Reduction in 2 h oral glucose tolerance test (OGTT) by 21.1 mg/dL	None
Angiotensin-converting enzyme inhibitors and angiotensin receptor blockers	Decreases conversion of angiotensin I to angiotensin II; Angiotensin receptor antagonist	6%–22% Reduction in T2D incidence	Hypotension Cough Acute kidney injury Angioedema

GIP, glucose-dependent insulinotropic polypepide; *GLP-1*, glucagon-like peptide-1; *SGLT2*, sodium glucose cotransporter 2.

two dietary groups in a 2-by-2 factorial design.[10] Over 10 years of follow-up, 15% of participants developed T2D, but neither the drug nor diet interventions reduced the progression to T2D. The Malmöhus trial of tolbutamide also studied in 147 men with IGT in Malmöhus County, Sweden. All study participants were given dietary advice and randomly assigned to tolbutamide, matching placebo, or neither medication. Tolbutamide was reported to prevent T2D when the trial was analyzed by estimated drug adherence[11] but not when analyzed by the more rigorous intention-to-treat principle.[12]

The Nateglinide and Valsartan in Impaired Glucose Tolerance Outcome Research (NAVIGATOR) was a 2-by-2 factorial 5-year RCT of the short-acting insulin secretagogue nateglinide of the meglitinide class and the angiotensin receptor blocker valsartan in 9306 participants with IGT, elevated fasting glucose, and CVD or CVD risk factors.[13] Nateglinide did not affect T2D incidence (HR = 1.07; 95% CI, 1.00–1.15) and was associated with increased frequency of hypoglycemia and modest weight gain. Based on these RCTs, it appears that sulfonylureas and nateglinide, aimed primarily at enhancing insulin secretion, have limited utility for preventing or delaying T2D in high-risk adults.

Impaired Insulin Action

METFORMIN

The Diabetes Prevention Program enrolled 3234 patients with IFG/IGT to placebo, metformin (850 mg twice/day), or lifestyle modifications (goal of 150 minutes of activity

TABLE 4.3 Surgical Interventions That Remit Type 2 Diabetes (*T2D*)

SURGICAL INTERVENTION	MECHANISM OF ACTION	EFFECT ON T2D	MAIN ADVERSE EFFECTS
Roux-en-Y gastric bypass (*RYGB*)	Decrease in energy intake	30%–81% T2D remission	Stomal stenosis, ulcers, cholelithiasis
Laparoscopic adjustable gastric banding (*LAGB*)	Decrease in energy intake	37%–73% T2D remission	Obstruction, port infection, band erosion
Laparoscopic sleeve gastrectomy (*LSG*)	Decrease in energy intake	60% T2D remission	Bleeding, stenosis, gastric leak
Biliopancreatic diversion (*BPD*) with or without duodenal switch	Decrease in energy intake and nutrient malabsorption	95% T2D remission	Electrolytes imbalance, protein/calorie malnutrition
Single anastomosis duodenal-ileal bypass with sleeve gastrectomy (*SADI-S*)	Decrease in energy intake and nutrient malabsorption	Similar or more effective than RYGB	Electrolytes imbalance, protein/calorie malnutrition

per week, and goal of 7% weight loss) over 2.8 years of follow-up[14] (see also Chapters 3 and 17). The metformin group had a 31% reduction in the incidence of diabetes (95% CI, 17%–43%) and the lifestyle group had a 58% reduction (95% CI, 48%–66%), compared to the placebo. The Diabetes Prevention Program Outcomes Study (DPPOS) evaluated continued follow-up of the DPP participants over a 10-year period. Eighty-eight percent of those enrolled in the DPP continued on to be part of the DPPOS. In this long-term follow-up cohort, diabetes incidence in the metformin group was reduced by 18% and in the lifestyle group by 34% when compared to the placebo.[15]

A review of the literature published between 1998 and 2017 on the use of metformin for diabetes prevention suggested that metformin is an effective tool to prevent or delay the development of T2D. They demonstrated that the relative risk reduction of T2D development was highest in patients with existing diabetes risk factors such as IGT, IFG, age $\leq$60 years, body mass index (BMI) $\geq$35 kg/m^2, and gestational diabetes.[16] Metformin was additionally noted to be cost-effective in 11 analyses and even demonstrated some cost savings.[16] Metformin for the prevention of T2D and its associated complications in persons at risk for increased risk for the development of T2D was recently systematically reviewed and meta-analyzed, including 20 RCTs randomizing 6774 participants.[17] One trial contributed 48% of all participants. The duration of intervention in the trials varied from 1 to 5 years. In the final analysis, metformin compared with placebo or diet and exercise reduced or delayed the risk of T2D in people at increased risk for the development of T2D (moderate-quality evidence). However, metformin compared to intensive diet and exercise did not reduce or delay the risk of T2D (moderate-quality evidence). Likewise, the combination of metformin and intensive diet and exercise compared to intensive diet and exercise only neither showed an advantage or disadvantage regarding the development of T2D (very low-quality evidence).

THIAZOLIDINEDIONES

TZDs improve cell responsiveness to insulin and are believed to also preserve insulin secretion. It is postulated that β-cell function improves with the intake of TZDs through a variety of mechanisms, such as decreasing glucotoxicity, lipotoxicity, inflammatory cytokines, oxidative damage, and lowering of free fatty acids, leading to prolonged survival of β-cells.[18–22] In the Diabetes Reduction Assessment with Ramipril and Rosiglitazone Medication (DREAM) Trial, 5269 patients with IGT and/or IFG were randomized to receive rosiglitazone or a placebo for 3 years. β-cell function was measured using the validated assessments of insulinogenic index and proinsulin concentration.[23] This international trial demonstrated that 25% of patients developed diabetes in the placebo arm compared with 10.6% in the rosiglitazone group (HR 0.38; $P < 0.0001$), a 62% reduction in the risk of progression to T2D with a daily intake of 8 mg of rosiglitazone.[24] The effects of rosiglitazone were not influenced by baseline glucose control.[25] The study also showed a 70% to 80% likelihood to revert from IFG/IGT to normal glucose tolerance during that time frame. This regression to normoglycemia, however, appeared to be similar to lifestyle modifications.[24] Though the waist:hip ratio was unchanged in the rosiglitazone group, there was a weight gain of 2.2 kg during the 3 years.[25] As expected, there did not seem to be a persistent effect of the TZD use 6 months after its discontinuation with the closure of the DREAM trial.[25]

The ACT NOW study evaluated 602 patients with IGT randomized to receive pioglitazone 30 mg per day or a placebo and followed for 2.4 years. Although there was significant weight gain and edema in the TZD group, there was a reduction of the progression to diabetes by 72%.[26] The PREVENT-J, Pioglitazone and Sulfonylurea Remission from Type 2 Diabetes Mellitus Development and Antiatherosclerosis in Japan, study evaluated patients with early-stage T2D and randomized them to lifestyle modifications, pioglitazone, or sulfonylurea treatment over an 18-month period (phase 1) and then subsequently discontinued the medications over the following 18-month period (phase 2).[27] Enrolled patients had diabetes duration for less than 5 years and had either an HbA1c < 7.9% or < 7.4% (with no prior diabetes treatment, or were on either metformin or alpha-glucosidase inhibitor, respectively). Throughout phase 2, the pioglitazone group had the highest proportion of patients who were able to maintain an $HbA_{1c} < 6.2\%$.[27] In this study, the remission of diabetes was best sustained after discontinuation of the TZD in comparison to the sulfonylurea and lifestyle modifications. In a Cochrane Systematic Review, pioglitazone reduced or delayed the development of T2D in people at increased risk of T2D compared with a placebo (low-certainty evidence) and compared with no intervention (moderate-certainty evidence).[28] It is unclear whether the effect of pioglitazone is sustained once discontinued. Pioglitazone compared with metformin neither showed advantage nor disadvantage regarding the development of

T2D in people at increased risk (low-certainty evidence). The data and reporting of all-cause mortality, serious adverse events, and micro- and macrovascular complications were generally sparse. None of the included studies reported on quality of life or socioeconomic effects.

Visceral Obesity

GLUCAGON-LIKE PEPTIDE-1 RECEPTOR AGONISTS

The incretins, including glucagon-like peptide-1 (GLP-1) and glucose-dependent insulinotropic polypeptide (GIP), are released in a glucose-dependent manner and behave as insulin secretagogues. GLP-1 also contributes to the inhibition of glucagon secretion, gastric emptying delays, and the promotion of centrally mediated appetite suppression, leading to sustained weight loss.[29] For example, high-dose injectable, once-weekly semaglutide (2.4 mg/wk) plus lifestyle intervention was shown to reduce weight by >12% over 68 weeks in individuals with obesity or overweight compared with lifestyle alone in STEP 1 (STEP 1: Research Study Investigating How Well Semaglutide Works in People Suffering From Overweight or Obesity).[30] In the STEP 2 trial assessing the efficacy of once weekly semaglutide in adults with overweight or obesity and T2D, the proportion of individuals in each group who achieved diabetes remission with HbA_{1c} levels of ≤6.5% at week 68 were 72.0%, 63.1%, and 14.2% for semaglutide 2.4, semaglutide 1.0, and a placebo, respectively; and the proportion of those achieving HbA_{1c} <7.0% at week 68 were 82.3%, 76.0%, and 25.8% for semaglutide 2.4, semaglutide 1.0, and a placebo, respectively.[31] Most recently, semaglutide 2.4 mg once weekly was seen to be superior to a placebo in reducing the incidence of death from cardiovascular causes, nonfatal myocardial infarction, or nonfatal stroke (hazard ratio, 0.80; 95% CI, 0.72–0.90; $P < .001$) in adults with preexisting cardiovascular disease and overweight or obesity but without diabetes in the SELECT trial. Novel agents targeting multiple obesogenic pathways thought to act synergistically are also in development and may offer even greater weight reduction. SURPASS-2 (a study of tirzepatide [LY3298176] vs. semaglutide once weekly as add-on therapy to metformin in participants with type 2 diabetes), testing treatment with the combined glucose-dependent insulinotropic polypeptide receptor agonist (RA)/GLP-1 RA tirzepatide compared with semaglutide 1.0 mg subcutaneous injection (SQ) weekly in patients with T2D,[32] showed that tirzepatide reduced body weight to a greater degree than the 1.0-mg dose of semaglutide as a secondary end point. In the SURPASS-1 study, tirzepatide treatment reduced HbA_{1c} to less than 6.5% in 81% to 86% of patients (compared with 10% on a placebo) and to an HbA_{1c} less than 5.7% in 31% to 52% of patients (compared with 1% on placebo).[33] The SURPASS-4 trial assessed glycemic efficacy and cardiovascular safety in patients with T2D and elevated cardiovascular risk and found that tirzepatide, compared with glargine, demonstrated greater and clinically meaningful HbA_{1c} reduction (−2.43% [SD 0.05] with 10 mg and −2.58% [0.05] with 15 mg, vs. −1.44% [0.03] with glargine) with a lower incidence of hypoglycemia at week 52 and was not associated with excess cardiovascular risk compared with glargine (HR, 0.74; 95% CI, 0.51–1.08).[34] Data from the pooled SURPASS clinical program in adults with T2D showed that diabetes remission was common with tirzepatide treatment, with 44% and 37% of individuals treated with tirzepatide achieving HbA_{1c} 5.7% to 6.5% and <5.7%, respectively.[35] GLP-1 RA effects on body weight are most prominent on visceral and ectopic body fat, with a two to threefold greater effect on reducing these diabesogenic risk factors compared with other body fat compartments.[36] GLP-1 RAs and related compounds are therefore highly promising agents for prevention and/or remission of T2D.

Liraglutide was evaluated in a 20-week European study where 564 patients with obesity but without T2D were randomized to placebo versus liraglutide versus orlistat.[37] Of these patients, 31% enrolled had IFG. At 20 weeks, those treated with liraglutide showed a decrease of 84% to 96% in the prevalence of prediabetes. HbA_{1c} also showed a reduction of 0.14% to 0.24% in the liraglutide group and the metabolic syndrome decreased by >60%.[37] The effect of liraglutide on fat distribution and β-cell function was assessed in a study looking at 62 metformin-treated patients with obesity and prediabetes or new-onset T2D. Patients were randomized to liraglutide or lifestyle modifications and both groups achieved comparable weight loss. Visceral adipose tissue was significantly reduced ($P = .028$) and β-cell function (measured as β-index) improved ($P = 0.021$) in the liraglutide group.[38] Since weight loss and HbA_{1c} reduction were the same in the liraglutide and lifestyle groups, the analysis described the β-cell function improvement in the treatment group as being an independent outcome.[38] Therefore early use of the GLP-1 agonist can diminish β-cell dysfunction in prediabetes and prevent progression to T2D.

As part of the SCALE Obesity and Prediabetes Study Group, patients with prediabetes and a BMI of 30 kg/m² or 27 kg/m² (with comorbidities) were randomized to either daily liraglutide 3 mg or placebo over a 160-week period. In this study, liraglutide reduced the risk of new-onset of T2D by 80% relative to placebo (HR, 0.21; 95% CI, 0.13–0.34) and 66% of individuals in the treatment group showed regression from prediabetes to normoglycemia. With liraglutide, the time to onset of T2D was 2.7 times longer than with placebo over the 160 weeks.[39]

Many other GLP-1 RA-based compounds that combine GLP-1 RA with other targets, such as glucose-dependent insulinotropic polypeptide (GIP) and glucagon receptor (GR) are currently in research and development (phase I/II/III) and hold additional promise for substantial cardiometabolic benefits. The triple agonist (GLP-1/GIP/GR) retatrutide recently demonstrated up to 24.2% body weight loss over 48 weeks in adults with overweight or obesity without diabetes[40] and significant reductions in HbA_{1c} in patients with T2D compared with dulaglutide (up to −2.02% [SD 0.11] for the 12 mg group vs. −1.41% [0.12] for the dulaglutide group, $P < .001$).[41] The dual GLP-1/GR agonist, survodutide, recently demonstrated significant efficacy for weight loss in a phase II study (up to −14.9% [−16.9 to −13.0] for 4.8 mg vs. −2.8% [−4.9 to −0.7] for a placebo). These compounds are also being tested for other conditions associated with obesity and diabetes including metabolic dysfunction-associated steatohepatitis (MASH), now the leading cause for liver transplantation. Both survodutide[42] and tirzepatide[43] recently showed improvement in MASH without worsening of fibrosis in patients with biopsy-confirmed MASH. Other compounds in development for obesity include oral agonists of GLP-1 such as orforglipron[44] and oral semaglutide (estimated mean body weight change from baseline to week 68%–15.1% [SE 0.5] with oral semaglutide 50 mg vs. −2.4% [0.5] with placebo),[45] as well as the GLP-1 RA/GIP antagonist, maridebart cafraglutide.[46]

SODIUM GLUCOSE COTRANSPORTER 2 INHIBITORS

Sodium glucose cotransporter 2 (SGLT2) inhibitors lower the plasma glucose concentration via a mechanism independent of insulin secretion and insulin action. By inhibiting renal glucose reabsorption, they cause glucosuria, leading to a decline in fasting and postprandial plasma glucose concentration. Despite the lack of a direct effect on the β-cell, preclinical studies in animal models of diabetes have demonstrated improved β-cell function secondary to reduction of the plasma glucose concentration and amelioration of glucotoxicity.[47] SGLT2i have been demonstrated to reduce markers of visceral adiposity[48] and improve adipose-tissue function.[49] Therefore SGLT2i have been postulated to prevent development of T2D.

The DAPA-CKD and DAPA-HF trials evaluated the effect of dapagliflozin on reduction of chronic kidney disease and heart failure as primary outcomes in patients with or without T2D. A pooled analysis from both trials demonstrated that dapagliflozin, compared with placebo, reduced the development of new-onset T2D (HR, 0.67; 95% CI, 0.51–0.88; p = .0040) with a greater effect in younger patients and those with elevated blood pressure.[50] Due to the minimal difference in mean HbA_{1c} between placebo and dapagliflozin in the trials, the mechanisms of benefit were suggested to be a potential direct positive impact of dapagliflozin on β-cell function as well as increased sensitivity of insulin in the periphery.[50] The PRE-D trial was a multiarm study comparing 1:1:1:1 randomization of patients with overweight/obesity and prediabetes to dapagliflozin, metformin, interval-based exercises, and a control arm over 13 weeks. The evaluation of glycemic variability was conducted using a continuous glucose monitor with a measurement of mean amplitude of glycemic excursions (MAGE). As compared to metformin, dapagliflozin yielded positive improvements in glycemic variability (dapagliflozin vs. metformin, MAGE reduction of 17.2% [p= 0.041], and lower incidence of diabetes [2.1% vs. 3.9%; HR, 0.53; 95% CI, 0.36–0.77]).[51]

However, the prevention of T2D development may not be universal among the SGLT2i. Studies of empagliflozin in heart failure did not individually reduce new diagnosis of T2D in those without diabetes. Neither the EMPEROR-reduced nor the EMPORER-preserved trial showed a reduction in new-onset T2D with empagliflozin (HR, 0.86; 95% CI, 0.62–1.19[52] and HR, 0.84; 95% CI, 0.65–1.07,[53] respectively). This might be due to inadequate power; therefore a pooled analysis might produce statistically significant results, as opposed to a difference in the SGLT2 inhibitors per se. Furthermore, much like other studies of diabetes prevention, the question remains whether the effects seen are due to masking or true prevention.

OTHER WEIGHT-MODIFYING MEDICATIONS

The XENDOS study was a 4-year double-blind RCT of 3305 patients with obesity (BMI ≥ 30 kg/m^2) with normoglycemia (79%) or IGT (21%) randomized to lifestyle modification with either orlistat 120 mg or a placebo three times daily. The incidence of T2D with orlistat was 6.2% compared with 9.0% with a placebo, resulting in a 37.3% reduced risk of progression to T2D in the orlistat group (HR, 0.63; 95% CI, 0.45–0.86).[54]

The progression of prediabetes to T2D has been shown to be preventable in patients with metabolic syndrome and obesity with weight loss of 5% to 10%. An RCT looked at overweight/obese patients with prediabetes and/or metabolic syndrome and randomized participants to Phentermine 7.5 mg/Topiramate ER 46 mg, Phen 15 mg/TPM ER 92 mg, or placebo plus lifestyle modifications for 108 weeks. The annualized incidence rate for T2D was reduced by 70.5% in those receiving 7.5/46 dosage, and by 78.7% in the 15/92 dosage, versus placebo ($P < .05$). The ability to prevent diabetes development in the treatment arms was related to the degree of weight loss.[55]

The effect of lorcaserin on the prevention and remission of T2D in patients with overweight and obesity was tested in the CAMELLIA-TIMI 61 trial.[56] Lorcaserin decreased the risk for incident diabetes, induced remission of hyperglycemia, and reduced the risk of microvascular complications in obese and overweight patients, supporting the role of lorcaserin as an adjunct to lifestyle modification for chronic management of weight and metabolic health. Unfortunately, in February 2020, the FDA requested that the manufacturer of lorcaserin voluntarily withdraw the drug from the US market because a safety clinical trial showed an increased occurrence of cancer, and the medication is no longer available for use.

Alternative Mechanisms

ALPHA-GLUCOSIDASE INHIBITORS

Alpha-glucosidase inhibitors have no known direct effects on insulin secretion or action, but lower postprandial hyperglycemia by slowing glucose absorption from the gut. They have been tested for T2D prevention under the hypothesis that dampening postprandial glucose excursions in persons with IGT may help preserve insulin secretion or action, thus preventing incident T2D. The STOP-NIDDM trial was a double-blind, placebo-controlled study that evaluated patients with IGT and randomized them either to acarbose or placebo for 3 years. Findings demonstrated that the intake of acarbose lowered the progression to T2D by 25% and fostered the reversion of IGT to normal glucose tolerance ($p < .0001$).[57] The voglibose Ph-3 Study Group evaluated the use of the alpha-glucosidase inhibitor voglibose in a high-risk Japanese population with IGT. The study demonstrated that in contrast to placebo, those treated with voglibose had a significantly reduced risk for progressing to T2D (50 of 897 vs. 106 of 881; HR, 0.59; 95% CI, 0.43–0.82; p = .001).[58] Also, they noted a statistically significant achievement of normoglycemia in the voglibose group compared with the placebo.[58]

A meta-analysis of acarbose monotherapy for prevention of T2D from prediabetes evaluated eight randomized controlled trials which included 2628 participants over at least 3 years. They demonstrated that patients randomized to acarbose had a decreased incidence of T2D (number needed to treat [NNT] to prevent one case of T2D was 6.7 over 3 years). Notably, the T2DM incidence was lower in the Eastern group (Asia) than in the Western group (North America and Europe) (NNT 5.9 Eastern, NNT 11.1 Western; $P < .0001$).[59] Alpha-glucosidase inhibitors work best on individuals who consume higher carbohydrate intake. The analysis suggested that the Eastern diet contained a greater proportion of starchy carbohydrates and therefore had a greater benefit from acarbose.[59] A recent systematic review concluded that alpha-glucosidase inhibitors may prevent or delay the development of T2D in people with IGT.[60] There is no firm evidence that alpha-glucosidase inhibitors have a beneficial effect on cardiovascular mortality or cardiovascular events.

VITAMIN D

Vitamin D deficiency and its role in the development of T2D is a controversial topic. Studies have shown that vitamin D is associated with improvement in β-cell function, reducing the risk of the metabolic syndrome and inflammation.[61] However, it is not known if supplementation with vitamin D actually prevents progression to T2D. The D2d Research Group randomized 2423 patients with prediabetes to 4000 IU of vitamin D_3 or placebo, regardless of their underlying vitamin D level. After a median of 2.5 years of follow-up, there was no statistically significant lowering of the risk of T2D in the vitamin D group (HR, 0.88; 95% CI, 0.75–1.04; $P = .12$).[62] A meta-analysis conducted in 2020 evaluated 10 studies with a total of 34,882 patients, analyzing both cross-sectional studies and RCTs. There was a significant association between lower vitamin D levels and T2D in the cross-sectional studies (pooled OR, 1.77 [1.51–2.07, $P < .001$] but a nonsignificant 11% [$P = 0.08$] decrease in risk of T2DM for patients receiving vitamin D was observed in the RCTs).[61] In contrast, a different meta-analysis evaluated eight randomized controlled studies with a total of 4896 patients with prediabetes who received vitamin D supplementation versus a placebo.[63] They detected a statistically significant reduction in the risk of T2DM development with supplementation of vitamin D (risk ratio [RR], 0.89; 95% CI, 0.80–0.99; $I^2 = 0\%$); however, this was significant only in patients without obesity. They also noted a 48% increase in reversion of prediabetes to a normal glucose state in the vitamin D supplementation groups (RR, 1.48; 95% CI, 1.14–1.92; $I^2 = 0\%$).[63]

ZINC

Zinc has been proposed to improve fasting blood glucose and insulin parameters. There are a few possible mechanisms of action of zinc that are beneficial. Zinc is involved in insulin action and its synthesis; it helps moderate cytokine levels and therefore helps decrease β-cell destruction in states of hyperglycemia, and it helps with oxidative stress, among other mechanisms.[64] A pilot study looking at patients with prediabetes was conducted in a 6-month double-blind randomized placebo-controlled trial, where patients received either zinc 30 mg per day or a placebo. At the end of the trial, the zinc treatment group demonstrated a statistically significant improvement in the homeostasis model (HOMA) parameters for insulin resistance, insulin sensitivity, and β-cell function and in the fasting blood glucose (5.37 ± 0.20 mmol/L vs. 5.69 ± 0.26, $p < .001$).[64]

Zinc and other micronutrients have been evaluated in their relationship with blood sugar control. One systematic review and meta-analysis looked at three studies with a pooled total of 265 participants with prediabetes who received supplementation with zinc (20–30 mg/day) over a 6- to 12-month period.[65] When given alone, zinc supplementation showed a statistically significant reduction in the fasting blood glucose (−10.86 mg/dL; 95% CI, −14.74 to −6.98; $p < .001$). Additionally, in the zinc alone and the zinc with other micronutrients pooled data, there was a significant reduction in the 2-hour oral glucose tolerance test by 21.08 mg/dL (95% CI, −40.05 to −2.11; $p = .03$).[65]

ANGIOTENSIN-CONVERTING ENZYME INHIBITORS AND ANGIOTENSIN RECEPTOR BLOCKERS

It is not clear that a reduction in diabetes incidence through blockade of the RAAS pathway observed in a number of randomized trials represents a truly preventive effect or simply a delay or a masking effect. Overall, diabetes incidence was not a prespecified, primary endpoint in any of these prior studies, and there was insufficient evidence to definitively recommend any given angiotensin-converting enzyme (ACE) inhibitors or angiotensin receptor blockers (ARBs) in patients at risk of developing T2D for the purpose of diabetes prevention. Nevertheless, in the Heart Outcomes Prevention Evaluation (HOPE) trial,[66] angiotensin converting enzyme (ACE) inhibitor therapy with ramipril lowered diabetes incidence from 5.4% to 3.6% overall, and in the Studies of Left Ventricular Dysfunction (SOLVD) trial of patients with systolic heart failure, enalapril reduced diabetes incidence from 22% to 6%.[67] The Prevention of Events with Angiotensin Converting Enzyme Inhibition (PEACE) study reported a significant reduction in the incidence of T2D from 11.5% to 9.8% in patients with stable coronary artery disease (CAD) treated with trandolapril.[68] ARB therapy significantly decreased diabetes incidence in the Candesartan in Heart Failure: Assessment of Reduction in Mortality and Morbidity (CHARM) study from 7% to 6%.[69] In the Valsartan Antihypertensive Long-Term Use Evaluation (VALUE) trial of 10,419 hypertensive patients at high cardiovascular risk, a valsartan-based treatment regimen was associated with a decrease in the incidence of T2D from 16% to 13% compared with an amlodipine-based regimen.[70]

SURGICAL INTERVENTIONS THAT PREVENT OR REMIT TYPE 2 DIABETES

Major, durable weight loss for remission of T2D is challenging with medical and/or behavioral approaches, and adequate glycemic control often remains elusive.[71] Bariatric procedures, especially intestinal-bypass variants, can dramatically resolve T2D, often long before and out of proportion to postoperative weight loss.[72] Surgical procedures performed to modify the gastrointestinal anatomy to result in weight loss and metabolic benefits (e.g., remission of T2D) is currently considered an appropriate option for patients with BMI >40 kg/m² or >35 mg/m² with serious comorbid conditions, including hypertension, T2D, sleep apnea, and cardiovascular disease.[73,74] Currently, five bariatric surgical procedures are considered acceptable therapy for appropriate patients: Roux-en-Y gastric bypass (RYGB), laparoscopic adjustable gastric banding (LAGB), laparoscopic sleeve gastrectomy (LSG), biliopancreatic diversion (BPD) with or without duodenal switch (-DS), and single anastomosis duodenal-ileal bypass with sleeve gastrectomy (SADI-S) (Fig. 4.2). SADI-S is the most recent procedure to be endorsed by the American Society for Metabolic and Bariatric Surgery. While similar to the BPD-DS, the SADI-S is simpler and takes less time to perform as there is only one surgical bowel connection. Weight loss after LAGB and LSG procedures is primarily caused by a decrease in energy intake because there is little or no malabsorption after these procedures, and weight loss after RYGB, BPD with or without duodenal switch, and SADI-S is a result of a combination of decreased energy intake and nutrient malabsorption.

Randomized Controlled Trials of Bariatric Surgery for Type 2 Diabetes Remission

The therapeutic superiority of bariatric surgery over medical therapy for T2D remission has been shown in several RCTs and has been recently reviewed.[75] Initially, three studies reported on 1-year or 2-year prospective outcomes. In a study by Dixon et al., 73% of patients who underwent LAGB surgery in contrast to only 13% in the medical-lifestyle therapy group achieved remission of T2D.[76] Relative risk of remission for the surgical group was 5.5 (95% CI, 2.2–14.0). Surgical and conventional-therapy groups lost a mean (SD) of 20.7% (8.6%) and 1.7% (5.2%) of weight, respectively, at 2 years ($P < .001$). Remission of T2D was related to weight loss (R2 = 0.46; $P < .001$) and lower baseline HbA_{1c} levels (combined R2 = 0.52; $P < .001$).

In a study by Schauer et al., the primary endpoint was the proportion of patients with a glycated hemoglobin level of 6.0% or less 12 months after treatment. In this study, 42% of patients who underwent RYGB surgery and 37% who underwent LSG, but only 12% treated with intensive medical therapy, achieved remission of T2D at 12 months.[77] Glycemic control improved in all three groups, with a mean glycated hemoglobin level of 7.5±1.8% in the medical-therapy group, 6.4±0.9% in the gastric-bypass group ($P < .001$), and 6.6±1.0% in the sleeve-gastrectomy group ($P = .003$). Weight loss was greater in the gastric-bypass group and sleeve-gastrectomy group (–29.4 ± 9.0 kg and –25.1 ± 8.5 kg, respectively) than in the medical-therapy group (–5.4 ± 8.0 kg) ($P < 0.001$ for both comparisons). The use of drugs to lower glucose, lipid, and blood-pressure levels decreased significantly after both surgical procedures but increased in patients receiving medical therapy only.

In a study by Mingrone et al., the primary endpoint was the rate of diabetes remission at 2 years (defined as a fasting glucose level of <100 mg/dL [5.6 mmol/L] and a glycated hemoglobin level of <6.5% in the absence of pharmacologic therapy). In this study, after 2 years, diabetes remission had occurred in no patients in the medical-therapy group versus 75% in the gastric-bypass group and 95% in the biliopancreatic-diversion group ($P < .001$ for both comparisons). Age, sex, baseline BMI, duration of diabetes, and weight changes were not significant predictors of diabetes remission at 2 years or of improvement in glycemia at 1 and 3 months. At 2 years, the average baseline glycated hemoglobin level (8.65±1.45%) had decreased in all groups, but patients in the two surgical groups had the greatest degree of improvement (average glycated hemoglobin levels, 7.69±0.57% in the medical-therapy group, 6.35±1.42% in the gastric-bypass group, and 4.95±0.49% in the biliopancreatic-diversion group).[78]

The between-trial heterogeneity observed is probably a result of differences in the primary endpoint, which in the study by Mingrone and colleagues was a glycated hemoglobin (HbA_{1c}) value below 6.5% in patients off all diabetes medications, as opposed to 6.0% or lower (with or without medications) in the study by Schauer and colleagues. Whereas fewer patients achieved the latter study's more stringent endpoint, the HbA_{1c} decrement after surgical procedures was noteworthy (from approximately 9.4% to approximately 6.5%), with an important decrease in glucose-lowering medication.

CLINICAL EFFECTIVENESS OF THE VARIOUS BARIATRIC PROCEDURES

Given an increasing number of studies in this area and potential heterogeneity noted here, several studies have evaluated the clinical effectiveness of one type of bariatric procedure versus another in order to aid clinicians and patients for informed decision-making. A recent study evaluated the comparative effectiveness of RYGB versus LSG for sustained remission of T2D.[79] Of 5119 patients studied, 81% experienced remission of T2D. Those who underwent RYGB had a 24% (HR = 1.24; 95% CI, 1.16, 1.32) increased probability of achieving remission compared with LSG. A higher number of diabetes medications at the time of surgery and a higher Charlson index score were associated with decreased probability of remission. The authors concluded that while both procedures are initially effective, RYGB may be superior to LSG at providing lasting remission of T2D. A systematic review and meta-analysis, using a random effects model, was performed to calculate relative risk of T2D remission between groups who underwent RYBG and LSG in contemporary RCTs.[80] Of 2650 records identified, 12 records from 10 different RCTs were finally included. The studies comprised 705 patients with follow-up from 1 to 5 years. The remission rate of T2D at 1 year was higher among those undergoing RYGB (156/276, 57%) compared with those undergoing LSG (128/275, 47%), RR 1.20 (95% CI, 1.00–1.45), $P = 0.047$, $I^2 = 24.9\%$, moderate-quality evidence. Among studies with 2- to 5-year follow-up, there was no difference in remission rates between the RYGB (132/263, 50%) and LSG (121/266, 46%) groups, RR 1.06 (0.94–1.20), $P = 0.34$, $I^2 = 0.0\%$, low-quality evidence. RYGB resulted in a higher rate of T2D remission compared with LSG after 1 year. The T2D remission rates did not differ in studies with 2- to 5-year follow-up. A further meta-analysis including 10 studies with a total of 778 patients demonstrated that the overall prevalence of achievement of broad and narrow criteria for T2D remission was 73% and 53% at the 1-year, 60% and 48% at the 3-year, and 51% and 43% at the 5-year assessment, respectively.[81] Compared to

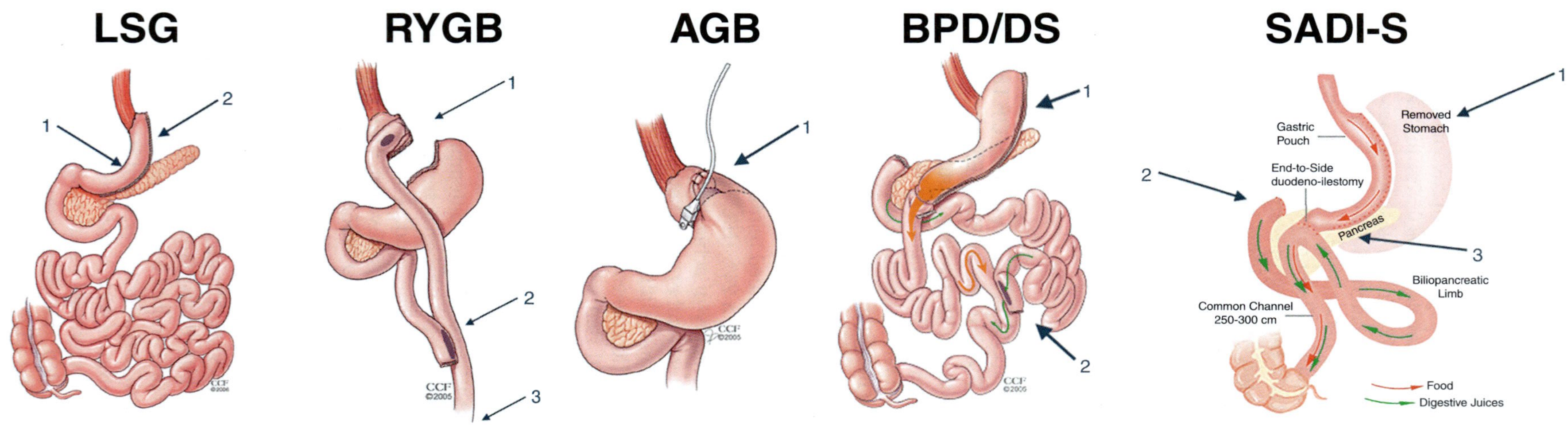

LSG — The Procedure

1. The stomach is freed from organs around it.
2. Surgical staplers are used to remove 80% of the stomach, making it much smaller.

RYGB — The Procedure

1. First, the stomach is divided into a smaller top portion (pouch) which is about the size of an egg. The larger part of the stomach is bypassed and no longer stores or digests food.
2. The small intestine is also divided and connected to the new stomach pouch to allow food to pass. The small bowel segment which empties the bypassed or larger stomach is connected into the small bowel approximately 3–4 feet downstream, resulting in a bowel connection resembling the shape of the letter Y.
3. Eventually the stomach acids and digestive enzymes from the bypassed stomach and first portion of the small intestine will mix with food that is eaten.

AGB — The Procedure

1. This device is placed and secured around the top part of the stomach creating a small pouch above the band.

BPD/DS — The Procedure

1. Following creation of the sleeve-like stomach, the first portion of the small intestine is separated from the stomach.
2. A part of the small intestine is then brought up and connected to the outlet of the newly created stomach, so that when the patient eats, the food goes through the sleeve pouch and into the latter part of the small intestine.

SADI-S — The Procedure

1. The operation starts the same way as the sleeve gastrectomy, making a smaller tube-shaped stomach.
2. The first part of the small intestine is divided just after the stomach.
3. A loop of intestine is measured several feet from its end and is then connected to the stomach. This is the only intestinal connection performed in this procedure.

FIG. 4.2 Bariatric surgery procedures and how they work. *LSG*, Laparoscopic sleeve gastrectomy, *RYGB*, roux-en-Y gastric bypass; *AGB,* adjustable gastric band; *BPD/DS*, biliopancreatic diversion with or without duodenal switch; *SADI-S*, single anastomosis duodeno-ileal bypass with sleeve gastrectomy. Courtesy and with permission from the American Society for Metabolic & Bariatric Surgery.

LSG, RYGB was associated with a higher chance of achieving remission at 1 year after surgery (RR = 1.34 vs. RR = 1.22) and at 5 years (RR = 1.18). These findings suggest a more favorable effect of RYGB than LSG on achieving T2D remission in the short term, although the evidence currently available does not clarify whether these differences are sustained long term. Within the LSG procedure itself, variation in the surgical approach may also influence T2D remission rates. In a recent study evaluating antrum preservation versus antrum resection in LSG, LSG with antrum resection (2 cm from the pylorus) had significantly lower postoperative BMI, better control of T2D, and more retention of gastric contents in patients with BMI 30 to 40 kg/m^2 in comparison with LSG with antral preservation with a nonsignificant increase in incidence of gastrointestinal esophageal reflux disease (GERD) symptoms.[82]

A recent systematic review and meta-analysis evaluated metabolic outcomes after SADI-S, the newest bariatric procedure available.[83] The meta-analysis included 16 studies of 3319 patients, with 1704 (51.3%) undergoing SADI-S. SADI-S patients had increased BMI (49.6 kg/m^2 vs. 48.8 kg/m^2) and weight (139.7 kg vs. 137.1 kg), were more likely to have T2D (46.3% vs. 42.1%), and dyslipidemia (36.6% SADI-S vs. 32.7%) compared with other bariatric procedures. SADI-S had a shorter operative duration than other procedures, a shorter postoperative stay ($p < .001$), and trended toward fewer complications (OR, 0.69; $p = .06$). Remission of T2D was similar between SADI-S and other procedures (OR, 0.07; $p = .1$) and subgroup analysis suggested greater T2D remission than RYGB (OR, 4.42; $p = .04$). Achieved weight loss was similar between procedures.

The impact of bariatric surgery on risk markers in T2D such as albuminuria and chronic kidney disease (CKD) stage has also been recently evaluated in 100 patients with early-stage CKD and T2D. After 24 months, remission of albuminuria occurred in 55% of patients (95% CI, 39%–70%) after the best medical treatment and 82% of patients (95% CI, 72%–93%) after RYGB ($P = 0.006$), resulting in CKD remission rates of 48% (95% CI, 32%–64%) after the best medical treatment and 82% (95% CI, 72%–92%) after RYGB ($P = 0.002$).[84] More recently, studies have reported longer-term outcomes of at least 3 years and beyond. One study evaluated outcomes of bariatric surgery versus lifestyle intervention for T2D treatment and reported that partial or complete T2DM remission was achieved by 40% of RYGB, 29% of LAGB, and no intensive lifestyle weight loss intervention participants ($P = 0.004$).[85] The use of diabetes medications was reduced more in the surgical groups than the lifestyle intervention-alone group, with 65% of RYGB, 33% of LAGB, and none of the intensive lifestyle weight loss intervention participants going from using insulin or oral medication at baseline to no medication at year 3 ($P < 0.001$).

FACTORS TO CONSIDER FOR SURGICAL INTERVENTION FOR REMISSION OF TYPE 2 DIABETES

Specific characteristics have been identified that predict the response of T2D to surgery-induced weight loss among patients undergoing RYGB surgery. Several factors have been associated with treatment failure: longer duration of T2D, inadequate postoperative weight loss, more severe diabetes requiring insulin therapy before surgery, and older age.[86] Of importance, early remission does not necessarily translate into long-term success, and relapse can occur. Remission scores and diabetes duration are good predictors of short-term diabetes remission; however, for durable remission and risk of complications, remission scores and diabetes duration alone have limited predictive ability.[87] Data from the Swedish Obese Subjects long-term observational study, which evaluated the effect of bariatric surgery in 4047 patients with T2D, found that one-half of the 72% of patients who had achieved diabetes remission at 2 years after surgery remained in remission at 10 years.[88] The precise reasons for recurrence of diabetes are not known but are likely related to recidivism of weight loss because relapse or worsening of T2D is associated with weight regain.

An important confounding factor in interpreting the efficacy of bariatric surgery in the management of T2D is the lack of a consistent, uniform definition of diabetes "remission" or "resolution" used in different studies. In the surgical literature, remission has most often been defined as the withdrawal of all diabetes medications, in conjunction with normal fasting plasma glucose levels (ranging from <100 to <126 mg/dL) and/or a normal HbA_{1c} level (ranging from <6% to <7%). Obviously, differences in the definition of remission among studies will lead to differences in estimated remission rates. Nevertheless, the T2D remission rate is not the same with all bariatric surgical procedures. Results from a meta-analysis involving approximately 8000 patients with T2D found that the rate of diabetes resolution was much greater in patients who underwent surgical procedures that involved anatomic diversion of the upper gastrointestinal tract (BPD and RYGB: 95% and 80% resolution rates, respectively) than in procedures that implied a restrictive approach (LAGB: 57% resolution rate).[89,90]

Medical costs for a patient with type 2 diabetes are greater than costs for a patient without diabetes. Estimated yearly costs of managing a patient with diabetes in the United States (US$13,243) are more than five times that of a patient without diabetes (US$2560).[91] The largest components of costs are hospital inpatient care (50%), medication and supplies (12%), retail prescriptions to treat complications (11%), and physician office visits (9%).[91] Advantages of bariatric surgery with regard to diabetes translate into considerable economic benefits. Surgery costs for laparoscopic surgery may fully be recovered after 26 months. These data suggest that surgical therapy is clinically more effective and ultimately less expensive than standard therapy for diabetes patients with a BMI of 35 kg/m^2 or higher.[92] This has also been reported in Canada, where health care system coverage differs from the United States. The initial costs of surgery can be amortized over 3.5 years.[93]

Observed metabolic effects following some procedures implicate weight-independent antidiabetes mechanisms. These benefits result in part from mechanisms beyond reduced food intake and body weight because glycemic improvements precede substantial weight loss. Mingrone and colleagues[78] found that all the surgical patients achieved glycemic control without diabetes medications within only

15 days after surgery. Schauer and colleagues reported that diabetes medication use decreased postoperatively, long before maximum weight loss occurred.[77] Recent studies corroborate a growing body of evidence showing that weight-independent mechanisms contribute to diabetes remission after some bariatric procedures.[94] This notion is based primarily on (1) the early postoperative effects of RYGB surgery on glycemic control; (2) the long-term efficacy of different surgical procedures on resolution of T2D; (3) the effect of duodenojejunal bypass (DJB) surgery, which bypasses the upper gastrointestinal tract but causes minimal weight loss; (4) the hormonal response to glucose or mixed-meal ingestion; and (5) upper gastrointestinal tract bypass in rodent models. Operations that reroute chyme in such a way that the duodenum and proximal jejunum are bypassed, resulting in chyme delivery directly to the jejunum, may be a promising pathophysiologic avenue in diabetes management.

There is a growing recognition that bariatric surgery, through its metabolic effects, including remission of T2D, may reduce the risk of CV events, both in the primary and secondary prevention populations. Although currently limited to observational studies (albeit with rigorous adjustment for propensity and potential confounders), the evidence suggests that bariatric surgery could reduce CV risk by 22% (for atrial fibrillation) to 62% (for heart failure).[95] In the SWEDEHEART registry, the 8-year cumulative probability of major adverse CV events was lower in patients undergoing metabolic surgery (18.7% [95% CI, 15.9%–21.5%] versus 36.2% [33.2%–39.3%], adjusted hazard ratio, 0.44 [95% CI, 0.32–0.61]). Patients undergoing metabolic surgery had also a lower risk of death (adjusted HR, 0.45 [95% CI, 0.29–0.70]; MI, 0.24 [0.14–0.41]) and new-onset heart failure, but there were no significant differences regarding stroke (0.91 [0.38–2.20]) and new-onset atrial fibrillation (0.56 [0.31–1.01]).[96] Similarly, in Canada, among 2638 patients with existing ischemic heart disease or heart failure undergoing metabolic surgery, the primary outcome of extended MACE (first occurrence of all-cause mortality, myocardial infarction, coronary revascularization, cerebrovascular events, and heart failure hospitalization) occurred in 11.5% of the surgery group and 19.6% of the controls (adjusted HR, 0.58 [95% CI, 0.48–0.71]; $P < .001$). The association was notable for those with heart failure (HR, 0.44 [95% CI, 0.31–0.62]; $P < .001$; absolute risk difference, 19.3% [95% CI, 12.0%–26.7%]) and in those with ischemic heart disease (HR, 0.60 [95% CI, 0.48–0.74]; $P < .001$; absolute risk difference, 7.5% [95% CI, 4.7%–10.5%]). Surgery was also associated with a lower incidence of cardiovascular mortality (HR, 0.35 [95% CI, 0.15–0.80]; $P = .001$).[97] Based on these data, there have been calls for a prospective, multicenter clinical trial with major adverse CV event end points for metabolic surgery, including a broad population.[98] Such a trial is currently being designed and, if successfully completed, the implications are profound. If such a study is positive, many doubts will be erased, and many more patients will benefit from greater use of a surgical approach to obesity and T2D. Furthermore, wider use of metabolic surgery (US$15,000–US$25,000 per procedure) might even result in relative cost savings in some populations because of medication reduction and reduced costs of treating CV morbidity. If such a study is negative, then perhaps a reassessment of the appropriate metabolic surgery use would be required.

NONSURGICAL DUODENAL EXCLUSION

An alternative approach would be to duplicate the effects of the gastric bypass or BPD procedure by diverting chyme from the proximal small intestine. The duodenojejunal bypass liner (DJBL) is an endoscopically placed and removable intestinal liner developed to achieve duodenal exclusion and promote significant weight loss beyond a minimal sham. The DJBL is a 60-cm impermeable fluoropolymer device, which, after endoscopic deployment in the proximal duodenum, functions to prevent partially digested food from contacting the proximal intestine, similar to RYGB but without gastric restriction. Bile and pancreatic secretions pass along the outer wall of the liner and mix with the chyme exiting distal to the liner into the jejunum. Mean weight loss averages approximately 10 kg after 12 weeks with diabetes remission observed in several studies.[99] Most DJBL-related adverse events are mild or moderate in implantation patients. Many of the adverse events occurring within the first 2 weeks likely reflect adaptation to the DJBL. Mild bleeding is an expected adverse event associated with the anchoring of the device in the gastric pylorus.

KEY POINTS SUMMARY

1. Prevention and remission of T2D is a major focus of cardiometabolic care management due to adverse outcomes related to T2D disease and complications.
2. Pharmacological interventions prevent or remit T2D through targeting insulin secretion, insulin action, or visceral obesity.
3. New and emerging pharmacological therapies, such as GLP-1 RAs and dual GIP-GLP-1 RAs show significant promise for T2D prevention or remission given their substantial effect on weight and visceral adiposity.
4. Surgical interventions are mostly focused on visceral obesity, although certain procedures can impact glucose and insulin metabolism very rapidly (within hours to days) long before substantial weight loss occurs.
5. Surgical interventions may remit T2D by up to 95% for malabsorptive procedures, although adverse effects increase with greater weight loss.

REFERENCES

1. Riddle MC, Cefalu WT, Evans PH, et al. Consensus report: definition and interpretation of remission in type 2 diabetes. *Diabetes Med*. 2022;39:e14669.
2. Knowler WC, Barrett-Connor E, Fowler SE, et al. Reduction in the incidence of type 2 diabetes with lifestyle intervention or metformin. *N Engl J Med*. 2002;346:393–403.
3. Diabetes Prevention Program Research Group Long-term effects of metformin on diabetes prevention: identification of subgroups that benefited most in the diabetes prevention program and diabetes prevention program outcomes study. *Diabetes Care*. 2019;42:601–608.
4. Weng J, Li Y, Xu W, et al. Effect of intensive insulin therapy on beta-cell function and glycaemic control in patients with newly diagnosed type 2 diabetes: a multicentre randomised parallel-group trial. *Lancet*. 2008;371:1753–1760.
5. Chen HS, Wu TE, Kuo CS. Long-term glycemic control after 6 months of basal insulin therapy. *Am J Manag Care*. 2014;20:e369–e379.
6. Investigators OT, Gerstein HC, Bosch J, et al. Basal insulin and cardiovascular and other outcomes in dysglycemia. *N Engl J Med*. 2012;367:319–328.
7. Bethel MA, Xu W, Theodorakis MJ. Pharmacological interventions for preventing or delaying onset of type 2 diabetes mellitus. *Diabetes Obes Metab*. 2015;17:231–244.

8. Khetan AK, Rajagopalan S. Prediabetes. *Can J Cardiol*. 2018;34:615–623.
9. Kramer CK, Zinman B, Retnakaran R. Short-term intensive insulin therapy in type 2 diabetes mellitus: a systematic review and meta-analysis. *Lancet Diabetes Endocrinol*. 2013;1:28–34.
10. Keen H, Jarrett RJ, McCartney P. The ten-year follow-up of the Bedford survey (1962-1972): glucose tolerance and diabetes. *Diabetologia*. 1982;22:73–78.
11. Sartor G, Schersten B, Carlstrom S, Melander A, Norden A, Persson G. Ten-year follow-up of subjects with impaired glucose tolerance: prevention of diabetes by tolbutamide and diet regulation. *Diabetes*. 1980;29:41–49.
12. Knowler WC, Sartor G, Melander A, Schersten B. Glucose tolerance and mortality, including a substudy of tolbutamide treatment. *Diabetologia*. 1997;40:680–686.
13. Group NS, Holman RR, Haffner SM, et al. Effect of nateglinide on the incidence of diabetes and cardiovascular events. *N Engl J Med*. 2010;362:1463–1476.
14. Knowler WC, Barrett-Connor E, Fowler SE, et al. Reduction in the incidence of type 2 diabetes with lifestyle intervention or metformin. *N Engl J Med*. 2002;346:393–403.
15. Knowler WC, Fowler SE, et al. Diabetes Prevention Program Research Group 10-year follow-up of diabetes incidence and weight loss in the Diabetes Prevention Program Outcomes Study. *Lancet*. 2009;374:1677–1686.
16. Moin T, Schmittdiel JA, Flory JH, et al. Review of metformin use for type 2 diabetes prevention. *Am J Prev Med*. 2018;55:565–574.
17. Madsen KS, Chi Y, Metzendorf MI, Richter B, Hemmingsen B. Metformin for prevention or delay of type 2 diabetes mellitus and its associated complications in persons at increased risk for the development of type 2 diabetes mellitus. *Cochrane Database Syst Rev*. 2019;12:CD008558.
18. Decker M, Hofflich H, Elias AN. Thiazolidinediones and the preservation of beta-cell function, cellular proliferation and apoptosis. *Diabetes Obes Metab*. 2008;10:617–625.
19. Bell DS. Beta-cell rejuvenation with thiazolidinediones. *Am J Med*. 2003;115(Suppl 8A):20S–23S.
20. Gastaldelli A, Ferrannini E, Miyazaki Y, Matsuda M, Mari A, DeFronzo RA. Thiazolidinediones improve beta-cell function in type 2 diabetic patients. *Am J Physiol Endocrinol Metab*. 2007;292:E871–E883.
21. Robertson RP, Harmon J, Tran PO, Poitout V. Beta-cell glucose toxicity, lipotoxicity, and chronic oxidative stress in type 2 diabetes. *Diabetes*. 2004;53(Suppl 1):S119–S124.
22. Haffner SM, Greenberg AS, Weston WM, Chen H, Williams K, Freed MI. Effect of rosiglitazone treatment on nontraditional markers of cardiovascular disease in patients with type 2 diabetes mellitus. *Circulation*. 2002;106:679–684.
23. Hanley AJ, Zinman B, Sheridan P, Yusuf S, Gerstein HC. Diabetes Reduction Assessment with R and Rosiglitazone Medication I. Effect of rosiglitazone and ramipril on {beta}-cell function in people with impaired glucose tolerance or impaired fasting glucose: the DREAM trial. *Diabetes Care*. 2010;33:608–613.
24. Investigators DT, Gerstein HC, Yusuf S, et al. Effect of rosiglitazone on the frequency of diabetes in patients with impaired glucose tolerance or impaired fasting glucose: a randomised controlled trial. *Lancet*. 2006;368:1096–1105.
25. Goldberg RB. The new clinical trials with thiazolidinediones—DREAM, ADOPT, and CHICAGO: promises fulfilled? *Curr Opin Lipidol*. 2007;18:435–442.
26. DeFronzo RA, Tripathy D, Schwenke DC, et al. Pioglitazone for diabetes prevention in impaired glucose tolerance. *N Engl J Med*. 2011;364:1104–1115.
27. Hirukawa H, Hashiramoto M, Tanizawa Y, Kaku K. Pioglitazone, Sulfonylurea Remission from Type 2 Diabetes M and Anti-Atherosclerosis in Japan Study Group Remission of hyperglycemia after withdrawal of oral antidiabetic drugs in Japanese patients with early-stage type 2 diabetes. *J Diabetes Investig*. 2018;9:1119–1127.
28. Ipsen EO, Madsen KS, Chi Y, et al. Pioglitazone for prevention or delay of type 2 diabetes mellitus and its associated complications in people at risk for the development of type 2 diabetes mellitus. *Cochrane Database Syst Rev*. 2020;11:CD013516.
29. DeFronzo RA, Abdul-Ghani MA. Preservation of beta-cell function: the key to diabetes prevention. *J Clin Endocrinol Metab*. 2011;96:2354–2366.
30. Wilding JPH, Batterham RL, Calanna S, et al. Once-weekly semaglutide in adults with overweight or obesity. *N Engl J Med*. 2021;384:989–1002.
31. Davies M, Faerch L, Jeppesen OK, et al. Semaglutide 2.4 mg once a week in adults with overweight or obesity, and type 2 diabetes (STEP 2): a randomised, double-blind, double-dummy, placebo-controlled, phase 3 trial. *Lancet*. 2021;397:971–984.
32. Frias JP, Davies MJ, Rosenstock J, et al. Tirzepatide versus semaglutide once weekly in patients with type 2 diabetes. *N Engl J Med*. 2021;385:503–515.
33. Rosenstock J, Wysham C, Frias JP, et al. Efficacy and safety of a novel dual GIP and GLP-1 receptor agonist tirzepatide in patients with type 2 diabetes (SURPASS-1): a double-blind, randomised, phase 3 trial. *Lancet*. 2021;398:143–155.
34. Del Prato S, Kahn SE, Pavo I, et al. Tirzepatide versus insulin glargine in type 2 diabetes and increased cardiovascular risk (SURPASS-4): a randomised, open-label, parallel-group, multicentre, phase 3 trial. *Lancet*. 2021;398:1811–1824.
35. Rosenstock J, Vazquez L, Del Prato S, et al. Achieving normoglycemia with tirzepatide: analysis of SURPASS 1-4 trials. *Diabetes Care*. 2023;46:1986–1992.
36. Neeland IJ, Marso SP, Ayers CR, et al. Effects of liraglutide on visceral and ectopic fat in adults with overweight and obesity at high cardiovascular risk: a randomised, double-blind, placebo-controlled, clinical trial. *Lancet Diabetes Endocrinol*. 2021;9:595–605.
37. Astrup A, Rossner S, Van Gaal L, et al. Effects of liraglutide in the treatment of obesity: a randomised, double-blind, placebo-controlled study. *Lancet*. 2009;374:1606–1616.
38. Santilli F, Simeone PG, Guagnano MT, et al. Effects of liraglutide on weight loss, Fat Distribution, and beta-cell function in obese subjects with prediabetes or early type 2 diabetes. *Diabetes Care*. 2017;40:1556–1564.
39. le Roux CW, Astrup A, Fujioka K, et al. 3 years of liraglutide versus placebo for type 2 diabetes risk reduction and weight management in individuals with prediabetes: a randomised, double-blind trial. *Lancet*. 2017;389:1399–1409.
40. Jastreboff AM, Kaplan LM, Frias JP, et al. Retatrutide Phase 2 Obesity Trial Investigators Triple-hormone-receptor agonist retatrutide for obesity—A phase 2 trial. *N Engl J Med*. 2023;389:514–526.
41. Rosenstock J, Frias J, Jastreboff AM, et al. Retatrutide, a GIP, GLP-1 and glucagon receptor agonist, for people with type 2 diabetes: a randomised, double-blind, placebo and active-controlled, parallel-group, phase 2 trial conducted in the USA. *Lancet*. 2023;402:529–544.
42. Sanyal AJ, Bedossa P, Fraessdorf M, et al. 1404-0043 Trial Investigators A phase 2 randomized trial of survodutide in MASH and fibrosis. *N Engl J Med*. 2024.
43. Loomba R, Hartman ML, Lawitz EJ, et al. Tirzepatide for metabolic dysfunction-associated steatohepatitis with liver fibrosis. *N Engl J Med*. 2024
44. Wharton S, Blevins T, Connery L, et al. Daily oral GLP-1 receptor agonist orforglipron for adults with obesity. *N Engl J Med*. 2023;389:877–888.
45. Knop FK, Aroda VR, do Vale RD, et al. Oral semaglutide 50 mg taken once per day in adults with overweight or obesity (OASIS 1): a randomised, double-blind, placebo-controlled, phase 3 trial. *Lancet*. 2023;402:705–719.
46. Veniant MM, Lu SC, Atangan L, et al. A GIPR antagonist conjugated to GLP-1 analogues promotes weight loss with improved metabolic parameters in preclinical and phase 1 settings. *Nat Metab*. 2024;6:290–303.
47. Rossetti L, Shulman GI, Zawalich W, DeFronzo RA. Effect of chronic hyperglycemia on in vivo insulin secretion in partially pancreatectomized rats. *J Clin Invest*. 1987;80:1037–1044.
48. Neeland IJ MD, Chilton B, Crowe S, et al. The sodium glucose cotransporter 2 inhibitor empagliflozin reduces weight and markers of visceral adiposity in type 2 diabetes in short and intermediate term. *Circulation*. 2014;130:A16518.
49. Neeland IJ, de Albuquerque Rocha N, Hughes C, Ayers CR, Malloy CR, Jin ES. Effects of empagliflozin treatment on glycerol-derived hepatic gluconeogenesis in adults with obesity: a randomized clinical trial. *Obesity (Silver Spring)*. 2020;28:1254–1262.
50. Rossing P, Inzucchi SE, Vart P, et al. Dapagliflozin and new-onset type 2 diabetes in patients with chronic kidney disease or heart failure: pooled analysis of the DAPA-CKD and DAPA-HF trials. *Lancet Diabetes Endocrinol*. 2022;10:24–34.
51. Faerch K, Blond MB, Bruhn L, et al. The effects of dapagliflozin, metformin or exercise on glycaemic variability in overweight or obese individuals with prediabetes (the PRE-D Trial): a multi-arm, randomised, controlled trial. *Diabetologia*. 2021;64:42–55.
52. Packer M, Anker SD, Butler J, et al. Cardiovascular and renal outcomes with empagliflozin in heart failure. *N Engl J Med*. 2020;383:1413–1424.
53. Anker SD, Butler J, Filippatos G, et al. Empagliflozin in heart failure with a preserved ejection fraction. *N Engl J Med*. 2021;385:1451–1461.
54. Torgerson JS, Hauptman J, Boldrin MN, Sjostrom L. XENical in the prevention of diabetes in obese subjects (XENDOS) study: a randomized study of orlistat as an adjunct to lifestyle changes for the prevention of type 2 diabetes in obese patients. *Diabetes Care*. 2004;27:155–161.
55. Garvey WT, Ryan DH, Henry R, et al. Prevention of type 2 diabetes in subjects with prediabetes and metabolic syndrome treated with phentermine and topiramate extended release. *Diabetes Care*. 2014;37:912–921.
56. Bohula EA, Scirica BM, Inzucchi SE, et al. Effect of lorcaserin on prevention and remission of type 2 diabetes in overweight and obese patients (CAMELLIA-TIMI 61): a randomised, placebo-controlled trial. *Lancet*. 2018;392:2269–2279.
57. Chiasson JL, Josse RG, Gomis R, Hanefeld M, Karasik A, Laakso M. and Group S-NTR. Acarbose for prevention of type 2 diabetes mellitus: the STOP-NIDDM randomised trial. *Lancet*. 2002;359:2072–2077.
58. Kawamori R, Tajima N, Iwamoto Y, Kashiwagi A, Shimamoto K, Kaku K. and Voglibose Ph-3 Study G. Voglibose for prevention of type 2 diabetes mellitus: a randomised, double-blind trial in Japanese individuals with impaired glucose tolerance. *Lancet*. 2009;373:1607–1614.
59. Hu R, Li Y, Lv Q, Wu T, Tong N. Acarbose monotherapy and type 2 diabetes prevention in Eastern and Western prediabetes: an ethnicity-specific meta-analysis. *Clin Ther*. 2015;37:1798–1812.
60. Moelands SV, Lucassen PL, Akkermans RP, De Grauw WJ, Van de Laar FA. Alpha-glucosidase inhibitors for prevention or delay of type 2 diabetes mellitus and its associated complications in people at increased risk of developing type 2 diabetes mellitus. *Cochrane Database Syst Rev*. 2018;12:CD005061.
61. Tabatabaeizadeh SA, Tafazoli N. The role of vitamin D in prevention of type 2 diabetes. A meta-analysis. *Clin Nutr ESPEN*. 2021;41:88–93.
62. Pittas AG, Dawson-Hughes B, Sheehan P, et al. Vitamin D supplementation and prevention of type 2 diabetes. *N Engl J Med*. 2019;381:520–530.
63. Zhang Y, Tan H, Tang J, et al. Effects of vitamin D supplementation on prevention of type 2 diabetes in patients with prediabetes: a systematic review and meta-analysis. *Diabetes Care*. 2020;43:1650–1658.
64. Islam MR, Attia J, Ali L, et al. Zinc supplementation for improving glucose handling in pre-diabetes: A double blind randomized placebo controlled pilot study. *Diabetes Res Clin Pract*. 2016;115:39–46.

65. Jayawardena R, Ranasinghe P, Kodithuwakku W, Dalpatadu C, Attia J. Zinc supplementation in pre-diabetes mellitus: a systematic review and meta-analysis. *Minerva Endocrinol (Torino)*. 2021
66. Yusuf S, Gerstein H, Hoogwerf B, et al. Ramipril and the development of diabetes. *JAMA*. 2001;286:1882–1885.
67. Vermes E, Ducharme A, Bourassa MG, et al. Studies of left ventricular D. Enalapril reduces the incidence of diabetes in patients with chronic heart failure: insight from the Studies Of Left Ventricular Dysfunction (SOLVD). *Circulation*. 2003;107:1291–1296.
68. Braunwald E, Domanski MJ, Fowler SE, et al. Angiotensin-converting-enzyme inhibition in stable coronary artery disease. *N Engl J Med*. 2004;351:2058–2068.
69. Pfeffer MA, Swedberg K, Granger CB, et al. Effects of candesartan on mortality and morbidity in patients with chronic heart failure: the CHARM-Overall programme. *Lancet*. 2003;362:759–766.
70. Julius S, Kjeldsen SE, Weber M, et al. Outcomes in hypertensive patients at high cardiovascular risk treated with regimens based on valsartan or amlodipine: the VALUE randomised trial. *Lancet*. 2004;363:2022–2031.
71. Poirier P, Cornier MA, Mazzone T, et al. American Heart Association Obesity Committee of the Council on Nutrition PA and Metabolism Bariatric surgery and cardiovascular risk factors: a scientific statement from the American Heart Association. *Circulation*. 2011;123:1683–1701.
72. Rubino F, Schauer PR, Kaplan LM, Cummings DE. Metabolic surgery to treat type 2 diabetes: clinical outcomes and mechanisms of action. *Annu Rev Med*. 2010;61:393–411.
73. Arterburn DE, Telem DA, Kushner RF, Courcoulas AP. Benefits and risks of bariatric surgery in adults: a review. *JAMA*. 2020;324:879–887.
74. Jensen MD, Ryan DH, Apovian CM, et al. 2013 AHA/ACC/TOS guideline for the management of overweight and obesity in adults: a report of the American College of Cardiology/American Heart Association Task Force on Practice Guidelines and The Obesity Society. *Circulation*. 2014;129:S102–S138.
75. Tsilingiris D, Koliaki C, Kokkinos A. Remission of type 2 diabetes mellitus after bariatric surgery: fact or fiction? *Int J Environ Res Public Health*. 2019:16.
76. Dixon JB, O'Brien PE, Playfair J, et al. Adjustable gastric banding and conventional therapy for type 2 diabetes: a randomized controlled trial. *JAMA*. 2008;299:316–323.
77. Schauer PR, Kashyap SR, Wolski K, et al. Bariatric surgery versus intensive medical therapy in obese patients with diabetes. *N Engl J Med*. 2012
78. Mingrone G, Panunzi S, De Gaetano A, et al. Bariatric surgery versus conventional medical therapy for type 2 diabetes. *N Engl J Med*. 2012;366:1577–1585.
79. Nudotor RD, Prokopowicz G, Abbey EJ, Gonzalez A, Canner JK, Steele KE. Comparative effectiveness of Roux-en Y gastric bypass versus vertical sleeve gastrectomy for sustained remission of type 2 diabetes mellitus. *J Surg Res*. 2021;261:407–416.
80. Borgeraas H, Hofso D, Hertel JK. and Hjelmesaeth J. Comparison of the effect of Roux-en-Y gastric bypass and sleeve gastrectomy on remission of type 2 diabetes: a systematic review and meta-analysis of randomized controlled trials. *Obes Rev*. 2020;21:e13011.
81. Castellana M, Procino F, Biacchi E, et al. Roux-en-Y gastric bypass vs sleeve gastrectomy for remission of type 2 diabetes. *J Clin Endocrinol Metab*. 2021;106:922–933.
82. Eskandaros MS. Antrum preservation versus antrum resection in laparoscopic sleeve gastrectomy with effects on gastric emptying, body mass index, and type II diabetes remission in diabetic patients with body mass index 30-40 kg/m(²): a randomized controlled study. *Obes Surg*. 2022;32:1412–1420.
83. Verhoeff K, Mocanu V, Zalasky A, et al. Evaluation of metabolic outcomes following SADI-S: a systematic review and meta-analysis. *Obes Surg*. 2022;32:1049–1063.
84. Cohen RV, Pereira TV, Aboud CM, et al. Effect of gastric bypass vs best medical treatment on early-stage chronic kidney disease in patients with type 2 diabetes and obesity: a randomized clinical trial. *JAMA Surg*. 2020;155:e200420.
85. Courcoulas AP, Belle SH, Neiberg RH, et al. Three-year outcomes of bariatric surgery vs lifestyle intervention for type 2 diabetes mellitus treatment: a randomized clinical trial. *JAMA Surg*. 2015;150:931–940.
86. Stenberg E, Olbers T, Cao Y, et al. Factors determining chance of type 2 diabetes remission after Roux-en-Y gastric bypass surgery: a nationwide cohort study in 8057 Swedish patients. *BMJ Open Diabetes Res Care*. 2021:9.
87. Sjoholm K, Carlsson LMS, Taube M, le Roux CW, Svensson PA, Peltonen M. Comparison of preoperative remission scores and diabetes duration alone as predictors of durable type 2 diabetes remission and risk of diabetes complications after bariatric surgery: a post hoc analysis of participants from the Swedish Obese Subjects Study. *Diabetes Care*. 2020;43:2804–2811.
88. Sjostrom L, Lindroos AK, Peltonen M, et al. Swedish Obese Subjects Study Scientific Group. Lifestyle, diabetes, and cardiovascular risk factors 10 years after bariatric surgery. *N Engl J Med*. 2004;351:2683–2693.
89. Buchwald H, Avidor Y, Braunwald E, et al. Bariatric surgery: a systematic review and meta-analysis. *JAMA*. 2004;292:1724–1737.
90. Buchwald H, Estok R, Fahrbach K, et al. Weight and type 2 diabetes after bariatric surgery: systematic review and meta-analysis. *Am J Med*. 2009;122:248–256. e5.
91. Campbell RK, Martin TM. The chronic burden of diabetes. *Am J Manag Care*. 2009;15:S248–S254.
92. Klein S, Ghosh A, Cremieux PY, Eapen S, McGavock TJ. Economic impact of the clinical benefits of bariatric surgery in diabetes patients with BMI >/=35 kg/m(2). *Obesity (Silver Spring)*. 2011;19:581–587.
93. Sampalis JS, Liberman M, Auger S, Christou NV. The impact of weight reduction surgery on health-care costs in morbidly obese patients. *Obes Surg*. 2004;14:939–947.
94. Laferrere B, Pattou F. Weight-independent mechanisms of glucose control after Roux-en-Y gastric bypass. *Front Endocrinol (Lausanne)*. 2018;9:530.
95. Aminian A, Zajichek A, Arterburn DE, et al. Association of metabolic surgery with major adverse cardiovascular outcomes in patients with type 2 diabetes and obesity. *JAMA*. 2019;322:1271–1282.
96. Naslund E, Stenberg E, Hofmann R, et al. Association of metabolic surgery with major adverse cardiovascular outcomes in patients with previous myocardial infarction and severe obesity: a nationwide cohort study. *Circulation*. 2021;143:1458–1467.
97. Doumouras AG, Wong JA, Paterson JM, et al. Bariatric surgery and cardiovascular outcomes in patients with obesity and cardiovascular disease: a population-based retrospective cohort study. *Circulation*. 2021;143:1468–1480.
98. Schauer PR, Nissen SE. After 70 years, metabolic surgery has earned a cardiovascular outcome trial. *Circulation*. 2021;143:1481–1483.
99. Tarnoff M, Rodriguez L, Escalona A, et al. Open label, prospective, randomized controlled trial of an endoscopic duodenal-jejunal bypass sleeve versus low calorie diet for pre-operative weight loss in bariatric surgery. *Surg Endosc*. 2009;23:650–656.

5 Type 1 Diabetes: Pathophysiology and Treatment Considerations for Cardiovascular Risk and Disease

KALIE L. TOMMERDAHL AND PETTER BJORNSTAD

INTRODUCTION

Type 1 diabetes (T1D) is one of the most prevalent chronic diseases of childhood, affecting more than 8.4 million people worldwide, 1.5 million of which are children.[1] Over the past 50 years, the incidence of T1D in children has increased at a rapid rate of up to 5% per year worldwide, with a doubling in prevalence seen approximately every 20 years.[2] The lifetime risk of developing T1D now exceeds 1% in North America and Europe. Whereas T1D only accounts for 5% to 20% of diabetes, it is associated with higher per person morbidity, mortality, and healthcare costs than type 2 diabetes (T2D).[3]

The incidence of T1D is trimodal and peaks at the ages of 2, 4 to 6, and 10 to 14 years. This pattern is hypothesized to be secondary to changes in trends of infections and increased insulin resistance of puberty. While children are most visibly affected, half of individuals with T1D are diagnosed after age 20 years. There is generally an equal male-to-female distribution of T1D; however, a slight male predominance has been reported in high-risk populations and a slight female predominance in low-risk ethnic groups.[4] Many factors are hypothesized to contribute to the autoimmune destruction of β-cells in T1D that results in progressive insulin deficiency, including genetic and environmental factors such as gestational environment, dietary intake, stressful life events, and infectious triggers.

Etiology

The etiology of T1D has still not been fully elucidated, but it is likely that both genetic and environmental factors contribute to the autoimmune destruction of pancreatic β-cells.[5]

PATHOGENESIS OF TYPE 1 DIABETES

T1D is characterized by a long preclinical period of autoimmune attack on the pancreatic β-cells, carried out by autoreactive T-cells and marked by the emergence of noncytopathic antibodies. The process appears to start as a loss of tolerance to β-cell autoantigens in genetically susceptible individuals. Several environmental triggers have also been implicated, yet none have been proven definitively.

The normal pancreas has a large reserve capacity and at least 75% of the functional capacity for the production and release of insulin from the β-cells must be lost before clinically evident T1D develops.[6] Studies of human pancreas cells in individuals with established T1D suggest that while multiple β-cells may be able to survive the autoimmune insult, the remaining β-cells are unable to secrete enough insulin to prevent hyperglycemia. Rodents, in contrast, may generate new β-cell progenitor cells which can assist in the continued production of insulin,[7] but there is no evidence for β-cell regeneration in humans with diabetes.

Selective destruction of pancreatic β-cells, as in the setting of autoimmune reactivity, results in insulinopenia. The impairment in insulin secretion is also partially functional and caused by the inhibition of insulin secretion by cytokines including interleukin-1, tumor necrosis factor–α, tumor necrosis factor–β, and interferon-γ, a finding which has been consistently demonstrated for decades.[8–10]

Autoimmunity

Autoimmunity is considered the hallmark of T1D pathogenesis. It is now generally accepted that T1D arises due to a breakdown in self-tolerance to β-cell-specific autoantigens. Chronic T-cell mediated inflammation of the pancreatic islets results in selective destruction of β-cells and sparing of the α, δ, and pancreatic polypeptide cells.[11–13] However, alternative scenarios are possible such as autoreactive T-cell activation due to molecular mimicry with viral antigens sharing structural features with β-cell antigens, bystander activation, or epitope spreading in the setting of inflammation.[14,15]

Autopsy data have shown that β-cell destruction is due to infiltration of the islets by macrophages, dendritic cells, natural killer cells, and lymphocytes.[16] T-cells are the key players in the autoimmune attack of β-cells, including helper T-cells, cytotoxic T-cells, and regulatory T-cells.[17] Humoral response and autoantibody production do not cause direct β-cell damage, but develop secondary to β-cell damage, and are useful disease markers.

Insulin Resistance

Insulin resistance may also play a role in the pathogenesis of T1D and cannot simply be ascribed to obesity or poor glycemic control. In fact, people with T1D demonstrate higher insulin resistance than people without T1D despite similar adiposity, body fat composition, and high-density lipoprotein cholesterol (HDL-C).[18] Furthermore, significant insulin resistance has been documented in people with T1D with relatively good glycemic control.[18,19] The impairment of glucose utilization and insulin-induced nonesterified fatty acid suppression appears to be largely independent of prevailing glycemic control.[18] The effects of puberty in adolescence on the development of insulin resistance must also be considered as it has been widely demonstrated that insulin resistance is accentuated in the setting of puberty, irrespective of diabetes status.[20–22]

The exact mechanism of insulin resistance in T1D is poorly understood. The most popular hypothesis is that insulin resistance occurs secondary to prolonged exposure to supraphysiologic concentrations of exogenous insulin. Exogenous insulin removes all physiologic fluctuations, circadian rhythms, and oscillations of endogenous insulin and has been shown to be associated with increased ectopic fat accumulation in liver and skeletal muscles, increased oxidative stress, and impaired mitochondrial biogenesis.[23–25] The inability of insulin to suppress adipocyte free fatty acid release causes delivery of high concentrations of free fatty acids to tissues and thereby results in an accumulation of intramyocellular lipids in hepatocytes and skeletal muscle.[18] The ectopically accumulated fat and its catabolites is thought to induce insulin resistance via various signaling pathways, including mitogen-activated protein kinase, protein kinase C, IkB kinases, S6 kinases, and endoplasmic reticulum stress.[26–30]

We now also recognize the importance of insulin resistance in the development of micro- and macrovascular complications secondary to diabetes, possibly via lipotoxicity and tissue hypoxia.[18,31] Estimated glucose disposal rate, as a surrogate marker for insulin resistance, has been shown to predict both hard coronary artery disease endpoints and microvascular complications, including diabetic retinopathy, diabetic neuropathy, and diabetic nephropathy.[32–36]

Environmental Factors

It is well accepted that environmental factors play an important role in the pathogenesis of T1D.[37] Potential mechanisms of environmental effects include direct β-cell toxicity, triggering of β-cell autoimmunity, molecular mimicry, and induction of insulin resistance.

DIETARY FACTORS

Islet autoantibodies may emerge during the first year of life,[38] suggesting that early life exposures may be pivotal. Consequently, infant and childhood dietary factors have been implicated as the vehicle for environmental triggers in the pathogenesis of the disease.[37,39]

Exposure to cow's milk in early neonatal life has received considerable attention in the pathogenesis of T1D.[40,41] In the "Childhood Diabetes in Finland (DiMe)" study, high consumption of cow's milk protein was strongly associated with the emergence of β-cell autoantibodies and progression to clinical T1D in initially unaffected siblings of children with T1D,[42] potentially secondary to a misdirected immune response to bovine serum albumin due to a shared structure with islet protein p69.[43] Alternatively, this process could be due to a higher titer of antibodies to bovine insulin, resulting in immunization to bovine insulin, a molecule that differs structurally from human insulin in only three amino acid positions.[44,45] However, more recent large-scale studies have been inconclusive. The "Trial to Reduce IDDM in Genetically at Risk (TRIGR)" randomized infants at increased risk of T1D to receive either an extensively hydrolyzed formula or a conventional cow milk–based formula and found that weaning to a hydrolyzed formula did not reduce the cumulative incidence of T1D after a median follow-up of 11.5 years.[46] In contrast, early reports have suggested that children who were exclusively breastfed for prolonged periods as infants are at lower risk of developing T1D[47] due to decreased gut permeability and enterovirus infection protection.[48,49] More recent studies have suggested that nonbreastfed children have a higher risk of developing T1D than infants who were breastfed; however, this association seems to be independent from breastfeeding duration.[50]

Gluten has also been incriminated as an important diabetes promoting agent.[51,52] Two prospective studies have shown an association between introduction of cereals in infancy, particularly within the first 3 months of life, and early β-cell autoimmunity,[53,54] possibly secondary to effects of gut and immune system immaturity in at-risk individuals.[39] Yet, delaying gluten exposure until 12 months of age in the "Primary Prevention of Type 1 Diabetes in Relatives at Increased Genetic Risk (BABYDIET)" study was safe but did not cause a substantial reduction in the risk for islet autoimmunity in children at risk.[55]

Vitamin D deficiency has also been implicated as a risk factor for T1D.[56,57] Results reported by a Finnish study found that regular, high-dose vitamin D supplements in infancy were associated with a decreased risk compared with no supplementation.[56] Yet, this could be influenced by additional genetic factors as there is also a striking difference in the annual incidence rate of T1D in the neighboring populations of Finland and Russian Karelia (42/100,000 vs. 7.8/100,000) with no difference reported in the circulating vitamin D concentrations in pregnant women and schoolchildren.[58] The "Diabetes Autoimmunity Study in the Young (DAISY)" found no association between vitamin D intake or 25-hydroxyvitamin D concentrations and islet autoimmunity and T1D in childhood,[59] although multiple vitamin D metabolism polymorphisms have been implicated in the risk of islet autoimmunity and progression to T1D.[60,61]

Omega-3 fatty acids have also been reported to play a protective role in the etiology of T1D and studies have shown that a higher omega-3 fatty acid intake is associated with lower risk of β-cell autoimmunity, particularly in young children.[62]

INFECTIOUS FACTORS

Viruses such as herpesviruses,[63] mumps,[64] rubella, rotavirus,[65] retroviruses,[66] and, in particular, enteroviruses[67–74] have long been implicated in the etiology of T1D. Viruses can initiate autoimmunity by at least four mechanisms: (1) molecular mimicry between viral proteins and autoantigens; (2) release of autoantigens following β-cell cytokine-induced injury; (3) cytokine-induced upregulation of major histocompatibility complexes and costimulatory molecules on antigen-presenting cells, enabling them to present self-peptides in immunogenic form to T-cells; and (4) interference with central and peripheral self-tolerance. Notably, in animal models, viral infections can both promote and diminish autoimmunity[75–78] which may have potential as a future prevention strategy.

Viral infections during childhood may also play a role in the development of immunoregulatory mechanisms which protect against diabetes.[78] The hygiene hypothesis proposes that improved hygiene in the Western world has led to a decline in immunity to common infections and increased incidence of autoimmunity.[79] Put another way, with early infectious exposures, young children build appropriate immune responses to pathogens. This idea is also supported by the findings that daycare attendance in early infancy confers protection against the development of childhood diabetes.[80] The relationship between viral infection and autoimmunity appears to be temporal, as studies have shown that enteroviral infections before weaning are beneficial and infections after are associated with susceptibility to T1D development.[81–83] Vaccinations have not been associated with the development of T1D.[84–87]

OTHER

There are many other environmental factors that have been proposed to be involved in the pathogenesis of T1D. Increased weight gain in infancy has been reported to be an important risk factor[88] but has not been confirmed in larger studies. Children who develop T1D have been shown to be both heavier and taller in infancy than their peers without diabetes.[89] Psychological stress may also constitute a trigger in the etiology of T1D. Children with T1D have been shown to be more frequently exposed to stressful situations than children without diabetes. Psychological stress is particularly frequent in the 2 years preceding T1D diagnosis, and stress-related changes in hormonal and neuronal signals may contribute to the development of T1D in genetically susceptible individuals.[90]

One potential protective factor is the microbiome, as a study in nonobese mice with diabetes demonstrated associations between T1D prevention and probiotic administration.[91] In another study, BioBreeding diabetes-prone rats were given lactobacillus strains isolated from BioBreeding diabetes-resistant rats and showed reduced rates of diabetes development.[92]

EPIDEMIOLOGY OF CARDIOVASCULAR DISEASE IN TYPE 1 DIABETES

Cardiovascular disease is the leading cause of mortality in T1D.[93] Premature arterial stiffening and atherosclerosis develop in people with T1D, and lesions are more diffuse than those found in people without T1D, thus leading to a higher case fatality rate.[94,95] Epidemiologic data from Scotland, Australia, and Finland suggest an 8- to 13-year shorter lifespan in people with T1D compared to their peers without diabetes.[96–98] This decrease in life expectancy is primarily ascribed to cardiovascular disease. Notably, a recent Finnish study showed that the cumulative incidence of cardiovascular disease was 7.4-fold greater in people with T1D compared to those without diabetes.[99] The "EURODIAB IDDM Complications Study," a study of >3200 individuals with T1D from 16 European countries, identified a 9% prevalence of cardiovascular disease in men with T1D and a 10% prevalence in women.[100] Increased diabetes duration and age are significant risk factors for disease progression and an increase in prevalence of cardiovascular disease from 6% in individuals aged 15 to 29 years to 25% in the 45- to 59-year age group has been observed.[100] Furthermore, subclinical cardiomyopathy secondary to diabetes, defined as diabetes-associated changes in the myocardium structure and function in the absence of coronary artery disease, hypertension, or valvular disease, occurs in 19% to 26% of people with T1D and may be related to myocardial fibrosis.[101–103] Silent myocardial ischemia has been found in 24% of asymptomatic individuals >35 years with T1D and 10% of those individuals demonstrated >50% coronary artery stenosis.[104] Although hard outcomes of cardiovascular disease are rarely detected until young adulthood, early markers of cardiovascular disease and pathologic changes typically manifest in adolescence.[105] Additionally, while important advances have been made in the management of microvascular complications in T1D, progress in the reduction of macrovascular complications is lacking.[105] Further, optimization of glycemic control (i.e., hemoglobin A1c <7%) decreases but does not fully abolish the risk of cardiovascular disease in T1D, and achievement of this goal is both difficult to obtain and maintain in adolescence.[106–108] Thus new therapies to mitigate cardiovascular disease in T1D are needed. In this chapter we will review the pathophysiology and treatment considerations for cardiovascular risk and disease in individuals with T1D.

Hyperglycemia

Hyperglycemia is strongly associated with the development of microvascular complications, including diabetic kidney disease, neuropathy, and retinopathy,[109] and higher glycemic concentrations have been directly associated with greater evidence of microvascular complications. The "Diabetes Control and Complications Trial/Epidemiology of Diabetes Interventions and Complications (DCCT/EDIC)" study has shown a consistent beneficial effect of intensive insulin therapy on the development of microvascular complications.[110] DCCT/EDIC has also extended these findings to investigations of macrovascular complications and found a 42% reduction in cardiovascular

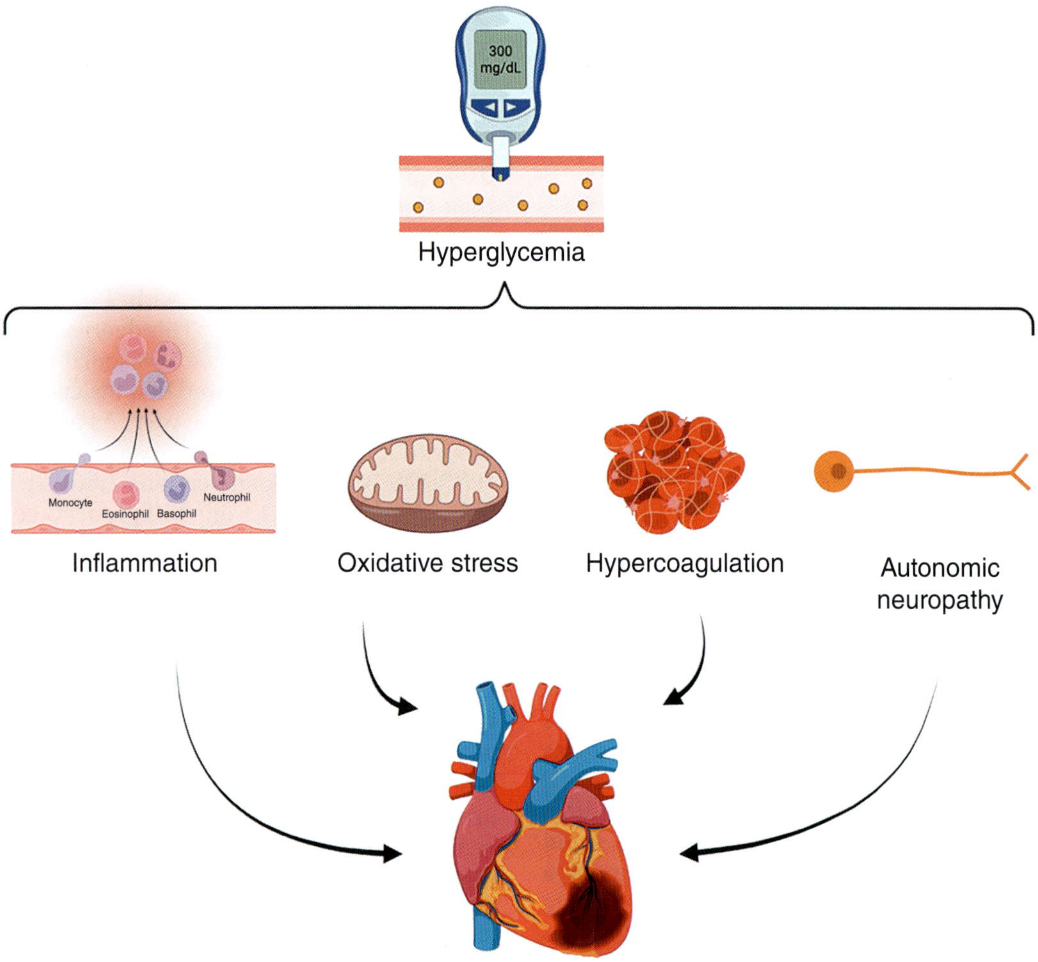

FIG. 5.1 Potential etiologies for the detrimental effects of hyperglycemia on the cardiovascular system.

events and a 57% reduction in the risk for severe clinical events, including myocardial infarction, stroke, or death secondary to cardiovascular disease with intensive insulin therapy when compared to conventional therapy in adults with T1D.[111] In a large Finnish database study, adults aged 45 to 64 years with T1D demonstrated a 50% increase in cardiovascular disease mortality with every 1% increase in hemoglobin A1c, as compared to an only 7.5% increase in adults with T2D.[112]

Hypothesized etiologies for the detrimental effects of hyperglycemia on the cardiovascular system are numerous and include oxidative stress, inflammation, hypercoagulability, and autonomic neuropathy (Fig. 5.1). Hyperglycemia-induced oxidative stress occurs secondary to a combination of factors, such as excess superoxide production and increased nitric oxide generation which leads to the formation of peroxynitrite, a strong oxidant which plays an important role in DNA damage and endothelial cell dysfunction.[113] Inflammatory cytokines, as evidenced by elevated inflammatory markers, including interleukin-6 and interleukin-8, C-reactive protein, endothelin-1, and tumor necrosis factor–α, are also elevated in the setting of hyperglycemia and induce both endothelial cell injury and hypercoagulability, thus contributing to plaque formation and instability.[114] Hypercoagulation poses an additional significant challenge for individuals with T1D as the hyperinsulinemia inherent to all current methods of insulin delivery in T1D results in increased prothrombotic factors including fibrinogen and plasma activator inhibitor-1 from the liver.[115] Counterregulatory fibrinolysis is also decreased in the setting of diabetes.[115]

Additionally, hyperglycemia contributes to the development of cardiac autonomic neuropathy, damage to the autonomic nerves innervating the heart and vasculature, resulting in clinical manifestations that vary from tachycardia and heart rate variability to orthostasis, exercise intolerance, myocardial infarction, and generalized cardiovascular compromise. Cardiac autonomic neuropathy is frequently underdiagnosed in individuals with diabetes and varies in prevalence from 2% to >90% in people with T1D,[116,117] with a high amount of variability due to a lack of consistent diagnostic criteria. The DCCT demonstrated a prevalence of approximately 60% for cardiac autonomic neuropathy in people with T1D of >15 years duration, with a 53% reduction in incidence in individuals undergoing intensive insulin therapy, as compared to conventional therapy.[118] Cardiac autonomic neuropathy has been associated with various cardiovascular disorders including hypertension,[119] increased arterial stiffness,[120] and QT prolongation.[121] Cardiac sympathetic dysinnervation has also been identified on scintigraphy in individuals newly diagnosed with T1D and defects progress with prolonged duration of T1D.[122]

HYPOGLYCEMIA

Yet, with intensive treatment of hyperglycemia also comes an increased risk of hypoglycemia which may play an equally important role in the development of cardiovascular disease in T1D. Due to the potential for severe neurological compromise (i.e., impaired cognition, seizures, coma) in the setting of severe hypoglycemia, the autonomic system activates multiple counterregulatory responses including stimulated release of glucagon and epinephrine and increased gluconeogenesis at the level of the liver to acutely raise blood glucose concentrations and improve blood flow to the brain to prevent neuroglycopenia.[123] Recurrent and severe hypoglycemia can lead to severe damage of cerebral tissues and a fine balance exists between prevention of longstanding hyperglycemia and recurrent hypoglycemia. In animal studies of hypoglycemia, rats exposed to recurrent hypoglycemic episodes exhibited a 44% increase in neuronal death when compared to rats exposed to insulin without hypoglycemia, demonstrating the potential for severe cerebral ischemia in the setting of low blood sugars.[124] Recurrent hypoglycemia has also been directly associated with an increased frequency of brain lesions on MRI in individuals with T1D,[125] as well as detrimental effects on cognitive function which can lead to an increased risk of cardiovascular events and mortality. Further, there is also evidence of structural white and gray matter changes in the brain in adults with T1D who exhibit impaired hypoglycemia awareness.[126]

Euglycemia is also an essential feature of normal cardiac function and hypoglycemic episodes can result in multiple features of cardiac dysfunction, such as a widened pulse pressure with reduction of myocardial perfusion in diastole and ECG changes including QT prolongation with ST changes and arrhythmias.[123,127] Catecholamine release in the setting of hypoglycemia, as well as an imbalance between insulin exposure and available carbohydrates, results in hypokalemia which may further result in ECG changes. These effects are most dangerous overnight in individuals with T1D as the altered mental status of sleep makes it difficult to assess for the effects of hypoglycemia and ensure swift treatment. Cardiac arrhythmias that occur secondary to severe hypoglycemia have resulted in a well-known complication entitled sudden cardiac death during hypoglycemia,[128] a condition that may be preventable with the more widespread use of continuous glucose monitors to alert people with T1D of impending hypoglycemia. Recent studies suggest diurnal differences in individual susceptibility to cardiac arrhythmias, with daytime episodes of acute hypo- and hyperglycemia presenting a greater risk for arrhythmia than nighttime episodes in people with T1D.[129] Lastly, individuals with recurrent hypoglycemia demonstrate greater endothelial dysfunction, as evidenced by flow-mediated dilatation and increased carotid intima-media thickness, an indicator of subclinical atherosclerosis.[130] This effect has been theorized to be more significant in the setting of poorly controlled diabetes of long duration as there is a greater risk of baseline vascular damage.

OBESITY

The incidence of obesity is rapidly increasing in both youth and adults with T1D. Central adiposity, an important risk factor that is worsened by intensive insulin therapy, is increasingly recognized in T1D.[19] The incidence of obesity was recently reported to be 37% in one cohort of adults with newly diagnosed T1D,[131] and 78% of men with T1D in the "Urologic EDIC (UroEDIC)" study were overweight or obese.[132] A similar trend has been observed worldwide[133–135] and also in young persons with T1D.[136–138] This trend is likely secondary to general population factors such as decreased physical activity and sleep and increased high-calorie food consumption, as well as T1D-specific factors such as an overemphasis on carbohydrate counting and/or aggressive insulin management strategies to target euglycemia, the need to treat hypoglycemia with food, disrupted sleep from device alarms and overnight hypoglycemia, and fear of hypoglycemia reducing physical activity. Indeed, the DCCT found that intensive insulin management improved glycemia and complications in T1D; however, it also resulted in weight gain, central adiposity, hypertension, dyslipidemia, and generalized inflammation, all factors associated with diabetic kidney disease and cardiovascular disease.[139,140]

DYSLIPIDEMIA

T1D is characterized by a distinct lipid profile including elevated triglycerides and a low HDL-C concentration which is exacerbated by elevated insulin resistance,[141] a finding that is shared with T2D. Adults with poorly controlled T1D exhibit increased triglyceride-rich lipoproteins and low-density lipoprotein cholesterol (LDL-C) particles, with a shift towards the more atherogenic small, dense LDL-C,[142] a finding that is also exhibited in youth with T1D.[143] Impaired cholesterol metabolism is also an important feature of T1D and youth with T1D demonstrate impaired fatty acid oxidation, increased free fatty acid uptake, and increased lipid accumulation in a variety of organ systems.[144] Insulin therapy and good glycemic control can help lower LDL-C and raise HDL-C concentrations,[143] improve lipoprotein concentrations,[145] reduce the rate of LDL-C production,[146] and improve lipid transfers.[147]

Although total LDL-C concentrations are often within the normal range in people with T1D, LDL-C remains a significant predictor of cardiovascular disease risk. LDL-C particles in T1D are increasingly pathogenic as they are smaller, denser particles than those found in healthy controls and are more prone to entry, oxidation, and retention in the arterial wall,[142] which may contribute to the development of early atherosclerosis. In fact, extensive evidence implicates the oxidation of LDL-C as a major player in atherosclerosis which may be compounded by the negative effects of hyperglycemia and other aspects inherent to diabetes that promote altered redox balance and increased oxidative stress. An intriguing more recent finding in this field has been the identification of autoantibodies to oxidized LDL-C which may be involved in atherosclerosis and coronary calcification, particularly in T1D.[148,149]

Central adiposity may further promote dyslipidemia, including the development of secondary factors such as increased generalized inflammation and inflammation localized to the adipose tissue, as well as through the development of higher free fatty acid concentrations.[150] Hypertriglyceridemia of diabetes involves changes in both the production and degradation of lipids, including a higher hepatic secretion of triglyceride-rich lipoproteins such as very low-density lipoproteins (VLDLs) and altered hydrolysis of these and other triglyceride-rich lipoproteins.[151–153] Another potential component of hypertriglyceridemia may be postprandial triglyceride excursions, which may be more predictive of cardiovascular disease risk than fasting triglyceride concentrations usually obtained in clinic settings for dyslipidemia screening.[154,155]

Lipoprotein lipase, a key enzyme involved in hydrolyzing fatty acids from triglycerides and delivering these fatty acids to tissues, may also be defective in T1D in a similar fashion as T2D. Notably, lipoprotein lipase-mediated hydrolysis of triglycerides has been identified as a mechanism for generating natural ligands for the nuclear receptor known as peroxisome proliferator-activated receptor alpha (PPAR-α), which, when activated by ligands, controls the expression of multiple genes involved in lipid metabolism, inflammation, and fatty acid oxidation.[156–158]

Hepatic dysregulation, a consequence of hyperinsulinemia and hyperglycemia,[159] may also impact lipid metabolism through the glycation of proteins and lipoproteins. In addition to altering the normal function of these entities, the breakdown of glycated proteins and lipoproteins, known as advanced glycation end products (AGEs), activates specific receptors for AGEs (RAGEs), resulting in responses closely linked to atherosclerotic complications, such as increases in matrix metalloproteinases thought to promote plaque destabilization and rupture.[160,161]

HDL-C concentrations are inversely associated with coronary heart disease risk and significant effort has been applied to elucidating the mechanisms underlying the low HDL-C commonly observed in people with diabetes.[162,163] Both abnormal production of HDL-C and remodeling of this lipid by plasma enzymes may contribute to the low concentration of circulating HDL-C observed in people with T1D. Expression and activity of endothelial lipase, a phospholipase that is synthesized in and expressed on the surface of vascular endothelium, catabolizes HDL-C, resulting in decreased concentrations of this putatively antiatherogenic lipoprotein. Elevated concentrations of endothelial lipase protein are significantly correlated with coronary artery calcification score as well as other features of metabolic syndrome including waist circumference, blood pressure, triglycerides, HDL-C, and fasting glucose in individuals with a family history of premature coronary heart disease.[164] In addition, direct correlations have been observed between endothelial lipase levels and circulating markers of inflammation including high-sensitivity C-reactive protein, interleukin-6, and soluble intercellular adhesion molecule. Low-dose endotoxemia in 20 research participants increased endothelial lipase concentrations 12 to 16 hours after injection, and this increase in endothelial lipase correlated with reductions in plasma HDL-C.[165–167]

Collectively these data suggest that low-intensity, generalized inflammation, a common feature of both T1D and T2D, controls HDL-C through effects on endothelial lipase, providing a possible mechanism for the low HDL-C in T1D and the exaggerated cardiovascular risk associated with insulin-resistant states such as T1D. Despite the clear epidemiologic inverse association between HDL-C and cardiovascular risk, the hypothesis that raising HDL-C can reduce cardiovascular events has not yet been proven. The recent failure of large randomized, placebo-controlled trials designed to test this hypothesis using cholesteryl ester transfer protein inhibitors and niacin, which both raise HDL-C concentrations, suggests that the biology of the athero-protective effects of HDL-C are likely very complex and cannot be ascribed exclusively to a single parameter such as HDL-C quantity, the current clinically monitored lipid parameter.[168,169]

The "Pittsburgh Epidemiology of Diabetes Complications Study," a 10-year prospective study in adults with T1D of childhood onset (<17 years of age), further identified strong relationships between elevated LDL-C, elevated triglycerides, and low HDL-C with both mortality and coronary artery disease in T1D (RR 1.8–12.1 for LDL-C >100 mg/dL, 2.0–7.1 for triglycerides >150 mg/dL, 0.4–0.7 for HDL-C <45 mg/dL).[170] Based on these results, it is recommended that the treatment goals for adults with T1D should be LDL-C <100 mg/dL (2.6 mmol/L), HDL cholesterol >45 mg/dL (1.1 mmol/L), and triglycerides <150 mg/dL (1.7 mmol/L)[170] to reduce long-term risk of cardiovascular disease.

INSULIN RESISTANCE

Insulin resistance is common in T1D and occurs independently from hyperglycemia. In studies using gold standard hyperinsulinemic-euglycemic clamps, both normal weight youth and adults with T1D demonstrate substantial whole body insulin resistance compared to their peers without diabetes of similar age and body mass index (BMI), and the degree of insulin resistance did not relate to hyperglycemia but instead related to hypoglycemia assessed via continuous glucose monitor, thus supporting the use of agents that may lessen hypoglycemia.[18,19,171] Moreover, normal weight youth and adults with T1D also have adipose-specific insulin resistance, as evidenced by failure to suppress free fatty acids during hyperinsulinemia, causing chronic exposure to increased free fatty acids, which can induce muscle insulin resistance and vascular dysfunction, and also exhibit hepatic insulin resistance, contributing to hyperglycemia.[171]

Insulin resistance is also a strong risk factor for cardiovascular disease in T1D. In adolescents with T1D, insulin resistance is associated with increased free fatty acids,[19] a more atherogenic lipoprotein profile, as well as vascular dysfunction, decreased maximal exercise capacity, and increased waist circumference.[172] In the "Coronary Artery Calcification in Type 1 Diabetes (CACTI)" study, skeletal muscle insulin resistance was also associated with a higher burden of coronary artery calcification in adults with T1D.[18] Orchard et al. have also demonstrated that insulin resistance, but not glycemia, was associated with higher rates of hard coronary artery disease and mortality in T1D.[19,173] Additionally, insulin resistance has been closely linked with markers of increased proximal vessel stiffness in the thoracic descending aorta on aortic MRI in adolescents with T1D.[174] In the "SEARCH for Diabetes in Youth" study, elevated estimated insulin resistance associated with arterial stiffness.[175] Thus insulin resistance may be a distinct metabolic complication of T1D that contributes to multiple aspects of cardiovascular disease risk, independent of glycemic control.

INFLAMMATION

Inflammation plays a key role in the progression of cardiovascular disease and T1D is closely associated with chronic systemic inflammation and macrophage reprogramming.[176] Atherosclerosis is also strongly driven by chronic inflammation. Significant inflammatory cell infiltrates have been found in atherosclerotic plaques[177] and proinflammatory cytokines released by macrophages lead to endothelial dysfunction and microcalcifications.[178] Systemic markers of inflammation (e.g., highly sensitive C-reactive protein) are strong predictors of future cardiovascular events.[179] Two of the greatest contributors to cardiovascular disease are the development of vascular endothelial dysfunction, most commonly assessed as brachial artery flow-mediated dilation (FMD_{BA}), and stiffening of the aorta and carotid arteries.[180]

Considerable evidence now points to chronic, low-grade inflammation as a factor for initiation and perpetuation of atherothrombosis and insulin resistance. In the "Physicians' Health Study" (n = 22,000 men) and the "Women's Health Study" (n = 38,000 women), the relative risk of future myocardial ischemia, stroke, and cardiovascular death in these otherwise healthy individuals at baseline was linearly associated with highly sensitive C-reactive protein across the normal range (≤3 mg/L).[181,182] Furthermore, this relationship was evident even after controlling for other risk factors. Similar findings have since been validated in other large cohorts, with only a few controversial exceptions. In a cross-sectional study of 48 people with T1D and 66 people without T1D from the DCCT, significantly higher concentrations of acute-phase proteins including alpha$_1$-acid glycoprotein and highly sensitive C-reactive protein were found in those with diabetes.[183] Other circulating inflammatory biomarkers including interleukin-6, matrix metalloproteinase-9, pentraxin-3, lipoprotein-associated phospholipase A_2, and soluble adhesion molecules have demonstrated similar results for predicting cardiovascular disease risk, albeit with different magnitudes and variable usefulness as clinical tools.[184,185] These results suggest that the clinical observations regarding highly sensitive C-reactive protein may reflect inflammatory responses in the vasculature.

Inflammatory changes have also been found in both adipose tissue and pancreatic β-cells, which may relate to subsequent development of insulin resistance and potential β-cell failure.[186] Notably, infiltration of visceral adipose tissue by macrophages and other leukocytes has been shown to contribute to the systemic proinflammatory state observed in insulin resistance. Moreover, studies with salicylates, thiazolidinediones, and other agents have raised the question of whether treating systemic inflammation can improve insulin resistance and ultimately the course of diabetes itself.[187] Hence, treatments that target chronic inflammation may have a significant impact on cardiovascular disease outcomes in T1D, but this has not yet been definitively proven.

ENDOTHELIAL DYSFUNCTION

The endothelium, a single cell layer lining the entire vascular tree, serves as a dynamic, reactive organ engaged in endocrine, paracrine, and autocrine function which also assists the body as a transducer of circulatory components including mediators of disease risk such as glucose, free fatty acids, and pathogenic lipoproteins. As the physical barrier separating flowing blood from the vessel wall, the endothelium is uniquely positioned to control homeostatic processes including blood pressure, hemostasis, and homing of immune cells to sites of inflammation. When dysregulated, each of these processes can contribute to the development of atherosclerosis and have been especially implicated in atherosclerosis secondary to diabetes.

The control of vascular resistance by the endothelium is essential for maintaining mean arterial pressure and autoregulating flow regionally to different tissues depending on metabolic demands. Endothelial cells synthesize nitric oxide from L-arginine by the action of the Ca^{2+}-dependent, endothelial-specific nitric oxide synthase isoform in response to changes in blood flow.[188] Once formed, nitric oxide activates soluble guanylate cyclase located in adjacent vascular smooth muscle cells, leading to increased cyclic guanosine monophosphate levels, smooth muscle cell relaxation, and functional vasodilation. This process is dependent on intact vascular endothelium and is a defining feature of normal endothelial function.[189,190] Endothelial dysfunction, among the earliest features of atherosclerosis, particularly in atherosclerosis due to diabetes and insulin resistance, manifests as loss of flow-mediated vasodilation, which can be measured noninvasively by brachial artery ultrasound. Endothelial cells produce other important vasoactive mediators, including prostacyclin and endothelium-derived hyperpolarizing factor, that couple tissue blood flow to metabolic demands. In response to stimuli, including proinflammatory cytokines, the vascular endothelium also elaborates vasoconstrictors, including endothelin-1, angiotensin-II, thromboxane A_2, and isoprostanes, that increase vascular tone, permeability, hemostasis, and inflammation. The balance of these vasodilator and vasoconstrictor factors is pivotal for maintaining arteriolar resistance and establishing mean arterial blood pressure. Nitric oxide also reduces platelet aggregation and leukocyte adhesion, thereby suppressing endogenous thrombus formation, maintaining blood rheology, and suppressing leukocyte accumulation in the vessel wall. As discussed further later, extensive evidence implicates shifts in all of these components of normal endothelial function in the setting of diabetes and its associated abnormalities.

In addition to helping control vascular homeostasis, the endothelium also plays a part in host response to inflammation by regulating leukocyte trafficking to sites of injury. Proinflammatory signals including interleukin-1β, tumor necrosis factor–α, and oxidized LDL-C induce endothelial cell expression of genes involved in leukocyte homing and diapedesis, a multistep and orchestrated process collectively known as the *leukocyte adhesion cascade*. The induction of specific endothelial gene networks, composed of key mediators of leukocyte adhesion, such as E-selectin, P-selectin, vascular adhesion molecule-1, and intercellular adhesion molecule-1, along with chemoattractants such as interleukin-8 and monocyte chemoattractant protein-1, coordinates leukocyte rolling, firm adhesion to endothelial cells, and transmigration into the vessel wall.[191] The ability of neutrophils, monocytes, and lymphocytes to attract to local areas of inflammation is vital to host defense during acute inflammatory responses. However, this endothelial activation becomes maladaptive in chronic states of inflammation, such as atherosclerosis, enabling monocytes or other immune cells to accumulate within the vessel wall and propagate atherosclerotic plaques as well as plaque rupture. Of note, most of the metabolic abnormalities associated with T1D, including hyperglycemia, elevated free fatty acids, hypertriglyceridemia, and hypertension, have all been linked to an activated endothelial state.

Endothelial dysfunction is a defining feature of early atherosclerosis in individuals with T1D[192] and also occurs in the presence of other traditional cardiovascular risk factors such as hypertension and hyperlipidemia.[193,194] Mechanistically, endothelial dysfunction results from a loss of nitric oxide bioavailability, which can occur through impaired production by endothelial nitric oxide synthase or increased degradation. Consequently, the atheroprotective effects of nitric oxide including vasodilation, inhibition of thrombosis formation or aggregation, and suppression of leukocyte adhesion to the vessel wall are lost. There are multiple metabolic derangements common to T1D and metabolic syndrome including insulin resistance, hyperglycemia, high circulating free fatty acid concentrations, and elevated reactive oxygen species that all contribute to loss of nitric oxide and endothelial dysfunction in people with T1D.[19,195,196]

Infusion of free fatty acids has been shown to reduce endothelium-dependent vasodilation in animal models and in humans.[197] Free fatty acids activate protein kinase C, driving signal transduction pathways that reduce nitric oxide production by endothelial nitric oxide synthase.[198] The accumulation of lipids in tissues and cells including free fatty acids, fatty acyl-coenzyme As, and others such as diacylglycerols is termed *lipotoxicity* because of the effect that these lipid mediators have on intracellular signal transduction pathways including insulin. Another major cause of reduced nitric oxide bioavailability is the formation of peroxynitrite (ONOO−) through the reaction of nitric oxide with superoxide anion. High intracellular free fatty acids result in uncoupling of fatty acid oxidation, which increases levels of free radicals such as superoxide anion ($O_2^{-\bullet}$). Normally, superoxide is rapidly removed by scavenging enzymes such as superoxide dismutase. When superoxide anion levels rise, as occurs in people with diabetes in response to elevated free fatty acids and hyperglycemia, peroxynitrite is formed nonenzymatically at high levels. Other enzymes that increase superoxide, including nicotinamide adenine dinucleotide phosphate, reduced form nicotinamide adenine dinucleotide phosphate oxidases, and xanthine oxidases, can also indirectly promote formation of peroxynitrite in the setting of diabetes. Once generated, peroxynitrite fosters endothelial dysfunction and vascular disease in several postulated ways.[199,200] Peroxynitrite can trigger apoptosis and cell death in endothelial cells and vascular smooth muscle cells, induce endothelial adhesion molecule expression, and disrupt the endothelial glycocalyx. In addition, peroxynitrite-dependent oxidation of tetrahydrobiopterin, a critical cofactor for endothelial nitric oxide synthase function, uncouples endothelial nitric oxide synthase, leading to production of superoxide instead of nitric oxide.[201,202] Lastly, reactive oxygen species can enhance proinflammatory gene expression leading to endothelial activation.

Recent preclinical work provides another perspective on endothelial dysfunction, namely that this dysfunction may extend beyond altered vasomotor function to include changes in metabolism. Several recent studies have reported pathway alterations that result in changes in glucose and free fatty acid handling. For example, a loss of PPAR-γ in the endothelium changes lipid metabolism, free fatty acid levels, and adiposity with concomitant changes in insulin sensitivity.[203] Other work has found that regulation of insulin receptor adaptor proteins in the endothelium (IRS1 and IRS2) by the Forkhead box proteins, a family of DNA binding transcription factors that regulate expression of genes involved in growth, proliferation, and metabolism, can mediate atherogenesis. In these studies, deletion of the three genes encoding Forkhead box protein isoforms conditionally in the endothelium protects against atherosclerosis while also promoting hepatic insulin sensitivity.[204,205] By establishing a role for endothelial cells directly in metabolism, these and other studies force a broader definition of what endothelial dysfunction might represent. Furthermore, these observations link to clinical studies which have identified changes in the endothelium as an early and important aspect of diabetes complication development, far earlier than clinically evident atherosclerosis.

Further evaluation of the effects of T1D on endothelial function is contingent on advancing our ability to measure endothelial function, either invasively in the cardiac catheterization laboratory or noninvasively with techniques such as brachial artery ultrasound. These techniques build on the seminal observation that after removal of the endothelium in arterial preparations, the normal vasodilatory response to substances such as acetylcholine becomes paradoxical, resulting in vasoconstriction.[190] Quantitative coronary angiography can document the change in vascular diameter in response to acetylcholine (or bradykinin, substance P, or serotonin). In people with endothelial dysfunction, the vasodilator response to acetylcholine is blunted or results in paradoxical vasoconstriction. In brachial artery ultrasound, forearm blood flow is occluded for 5 minutes with use of a sphygmomanometer and subsequently maintained at constant pressure. After release of the cuff, reactive hyperemia ensues, leading to endothelium-dependent, flow-mediated nitric oxide production and vasodilation, measured by an increase in artery diameter on ultrasound. In individuals with endothelial dysfunction, these responses are severely blunted.

ENDOTHELIAL ADHESION AND INFLAMMATION

Endothelial dysfunction is also associated with increased adhesiveness of the endothelium. Indeed, the induction of vascular cell adhesion molecule–1 (VCAM-1) messenger RNA and VCAM-1 protein in vascular endothelial cells is one of the earliest molecular events in experimental models of atherosclerosis such as the Watanabe heritable hyperlipidemic rabbit model.[206,207] In humans, adhesion molecule expression can also be detected in atherosclerotic plaques, and circulating levels of soluble adhesion molecules such as VCAM-1 and intracellular adhesion molecule–1 (ICAM-1) positively predict future risk of cardiovascular disease.[185] Aortic endothelium from genetic models of hyperlipidemia such as the LDL receptor null mouse supports greater leukocyte rolling and firm adhesion of leukocytes, as determined by mononuclear cell adhesion assays versus aortas from animals with normal lipid concentrations.[208] Studies in individuals with T1D have shown enhanced in vivo leukocyte activation and platelet-leukocyte aggregation, as well as enhanced in vitro platelet and leukocyte responsiveness to stimulation by agonists.[209] In diabetes, this activation of the endothelium occurs secondary to factors including reduced nitric oxide bioavailability and the chronic proinflammatory state within the vasculature. Recent work identifies Toll-like receptors as proteins on the surface of endothelial cells and macrophages that bind circulating free fatty acids and propagate signal transduction cascades that promote proinflammatory gene expression in T1D.[210,211] The master transcription factor, nuclear factor-κB, mediates multiple proinflammatory responses, including those in the endothelium, enhancing expression of adhesion molecules and chemoattractant cytokines, or chemokines, that call monocytes to sites of injury.[212] Chemokines such as monocyte chemoattractant protein-1 have been strongly implicated as integral signals in atherosclerosis, particularly diabetic atherosclerosis. Thus one can understand endothelial activation as enabling a series of steps in response to injury, whether as a result of hyperglycemia, elevated free fatty acids, hypertension, smoking, or other noxious stimuli, that promote multiple steps of leukocyte trafficking into the vessel wall.[213] While in other settings such responses are integral to host defenses and healing, in the setting of atherosclerosis such important responses may ultimately prove maladaptive. The influx of leukocytes including monocytes and lymphocytes increases plaque cellularity. Lipid-laden macrophages, termed *foam cells*, phagocytose necrotic cells and free cholesterol in the vessel wall, forming the characteristic atherosclerotic plaque and promoting plaque disruption.[214] Aside from these classic models of atherogenesis, loss of the endothelial cells, known as *superficial erosion*, has been identified as another pathologic mechanism that can also lead to atherosclerotic plaque formation and its complications.[215,216]

Hemodynamic Forces

Early atherosclerotic lesions, known as "fatty streaks," typically form at branch points in the aorta. These regions are characterized by a disturbed blood flow profile that is distinct from the physiologic laminar shear stress in other regions of the aorta. Silver staining of aortic endothelium has revealed that the endothelial cells at these branch points appear irregular in shape, whereas endothelial cells from other regions align in the direction of blood flow. Pioneering research using flow models to study vascular endothelium in vitro has revealed that shear stress forces not only alter endothelial cell shape, but also modulate endothelial cell gene expression, with the identification of gene regulatory regions modulated in response to distinct patterns of flow.[217] Exposure of static monolayers of cultured endothelial cells to physiologic levels of shear stress results in dynamic induction of genes known to suppress atherogenesis including endothelial nitric oxide synthase, superoxide dismutase, catalase, and transforming growth factor-β signaling molecules.[218,219] Endothelial cells exposed to disturbed, nonlaminar shear stress fail to express these athero-protective gene programs. In addition to regulating nitric oxide bioavailability by endothelial nitric oxide synthase and the enzymes involved in reducing reactive oxygen species generation (i.e., superoxide dismutase, catalase), shear stress also alters nuclear factor-κB tissue levels and activation. Confocal microscopy has demonstrated that lesion-prone regions of the aorta, including branch points, are associated with higher levels of nuclear localized, active nuclear factor-κB in the endothelium.[220] In addition, the nuclear factor-κB–dependent transcriptional responses at these branch points are significantly higher when stimulated by low-level, proinflammatory stimuli, including factors common in individuals with hyperglycemia, insulin resistance, and diabetes.[220] Enhanced inflammatory signaling through altered nuclear factor-κB activation and loss of nitric oxide results in heightened endothelial activation and contributes to the endothelial dysfunction observed in early atherosclerosis in the setting of diabetes. Collectively, these studies reveal that hemodynamic forces have broad effects on endothelial function and inflammation that contribute to early atherosclerotic plaque formation. Given the elevated frequency of hypertension in T1D, many of these mechanisms are activated, if not augmented, in people with T1D.

HYPERTENSION

Elevated blood pressure and hypertension are strong risk factors for both microvascular complications and macrovascular complications of diabetes including atherosclerotic cardiovascular disease and heart failure. Atherosclerotic cardiovascular disease, a group of cardiovascular complications including acute coronary syndrome, coronary or arterial revascularization, angina, transient ischemic attack, myocardial infarction, and peripheral arterial disease that develop secondary to atherosclerosis, is the leading cause of morbidity and mortality in people with T1D and T2D[221] and is directly related to elevations in average blood pressure. Notably, numerous studies have demonstrated strong associations with the consistent use of antihypertensive therapy and a reduction in micro- and macrovascular complications, including atherosclerotic cardiovascular disease and heart failure.[222,223]

The American Diabetes Association recommends a goal blood pressure of <140/90 mm Hg for individuals with both diabetes and high blood pressure, with a stricter goal of <130/80 mm Hg for people with additional risk factors that place them at higher risk of cardiovascular disease.[221] Initial antihypertensive treatments include angiotensin-converting enzyme inhibitors (ACEis), angiotensin II receptor blockers

(ARBs), thiazide diuretics, or Ca^{2+} channel blockers, with an emphasis on personalized medicine unless present with other indicators of diabetic kidney disease, when ACEis and ARBs are preferred.[221] Albuminuria and impaired glomerular filtration rate are each independent risk factors for cardiovascular disease; thus it is imperative to target treatment of both hypertension and diabetic kidney disease with complementary medications, if possible.[224]

Stricter blood pressure goals for the prevention of future cardiovascular disease may be indicated in the setting of youth-onset diabetes due to a combination of factors including a more aggressive diabetes phenotype and longer diabetes duration. In the "Pittsburgh Epidemiology of Diabetes Complications Study," a 10-year prospective study in adults with T1D of childhood onset (<17 years of age), the goal blood pressure range for adults with T1D was determined to be a systolic blood pressure <120 mm Hg and a diastolic blood pressure <80 mm Hg due to significantly elevated age-adjusted relative risk for mortality, coronary artery disease, lower extremity arterial disease, diabetic kidney disease, neuropathy, and retinopathy.[170]

TREATMENTS

Current therapies to prevent and treat cardiovascular disease in T1D remain limited. Intensive glycemic control is the only specific therapy known to prevent cardiovascular disease in T1D.[108,225,226] Yet, despite modern advances in glycemic monitoring through continuous glucose monitors and insulin delivery through automated insulin delivery-enabled pumps, euglycemia remains elusive and substantial residual risk remains, requiring complementary therapies.[105] Further, intensive glycemic control in the DCCT was associated with weight gain in a subset of participants, including women, along with worsening insulin resistance, central obesity, lipids, blood pressure, inflammation, and albuminuria, all of which increase cardiovascular disease risk.[139,227–229] Accordingly, further investigation into the use of ancillary medications traditionally used in the treatment of T2D, including metformin, bromocriptine, glucagon-like peptide–1 receptor agonists (GLP1-RAs), sodium glucose cotransporter–2 inhibitors (SGLT2is), and pioglitazone for cardiorenal protection in T1D, is necessary. Blood pressure, lipid, and weight-modifying agents must also be strongly considered as hypertension, dyslipidemia, and obesity are known risk factors for cardiovascular disease.

Glucose-Modifying Agents

Studies to date suggest that mechanisms of kidney and heart damage in T1D may parallel those in T2D, and drugs that target diabetic kidney disease and cardiovascular disease outcomes in T2D may also be beneficial in T1D. Multiple drugs designed to lower blood glucose concentrations in T2D have been found to reduce risks of macrovascular complications in T1D, including metformin, bromocriptine, SGLT2is, and GLP1-RAs.[230–233]

METFORMIN

Metformin is an oral antihyperglycemic agent from the biguanide class that acts through both inhibition of complex 1 in the mitochondrial electron transport chain to activate 5′-adenosine monophosphate-activated protein kinase dependent and independent mechanisms in a tissue-specific manner to produce a variety of effects that are beneficial for individuals with diabetes.[234] Available since the 1950s, metformin remains a first-line therapy for the treatment of T2D due to important systemic effects including inhibition of intestinal glucose absorption, suppression of gluconeogenesis in the liver, reduction of hepatic glucose output, facilitation of glucose uptake into the tissues, and improvement in insulin sensitivity and inflammation.[235] Metformin has been shown to consistently improve body composition and reduce the risk for cardiovascular disease in adults with T2D;[236] yet, less is known about the effects of metformin as an ancillary agent in T1D.

Among 50 participants aged 12 to 21 years with T1D in the randomized, placebo-controlled "Effects of MEtformin on cardiovasculaR function in AdoLescents with type 1 Diabetes (EMERALD)" study, metformin significantly attenuated vascular abnormalities detected with phase-contrast and 4-D flow MRI, including reductions in ascending aorta pulse wave velocity, wall shear stress, and carotid intima-media thickness-assessed atherosclerosis.[237] These findings are clinically significant, as arterial stiffness and carotid intima-media thickness predict mortality in T1D.[238] Additionally, reduced left ventricular contractile efficiency and discoordinated myocardial relaxation were identified in adolescents and young adults with T1D versus healthy controls along with improvements in left ventricular end-systolic and end-diastolic volume, dissynchrony, and longitudinal strain.[239] Moreover, metformin significantly attenuated insulin resistance by hyperinsulinemic-euglycemic clamp.[237] However, it is notable that the effects of metformin on BMI and insulin resistance were modest and glycemia did not significantly improve in T1D. In the "Reversing with Metformin Vascular Adverse Lesions (REMOVAL)" trial, a randomized, double-blind, placebo-controlled study of metformin in 428 adults with T1D with a median follow-up duration of 5 years, atherosclerosis progression, as measured by averaged maximal carotid intima-media thickness, was significantly reduced with metformin (–0.013 mm/year, –0.024 to –0.003 mm/year, $P = .0093$).[240] However, it is notable that the hemoglobin A1c was minimally reduced in the metformin group versus placebo and the effect was not sustained beyond the initial 3-month treatment period.[240] Taken together, the cardioprotective effects of metformin appear to be separate from effects on glycemia and warrant further study.

BROMOCRIPTINE

Bromocriptine, a dopamine agonist that has been widely used in the treatment of both Parkinson's disease and prolactin-secreting adenomas, was approved by the Food and Drug Administration in 2009 for the treatment of T2D in a quick release formulation.[241] Postulated mechanisms for the positive effects of bromocripine quick release on glycemic control in T2D include targeting of the attenuated morning dopaminergic signaling seen in T2D that helps to reset the circadian neuronal activities in the hypothalamus that increase overnight plasma glucose, free fatty acids, and triglycerides.[242] If administered within 2 hours of wakening, bromocriptine quick release is hypothesized to result in a reduction of postprandial glycemia due to suppression of hepatic gluconeogenesis[243] and reduction of sympathetic nervous system and renin-angiotensin system activity and may result in decreased micro- and macrovascular complications.

Bromocriptine quick release warrants further study in the T1D population as the "Cycloset Safety Trial," a study of 1834 people with well-controlled T2D (hemoglobin A1c ≤7.0%) resulted in a 48% reduction in a composite cardiovascular disease endpoint (i.e., first myocardial infarction, stroke, coronary revascularization, or hospitalization for angina/congestive heart failure) after 12 months of treatment in an intention-to-treat analysis.[244] Additionally, bromocriptine quick release reduced the odds of loss of glycemic control (OR: 0.63 [0.47–0.85]) and the need for therapy intensification to maintain a hemoglobin A1c ≤7.0% (OR: 0.46 [0.31–0.69]).[244] Studies evaluating the application of bromocriptine quick release in people with T1D are ongoing. In a study of 40 adolescents and 40 adults with T1D, a 4-week treatment course of bromocriptine quick release titrated to 3.2 mg once daily was associated with a significant decrease in systolic and diastolic blood pressure in the adolescent population with T1D and a decrease in systolic blood pressure, mean arterial pressure, systemic vascular resistance, and orthostatic drop in blood pressure in the adult population with T1D, despite having a minimal overall effect on glycemia or insulin sensitivity.[245] Analyses of the effects of bromocriptine quick release on central aortic stiffness, as evidenced by changes in aortic MRI, are forthcoming and hold promise that bromocriptine quick release may represent a treatment that could target the prevention of cardiovascular disease independent of effects on both glycemia and insulin sensitivity in T1D.

SODIUM GLUCOSE COTRANSPORTER–2 INHIBITORS

Sodium glucose cotransporter-2 inhibitor (SGLT2i) is a glucose transporter expressed primarily in the proximal tubules of the renal cortex that is sodium-dependent and serves as the primary site for glucose reabsorption in the kidney.[246] SGLT2is inhibit this protein and represent a therapeutic target for glycemic control in diabetes while having a low risk of hypoglycemia secondary to an intact compensatory mechanism through the use of the SGLT1 glucose transporter located in the late proximal renal tubules which are unaffected by SGLT2is.[247] Due to the prevention of glucose reabsorption in the kidney, SGLT2is have consistently demonstrated a reduction in hemoglobin A1c, a reduction in total daily insulin dose, and weight loss when compared to placebo,[248–250] which may all translate to prevention against future cardiovascular disease. Treatment with SGLT2is encourages a shift from utilization of carbohydrates for energy to lipids secondary to the reduction of reabsorbed glucose and this results in a combination of lipolysis and weight loss.[251] However, the impact of SGLT2is on insulin resistance and BMI is modest,[252–255] and importantly, SGLT2is are associated with ketogenesis in the setting of lipolysis and thus portend a higher risk of diabetic ketoacidosis in T1D, a potentially fatal complication.[255,256] Consequently, SGLT2is are not frequently considered as adjunctive therapies in T1D, particularly in adolescents with T1D who are at higher risk of diabetic ketoacidosis secondary to increased insulin resistance in the setting of puberty and poor baseline glycemic control. In the recently published "Adolescent Type 1 Diabetes Treatment with SGLT2i for Hyperglycemia and Hyperfiltration (ATTEMPT)" trial, a 22-week, double-blind, randomized, placebo-controlled study of dapagliflozin 5 mg once daily in adolescents with T1D, dapagliflozin was associated with a reduction in measured GFR as well as a 0.47% decrease in hemoglobin A1c and a 9.0% increase in glycemic time in range. Furthermore, adverse events were similar between groups and only one episode of mild diabetic ketoacidosis was reported, demonstrating both safety and efficacy of SGLT2i treatment in adolescents with T1D.[257] Further study of SGLT2is with close attention to frequent screening for ketosis is necessary in youth and adults with T1D is needed. Continuous ketone monitoring also holds promise to mitigate the risk of diabetic ketoacidosis and may facilitate safe use of SGLT2is in T1D.

GLUCAGON-LIKE PEPTIDE–1 RECEPTOR AGONISTS

The L-cells of the distal ileum release an incretin hormone called glucagon-like peptide–1 (GLP-1) in response to ingestion of glucose which binds to a 7-transmembrane G-protein-coupled receptor (GLP-1R) and induces a variety of downstream effects in the pancreas, heart, gastrointestinal tract, and kidneys[258] before being quickly degraded over 2 to 3 minutes by dipeptidyl peptidase-4 (DPP-4).[259] While multiple known beneficial effects of GLP-1 are pancreatic in origin and thus are less likely to be stimulated in T1D (i.e., β-cell proliferation, decreased β-cell apoptosis, postprandial secretion of insulin), multiple gastrointestinal, immune, and kidney effects remain in play in T1D. These effects include postprandial secretion of somatostatin, inhibition of glucagon secretion, decreased gastric emptying and motility, decreased gluconeogenesis and steatosis, increased natriuresis, increased lipolysis and glucose uptake in the adipose and muscle, decreased generalized inflammation, increased muscle perfusion, and increased satiety.[260]

In animal models, GLP-1Rs are not only present in the heart and endothelial tissue,[261–263] but also in the kidney[264] and central nervous system[265] where they may exert direct effects. Consequently, GLP-1RAs hold significant promise in the treatment of diabetes, particularly in the setting of metabolic features including overweight and obesity. Substantial weight loss (i.e., 3–9%) and reduction in insulin resistance have been reported following treatment with GLP-1RAs in adults with T2D.[266,267] Similar weight loss as well as a reduction in fat mass have been demonstrated in adults with T1D in response to the GLP-1RAs exenatide and liraglutide, without increased frequency of hypoglycemia.[268–270] Indeed, liraglutide has been shown to decrease hypoglycemic events in T1D, with no increased risk of diabetic ketoacidosis.[271] In adults with T1D, an infusion of GLP-1 in the setting of both hyperglycemia and hypoglycemia has also resulted in attenuation of systemic inflammation, oxidative stress, and endothelial dysfunction,[272] potentially lessening the risk of inflammation-induced cardiovascular disease and diabetic kidney disease progression. While a study of liraglutide in overweight adults with T1D found no significant effect on carotid intima-media thickness and peripheral pulse wave velocity, carotid intima-media thickness may take considerable time to change, and peripheral measures of arterial stiffness may be insensitive to early hemodynamic changes.[273] Despite their minimal effects on glycemia, GLP-1RAs remain a promising avenue for adjunctive therapy for T1D due to their positive effects on weight, inflammation, and endothelial dysfunction, and further studies of cardiovascular function are needed.

PIOGLITAZONE

Pioglitazone, an oral antihyperglycemic medication from the thiazolidinedione class, works to improve insulin sensitivity through activation of the λ isoform of the peroxisome proliferator-activated receptor to increase peripheral glucose utilization at the level of the muscle, adipose, and liver, and decrease hepatic gluconeogenesis.[274] To date, the effects of pioglitazone on glycemia and weight in T1D are mixed. In a small cohort of 35 pubertal adolescents with T1D, a 6-month course of adjunctive pioglitazone titrated to 30 mg once daily was not associated with a significant difference in hemoglobin A1c or total daily insulin dose when compared to the placebo, but it was associated with a significant increase in BMI z-score (pioglitazone: 0.3 ± 0.3 kg/m² [95% CI, –1.4, +1.9 kg/m²] vs. placebo: 0 ± 0.3 kg/m² [95% CI, –1.4, +1.4 kg/m²], $P = .01$).[275] In contrast, a study in 60 lean (BMI 18–24.9 kg/m²) youth with T1D showed a significant decrease in hemoglobin A1c in the pioglitazone treated group versus placebo after 6 months of therapy (–0.22 ± 0.29 vs. –0.06 ± 0.49, $P = .03$) with no change in body weight, BMI, insulin requirement, blood pressure, or lipids over time.[276] Rosiglitazone, another drug in the thiazolidinedione class, has been associated with a significant decrease in total daily insulin dose (–5.8% vs. –9.4%, $P = .02$) and an increase in serum adiponectin (+0.05 mmol/L vs. 0.0 mmol/L, $P = .02$), but has shown no change in hemoglobin A1c or BMI in adolescents with T1D.[277] Additional cardiovascular effects of adjunctive treatment with thiazolidinediones remain largely unstudied in individuals with T1D and warrant further evaluation.

Blood Pressure Management

ANGIOTENSIN-CONVERTING ENZYME INHIBITORS/ ANGIOTENSIN II RECEPTOR BLOCKERS

ACEis modulate blood pressure by inhibiting the conversion of angiotensin I to angiotensin II at the level of the angiotensin-converting enzyme. Angiotensin II plays an important role in blood pressure regulation through activation of the angiotensin II type 1 receptor which promotes vasoconstriction, sodium and water retention, sympathetic activation, and cell growth.[278] Interestingly, ACEis also prevent activation of the angiotensin II type 2 receptor and inhibit breakdown of bradykinin which both result in incremental vasodilation and antiproliferation.[279] Higher bradykinin concentrations thereby result in increased prostaglandin synthesis and nitric oxide release which have important dilatory effects on the vasculature.[279] ARBs, in contrast, work to displace angiotensin II from the angiotensin II type 1 receptor and in doing so may stimulate the angiotensin II type 2 receptor, thus triggering both vasodilation and natriuresis; however, this effect is considerably less significant than that seen with ACEis.[280] In the setting of T1D and albuminuria, as evidenced by a urine albumin to creatinine ratio ≥30 mg/g, initial treatment should include either an ACEi or an ARB to reduce the risk for progression of diabetic kidney disease as this is a strong risk factor for future cardiovascular disease. In the "ACE Inhibitors in Diabetic Nephropathy Trial," a meta-analysis of 12 trials involving 698 individuals with T1D and microalbuminuria, treatment with an ACEi reduced the odds of progression to macroalbuminuria (i.e., urine albumin to creatinine ratio ≥300 mg/g) (OR 0.38 [95% CI, 0.25–0.57][281]) and increased the odds of regression to normalbuminuria (OR 3.07 [95% CI, 2.15–4.44]), with a significant decrease in urine albumin excretion by 50.5% [95% CI, 29.2–65.5%] in individuals receiving treatment with an ACEi versus placebo ($P < .001$).[281] In the absence of early diabetic kidney disease, treatment with ACEis and/or ARBs for blood pressure modification is equivalent to other antihypertensive agents.[282]

THIAZIDES

Thiazide diuretics promote natriuresis and diuresis through inhibition of the sodium/chloride channel in the proximal segment of the distal convoluted tubule in the nephron, resulting in prevention of up to 3% to 5% reabsorption of luminal sodium.[283] In the "Antihypertensive and Lipid Lowering Treatment to Prevent Heart Attack (ALLHAT)" trial, there was no evidence of treatment superiority with thiazide diuretics versus ACEis versus Ca^{2+} channel blockers for treatment of hypertension in individuals with diabetes, impaired fasting glucose, or normoglycemia.[284] Similar rates of cardiovascular events were also seen in individuals with diabetes receiving treatment with thiazide diuretics when compared to either ACEis or Ca^{2+} channel blockers.[284] However, potential side effects of treatment should be considered when selecting a thiazide diuretic as a primary or secondary agent for blood pressure management. Thiazide diuretics exhibit a well-characterized relationship with hypokalemia[285] due to increased renal potassium excretion as a function of effects on the sodium/chloride channel in the distal convoluted tubule of the nephron. It is estimated that up to 50% of individuals receiving treatment with thiazide diuretics will develop some degree of hypokalemia[286] while on treatment. Additionally, at the level of the β-cells in the pancreas, hypokalemia also causes cellular hyperpolarization and this subsequently results in decreased insulin secretion and potential hyperglycemia.[287] This effect is most important to consider in the setting of T2D and early T1D when residual β-cell function and associated insulin secretion is retained. Furthermore, historical observational studies have proposed an association between diuretic-induced hypokalemia and cardiac arrhythmias,[288–290] although this has not been conclusively proven and is likely a dose-dependent effect.

β-BLOCKERS

The term "β-blockers" refers to a group of drugs which act to block the action of endogenous catecholamines on multiple different types of β-adrenergic receptors which function as a part of the autonomic nervous system.[291] First-generation β-blockers are nonselective and exhibit affinity for both the β1 and β2 receptors (i.e., propranolol) while second-generation β-blockers more selectively block the β1 receptor over the β2 receptor (i.e., atenolol).[292]

Third-generation β-blockers are further advanced and demonstrate more intrinsic vasodilation (i.e., nebivolol).[292] β-blockers have been associated with long-term improvements in both mortality and cardiovascular disease in people with either heart failure or acute myocardial infarction but a reduction in mortality has not been shown in the absence of these conditions. In the "Action to Control Cardiovascular Risk in Diabetes (ACCORD)" trial, cardiovascular event rates in people with T2D on β-blockers were significantly lower in people receiving intensive therapy (i.e., metformin, short- and long-acting insulin, sulfonylureas, acarbose, meglitinides, thiazolidinediones) to target a hemoglobin A1c <6.0% versus people on standard therapy to target a hemoglobin A1c 7.0% to 7.9%.[293] In that same study, targeting a systolic blood pressure of <120 mm Hg did not reduce the rate of a composite cardiovascular outcome after 4.7 years of follow-up as compared to targeting a systolic blood pressure of <140 mm Hg after a mean follow-up of 4.7 years in people with T2D at high risk for cardiovascular disease.[294]

However, β-blockers have been reported to increase the risk for severe hypoglycemia by blunting the adrenergic symptoms that are earliest warning sign of impending hypoglycemia.[295,296] Nonselective β-blockers act on the β2 receptor, thereby blocking catecholamine-induced arterial vasodilation and allowing α-stimulation that is unopposed in the setting of hypoglycemia.[297,298] However, β1-selective blockade in people with diabetes has been shown to prevent the hypoglycemia-induced impairment in autonomic response that follows a hypoglycemic event[299,300] and β-blockers decrease the risk of hypoglycemia-associated cardiac arrhythmias and death.[293] Further studies evaluating the use of β-blockers in individuals with T1D are needed.

Ca^{2+} CHANNEL BLOCKERS

Calcium channel blockers are a group of heterogeneous organic compounds that block the calcium channel, thereby preventing the transit of Ca^{2+} into the cell and thus reducing subsequent cellular excitability. Ca^{2+} channel blockers can be stratified into the following three categories: (1) dihydropyridinic agents which act as vasodilators in the periphery, (2) phenilalchilaminic agents which are cardiac negative inotropes and chronotropes, and (3) benzothiazepinic agents which are intermediate in their action profile.[301] An abundance of randomized controlled trials have demonstrated the safety and efficacy of dihydropyridinic Ca^{2+} channel blockers in the management of hypertension and the prevention of cardiovascular events,[302–304] further supporting the use of Ca^{2+} channel blockers as a first-line therapy in individuals with T1D and an ideal agent in dual and triple combination therapy regimens. However, Ca^{2+} channel blockers have also been shown to have blood pressure–independent effects on glycemic control in people with T1D, particularly in the earliest phase of T1D after diagnosis. In a phase 2, randomized, placebo-controlled trial of individuals with recently diagnosed T1D, administration of a 12-month course of the Ca^{2+} channel blocker verapamil resulted in improvements in area under the curve for a 2-hour mixed-meal tolerance test c-peptide, a marker of endogenous β-cell function, as well as lower insulin requirements and decreased hypoglycemia when compared to placebo.[305] Of note, in this trial, verapamil was not associated with any adverse events or episodes of hypotension.[305] To further evaluate the molecular basis for these glycemic changes in T1D, a study of human islet cells and murine models for T1D showed that verapamil inhibited the expression of proapoptotic β-cell thioredoxin-interacting protein (TXNIP) in human islets and INS-1 cells to improve the survival and function of residual β-cells.[306] Additionally, a global serum proteomics analysis in T1D identified the T1D autoantigen chromogranin A as the primary protein that is altered by verapamil to reduce elevations in circulating proinflammatory T-follicular-helper cell markers, thereby promoting β-cell health and function and delaying T1D progression for the duration of treatment.[307] Consequently, chromogranin A remains a potential therapeutic target to further prevent T1D progression and verapamil may represent an important avenue for both T1D prevention and delay of progression.

Lipid Management

STATINS

Statins primarily work by inhibiting the hydroxymethylglutaryl coenzyme A (HMG-CoA), the first and rate-limiting step of the cholesterol biosynthesis pathway, thereby preventing HMG-CoA from converting into mevalonic acid.[308] Not only does inhibition of this step in the cholesterol biosynthesis pathway result in 20% to 55% reductions in serum LDL-C concentrations, it also upregulates cell surface LDL-C receptor expression to promote LDL-C clearance and may also improve endothelial cell function, decrease generalized inflammation, stabilize atherosclerotic plaques, exhibit antithrombotic effects, and reduce the risk for dementia secondary to inhibition of additional isoprenoid intermediates as a part of the mevalonate pathway.[309]

The American Diabetes Association recommends consideration of moderate-dose statin therapy, in addition to lifestyle modification, for all individuals with T1D aged 40 years and older, and in individuals less than 40 years of age in the setting of cardiovascular risk factors.[310] High-dose statin therapy is recommended for any individual, regardless of age, in the setting of known cardiovascular disease.[310] The American Heart Association mirrors these recommendations and recommends moderate-intensity statin therapy in all individuals with diabetes who are age 40 to 75 years of age and have an LDL-C of ≥70 mg/dL, with a titration to a high-intensity statin to reduce the LDL-C by ≥50% in people with diabetes who are at high risk.[311] T1D is considered a "risk enhancer" for cardiovascular disease for all individuals who have had diabetes for ≥20 years with at least one additional risk factor for cardiovascular disease and initiation of a statin for cardiovascular protection should be considered at an earlier age in this population.[311] Of note, analyses suggest a 22% relative risk reduction in major vascular and coronary artery events with every 38.7 mg/dL (1 mmol/L) reduction in LDL-C in all adults,[312] making initiation and maintenance of statin therapy an excellent tool in the prevention of cardiovascular disease in T1D, despite the risk for potential side effects, including arthralgias, myalgias, myopathy, myositis, rhabdomyolysis, etc.[308]

FIBRATES

Fibrates, lipid-lowering agents used to treat hypertriglyceridemia, are thought to work as PPAR-α agonists.[313,314] Of note, other endogenous lipolytic pathways including adipose tissue triglyceride lipase and hepatic lipase as well as fatty acid synthase can generate PPAR ligands in different physiologic contexts as well.[158,315,316] These lines of evidence suggest that in diabetes, loss of endogenous lipoprotein lipase action decreases activation of the PPAR-α–regulated gene cassette, which would be predicted to result in decreased expression of apolipoprotein (apo) A-I, which is involved in HDL function, and increased endothelial inflammation. It is important to note that fibrates, as synthetic PPAR-α agonists, may not faithfully replicate cellular responses to natural PPAR-α ligands. Of interest, the potential role of lipoprotein lipase has expanded to include other proteins involved in lipoprotein lipase action. For example, apolipoprotein C-III is an endogenous inhibitor of lipoprotein lipase activity. Recent studies implicate apo C-III in promoting proatherogenic, proinflammatory responses, which may occur through various mechanisms, including potential modulation of endogenous PPAR responses, as outlined previously, as well as other means.[317]

SUMMARY

Diabetes is a complex condition with a pathogenesis, like atherosclerosis, that involves multiple different processes and likely represents distinct forms even beyond the typical T1D or T2D designation. The intricacies of this picture are evident in attempts to deconvolute the nature of the vascular biology of atherosclerosis in the setting of diabetes—the factors that drive the disorder, determine outcomes, and provide opportunities for interrupting the natural history. The challenges in understanding the molecular basis of the intersection of diabetes and atherosclerosis are many, given overlapping issues between these two diseases such as very long subclinical phases, a frequency in the population that sets up multiple confounding variables, shared mechanistic underpinnings, and cellular players such as adipocytes and macrophages with many similar characteristics. These issues combine with clinical experience to frame a fundamental question in this field—to what extent is diabetic atherosclerosis unique and distinct from general atherosclerosis, or is it simply the same disease accelerated in the context of hyperglycemia, insulin resistance, and other factors? It is frustrating that, despite intense efforts by many groups using different approaches over many years, this question remains unresolved. Clearly the issues considered here are important in diabetic atherosclerosis independent of whether they are unique to T1D or not. Diabetic dyslipidemia is a central part of the clinical picture, with all the key components of the arterial wall and the inflammatory system altered by interaction with the altered lipid metabolism of T1D. Increased thrombogenicity clearly contributes to cardiovascular outcomes in people with diabetes and the extent to which all aspects of coagulation are shifted in diabetes is impressive. Endothelial dysfunction is an early part of the disease even before diabetes or cardiovascular complications become apparent. Ultimately, the inflammatory responses generated by core elements of T1D, such as hyperglycemia, elevated free fatty acids, and increased reactive oxygen species, may be pointing us in the direction we must head if we are to understand better diabetic atherosclerosis, identify the problems earlier, and further improve outcomes.

REFERENCES

1. Gregory GA, et al. Global incidence, prevalence, and mortality of type 1 diabetes in 2021 with projection to 2040: a modelling study. *Lancet Diabetes Endocrinol*. 2022;10(10):741–760.
2. Forlenza GP, Rewers M. The epidemic of type 1 diabetes: what is it telling us? *Curr Opin Endocrinol Diabetes Obes*. 2011;18(4):248–251.
3. Ruiz PLD, et al. Mortality trends in type 1 diabetes: a multicountry analysis of six population-based cohorts. *Diabetologia*. 2022;65(6):964–972.
4. Gale EA, Gillespie KM. Diabetes and gender. *Diabetologia*. 2001;44(1):3–15.
5. Houeiss P, Luce S, Boitard C. Environmental triggering of type 1 diabetes autoimmunity. *Front Endocrinol (Lausanne)*. 2022;13:933965.
6. Flatt AJS, et al. Pancreatic islet reserve in type 1 diabetes. *Ann N Y Acad Sci*. 2021;1495(1):40–54.
7. Zhong F, Jiang Y. Endogenous pancreatic β cell regeneration: a potential strategy for the recovery of β cell deficiency in diabetes. *Front Endocrinol (Lausanne)*. 2019;10:101.
8. Davies JL, et al. A genome-wide search for human type 1 diabetes susceptibility genes. *Nature*. 1994;371(6493):130–136.
9. Rabinovitch A. An update on cytokines in the pathogenesis of insulin-dependent diabetes mellitus. *Diabetes Metab Rev*. 1998;14(2):129–151.
10. Demine S, et al. Pro-inflammatory cytokines induce cell death, inflammatory responses, and endoplasmic reticulum stress in human iPSC-derived beta cells. *Stem Cell Res Ther*. 2020;11(1):7.
11. Hanafusa T, et al. Examination of islets in the pancreas biopsy specimens from newly diagnosed type 1 (insulin-dependent) diabetic patients. *Diabetologia*. 1990;33(2):105–111.
12. Foulis AK, Stewart JA. The pancreas in recent-onset type 1 (insulin-dependent) diabetes mellitus: insulin content of islets, insulitis and associated changes in the exocrine acinar tissue. *Diabetologia*. 1984;26(6):456–461.
13. Bottazzo GF, et al. In situ characterization of autoimmune phenomena and expression of HLA molecules in the pancreas in diabetic insulitis. *N Engl J Med*. 1985;313(6):353–360.
14. Cusick MF, Libbey JE, Fujinami RS. Molecular mimicry as a mechanism of autoimmune disease. *Clin Rev Allergy Immunol*. 2012;42(1):102–111.
15. Shim CH, et al. Emerging role of bystander T cell activation in autoimmune diseases. *BMB Rep*. 2022;55(2):57–64.
16. Foulis AK, et al. The histopathology of the pancreas in type 1 (insulin-dependent) diabetes mellitus: a 25-year review of deaths in patients under 20 years of age in the United Kingdom. *Diabetologia*. 1986;29(5):267–274.
17. Bluestone JA, Herold K, Eisenbarth G. Genetics, pathogenesis and clinical interventions in type 1 diabetes. *Nature*. 2010;464(7293):1293–1300.
18. Schauer IE, et al. Insulin resistance, defective insulin-mediated fatty acid suppression, and coronary artery calcification in subjects with and without type 1 diabetes: The CACTI study. *Diabetes*. 2011;60(1):306–314.
19. Nadeau KJ, et al. Insulin resistance in adolescents with type 1 diabetes and its relationship to cardiovascular function. *J Clin Endocrinol Metab*. 2010;95(2):513–521.
20. Moran A, et al. Insulin resistance during puberty: results from clamp studies in 357 children. *Diabetes*. 1999;48(10):2039–2044.
21. Moran A, et al. Association between the insulin resistance of puberty and the insulin-like growth factor-I/growth hormone axis. *J Clin Endocrinol Metab*. 2002;87(10):4817–4820.
22. Reinehr T, et al. Strong effect of pubertal status on metabolic health in obese children: a longitudinal study. *J Clin Endocrinol Metab*. 2015;100(1):301–308.
23. Asrih M, Jornayvaz FR. Metabolic syndrome and nonalcoholic fatty liver disease: Is insulin resistance the link? *Mol Cell Endocrinol*. 2015;418:55–65. Pt 1.
24. Mäkinen VP, et al. Triglyceride-cholesterol imbalance across lipoprotein subclasses predicts diabetic kidney disease and mortality in type 1 diabetes: the FinnDiane Study. *J Intern Med*. 2013;273(4):383–395.
25. Chen J, et al. Mitochondrial reactive oxygen species and type 1 diabetes. *Antioxid Redox Signal*. 2018;29(14):1361–1372.
26. Ye J. Role of insulin in the pathogenesis of free fatty acid-induced insulin resistance in skeletal muscle. *Endocr Metab Immune Disord Drug Targets*. 2007;7(1):65–74.
27. Wullaert A, et al. Hepatic tumor necrosis factor signaling and nuclear factor-kappaB: effects on liver homeostasis and beyond. *Endocr Rev*. 2007;28(4):365–386.
28. Kaneto H, et al. Oxidative stress and the JNK pathway are involved in the development of type 1 and type 2 diabetes. *Curr Mol Med*. 2007;7(7):674–686.
29. Manning BD. Balancing Akt with S6K: implications for both metabolic diseases and tumorigenesis. *J Cell Biol*. 2004;167(3):399–403.
30. Gregor MF, Hotamisligil GS. Thematic review series: adipocyte biology. Adipocyte stress: the endoplasmic reticulum and metabolic disease. *J Lipid Res*. 2007;48(9):1905–1914.
31. Rodrigues TC, et al. Obesity and coronary artery calcium in diabetes: the coronary artery calcification in type 1 diabetes (CACTI) study. *Diabetes Technol Ther*. 2011;13(10):991–996.

32. Girgis CM, Scalley BD, Park KE. Utility of the estimated glucose disposal rate as a marker of microvascular complications in young adults with type 1 diabetes. *Diabetes Res Clin Pract.* 2012;96(3):e70–e72.
33. Nadeau KJ, et al. Insulin resistance in adolescents with type 2 diabetes is associated with impaired exercise capacity. *J Clin Endocrinol Metab.* 2009;94(10):3687–3695.
34. Karamanakos G, et al. The association of insulin resistance measured through the estimated glucose disposal rate with predictors of micro-and macrovascular complications in patients with type 1 diabetes. *Prim Care Diabetes.* 2022;16(6):837–843.
35. Chillarón JJ, et al. Estimated glucose disposal rate in assessment of the metabolic syndrome and microvascular complications in patients with type 1 diabetes. *J Clin Endocrinol Metab.* 2009;94(9):3530–3534.
36. Linn W, et al. Estimated glucose disposal rate is associated with retinopathy and kidney disease in young people with type 1 diabetes: a nationwide observational study. *Cardiovasc Diabetol.* 2023;22(1):61.
37. Rewers M, Ludvigsson J. Environmental risk factors for type 1 diabetes. *Lancet.* 2016;387(10035):2340–2348.
38. Kimpimaki T, et al. The first signs of beta-cell autoimmunity appear in infancy in genetically susceptible children from the general population: the Finnish Type 1 Diabetes Prediction and Prevention Study. *J Clin Endocrinol Metab.* 2001;86(10):4782–4788.
39. Norris JM. Infant and childhood diet and type 1 diabetes risk: recent advances and prospects. *Curr Diab Rep.* 2010;10(5):345–349.
40. Chia JSJ, et al. A1 beta-casein milk protein and other environmental predisposing factors for type 1 diabetes. *Nutr Diabetes.* 2017;7(5):e274.
41. Lamminsalo A, et al. Cow's milk allergy in infancy and later development of type 1 diabetes-nationwide case-cohort study. *Pediatr Diabetes.* 2021;22(3):400–406.
42. Virtanen SM, et al. Cow's milk consumption, disease-associated autoantibodies and type 1 diabetes mellitus: a follow-up study in siblings of diabetic children. Childhood Diabetes in Finland Study Group. *Diabet Med.* 1998;15(9):730–738.
43. Karjalainen J, et al. A bovine albumin peptide as a possible trigger of insulin-dependent diabetes mellitus. *N Engl J Med.* 1992;327(5):302–307.
44. Vaarala O, et al. Cow milk feeding induces antibodies to insulin in children – a link between cow milk and insulin-dependent diabetes mellitus? *Scand J Immunol.* 1998;47(2):131–135.
45. Vaarala O, et al. Cow's milk formula feeding induces primary immunization to insulin in infants at genetic risk for type 1 diabetes. *Diabetes.* 1999;48(7):1389–1394.
46. Knip M, et al. Writing Group for the TRIGR Study Group. Effect of hydrolyzed infant formula vs conventional formula on risk of type 1 diabetes: the TRIGR randomized clinical trial. *JAMA.* 2018;319(1):38–48.
47. Kimpimaki T, et al. Short-term exclusive breastfeeding predisposes young children with increased genetic risk of type I diabetes to progressive beta-cell autoimmunity. *Diabetologia.* 2001;44(1):63–69.
48. Jenista JA, Powell KR, Menegus MA. Epidemiology of neonatal enterovirus infection. *J Pediatr.* 1984;104(5):685–690.
49. Sadeharju K, et al. Maternal antibodies in breast milk protect the child from enterovirus infections. *Pediatrics.* 2007;119(5):941–946.
50. Lund-Blix NA, et al. Infant feeding and risk of type 1 diabetes in two large scandinavian birth cohorts. *Diabetes Care.* 2017;40(7):920–927.
51. Antvorskov JC, et al. Dietary gluten and the development of type 1 diabetes. *Diabetologia.* 2014;57(9):1770–1780.
52. Serena G, et al. The role of gluten in celiac disease and type 1 diabetes. *Nutrients.* 2015;7(9):7143–7162.
53. Norris JM, et al. Timing of initial cereal exposure in infancy and risk of islet autoimmunity. *JAMA.* 2003;290(13):1713–1720.
54. Ziegler AG, et al. Early infant feeding and risk of developing type 1 diabetes-associated autoantibodies. *JAMA.* 2003;290(13):1721–1728.
55. Hummel S, et al. Primary dietary intervention study to reduce the risk of islet autoimmunity in children at increased risk for type 1 diabetes: the BABYDIET study. *Diabetes Care.* 2011;34(6):1301–1305.
56. Hypponen E, et al. Intake of vitamin D and risk of type 1 diabetes: a birth-cohort study. *Lancet.* 2001;358(9292):1500–1503.
57. Zipitis CS, Akobeng AK. Vitamin D supplementation in early childhood and risk of type 1 diabetes: a systematic review and meta-analysis. *Arch Dis Child.* 2008;93(6):512–517.
58. Viskari H, et al. Circulating vitamin D concentrations in two neighboring populations with markedly different incidence of type 1 diabetes. *Diabetes Care.* 2006;29(6):1458–1459.
59. Simpson M, et al. No association of vitamin D intake or 25-hydroxyvitamin D levels in childhood with risk of islet autoimmunity and type 1 diabetes: the Diabetes Autoimmunity Study in the Young (DAISY). *Diabetologia.* 2011;54(11):2779–2788.
60. Frederiksen BN, et al. Association between vitamin D metabolism gene polymorphisms and risk of islet autoimmunity and progression to type 1 diabetes: the diabetes autoimmunity study in the young (DAISY). *J Clin Endocrinol Metab.* 2013;98(11):E1845–E1851.
61. Najjar L, et al. Vitamin D and type 1 diabetes risk: a systematic review and meta-analysis of genetic evidence. *Nutrients.* 2021;13(12):4260.
62. Norris JM, et al. Omega-3 polyunsaturated fatty acid intake and islet autoimmunity in children at increased risk for type 1 diabetes. *JAMA.* 2007;298(12):1420–1428.
63. Sairenji T, et al. Relating homology between the Epstein-Barr virus BOLF1 molecule and HLA-DQw8 beta chain to recent onset type 1 (insulin-dependent) diabetes mellitus. *Diabetologia.* 1991;34(1):33–39.
64. Hyoty H, et al. Decline of mumps antibodies in type 1 (insulin-dependent) diabetic children and a plateau in the rising incidence of type 1 diabetes after introduction of the mumps-measles-rubella vaccine in Finland. Childhood Diabetes in Finland Study Group. *Diabetologia.* 1993;36(12):1303–1308.
65. Couper JJ. Environmental triggers of type 1 diabetes. *J Paediatr Child Health.* 2001;37(3):218–220.
66. Conrad B, et al. Evidence for superantigen involvement in insulin-dependent diabetes mellitus aetiology. *Nature.* 1994;371(6495):351–355.
67. Yin H, et al. Enterovirus RNA is found in peripheral blood mononuclear cells in a majority of type 1 diabetic children at onset. *Diabetes.* 2002;51(6):1964–1971.
68. Craig ME, et al. Reduced frequency of HLA DRB1*03-DQB1*02 in children with type 1 diabetes associated with enterovirus RNA. *J Infect Dis.* 2003;187(10):1562–1570.
69. Jaidane H, Hober D. Role of coxsackievirus B4 in the pathogenesis of type 1 diabetes. *Diabetes Metab.* 2008;34(6 Pt 1):537–548.
70. Hyoty H. Enterovirus infections and type 1 diabetes. *Ann Med.* 2002;34(3):138–147.
71. Haverkos HW, et al. Enteroviruses and type 1 diabetes mellitus. *Biomed Pharmacother.* 2003;57(9):379–385.
72. Hyoty H, Taylor KW. The role of viruses in human diabetes. *Diabetologia.* 2002;45(10):1353–1361.
73. Moya-Suri V, et al. Enterovirus RNA sequences in sera of schoolchildren in the general population and their association with type 1-diabetes-associated autoantibodies. *J Med Microbiol.* 2005;54(Pt 9):879–883.
74. Sarmiento L, et al. Occurrence of enterovirus RNA in serum of children with newly diagnosed type 1 diabetes and islet cell autoantibody-positive subjects in a population with a low incidence of type 1 diabetes. *Autoimmunity.* 2007;40(7):540–545.
75. Jaidane H, et al. Coxsackievirus B4 and type 1 diabetes pathogenesis: contribution of animal models. *Diabetes Metab Res Rev.* 2009;25(7):591–603.
76. Bach JF. The effect of infections on susceptibility to autoimmune and allergic diseases. *N Engl J Med.* 2002;347(12):911–920.
77. Goldberg E, Krause I. Infection and type 1 diabetes mellitus—a two edged sword? *Autoimmun Rev.* 2009;8(8):682–686.
78. Bach JF. Infections and autoimmune diseases. *J Autoimmun.* 2005;25 (Suppl):74–80.
79. Bach JF. Revisiting the hygiene hypothesis in the context of autoimmunity. *Front Immunol.* 2020;11:615192.
80. McKinney PA, et al. Early social mixing and childhood type 1 diabetes mellitus: a case-control study in Yorkshire, UK. *Diabet Med.* 2000;17(3):236–242.
81. Tracy S, Drescher KM. Coxsackievirus infections and NOD mice: relevant models of protection from, and induction of, type 1 diabetes. *Ann N Y Acad Sci.* 2007;1103:143–151.
82. Lonnrot M, et al. Enterovirus infection as a risk factor for beta-cell autoimmunity in a prospectively observed birth cohort: the Finnish Diabetes Prediction and Prevention Study. *Diabetes.* 2000;49(8):1314–1318.
83. Hyoty H, et al. A prospective study of the role of coxsackie B and other enterovirus infections in the pathogenesis of IDDM. Childhood Diabetes in Finland (DiMe) Study Group. *Diabetes.* 1995;44(6):652–657.
84. EURODIAB Substudy 2 Study Group. Infections and vaccinations as risk factors for childhood type I (insulin-dependent) diabetes mellitus: a multicentre case-control investigation. *Diabetologia.* 2000;43(1):47–53.
85. Blom L, Nyström L, Dahlquist G. The Swedish childhood diabetes study. Vaccinations and infections as risk determinants for diabetes in childhood. *Diabetologia.* 1991;34(3):176–181.
86. Graves PM, et al. Lack of association between early childhood immunizations and beta-cell autoimmunity. *Diabetes Care.* 1999;22(10):1694–1697.
87. Hummel M, et al. No major association of breast-feeding, vaccinations, and childhood viral diseases with early islet autoimmunity in the German BABYDIAB Study. *Diabetes Care.* 2000;23(7):969–974.
88. Beyerlein A, et al. Early infant growth is associated with the risk of islet autoimmunity in genetically susceptible children. *Pediatr Diabetes.* 2014;15(7):534–542.
89. Pacaud D, et al. Association between family history, early growth and the risk of beta cell autoimmunity in children at risk for type 1 diabetes. *Diabetologia.* 2021;64(1):119–128.
90. Karavanaki K, et al. Psychological stress as a factor potentially contributing to the pathogenesis of type 1 diabetes mellitus. *J Endocrinol Invest.* 2008;31(5):406–415.
91. Calcinaro F, et al. Oral probiotic administration induces interleukin-10 production and prevents spontaneous autoimmune diabetes in the non-obese diabetic mouse. *Diabetologia.* 2005;48(8):1565–1575.
92. Valladares R, et al. Lactobacillus johnsonii N6.2 mitigates the development of type 1 diabetes in BB-DP rats. *PLoS One.* 2010;5(5):e10507.
93. Manrique-Acevedo C, Hirsch IB, Eckel RH. Prevention of cardiovascular disease in type 1 diabetes. *N Engl J Med.* 2024;390(13):1207–1217.
94. Urbina EM, et al. Burden of cardiovascular risk factors over time and arterial stiffness in youth with type 1 diabetes mellitus: the SEARCH for diabetes in youth study. *J Am Heart Assoc.* 2019;8(13):e010150.
95. Bishop FK, et al. Lifestyle risk factors for atherosclerosis in adults with type 1 diabetes. *Diab Vasc Dis Res.* 2009;6(4):269–275.
96. Huo L, et al. Burden of diabetes in Australia: life expectancy and disability-free life expectancy in adults with diabetes. *Diabetologia.* 2016;59(7):1437–1445.
97. Livingstone SJ, et al. Estimated life expectancy in a Scottish cohort with type 1 diabetes, 2008–2010. *JAMA.* 2015;313(1):37–44.

98. Harjutsalo V, Pongrac Barlovic D, Groop PH. Long-term population-based trends in the incidence of cardiovascular disease in individuals with type 1 diabetes from Finland: a retrospective, nationwide, cohort study. *Lancet Diabetes Endocrinol*. 2021.
99. Harjutsalo V, et al. Presence and determinants of cardiovascular disease and mortality in individuals with type 1 diabetes of long duration: the FinnDiane 50 Years of Diabetes Study. *Diabetes Care*. 2021;44(8):1885–1893.
100. Koivisto VA, et al. Cardiovascular disease and its risk factors in IDDM in Europe. EURODIAB IDDM Complications Study Group. *Diabetes Care*. 1996;19(7):689–697.
101. Miki T, et al. Diabetic cardiomyopathy: pathophysiology and clinical features. *Heart Fail Rev*. 2013;18(2):149–166.
102. Armstrong AC, et al. Association of cardiovascular risk factors and myocardial fibrosis with early cardiac dysfunction in type 1 diabetes: the diabetes control and complications trial/epidemiology of diabetes interventions and complications study. *Diabetes Care*. 2017;40(3):405–411.
103. Lam B, et al. Myocardial native-T1 times are elevated as a function of hypertrophy, HbA1c, and heart rate in diabetic adults without diffuse fibrosis. *Magn Reson Imaging*. 2019;61:83–89.
104. Llaurado G, et al. Type 1 diabetes: developing the first risk-estimation model for predicting silent myocardial ischemia. The potential role of insulin resistance. *PLoS One*. 2017;12(4):e0174640.
105. Bjornstad P, Donaghue KC, Maahs DM. Macrovascular disease and risk factors in youth with type 1 diabetes: time to be more attentive to treatment? *Lancet Diabetes Endocrinol*. 2018;6(10):809–820.
106. Orchard TJ, et al. Writing Group for the DCCT/EDIC Research Group. Association between 7 years of intensive treatment of type 1 diabetes and long-term mortality. *JAMA*. 2015;313(1):45–53.
107. Lind M, et al. Glycemic control and excess mortality in type 1 diabetes. *N Engl J Med*. 2014;371(21):1972–1982.
108. Lachin JM, Nathan DM. DCCT/EDIC Research Group. Understanding metabolic memory: the prolonged influence of glycemia during the diabetes control and complications trial (DCCT) on future risks of complications during the study of the epidemiology of diabetes interventions and complications (EDIC). *Diabetes Care*. 2021;44(10):2216–2224.
109. Nathan DM. Long-term complications of diabetes mellitus. *N Engl J Med*. 1993;328(23):1676–1685.
110. Diabetes Control and Complications Trial Research Group. Effect of intensive diabetes treatment on the development and progression of long-term complications in adolescents with insulin-dependent diabetes mellitus: Diabetes Control and Complications Trial. *J Pediatr*. 1994;125(2): 177–188.
111. Nathan DM, et al. Intensive diabetes treatment and cardiovascular disease in patients with type 1 diabetes. *N Engl J Med*. 2005;353(25):2643–2653.
112. Juutilainen A, et al. Similarity of the impact of type 1 and type 2 diabetes on cardiovascular mortality in middle-aged subjects. *Diabetes Care*. 2008;31(4):714–719.
113. González P, et al. Hyperglycemia and oxidative stress: an integral, updated and critical overview of their metabolic interconnections. *Int J Mol Sci*. 2023;24(11):9352.
114. Desouza CV, Bolli GB, Fonseca V. Hypoglycemia, diabetes, and cardiovascular events. *Diabetes Care*. 2010;33(6):1389–1394.
115. Alzahrani SH, Ajjan RA. Coagulation and fibrinolysis in diabetes. *Diab Vasc Dis Res*. 2010;7(4):260–273.
116. Vinik AI, Ziegler D. Diabetic cardiovascular autonomic neuropathy. *Circulation*. 2007;115(3):387–397.
117. Dimitropoulos G, Tahrani AA, Stevens MJ. Cardiac autonomic neuropathy in patients with diabetes mellitus. *World J Diabetes*. 2014;5(1):17–39.
118. Pop-Busui R, et al. Effects of prior intensive insulin therapy on cardiac autonomic nervous system function in type 1 diabetes mellitus: the Diabetes Control and Complications Trial/Epidemiology of Diabetes Interventions and Complications study (DCCT/EDIC). *Circulation*. 2009;119(22):2886–2893.
119. Ayad F, et al. Association between cardiac autonomic neuropathy and hypertension and its potential influence on diabetic complications. *Diabet Med*. 2010;27(7):804–811.
120. Prince CT, et al. Cardiovascular autonomic neuropathy, HDL cholesterol, and smoking correlate with arterial stiffness markers determined 18 years later in type 1 diabetes. *Diabetes Care*. 2010;33(3):652–657.
121. Spallone V, et al. Cardiovascular autonomic neuropathy in diabetes: clinical impact, assessment, diagnosis, and management. *Diabetes Metab Res Rev*. 2011;27(7):639–653.
122. Schnell O, et al. Scintigraphic evidence for cardiac sympathetic dysinnervation in long-term IDDM patients with and without ECG-based autonomic neuropathy. *Diabetologia*. 1995;38(11):1345–1352.
123. Frier BM, Schernthaner G, Heller SR. Hypoglycemia and cardiovascular risks. *Diabetes Care*. 2011;34(suppl 2):S132–S137.
124. Dave KR, et al. Recurrent hypoglycemia exacerbates cerebral ischemic damage in streptozotocin-induced diabetic rats. *Stroke*. 2011;42(5):1404–1411.
125. Perros P, et al. Brain abnormalities demonstrated by magnetic resonance imaging in adult IDDM patients with and without a history of recurrent severe hypoglycemia. *Diabetes Care*. 1997;20(6):1013–1018.
126. Stantonyonge N, et al. Structural gray and white matter differences in patients with type 1 diabetes and impaired awareness of hypoglycemia. *J Clin Endocrinol Metab*. 2021;106(2):450–458.
127. Gill GV, et al. Cardiac arrhythmia and nocturnal hypoglycaemia in type 1 diabetes–the 'dead in bed' syndrome revisited. *Diabetologia*. 2009;52(1): 42–45.
128. Tu E, et al. Post-mortem pathologic and genetic studies in "dead in bed syndrome" cases in type 1 diabetes mellitus. *Hum Pathol*. 2010;41(3):392–400.
129. Hagelqvist PG, et al. Glycaemia and cardiac arrhythmias in people with type 1 diabetes: a prospective observational study. *Diabetes Obes Metab*. 2023;25(8):2300–2309.
130. Gimenez M, et al. Repeated episodes of hypoglycemia as a potential aggravating factor for preclinical atherosclerosis in subjects with type 1 diabetes. *Diabetes Care*. 2011;34(1):198–203.
131. Fourlanos S, et al. Higher body mass index in adults at diagnosis of the slowly progressive form of type 1 diabetes mellitus is associated with lower risk HLA genes. *Diabetes Res Clin Pract*. 2014;104(3):e69–e71.
132. Holt SK, et al. Prevalence of low testosterone and predisposing risk factors in men with type 1 diabetes mellitus: findings from the DCCT/EDIC. *J Clin Endocrinol Metab*. 2014;99(9):E1655–E1660.
133. Price SA, et al. Obesity is associated with retinopathy and macrovascular disease in type 1 diabetes. *Obes Res Clin Pract*. 2014;8(2):e178–e182.
134. Pinhas-Hamiel O, et al. Prevalence of overweight, obesity and metabolic syndrome components in children, adolescents and young adults with type 1 diabetes mellitus. *Diabetes Metab Res Rev*. 2015;31(1):76–84.
135. Kapellen TM, et al. Children and adolescents with type 1 diabetes in Germany are more overweight than healthy controls: results comparing DPV database and CrescNet database. *J Pediatr Endocrinol Metab*. 2014;27(3-4):209–214.
136. Liu LL, et al. Prevalence of overweight and obesity in youth with diabetes in USA: the SEARCH for Diabetes in Youth study. *Pediatr Diabetes*. 2010;11(1):4–11.
137. Libman IM, et al. Changing prevalence of overweight children and adolescents at onset of insulin-treated diabetes. *Diabetes Care*. 2003;26(10):2871–2875.
138. Lipman TH, et al. Increasing incidence of type 1 diabetes in youth: twenty years of the Philadelphia Pediatric Diabetes Registry. *Diabetes Care*. 2013;36(6):1597–1603.
139. Purnell JQ, et al. Effect of excessive weight gain with intensive therapy of type 1 diabetes on lipid levels and blood pressure: results from the DCCT. Diabetes Control and Complications Trial. *JAMA*. 1998;280(2):140–146.
140. Parente EB, et al. The relationship between body fat distribution and nonalcoholic fatty liver in adults with type 1 diabetes. *Diabetes Care*. 2021;44(7):1706–1713.
141. Hager MR, Narla AD, Tannock LR. Dyslipidemia in patients with chronic kidney disease. *Rev Endocr Metab Disord*. 2017;18(1):29–40.
142. James RW, Pometta D. Differences in lipoprotein subfraction composition and distribution between type I diabetic men and control subjects. *Diabetes*. 1990;39(10):1158–1164.
143. Guy J, et al. Lipid and lipoprotein profiles in youth with and without type 1 diabetes: the SEARCH for Diabetes in Youth case-control study. *Diabetes Care*. 2009;32(3):416–420.
144. Mitrofanova A, et al. New insights into renal lipid dysmetabolism in diabetic kidney disease. *World J Diabetes*. 2021;12(5):524–540.
145. Bagdade JD, Dunn FL. Effects of insulin treatment on lipoprotein composition and function in patients with IDDM. *Diabetes*. 1992;41(suppl 2):107–110.
146. Rosenstock J, Vega GL, Raskin P. Effect of intensive diabetes treatment on low-density lipoprotein apolipoprotein B kinetics in type I diabetes. *Diabetes*. 1988;37(4):393–397.
147. Bagdade JD, et al. Intraperitoneal insulin therapy corrects abnormalities in cholesteryl ester transfer and lipoprotein lipase activities in insulin-dependent diabetes mellitus. *Arterioscler Thromb*. 1994;14(12):1933–1939.
148. Lichtman AH, et al. Adaptive immunity in atherogenesis: new insights and therapeutic approaches. *J Clin Invest*. 2013;123(1):27–36.
149. Lopes-Virella MF, et al. Immune complexes and the risk of CVD in type 1 diabetes. *Diabetes*. 2019;68(9):1853–1860.
150. Neeland IJ, et al. Dysfunctional adiposity and the risk of prediabetes and type 2 diabetes in obese adults. *JAMA*. 2012;308(11):1150–1159.
151. Adiels M, et al. Overproduction of very low-density lipoproteins is the hallmark of the dyslipidemia in the metabolic syndrome. *Arterioscler Thromb Vasc Biol*. 2008;28(7):1225–1236.
152. Adiels M, et al. Overproduction of VLDL1 driven by hyperglycemia is a dominant feature of diabetic dyslipidemia. *Arterioscler Thromb Vasc Biol*. 2005;25(8):1697–1703.
153. Barrera Echegoyen FX, et al. The nature and characteristics of hypertriglyceridemia in a large cohort with type 2 diabetes. *J Diabetes Complications*. 2023;37(2):108387.
154. Chan DC, et al. Postprandial hypertriglyceridemia and cardiovascular disease: current and future therapies. *Curr Atheroscler Rep*. 2013;15(3):309.
155. Pang J, et al. Postprandial dyslipidaemia and diabetes: mechanistic and therapeutic aspects. *Curr Opin Lipidol*. 2012;23(4):303–309.
156. Ruby MA, et al. VLDL hydrolysis by LPL activates PPAR-alpha through generation of unbound fatty acids. *J Lipid Res*. 2010;51(8):2275–2281.
157. Grabner GF, et al. Lipolysis: cellular mechanisms for lipid mobilization from fat stores. *Nat Metab*. 2021;3(11):1445–1465.
158. Brown JD, et al. VLDL hydrolysis by hepatic lipase regulates PPARdelta transcriptional responses. *PLoS One*. 2011;6(7):e21209.
159. Adiels M, Taskinen MR, Boren J. Fatty liver, insulin resistance, and dyslipidemia. *Curr Diab Rep*. 2008;8(1):60–64.
160. Barlovic DP, Soro-Paavonen A, Jandeleit-Dahm KA. RAGE biology, atherosclerosis and diabetes. *Clin Sci (Lond)*. 2011;121(2):43–55.
161. Egaña-Gorroño L, et al. Receptor for advanced glycation end products (RAGE) and mechanisms and therapeutic opportunities in diabetes and

cardiovascular disease: insights from human subjects and animal models. *Front Cardiovasc Med*. 2020;7:37.

162. Asztalos BF, et al. LpA-I, LpA-I:A-II HDL and CHD-risk: the Framingham Offspring Study and the Veterans Affairs HDL Intervention Trial. *Atherosclerosis*. 2006;188(1):59–67.
163. Femlak M, et al. The role and function of HDL in patients with diabetes mellitus and the related cardiovascular risk. *Lipids Health Dis*. 2017;16(1):207.
164. Badellino KO, et al. Endothelial lipase concentrations are increased in metabolic syndrome and associated with coronary atherosclerosis. *PLoS Med*. 2006;3(2):e22.
165. Paradis ME, et al. Endothelial lipase is associated with inflammation in humans. *J Lipid Res*. 2006;47(12):2808–2813.
166. Paradis ME, et al. Visceral adiposity and endothelial lipase. *J Clin Endocrinol Metab*. 2006;91(9):3538–3543.
167. Badellino KO, et al. Endothelial lipase is increased in vivo by inflammation in humans. *Circulation*. 2008;117(5):678–685.
168. Li C, et al. Cholesteryl ester transfer protein inhibitors in the treatment of dyslipidemia: a systematic review and meta-analysis. *PLoS One*. 2013;8(10):e77049.
169. Investigators A-H, et al. Niacin in patients with low HDL cholesterol levels receiving intensive statin therapy. *N Engl J Med*. 2011;365(24):2255–2267.
170. Orchard TJ, et al. Lipid and blood pressure treatment goals for type 1 diabetes: 10-year incidence data from the Pittsburgh Epidemiology of Diabetes Complications Study. *Diabetes Care*. 2001;24(6):1053–1059.
171. Cree-Green M, et al. Youth with type 1 diabetes have adipose, hepatic, and peripheral insulin resistance. *J Clin Endocrinol Metab*. 2018;103(10):3647–3657.
172. Cree-Green M, et al. Metformin improves peripheral insulin sensitivity in youth with type 1 diabetes. *J Clin Endocrinol Metab*. 2019;104(8):3265–3278.
173. Orchard TJ, et al. Insulin resistance-related factors, but not glycemia, predict coronary artery disease in type 1 diabetes: 10-year follow-up data from the Pittsburgh Epidemiology of Diabetes Complications Study. *Diabetes Care*. 2003;26(5):1374–1379.
174. McCulloch MA, et al. Magnetic resonance imaging measures of decreased aortic strain and distensibility are proportionate to insulin resistance in adolescents with type 1 diabetes mellitus. *Pediatr Diabetes*. 2015;16(2):90–97.
175. Bjornstad P, et al. Estimated insulin sensitivity predicts incident micro- and macrovascular complications in adults with type 1 diabetes over 6 years: the coronary artery calcification in type 1 diabetes study. *J Diabetes Complications*. 2016;30(4):586–590.
176. Skyler JS, et al. Differentiation of diabetes by pathophysiology, natural history, and prognosis. *Diabetes*. 2017;66(2):241–255.
177. Ajoolabady A, et al. Inflammation in atherosclerosis: pathophysiology and mechanisms. *Cell Death Dis*. 2024;15(11):817.
178. Alfaddagh A, et al. Inflammation and cardiovascular disease: from mechanisms to therapeutics. *Am J Prev Cardiol*. 2020;4:100130.
179. Ridker PM, et al. Inflammation and cholesterol as predictors of cardiovascular events among 13970 contemporary high-risk patients with statin intolerance. *Circulation*. 2024;149(1):28–35.
180. Hooglugt A, Klatt O, Huveneers S. Vascular stiffening and endothelial dysfunction in atherosclerosis. *Curr Opin Lipidol*. 2022;33(6):353–363.
181. Ridker PM, et al. Prospective study of C-reactive protein and the risk of future cardiovascular events among apparently healthy women. *Circulation*. 1998;98(8):731–733.
182. Ridker PM, et al. Inflammation, aspirin, and the risk of cardiovascular disease in apparently healthy men. *N Engl J Med*. 1997;336(14):973–979.
183. Gomes MB, et al. Acute-phase proteins among patients with type 1 diabetes. *Diabetes Metab*. 2003;29(4 Pt 1):405–411.
184. Ridker PM, et al. Relationship of lipoprotein-associated phospholipase A(2) mass and activity with incident vascular events among primary prevention patients allocated to placebo or to statin therapy: an analysis from the JUPITER trial. *Clin Chem*. 2012;58(5):877–886.
185. de Lemos JA, Hennekens CH, Ridker PM. Plasma concentration of soluble vascular cell adhesion molecule-1 and subsequent cardiovascular risk. *J Am Coll Cardiol*. 2000;36(2):423–426.
186. Despres JP. Abdominal obesity and cardiovascular disease: is inflammation the missing link? *Can J Cardiol*. 2012;28(6):642–652.
187. Tsalamandris S, et al. The role of inflammation in diabetes: current concepts and future perspectives. *Eur Cardiol*. 2019;14(1):50–59.
188. Moncada S, Higgs A. The L-arginine-nitric oxide pathway. *N Engl J Med*. 1993;329(27):2002–2012.
189. Furchgott RF, Zawadzki JV. The obligatory role of endothelial cells in the relaxation of arterial smooth muscle by acetylcholine. *Nature*. 1980;288(5789):373–376.
190. Kinlay S, Libby P, Ganz P. Endothelial function and coronary artery disease. *Curr Opin Lipidol*. 2001;12(4):383–389.
191. Gerszten RE, et al. MCP-1 and IL-8 trigger firm adhesion of monocytes to vascular endothelium under flow conditions. *Nature*. 1999;398(6729):718–723.
192. Jarvisalo MJ, et al. Endothelial dysfunction and increased arterial intima-media thickness in children with type 1 diabetes. *Circulation*. 2004;109(14):1750–1755.
193. Johnstone MT, et al. Impaired endothelium-dependent vasodilation in patients with insulin-dependent diabetes mellitus. *Circulation*. 1993;88(6):2510–2516.
194. Williams SB, et al. Impaired nitric oxide-mediated vasodilation in patients with non-insulin-dependent diabetes mellitus. *J Am Coll Cardiol*. 1996;27(3):567–574.
195. Takaya T, et al. A specific role for eNOS-derived reactive oxygen species in atherosclerosis progression. *Arterioscler Thromb Vasc Biol*. 2007;27(7):1632–1637.
196. Tommerdahl KL, et al. Impact of obesity on measures of cardiovascular and kidney health in youth with type 1 diabetes as compared with youth with type 2 diabetes. *Diabetes Care*. 2021;44(3):795–803.
197. Steinberg HO, et al. Elevated circulating free fatty acid levels impair endothelium-dependent vasodilation. *J Clin Invest*. 1997;100(5):1230–1239.
198. Griffin ME, et al. Free fatty acid-induced insulin resistance is associated with activation of protein kinase C theta and alterations in the insulin signaling cascade. *Diabetes*. 1999;48(6):1270–1274.
199. Dickhout JG, et al. Peroxynitrite causes endoplasmic reticulum stress and apoptosis in human vascular endothelium: implications in atherogenesis. *Arterioscler Thromb Vasc Biol*. 2005;25(12):2623–2629.
200. Zou MH, Shi C, Cohen RA. High glucose via peroxynitrite causes tyrosine nitration and inactivation of prostacyclin synthase that is associated with thromboxane/prostaglandin H(2) receptor-mediated apoptosis and adhesion molecule expression in cultured human aortic endothelial cells. *Diabetes*. 2002;51(1):198–203.
201. Bauersachs J, Schafer A. Tetrahydrobiopterin and eNOS dimer/monomer ratio–a clue to eNOS uncoupling in diabetes? *Cardiovasc Res*. 2005;65(4):768–769.
202. Kar S, Bhandar B, Kavdia M. Impact of SOD in eNOS uncoupling: a two-edged sword between hydrogen peroxide and peroxynitrite. *Free Radic Res*. 2012;46(12):1496–1513.
203. Kanda T, et al. PPARgamma in the endothelium regulates metabolic responses to high-fat diet in mice. *J Clin Invest*. 2009;119(1):110–124.
204. Tsuchiya K, et al. FoxOs integrate pleiotropic actions of insulin in vascular endothelium to protect mice from atherosclerosis. *Cell Metab*. 2012;15(3):372–381.
205. Qiang L, et al. Increased atherosclerosis and endothelial dysfunction in mice bearing constitutively deacetylated alleles of Foxo1 gene. *J Biol Chem*. 2012;287(17):13944–13951.
206. Li H, et al. An atherogenic diet rapidly induces VCAM-1, a cytokine-regulatable mononuclear leukocyte adhesion molecule, in rabbit aortic endothelium. *Arterioscler Thromb*. 1993;13(2):197–204.
207. Cybulsky MI, Gimbrone Jr. MA. Endothelial expression of a mononuclear leukocyte adhesion molecule during atherogenesis. *Science*. 1991;251(4995):788–791.
208. Maganto-Garcia E, et al. Dynamic changes in regulatory T cells are linked to levels of diet-induced hypercholesterolemia. *Circulation*. 2011;124(2):185–195.
209. Hu H, et al. Enhanced leukocyte-platelet cross-talk in type 1 diabetes mellitus: relationship to microangiopathy. *J Thromb Haemost*. 2004;2(1):58–64.
210. Devaraj S, et al. Demonstration of increased toll-like receptor 2 and toll-like receptor 4 expression in monocytes of type 1 diabetes mellitus patients with microvascular complications. *Metabolism*. 2011;60(2):256–259.
211. Devaraj S, Tobias P, Jialal I. Knockout of toll-like receptor-4 attenuates the pro-inflammatory state of diabetes. *Cytokine*. 2011;55(3):441–445.
212. Liu T, et al. NF-κB signaling in inflammation. *Signal Transduct Target Ther*. 2017;2:17023.
213. Ley K, et al. Getting to the site of inflammation: the leukocyte adhesion cascade updated. *Nat Rev Immunol*. 2007;7(9):678–689.
214. Lee-Rueckert M, et al. Lipid-laden macrophages and inflammation in atherosclerosi s and cancer: an integrative view. *Front Cardiovasc Med*. 2022;9:777822.
215. Farb A, et al. Coronary plaque erosion without rupture into a lipid core. A frequent cause of coronary thrombosis in sudden coronary death. *Circulation*. 1996;93(7):1354–1363.
216. Arbustini E, et al. Plaque erosion is a major substrate for coronary thrombosis in acute myocardial infarction. *Heart*. 1999;82(3):269–272.
217. Gimbrone Jr. MA, et al. Endothelial dysfunction, hemodynamic forces, and atherogenesis. *Ann N Y Acad Sci*. 2000;902:230–239. discussion 239-40.
218. Topper JN, et al. Vascular MADs: two novel MAD-related genes selectively inducible by flow in human vascular endothelium. *Proc Natl Acad Sci U S A*. 1997;94(17):9314–9319.
219. Topper JN, et al. Expression of the bumetanide-sensitive Na-K-Cl cotransporter BSC2 is differentially regulated by fluid mechanical and inflammatory cytokine stimuli in vascular endothelium. *J Clin Invest*. 1997;99(12):2941–2949.
220. Hajra L, et al. The NF-kappa B signal transduction pathway in aortic endothelial cells is primed for activation in regions predisposed to atherosclerotic lesion formation. *Proc Natl Acad Sci U S A*. 2000;97(16):9052–9057.
221. de Boer IH, et al. Diabetes and hypertension: a position statement by the American Diabetes Association. *Diabetes Care*. 2017;40(9):1273–1284.
222. Brunstrom M, Carlberg B. Effect of antihypertensive treatment at different blood pressure levels in patients with diabetes mellitus: systematic review and meta-analyses. *BMJ*. 2016;352:i717.
223. Ettehad D, et al. Blood pressure lowering for prevention of cardiovascular disease and death: a systematic review and meta-analysis. *Lancet*. 2016;387(10022):957–967.
224. Matsushita K, et al. Chronic Kidney Disease Prognosis Consortium. Association of estimated glomerular filtration rate and albuminuria with all-cause and cardiovascular mortality in general population cohorts: a collaborative meta-analysis. *Lancet*. 2010;375(9731):2073–2081.
225. de Boer IH, et al. DCCT/EDIC Research Group. Intensive diabetes therapy and glomerular filtration rate in type 1 diabetes. *N Engl J Med*. 2011;365(25):2366–2376.
226. DCCT/EDIC research group. Effect of intensive diabetes treatment on albuminuria in type 1 diabetes: long-term follow-up of the Diabetes Control

and Complications Trial and Epidemiology of Diabetes Interventions and Complications study. *Lancet Diabetes Endocrinol.* 2014;2(10):793–800.
227. Rapaport R, Sills IN. Implications of the DCCT for children and adolescents with IDDM. *N J Med.* 1994;91(4):227–228.
228. Purnell JQ, et al. Impact of excessive weight gain on cardiovascular outcomes in type 1 diabetes: results from the Diabetes Control and Complications Trial/Epidemiology of Diabetes Interventions and Complications (DCCT/EDIC) study. *Diabetes Care.* 2017;40(12):1756–1762.
229. de Boer IH, et al. Central obesity, incident microalbuminuria, and change in creatinine clearance in the epidemiology of diabetes interventions and complications study. *J Am Soc Nephrol.* 2007;18(1):235–243.
230. Bhatt DL, et al. Sotagliflozin in patients with diabetes and chronic kidney disease. *N Engl J Med.* 2021;384(2):129–139.
231. Perkovic V, et al. Canagliflozin and renal outcomes in type 2 diabetes and nephropathy. *N Engl J Med.* 2019;380(24):2295–2306.
232. Mann JFE, et al. Liraglutide and renal outcomes in type 2 diabetes. *N Engl J Med.* 2017;377(9):839–848.
233. Wanner C, et al. Empagliflozin and progression of kidney disease in type 2 diabetes. *N Engl J Med.* 2016;375(4):323–334.
234. Owen MR, Doran E, Halestrap AP. Evidence that metformin exerts its anti-diabetic effects through inhibition of complex 1 of the mitochondrial respiratory chain. *Biochem J.* 2000;348(Pt 3):607–614.
235. Duca FA, et al. Metformin activates a duodenal Ampk-dependent pathway to lower hepatic glucose production in rats. *Nat Med.* 2015;21(5):506–511.
236. UK Prospective Diabetes Study (UKPDS) Group. Effect of intensive blood-glucose control with metformin on complications in overweight patients with type 2 diabetes (UKPDS 34). *Lancet.* 1998;352(9131): 854–865.
237. Bjornstad P, et al. Metformin improves insulin sensitivity and vascular health in youth with type 1 diabetes mellitus. *Circulation.* 2018;138(25):2895–2907.
238. Tynjala A, et al. Arterial stiffness predicts mortality in individuals with type 1 diabetes. *Diabetes Care.* 2020;43(9):2266–2271.
239. Schafer M, et al. Frequency of reduced left ventricular contractile efficiency and discoordinated myocardial relaxation in patients aged 16 to 21 years with type 1 diabetes mellitus (from the Emerald Study). *Am J Cardiol.* 2020;128:45–53.
240. Petrie JR, et al. Cardiovascular and metabolic effects of metformin in patients with type 1 diabetes (REMOVAL): a double-blind, randomised, placebo-controlled trial. *Lancet Diabetes Endocrinol.* 2017;5(8):597–609.
241. Shivaprasad C, Kalra S. Bromocriptine in type 2 diabetes mellitus. *Indian J Endocrinol Metab.* 2011;15(suppl 1):S17–S24.
242. Via MA, et al. Bromocriptine approved as the first medication to target dopamine activity to improve glycemic control in patients with type 2 diabetes. *Diabetes Metab Syndr Obes.* 2010;3:43–48.
243. Defronzo RA. Bromocriptine: a sympatholytic, D2-dopamine agonist for the treatment of type 2 diabetes. *Diabetes Care.* 2011;34(4):789–794.
244. Chamarthi B, et al. Timed bromocriptine-QR therapy reduces progression of cardiovascular disease and dysglycemia in subjects with well-controlled type 2 diabetes mellitus. *J Diabetes Res.* 2015;2015:157698.
245. Tell SS, Schafer M, Vigers T, Baumgartner AD, et al. Bromocriptine quick-release as adjunct therapy in youth and adults with type 1 diabetes: a randomized, placebo-controlled crossover study. *Diabetes, Obesity, Metab.* 2022;24(11):2148–2158.
246. Cherney DZ, Kanbay M, Lovshin JA. Renal physiology of glucose handling and therapeutic implications. *Nephrol Dial Transplant.* 2020;35(suppl 1):i3–i12.
247. Vallon V, Thomson SC. Targeting renal glucose reabsorption to treat hyperglycaemia: the pleiotropic effects of SGLT2 inhibition. *Diabetologia.* 2017;60(2):215–225.
248. Henry RR, et al. Efficacy and safety of canagliflozin, a sodium-glucose cotransporter 2 inhibitor, as add-on to insulin in patients with type 1 diabetes. *Diabetes Care.* 2015;38(12):2258–2265.
249. Dandona P, et al. Efficacy and safety of dapagliflozin in patients with inadequately controlled type 1 diabetes: the DEPICT-1 52-week study. *Diabetes Care.* 2018;41(12):2552–2559.
250. Garg SK, Strumph P. Effects of sotagliflozin added to insulin in type 1 diabetes. *N Engl J Med.* 2018;378(10):967–968.
251. Yokono M, et al. SGLT2 selective inhibitor ipragliflozin reduces body fat mass by increasing fatty acid oxidation in high-fat diet-induced obese rats. *Eur J Pharmacol.* 2014;727:66–74.
252. Scholtes RA, et al. Renal haemodynamic and protective effects of renoactive drugs in type 2 diabetes: Interaction with SGLT2 inhibitors. *Nephrology (Carlton).* 2021;26(5):377–390.
253. Hesp AC, et al. The role of renal hypoxia in the pathogenesis of diabetic kidney disease: a promising target for newer renoprotective agents including SGLT2 inhibitors? *Kidney Int.* 2020;98(3):579–589.
254. Bjornstad P, et al. The potential roles of osmotic and nonosmotic sodium handling in mediating the effects of sodium-glucose cotransporter 2 inhibitors on heart failure. *J Card Fail.* 2021;27(12):1447–1455.
255. van Raalte DH, Bjornstad P. Role of sodium-glucose cotransporter 2 inhibition to mitigate diabetic kidney disease risk in type 1 diabetes. *Nephrol Dial Transplant.* 2020;35(suppl 1):i24–i32.
256. Scholtes RA, et al. Sodium glucose cotransporter (SGLT)-2 inhibitors: do we need them for glucose-lowering, for cardiorenal protection or both? *Diabetes Obes Metab.* 2019;21(suppl 2):24–33.
257. Mahmud FH, et al. Adjunct-to-insulin therapy using SGLT2 inhibitors in youth with type 1 diabetes: a randomized controlled trial. *Nat Med.* 2025. https://doi.org/10.1038/s41591-025-03723-6. Epub ahead of print. PMID: 40481206.
258. Anandhakrishnan A, Korbonits M. Glucagon-like peptide 1 in the pathophysiology and pharmacotherapy of clinical obesity. *World J Diabetes.* 2016;7(20):572–598.
259. Meier JJ. GLP-1 receptor agonists for individualized treatment of type 2 diabetes mellitus. *Nat Rev Endocrinol.* 2012;8(12):728–742.
260. Kalra S, et al. Consensus recommendations on GLP-1 RA use in the management of type 2 diabetes mellitus: South Asian Task Force. *Diabetes Ther.* 2019;10(5):1645–1717.
261. Baggio LL, et al. GLP-1 receptor expression within the human heart. *Endocrinology.* 2018;159(4):1570–1584.
262. Bethel MA, et al. Cardiovascular outcomes with glucagon-like peptide-1 receptor agonists in patients with type 2 diabetes: a meta-analysis. *Lancet Diabetes Endocrinol.* 2018;6(2):105–113.
263. Marso SP, et al. Semaglutide and cardiovascular outcomes in patients with type 2 diabetes. *N Engl J Med.* 2016;375(19):1834–1844.
264. Kim M, et al. GLP-1 receptor activation and Epac2 link atrial natriuretic peptide secretion to control of blood pressure. *Nat Med.* 2013;19(5): 567–575.
265. Yamamoto H, et al. Glucagon-like peptide-1-responsive catecholamine neurons in the area postrema link peripheral glucagon-like peptide-1 with central autonomic control sites. *J Neurosci.* 2003;23(7):2939–2946.
266. Fonseca VA, et al. Reductions in insulin resistance are mediated primarily via weight loss in subjects with type 2 diabetes on semaglutide. *J Clin Endocrinol Metab.* 2019;104(9):4078–4086.
267. Davies M, et al. Semaglutide 2.4 mg once a week in adults with overweight or obesity, and type 2 diabetes (STEP 2): a randomised, double-blind, double-dummy, placebo-controlled, phase 3 trial. *Lancet.* 2021;397(10278): 971–984.
268. Johansen NJ, et al. Effect of short-acting exenatide administered three times daily on markers of cardiovascular disease in type 1 diabetes: A randomized double-blind placebo-controlled trial. *Diabetes Obes Metab.* 2020;22(9):1639–1647.
269. Dube MC, D.'Amours M, Weisnagel SJ. Beyond glycaemic control: a crossover, double-blinded, 24-week intervention with liraglutide in type 1 diabetes. *Diabetes Obes Metab.* 2018;20(1):178–184.
270. Frandsen CS, et al. Liraglutide as adjunct to insulin treatment in type 1 diabetes does not interfere with glycaemic recovery or gastric emptying rate during hypoglycaemia: a randomized, placebo-controlled, double-blind, parallel-group study. *Diabetes Obes Metab.* 2017;19(6):773–782.
271. Dejgaard TF, et al. Efficacy and safety of liraglutide for overweight adult patients with type 1 diabetes and insufficient glycaemic control (Lira-1): a randomised, double-blind, placebo-controlled trial. *Lancet Diabetes Endocrinol.* 2016;4(3):221–232.
272. Ceriello A, et al. Glucagon-like peptide 1 reduces endothelial dysfunction, inflammation, and oxidative stress induced by both hyperglycemia and hypoglycemia in type 1 diabetes. *Diabetes Care.* 2013;36(8):2346–2350.
273. Dejgaard TF, et al. Effects of liraglutide on cardiovascular risk factors in patients with type 1 diabetes. *Diabetes Obes Metab.* 2017;19(5):734–738.
274. Singh G, Can AS, Correa R. Pioglitazone. In: *StatPearls.* StatPearls Publishing; 2022.
275. Zdravkovic V, et al. Pioglitazone as adjunctive therapy in adolescents with type 1 diabetes. *J Pediatr.* 2006;149(6):845–849.
276. Bhat R, et al. Effect of pioglitazone therapy in lean type 1 diabetes mellitus. *Diabetes Res Clin Pract.* 2007;78(3):349–354.
277. Stone ML, et al. The addition of rosiglitazone to insulin in adolescents with type 1 diabetes and poor glycaemic control: a randomized-controlled trial. *Pediatr Diabetes.* 2008;9(4 Pt 1):326–334.
278. Messerli FH, et al. Angiotensin-converting enzyme inhibitors in hypertension: to use or not to use? *J Am Coll Cardiol.* 2018;71(13):1474–1482.
279. Hornig B, Kohler C, Drexler H. Role of bradykinin in mediating vascular effects of angiotensin-converting enzyme inhibitors in humans. *Circulation.* 1997;95(5):1115–1118.
280. Messerli FH, Weber MA, Brunner HR. Angiotensin II receptor inhibition. A new therapeutic principle. *Arch Intern Med.* 1996;156(17):1957–1965.
281. ACE Inhibitors in Diabetic Nephropathy Trialist Group. Should all patients with type 1 diabetes mellitus and microalbuminuria receive angiotensin-converting enzyme inhibitors? A meta-analysis of individual patient data. *Ann Intern Med.* 2001;134(5):370–379.
282. Bangalore S, et al. Diabetes mellitus as a compelling indication for use of renin angiotensin system blockers: systematic review and meta-analysis of randomized trials. *BMJ.* 2016;352:i438.
283. Akbari P, Khorasani-Zadeh A. Thiazide diuretics. In: *StatPearls.* StatPearls Publishing; 2022.
284. Whelton PK, et al. Clinical outcomes in antihypertensive treatment of type 2 diabetes, impaired fasting glucose concentration, and normoglycemia: Antihypertensive and Lipid-Lowering Treatment to Prevent Heart Attack Trial (ALLHAT). *Arch Intern Med.* 2005;165(12):1401–1409.
285. Morgan DB, Davidson C. Hypokalaemia and diuretics: an analysis of publications. *Br Med J.* 1980;280(6218):905–908.
286. Bloomfield RL, Wilson DJ, Buckalew Jr. VM. The incidence of diuretic-induced hypokalemia in two distinct clinic settings. *J Clin Hypertens.* 1986;2(4):331–338.
287. Rowe JW, et al. Effect of experimental potassium deficiency on glucose and insulin metabolism. *Metabolism.* 1980;29(6):498–502.
288. Siscovick DS, et al. Diuretic therapy for hypertension and the risk of primary cardiac arrest. *N Engl J Med.* 1994;330(26):1852–1857.
289. Siegel D, et al. Diuretics, serum and intracellular electrolyte levels, and ventricular arrhythmias in hypertensive men. *JAMA.* 1992;267(8):1083–1089.
290. Myers MG. Diuretic therapy and ventricular arrhythmias in persons 65 years of age and older. *Am J Cardiol.* 1990;65(9):599–603.
291. Wiysonge CS, Volmink J, Opie LH. Beta-blockers and the treatment of hypertension: it is time to move on. *Cardiovasc J Afr.* 2007;18(6):351–352.

292. Weber MA. The role of the new beta-blockers in treating cardiovascular disease. *Am J Hypertens*. 2005;18(12 Pt 2):169S–176S.
293. Tsujimoto T, et al. Intensive glycemic therapy in patients with type 2 diabetes on beta-blockers. *Diabetes Care*. 2016;39(10):1818–1826.
294. Cushman WC, et al. ACCORD Study Group Effects of intensive blood-pressure control in type 2 diabetes mellitus. *N Engl J Med*. 2010;362(17): 1575–1585.
295. Hirsch IB, et al. Higher glycemic thresholds for symptoms during beta-adrenergic blockade in IDDM. *Diabetes*. 1991;40(9):1177–1186.
296. Tsujimoto T, et al. Risk of cardiovascular events in patients with diabetes mellitus on beta-blockers. *Hypertension*. 2017;70(1):103–110.
297. Lager I, Blohme G, Smith U. Effect of cardioselective and non-selective beta-blockade on the hypoglycaemic response in insulin-dependent diabetics. *Lancet*. 1979;1(8114):458–462.
298. Kerr D, et al. Beta-adrenoceptor blockade and hypoglycaemia. A randomised, double-blind, placebo controlled comparison of metoprolol CR, atenolol and propranolol LA in normal subjects. *Br J Clin Pharmacol*. 1990;29(6):685–693.
299. Ramanathan R, Cryer PE. Adrenergic mediation of hypoglycemia-associated autonomic failure. *Diabetes*. 2011;60(2):602–606.
300. Farhat R, et al. Carvedilol prevents counterregulatory failure and impaired hypoglycaemia awareness in non-diabetic recurrently hypoglycaemic rats. *Diabetologia*. 2019;62(4):676–686.
301. Tocci G, et al. Calcium channel blockers and hypertension. *J Cardiovasc Pharmacol Ther*. 2015;20(2):121–130.
302. Pepine CJ, et al. A calcium antagonist vs a non-calcium antagonist hypertension treatment strategy for patients with coronary artery disease. The International Verapamil-Trandolapril Study (INVEST): a randomized controlled trial. *JAMA*. 2003;290(21):2805–2816.
303. Liu L, et al. The Felodipine Event Reduction (FEVER) Study: a randomized long-term placebo-controlled trial in Chinese hypertensive patients. *J Hypertens*. 2005;23(12):2157–2172.
304. ALLHAT Officers and Coordinators for the ALLHAT Collaborative Research Group. The Antihypertensive and Lipid-Lowering Treatment to Prevent Heart Attack Trial Major outcomes in high-risk hypertensive patients randomized to angiotensin-converting enzyme inhibitor or calcium channel blocker vs diuretic: The Antihypertensive and Lipid-Lowering Treatment to Prevent Heart Attack Trial (ALLHAT). *JAMA*. 2002;288(23):2981–2997.
305. Ovalle F, et al. Verapamil and beta cell function in adults with recent-onset type 1 diabetes. *Nat Med*. 2018;24(8):1108–1112.
306. Xu G, et al. Preventing beta-cell loss and diabetes with calcium channel blockers. *Diabetes*. 2012;61(4):848–856.
307. Xu G, et al. Exploratory study reveals far reaching systemic and cellular effects of verapamil treatment in subjects with type 1 diabetes. *Nat Commun*. 2022;13(1):1159.
308. Ward NC, Watts GF, Eckel RH. Statin toxicity. *Circ Res*. 2019;124(2):328–350.
309. Buhaescu I, Izzedine H. Mevalonate pathway: a review of clinical and therapeutical implications. *Clin Biochem*. 2007;40(9–10):575–584.
310. American Diabetes Association. 10. Microvascular Complications and Foot Care: Standards of Medical Care in Diabetes-2018. *Diabetes Care*. 2018;41(Supplement 1):S105–S118.
311. Grundy SM, et al. 2018 AHA/ACC/AACVPR/AAPA/ABC/ACPM/ADA/AGS/APhA/ASPC/NLA/PCNA Guideline on the Management of Blood Cholesterol: a report of the American College of Cardiology/American Heart Association Task Force on Clinical Practice Guidelines. *Circulation*. 2019;139(25):e1082–e1143.
312. Silverman MG, et al. Association between lowering LDL-C and cardiovascular risk reduction among different therapeutic interventions: a systematic review and meta-analysis. *JAMA*. 2016;316(12):1289–1297.
313. Brown JD, Plutzky J. Peroxisome proliferator-activated receptors as transcriptional nodal points and therapeutic targets. *Circulation*. 2007; 115(4):518–533.
314. Rosenson RS, et al. Modulating peroxisome proliferator-activated receptors for therapeutic benefit? Biology, clinical experience, and future prospects. *Am Heart J*. 2012;164(5):672–680.
315. Chakravarthy MV, et al. Identification of a physiologically relevant endogenous ligand for PPARalpha in liver. *Cell*. 2009;138(3):476–488.
316. Haemmerle G, et al. ATGL-mediated fat catabolism regulates cardiac mitochondrial function via PPAR-alpha and PGC-1. *Nat Med*. 2011;17(9): 1076–1085.
317. Zheng C, et al. Statins suppress apolipoprotein CIII-induced vascular endothelial cell activation and monocyte adhesion. *Eur Heart J*. 2013;34(8):615–624.

PART II CARDIOVASCULAR COMPLICATIONS OF TYPE 2 DIABETES

6 Epidemiology of Diabetes Mellitus and Atherosclerotic Cardiovascular Disease

NATHAN D. WONG AND WENJUN FAN

KEY POINTS

- Diabetes mellitus (DM) is associated with approximately a **2–4 times higher risk** of coronary artery disease (CAD), stroke, peripheral artery disease (PAD), and heart failure. These conditions are leading causes of death among people with diabetes, especially in those with coexisting atherosclerotic cardiovascular disease (ASCVD).
- Subclinical markers including **coronary artery calcium (CAC)** and **carotid intimal medial thickness (IMT)** are prevalent in people with diabetes and predict future cardiovascular events. CAC scoring is especially valuable in identifying high risk but asymptomatic individuals with diabetes.
- Mortality and event rates from CAD, CVD, and all causes increase progressively across disease states, from metabolic syndrome to diabetes without CVD, to CVD alone, and are **highest in those with both diabetes and CVD**.
- While previous studies classified diabetes as a "coronary heart disease risk equivalent," **recent evidence shows heterogeneity** in cardiovascular risk among people with diabetes. Factors like duration of diabetes, HbA_{1c}, and kidney function strongly influence whether an individual reaches this equivalence.
- People with diabetes often exhibit coexisting **hypertension, dyslipidemia, obesity**, and **unhealthy lifestyle habits**, amplifying their ASCVD risk. However, **risk factor control is generally suboptimal**, with less than 20% achieving combined targets for HbA_{1c}, BP, and LDL-C.
- Several tools like **UKPDS, TIMI, and SCORE2-Diabetes** offer tailored risk prediction for individuals with diabetes. Newer models integrate diabetes-specific factors such as duration, HbA_{1c}, and eGFR to improve accuracy.
- Achieving control of multiple risk factors significantly reduces cardiovascular event rates. Clinical trials like **Steno-2** demonstrate that **intensive therapy** targeting glucose, BP, and lipids can reduce cardiovascular morbidity and mortality in people with type 2 diabetes.

Diabetes mellitus (DM) is characterized by hyperglycemia as a result of insulin secretion, excessive glucagon secretion, or insulin resistance.[1,2] Globally, DM prevalence was estimated to be 9.3% (463 million people) in 2019, predicted to increase to 10.2% (578 million) by 2030 and 10.9% (700 million) by 2045.[3] Overall, 38.4 million persons (11.6%) in the United States of all ages had DM in 2021, including 38.1 million adults $\geq$18 years of age (14.7%), with an additional 97.6 million (38.0%) having pre-DM.[4]

Atherosclerotic cardiovascular diseases (ASCVD), i.e., coronary artery disease (CAD), cerebrovascular disease, and peripheral artery disease (PAD), are the most important complications in those with DM,[5] representing the main causes of morbidity and mortality in subjects with type 2 DM, where it occurs approximately 15 years earlier than in people without DM[6] and affecting about one-third of patients with type 2 DM.[7] The risk for developing ASCVD is two to four times higher in patients with versus without DM.[8] Half or more of medical costs of DM in the United States are attributed to treating cardiovascular complications.[9]

Atherosclerosis is accelerated in type 2 DM[10] and involves progression from the fatty streak to the formation of more complex atherosclerotic plaques that can rupture, resulting in myocardial infarction (MI), unstable angina, or strokes.[11] Patients with DM who have microvascular complications are also at higher risk of accelerated atherosclerosis, ultimately resulting in cerebrovascular and cardiovascular events and premature mortality.[10]

This chapter describes the epidemiology of ASCVD in persons with DM, including major complications, ASCVD risk assessment, as well as the major cardiovascular disease risk factors in those with DM and the current state of their control and relation to cardiovascular outcomes.

DIABETES IN PERSONS WITH PREEXISTING ATHEROSCLEROTIC CARDIOVASCULAR DISEASE

ASCVD are the leading causes of death in persons with DM.[12] Multiple indirect or direct pathways resulting in accelerated atherosclerosis have been proposed to explain the deleterious effects of hyperglycemia on the cardiovascular system. Indirect pathways promoted by hyperglycemia include worsening of dyslipidemia, especially the development of atherogenic dyslipidemia and sympathetic nervous system dysfunction. Direct acceleration of the atherosclerotic process by hyperglycemia may be in part related to endothelial dysfunction that in turn promotes vasoconstrictive, proinflammatory, and prothrombotic processes that contribute to plaque development and rupture.[13] Among several large studies of persons with established CAD, 18% to 31% already have DM and more than a third have pre-DM.[14] From the Ludwigshafen Risk and Cardiovascular Health Study, approximately 20% of males and 25% of females had previously diagnosed DM.[15] Among the Euro Heart Survey on Diabetes and the Heart of more than 4000 patients referred to a cardiologist because of suspected CAD, 31% had manifest DM.[16] And in another study from Spain, among 662 consecutive patients admitted to the hospital without a previous diagnosis of DM who were referred for coronary intervention, the prevalence of DM was 45%.[17]

SUBCLINICAL ATHEROSCLEROSIS IN DIABETES MELLITUS

Prior to the development of clinical events, subclinical atherosclerosis is normally present and identifies those at greater risk for the development of clinical events. Most data on subclinical atherosclerosis derives from carotid ultrasonography measuring carotid intimal medial thickness and plaque for examining carotid atherosclerosis, coronary artery calcium (CAC) scanning for examining coronary atherosclerosis, and ankle-brachial index (ABI) screening for evaluation of peripheral arterial disease. In the Cardiovascular Health Study (CHS), 1343 patients with DM, 1432 patients with impaired glucose tolerance (IGT), and 2421 normoglycemic patients were followed on average for 6.4 years. Those with DM had a higher prevalence of clinical and subclinical cardiovascular disease (CVD) (assessed by several measures) that was strongly associated with subsequent coronary heart disease (CHD), stroke, and heart failure (Fig. 6.1).[18]

In a systematic review[19] of the relevance of carotid IMT in patients with type 2 DM and IGT comprising 23 studies with 20,111 patients, including 4019 with DM and 1110 with IGT, showed those with DM to have increases in IMT approximately three times that of those with IGT, as well

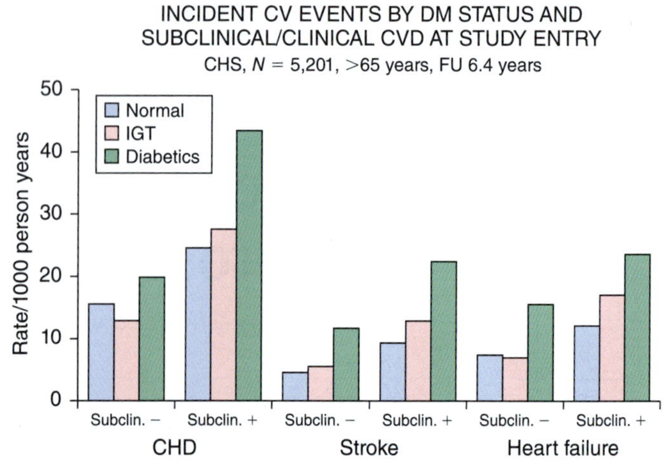

FIG. 6.1 Diabetes status and presence of subclinical and clinical CVD at baseline and incidence of specific events among males and females in the CHS. *CHD*, Coronary heart disease; *CVD*, cardiovascular disease; *DM*, diabetes mellitus; *IGT*, impaired glucose tolerance. Modified from Kuller LH, Velentgas P, Barzilay J, et al. Diabetes mellitus: subclinical cardiovascular disease and risk of incident cardiovascular disease and all-cause mortality, *Arterioscler Thromb Vasc Biol*. 2000;20:823–829.

as an increased risk of MI and stroke in those with DM of nearly 40%. Moreover, the Bruneck study[20] examined patients with metabolic syndrome who had an increased 5-year incidence and progression of carotid atherosclerosis as well as clinical events compared with controls.

Both low (<0.9) and high (>1.3) ABI as a measure of PAD has been associated with increased cardiovascular and other complications in persons with type 2 DM among a large cohort study of 34,689 persons, with increases in incidence (per 1000 person-years) for mortality and acute MI of 15.4 and 4.1, respectively, with risks rising steeply below 0.9.[21] A cohort study from China also recently showed low ABI (<0.9) as well as ankle-brachial pulse wave velocity (highest quartile) to be independently associated with cardiovascular and total mortality, with the combination of the two being associated with the highest risks (relative risks of 4.5 for all-cause and 9.7 for cardiovascular mortality).[22] Finally, a Brazilian study of persons with type 2 DM showed after 10 years of follow-up, those with a baseline ABI of ≤0.90 have a 2.1-fold increased risk of all-cause mortality, 2.7-fold excess risk of cardiovascular mortality, and a 2.5-fold increased risk of major adverse cardiovascular events.[23]

Several studies have also assessed the prevalence and progression of CAC and its prognostic significance for ASCVD events in persons with DM. Wong et al.[24] reported in a study of 1823 individuals aged 23 to 79 years that the prevalence of CAC increased progressively across metabolic risk groups: among men, CAC prevalence was 53.5% in those without metabolic syndrome or diabetes, 58.8% in those with metabolic syndrome, and 75.3% in those with diabetes; among women, the corresponding prevalences were 37.6%, 50.8%, and 52.6%, respectively. CAC prevalence also rose with the number of metabolic syndrome components, increasing from 34% in those with none to 58% in those with all five components. Moreover, data from the Multi-Ethnic Study of Atherosclerosis (MESA) showed a greater prevalence of CAC in those with metabolic syndrome and especially DM, with an approximate 10-fold increase in CHD events across CAC scores ranging from 0 to ≥400; annual CHD event rates in those with DM ranged from 0.4% per year in those with CAC scores of 0%

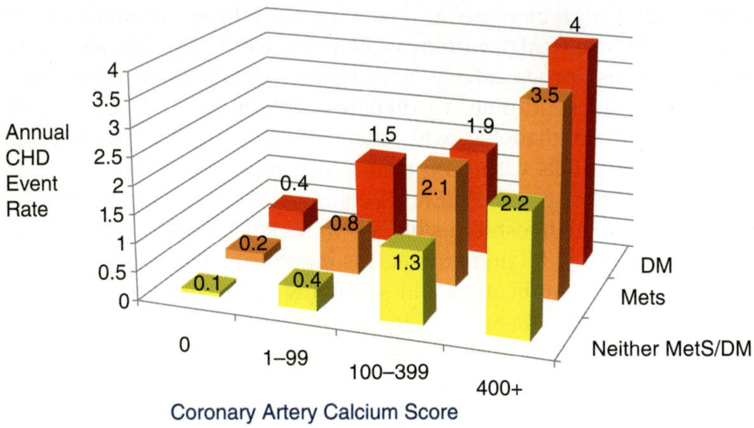

FIG. 6.2 Annual CHD event rates (%) by calcium score categories in subjects with diabetes, metabolic syndrome (*MetS*), or neither condition. *CHD*, Cardiovascular Health Study; *DM*, diabetes mellitus. Adapted from Malik S, Budoff MJ, Katz R, et al. Impact of subclinical atherosclerosis on cardiovascular disease events in individuals with metabolic syndrome and diabetes: the multi-ethnic study of atherosclerosis. *Diabetes Care*. 2011;34(10):2285–2290.

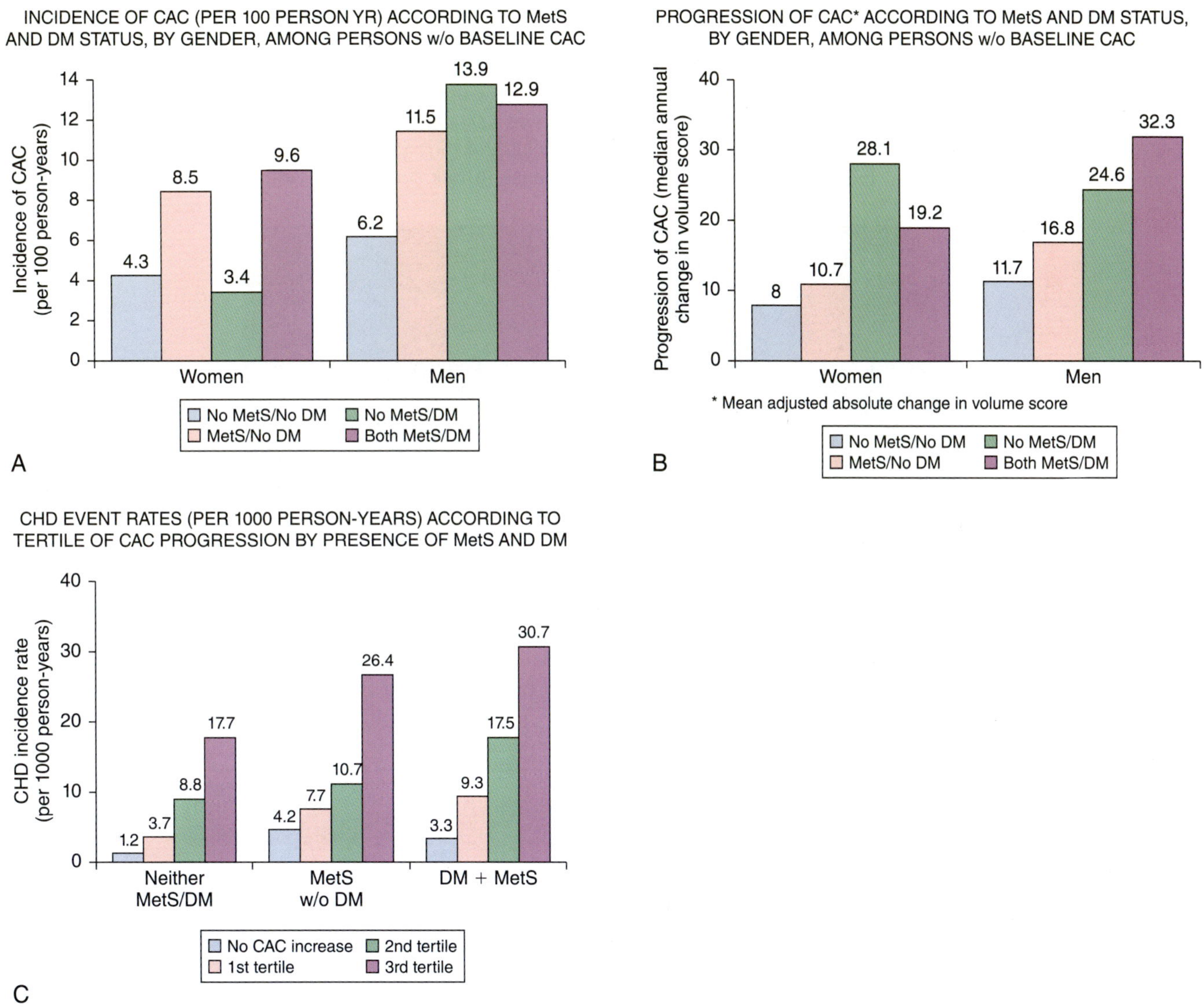

FIG. 6.3 **A**, Incidence of CAC (per 100 person-years) according to metabolic syndrome (*MetS*) and diabetes (*DM*) status by gender among persons without baseline CAC. **B**, Progression of CAC (mean unadjusted absolute change in volume score) according to MetS and DM status by gender in persons without baseline CAC. **C**, CHD event rates (per 1000 person-years) according to tertile of CAC progression by presence of MetS and DM. Data are not shown for persons with DM without MetS because of an insufficient number of CHD events. *CHD*, Cardiovascular Health Study; *CAD*, coronary artery disease; *DM*, diabetes mellitus. From Wong ND, Nelson JC, Granston T, et al. Metabolic syndrome, diabetes, and incidence and progression of coronary calcium: the Multiethnic Study of Atherosclerosis study. *JACC Cardiovasc Imaging.* 2012;5:358–366.

to 4% per year with CAC scores of ≥400 (Fig. 6.2), with CAC providing significant improvements in the C-statistic beyond risk factors.[25] In a follow-up study from MESA, those with metabolic syndrome or DM had a higher incidence and absolute progression of CAC compared with patients without DM. In addition, CAC progression predicted future CHD events (Fig. 6.3).[26] Moreover, data from the Dallas Heart Study showed that both MetS and DM were independently associated with a greater prevalence of atherosclerosis evaluated by CAC, with the highest prevalence seen in those fulfilling both criteria.[27]

Elkeles et al.[28] prospectively evaluated CAC score as a predictor for CVD events in 589 patients with type 2 DM, finding that after 4 years first CHD and stroke events were 32% greater for every doubling of CAC score. CAC scoring improved discrimination over and above the Framingham CHD risk score and the United Kingdom Prospective Diabetes Study (UKPDS) risk score. Finally, in a recent meta-analysis of 10 studies (n = 110,396 person-years) with prognostic data, the pooled relative risks for the incidence of all-cause death and/or cardiovascular events were 4.03 (95% CI, 3.04–5.34), 5.87 (95% CI, 4.32–7.99), and 9.04 (95% CI, 5.81–14.06), respectively, for CAC scores >0 versus 0, CAC scores ≥100 versus 0.[29] These data support the important role of CAC scoring as the most valuable subclinical disease measure to improve risk prediction in asymptomatic patients with DM.

CARDIOVASCULAR OUTCOMES IN PERSONS WITH DIABETES

Using data from the US National Health and Nutrition Examination Survey (NHANES), we initially demonstrated a stepwise increase in mortality rates from coronary artery disease (CAD), cardiovascular disease (CVD), and all causes across progressively more severe disease states: from metabolic syndrome, to diabetes without prior CVD, to CVD without diabetes, with the highest mortality observed in individuals with both prior CVD and diabetes[30] (Fig. 6.4). In addition, the CALIBER UK cohort showed the most common initial manifestations of CVD to be PAD and heart failure, followed by MI and stroke; this emphasizes the importance of early identification and screening of these conditions (Fig. 6.5).[31] A meta-analysis involving nearly 700,000 patients and over 50,000 vascular outcomes from the Emerging Risk Factors Collaboration (Fig. 6.6)[32] showed DM to be associated with a two- to threefold excess risk for a wide range of vascular diseases independently from conventional risk factors, including MI, coronary death, hemorrhagic stroke, and other vascular deaths. From the UK Clinical Practice Research Datalink of over 700,000 adults with and without type 2 DM with follow-up for first CVD events over 11 years, while type 2 DM was associated with a small increase in CVD events (HR, 1.06 [1.02–1.09]) in White individuals, there was a greater increase in risk seen in individuals of South Asian ethnicity

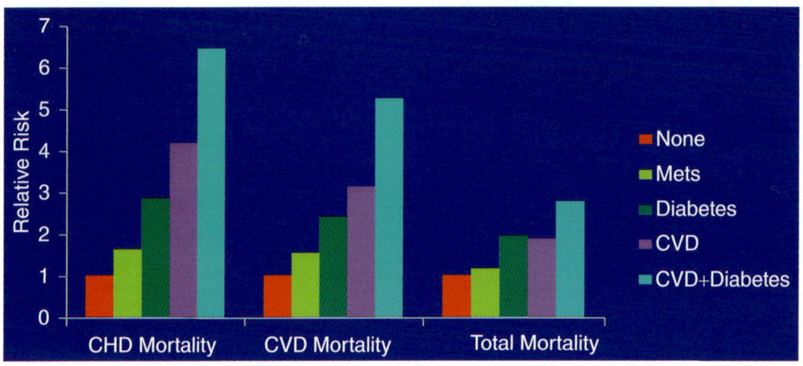

FIG. 6.4 Metabolic syndrome and diabetes in relation to CHD, CVD, and total mortality: US mention and female ages 30–74 (risk factor-adjusted Cox regression): NHANES II follow-up (n = 6255). *CHD*, Cardiovascular Health Study; *CVD*, Cardiovascular disease; *MetS*, metabolic syndrome. Adapted from Malik S, Wong ND, Franklin SS, Kamath TV, L'Italien GJ, Pio JR, Williams GR. Impact of the metabolic syndrome on mortality from coronary heart disease, cardiovascular disease, and all causes in United States adults. *Circulation*. 2004;110(10):1245–50.

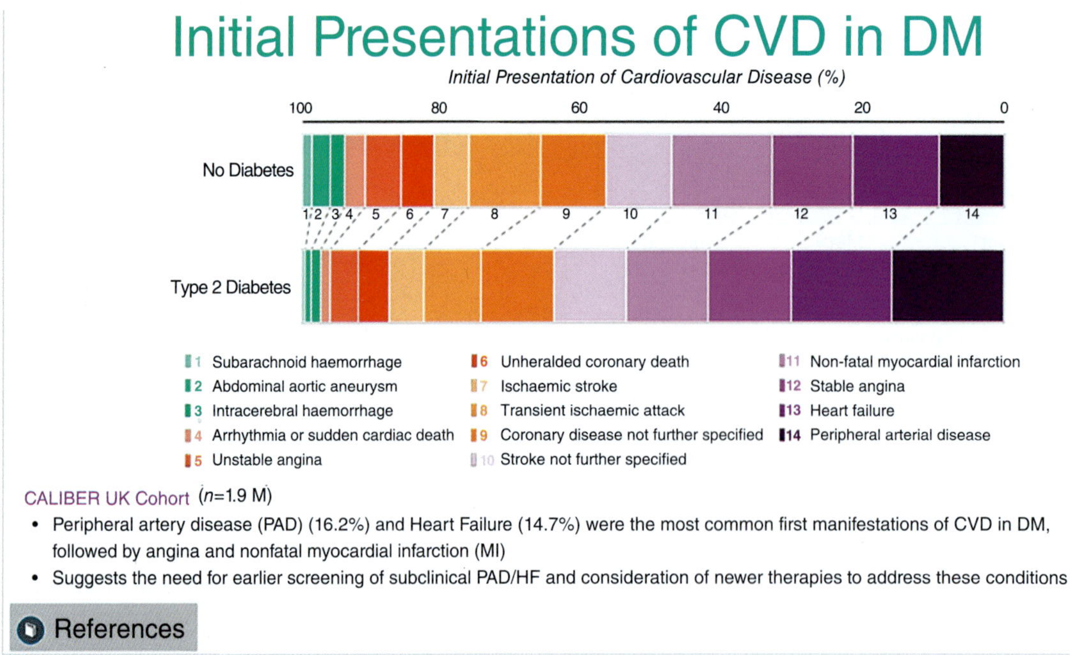

FIG. 6.5 CALIBER UK cohort (n = 1.9 million) most common initial presentations of cardiovascular disease (*CVD*) in diabetes mellitus (*DM*). Adapted from Shah AD, Langenberg C, Rapsomaniki E, et al. Type 2 diabetes and incidence of cardiovascular diseases: a cohort study in 1.9 million people. *Lancet Diabetes Endocrinol*. 2015;3(2):105–113.

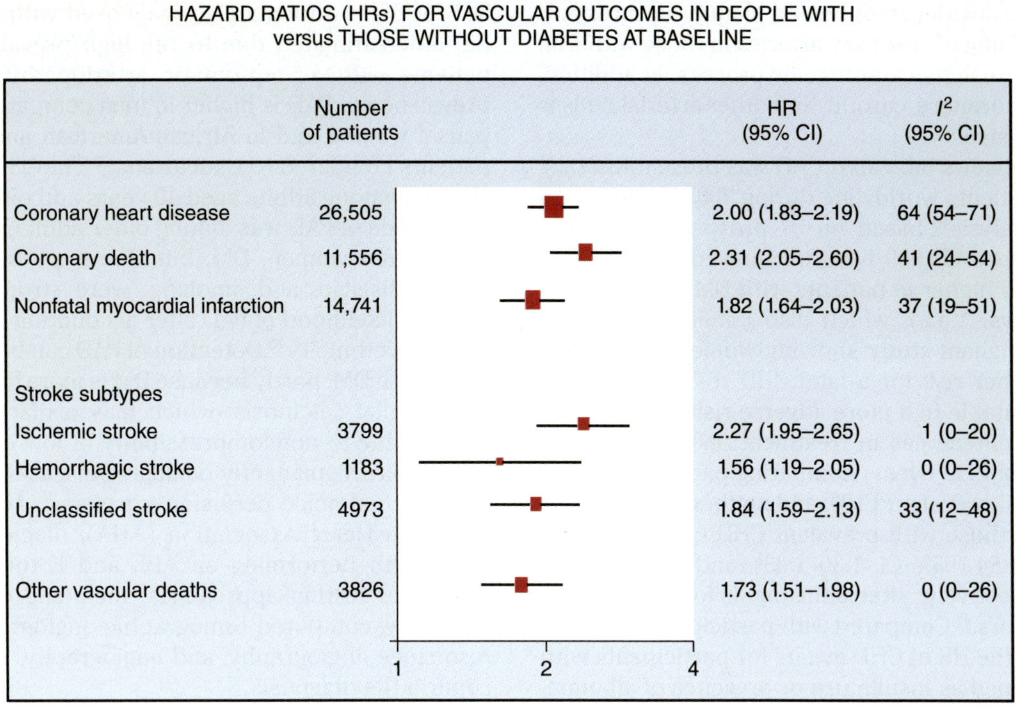

FIG. 6.6 Hazard ratios (*HRs*) for vascular outcomes in people with versus those without diabetes at baseline. *CI*, Confidence interval; I^2, statistic for heterogeneity. From Emerging Risk Factors Collaboration; Sarwar N, Gao P, Seshasai SR, et al. Diabetes mellitus, fasting blood glucose concentration, and risk of vascular disease: a collaborative meta-analysis of 102 prospective studies. *Lancet* 2010;375:2215–2222.

(1.28 [1.09–1.51]), primarily due to an increased risk of MI (1.53 [1.08–2.18]).[33] In a systematic review and meta-analysis from 26 observational studies among over 1.3 million persons across 30 countries, the age at DM diagnosis was inversely associated with all-cause mortality and macrovascular and microvascular disease risk (all $P<0.001$).[34] Each 1-year increase in age at DM diagnosis was associated with a 4%, 3%, and 5% decreased risk of all-cause mortality, macrovascular disease, and microvascular disease, respectively, adjusted for age.

There is also a wealth of data regarding long-term glycemic control in patients with DM and its association with macrovascular complications such as MI, stroke, amputation, and total mortality. In the UKPDS 35[35] each 1% reduction in mean hemoglobin A1c (HbA_{1c}) was associated with reductions in risk of 21% for any endpoint related to DM, 21% for deaths, and 40% for MI. The European Prospective Investigation into Cancer and Nutrition (EPIC)[36] study comprising 4662 males aged 45 to 79 years showed those with manifest DM had a 3.5-fold increased risk of death from all causes, more than an 8-fold increased risk of cardiovascular mortality, and a 10-fold increased risk for CHD compared with patients with an HbA_{1c} of less than 5%. However, from an HbA_{1c} from below 5% to above 7%, there was a gradual increase for all of the above-mentioned endpoints, suggesting that even in the normal upper range of HbA_{1c} an increased risk of death or nonfatal coronary complications was present.

Significant data also support DM as a stronger risk factor for CVD outcomes in females compared to males. A 36-year follow-up in the Framingham Heart Study initially showed DM to be associated with a 3.7-fold greater risk of all CVD events in females compared to 2.2-fold in men. There was a 6.4-fold greater risk of PAD in females with DM compared to 3.4-fold in men with DM; for heart failure these risks were 7.8-fold and 4.4-fold, respectively.[37] Moreover, the Interheart Study showed DM to be a stronger risk factor for CVD in females than in men.[38] The British Regional Heart Study and British Women's Heart Health Study[39] examined a large panel of traditional and more novel risk markers, such as insulin resistance, inflammation, activated coagulation, and endothelial dysfunction, in 7529 men and females aged 60 to 79 years with no previous MI showed greater differences in several of these factors among females compared to men with DM versus without DM, potentially explaining their greater CVD risk. There also was an increased risk of death in females with DM who developed complications after MI, such as congestive heart failure.[40] However, in the TECOS trial of adults with type 2 DM and ASCVD, females with DM had a lower risk of secondary MI (HR, 0.70 [95% CI, 0.55–0.90]) and stroke (HR, 0.52 [95% CI, 0.38–0.71]) than males with DM.[41] In the UK Biobank, the association between previously diagnosed DM and MI was stronger in females (HR, 2.33 [95% CI, 1.96–2.78]) than in males (HR, 1.81 [95% CI, 1.63–2.02]).[42] Among male National Health Interview Study participants enrolled in 2000 to 2009 and followed up through 2011, DM was associated with increased risk for heart disease mortality (HR, 1.72 [95% CI, 1.53–1.93]), cerebrovascular mortality (HR, 1.48 [95% CI, 1.18–1.85]), and CVD mortality (HR, 1.67 [95% CI, 1.51–1.86]). Among female participants, DM was also associated with increased risk for heart disease mortality (HR, 2.02 [95% CI, 1.81–2.25]), cerebrovascular mortality (HR, 1.43 [95% CI, 1.15–1.77]), and CVD mortality (HR, 1.85 [95% CI, 1.69–1.96]).[43]

Coronary Artery Disease

In patients with DM, coronary artery plaques generally exhibit larger necrotic cores and significantly greater inflammation relative to patients without DM. Moreover, there is a higher incidence of healed plaque ruptures and positive remodeling of coronary arteries in those with DM, suggesting a more active atherogenic process. In addition, calcification of coronary, carotid, and other arterial beds is also more extensive.[44]

Systematic reviews indicated CAD was present in 21.2% of type 2 DM patients worldwide during 2007 to 2017.[45] An earlier meta-analysis[46] based on 37 prospective cohorts comprising almost 450,000 patients showed that the rate of fatal CHD was higher in patients with DM than in those without (5.4% vs. 1.6%), which also confirmed findings from the Framingham study showing women with DM to have a 50% higher risk for a fatal CHD than men, which might be attributable to a more adverse risk factor profile in women and differences in treatment. In the REGARDS study, the HRs of CHD events comparing participants with DM only, DM and prevalent CHD, and neither DM nor prevalent CHD with those with prevalent CHD were 0.65 (95% CI, 0.54–0.77), 1.54 (95% CI, 1.30–1.83), and 0.41 (95% CI, 0.35–0.47), respectively, after adjustment for demographics and risk factors.[47] Compared with participants who had prevalent CHD, the HR of CHD events for participants with severe DM (defined as insulin use or presence of albuminuria) was 0.88 (95% CI, 0.72–1.09).

Cerebrovascular Diseases

DM is also strongly associated with increased risk of cerebrovascular outcomes. In a large, international, multicenter case-control study across 32 countries (n = 26,919) DM defined by an HbA_{1c} of ≥6.5% (48 mmol/mol) was found in 26% of acute stroke inpatients compared with 22% of nonstroke controls.[48] In addition, those with DM are more likely to develop ischemic stroke than hemorrhagic stroke.[48] Among stroke patients, those who also have DM have longer hospital stays[49–51] and increased hospital readmission and stroke recurrence at 3 months,[52] 6 months,[53] and 1 year[54] after the index stroke.

Those with a stroke who also have DM compared to those without DM also have greater postdischarge mortality and reduced median survival time.[55,56] Greater levels of HbA_{1c} are also associated with worse stroke outcomes, increased stroke severity, mortality rates, and stroke recurrence[52,55,57,58] in both those with and without DM. HbA_{1c} has been shown to be a good predictor of acute (HR, 1.45; 95% CI, 1.09–1.93, $P = 0.011$) and long-term mortality (HR, 1.29; 95% CI, 1.03–1.62; $P = 0.029$); subjects with HbA_{1c} >6% had a 29% higher risk of severe acute stroke severity and were more likely to experience worse functional outcomes.[57] Moreover, DM is associated with poorer recovery after rehabilitation,[59] higher risk of mortality,[60] and a greater risk of recurrent ischemic stroke.[52,54] Also, among those with a prior ischemic stroke, the risk of mortality and poor outcomes increases with elevated HbA_{1C}, both in those with DM and without DM.

Peripheral Artery Disease in Diabetes Mellitus

Like the other manifestations of atherosclerosis, PAD is linked strongly to DM as well. Studies report more than 12 million people in the United States and over 200 million people worldwide have PAD, with approximately 20% to 30% of these patients also diagnosed with DM that could be underestimated due to the high prevalence of DM in patients with asymptomatic arteriopathy.[61] Overall, the prevalence of PAD is higher in men compared to premenopausal women and in African-American and Hispanic DM patients compared to Caucasians.[62] The US NHANES study showed among adults aged 40 years and older, the highest prevalence of PAD was among older adults, non-Hispanics, Blacks, and women. DM, but also hypertension, chronic kidney disease, and smoking, were strongly associated with the likelihood of PAD after accounting for age, gender, and race/ethnicity.[63] Detection of PAD can be challenging in those with DM, partly because DM is more likely associated with medial calcinosis, which may artifactually increase the ABI due to noncompressibility of low extremity arteries, despite significantly occlusive disease and reductions in the actual ankle perfusion pressure.[64] According to the American Heart Association (AHA), diagnosing PAD can begin with performing an ABI, and if this is abnormal, additional testing approaches, including duplex ultrasonography, computed tomographic angiography, magnetic resonance angiography, and angiography, can be used to confirm the diagnosis.[65]

Several epidemiological studies have suggested a strong association between DM and PAD; thus patients affected by both conditions are at very high risk for major adverse cardiovascular events (MACE) in the future.[64] The Framingham study showed a strong association between DM and PAD.[66] The risk for PAD has been noted to be two to four times greater in those with DM versus without DM.[67] Among patients in Denmark undergoing coronary angiography, those with DM but not CAD had a 1.7-fold increased risk of PAD and lower limb revascularization compared with those without these conditions. Those with both DM and CAD also had a 3.9-fold greater increased risk of PAD and a 4.6-fold greater risk of lower limb revascularization (HR, 4.61 [95% CI, 3.85–5.52]).[68]

In addition, the duration and severity of DM as measured by glycemic control are associated with the incidence and extent of PAD.[69,70] PAD associated with DM often is associated with diffuse and more distal lesions than in those without DM. Evaluation with an ABI shows 20% to 30% of those with DM are diagnostic of PAD based on an ABI <0.9, but among those who have PAD, only about 20% are symptomatic. Although PAD may often be asymptomatic or stable, CHD events often are dramatically increased, with a 20% nonfatal MI and stroke rate and a 30% death rate.[71] Even in the absence of symptomatic PAD, worsening of PAD is associated with a three- to fourfold increased risk of MACE.[72] Atherosclerosis is also most common cause of PAD in patients with DM.[64]

IS DIABETES A CORONARY OR CARDIOVASCULAR DISEASE RISK EQUIVALENT?

In a study by Haffner et al. had found that among a Finnish male population, DM alone carried the equivalent risk of future MI and fatal CVD as patients without DM but a previous MI[73] (Fig. 6.7). But more recently a meta-analysis of nearly 40,000 patients with a follow-up of up to 25 years showed the risk of CAD events to be over 40% lower in those with DM but no prior MI compared to patients with a prior MI but no DM (Fig. 6.8).[74] More recent differences in the DM definition and the extent of comorbidities in the different studies may explain these differences. In the Finnish study, DM diagnosis was based on higher glucose cutpoints used in the past. However, more recent studies using more rigorous definitions of MI and lower thresholds of glucose for defining DM have shown lower risk in patients with DM but without CVD compared with patients after MI but without DM. Evans et al.[75] showed among 3402 patients with newly diagnosed type 2 DM and 5350 post-MI patients, the post-MI group had a nearly threefold greater risk of death and threefold greater risk of recurrent MI over follow-up of more than 10 years. Also, the ARIC study[76] showed those with a history of MI without DM had a 1.9-times greater risk of fatal and nonfatal MI and a 1.8-times greater risk of CHD mortality compared to those with DM without a history of MI, although a similar risk of stroke. Wannamethee et al.[77] showed that patients with both early and late onset of DM had a significantly greater risk of major CHD and CVD events and all-cause mortality compared to those without DM or prior MI, but those diagnosed before age 60 who had a duration of DM of more than 30 years had a similar risk as those with a prior MI without DM. More recent data from Rana et al. from Kaiser Permanente Northern California corroborate these results, showing persons with DM with 10 years or longer duration have a similar risk of future CHD events compared to those with a prior MI.[78] Imaging studies have also shown patients with a DM duration of 10 years or longer showed a greater plaque burden in most diseased segments; also, the proportion of intravascular ultrasound (IVUS)-defined thin-cap fibroatheroma in those with long-standing DM was greater than in those with a DM duration of less than 10 years.[79] Finally, in a recent pooling of four US cohorts Atherosclerosis Risk in Communities [ARIC], Jackson Heart Study [JHS], Multi-Ethnic Study of Atherosclerosis [MESA], Framingham Heart Study-Offspring [FHS-OS]) comprising over 27,000 adults, classifying persons according to the presence or absence of DM and CVD, DM was identified to be a cardiovascular disease

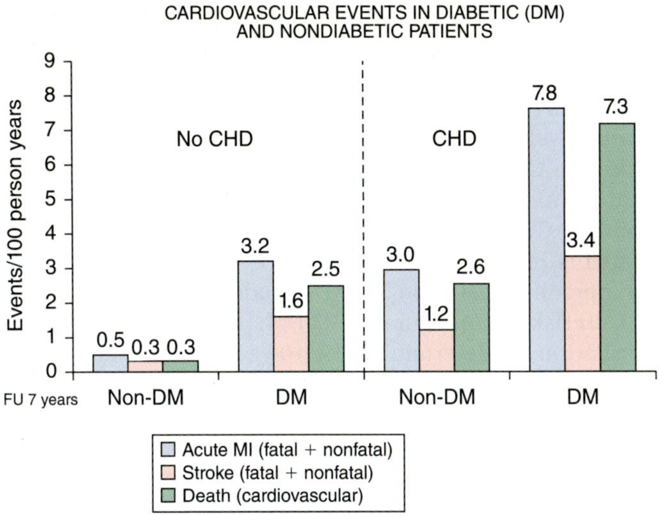

FIG. 6.7 Incidence of cardiovascular events during a 7-year follow-up in relation to history of MI in patients with type 2 diabetes and in nondiabetic patients. *CHD*, Coronary heart disease; *DM*, diabetes mellitus; *MI*, myocardial infarction. Data from Haffner SM, Lehto S, Rönnemaa T, et al. Mortality from coronary heart disease in patients with type 2 diabetes and in nondiabetic patients with and without prior myocardial infarction. *N Engl J Med.* 1998;339:229–234.

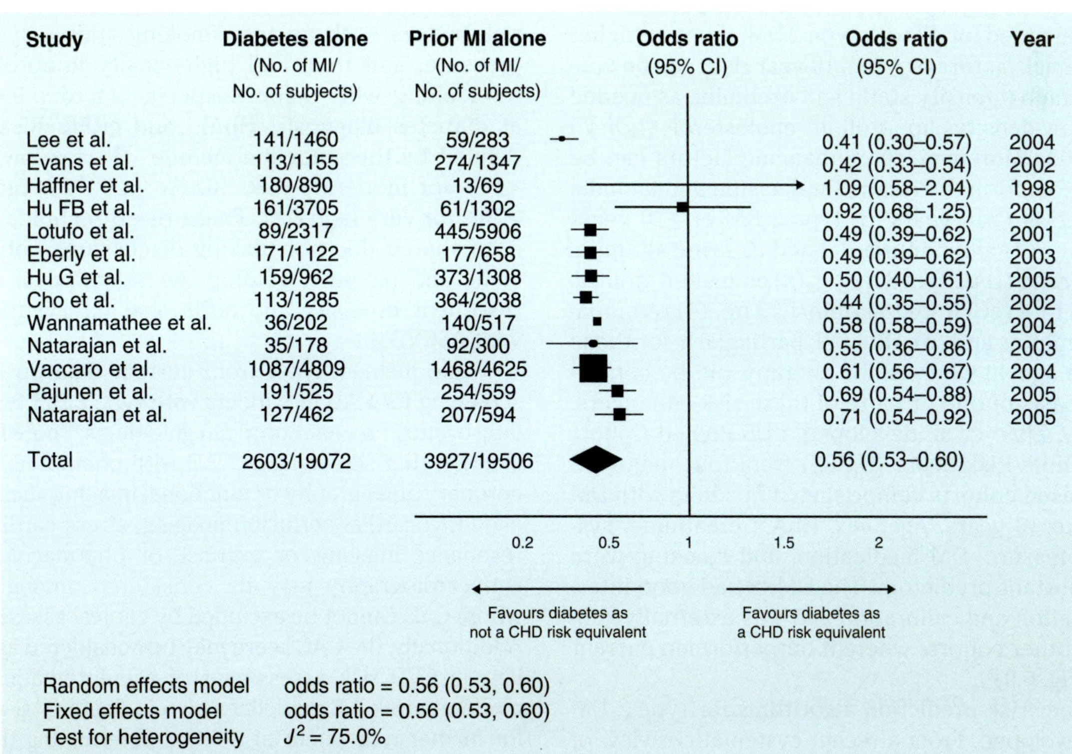

FIG. 6.8 Odds of coronary heart disease according to presence of diabetes or myocardial infarction alone: meta-analysis of 38,578 subjects. *CI*, Confidence interval; *MI*, myocardial infarction. From Bulugahapitiya U, Siyambalapitiya S, Sithole J, Idris I. Is diabetes a coronary risk equivalent? Systematic review and meta-analysis. *Diabet Med.* 2009;26(2):142–148.

risk equivalent in only one-fifth of CVD-free adults. High HbA_{1c}, long DM duration, and DM medication use were the most important predictors of CVD risk equivalence. DM is a CVD risk equivalent for women, white people, those of younger age, with higher triglycerides or CRP, or reduced kidney function.[80]

CARDIOVASCULAR DISEASE RISK ASSESSMENT IN DIABETES MELLITUS

DM is associated with great heterogeneity in risk of CVD and many persons with DM are no longer considered CHD risk equivalents. Persons with DM have a wide heterogeneity of risk of CVD based on Framingham risk scores, with approximately half of women and a third of men with DM being without known CVD or with 10-year risk <20%, the cutpoint generally considered to be a CVD risk equivalent.[81] This emphasizes the importance of risk stratification in persons with DM. Assessment of CVD risk is the first step for guiding the intensity of preventive treatments for CVD in persons with DM (see also Chapter 8).

The American College of Cardiology/American Heart Association (ACC/AHA) ASCVD risk estimator can be used to estimate the 10-year risk and lifetime risk of a first ASCVD event both in those with DM and without DM.[82] Since the calculator includes DM as a binary risk factor, it does not account for DM-specific risk factors such as duration or HbA_{1c} levels. Although some variability in calibration exists in various subgroups by gender and race, the precision of risk prediction is similar in those with or without DM. The US 2018 cholesterol management recommendations[83] call for the use of the pooled cohort risk score in all persons with DM aged 40 to 79 years. While statin therapy is recommended for all with type 2 DM, those at higher risk (multiple risk factors or ≥20% 10-year risk) can be considered for a high-intensity statin and ezetimibe as needed to reduce low-density lipoprotein cholesterol (LDL-C) by at least 50%. Moreover, risk-enhancing factors can be further used to inform the treatment decision and include: (1) long duration (≥10 years for type 2 DM or ≥20 years for type 1 DM), (2) albuminuria defined as urine albumin-to-creatinine ratio (UACR) of 30 mg/g, (3) estimated glomerular filtration rate (eGFR <60 mL/min/1.73 m^2, (4) retinopathy, (5) neuropathy, and (6) ABI <0.9, particularly for those younger than age 40 where statin therapy can be considered on the basis of one or more of these risk enhancers. Most recently, Zhao et al. developed a US Pooled Cohort Diabetes Mellitus Risk Score (DMRS) from four major US population-based cohorts comprising 2174 adults with DM followed up to 10 years. Age, sex, HbA_{1c}, creatinine, systolic blood pressure, DM medication, and smoking were the most important predictors. The DMRS had good internal discrimination and calibration and was externally validated in two other cohorts where it outperformed current risk scores (Fig. 6.9)[84].

Several other risk prediction algorithms for type 2 DM have been developed. From a recent systematic review of 15 observational studies reporting on seven risk models with >1 validation cohort, the Risk Equations for Complications of Type 2 Diabetes had the best calibration in primary studies with the greatest discrimination measures for all-cause mortality (C-statistics, 0.75 [95% CI, 0.70–0.80]; high certainty), cardiovascular mortality (0.79 [95% CI, 0.75–0.84]; low certainty), end-stage kidney disease (ESKD) (0.73 [95% CI, 0.52–0.94]; low certainty), MI (0.72 [95% CI, 0.69–0.74]; moderate certainty), and stroke (0.71 [95% CI, 0.68–0.74]; moderate certainty).[85] The updated version of the QDiabetes risk prediction algorithm had C statistics between 0.81 and 0.89.[86] Risk prediction algorithms for CVD among individuals with DM have also been developed.[87-89] A meta-analysis found an overall pooled C statistic of 0.67 for 15 algorithms developed in populations with DM and 0.64 for 11 algorithms originally developed in a general population.[88] The Thrombolysis In Myocardial Infarction (TIMI) risk score for CVD events performed moderately well among adults with type 2 DM and high CVD risk. The C statistic was 0.71 (95% CI, 0.69–0.73) for CVD death and 0.66 (95% CI, 0.64–0.67) for a composite endpoint of CVD death, MI, or stroke.[90] The UK Prospective Diabetes Study (UKPDS) risk score (Fig. 6.10) developed for persons with type 2 DM includes, along with major ASCVD risk factors, duration of DM, HbA_{1c} levels, and atrial fibrillation for determining the 10-year risk of fatal or nonfatal CAD or stroke.[91,92] The MESA-HNR CAD risk estimator for patients with type 2 DM is based on patients from the MESA and Heinz Nixdorf Recall (HNR) studies and includes both conventional and novel clinical risk factors, as well as CAC and shows improved discrimination for incident CAD over several other risk scores.[93]

The European Society of Cardiology guideline for DM patients has recently recommended the use of newly developed SCORE2-Diabetes algorithm (Fig. 6.11) to assess the 10-year CVD risk in individuals aged 40 years and older who have T2DM without ASCVD or severe target-organ damage.[94] SCORE2-Diabetes incorporates traditional CVD risk factors such as age, smoking status, systolic blood pressure, and total and high-density lipoprotein cholesterol along with diabetes-specific factors including age at diabetes diagnosis, HbA_{1c}, and eGFR. Risk categories defined by the guideline include <5% for low risk, 5% to <10% for moderate risk, 10% to <20% for high risk, and ≥20% for very high risk. These risk thresholds aim to facilitate shared decision-making discussions between physicians and patients, guiding the selection of appropriate treatment intensity and additional interventions to prevent ASCVD.

While meta-analyses from current data do not support screening for CAD in patients with type 2 DM for preventing fatal events,[95] recent European guidelines,[96] note for risk stratification that screening of CAD with computed tomography coronary angiography or functional imaging such as radionuclide myocardial perfusion imaging, stress cardiac magnetic resonance imaging, or exercise or pharmacological stress echocardiography may be considered among patients in whom CAD cannot be excluded by clinical assessment alone. Additionally, the CAC score may be considered as a risk modifier in CVD risk assessment of asymptomatic patients at moderate risk. US guidelines also indicate CAC as an option for further refinement of risk for determining the appropriateness of statin therapy after consideration of global risk assessment and risk-enhancing factors, although not specifically in those with DM, and in fact, for those with DM, statin therapy should not be withheld or delayed in those with a

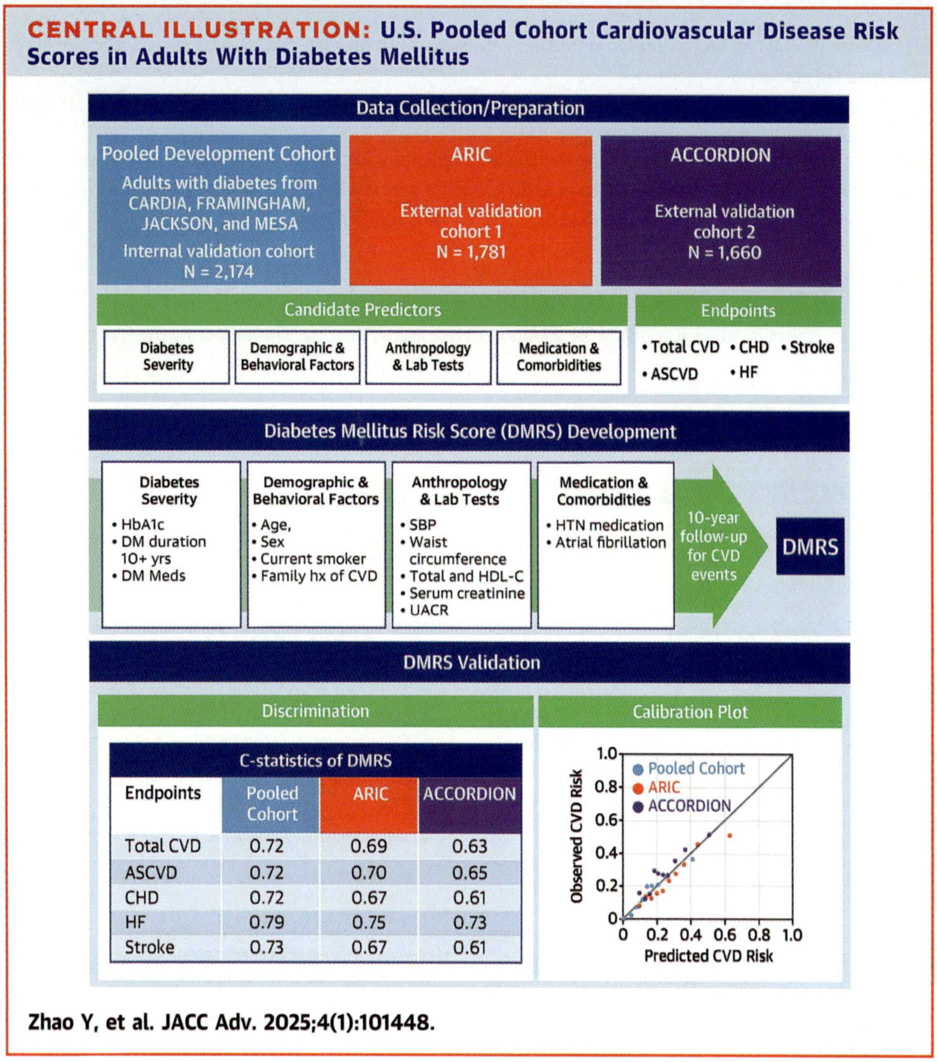

FIG. 6.9 US Pooled Cohort Cardiovascular Disease Risk Scores for Adults with Diabetes Mellitus. From Zhao Y, D'Agostino RB Sr, Malik S, et al. United States Cardiovascular Disease Risk Scores in adults with diabetes mellitus. *JACC Adv*, 2004;4(1):101–448.

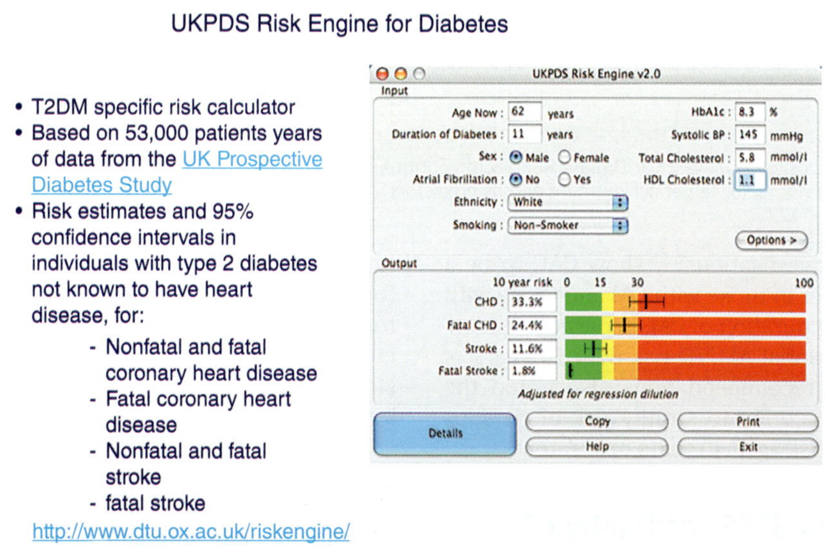

FIG. 6.10 UKPDS risk engine for diabetes. From Stevens RJ, Kothari V, Adler AI, Stratton IM; United Kingdom Prospective Diabetes Study (*UKPDS*) Group. The UKPDS risk engine: a model for the risk of coronary heart disease in type II diabetes (UKPDS 56).

Key Question

Can cardiovascular disease (CVD) risk prediction for individuals with type-2 diabetes be improved to reflect substantial regional variation in CVD incidence across Europe?

Key Finding

The SCORE2-Diabetes algorithms were developed by extending SCORE2, using data from >220,000 individuals with type 2 diabetes. Recalibration accounted for three- to four-fold variation in CVD incidence across Europe. SCORE2-Diabetes showed good external validation in >210,000 individuals from four countries (Sweden, Spain, Malta and Croatia).

Take Home Message

SCORE2-Diabetes accurately estimates CVD risk in individuals with type-2 diabetes. It extends SCORE2, aligning CVD risk prediction for those with and without diabetes, while accounting for variation in risk across Europe. This facilitates the identification of individuals at high CVD risk.

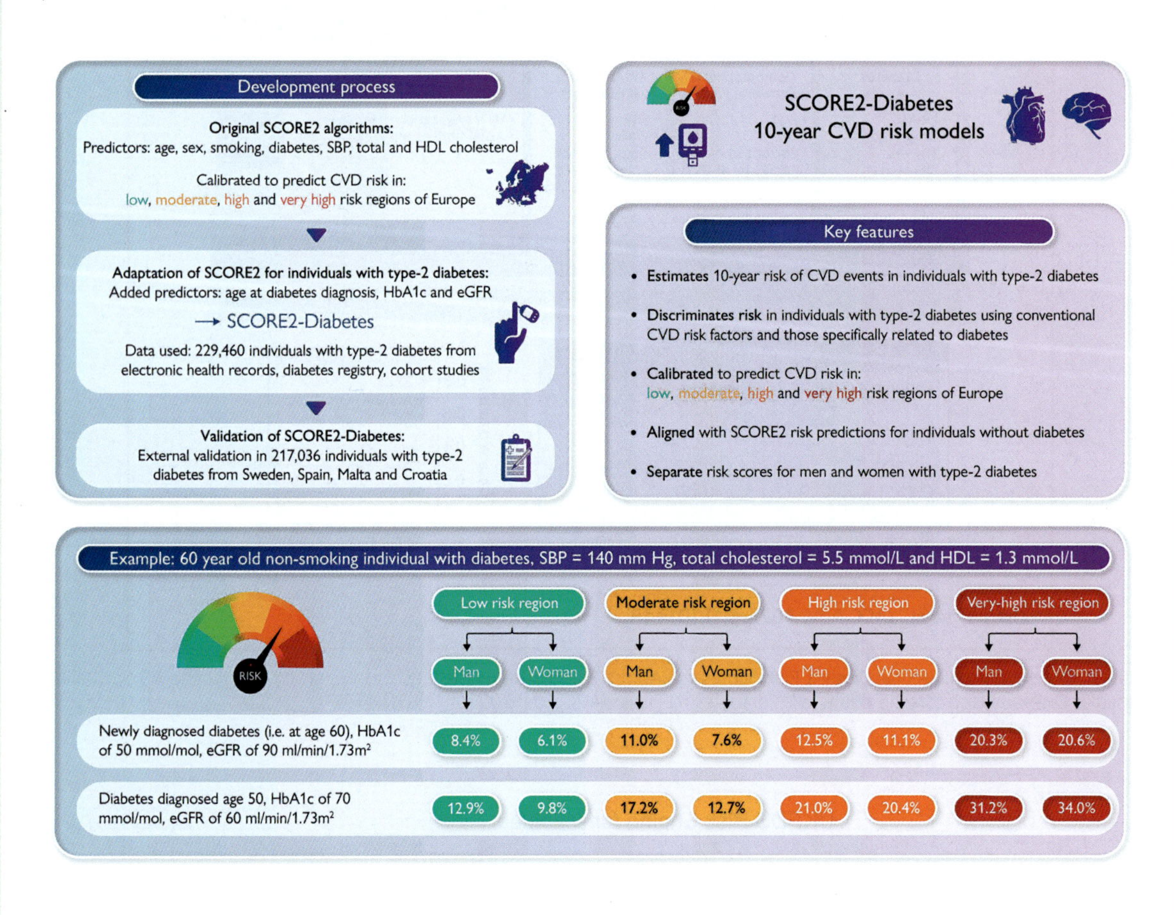

FIG. 6.11 Individual and Composite Cardiovascular Disease Risk Factor Control in US Adults with Diabetes. Adapted from Fan W, Song Y, Inzucchi SE, et al. Composite cardiovascular risk factor target achievement and its predictors in US adults with diabetes: The Diabetes Collaborative Registry. *Diabetes Obes Metab*. 2019;21(5):1121–1127.

CAC score of 0.[83] Prior investigations[25,97] show CAC to be a very effective risk stratifier in those with DM and those with high CAC scores and long duration of DM, in particular, identifies persons with substantial ASCVD risk over 10 years of follow-up.[97] Earlier AHA recommendations also noted the appropriateness of CAC scoring to stratify risk of persons with DM at intermediate risk aged 40 years or greater.[98]

RISK FACTORS IN DIABETES AND IMPACT ON ATHEROSCLEROTIC CARDIOVASCULAR DISEASE

Multiple cardiovascular risk factors are commonly seen in those with DM. NHANES has shown 21% of adults with type 2 DM had hypertension, hyperlipidemia, and obesity together, with another 36% having two of these risk factors.[99] We review here the most common risk factors that cluster in those with DM: obesity, dyslipidemia, hypertension, and lifestyle factors and their impact on cardiovascular disease risk.

Obesity

Obesity globally impacts more than 600 million people around the world and is associated with nearly 50 comorbidities, including metabolic syndrome, DM, and cardiovascular disease.[100] An estimated 90% of type 2 DM is attributable to excess body weight.[101] The relationship of obesity with type 2 DM has been long established and while obesity is often accompanied with other chronic conditions, including hypertension and dyslipidemia, many patients with DM who have obesity have a clustering of multiple metabolic and cardiovascular risk factors.

While BMI is often used to determine obesity, the distribution of excess body fat determines its impact on cardiovascular risk factor alterations.[102] Patients with type 2 DM have greater visceral adipose tissue than BMI-matched individuals without type 2 DM that contributes further to the risk of adverse cardiovascular outcomes.[103] A strong gradient in risk of developing DM is noted in women beginning at a waist circumference of 30 inches (76 cm), with risks more than 10-fold higher for those with waist circumferences of ≥38 inches (~97 cm) compared to <30 inches.[104] The Women's Health Initiative among postmenopausal women showed the risk of DM, compared to those who were metabolically healthy and normal weight, was increased 4.5-fold among those who were metabolically unhealthy and obese, 2.2-fold among those who were metabolically unhealthy and normal weight, and 1.7-fold among those who were metabolically healthy and obese,[105] and in those with DM, metabolically unhealthy normal weight or overweight/obesity to be associated with subsequent increases in risk of heart failure.[106] Moreover, among African-American adults in the JHS, the risk of DM was increased 2.4-fold for those with obesity who were insulin resistant, 1.6-fold for those without obesity who were insulin resistant, and 1.7-fold for those with obesity who were insulin sensitive compared with those without obesity and who were insulin sensitive.[107]

Dyslipidemia

Characteristics of dyslipidemia in persons with DM include not only elevated LDL-C but also elevated triglycerides and decreased HDL-C (see also Chapter 19). Insulin resistance not only plays an important role in the onset and progression of DM, it also is closely related to DM dyslipidemia.[108] The development of atherosclerotic lesions is promoted by local inflammation in the vascular wall that is induced by dyslipidemia, particularly high LDL-C levels. Moreover, levels of small dense LDL-C are higher in patients with versus without DM. Small dense LDL-C particles are more atherogenic with a greater propensity for transport into the subendothelial space and propensity to be oxidized, helping to explain in part how dyslipidemia promotes ASCVD risk in persons with DM.[109]

While LDL-C remains among the most important risk factors for ASCVD in persons with DM, hypertriglyceridemia and low HDL-cholesterol levels are often at least as common in those with DM. A Japanese cohort study of patients with type 2 DM showed that serum triglyceride levels were a leading predictor of CVD, comparable to LDL-C, both of which were greater than the predictive value from HbA_{1c}.[110] Hypertriglyceridemia is present in over one-fifth (~5.5 million) of US adults with DM, even among those on statin therapy and with well-controlled LDL-C levels; over 75% of those with DM and hypertriglyceridemia are at moderate or high 10-year risk for ASCVD.[111] Finally, lipoprotein(a), included as a risk-enhancing factor in US guidelines[83] and recently recommended by the US National Lipid Association for measurement in all adults,[112] predicts future ASCVD risk in persons with or without DM, with recent evidence indicating higher levels of lipoprotein(a) predict ASCVD events more strongly in those with DM versus without DM, despite a modestly increased risk of developing DM among those with the lowest lipoprotein(a) levels.[113]

Hypertension

Hypertension is twice as common in persons with DM versus without DM, with approximately two-thirds of patients with type 2 DM also being affected by hypertension[114] (see also Chapter 18). Insulin resistance among patients with DM is associated with increased oxidative stress, inflammation, and decreased vascular nitric oxide levels, which in turn promote vascular stiffness, resulting in persistent hypertension.

Hypertension contributes to increased incidence of cardiovascular and other macrovascular complications in patients with type 2 DM; the presence of two additional major risk factors is associated with a fourfold increased risk for CVD as compared to normotensive nondiabetic controls. The magnitude of risk conferred by type 2 DM and hypertension depends on age, BMI, and ethnicity.[115] Increases in blood pressure (BP) beginning at 115/75 mm Hg are associated with increased cardiovascular event rates and mortality in DM patients.[116] Moreover, uncontrolled hypertension is associated with increased risk for developing DM, independently of age, BMI, baseline BP, or fasting glucose levels.[117]

LIFESTYLE FACTORS

A variety of lifestyle factors (higher alcohol consumption, lower physical activity [PA], higher sedentary time, and unhealthy diet) has also been shown to be associated with DM risk in adults over a median 3.8 years of follow-up and may thus further affect cardiovascular disease risk (see also Chapters 3 and 17.). Those with the least favorable lifestyle profile had an increased risk for DM compared with those with the most favorable lifestyle profile.[118] A meta-analysis of 14 studies also showed those with the most favorable combined lifestyle factors had a lower DM risk compared to those with the least favorable combined lifestyle factors.[119] Sedentary behavior, including television viewing, has also been shown to be associated with DM risk in a systematic review and meta-analysis.[120] Among a meta-analysis of 39 cohort studies, sugar-sweetened and artificially sweetened beverage intake show an association with increased type 2 DM risk.[121] In a systematic review and meta-analysis of five eligible prospective studies of 22,591 subjects with DM followed for an average of 9.8 years showed reduced cardiovascular outcomes from replacement analyses of saturated fat with polyunsaturated fat (RR for 2% energy replacement, 0.87 [95% CI, 0.77–0.99]) or carbohydrate (RR for 5% energy replacement, 0.82 [95% CI, 0.67–1.00]).[122]

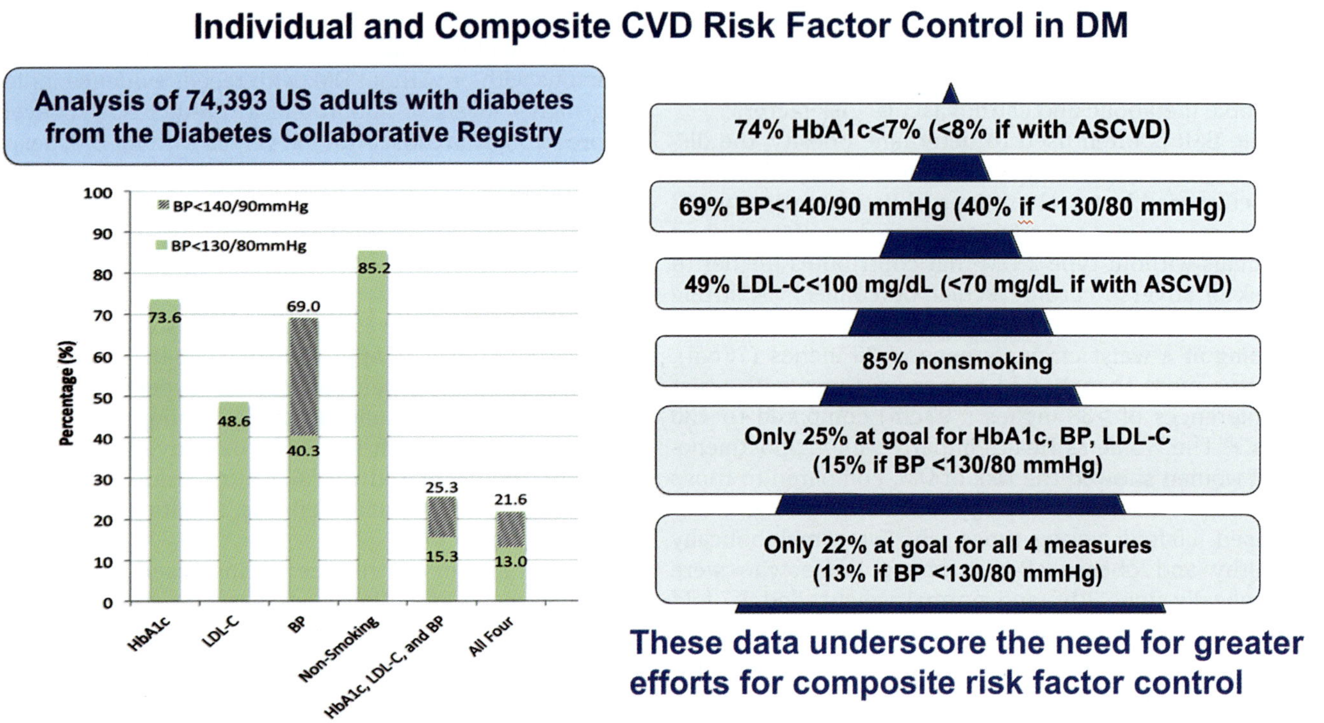

FIG. 6.12 Cardiovascular Disease (CVD) and Coronary Heart Disease (CHD) Event Rates by Number of Diabetes Risk Factors Controlled: Pooling of ARIC, JACKSON and MESA Diabetes Subjects. *ASCVD*, Atherosclerotic cardiovascular diseases; *CVD*, cardiovascular disease; *DM*, diabetes mellitus. Adapted from Wong ND, Zhao Y, Patel R, et al. Cardiovascular Risk Factor Targets and Cardiovascular Disease Event Risk in Diabetes: A Pooling Project of the Atherosclerosis Risk in Communities Study, Multi-Ethnic Study of Atherosclerosis, and Jackson Heart Study. *Diabetes Care*. 2016;39(5):668–676.

CARDIOVASCULAR RISK FACTOR CONTROL AND RELATION TO CARDIOVASCULAR OUTCOMES IN DIABETES

Despite modest improvements in cardiovascular risk factor control over years among those with DM,[123] many are insufficiently controlled for multiple risk factors needed to achieve meaningful reductions in CVD risk. We showed from the Diabetes Collaborative Registry individual target attainment for HbA_{1c}, BP, LDL-C, and nonsmoking status to be 73.6%, 69.0% (40.3% for BP <130/80 mm Hg), 48.6%, and 85.2%, respectively. However, only 21.6% (13.0% with BP <130/80 mm Hg) were at target for all four measures (Fig. 6.12), with multiple target attainment higher in men (23.6%) versus women (18.6%) and in white people (22.5%) versus African-American people (14.7%) and people of other races (20.8%; $P < 0.01$).[124] Moreover, recent data from the NHANES indicated that among adults with type 2 DM, approximately half met individual targets for HbA_{1c} (55.8%), blood pressure (51.3%), and LDL cholesterol (49.3%), while a higher proportion were nonsmokers (84.3%). However, only 17.3% achieved combined control of HbA_{1c}, blood pressure, and LDL cholesterol, and this dropped to 16.0% when nonsmoking was included, and to under 10% when BMI targets were also considered.[125] These data demonstrate the need to reduce clinical inertia among healthcare providers to ensure the composite of these risk factors is addressed with appropriate lifestyle interventions and pharmacologic therapies.

Several studies demonstrate the importance of multiple risk factor controls for reducing cardiovascular risk, among those with DM. Among patients with DM without prior CVD from the ARIC study, MESA, and JHS, we have observed CVD

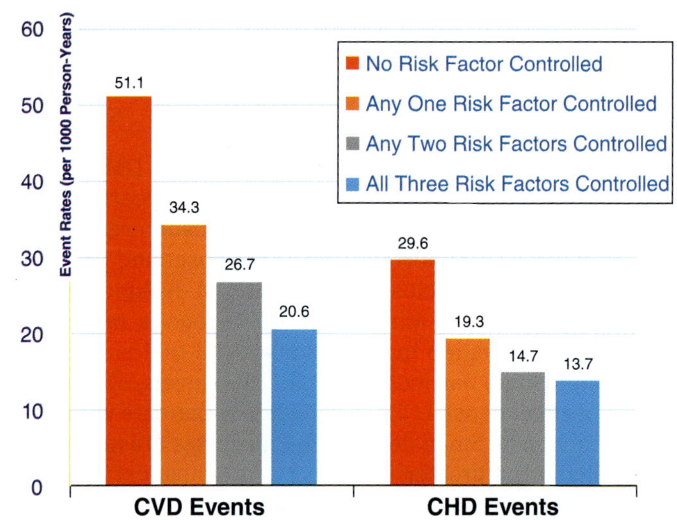

FIG. 6.13 Cardiovascular disease (*CVD*) and coronary heart disease (*CHD*) event rates by number of diabetes risk factors controlled: pooling of ARIC, JACKSON, and MESA diabetes subejcts. From Wong ND, Zhao Y, Patel R, et al. Cardiovascular risk factor targets and cardiovascular disease event risk in diabetes: a pooling project of the Atherosclerosis Risk in Communities Study, Multi-Ethnic Study of Atherosclerosis, and Jackson Heart Study. *Diabetes Care*. 2016;39(5):668–676.

event rates to be 51.1%, 34.3%, 26.7%, and 20.6% among those with none, any single, any two, or all three risk factor controls of BP, LDL-C, and HbA_{1c}, respectively. Those with one, two, or all three risk factors at target levels (vs. none) had incrementally lower adjusted relative risks of CVD events of 36%, 52%, and 62%, respectively (Fig. 6.13).[126] In addition, the UK Clinical Practice Research Datalink (CPRD) and the Scottish Care Information-Diabetes (SCI-Diabetes) dataset showed multiple uncontrolled risk factors (smoking, total cholesterol, triglyceride, HbA_{1c}, systolic BP) conferred more than twofold greater risks for CAD and heart failure, with more than a threefold risk of stroke among those with DM versus without DM.[127] From a study calculating the 10-year risk of CAD based on the UKPDS risk engine, controlling all risk factors (smoking, HbA_{1c}, systolic BP, and total and HDL cholesterol) to the goal can be projected to prevent 35% and 45% of CAD events in men and women, respectively, with further aggressive risk factor controls projected to prevent 51% and 61% of CAD events, respectively.[128] For those with both DM and CVD, simultaneous control of multiple risk factors through protocol-guided intensive medical therapy is feasible and relates to lower cardiovascular morbidity and mortality. And from an analysis of a number of controlled risk factors in relation to cardiovascular events (among the following risk factors: nonsmoking, HDL-C <130 mg/dL [<3.4 mmol/L], TG <150 mg/dL [<1.7 mmol/L], systolic BP <130 mm Hg; DBP <80 mm Hg; HbA_{1c} <7% [<53 mmol/mol]) in the Bypass Angioplasty Investigation Revascularization 2 Diabetes (BARI 2D) trial, involving over 2200 patients with 5 years follow-up, the number of risk factors in the control was strongly related to death ($p = 0.0010$) and the composite of death, MI, and stroke ($p = 0.0035$) in fully adjusted models.[129] Those with zero to two risk factors in the control during follow-up had a twofold higher risk of death (HR, 2.0; 95% CI, 1.3–3.3; $p = 0.0031$) and a 1.7-fold higher risk of the composite cardiovascular endpoint (HR, 1.7; 95% CI, 1.2–2.5; $p = 0.0043$), compared with those with all six risk factors in control.

Clinical trials have also examined the effect of composite risk factor control in CVD prevention among those with DM. The Steno-2 Study[130] randomly assigned 160 patients with type 2 DM and microalbuminuria to receive either intensive therapy or conventional therapy. Intensive therapy (targets included an HbA_{1c}< 6.5% [<48 mmol/mol], a fasting serum total cholesterol <175 mg/dL [<4.5 mmol/L], a fasting serum TG < 150 mg /dL [<1.7 mmol/L], systolic BP <130 mm Hg, and diastolic BP <80 mm Hg) was associated with a lower risk of death from cardiovascular causes (HR, 0.43; 95% CI, 0.19–0.94; $p = 0.04$) and of cardiovascular events (HR, 0.41; 95% CI, 0.25–0.67; $p < 0.001$). In Japan, a multicenter, open-label, randomized, parallel group that randomly assigned (1:1) patients with type 2 DM aged 45 to 69 years with hypertension, dyslipidemia, or both, and an HbA_{1c} of 6.9% or higher, to receive conventional therapy for glucose, BP, and lipid control (targets: HbA_{1c} <6.9% [<52 mmol/mol], BP <130/80 mm Hg, LDL-C cholesterol <120 mg/dL [<3.1 mmol/L] or 100 mg/dL [<2.6 mmol/L] in patients with a history of CAD) or intensive therapy (HbA_{1c} <6.2% [<44 mmol/mol], BP <120/75 mm Hg, LDL-C <80 mg/dL <2.1 mmol/L] [or 70 mg/dL [1.8 mmol/l] in patients with a history of CAD]). While the primary composite CVD outcome was not significantly reduced, cerebrovascular events (stroke, carotid endarterectomy, percutaneous transluminal cerebral angioplasty, and carotid artery stenting) were significantly less frequent in the intensive therapy group (HR, 0.42; 95% CI, 0.24–0.74; $p = 0.002$).[131]

SUMMARY

There is a consistent upward trend of DM prevalence worldwide, with macrovascular diseases, primarily CAD, stroke, and PAD, being the most common and fatal comorbidities. There is clear evidence from a large number of well-controlled prospective epidemiologic studies, that the presence of type 2 DM is associated with an approximately two-fold increased risk for various cardiovascular complications. In those with DM, the long-term control of glucose metabolism seems to play an important role because a strong relationship has been seen in several studies between HbA_{1c} levels and cardiovascular outcome as well as total mortality. Appropriate cardiovascular risk assessment using scores developed for those with DM together with consideration of risk-enhancing factors and subclinical atherosclerosis, as well as strategic multifactorial controls, are key approaches for macrovascular disease prevention among patients with diabetes.

REFERENCES

1. Blair M. Diabetes mellitus review. *Urol Nurs.* 2016;36(1):27–36.
2. American Diabetes Association Classification and diagnosis of diabetes: Standards of Medical Care in Diabetes-2020. *Diabetes Care.* 2020;43(Suppl 1): S14–S31.
3. Saeedi P, Petersohn I, Salpea P, et al. Global and regional diabetes prevalence estimates for 2019 and projections for 2030 and 2045: results from the International Diabetes Federation Diabetes Atlas, 9th edition. *Diabetes Res Clin Pract.* 2019;157:107843.
4. Centers for Disease Control and Prevention. *National Diabetes Statistics* https://www.cdc.gov/diabetes/php/data-research/index.html.
5. Carracher AM, Marathe PH, Close KL. International Diabetes Federation 2017. *J Diabetes.* 2018;10(5):353–356.
6. Booth GL, Kapral MK, Fung K, Tu JV. Relation between age and cardiovascular disease in men and women with diabetes compared with non-diabetic people: a population-based retrospective cohort study. *Lancet.* 2006;368(9529):29–36.
7. Litwak L, Goh SY, Hussein Z, Malek R, Prusty V, Khamseh ME. Prevalence of diabetes complications in people with type 2 diabetes mellitus and its association with baseline characteristics in the multinational A1chieve study. *Diabetol Metab Syndr.* 2013;5(1):57.
8. Gregg EW, Sattar N, Ali MK. The changing face of diabetes complications. *Lancet Diabetes Endocrinol.* 2016;4(6):537–547.
9. Zhuo X, Zhang P, Hoerger TJ. Lifetime direct medical costs of treating type 2 diabetes and diabetic complications. *Am J Prev Med.* 2013;45(3):253–261.
10. Kalofoutis C, Piperi C, Kalofoutis A, Harris F, Phoenix D, Singh J. Type II diabetes mellitus and cardiovascular risk factors: current therapeutic approaches. *Exp Clin Cardiol.* 2007;12(1):17–28.
11. Chawla A, Chawla R, Jaggi S. Microvasular and macrovascular complications in diabetes mellitus: distinct or continuum? *Indian J Endocrinol Metab.* 2016;20(4):546–551.
12. American Diabetes Association Cardiovascular disease and risk management: Standards of Medical Care in Diabetes. *Diabetes Care.* 2021;44(Suppl 1): S125–S150.
13. Hewitt J, Castilla Guerra L, Fernández-Moreno Mdel C, Sierra C. Diabetes and stroke prevention: a review. *Stroke Res Treat.* 2012;2012:673187.
14. Zhang H, Dellsperger KC, Zhang C. The link between metabolic abnormalities and endothelial dysfunction in type 2 diabetes: an update. *Basic Res Cardiol.* 2012;107(1):237.
15. Winkelmann BR, Marz W, Boehm BO, et al. Rationale and design of the LURIC study–a resource for functional genomics, pharmacogenomics and long-term prognosis of cardiovascular disease. *Pharmacogenomics.* 2001;2:S1.
16. Bartnik M, Ryden L, Ferrari R, et al. The prevalence of abnormal glucose regulation in patients with coronary artery disease across Europe. The Euro Heart Survey on diabetes and the heart. *Eur Heart J.* 2004;25:1880.
17. de la Hera JM, Delgado E, Hernandez E, et al. Prevalence and outcome of newly detected diabetes in patients who undergo percutaneous coronary intervention. *Eur Heart J.* 2009;30:261.
18. Kuller LH, Velentgas P, Barzilay J, et al. Diabetes mellitus: subclinical cardiovascular disease and risk of incident cardiovascular disease and all-cause mortality. *Arterioscler Thromb Vasc Biol.* 2000;20:823.
19. Brohall G, Oden A, Fagerberg B. Carotid artery intima-media thickness in patients with type 2 diabetes mellitus and impaired glucose tolerance: a systematic review. *Diabet Med.* 2006;23:609.
20. Bonora E, Kiechl S, Willeit J, et al. Carotid atherosclerosis and coronary heart disease in the metabolic syndrome: prospective data from the Bruneck study. *Diabetes Care.* 2003;26:1251.
21. Alves-Cabratosa L, Comas-Cufí M, Ponjoan A, et al. Levels of ankle-brachial index and the risk of diabetes mellitus complications. *BMJ Open Diabetes Res Care.* 2020;8(1):e000977. https://doi.org/10.1136/bmjdrc-2019-000977. PMID: 32144131; PMCID: PMC7059529.

22. Lin CC, Li CI, Liu CS, Lin CH, Yang SY, Li TC. Prediction of all-cause and cardiovascular mortality using ankle-brachial index and brachial-ankle pulse wave velocity in patients with type 2 diabetes. *Sci Rep*. 2022;12(1):11053. https://doi.org/10.1038/s41598-022-15346-9. PMID: 35773381; PMCID: PMC9247028.
23. Cardoso CRL, Melo JV, Salles GC, Leite NC, Salles GF. Prognostic impact of the ankle-brachial index on the development of micro- and macrovascular complications in individuals with type 2 diabetes: the Rio de Janeiro Type 2 Diabetes Cohort Study. *Diabetologia*. 2018;61(11):2266–2276. https://doi.org/10.1007/s00125-018-4709-9. Epub 2018 Aug 15. PMID: 30112690.
24. Wong ND, Sciammarella MG, Polk D, et al. The metabolic syndrome, diabetes, and subclinical atherosclerosis assessed by coronary calcium,. *J Am Coll Cardiol*. 2003;1547:41.
25. Malik S, Budoff MJ, Katz R, et al. Impact of subclinical atherosclerosis on cardiovascular disease events in individuals with metabolic syndrome and diabetes: the multi-ethnic study of atherosclerosis. *Diabetes Care*. 2011;34(10):2285–2290.
26. Wong ND, Nelson JC, Granston T, et al. Metabolic syndrome, diabetes, and incidence and progression of coronary calcium: the Multiethnic Study of Atherosclerosis Study. *JACC Cardiovasc Imaging*. 2012;5:358.
27. Chen K, Lindsey JB, Khera A, et al. Independent associations between metabolic syndrome, diabetes mellitus and atherosclerosis: observations from the Dallas Heart study. *Diab Vasc Dis Res*. 2008;5:96.
28. Elkeles RS, Godsland IF, Feher MD, et al. Coronary calcium measurement improves prediction of cardiovascular events in asymptomatic patients with type 2 diabetes: the PREDICT study. *Eur Heart J*. 2008;29:2244.
29. Sow MA, Magne J, Salle L, Nobecourt E, Preux PM, Aboyans V. Prevalence, determinants and prognostic value of high coronary artery calcium score in asymptomatic patients with diabetes: a systematic review and meta-analysis. *J Diabetes Complications*. 2022:108237. Epub ahead of print. PMID: 35773171.
30. Malik S, Wong ND, Franklin SS, et al. Impact of the metabolic syndrome on mortality from coronary heart disease, cardiovascular disease, and all causes in United States adults. *Circulation*. 2004;110(10):1245–1250.
31. Shah AD, Langenberg C, Rapsomaniki E, et al. Type 2 diabetes and incidence of cardiovascular diseases: a cohort study in 1.9 million people. *Lancet Diabetes Endocrinol*. 2015;3(2):105–113.
32. Emerging Risk Factors Collaboration, et al.Sarwar N, Gao P, et al. Diabetes mellitus, fasting blood glucose concentration, and risk of vascular disease: a collaborative meta-analysis of 102 prospective studies. *Lancet*. 2010;375:2215.
33. Coles B, Zaccardi F, Ling S, Davies MJ, Samani NJ, Khunti K. Cardiovascular events and mortality in people with and without type 2 diabetes: an observational study in a contemporary multi-ethnic population. *J Diabetes Investig*. 2021;12:1175–1182.
34. Nanayakkara N, Curtis AJ, Heritier S, et al. Impact of age at type 2 diabetes mellitus diagnosis on mortality and vascular complications: systematic review and meta-analyses. *Diabetologia*. 2021;64:275–287.
35. Stratton IM, Adler AI, Neil HA, et al. Association of glycaemia with macrovascular and microvascular complications of type 2 diabetes (UKPDS 35): prospective observational study. *BMJ*. 2000;321:405.
36. Khaw KT, Wareham N, Luben R, et al. Glycated haemoglobin, diabetes, and mortality in men in Norfolk cohort of European prospective investigation of cancer and nutrition (EPIC-Norfolk). *BMJ*. 2001;322:1.
37. Fox CS. Cardiovascular disease risk factors, type 2 diabetes mellitus, and the Framingham Heart Study. *Trends Cardiovasc Med*. 2010;20(3): 90–95.
38. Yusuf S, Hawken S, Ounpuu S, et al. Effect of potentially modifiable risk factors associated with myocardial infarction in 52 countries (the INTERHEART study): case-control study. *Lancet*. 2004;364(9438):937–952.
39. Wannamethee SG, Papacosta O, Lawlor DA, et al. Do women exhibit greater differences in established and novel risk factors between diabetes and non-diabetes than men? The British Regional Heart Study and British Women's Heart Health Study. *Diabetologia*. 2012;55:80.
40. Gustafsson I, Brendorp B, Seibaek M, et al. Influence of diabetes and diabetes-gender interaction on the risk of death in patients hospitalized with congestive heart failure. *J Am Coll Cardiol*. 2004;43:771.
41. Alfredsson J, Green JB, Stevens SR, et al. Sex differences in management and outcomes of patients with type 2 diabetes and cardiovascular disease: a report from TECOS. *Diabetes, Obesity and Metabolism*. 2018;20:2379–2388.
42. de Jong M, Woodward M, Peters SAE. Diabetes, glycated hemoglobin, and the risk of myocardial infarction in women and men: a prospective cohort study of the UK Biobank. *Diabetes Care*. 2020;43:2050–2059.
43. Liu L, Simon B, Shi J, Mallhi AK, Eisen HJ. Impact of diabetes mellitus on risk of cardiovascular disease and all-cause mortality: evidence on health outcomes and antidiabetic treatment in United States adults. *World J Diabetes*. 2016;7:449–461.
44. Yahagi K, Kolodgie FD, Lutter C, et al. Pathology of human coronary and carotid artery atherosclerosis and vascular calcification in diabetes mellitus. *Arterioscler Thromb Vasc Biol*. 2017;37(2):191–204.
45. Einarson TR, Acs A, Ludwig C, Panton UH. Prevalence of cardiovascular disease in type 2 diabetes: a systematic literature review of scientific evidence from across the world in 2007-2017. *Cardiovasc Diabetol*. 2018;17(1):83.
46. Huxley R, Barzi F, Woodward M. Excess risk of fatal coronary heart disease associated with diabetes in men and women: meta-analysis of 37 prospective cohort studies. *BMJ*. 2006;332:73.
47. Mondesir FL, Brown TM, Muntner P, et al. Diabetes, diabetes severity, and coronary heart disease risk equivalence: REasons for Geographic and Racial Differences in Stroke (REGARDS). *Am Heart J*. 2016;181:43–51.
48. O'Donnell MJ, Chin SL, Rangarajan S, et al. Global and regional effects of potentially modifiable risk factors associated with acute stroke in 32 countries (INTERSTROKE): a case-control study. *Lancet*. 2016;388(10046):761–775.
49. Gofir A, Mulyono B, Sutarni S. Hyperglycemia as a prognosis predictor of length of stay and functional outcomes in patients with acute ischemic stroke. *Int J Neurosci*. 2017;127(10):923–929.
50. Nakagawa K, Vento MA, Ing MM, Asai SM. Impact of diabetes on prolonged hospital stay among Native Hawaiians and other Pacific Islanders with ischemic stroke. *Hawaii J Med Public Health*. 2014;73(12 Suppl 3):4–7.
51. Delbari A, Salman Roghani R, Tabatabaei SS, Lökk J. A stroke study of an urban area of Iran: risk factors, length of stay, case fatality, and discharge destination. *J Stroke Cerebrovasc Dis*. 2010;19(2):104–109.
52. Wu S, Shi Y, Wang C, et al. Glycated hemoglobin independently predicts stroke recurrence within one year after acute first-ever non-cardioembolic strokes onset in A Chinese cohort study. *PLoS One*. 2013;8(11):e80690.
53. Li HW, Yang MC, Chung KP. Predictors for readmission of acute ischemic stroke in Taiwan. *J Formos Med Assoc*. 2011;110(10):627–633.
54. Sun Y, Toh MP. Impact of diabetes mellitus (DM) on the health-care utilization and clinical outcomes of patients with stroke in Singapore. *Value Health*. 2009;12(Suppl 3):S101–S105.
55. Lei C, Wu B, Liu M, Chen Y. Association between hemoglobin A1C levels and clinical outcome in ischemic stroke patients with or without diabetes. *J Clin Neurosci*. 2015;22(3):498–503.
56. Eriksson M, Carlberg B, Eliasson M. The disparity in long-term survival after a first stroke in patients with and without diabetes persists: the Northern Sweden MONICA study. *Cerebrovasc Dis*. 2012;34(2):153–160.
57. Hjalmarsson C, Manhem K, Bokemark L, Andersson B. The role of prestroke glycemic control on severity and outcome of acute ischemic stroke. *Stroke Res Treat*. 2014;2014:694569.
58. Xu L, Chan WM, Hui YF, Lam TH. Association between HbA_{1c} and cardiovascular disease mortality in older Hong Kong Chinese with diabetes. *Diabet Med*. 2012;29(3):393–398.
59. Piernik-Yoder B, Ketchum N. Rehabilitation outcomes of stroke patients with and without diabetes. *Arch Phys Med Rehabil*. 2013;94(8):1508–1512.
60. Masrur S, Cox M, Bhatt DL, et al. Association of acute and chronic hyperglycemia with acute ischemic stroke outcomes post-thrombolysis: findings from get with the guidelines-stroke. *J Am Heart Assoc*. 2015;4(10):e002193.
61. Shu J, Santulli G. Update on peripheral artery disease: Epidemiology and evidence-based facts. *Atherosclerosis*. 2018;275:379–381.
62. Kullo IJ, Bailey KR, Kardia SL, Mosley Jr TH, Boerwinkle E, Turner ST. Ethnic differences in peripheral arterial disease in the NHLBI Genetic Epidemiology Network of Arteriopathy (GENOA) study. *Vasc Med*. 2003;8(4):237–242.
63. Eraso LH, Fukaya E, Mohler III ER, et al. Peripheral arterial disease, prevalence and cumulative risk factor profile analysis. *Eur J Prev Cardiol*. 2012
64. Thiruvoipati T, Kielhorn CE, Armstrong EJ. Peripheral artery disease in patients with diabetes: epidemiology, mechanisms, and outcomes. *World J Diabetes*. 2015;6(7):961–969.
65. Gerhard-Herman MD, Gornik HL, Barrett C, et al. 2016 AHA/ACC Guideline on the management of patients with lower extremity peripheral artery disease: executive summary: a report of the American College of Cardiology/American Heart Association Task Force on Clinical Practice Guidelines. *Circulation*. 2017;135(12):e686–e725.
66. Kannel WB, McGee DL. Diabetes and cardiovascular disease. The Framingham study. *JAMA*. 1979;241:2035.
67. Newman AB, Siscovick DS, Manolio TA, et al. Ankle-arm index as a marker of atherosclerosis in the Cardiovascular Health Study. Cardiovascular Heart Study (CHS) Collaborative Research Group. *Circulation*. 1993; 88:837.
68. Olesen KKW, Gyldenkerne C, Thim T, Thomsen RW, Maeng M. Peripheral artery disease, lower limb revascularization, and amputation in diabetes patients with and without coronary artery disease: a cohort study from the Western Denmark Heart Registry. *BMJ Open Diabetes Res Care*. 2021:9.
69. Jude EB, Oyibo SO, Chalmers N, et al. Peripheral arterial disease in diabetic and nondiabetic patients: a comparison of severity and outcome. *Diabetes Care*. 2001;24:1433.
70. Chen J, Spracklen CN, Marenne G, et al. Meta-Analysis of G and Insulin-related Traits C. The trans-ancestral genomic architecture of glycemic traits. *Nat Genet*. 2021;53:840–860.
71. Weitz JI, Byrne J, Clagett GP, et al. Diagnosis and treatment of chronic arterial insufficiency of the lower extremities: a critical review. *Circulation*. 1996;94:3026.
72. Das JR, Eberhardt RT. Contemporary risk assessment and cardiovascular outcomes in peripheral arterial disease. *Cardiovasc Hematol Disord Drug Targets*. 2013;13(3):185–196.
73. Haffner SM, Lehto S, Rönnemaa T, Pyörälä K, Laakso M. Mortality from coronary heart disease in subjects with type 2 diabetes and in nondiabetic subjects with and without prior myocardial infarction. *N Engl J Med*. 1998;339(4):229–234.
74. Bulugahapitiya U, Siyambalapitiya S, Sithole J, Idris I. Is diabetes a coronary risk equivalent? Systematic review and meta-analysis. *Diabet Med*. 2009;26(2):142–148.
75. Evans JM, Wang J, Morris AD. Comparison of cardiovascular risk between patients with type 2 diabetes and those who had had a myocardial infarction: cross sectional and cohort studies. *BMJ*. 2002;324:939.
76. Lee CD, Folsom AR, Pankow JS, et al. Cardiovascular events in diabetic and nondiabetic adults with or without history of myocardial infarction. *Circulation*. 2004;109:855.

77. Wannamethee SG, Shaper AG, Whincup PH, et al. Impact of diabetes on cardiovascular disease risk and all-cause mortality in older men: influence of age at onset, diabetes duration, and established and novel risk factors. *Arch Intern Med*. 2011;171:404.
78. Rana JS, Liu JY, Moffet HH, Jaffe M, Karter AJ. Diabetes and prior coronary heart disease are not necessarily risk equivalent for future coronary heart disease events. *J Gen Intern Med*. 2016;31(4):387–393. https://doi.org/10.1007/s11606-015-3556-3. Epub 2015 Dec 14. PMID: 26666660; PMCID: PMC4803685.
79. Lindsey JB, House JA, Kennedy KF, et al. Diabetes duration is associated with increased thin-cap fibroatheroma detected by intravascular ultrasound with virtual histology. *Circ Cardiovasc Interv*. 2009;2:543.
80. Zhao Y, Malik S, Budoff MJ, et al. Identification and predictors for cardiovascular disease risk equivalents among adults with diabetes mellitus. *Diabetes Care*. 2021:dc210431. https://doi.org/10.2337/dc21-0431. Epub ahead of print. PMID: 34380703.
81. Wong ND, Glovaci D, Wong K, et al. Global cardiovascular disease risk assessment in United States adults with diabetes. *Diab Vasc Dis Res*. 2012;9(2):146–152.
82. Arnett DK, Blumenthal RS, Albert MA, et al. 2019 ACC/AHA Guideline on the primary prevention of cardiovascular disease: a report of the American College of Cardiology/American Heart Association Task Force on Clinical Practice Guidelines. *Circulation*. 2019;140(11):e596–e646.
83. Grundy SM, Stone NJ, Bailey AL, et al. 2018 AHA/ACC/AACVPR/AAPA/ABC/ACPM/ADA/AGS/APhA/ASPC/NLA/PCNA Guideline on the management of blood cholesterol: a report of the American College of Cardiology/American Heart Association Task Force on Clinical Practice Guidelines. *Circulation*. 2019;139(25):e1082–e1143.
84. Zhao Y, D'Agostino RB Sr, Malik S, et al. United States Cardiovascular Disease Risk Scores in Adults With Diabetes Mellitus. *JACC Adv*, 2004;4(1): 101–448.
85. Buchan TA, Malik A, Chan C, et al. Predictive models for cardiovascular and kidney outcomes in patients with type 2 diabetes: systematic review and meta-analyses. *Heart*. 2021;107:1962–1973.
86. Hippisley-Cox J, Coupland C. Development and validation of QDiabetes-2018 risk prediction algorithm to estimate future risk of type 2 diabetes: cohort study. *BMJ*. 2017;359:j5019.
87. Read SH, van Diepen M, Colhoun HM, et al. Scottish Diabetes Research Network Epidemiology Group Performance of cardiovascular disease risk scores in people diagnosed with type 2 diabetes: external validation using data from the National Scottish Diabetes Register. *Diabetes Care*. 2018;41:2010–2018.
88. Chowdhury MZI, Yeasmin F, Rabi DM, Ronksley PE, Turin TC. Prognostic tools for cardiovascular disease in patients with type 2 diabetes: A systematic review and meta-analysis of C-statistics. *J Diabetes Complications*. 2019;33:98–111.
89. Hippisley-Cox J, Coupland C, Brindle P. Development and validation of QRISK3 risk prediction algorithms to estimate future risk of cardiovascular disease: prospective cohort study. *BMJ*. 2017;357:j2099.
90. Bergmark BA, Bhatt DL, Braunwald E, et al. Risk assessment in patients with diabetes with the TIMI risk score for atherothrombotic disease. *Diabetes Care*. 2018;41:577–585.
91. Stevens RJ, Kothari V, Adler AI, Stratton IM. United Kingdom Prospective Diabetes Study (UKPDS) Group The UKPDS risk engine: a model for the risk of coronary heart disease in Type II diabetes (UKPDS 56). *Clin Sci (London)*. 2001;101(6):671–679.
92. Kothari V, Stevens RJ, Adler AI, et al. UKPDS 60: risk of stroke in type 2 diabetes estimated by the UK Prospective Diabetes Study risk engine. *Stroke*. 2002;33(7):1776–1781.
93. Yeboah J, Erbel R, Delaney JC, et al. Development of a new diabetes risk prediction tool for incident coronary heart disease events: the Multi-Ethnic Study of Atherosclerosis and the Heinz Nixdorf Recall Study. *Atherosclerosis*. 2014;236(2):411–417.
94. SCORE2-Diabetes Working Group and the ESC Cardiovascular Risk Collaboration. SCORE2-Diabetes: 10-year cardiovascular risk estimation in type 2 diabetes in Europe. *Eur Heart J*. 2023;21;44(28):2544–2556.
95. Rados DV, Pinto LC, Leitão CB, Gross JL. Screening for coronary artery disease in patients with type 2 diabetes: a meta-analysis and trial sequential analysis. *BMJ Open*. 2017;7(5):e015089.
96. Knuuti J, Wijns W, Saraste A, et al. 2019 ESC Guidelines for the diagnosis and management of chronic coronary syndromes. *Eur Heart J*. 2020;41(3):407–477.
97. Malik S, Zhao Y, Budoff M, et al. Coronary artery calcium score for long-term risk classification in individuals with type 2 diabetes and metabolic syndrome from the multi-ethnic study of atherosclerosis. *JAMA Cardiol*. 2017;2(12):1332–1340.
98. Greenland P, Alpert JS, Beller GA, et al. 2010 ACCF/AHA guideline for assessment of cardiovascular risk in asymptomatic adults: executive summary: a report of the American College of Cardiology Foundation/American Heart Association Task Force on Practice Guidelines. *Circulation*. 2010;122(25):2748–2764.
99. Suh DC, Choi IS, Plauschinat C, Kwon J, Baron M. Impact of comorbid conditions and race/ethnicity on glycemic control among the US population with type 2 diabetes, 1988-1994 to 1999-2004. *J Diabetes Complications*. 2010;24(6):382–391.
100. World Health Organization. *Obesity and Overweight*. https://www.who.int/news-room/fact-sheets/detail/obesity-and-overweight.
101. Bhupathiraju SN, Hu FB. Epidemiology of obesity and diabetes and their cardiovascular complications. *Circ Res*. 2016;118(11):1723–1735.
102. Gómez-Ambrosi J, Silva C, Galofré JC, et al. Body mass index classification misses subjects with increased cardiometabolic risk factors related to elevated adiposity. *Int J Obes (Lond)*. 2012;36(2):286–294.
103. Després JP, Lemieux I, Bergeron J, et al. Abdominal obesity and the metabolic syndrome: contribution to global cardiometabolic risk [published correction appears in. *Arterioscler Thromb Vasc Biol*. 2008;28(7):1039–1049.
104. Martín-Timón I, Sevillano-Collantes C, Segura-Galindo A, Del Cañizo-Gómez FJ. Type 2 diabetes and cardiovascular disease: have all risk factors the same strength? *World J Diabetes*. 2014;5(4):444–470.
105. Cordola Hsu AR, Ames SL, Xie B, et al. Incidence of diabetes according to metabolically healthy or unhealthy normal weight or overweight/obesity in postmenopausal women: the Women's Health Initiative. *Menopause*. 2020;27:640–647.
106. Cordola Hsu AR, Xie B, Peterson DV, et al. WHI Investigators Metabolically healthy/unhealthy overweight/obesity associations with incident heart failure in postmenopausal women:. *Circ Heart Fail*. 2021;14(4):e007297. https://doi.org/10.1161/CIRCHEARTFAILURE.120.007297. Epub 2021 Mar 29. PMID: 33775111.
107. Lee S, Lacy ME, Jankowich M, Correa A, Wu WC. Association between obesity phenotypes of insulin resistance and risk of type 2 diabetes in African Americans: The Jackson Heart Study. *J Clin Transl Endocrinol*. 2020;19:100210.
108. Katakami N. Mechanism of development of atherosclerosis and cardiovascular disease in diabetes mellitus. *J Atheroscler Thromb*. 2018;25(1):27–39.
109. Berneis KK, Krauss RM. Metabolic origins and clinical significance of LDL heterogeneity. *J Lipid Res*. 2002;43(9):1363–1379.
110. Sone H, Tanaka S, Tanaka S, et al. Serum level of triglycerides is a potent risk factor comparable to LDL cholesterol for coronary heart disease in Japanese patients with type 2 diabetes: subanalysis of the Japan Diabetes Complications Study (JDCS). *J Clin Endocrinol Metab*. 2011;96(11):3448–3456.
111. Fan W, Philip S, Granowitz C, Toth PP, Wong ND. Residual hypertriglyceridemia and estimated atherosclerotic cardiovascular disease risk by statin use in U.S. adults with diabetes: National Health and Nutrition Examination Survey 2007-2014. *Diabetes Care*. 2019;42(12):2307–2314.
112. Koschinsky ML, Bajaj A, Boffa MB, et al. A focused update to the 2019 NLA scientific statement on use of lipoprotein(a) in clinical practice. *J Clin Lipidol*. 2024;18(3):e308–e319.
113. Wong ND, Fan W, Hu X, et al. Lipoprotein(a) and long-term cardiovascular risk in a multi-ethnic pooled prospective cohort. *J Am Coll Cardiol*. 2024 Apr 23;83(16):1511–1525.
114. Rizvi AA. Addressing hypertension in the patient with type 2 diabetes mellitus: pathogenesis, goals, and therapeutic approach. *Eur Med J Diabetes*. 2017;5(1):84–92.
115. Song Y, Liu X, Zhu X, et al. Increasing trend of diabetes combined with hypertension or hypercholesterolemia: NHANES data analysis 1999-2012. *Sci Rep*. 2016;6:36093.
116. Lewington S, Clarke R, Qizilbash N, Peto R, Collins R. Prospective Studies Collaboration Age-specific relevance of usual blood pressure to vascular mortality: a meta-analysis of individual data for one million adults in 61 prospective studies. *Lancet*. 2002;360:1903–1913.
117. Long AN, Dagogo-Jack S. Comorbidities of diabetes and hypertension: mechanisms and approach to target organ protection. *J Clin Hypertens (Greenwich)*. 2011;13(4):244–251.
118. Li M, Xu Y, Wan Q, et al. Individual and combined associations of modifiable lifestyle and metabolic health status with new-onset diabetes and major cardiovascular events: the China Cardiometabolic Disease and Cancer Cohort (4C) Study. *Diabetes Care*. 2020;43:1929–1936.
119. Zhang Y, Pan XF, Chen J, et al. Combined lifestyle factors and risk of incident type 2 diabetes and prognosis among individuals with type 2 diabetes: a systematic review and meta-analysis of prospective cohort studies. *Diabetologia*. 2020;63:21–33.
120. Patterson R, McNamara E, Tainio M, et al. Sedentary behaviour and risk of all-cause, cardiovascular and cancer mortality, and incident type 2 diabetes: a systematic review and dose response meta-analysis. *Eur J Epidemiol*. 2018;33:811–829.
121. Qin P, Li Q, Zhao Y, et al. Sugar and artificially sweetened beverages and risk of obesity, type 2 diabetes mellitus, hypertension, and all-cause mortality: a dose-response meta-analysis of prospective cohort studies. *Eur J Epidemiol*. 2020;35:655–671.
122. Schwab U, Reynolds AN, Sallinen T, Rivellese AA, Riserus U. Dietary fat intakes and cardiovascular disease risk in adults with type 2 diabetes: a systematic review and meta-analysis. *Eur J Nutr*. 2021;60:3355–3363.
123. Rana JS, Karter AJ, Liu JY, Moffet HH, Jaffe MG. Improved cardiovascular risk factors control associated with a large-scale population management program among diabetes patients. *Am J Med*. 2018;131(6):661–668.
124. Fan W, Song Y, Inzucchi SE, et al. Composite cardiovascular risk factor target achievement and its predictors in US adults with diabetes: The Diabetes Collaborative Registry. *Diabetes Obes Metab*. 2019;21(5):1121–1127.
125. Andary R, Fan W, Wong ND. Control of cardiovascular risk factors among us adults with type 2 diabetes with and without cardiovascular disease. *Am J Cardiol*. 2019;124(4):522–527.
126. Wong ND, Zhao Y, Patel R, et al. Cardiovascular risk factor targets and cardiovascular disease event risk in diabetes: a pooling project of the Atherosclerosis Risk in Communities Study, Multi-Ethnic Study of Atherosclerosis, and Jackson Heart Study. *Diabetes Care*. 2016;39(5):668–676.
127. Wright AK, Suarez-Ortegon MF, Read SH, et al. Risk factor control and cardiovascular event risk in people with type 2 diabetes in primary and secondary prevention settings. *Circulation*. 2020;142(20):1925–1936.

128. Wong ND, Patao C, Malik S, Iloeje U. Preventable coronary heart disease events from control of cardiovascular risk factors in US adults with diabetes (projections from utilizing the UKPDS risk engine). *Am J Cardiol*. 2014 Apr 15;113(8):1356–1361. https://doi.org/10.1016/j.amjcard.2013.12.042. Epub 2014 Jan 31. PMID: 24581920.

129. Chaitman BR, Hardison RM, Adler D, et al. The Bypass Angioplasty Revascularization Investigation 2 Diabetes randomized trial of different treatment strategies in type 2 diabetes mellitus with stable ischemic heart disease: impact of treatment strategy on cardiac mortality and myocardial infarction. *Circulation*. 2009;120(25):2529–2540.

130. Gaede P, Lund-Andersen H, Parving HH, Pedersen O. Effect of a multifactorial intervention on mortality in type 2 diabetes. *N Engl J Med*. 2008;358(6):580–591.

131. Ueki K, Sasako T, Okazaki Y, et al. Effect of an intensified multifactorial intervention on cardiovascular outcomes and mortality in type 2 diabetes (J-DOIT3): an open-label, randomised controlled trial. *Lancet Diabetes Endocrinol*. 2017;5(12):951–964.

7 Pathology and Vascular Biology of Atherosclerosis in Patients With Type 2 Diabetes

JORGE PLUTZKY, RENU VIRMANI, AND ANN MARIE SCHMIDT

KEY POINTS

- Multiple factors promote atherosclerosis in diabetes. Hyperglycemia itself exerts direct effects through reprogramming of fundamental biochemical mechanisms, such as the polyol pathway, hexosamine pathway, and protein kinase C.
- Hyperglycemia accelerates the formation of advanced glycation end-products (AGEs), which are irreversible products of glucose reactions with proteins and lipids.
- AGEs may exert their effects by multiple mechanisms, such as the crosslinking of proteins in the vessel wall, and through AGEs interaction with cell surface receptors, the best-characterized of which is the receptor for advanced glycation end products (RAGE).
- Antagonism of RAGE demonstrates benefit in assuaging accelerated diabetic atherosclerosis in preclinical models, at least in part through reduction of inflammation and oxidative stress.
- The patho-biology of diabetic atherosclerosis involves all major intrinsic cellular components of the arterial wall including endothelial cells and vascular smooth muscle cells as well as extrinsic cells including ones involved in inflammation, like monocyte/macrophages, lymphocytes, and neutrophils and in coagulation, like platelets.
- Mechanisms involved in diabetic atherosclerosis and its complications include alterations in coagulation, fibrinolysis, shear stress, and inflammation, with many of these responses activated by clinical parameters associated with diabetes, like hypertension, dyslipidemia, obesity and insulin resistance.
- Pathologic studies in arterial samples from patients with major cardiovascular events in the setting of diabetes supports many of the findings outlined in this chapter, including plaque disruption and superficial erosion as mechanisms involved with acute ischemic events.

OVERVIEW

The interaction between diabetes and atherosclerosis is complex and multifactorial: two particularly common diseases, often encountered in the same patients, both involving long, chronic subclinical phases, with clinical events within each that are distinct but often overlapping, involving serious complications, that impact life expectancy, and driven by shared as well as unique pathogenic mechanisms.[1] Perhaps this complexity helps explain the long-standing and only recently resolved glucose paradox—the long-standing conundrum that despite unequivocal evidence for increased cardiovascular disease (CVD) risk in patients with diabetes, prior trials using older agents that lowered glucose or different hyperglycemia management strategies failed to improve cardiovascular (CV) outcomes.[2] Challenges in this area begin with simple issues regarding definitions and expand quickly into problems of epistemology. Type 1 diabetes mellitus (T1DM) and type 2 diabetes mellitus (T2DM) differ fundamentally in their root causes but share increased risk of micro-CVD and macro-CVD as compared with those without diabetes.[3,4] The nature of the continuous relationship between CV risk issues and diabetes may well extend to prediabetes as well. Although the disease of diabetes is defined clinically by hyperglycemia, the pathologic picture of diabetes in all of its forms extends far beyond glucose and glucose homeostasis to involve multiple other organs and their distinct cellular components, including skeletal muscle, adipose tissue, the liver, lipid metabolism, blood pressure control, renal function, among many others, and ultimately how these organs and pathways that are integral to diabetes impact the vasculature and how the pathogenesis of atherosclerosis is shifted in the broad context of diabetes (Fig. 7.1). The nature of these forces in promoting diabetes,

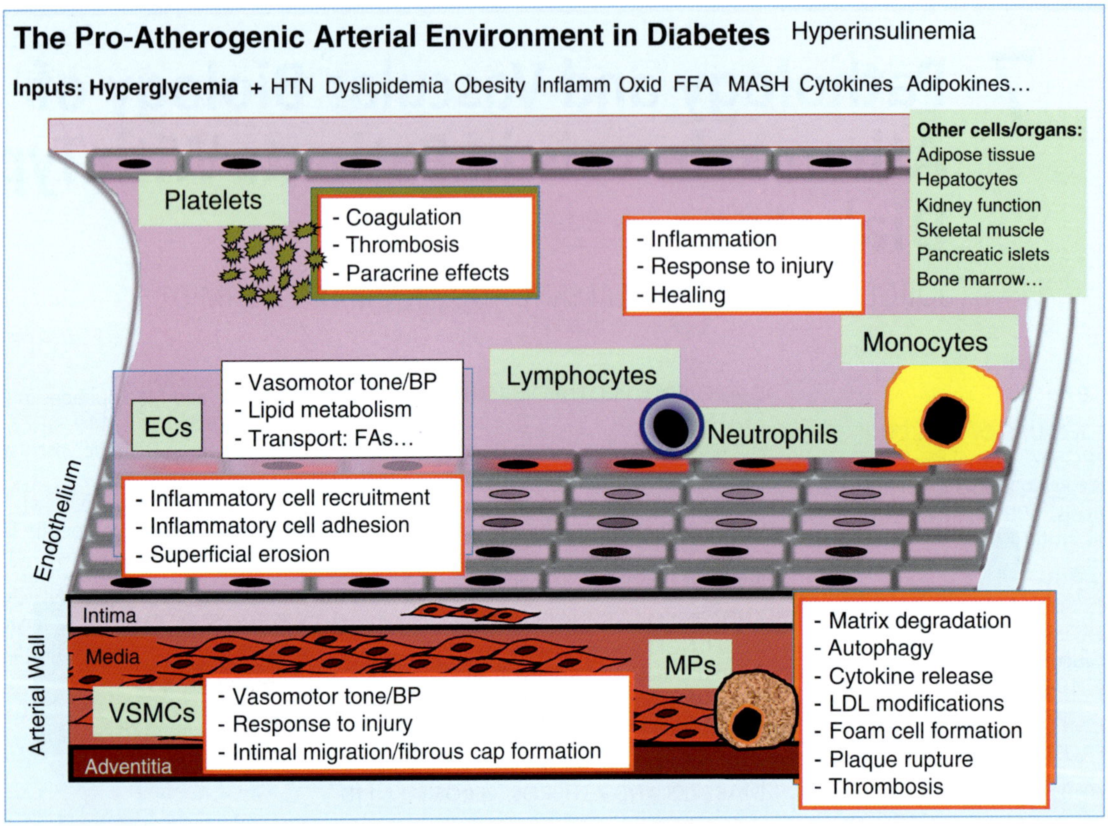

FIG. 7.1 The proatherogenic arterial environment in diabetes. Although diabetes is defined by hyperglycemia, the key cellular players in the vasculature, such as endothelial cells (ECs) and vascular smooth muscle cells (VSMCs), as well as inflammatory cells including lymphocytes and monocytes and macrophages (MPs) encounter multiple pathogenic inputs in the patient with diabetes, including elevated free fatty acids (FFAs), dyslipidemia, hyperinsulinemia, hypertension (HTN), increased cytokines, and altered adipokine levels. As such, resolving whether diabetic atherosclerosis represents unique pathogenic mechanisms or similar proatherosclerotic responses amplified by these stimuli remains unclear. Central issues related to diabetic atherosclerosis focused on in this chapter are schematized here. The dyslipidemia of diabetes is characterized by elevated triglycerides, decreased high-density lipoprotein (HDL), and low-density lipoproteins (LDLs) that may be smaller, denser, and more pathogenic. Diabetes involves a fundamental shift to a more prothrombotic state, as evident in platelet biology. The endothelium is an integral player in vascular health; endothelial dysfunction often characterizes diabetes and involves both abnormal vasomotor function and metabolic abnormalities. Inflammatory responses (highlighted in red) appear particularly involved in diabetic atherosclerosis, with inflammatory changes evident in the endothelium and in lymphocytes (T cells, B cells), monocytes, and monocyte-derived macrophages. In addition to these complexities, it is also important to note that atherosclerosis in diabetes is also influenced by "far-field" effects from other organs, including adipocytes and adipose tissue (e.g., adipokines, FFA release), hepatocytes (coagulation factor production, very low-density lipoprotein [VLDL] secretion), skeletal muscle (insulin resistance), pancreatic islets (insulin release), and bone marrow (progenitor cells). *BP*, Blood pressure.

atherosclerosis, and their intersection thus involve their inherent complexity. The pathogenic components of diabetes and atherosclerosis that are both shared and distinct, along with clinical characteristics of both conditions that involve long preclinical phases, help explain the fundamental observation of increased CAD and atherosclerotic complications, including sudden death, in those with T2DM versus those without diabetes, as seen in data from autopsy studies (Fig. 7.2).

This underlying complexity of diabetic atherosclerosis may underlie the prior challenges of demonstrating clinical CV benefit in treating diabetes. Recent impressive, positive clinical trial data demonstrating a reduction in CV events using sodium-glucose cotransporter-2 inhibitors (SGLT2is) and glucagon-like peptide-1 receptor agonists (GLP-1 RAs) usher in a new, exciting next stage regarding diabetes and CVD while also prompting more questions, such as how such agents exert CV benefit, the prior focus on glucose as a primary therapeutic target for improving CV outcomes in diabetes, the use of such agents in those with various prediabetic states, and how subspecialities define themselves and the diseases they must actively manage. These issues also force further consideration of the nature of diabetic atherosclerosis itself, including the mechanisms, inputs, factors, and biology of atherosclerosis in the context of diabetes, as discussed here, as well as in other chapters.

Although no one single pathway can be seen as accounting for how diabetes promotes atherogenesis, atherosclerosis, and atherothrombotic complications, various mediators and pathogenic forces help explain how diabetes and even the continuum of risk found in prediabetes, modulate atherosclerosis and atherosclerotic complications. Any consideration of mechanisms of CVD in diabetes begins with and is informed by our current state of answers to the fundamental question of what defines the pathology of diabetic atherosclerosis? This chapter will begin with the evidence for the pathologic nature of atherosclerosis in diabetes before using this as a basis for considering the vascular biology of diabetic atherosclerosis and integrated perspectives on the multiple inputs into CVD in diabetes and their clinical relevance in the new era we find ourselves in regarding CVD in the context of diabetes.

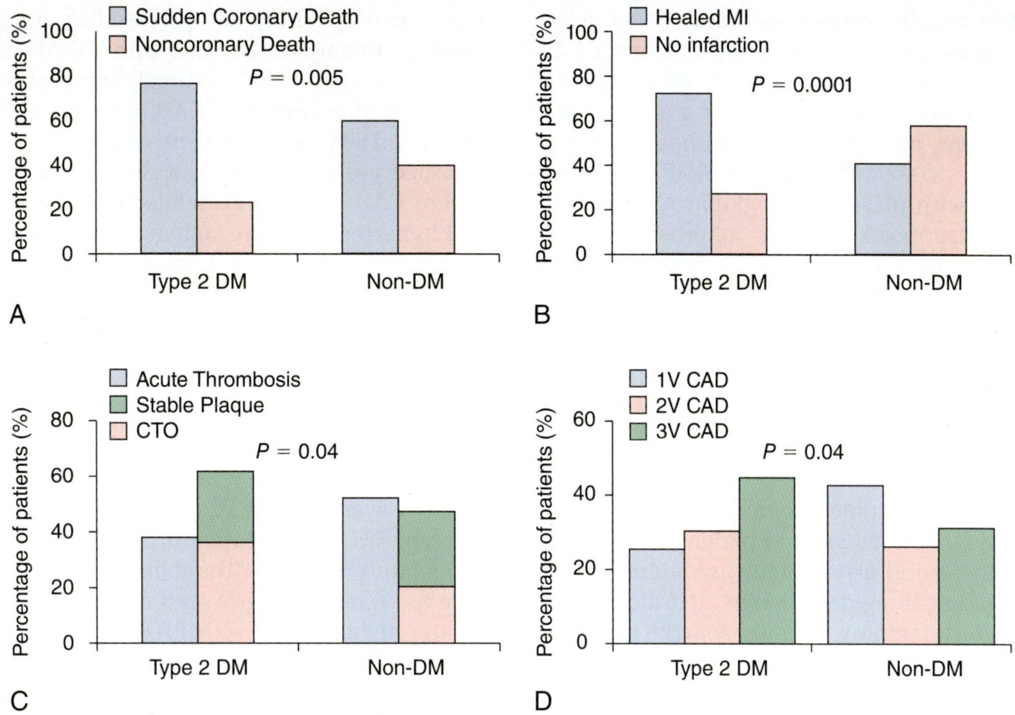

FIG. 7.2 Extent of coronary artery disease (CAD) in sudden death victims with and without diabetes mellitus (DM). A, Cause of death in sudden death victims with type 2 diabetes is more frequently attributed to coronary atherosclerotic disease than in those without diabetes. **B**, Healed myocardial infarction (MI) is more prevalent in patients with type 2 diabetes than in those without diabetes. **C**, The incidence of acute thrombi in patients with type 2 diabetes was lower than in those without diabetes, whereas stable severe coronary artery disease (CAD) and chronic total occlusion (CTO) were more frequently observed in patients with type 2 diabetes than in those without diabetes. **D**, Coronary atherosclerosis in patients with type 2 diabetes was more extensive than in those without diabetes. Approximately half of patients with diabetes showed triple vessel disease, whereas in those without diabetes, single-vessel disease was more frequent than double- or triple-vessel disease.

PATHOLOGIC NATURE OF DIABETIC ATHEROSCLEROSIS

Diabetes mellitus is associated with the development of accelerated atherosclerotic coronary artery disease, which results in significantly increased morbidity and mortality from CV complications including acute myocardial infarction (MI), stroke and peripheral arterial disease (PAD).[5,6] Multiple characteristics of atherosclerosis in diabetes have been proposed including ones considered more unique to diabetes as well as others common to atherosclerosis in general, even if accelerated and/or amplified in those carrying a diagnosis of diabetes. Diabetic atherosclerosis has been reported as being more diffuse, involving smaller arteries predominately, and also altered functional properties, including decreased vessel reactivity, distinct forms of dyslipidemia, inflammation, angiogenesis, and/or impaired reparative responses, among others. Such discussions return to the fundamental pathologic question: What characterizes vessels and specifically atherosclerotic plaque in those with diabetes?

Plaque Morphology in Diabetic Atherosclerosis

Diabetes is associated with an increased prevalence of hyperlipidemia, hypertension, obesity, and a hypercoagulable state, all of which contribute to higher incidence of coronary, carotid, and peripheral artery diseases as well as associated increases in mortality and morbidity.[7] Some risk factors, like lower HDL as well as hyperglycemia itself, have been independently associated with rapid plaque progression, as seen on imaging studies on patients with stable CAD.[8] Diabetic atherosclerotic lesions include pathologic characteristics associated with atherosclerosis and atherosclerotic complications in general as well as ones more linked specifically to diabetes.[9,10]

Coronary and Carotid Artery Disease

Moreno et al. evaluated coronary atherectomy specimens obtained from 47 patients with T2DM, comparing them with specimens from 48 nondiabetic individuals, and demonstrated that patients with diabetes exhibited a larger content of lipid-rich atheroma (7% ± 2%) than those without diabetes (2 ± 1%).[11] In addition, macrophage infiltration was significantly greater in patients with diabetes (22 ± 3%) than in those without diabetes (12 ± 1%) while the incidence of thrombus was higher in individuals with diabetes (62%) versus those without diabetes (40%). Cipollone and colleagues examined carotid endarterectomy specimens from patients with and without T2DM (n = 30/group) and found that plaques from those with diabetes were richer in macrophages and T lymphocytes while manifesting higher human leukocyte antigen–DR (HLA-DR) expression.[12] Immunohistochemistry revealed greater reactivity of the receptor for advanced glycation endproducts (RAGEs; discussed further below) in patients with diabetes versus those without diabetes, especially in macrophage-rich and angiogenic areas. In the diabetes samples, activity of the master proinflammatory transcription factor nuclear factor kappa B (NF-κB) was increased, which corresponded to RAGE expression. Also, cyclooxygenase 2 (COX-2) membrane-associated protein eicosanoid and glutathione metabolism synthase 1 (mPGES-1), matrix metalloproteinases (MMPs), and gelatinolytic activity, activities associated with plaque destabilization, were increased in patients with diabetes, who also had reduced collagen content and increased lipid and oxidized LDL content, all versus those without diabetes. In this study, RAGE, COX-2/mPGES-1, and MMP expression correlated linearly with plasma hemoglobin A1c (HbA1c) levels.[12] This data supports diabetic atherosclerosis as being characterized pathologically by pathways involving enhanced inflammation, RAGE, macrophage infiltration, and plaque destabilization (see Fig. 7.1); other work suggests distinct pathologic characteristics of atherosclerosis in diabetes when specific risk issues are present, as reported with microcalcifications in patients with diabetes, albuminuria, but not yet clinical CV disease.[13] These pathogenic signatures may represent targets whose modification would improve clinical outcomes. For example, statins may decrease levels of RAGE,[14] as seen in patients with T2DM and asymptomatic carotid artery stenosis randomized to diet plus simvastatin (40 mg/day) versus diet alone for 4 months before endarterectomy. Plaques from the simvastatin group showed significant decreases in immunoreactivity for RAGE and advanced glycation endproducts (AGEs) as well as other proinflammatory and proatherosclerotic signals, including myeloperoxidase (MPO); p65; COX-2; mPGES-1; MMP-2; MMP-9; oxidized LDL; and the number of macrophages, T lymphocytes, and HLA-DR–positive cells. In plaque-derived macrophages, simvastatin-mediated decreases in RAGE levels were reversed by AGE stimulation. Thus statin benefits on diabetic atherosclerosis may include reduced RAGE expression and MPO-mediated AGE generation, fostering plaque stabilization.

Additional insights into the pathology of diabetic atherosclerosis derive from autopsy studies. An analysis of morphologic findings in patients with T1DM and T2DM versus age- and sex-matched individuals was performed in a cohort who died suddenly from CAD.[15] A total of 16 patients with T1DM and 50 with T2DM were compared to 66 age- and sex-matched individuals without diabetes who also died from severe CAD (Table 7.1). While the prevalence of smoking and hypertension were similar among all groups, the body mass index (BMI) in individuals with T2DM (30.5 ± 7.4 kg/m^2) was significantly greater than in those without diabetes (26.6 ± 5.4 kg/m^2, $P = 0.001$) or T1DM BMI (25.6 ± 6.4 kg/m^2, $P = 0.7$). The ratio of total cholesterol (TC) to HDL-C was significantly higher in individuals with T2DM than in those without diabetes (7.9 ± 3.9 vs. 6.3 ± 3.4, $P = 0.02$), with trends for higher TC and lower HDL-C, as often encountered in T2DM. On the contrary, individuals with T1DM had a trend toward lower levels of TC (183 ± 52 mg/dL) and comparable levels of HDL-C (37 ± 14 mg/dL) and TC-to–HDL-C ratio (5.8 ± 2.9) relative to those without diabetes. The percent necrotic core area (necrotic core area divided by plaque area) was greater in individuals with T1DM (12.0% ± 5.7%) and T2DM (11.6% ± 8.4%) than those without diabetes (9.4% ± 9.3%; $P = 0.05$ vs. T1DM, $P = 0.004$ vs. T2DM) (Table 7.2). Those with T2DM had greater percent calcified area (12.1% ± 11.2%) than those without diabetes (11.4% ± 13.5%, $P = 0.05$) while those with T1DM and those without diabetes had a comparable percent calcified area (7.8% ± 9.1%). The number of fibroatheromas was greater in individuals with T2DM (8.8 ± 4.3) than in those without diabetes (6.9 ± 4.7, $P = 0.02$) or with T1DM (7.1 ± 5.0); healed plaque ruptures but not thin-cap fibroatheromas were also higher in T2DM versus those without diabetes.

TABLE 7.1 Sudden Coronary Death Registry: Demographics, Risk Factors, and Cardiac Findings in Patients With Type 1 Diabetes, Type 2 Diabetes, or No Diabetes

	TYPE 1 DM (N = 16)	TYPE 2 DM (N = 50)	NON-DM (N = 66)	*P* VALUE (TYPE 1 DM VS. NON-DM)	*P* VALUE (TYPE 2 DM VS. NON-DM)
Age (year)	50.3 ± 13.2	50.2 ± 11.0	50.6 ± 12.3	0.9	0.9
Women	25%	30%	29%	0.8	0.9
Blacks	20%	30%	29%	0.7	0.9
HbA1c (%)	12.2 ± 2.5	10.7 ± 2.6	6.2 ± 0.6	0.0001	0.0001
Smokers	42%	58%	55%	0.4	0.8
Hypertension	29%	35%	30%	0.9	0.6
Body mass index (kg/m^2)	25.6 ± 6.4	30.5 ± 7.4	26.6 ± 5.4	0.7	0.001
TC (mg/dL)	183 ± 52	227 ± 83	211 ± 79	0.3	0.3
HDL cholesterol (mg/dL)	37 ± 14	33 ± 16	38 ± 18	0.8	0.1
TC/HDL cholesterol	5.8 ± 2.9	7.9 ± 3.9	6.3 ± 3.4	0.7	0.02
Heart weight (g)	425 ± 119	524 ± 140	434 ± 121	0.7	0.004
Corrected heart weight (g)[a]	428 ± 94	508 ± 134	460 ± 106	0.3	0.03
Healed infarcts	33%	73%	37%	0.7	0.0001

[a]Corrected for body weight.
Values are expressed as mean ± standard deviation or percentage. *DM*, Diabetes mellitus; *HDL*, high-density lipoprotein; *TC*, total cholesterol.
Data from Burke AP, Kolodgie FD, Zieske A, et al. Morphologic findings of coronary atherosclerotic plaques in diabetics: a postmortem study. *Arterioscler Thromb Vasc Biol.* 2004;24:1266–1271.

TABLE 7.2 Sudden Coronary Death Registry: Plaque Characteristics in Patients With Type 1 Diabetes, Type 2 Diabetes, or No Diabetes

	TYPE 1 DM (N = 16)	TYPE 2 DM (N = 50)	NON-DM (N = 66)	*P* VALUE (TYPE 1 DM VS. NON-DM)	*P* VALUE (TYPE 2 DM VS. NON-DM)
Acute coronary thrombi	21%	42%	51%	0.03	0.2
Acute plaque rupture	6%	32%	27%	0.09	0.6
Plaque erosion	6%	12%	29%	0.02	0.04
Necrotic core area (%)[a]	12.0 ± 5.7	11.6 ± 8.4	9.4 ± 9.3	0.05[b]	0.004[b]
Calcified matrix area (%)[a]	7.8 ± 9.1	12.1 ± 11.2	11.4 ± 13.5	0.9[b]	0.05[b]
Fibroatheroma (n)	7.1 ± 5.0	8.8 ± 4.3	6.9 ± 4.7	0.9	0.02
Thin-cap fibroatheroma (n)	1.0 ± 1.3	0.8 ± 0.8	0.7 ± 0.8	0.5	0.8
Healed plaque rupture (n)	2.6 ± 2.1	2.6 ± 1.8	1.9 ± 1.8	0.2	0.04
Total plaque burden (%)	275 ± 129	358 ± 114	232 ± 128	0.04	0.0001
Distal plaque burden (%)	310 ± 114	630 ± 263	331 ± 199	0.8	0.0001
Macrophage area (mm^2)	0.15 ± 0.02	0.13 ± 0.03	0.10 ± 0.02[c]	0.03[b]	0.03[b]

[a]Divided by plaque area.
[b]*P* values calculated using log-normalized data.
[c]*P* = 0.006 versus type 1 and 2 diabetes combined.
Values are expressed as mean ± standard deviation or percentage. *DM*, Diabetes mellitus.
Data from Burke AP, Kolodgie FD, Zieske A, et al. Morphologic findings of coronary atherosclerotic plaques in diabetics: a postmortem study. *Arterioscler Thromb Vasc Biol.* 2004;24:1266–1271.

TABLE 7.3 Relationship Between Risk Factors, Including Diabetes and Plaque Characteristics: A Multivariate Analysis

INDEPENDENT VARIABLES	% NECROTIC CORE AREA[a]		NUMBER OF FIBROATHEROMAS[b]		% MACROPHAGE AREA[c]	
(RISK FACTORS)	T	*P* VALUE	T	*P* VALUE	T	*P* VALUE
Glycohemoglobin (%)	2.8	0.005	1.7	0.09	2.9	0.004
TC/HDL cholesterol	2.5	0.01	3.0	0.0003	1.3	0.19
Body mass index	3.5	0.006	0.57	0.57	1.5	0.14
Smoking	−0.4	0.7	−1.1	0.24	−0.6	0.5
Age	−1.2	0.2	−1.2	0.2	−5.4	0.0001

[a]Mean percent necrotic core area (of the four arteries studies per patient).
[b]Mean number of fibroatheromas per heart.
[c]Mean macrophage area (of the four arteries per patient).
The population for this table is the 132 patients with three separate one-way analysis of variance (ANOVA) analyses correlating three dependent variables (mean % necrotic core area, mean % macrophage area).
Data from Burke AP, Kolodgie FD, Zieske A, et al. Morphologic findings of coronary atherosclerotic plaques in diabetics: a postmortem study. *Arterioscler Thromb Vasc Biol.* 2004;24:1266–1271.

By multivariable analysis (Table 7.3), a positive correlation was found between mean percent necrotic core area and glycohemoglobin, independent of HDL-C, ratio of TC to HDL-C, age, smoking, and sex (T = 2.8, *P* = 0.005). Similarly, the ratio of TC to HDL-C (T = 2.5, *P* = 0.01) and BMI (T = 3.5, *P* = 0.006) correlated positively with percent necrotic core area. There was a significant relationship between numbers of fibroatheroma and ratio of TC to HDL-C (T = 3.0, *P* = 0.0003). Glycohemoglobin correlated positively with number of fibroatheromas, although not with statistical significance (T = 1.7, *P* = 0.09).

Observations within this cohort also pointed to inflammatory mechanisms in diabetes. Macrophage plaque area and T-cell infiltration were significantly greater in individuals with diabetes versus those without diabetes (*P* = 0.03, see Table 7.2; Fig. 7.3). T-cell infiltration was greater in individuals with T1DM, potentially consistent with T1DM as an autoimmune disease with a common genetic susceptibility to other disorders, like autoimmune thyroiditis, of potential pathophysiological significance in coronary plaque pathology.[16] The incidence of acute thrombi was significantly less in individuals with T1DM (21%) than in those without diabetes (51%, *P* = 0.03) in sudden coronary death victims (see Table 7.2). Individuals with T1DM showed a lower incidence of acute plaque rupture than those without diabetes (6% vs. 27%, *P* = 0.09) while plaque erosion was significantly less frequent in individuals with diabetes versus those without diabetes (6%, 12% vs. 29%, *P* = 0.02 and *P* = 0.04). Acute thrombi were found less in specimens from individuals with T2DM than in those without diabetes, whereas stable severe CAD and chronic total occlusion were more frequently observed in individuals with T2DM than in those without diabetes (see Fig. 7.2C). The incidence of acute plaque rupture was similar in those with (32%) or without T2DM (27%).

In sudden death victims, approximately half of individuals with diabetes showed triple-vessel disease, whereas those without diabetes more often had single-vessel disease (see Fig. 7.2D), in line with total plaque burden being significantly greater in those with T2DM than in those

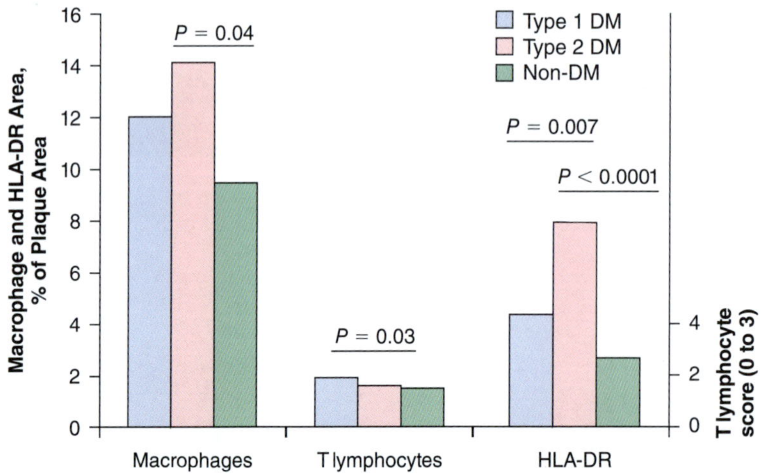

FIG. 7.3 Comparison of inflammatory infiltrate in patients with diabetes versus those without diabetes in autopsy samples. Bar graph showing quantitative and semiquantitative comparisons of the extent of macrophages, T lymphocytes, and human leukocyte antigen–DR (HLA-DR) expression in coronary arteries from patients with diabetes and those without diabetes. Plaque macrophages and HLA expression were greater in patients with diabetes (type 1 and 2) than in those without diabetes, whereas T-cell infiltration was maximal in patients with type 1 diabetes. (Modified from Burke AP, Kolodgie FD, Zieske A, et al. Morphologic findings of coronary atherosclerotic plaques in diabetics: a postmortem study. *Arterioscler Thromb Vasc Biol.* 2004;24:1266–1271.)

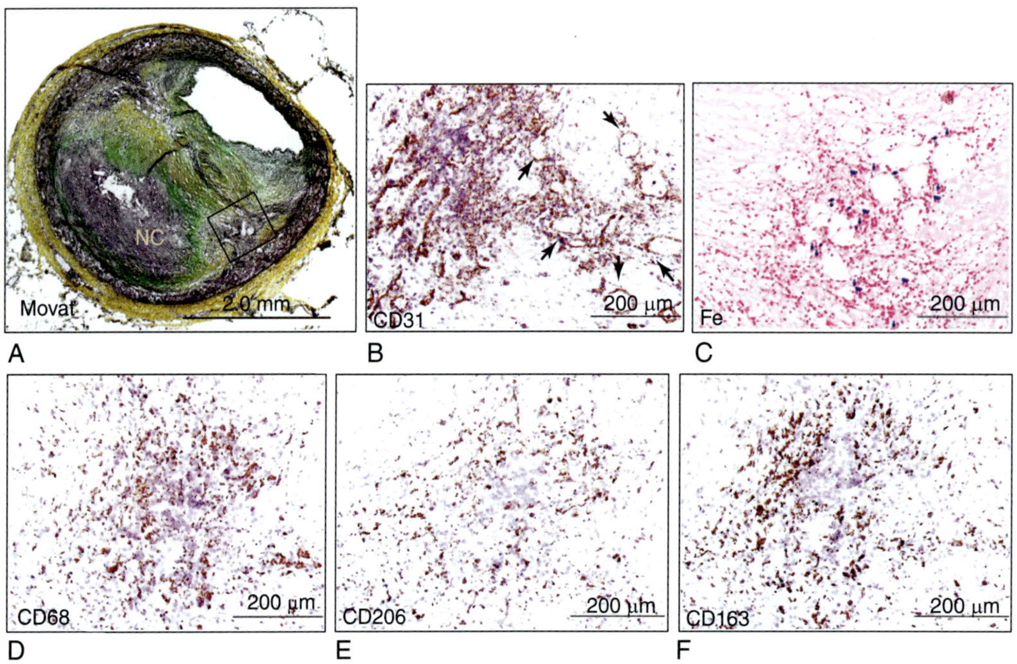

FIG. 7.4 Angiogenesis, hemorrhage, iron deposition, and inflammation in diabetic coronary plaques. Histologic sections from a 48-year-old black man with history of hypertension and diabetes who died suddenly. **A**, A low-power image shows fibroatheroma with severe luminal narrowing and angiogenesis. **B–F**, High-power images of the black box in **A. B**, Note abundant CD31 (platelet endothelial cell adhesion molecule 1 [PECAM-1]) staining that indicates the presence of angiogenesis (arrows). **C**, The same area shows abundance of iron (blue), suggestive of hemorrhage. **D–F**, There are also abundant macrophages that are detected by CD68, CD206 (mannose receptor), and CD163 (Hb-haptoglobin receptor) staining.

without diabetes (358 ± 114 vs. 232 ± 128, $P = 0.0001$; see Table 7.2). Increased plaque burden may involve a higher rate of healed plaque ruptures, which can promote plaque progression.[17] Diabetes is also linked to late complications following coronary artery bypass graft surgery, including acute MI and graft failure.[18–20] while greater plaque burden in diabetes may underlie evidence suggesting worse outcomes, including mortality, after percutaneous intervention versus bypass surgery in diabetes.[21]

Plaque hemorrhage is associated with intraplaque angiogenesis. Increased intraplaque hemorrhage, as assessed by glycophorin A staining of red cell membranes, has been linked with plaque progression, enlarging necrotic core, greater macrophage infiltration, and iron deposition within coronary atherosclerotic plaques.[22] In T2DM, plaque pathology has been reported to contain increased angiogenesis, plaque hemorrhage and rupture,[23] with similar findings in abdominal and thoracic aortas in T2DM[11] (Fig. 7.4). The extent of neovascularization correlates with macrophage and T-cell infiltration and plaque hemorrhage, which were greater in individuals with diabetes than in those without diabetes (Fig. 7.5).[24]

Advances in coronary imaging now offers this modality as an additional means of characterizing atherosclerotic plaque in diabetes outside of performing autopsies. In the Computed TomogRaphic Evaluation of Atherosclerotic Determinants

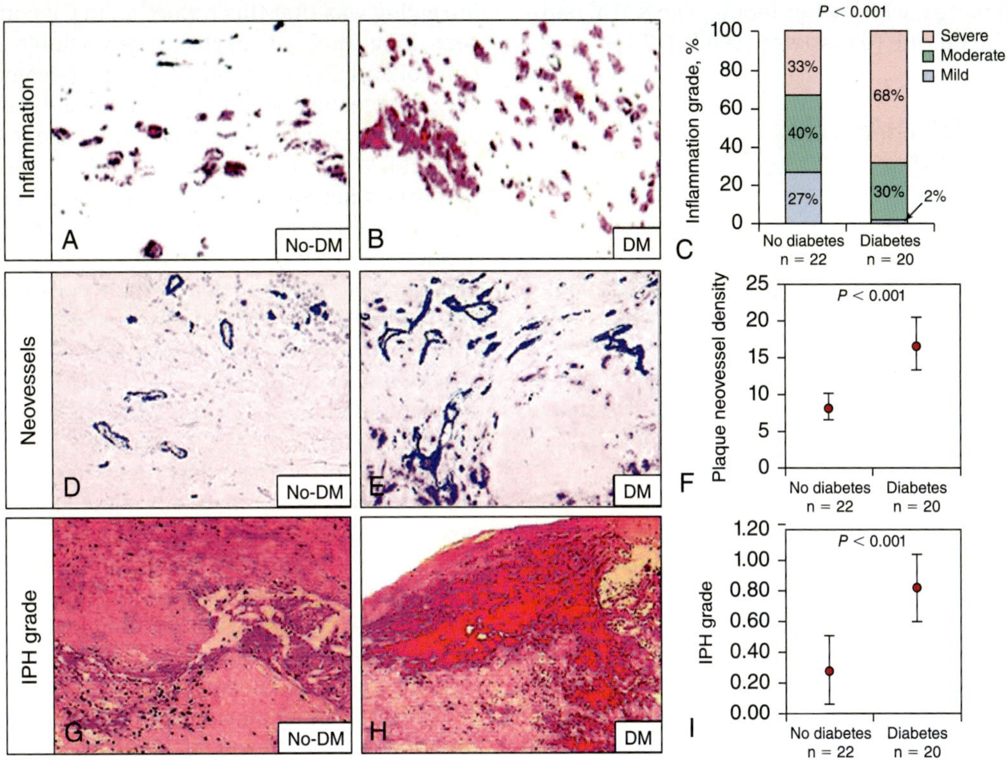

FIG. 7.5 Inflammation, neovascularization, and intraplaque hemorrhage in aortic atherosclerosis from patients with and without diabetes. **A**, Nondiabetic atherosclerotic plaque cap stained with CD68/CD3 in red chromogen shows mild inflammation in high-power field, 40 × (grade 1); less than 25 macrophages in the view. **B**, Diabetic plaque cap shows severe inflammation in high-power field, 40 × (grade 2); more than 25 macrophages per field are depicted in diabetic plaque. **C**, Distribution of inflammation grade in nondiabetic and diabetic plaques. **D**, Double-label immunohistochemistry with neovessels stained by CD34 in blue chromogen and inflammatory cells stained with CD68/CD3 in red chromogen. Nondiabetic plaque shows fewer dense neovessels and inflammatory cells in the high-power field, 40 ×. **E**, Diabetic plaque showing denser neovessels with tubuloluminal spaces surrounded by inflammatory cells seen in high-power field, 40 ×. **F**, Mean and 95% confidence interval for plaque neovessel density in nondiabetic and diabetic plaques. **G**, Nondiabetic plaque with less than 25% hemorrhage seen in high-power field (grade 1). **H**, Hematoxylin-eosin–stained diabetic plaque showing severe intraplaque hemorrhage occupying more than 75% of the plaque core seen in high-power field, 40 × (grade 3). **I**, Mean and 95% confidence interval for intraplaque hemorrhage (IPH) grade in nondiabetic and diabetic plaques. (Reproduced with permission from Purushothaman KR, Purushothaman M, Muntner P, et al. Inflammation, neovascularization and intra-plaque hemorrhage are associated with increased reparative collagen content: implication for plaque progression in diabetic atherosclerosis. *Vasc Med.* 2011;16:103–108.)

of Myocardial IsChEmia (CREDENCE) trial, patients (n = 303 subjects) referred for invasive coronary angiography also underwent coronary computed tomographic angiography (CCTA).[25] An analysis of CREDENCE participants with diabetes (n = 95, 31%) found that those with diabetes had greater plaque burden than those without diabetes, with lesions that were often obstructive (58.1%).[26] Patients with diabetes and nonobstructive disease had statistically significant increases in percentage of atheroma volume, PAV, noncalcified plaque, number of diseased vessels, and maximum stenosis compared to those without diabetes—findings that align with pathologic studies discussed previously. Another reported characteristic of coronary arteries in T2DM is a higher coronary calcium score.[27] A three-vessel optical coherence tomography study in nonculprit plaques found that patients with diabetes had a higher prevalence of calcification, along with lipid index and thrombus, than those without diabetes.[28] Imaging studies have also found increasing prevalence and extent of coronary plaque across a range of glucose from euglycemia to prediabetes to diabetes in asymptomatic patients undergoing coronary CT angiography.[29] This glycemia range also aligned in a stepwise manner with increases in the presence of any coronary plaque, noncalcified plaque, and plaque with ≥1 high-risk features. Among participants with diabetes and a coronary calcium score of zero, 30% had coronary plaque. In another study of 898 patients with acute MI (with or without ST-segment elevation) who underwent successful percutaneous coronary intervention (PCI), three-vessel quantitative coronary angiography, and coregistered near-infrared spectroscopy, and intravascular ultrasound imaging were also performed before these subjects were followed for subsequent major adverse cardiovascular event (MACE) occurrence (3.7 years).[30] These subsequent MACEs were adjudicated as to whether the recurrent event involved previously treated lesions and the associated characteristics of the previously obtained coronary imaging. In patients with diabetes (n = 109, 12.1%), recurrent events were more common and primarily involved the initial culprit lesion restenosis or prior nonculprit lesions that underwent spontaneous MI than those without diabetes. However, there was no difference between those with and without diabetes in regard to the extent of high-risk plaque characteristics seen at the start of the study. Although many interpretations of this data exist, it does suggest ongoing limitations in what imaging can inform us of regarding the nature of specific lesions and future events in those with diabetes.

Taken together, these and other studies underscore the complex pathologic state of diabetic atherosclerosis that overlap with nondiabetic atherosclerosis, even if augmented in diabetes, while other inputs, like RAGE pathways, that may be unique to diabetes (see Fig. 7.1).[1]

MECHANISMS OF DIABETIC ATHEROSCLEROSIS

Glucose and Glucose-Related Pathways

These findings on the nature of atherosclerotic plaque in diabetes prompt the fundamental issue of what mechanisms drive this augmented pathology. Hyperglycemia defines the presence of diabetes, raising the key question of how glucose itself promotes atherosclerosis. Extensive evidence supports the relationship between diabetes and atherosclerosis, even extending to dysglycemic states in the absence of frank diabetes. Such data only fueled the frustration that despite this strong, direct, continuous relationship between hyperglycemia and atherosclerosis, treating hyperglycemia, including the use of many different strategies—earlier intervention, tighter glucose control, insulin-providing versus insulin-sensitizing strategies—all failed to decease atherosclerotic complications even while improving hyperglycemia. The landmark positive clinical CV outcome trials with GLP-1 RAs and SGLT2i in reducing adverse CV outcomes does suggest that the prior therapeutic failures may have derived in part to older antidiabetic agents not targeting mechanisms of potential CV benefit and/or involved offsetting adverse CV effects, as discussed elsewhere in this textbook. This positive data with GLP-1 RAs and SGLT2is also provide new opportunities for insights into modifiable mechanisms in atherosclerotic complications. While evidence that the CV benefit of these agents involved primarily their glucose-lowering properties has been largely lacking, with subsequent data indicating their benefits in those without diabetes, decreases in hyperglycemia may still have an interactive effect with other actions. Despite these questions about hyperglycemia in macrovascular disease, elevated glucose both contributes to vascular pathogenesis and is established as a modifiable factor for improving outcomes in microvascular disease, including neuropathy, retinopathy, and nephropathy. Together these various factors argue for detailed consideration of glucose effects on the vasculature.

Long-term intervention studies have tested if strict glucose control reduces CV consequences in diabetes. In T1DM, as reviewed more extensively elsewhere, the Diabetes Control and Complications Trial (DCCT) randomized adolescents age 15 years (87 patients) or young adults, average age 28 years (191 patients), to either strict versus standard glycemic control.[31] Strict control of hyperglycemia reduced microvascular complications of diabetes compared with standard regimens of glycemic control.[32] No difference in CV events was noted, although study participants were younger. However, in the Epidemiology of Diabetes Interventions and Complications (EDIC) study, a longer-term follow-up of DCCT, both the atherosclerosis surrogate of carotid intimamedia thickness and the clinical combined endpoint of MI, stroke, and CV death were reduced in those who had earlier received strict glucose control as compared to standard regiments.[33,34] Particularly intriguing was that this reduction in CV complications was seen long after glycosylated hemoglobin levels between control and strict treatment groups became indistinguishable, suggesting a "legacy" effect and raising questions about the mechanisms underlying these results.

In T2DM, the mechanisms underlying the estimated two- to fourfold increase in CV risk are confounded by the overlapping, intertwined nature of risk factors in such patients, including obesity, hypertriglyceridemia, hypercholesterolemia, and hypertension, which coexist with hyperglycemia. The United Kingdom Prospective Diabetes Study (UKPDS) involved 3867 subjects with T2DM randomized to strict versus standard glycemic control. After 10 years, glycosylated hemoglobin levels were significantly lower in the strict control group (7.0%) versus standard (7.9%), with the strict control group having a 16% reduction in risk of MI, which was not statistically significant.[35] Notably, in the posttrial monitoring program, those randomized to standard control group had significantly fewer MIs than the strict glycemic control group, despite their convergence to similar glycosylated hemoglobin levels after the study,[36] another potential legacy effect raising further questions regarding glucose control in CV risk reduction.

Several large clinical trials offer insight into hyperglycemia as a mechanism in atherosclerotic complications and provide a broader context about this interaction. In the Action to Control Cardiovascular Risk in Diabetes (ACCORD) trial, stricter glycemic control was associated with higher CV and all-cause mortality versus the standard regimen, prompting early study discontinuation after a mean 3.5 years of follow-up.[37] There was, however, a nonstatistically significant trend toward fewer nonfatal MI, nonfatal stroke, or death from CV causes among those in the tighter glycemic control groups. Subsequent analyses suggested more hypoglycemia in the glycemic control arms may have contributed to the increased mortality. Separately, two important trials—the Action in Diabetes and Vascular Disease: Preterax and Diamicron Modified Release Controlled Evaluation (ADVANCE)[38] and the Veterans Affairs Diabetes Trial (VADT)[39]—also studied glycemic control in T2DM; both trials showed neither CV benefit nor harm. Despite the failure of better glucose control to improve macrovascular complications, considerable work has investigated how hyperglycemia alters microvasculature responses, even if questions about the relationship between hyperglycemia, glucose control, and macrovascular disease persist. In this regard, other more subtle factors are noteworthy as to hyperglycemia as a factor in vascular biology and CV outcomes. Even if glucose control does not decrease MACE directly, improvements in glycemia and/or the glucose-lowering agents in use may help decrease pathologic parameters of a given ischemic event or enhance other effects of the agent. As an illustrative example of this concept, considerable preclinical and clinical data indicate that cerebrovascular events while on statin treatment are smaller than without statin treatment, a potentially distinct outcome than preventing the event completely. Separately, among glucose-lowering agents with established CV benefits, improved glucose levels may help augment the agents beneficial mechanisms and/ or decrease pathologic parameters. Taking these issues together, reviewing the data for mechanisms that connect glucose metabolism and hyperglycemia to vascular responses is important.

POLYOL PATHWAY

The two major enzymes of the polyol pathway are aldose reductase (AR), the first and rate-limiting step that metabolizes glucose to sorbitol, and sorbitol dehydrogenase (SDH), which converts glucose to fructose. AR actions involve converting nicotinamide adenine dinucleotide phosphate, reduced form (NADPH) to nicotinamide adenine dinucleotide phosphate ($NADP^+$) with SDH consuming nicotinamide adenine dinucleotide (NAD^+) to yield NADH.[40] Globally AR-overexpressing transgenic mice, which have human-relevant AR levels, worsen atherosclerosis in the Apo E-deficient proatherosclerotic mouse model, with effects that may also involve inflammation (Fig. 7.6A and B)[42]; similar data are seen in the low-density lipoprotein (LDL) receptor-deficient atherosclerosis model with streptozotocin-induced diabetes, effects not due to altered lipid parameters. Other work implicates endothelial hAR in promoting atherosclerosis.[43] Of note, these transgenic hAR models of the polyol pathway increased proatherosclerotic changes in the presence of diabetes while administration of the AR inhibitor zopolrestat decreased the augmented atherosclerosis in the diabetic transgenic hAR/apoE-deficient mice (Fig. 7.6C). Together, these data implicate glucose flux via the polyol pathway in promoting diabetic atherosclerosis.

Of note, in contrast to these transgenic studies, an earlier report found that distinct AR inhibitors (ARIs, tolrestat and sorbinil) and genetic ablation of AR in diabetic apoE-deficient mice increased early lesion formation through increased levels of toxic aldehydes in lipid particles, suggesting AR might limit atherosclerosis.[44] Experimental differences, specifically genetic overexpression of AR to human-relevant levels, compensatory responses to complete genetic AR deletion, as well as potential ARI off-target effects may underlie these discrepancies. In humans with diabetes and neuropathy, 1 year of ARI zopolrestat treatment improved cardiac function, as measured by echocardiography while vehicle-treated patients with diabetes demonstrated ongoing reduction in cardiac function.[45] This study, which did not directly address diabetic atherosclerosis, suggested pharmacologic AR inhibition by zopolrestat did not worsen diabetic CV complications. Perhaps more potent and specific ARIs may hold promise for treating atherosclerosis in diabetes. Finally, it is worth noting that increased polyol pathway activity may increase oxidative stress.[41] NADPH is a cofactor of glutathione production; consumption of glutathione through polyol pathway activity may reduce the availability of this antioxidant mechanism.[46] These findings may align with data from mouse models and human macrophages that AR activity increases oxidative stress after high glucose and oxidized LDL exposure.

HEXOSAMINE PATHWAY

When excess glucose is shunted into the hexosamine biosynthetic pathway (HBP), the resulting products can cause endoplasmic reticulum stress and promote transcription of key proatherosclerotic molecules. In HBP, fructose-6-phosphate is converted to glucosamine-6-phosphate and uridine diphosphate (UDP)–*N*-acetyl glucosamine via the actions of the rate-limiting enzyme of the HBP, namely L-glutamine:D-fructose-6-phosphate amidotransferase (GFAT).[47] Various proposed mechanisms may explain how HBP may exacerbate atherosclerosis in diabetes. First, in a manner dependent on mitochondrial superoxide production, hyperglycemia increases hexosamine biosynthesis and *O*-glycosylation of the transcription factor Sp1 in bovine aortic endothelial cells (ECs). This Sp1 modification can increase expression of plasminogen activator inhibitor type 1 (PAI-1) and transforming growth factor beta 1 (TGF-β1).[48] Second, like ECs, hyperglycemia-induced PAI-1 via HBP is also reported in adipose tissue.[49] Third, in bovine aortic ECs, endothelial nitric oxide synthase (eNOS) activity was inhibited by HBP-mediated increases in *O*-linked *N*-acetylglucosamine modification of eNOS and a decrease in *O*-linked serine phosphorylation at residue 1177.[50] In the aortas of diabetic mice, similar changes in eNOS activity and these posttranslational modifications were also observed. Because reduced eNOS activity is found in diabetes and linked to endothelial dysfunction, HBP-mediated reductions in eNOS activity spurred by hyperglycemia may foster endothelial dysfunction, which then accelerates atherosclerosis.

PROTEIN KINASE C

Hyperglycemia stimulates the generation of diacylglycerol (DAG), which activates certain isoforms of protein kinase C (PKC), a family of at least 12 members.[51,52] PKCs participate in multiple, diverse cellular functions, many of which are implicated in diabetic atherosclerosis, including cellular proliferation, signal transduction, cell fate, and transcription factor modulation (e.g., Egr1, NF-κB, Sp1); cytokine expression; and oxidative stress in ECs, smooth muscle cells (SMCs), and monocytes/macrophages.[53]

Multiple studies implicate PKC isoforms in the pathogenesis of atherosclerosis. First, global deletion of the PKCβ isoform significantly reduced atherosclerosis in apoE null mice, even without diabetes.[54] In parallel, these researchers showed that PKCβ isoform deletion may have been atheroprotective by reducing vascular levels of the key transcription factor, Egr1, which promotes proinflammatory and prothrombotic gene expression in atherosclerosis. Furthermore, treating apoE null mice with the PKCβ inhibitor ruboxistaurin (also known as LY333531) decreased atherosclerosis. Although not performed in diabetic animals, this work does support PKCβ involvement in promoting diabetic atherosclerosis. Indeed, administration of ruboxistaurin to T2DM patients improved brachial artery flow-mediated dilation compared with vehicle treatment.[54] In addition to PKCβ, the PKCδ isoform may limit atherosclerosis through effects on SMC survival. In a model of vein graft atherosclerosis in nondiabetic mice, PKCδ deletion resulted in more severe atherosclerosis.[55] Further studies are needed to define specific PKC isoform roles in diabetic atherosclerosis. Other studies suggest that AGE pathways may contribute to activation of PKC isoforms—for example, in bovine retinal ECs.[56]

Oxidative stress has been extensively implicated in diabetic atherosclerosis. Samples from humans and diabetic

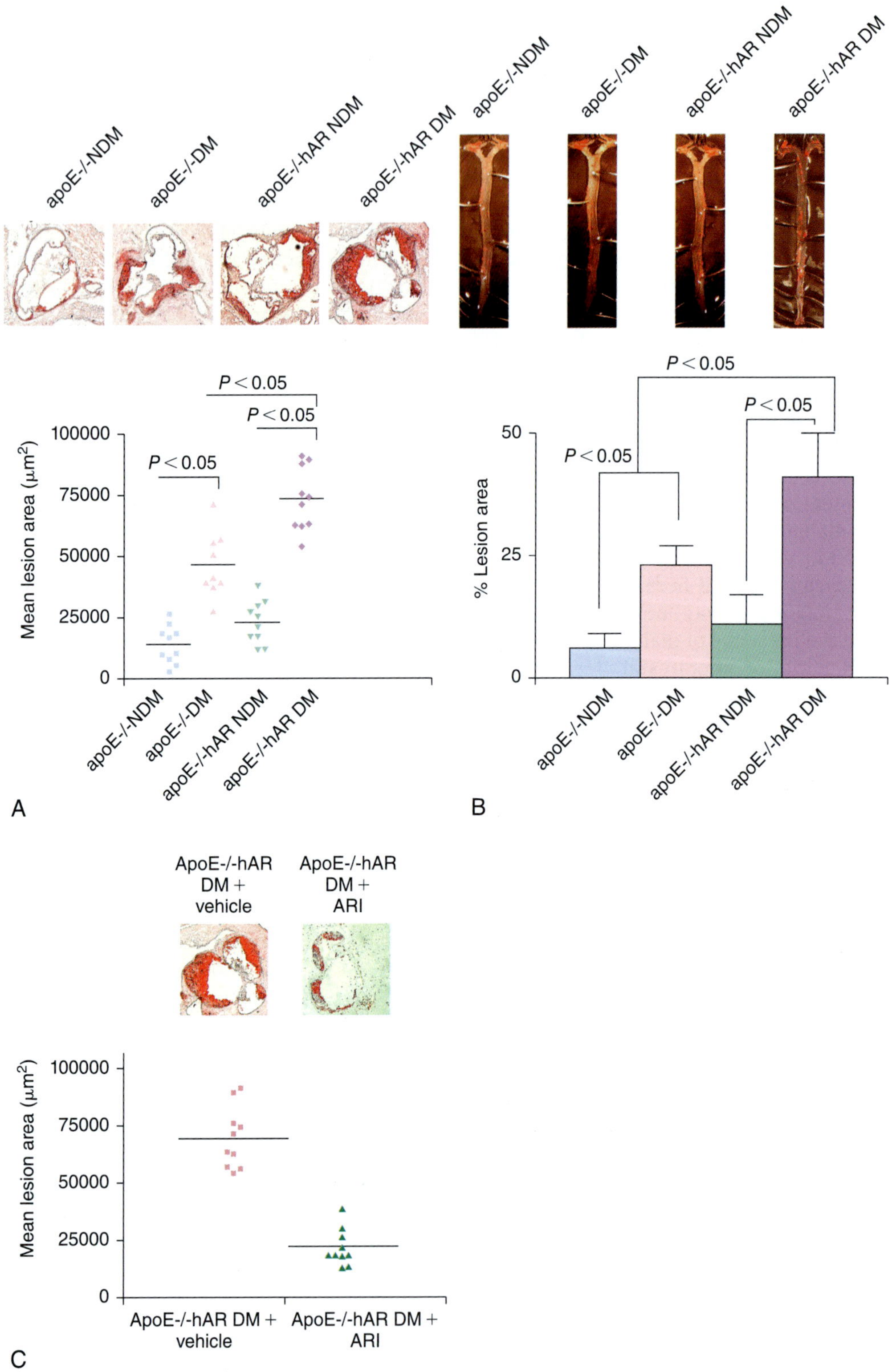

FIG. 7.6 Impact of diabetes and aldose reductase (AR) expression on atherosclerosis at 14 weeks after induction of diabetes. Representative images of aortic root sections stained with oil red O (**A**) and aorta specimens stained en face with Sudan IV (**B**). Hearts were retrieved from nondiabetic and diabetic apoE −/− (n = 10 and 9, respectively) mice, nondiabetic and diabetic apoE −/− hAR + (n = 10 in each group) mice, and diabetic apoE −/− hAR + mice treated with and without aldose reductase inhibitor (ARI) (n = 10 and 10, respectively) (**C**), and mean atherosclerotic lesion areas were determined. (Reprinted from Vedantham S, Ananthakrishnan R, Schmidt AM, Ramasamy R. Aldose reductase, oxidative stress and diabetic cardiovascular complications. *Cardiovasc Hematol Agents Med Chem*. 2012;10:234–240.)

animals show increased levels of oxidative stress markers such as plasma and urinary F2-isoprostanes and 8-hydroxydeoxyguanosine.[57] Such oxidative stress markers have been linked to diabetic complications, and in aortic rings retrieved from T1DM or T2DM animals, oxidative stress appears to increase endothelial dysfunction.[58] Specific roles for oxidative stress in diabetes are suggested by experiments in which heterozygous deletion of the lipoic acid synthase gene in streptozotocin-induced diabetic apoE null mice markedly increased atherosclerosis compared with diabetic mice with intact lipoic acid synthase.[59] The atherosclerotic lesions of these heterozygous lipoic acid synthase–deficient mice had more macrophages and cellular apoptosis along with increased indicators of oxidative stress and inflammation (e.g., interleukin 6 [IL-6]). These and other studies implicate oxidative stress as an important contributing mechanism to diabetes-associated accelerated atherosclerosis.

Despite the extensive data for oxidative stress in atherosclerosis, clinical trials with antioxidant therapies have been disappointing, such as the use of vitamin E (400 IU/day) alone or in combination with vitamin C, which may determine the potency and/or half-life of available antioxidants,[60] or be of greater relevance in those with specific high-risk oxidation issues, like individuals with the haptoglobin (Hp) 2-2 genotype.[61]

In diabetes, experimental models suggest two major sources of oxidative stress. In the first, hyperglycemia may drive overproduction of mitochondrial reactive oxygen species (ROS) in ECs and elsewhere, with adverse consequences in the vasculature, such as PARP activation (poly [ADP-ribose] polymerase) and increased levels of multiple prothrombotic and proinflammatory mediators.[62,63] Overproduction of mitochondrial ROS may also activate other pathways implicated in diabetic CVD, including the HBP pathway, PKCs, and glycation and RAGE activation. Whether increased oxidative stress-derived ROS, including those generated in the mitochondria, can be targeted therapeutically remains to be seen but continues to be pursued, despite prior failures, as with benfotiamine.[64]

In addition to increased mitochondrial sources of ROS in hyperglycemia and diabetes, ROS derived from NADPH oxidase have also been extensively studied.[65] Nox, a six-transmembrane domain family with multiple members, is a binding site for NADPH, flavin adenine dinucleotide (FAD), and two heme groups.[66] Hyperglycemia may activate Nox isoforms as well as by AGE and RAGE pathways.[67] Thus hyperglycemia may fuel multiple feed-forward mechanisms that involve the generation and maintenance of ROS. In specific Nox-modified animals, deletion of the p47phox subunit of the Nox1 and Nox2 complex in apoE null mice (without diabetes) decreased atherosclerosis independent of serum lipid levels or other factors. Superoxide production in the vessel wall was reduced by this genetic modification, along with decreased smooth muscle proliferation.[68] Mice lacking both Nox1 and apoE demonstrated reduced atherogenesis in parallel with decreased macrophage lesion infiltration.[69] Similar effects occurred in nondiabetic Nox2 null/apoE null mice fed a high-fat diet, with concomitant decreased aortic ROS production.[70] Further work is needed to know if such findings relate to diabetes-accelerated atherosclerosis.

Other studies supporting oxidative stress in atherosclerosis were performed in diabetic LDL receptor mice lacking glutathione peroxidase, resulting in increased atherosclerosis and inflammation.[71] Of note, in transgenic human aldose reductase (hAR) overexpressing mice in the LDL receptor null background who then undergo streptozotocin-induced type 1 diabetes, glutathione peroxidase levels in the aorta were significantly lower as compared to the diabetic LDL receptor null mice not expressing hAR.[42]

These and other preclinical data suggest that loss of key antioxidant protective enzymes worsens atherosclerosis.

Association studies in human aortas suggested that expression of Nox4 was decreased in regions of the aorta with dedifferentiated SMCs. In contrast, strong expression of Nox4 was observed in SMCs within the aorta that retained the contractile phenotype.[72] Of note, various classes of compounds are being developed for isoform-specific inhibition of different Nox forms. These advances warrant a cautionary note, because isoform-specific Nox inhibitors may not be possible while ROS production is necessary in certain scenarios in vivo, such as responses to infectious challenges.[73] Whether Nox inhibitors of any kind find utility in treating diabetes or other chronic diseases remains uncertain.

GLYCATION: RECEPTOR-DEPENDENT AND INDEPENDENT MECHANISMS IN DIABETIC ATHEROSCLEROSIS

Indirect consequences of hyperglycemia include the nonenzymatic glycation and oxidation of proteins and lipids to form AGEs, which also include key "intermediates" of dicarbonyl compounds (e.g., methylglyoxal [MG], glyoxal, and 3-deoxyglucone [3-DG])[74] (Fig. 7.7). AGE formation involves multiple mechanisms: (1) aldehydic group of reducing sugars interacting with proteins or lipids, forming Schiff bases and Amadori products; (2) glucose flux via the polyol pathway; (3) lipid and sugar oxidation, with resulting dicarbonyl intermediates that ultimately yield AGEs after further modification.[75] AGEs are heterogeneous compounds that include the highly cross-linked "brown" fluorescent AGEs (e.g., pentosidine and crosslines), nonfluorescent cross-linking AGEs (e.g., arginine-lysine imidazole), and noncross-linking AGEs (e.g., carboxymethyl lysine [CML]–AGEs).[76]

AGEs may form in diabetic tissues, exacerbating complications. For example, aging may promote AGE formation, particularly on long-lived proteins whose exposure to even normal glucose levels may gradually increase AGE

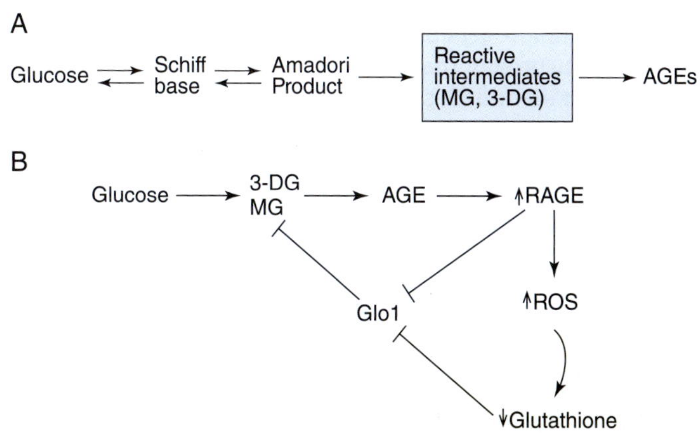

FIG. 7.7 Advanced glycation endproduct (AGE)/receptor for advanced glycation endproduct (RAGE): generation and interactions. (**A**) Chemical reactions leading to hyperglycemia-induced AGE generation are shown. Reactive intermediates include methylglyoxal (MG) and 3-deoxyglucone (3-DG). (**B**) Glucose-driven increases in intermediates and ultimately RAGE can increase reactive oxidative species (ROS), resulting in glutathione depletion and RAGE-dependent repression of the transcription of glyoxylase 1 (Glo1).

formation. Hypoxia and ischemia/reperfusion (I/R) may generate AGEs, thereby increasing AGE damage in settings such as MI, stroke, or PAD.[77] Renal failure significantly accelerates AGE formation; in patients with diabetes and severe nephropathy, increased AGE formation added to diabetes-associated glycation may significantly augment production and accumulation of these damaging species.[78] In other settings, myeloperoxidase enzymatic activity reportedly generates CML-AGEs.[79] Hence, in infectious or inflamed environments, AGE formation via inflammatory cell myeloperoxidase may further increase tissue stress, perhaps impairing effective wound healing, a major issue in diabetes.

Interestingly, food-derived AGEs may form during high temperatures[80] while environmental pollutants (e.g., fly ash particles) may promote AGE formation.[81] Of note, endogenous AGE detoxification mechanisms may exist, as suggested for the toxic AGE precursor MG dicarbonyl through the glutathione-dependent glyoxalase 1 (Glo1) enzyme system. Glo1 blocks MG formation into AGEs, producing lactate instead.[82] In RAGE-deficient mice, Glo1 mRNA and protein levels are significantly higher in the kidneys versus those in diabetic wild-type RAGE-expressing mice,[83] perhaps due to (1) decreased RAGE-dependent generation of ROS, which depletes glutathione and (2) RAGE-dependent transcriptional regulation of Glo1 (Fig. 7.7).

Receptor-Independent Pathways

One significant consequence of cross-linking AGEs is the formation of intermolecular bonds between extracellular matrix (ECM) elements. In the vasculature, such interactions may increase arterial stiffness and molecular trapping, for example, of oxidized lipoproteins, promoting atherogenesis in diabetic macrovessels.[84] Oxidized LDL contains significant amounts of AGE.[85] Furthermore, AGE-induced ECM formation in micro- and/or macrovessels may increase vascular permeability, thereby facilitating inflammatory or other cells migration into the perturbed vessel wall.[86]

Receptor-Dependent Pathways

Given the heterogeneous nature and diverse effects of AGEs, it is not surprising that multiple different AGE "receptors" have been identified, such as AGE-R1 (an antiinflammatory AGE receptor),[87] members of the scavenger receptor families such as CD36,[88] and the macrophage scavenger receptor.[89] Among AGE receptors, the receptor for AGEs (RAGE) is a well-characterized signal transduction receptor of the immunoglobulin superfamily.[90] RAGE binds AGEs such as CML-AGE and possibly hydroimidazolone AGEs. It is likely that other distinct AGEs exist and can also bind to RAGE.

RAGE is characterized by the presence of three extracellular domains, an N-terminal V-type Ig domain and two distinct C-type Ig domains, with the V-C1 domain reported as the chief ligand binding unit.[91] The extracellular portion of RAGE is composed of a large hydrophobic patch and a large negative patch, which modulate RAGE ligand binding patterns.[92,93]

In addition to AGEs, RAGE also binds other distinct ligands, as established for the S100/calgranulin family members.[94] Although RAGE was first described as a S100A12 receptor, other work reveals S100B, S100P, S100A8/A9, S100A4, and S100A6, as examples, may bind to and signal via RAGE.[95] S100 family members exert multiple pathogenic effects, including inducing and sustaining inflammatory reactions, promoting tumor cell proliferation, migration, induction of MMP expression and activity, and regulating cell survival.[96] RAGE also transduces signals for high-mobility group box 1 (HMGB1).[97] Like many RAGE ligand families, HMGB1 is also promiscuous, binding to RAGE and also certain toll-like receptor (TLR) signaling family members.[98] HMGB1, like S100/calgranulins, exerts both proinflammatory and protumor properties. In tumor cells, HMGB1 binding to RAGE mediates increased pancreatic tumor cell autophagy and decreased apoptosis, which together enhances tumor cell survival.[99] RAGE is also a receptor for amyloid-β peptide, among other amyloidogenic polypeptides,[100] complement-related factor C1q[101] and lysophosphatidic acid (LPA).[102] These findings underscore RAGE complexity, defining it as not a "one ligand–one disease" molecule. Rather, multiple ligands of RAGE may converge in distinct settings and across different timelines, mediating pathogenic inputs like hyperglycemia and inflammation, effecting chronic disease pathogenesis, like diabetic atherosclerosis and cancer.

Considerable evidence links RAGE ligands to diabetes and atherosclerosis in animal models and humans. Immunohistochemical studies in human atherosclerosis reveal RAGE expression in atherosclerotic plaques from carotid[12] and coronary artery lesions,[15] with higher levels in samples from those with diabetes versus nondiabetic patients. RAGE expression in lesions in those with diabetes showed increased inflammation (higher macrophages and T-cell numbers), increased NF-κB activation and expression of COX-2/mPGES-1, increased MMP expression and activity, more apoptotic SMCs, and higher RAGE ligand S100A12 levels. Notably, RAGE expression in diabetic carotid plaques correlated with glycosylated hemoglobin values. Indeed, at the level of the RAGE (*AGER*) gene, RAGE ligands such as AGEs induce RAGE expression itself, at least in part via NF-κB binding elements within the RAGE promoter.[103] RAGE is present in multiple cell types relevant to atherosclerosis, including ECs, monocytes/ macrophages, SMCs, and T lymphocytes. In these cell types, RAGE ligands mediate the induction of inflammatory signals and key transcription factors, such as NF-κB and Egr-1, and proatherogenic pathways, including in diabetes.[104]

Preclinical in vivo studies have used various approaches to investigate RAGE in diabetic atherosclerosis. ApoE-deficient mice with streptozotocin-induced diabetes demonstrated increased atherosclerosis and increased vascular inflammation versus vehicle-treated normoglycemic mice. The role of RAGE was initially tested using soluble RAGE (sRAGE), the extracellular ligand-binding domain of RAGE. Administering sRAGE to diabetic apoE null mice decreased early atherosclerosis in a concentration-dependent manner and in other studies, atherosclerosis progression.[105,106] Although streptozotocin-treated demonstrated higher plasma cholesterol, sRAGE administration reduced aortic inflammation, even in tissues without vascular lesions, but without altering cholesterol levels. Similar findings were observed in the T2DM-like *db/db* mouse model in the apoE null background, with sRAGE administration reducing atherosclerosis.[107] In additional approaches, mice with global RAGE deficiency or specific endothelial deletion of the RAGE cytoplasmic domain (and other cell types in which the preproendothelin-1 promoter is active) demonstrated significantly reduced atherosclerosis, including in diabetes, with cholesterol or lipid-independent effects.[85,108]

Studies reveal that the RAGE cytoplasmic domain binds to the formin family molecule diaphanous-1 (DIAPH1, also known as mDia1).[109] The formin family regulates cellular signaling via effectors of Rho GTPase protein while also influencing cellular migration and cytokinesis.[110] Studies to date in transformed cells, SMCs, and macrophages indicate that RAGE ligand-dependent signaling in these cell types is blocked after siRNA-knockdown of DIAPH1 or in DIAPH1 null cells.[109] In vivo, nondiabetic mice undergoing guidewire-induced femoral artery endothelial injury displayed significant DIAPH1 induction, especially in SMCs (Fig. 7.8A–I). Furthermore, DIAPH1-deficient mice were protected from aberrant neointimal expansion (Fig. 7.8J). In keeping with DIAPH1 transducing RAGE signaling in SMCs, DIAPH1 null-injured vessels and isolated aortic SMCs displayed reduced oxidative stress, cell signaling via GSK-3β, and cellular migration compared with wild-type counterparts with intact DIAPH1 (Fig. 7.8K),[111,112] data implicating DIAPH1 in transducing RAGE ligand effects on key signaling mediators, like activation of P-c-Src, Rac1, and Nox1, with subsequent AKT/GSK3β ser 9 phosphorylation (Fig. 7.8L), essential steps for RAGE ligand-induced vascular SMC migration in neointimal formation and atherosclerosis. Indeed, recent studies reveal that global deletion of DIAPH1 significantly attenuated atherosclerosis in male and female mice the LDL receptor null background.[113]

Although RAGE antagonists have not yet been tested in humans with diabetic atherosclerosis, ongoing evidence links RAGE to this disease. Single-nucleotide polymorphisms (SNPs) of RAGE are associated with human diabetic atherosclerosis.[112] Multiple studies report sRAGE levels correlate with human diabetic CV disease in humans.[114,115] Hence, in diabetic atherosclerosis, RAGE may serve as both a biomarker and a therapeutic target.

Importantly, in addition to glycation, RAGE involvement in diabetic atherosclerosis also involves inflammatory mechanisms. Given that multiple RAGE ligands are expressed in diabetic macrovessels and largely converge on this specific receptor, identifying specific effects of different ligand classes for RAGE is challenging. Clinical translation involving RAGE may well require identification and study of more specific RAGE inhibitors.

ADDITIONAL MECHANISMS OF DIABETIC ATHEROSCLEROSIS

While AGE formation and RAGE activation are compelling factors linking hyperglycemia to atherosclerosis and pathologic complications of diabetic atherosclerosis, additional important inputs in promoting diabetic atherosclerosis also exist. A fundamental issue encountered in understanding diabetic atherosclerosis is the many shared mechanisms involved in nondiabetic and diabetic atherosclerosis, even if accelerated in those with diabetes, as opposed to unique proatherosclerotic factors specific to diabetes. Support for diabetic atherosclerosis as a multifactorial disease has long existed, as initially supported by the landmark Steno-2 trial, which showed that T2DM management strategies targeting control of multiple factors—glycemic control, lipid levels, blood pressure, and microalbuminuria—exerted CV benefit, including a reduction in CV mortality by 50%.[116,117] While more recent studies with novel therapies like SGLT2is and GLP-1 RAs have greatly advanced T2DM management, the Steno-2 studies remain an important frame of reference, underscoring attention to other CV risk mechanisms in diabetic atherosclerosis and its complications. T2DM is typically characterized by a dyslipidemia involving elevated triglycerides (TGs), lower high-density lipoprotein (HDL) levels, and LDL levels that are not markedly elevated but are considered especially atherogenic. Diabetic atherosclerosis can involve a prothrombotic state, with an altered coagulation balance. Inflammation may be a central driver in the pathogenesis of diabetes, atherosclerosis, and their intersection, affecting all arterial cellular components. The breadth of abnormalities, whether molecular or clinical, implicated in T2DM and atherosclerosis independent of hyperglycemia is impressive and beyond the scope of any one summary, especially given ongoing rapid advances in this area. Here we build upon the evidence for AGEs and RAGEs as potential specific diabetes-related mechanisms to review key concepts regarding dyslipidemia, hypercoagulability, endothelial dysfunction, and inflammation in diabetic atherosclerosis and how such forces alter cellular responses, with an emphasis on emerging concepts, novel targets, and clinical relevance.

DIABETIC DYSLIPIDEMIA

T2DM is characterized by a distinct lipid profile involving LDL cholesterol (LDL-C) levels that are often not particularly elevated, higher triglyceride (TG) values, and lower HDL cholesterol (HDL-C) concentrations, with additional abnormalities such as elevated circulating FFAs.[118] This constellation of lipid abnormalities can arise early in T2DM, including prediabetes, drawing further attention to diabetic dyslipidemia in promoting diabetic atherosclerosis and its complications.[119] Multiple inputs underlie the dyslipidemia of T2DM. Central adiposity may promote dyslipidemia and increased FFAs, which can also increase secondary pathogenic responses, such as increased inflammation locally, within adipose, perivascular, and pericardial tissue as well as systemically.[119] Diabetic hypertriglyceridemia involves changes in the production, lipolysis, and clearance of TGs: the hepatic secretion of the TG-rich lipoprotein very low-density lipoproteins (VLDLs) and altered hydrolysis of these and other TG-rich lipoproteins through lipases.[120] Hypertriglyceridemia in diabetes can also involve abnormal postprandial TG excursions, which may predict CV risk more than the fasting levels usually obtained in the clinic.[121–124]

Lipoprotein lipase (LPL), a key enzyme involved in FA hydrolysis from TG-rich lipoproteins and subsequent

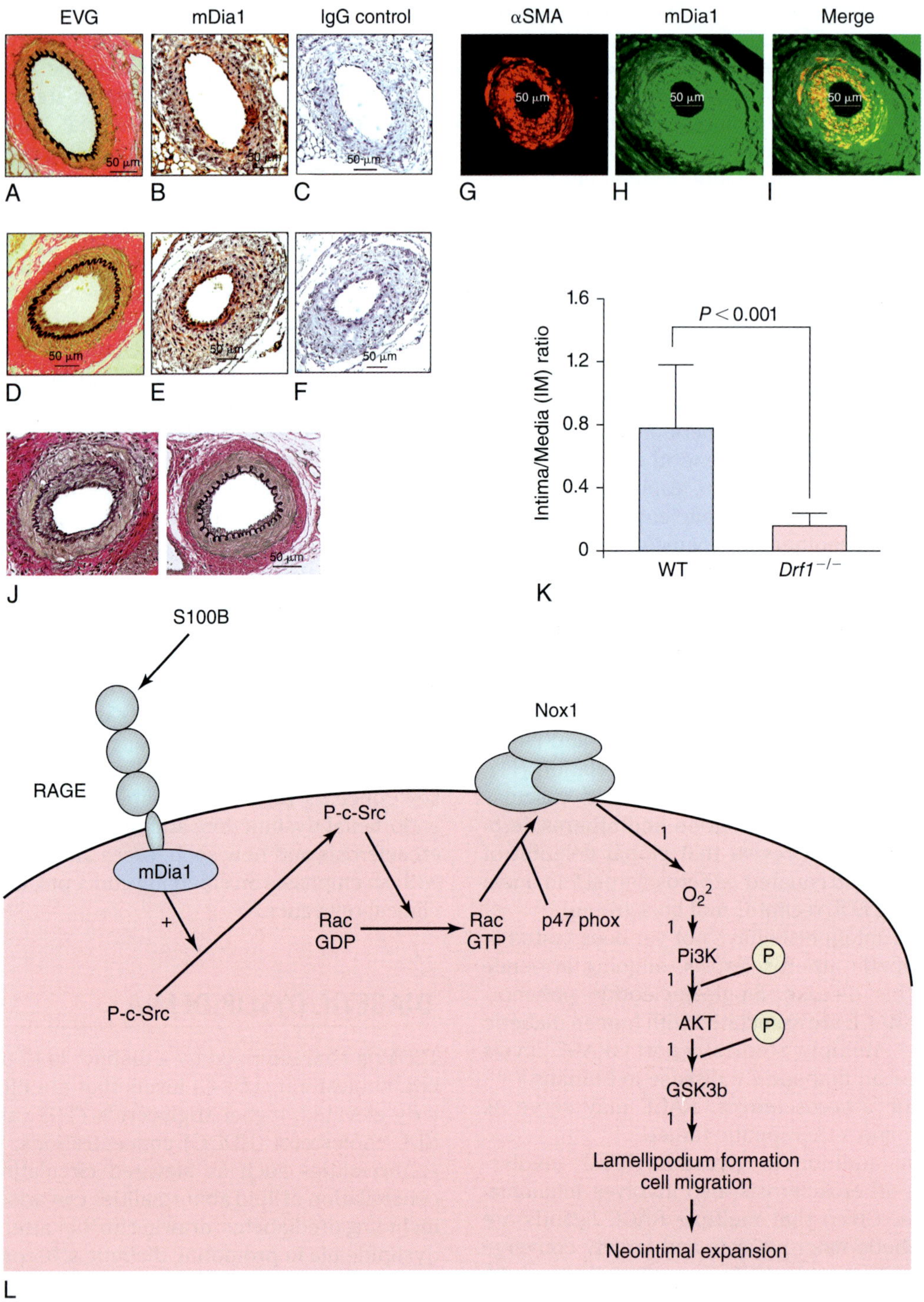

FIG. 7.8 Diaphanous-1 (mDia1) in vascular responses after endothelial denudation injury. Wild-type (WT), *Drf1*$^{-/-}$, and *RAGE*$^{-/-}$ mice subjected to femoral artery endothelial denudation or sham, and tissues were analyzed at the indicated times. **A** and **D**, Assessment of neointimal expansion by elastic–van Gieson (E-VG) staining on day 21 after injury in WT mice (**A**, sham and **D**, injury). **B, C, E,** and **F**, Immunostaining for mDia1 or isotype IgG control in WT mice on day 21 after injury (**E** and **F**) or sham (**B** and **C**). **G–J**, Immunofluoresence staining for mDia1 and α-smooth muscle cell actin (SMA) in sections of injured vessels revealed these two molecules colocalize in the neointima on day 21. **K**, Intima/Media (I/M) ratio measurement based on morphometric analysis of the vessels of WT and aged-sex-matched *Drf1*$^{-/-}$ mice (n = 11/group) was performed 21 days after guidewire-induced femoral artery denudation. Representative images are shown. $P < 0.001$. **L**, Proposed mechanism of the role of mDia1 in receptor for advanced glycation endproduct (RAGE)-induced redox signaling smooth muscle cell (SMC) migration and neointimal expansion. The data supports a critical role for mDia1 in transducing the effects of RAGE ligands on P-c-Src, Rac1, and Nox1 activation and consequent phosphorylation of AKT/GSK3β ser 9 processes essential for RAGE ligand-induced vascular SMC migration. (Reprinted from Toure F, Fritz G, Li Q, et al. Formin mDia1 mediates vascular remodeling via integration of oxidative and signal transduction pathways. *Circ Res.* 2012;110:1279–1293.)

delivery of FAs to tissues may be defective in T2DM.[125,126] Of note, LPL-mediated TG hydrolysis is an established mechanism for generating natural ligands for the nuclear receptor peroxisome proliferator-activated receptor alpha (PPAR-α), which, when activated by these natural LPL-derived ligands, regulates expression of multiple genes involved in lipid metabolism, fatty acid oxidation, inflammation, and atherosclerosis.[127–129] As such, the clinical picture of diabetic atherosclerosis may involve the loss of endogenous LPL action and a subsequent decrease in physiologic PPAR-α activation and its defined transcriptional gene cassette, including decreases in apolipoprotein (apo) A-I, which is integral to HDL function, and increasing endothelial inflammation, through increases in the leukocyte adhesion protein VCAM1, which is repressed by PPAR-α activation.[130] Other endogenous lipolytic pathways exist aside from LPL, including adipose tissue TG lipase (ATGL), hepatic lipase, and fatty acid synthase, with these pathways also generates distinct PPAR ligands in different physiologic contexts.[131–133] LPL's role in lipid metabolism includes other proteins involved in LPL action. For example, Apo C-III, an endogenous inhibitor of LPL activity, may promote proatherogenic, proinflammatory responses through various mechanisms,[134] including modulating endogenous LPL-mediated PPAR responses as above. Agents that target Apo C-III have been pursued as a means of treating lipids, now reaching the late stages of approval.

Fibrates, lipid-lowering agents used to treat hypertriglyceridemia, are considered pharmacologic PPAR-α agonists.[135] PPARα-activating agents, which themselves induce different cellular responses, have had mixed effectiveness in reducing CV events, ranging on primary endpoint from positive CV outcome trials (VA-HIT, gemfibrozil) to negative (FIELD, fenofibrate; PROMINENT, pemafibrate).[136,137] Importantly, drugs that activate PPAR-α manifest distinct characteristics and functional effects from endogenous PPAR-α ligands, as supported by the evidence that genetic variants predicted to increase generation of natural PPAR-α ligands have been found to be atheroprotective and without the issues seen with PPAR-α activating drugs.[138–140] Omega-3 FAs are also purported PPAR-α ligands, again with a mixed picture that varies depending on the specific omega-3 FA; icosopent ethyl has had a positive CV outcome trial (REDUCE-IT) while other omega-3 FAs have failed in achieving positive primary CV endpoints, including the omega-3 carboxylic acid formulation of eicosapentaenoic acid (EPA) and docosahexaenoic acid (DHA), which failed to improve outcomes in the STRENGTH trial.[141,142] Questions have been raised if the mineral oil used as the control in REDUCE-IT may have exerted adverse effects and an increase in CV outcomes in the control group, enhancing the signal for benefit with icosapent ethyl as compared to STRENGTH, which used the more neutral corn oil for its control group.[143]

Together, these data highlight the specificity and complexity of this TG-lipolytic network, the effects of these pathways including generation of biologically active molecules, and differences among specific therapeutic agents that target proteins involved in both endogenous as well as pathogenic responses. LPL's role in lipid metabolism has expanded to include other proteins involved in LPL action. For example, Apo C-III, an endogenous inhibitor of LPL activity, is implicated in promoting proatherogenic, proinflammatory responses through various mechanisms,[134] including modulating endogenous LPL-mediated PPAR responses as above while Apo C-III itself is also pursued as a drug target for treating lipids.[139,144,145]

Given that HDL-C levels were reported as being inversely associated with coronary heart disease (CHD) risk, significant efforts focused on mechanisms underlying low HDL seen in T2DM and pursuing HDL-C as a drug target.[146] Both abnormal production, remodeling of HDL-C by plasma enzymes and HDL-C clearance may underlie the low circulating HDL-C observed in T2DM. Expression and activity of endothelial lipase (EL), a phospholipase synthesized in and expressed on the endothelial surface, catabolizes HDL, decreasing levels of HDL-C. Elevated concentrations of EL protein correlate with coronary artery calcification as well as other features of metabolic syndrome/prediabetes/T2DM including waist circumference, blood pressure, TGs, HDL levels, and fasting glucose in individuals with a family history of premature CHD.[147] In addition, direct correlations may exist between EL levels and circulating inflammatory markers including high-sensitivity C-reactive protein (hsCRP), interleukin 6 (IL-6), and soluble intercellular adhesion molecule (sICAM). Low-dose endotoxemia in 20 subjects increased EL concentrations 12 to 16 hours after injection, which correlated with plasma HDL reductions.[148–150] Collectively, these data suggest that low-intensity inflammation, a common feature of T2DM, controls HDL through effects on EL. Despite this, attempts at EL inhibition for therapeutic purposes have not been successful,[151] perhaps because of beneficial effects of EL-dependent metabolites.[152] Despite the epidemiologic inverse association between HDL and CV risk, the prospect of raising HDL to reduce CV events remains unproven. Large randomized, placebo-controlled trials designed to raise HDL using cholesteryl ester transfer protein (CETP) inhibitors and niacin have failed for various reasons,[153] suggesting that the biology of HDL's atheroprotective effects is complex and not simply involves HDL-C quantity as opposed to function. More recent efforts to target CETP continue with obicetrapib, a unique agent that lacks the prior issues of other CETP inhibitors and whose benefit is centered on lowering LDL, with encouraging results seen in clinical trials.[154]

Another input into diabetic dyslipidemia is hepatic dysfunction involving various stages of fatty liver, now referred to as metabolic dysfunction-associated steatotic liver disease (MASLD) and metabolic dysfunction-associated steatohepatitis (MASH).[155,156] Hyperglycemia can alter lipid metabolism, as, for example, through the glycation of proteins and lipoproteins, altering their function, while the breakdown of glycated proteins and lipoproteins, through AGEs and their associated RAGE receptors, which promote atherosclerosis and plaque destabilization, as discussed.[109]

Although total LDL-C levels are often average in patients with T2DM, LDL still predicts CV risk in this patient population. As associated hypertriglyceridemia, LDL particles in T2DM are smaller, denser, and more prone to arterial wall entry, oxidation, and retention, and this is more pathogenic,[157] as can be tracked clinically by measuring apolipoprotein B (apoB) levels or also approximated by calculating non-HDL levels.[158] The concept that subendothelial lipoprotein retention may promote atherosclerosis may be especially relevant in diabetes. Extensive evidence implicates LDL oxidation in atherosclerosis. Given that hyperglycemia and other aspects of diabetes may promote altered redox balance and increased oxidative stress, increased LDL oxidation in diabetes may help drive diabetic atherosclerosis. An intriguing direction for this field involves using autoantibodies to oxidized LDL (oxLDL) to treat atherosclerosis, which may extend to diabetes.[159,160]

Placing lipid metabolism in diabetes into a broader context, lipoprotein particles are circulating, biologically active entities whose nature and function alter local and systemic responses in health and disease through their interaction with other cells, proteins, the vasculature, and organs. For example, lipoproteins interact with the coagulation system, including platelets. Increased platelet reactivity and thrombogenicity in response to VLDL and TG-rich lipoproteins has been reported.[161] Such potential interactions connect dysregulated lipid metabolism in diabetes to the coagulation system, a potent factor implicated in atherosclerosis and diabetic atherosclerosis.

DIABETES: A PROTHROMBOTIC STATE

T2DM can be characterized as a prothrombotic state, another contributor to diabetic vascular complications.[162] Multiple factors underlie this prothrombotic imbalance in diabetes, including platelet hyperreactivity, increased procoagulant proteins, and impaired fibrinolysis. Although hyperglycemia itself may promote these procoagulant shifts, other factors, such as dyslipidemia, obesity, and inflammation, as well as more specific pathogenic mechanisms, like oxidative stress, may also contribute to the prothrombotic, procoagulant state in diabetes, as considered here.

Altered Platelet Function in Diabetes

Platelets of patients with T2DM manifest dysregulation of several signaling pathways, resulting in enhanced platelet adhesion, aggregation, and activation (Fig. 7.9). Hyperglycemia, insulin resistance, dyslipidemia, inflammation, and increased oxidation may all increase diabetic platelet hyperactivity. Hyperglycemia increases platelet reactivity by altering different biochemical pathways, including PKC activation, with subsequent increased platelet granule release and aggregation.[163,164] Glucose may also increase platelet reactivity through direct osmotic effects.[165] In addition, by inducing nonenzymatic glycation of platelet surface proteins, hyperglycemia may decrease membrane fluidity while increasing platelet adhesion and activation.[166] Consistent with these findings, acute hyperglycemia can increase platelet activation markers like P-selectin and CD40 ligand (CD40L), while improved glycemic control may decrease platelet reactivity.[167,168]

Platelet aggregation is mediated by platelet surface receptors and adhesive proteins such as glycoproteins GPIIb/IIIa, GPIb, and P2Y12, each of which is altered in T2DM. Platelet turnover in T2DM appears accelerated. Hyperglycemia increases the release of reticulated, larger, and thus more reactive platelets, including a higher production of the potent vasoconstrictor, proaggregant thromboxane. Diabetic platelets may also have altered P2Y12 signaling, which increases adhesion, aggregation, and procoagulant activity.[169] Increased levels of circulating microparticles,

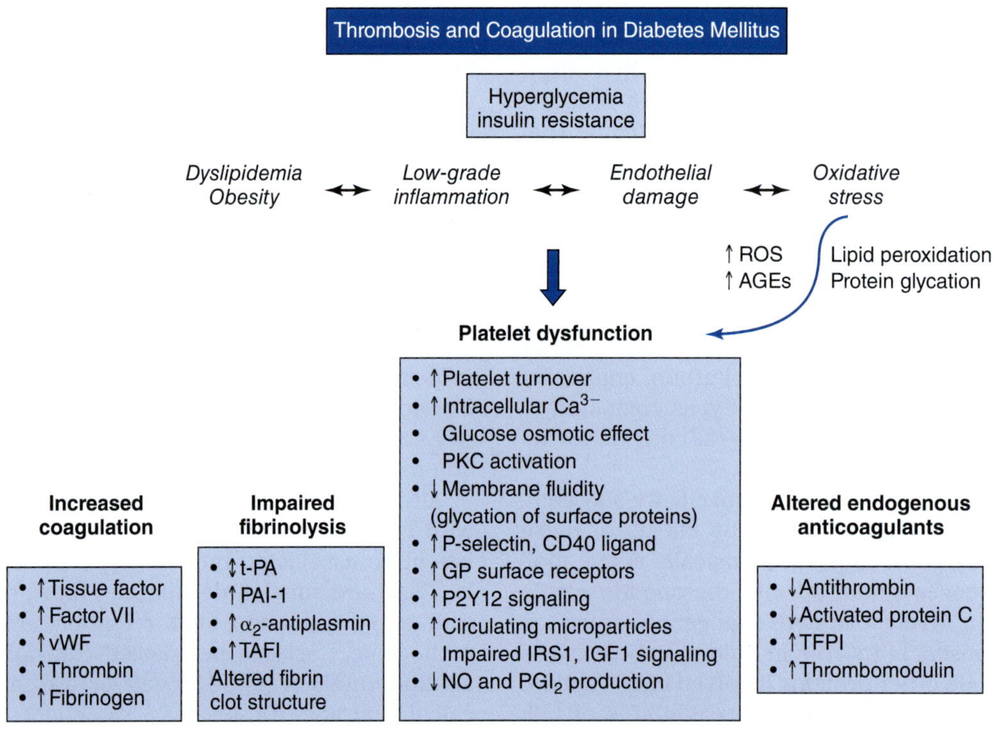

FIG. 7.9 Abnormal thrombosis and coagulation in diabetes. Many pathologic inputs in diabetes promote platelet dysfunction and hypercoagulability, all thus contributing to a prothrombotic phenotype in patients with diabetes. Hyperglycemia and insulin resistance, a fundamental pathophysiologic feature of T2DM, drives inflammation, dyslipidemia, endothelial dysfunction, and oxidative stress. Each of these stimuli activates platelets by increasing expression of surface receptors for aggregation, increasing production of vasoactive molecules, reducing nitric oxide bioavailability. Simultaneously, production of coagulation factors by ECs including von Willebrand factor (vWF) and tissue factor, along with fibrinogen and factor VII from other sources, enhances coagulation. Lastly, a defect in endogenous fibrinolysis through increased PAI-1 expression tPA all conspire to heighten thrombosis in diabetes. *AGEs*, Advanced glycation end products; *GP*, glycoprotein; *IGF-1*, insulin-like growth factor 1; *IRS-1*, insulin substrate receptor 1; *NO*, nitric oxide; *PAI-1*, plasminogen activator inhibitor 1; PGI_2, prostaglandin I_2; *PKC*, protein kinase C; *ROS*, reactive oxygen species; *TAFI*, thrombin-activatable fibrinolysis inhibitor; *TFPI*, tissue factor pathway inhibitor; *t-PA*, tissue plasminogen activator.

derived from platelets and various stimulated cell types, may also promote coagulation in diabetes.[170] Microparticle size is larger in those with T2DM than in normal subjects, with an increased microparticle number being associated with increased diabetic complications.[171]

Intracellular calcium flux helps regulate platelet function. Platelets in patients with diabetes contain lower cyclic adenosine monophosphate (cAMP) levels and higher intracellular calcium levels than nondiabetic patients, contributing to hyperreactivity, increased aggregation and activation, and stimulation of thromboxane synthesis.[172] Altered calcium homeostasis may involve changes in the activity of calcium ATPases, which are highly sensitive to oxidative damage.[173,174] The activity of calcium-activated proteases known as calpains is increased in platelets from those with diabetes, contributing to dysregulated platelet calcium signaling and hyperreactivity.[175]

Insulin resistance and insulin deficiency can both alter platelet reactivity. Insulin opposes the effects of platelet agonists through activation of an inhibitory G protein by insulin receptor substrate 1 (IRS-1); during insulin resistance, impaired insulin receptor signaling attenuates insulin-mediated antagonism of platelet activation, thus increasing platelet reactivity.[176] Insulin-like growth factor 1 (IGF-1), which is present in platelet granules while IGF-1 receptors are present on the platelet surface, stimulates tyrosine phosphorylation of IRS, potentiating platelet activation.[177] Reduced insulin sensitivity in platelets lowers cAMP levels and increases intracellular calcium levels, enhancing platelets degranulation and aggregation, with platelets from insulin-resistant patients displaying diminished nitric oxide (NO), prostacyclin sensitivity, and platelet NO-synthase activity.[178]

As noted, some other systemic abnormalities in diabetes may also alter platelet biology. Hypertriglyceridemia increases platelet reactivity, perhaps in part through apo E.[161] Glycation of LDL particles may also impair NO production and increased intraplatelet calcium concentration, with subsequent increased platelet hyperreactivity and microparticle formation.[179] Central obesity is linked to platelet dysfunction, with reduced responses to insulin, nitrates, and prostacyclin; elevated platelet count and volume; increased cytosolic calcium concentration; and increased oxidative stress.[180] Interestingly, weight loss reverses some of these changes, decreasing platelet activation,[181] as may be relevant to the CV benefits of GLP-1 RAs, as discussed elsewhere. Increased oxidative stress found in T2DM increases platelet reactivity.[182,183] Lipid peroxidation and protein glycation may also affect platelet activation.[184] Inflammation may promote platelet reactivity by increasing the expression of platelet activation mediators, such as CD40L, which also has proinflammatory properties and whose plasma-soluble levels are increased in T2DM.[185]

Increased Coagulation Factors in Diabetes

T2DM has been associated with increased activity of the complex coagulation cascade that helps generate thrombin, converts fibrinogen to fibrin, and enables fibrin clot formation (Fig. 10.2). For example, in healthy individuals, synthesis of the potent procoagulant protein tissue factor, expressed by ECs and vascular smooth muscle cells (VSMCs), is inhibited by insulin; platelets from T2DM patients have a significant increase in tissue factor levels versus matched controls, a shift promoted by both hyperglycemia and hyperinsulinemia.[186] AGEs can also contribute to the activation of surface clotting factors.[187] AGEs and ROS can promote tissue factor expression by activating NF-κB transcription factors.

In addition to tissue factor, many other coagulant proteins are implicated in T2DM's prothrombotic state. Factor VII, linked to increased CV mortality, is elevated with hyperglycemia, insulin resistance, and T2DM.[188,189] Hyertriglyceridemia is independently associated with Factor VII activity levels in patients with diabetes.[190] Factor XIII, activated by thrombin, produces multiple cross-links in the fibrin clot, increasing resistance to lysis. Factor XIII subunit levels correlate with metabolic syndrome components and insulin resistance with evidence for an association between Factor XIII polymorphisms and thrombotic CVD risk. Von Willebrand factor (vWF), which promotes platelet adhesion by binding to the platelet glycoprotein GPIb receptor, has been linked to endothelial damage, atherosclerosis, and future CV events as well as specifically insulin resistance and T2DM.[191] Increased platelet thrombin, which converts fibrinogen to fibrin, is associated with hyperglycemia. Thrombin is increased in patients with diabetes, including as a function of glucose control.[192] Given the connection of hyperglycemia and many of these responses, improved glucose control may help reduce thrombogenicity.[193] Fibrinogen, an acute-phase protein that independently predicts future CV events, is elevated in patients with diabetes and associated with microvascular and macrovascular complications.[194,195] Glycemia and insulin resistance correlate with increased fibrinogen levels,[196] perhaps through enhanced fibrinogen production stimulated by diabetes-associated hyperinsulinemia and inflammation.[197] IL-6 cytokine levels, which are elevated in T2DM, can stimulate hepatic fibrinogen production, further connecting inflammation to prothrombotic states.[198] Despite these myriad findings, questions persist regarding the extent to which glycemic control is involved in coagulation balance, especially given the question of CV risk reduction with prior clinical trials in diabetes; perhaps studies with the new agents with CV benefit will change this.

Changes in Endogenous Anticoagulants in Diabetes

The prothrombotic state of T2DM involves not only increases in procoagulant factors, but also changes in endogenous anticoagulants, such as antithrombin, tissue factor pathway inhibitor (TFPI), protein C, and thrombomodulin, all part of physiologic coagulation balance. Antithrombin forms a stable complex with thrombin, limiting its action, as it does with other coagulation factors, like inhibiting Factor VII bound to tissue factor. Patients with diabetes reportedly have reduced antithrombin anticoagulant activity.[199] Hyperglycemia may also induce conformational changes in antithrombin, prompting its retention and aggregation, perhaps through nonenzymatic glycation or endoplasmic reticulum (ER) stress.[200] The endogenous anticoagulant TFPI, produced mainly by ECs and associated with atherosclerosis, inhibits tissue factor–initiated coagulation by binding with activated Factor X and modifying Factor VII–tissue factor catalytic complex activity.[201,202] TFPI circulates primarily bound to circulating lipoproteins, with increased atherogenic lipoprotein levels associated with shifting tissue factor–TFPI balance toward plaque thrombogenicity.[203] Other identified noncoagulant roles of TFPI, including inflammation, angiogenesis, and lipid metabolism, may also occur with diabetic vascular damage.[204]

Activated protein C (APC), converted from protein C through endothelial thrombin-thrombomodulin complex action, inactivates the coagulation Factors V and VIII as well as PAI-1, thus promoting fibrinolysis and limiting inflammation, oxidation, and cellular damage.[205,206] Low protein C levels are a reported risk factor for incident ischemic stroke but not CHD,[207] while decreased APC generation is associated with progressive atherosclerosis in T2DM.[208]

As noted, endothelial thrombomodulin also reduces procoagulant activities such as fibrinogen clotting, Factor V, and platelets while also modulating cellular proliferation, adhesion, and inflammation, and revealing endothelial damage.[209] However, the association between circulating thrombomodulin levels and incident CHD is controversial.[210,211] In healthy individuals, an inverse association between soluble thrombomodulin levels and risk for future T2DM is reported,[212] while in patients with T2DM, plasma thrombomodulin levels were increased and positively correlated with metabolic syndrome components.[213] Elevated plasma soluble thrombomodulin in T2DM levels may reflect enhanced hypercoagulability and altered fibrinolysis.[214]

Impaired Fibrinolysis in Diabetes

Blood flow involves a coordinated balance between thrombus formation and its dissolution. Fibrinolysis, the process of clot dissolution and removal, involves multiple interacting proenzymes and enzymes while inhibition of fibrinolytic pathways promotes thrombus formation; shifts in this fibrinolytic balance are strongly implicated in atherothrombosis. Impaired fibrinolysis has been noted in T2DM and is cited as a risk for CV complications. Altered glucose concentrations can induce fibrin network modifications that promote thrombosis.[215] Fibrin clots in patients with diabetes are more compact, with decreased clot matrix pore size and more resistance to fibrinolysis, as compared to healthy controls.[216] Indeed, improving glycemic control in T2DM may foster a more benign clot structure.[217] The balance between thrombus formation and dissolution involves tissue plasminogen activator (t-PA) and PAI-1 as offsetting mediators. t-PA, produced by ECs, mediates plasminogen to plasmin conversion, initiating fibrinolysis. By binding to t-PA, PAI-1 blocks plasminogen conversion into active plasmin, thus inhibiting fibrinolysis. Adipocytes also produce PAI-1, a potential link between obesity in diabetes and CVD. In general, both t-PA and PAI-1 are reported to predict an increased CV risk and a worse prognosis,[218,219] although still debated.[220] PAI-1 is elevated in insulin resistance, correlates strongly with metabolic syndrome components, and may predict future T2D.[221,222]

Hyperglycemia and hyperinsulinemia, by increasing expression and activation of proinflammatory mediators (e.g., NF-κB and PAI-1), reduce t-PA activity, shifting fibrinolytic balance toward thrombosis while glucose lowering may reduce PAI-1 levels.[223]

Although t-PA, and its relationship with PAI-1, are key for thrombosis, other endogenous anticoagulants are implicated in diabetic atherothrombosis.[224] For example, thrombin-activatable fibrinolysis inhibitor (TAFI) inhibits fibrinolysis by cleaving lysine residues on fibrin, interfering with t-PA and plasminogen binding. Increased plasma TAFI levels were reported in insulin resistance and T2DM patients.[225,226] However, inconsistent results exist regarding TAFI levels and activation in thrombosis, especially in CAD.[227] Alpha$_2$-antiplasmin, the main physiologic inhibitor of plasmin, may correlate with MI risk[228] while the plasmin–alpha$_2$-antiplasmin complex formation, which indicates reactive fibrinolysis, may associate with subclinical atherosclerosis and CAD, with some questions as to gender-specific effects.[229,230] Specific involvement of alpha$_2$-antiplasmin in diabetes-related pathology has been suggested but remains unresolved.[231] More global assessment of whole-plasma fibrinolytic potential may better link fibrinolysis to arterial thrombosis than studies on specific fibrinolytic factors, especially in T2DM[232] (Table 7.4).

TABLE 7.4 Impaired Fibrinolysis in Diabetes

FIBRINOLYTIC FACTORS	FUNCTION	ALTERATION IN DIABETES	POTENTIAL UNDERLYING MECHANISMS FOR IMPAIRED FIBRINOLYSIS
Tissue-plasminogen activator (t-PA)	Clot lysis (converts plasminogen to plasmin)	↕	Endothelial cell dysfunction (t-PA)
Plasminogen activator inhibitor-1 (PAI-1)	Inhibition of clot lysis (binding to t-PA, blocking the conversion of plasminogen into plasmin)	↑	Inflammatory response; Protein glycation (plasminogen)
Thrombin Activatable Fibrinolysis Inhibitor (TAFI)	Attenuation of fibrinolysis; Proenzyme, cleaving fibrin, preventing t-PA and plasminogen binding activated by thrombin, plasmin, or thrombin/thrombomodulin complex	↑	Hyperglycemia; insulin resistance
Alpha$_2$-antiplasmin	Physiologic inhibitor of plasmin	↑	Increased secretion by adipocytes (PAI-1); Altered clot structure, ↓ pore size, ↑ clot-lysis time

ENDOTHELIAL FUNCTION AND DYSFUNCTION IN DIABETES

The multiple processes discussed here in initiating and/or promoting atherosclerosis in diabetes often involve the endothelial surface, if not endothelial function/dysfunction. Given its anatomic position, the single-cell-thick endothelium transduces many inputs, including circulating risk mediators such as glucose, FFAs, distinct lipoproteins, and inflammatory signals, in line with the modern understanding of the endothelium as a dynamic, reactive organ exerting local and systemic effects, including endocrine, paracrine, and autocrine action. As this circulatory-tissue interface, the endothelium is positioned to control homeostatic processes, including blood pressure; hemostasis; and adaptive, inflammatory responses to injury. When dysregulated, all these processes can promote atherosclerosis, including diabetic atherosclerosis (Table 7.5). Intriguingly, abnormal endothelial responses are among the earliest abnormalities found in seemingly healthy individuals destined to develop diabetes. In one clinical study, flow-mediated endothelium-dependent vasodilation (EDV) was 38% lower in patients without diabetes but a family history of T2DM in both parents versus those with no such history; those with a T2DM family history did have slightly higher fasting glucoses (5.3 vs. 4.9 mmol/L).[233]

Endothelial control of vascular resistance is essential for maintaining mean arterial pressure and for autoregulating flow regionally to different tissues depending on metabolic demands. ECs synthesize NO from L-arginine through the Ca^{2+}-dependent, endothelial-specific nitric oxide synthase isoform (eNOS) in response to flow dynamics.[234] Once formed, NO activates soluble guanylate cyclase located in adjacent VSMCs, increasing cyclic guanosine monophosphate (cGMP) levels, SMC relaxation, and vasodilation, processes dependent on intact vascular endothelium that help define normal endothelial function; indeed, in landmark aortic ring experiments, removing the endothelial layer induced paradoxical vasomotor responses to norepinephrine (Fig. 7.10).[235] Endothelial dysfunction manifests as a loss of flow-mediated vasodilation, as seen in arterial ultrasound studies.[236] ECs produce other important vasoactive mediators, including prostacyclin and endothelium-derived hyperpolarizing factor (EDHF), which couple tissue blood flow to metabolic demands. In response to stimuli including proinflammatory cytokines, the vascular endothelium also elaborates vasoconstrictors including endothelin-1, angiotensin II, thromboxane A_2, and isoprostanes that increase vascular tone, permeability, hemostasis, and inflammation. The balance of these vasodilator and vasoconstrictor factors is pivotal for maintaining arteriolar resistance and establishing mean arterial blood pressure. NO also reduces platelet aggregation and leukocyte adhesion, thereby suppressing endogenous thrombus formation, maintaining blood rheology, and suppressing leukocyte accumulation in the vessel wall. Extensive evidence implicates shifts in all these components of normal endothelial function in diabetes as well as abnormalities associated with diabetes in predicting, promoting, and treating CVD.[237]

In addition to helping control vascular homeostasis, the endothelium is also involved in the host response to inflammation, regulating leukocyte trafficking to sites of injury. Proinflammatory signals, including interleukin 1-beta (IL-1β), tumor necrosis factor α (TNF-α), and oxLDL, induce EC expression of genes involved in leukocyte homing and diapedesis, a multistep, orchestrated process

TABLE 7.5 Key Examples of Resident Vascular Cells, Cells of Innate and Adaptive Immunity, and the Pathways and Mediators Dysregulated in Diabetes

VASCULAR CELL	PATHWAYS	MEDIATORS
Endothelium	Leukocyte trafficking Vascular reactivity Inflammation Metabolism Redox signaling Biomechanical forces Apoptosis Thrombosis and fibrinolysis	E-selectin P-selectin VCAM-1 ICAM-1 NF-κB eNOS, nitric oxide EDHF FoxO PPAR-γ, PPAR-α SOD PAI-1, t-PA Thrombomodulin vWF Tissue factor
VSMCs	Inflammation Vascular reactivity Matrix remodeling Proliferation and migration	iNOS, nitric oxide MCP-1 IL-6 TGF-β Collagen MMPs PDGF
Monocyte/ Macrophages	Inflammation NLRP3 inflammasome Matrix remodeling Autophagy ER stress, UPR Lipid transport	IL-6 TNF-α IL-1β MMP COX-2 Toll-like receptors CHOP/caspase/JNK PPAR-α, PPAR-γ, PPAR-δ FABPs
Lymphocyte	Inflammation T- and B-cell proliferation Autoimmunity	IFN-γ IL-17 LDL autoantibodies
Platelet	Thrombosis Microparticles	Nitric oxide Thromboxane A_2 IGF-1 Calpains P-selectin Protein kinase C P2Y12

Endothelial dysfunction, a seminal event in diabetic atherogenesis, involves the loss of nitric oxide and induction of proinflammatory gene expression, including adhesion molecule expression essential for leukocyte homing to nascent plaque. Activation of master proximal transcription factors, including NF-κB and Forkheads (FoxO) by glucose, lipoproteins, FFAs, and insulin, drive this phenotypic change that encompasses endothelial dysfunction. VSMCs proliferate and secrete matrix proteins in response to similar stimuli in diabetes, enlarging the neointima. Monocyte recruitment through chemokines (e.g., MCP-1 among others) and the adhesion and entry of these cells results in macrophage foam cell formation in the growing plaque. Studies also demonstrate an important role for autophagy and ER stress responses in regulating macrophage inflammation, apoptosis, and plaque stability in atherosclerosis. As part of this process, lymphocytes are primed to produce autoantibodies and secrete proinflammatory cytokines including IFN-γ and interleukin-6 that further increase inflammation and plaque formation. Patients with diabetes also have higher thrombosis risk. Platelet dysfunction occurs through activation of multiple pathways including calpains, PKC, IGF-1, and enhanced production of vasoconstrictor lipids such as thromboxane. *CHOP*, C/EBP homologous protein; *COX-2*, cyclooxygenase 2; *EDHF*, endothelium-derived hyperpolarizing factor; *eNOS*, endothelial isoform of nitric oxide synthase; *ER*, endoplastic reticulum; *FABPs*, fatty acid binding proteins; *ICAM-1*, intercellular adhesion molecule-1; *IFN-γ*, interferon gamma; *iNOS*, inducible macrophage-type nitric oxide synthase; *JNF*, c-Jun N-terminal kinase; *MCP-1*, monocyte chemoattractant protein 1; *NLRP3*, Nod-like receptor protein 3; *PDGF*, platelet derived growth factor; *SOD*, superoxide dismutase; *TGF-β*, transforming growth factor beta; *TNF-α*, tumor necrosis factor alpha; *UPR*, unfolded protein response; *VCAM-1*, vascular adhesion molecule-1; *VSMCs*, vascular smooth muscle cells.

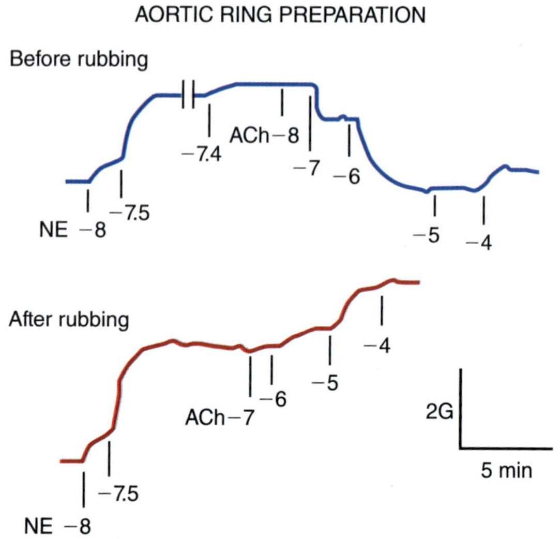

FIG. 7.10 Endothelial-dependent vasodilation in endothelial function. Nobel Prize–winning work by Furchgott and colleagues identified the critical importance of endothelial cells, the single-cell-thick layer lining the vascular tree, in maintaining vasomotor tone. These investigators discovered that acetylcholine treatment of isolated rabbit aortic rings induced vasodilation unless the intimal cell layer had been accidentally rubbed off during the tissue preparation, in which case vasoconstriction occurred. This observation identified a novel role for endothelium, at the time considered only a passive cell layer, ushering in a new era in vascular biology and leading to the eventual discovery of nitric oxide, a key regulator of vascular homeostasis. Now, the vascular endothelium is understood to be a dynamic organ that regulates (1) vascular tone, (2) inflammatory responses through recruitment of leukocytes to sites of injury including in atherosclerosis, (3) nutrient availability for metabolically active tissues such as fat and muscle, (4) resident vascular cell proliferation, and (5) thrombosis and platelet aggregation. Endothelial dysfunction is one of the earliest features of diabetic (and nondiabetic) atherosclerosis and can be measured noninvasively with brachial artery ultrasound, or invasively with acetylcholine (Ach) infusion during coronary artery angiography. Normal endothelial function results in vasodilation after Ach, whereas endothelial dysfunction results in paradoxical vasoconstriction. More recent work suggests that endothelial function may more broadly encompass regulation of systemic metabolic responses including fatty acid transport and adiposity. *NE*, Norepinephrine. (From Furchgott RF, Zawadzki JV. The obligatory role of endothelial cells in the relaxation of arterial smooth muscle by acetylcholine. *Nature*. 1980;288:373–376.)

collectively known as the *leukocyte adhesion cascade*. The induction of specific endothelial gene networks, composed of key mediators of leukocyte adhesion, such as E-selectin, P-selectin, vascular adhesion molecule–1 (VCAM-1), and intercellular adhesion molecule-1 (ICAM-1), along with chemoattractants such as IL-8 and monocyte chemoattractant protein 1 (MCP-1), coordinate leukocyte rolling, firm adhesion to ECs, and transmigration into the vessel wall.[238] The ability of neutrophils, monocytes, and lymphocytes to home to local areas of inflammation is vital to the host defense during acute inflammation. However, this endothelial activation becomes maladaptive in chronic states of inflammation, as occurs in atherosclerosis and diabetic atherosclerosis, promoting monocytes or other immune cell accumulation within the vessel wall, propagating atherosclerosis and its complications. Most T2DM-associated abnormalities—hyperglycemia, elevated FFAs, hypertriglyceridemia, hypertension—have been linked to an activated endothelial state.[237]

The ability to assess endothelial function, either in the cardiac catheterization laboratory or noninvasively with techniques such as brachial artery ultrasound, has advanced insight into endothelial function and its impact on vasomotor function and pathogenesis (Fig. 7.10). In patients with endothelial dysfunction, the normal vasodilator response to acetylcholine is blunted or causes paradoxical vasoconstriction. Using brachial artery ultrasound, after sphygmomanometer-mediated forearm blood flow occlusion (5 minutes) is released, reactive hyperemia ensues, causing endothelium-dependent, flow-mediated NO production and vasodilation, measured by ultrasound as an increased arterial diameter. In patients with endothelial dysfunction, these responses are severely blunted.[239]

Endothelial dysfunction is a defining feature of early atherosclerosis in patients with diabetes and is also associated with other traditional CV risk factors such as hypertension and dyslipidemia.[240,241] Mechanistically, endothelial dysfunction involves a loss of NO bioavailability through impaired production by eNOS or increased NO degradation, a consequence of multiple factors (Fig. 7.11). As a consequence, the atheroprotective effects of NO, including vasodilation, inhibition of thrombosis or aggregation, and suppression of leukocyte adhesion to the vessel wall, are lost. Multiple T2DM and prediabetic metabolic derangements all contribute to a loss of NO and endothelial dysfunction.[243,244] The specific role of hyperglycemia and insulin resistance in vascular function is discussed elsewhere. FFA infusion reduces endothelial dysfunction in animal models and in humans.[245] FFAs activate PKC, driving signal transduction pathways that reduce NO production by eNOS.[246] The accumulation of lipids in tissues and cells, including FFAs, fatty acetyl-coenzyme As, diacylglycerols, and other factors, referred to in general as *lipotoxicity*, involves the effects of these mediators on intracellular signal transduction pathways.

Another major cause of reduced NO bioavailability is peroxynitrite (ONOO–) formation through NO's reaction with superoxide anion, as implicated in atherosclerosis, diabetic atherosclerosis, and associated conditions like obesity.[247] Among mechanisms associated with peroxynitrite, high intracellular FFAs help uncouple fatty acid oxidation, increasing levels of free radicals, including superoxide anion (O_2^-). Normally, superoxide is rapidly cleared by scavenging enzymes such as superoxide dismutase. When superoxide anion levels rise, as occurs in patients with diabetes, through elevated FFAs and hyperglycemia, high peroxynitrite levels form nonenzymatically. Other enzymes that increase superoxide, including nicotinamide adenine dinucleotide phosphate, reduced form (NADPH) oxidases and xanthine oxidase, may also indirectly promote peroxynitrite formation. Once generated, peroxynitrite promotes endothelial dysfunction and vascular disease in several postulated ways, triggering apoptosis and cell death in ECs and VSMCs, inducing endothelial adhesion molecule expression, and disrupting the endothelial glycocalyx, among others.[248–250] In addition, peroxynitrite-dependent oxidation of tetrahydrobiopterin, a critical cofactor for eNOS function, uncouples eNOS, increasing production of superoxide instead of NO while the ROS generated can also promote inflammation, all as proposed to be at work in diabetes[251,252] (Fig. 7.11).

Alterations in NO bioavailability and the increased nitrosative stress in the form of greater peroxynitrite production and protein nitrosylation are also thought to contribute to

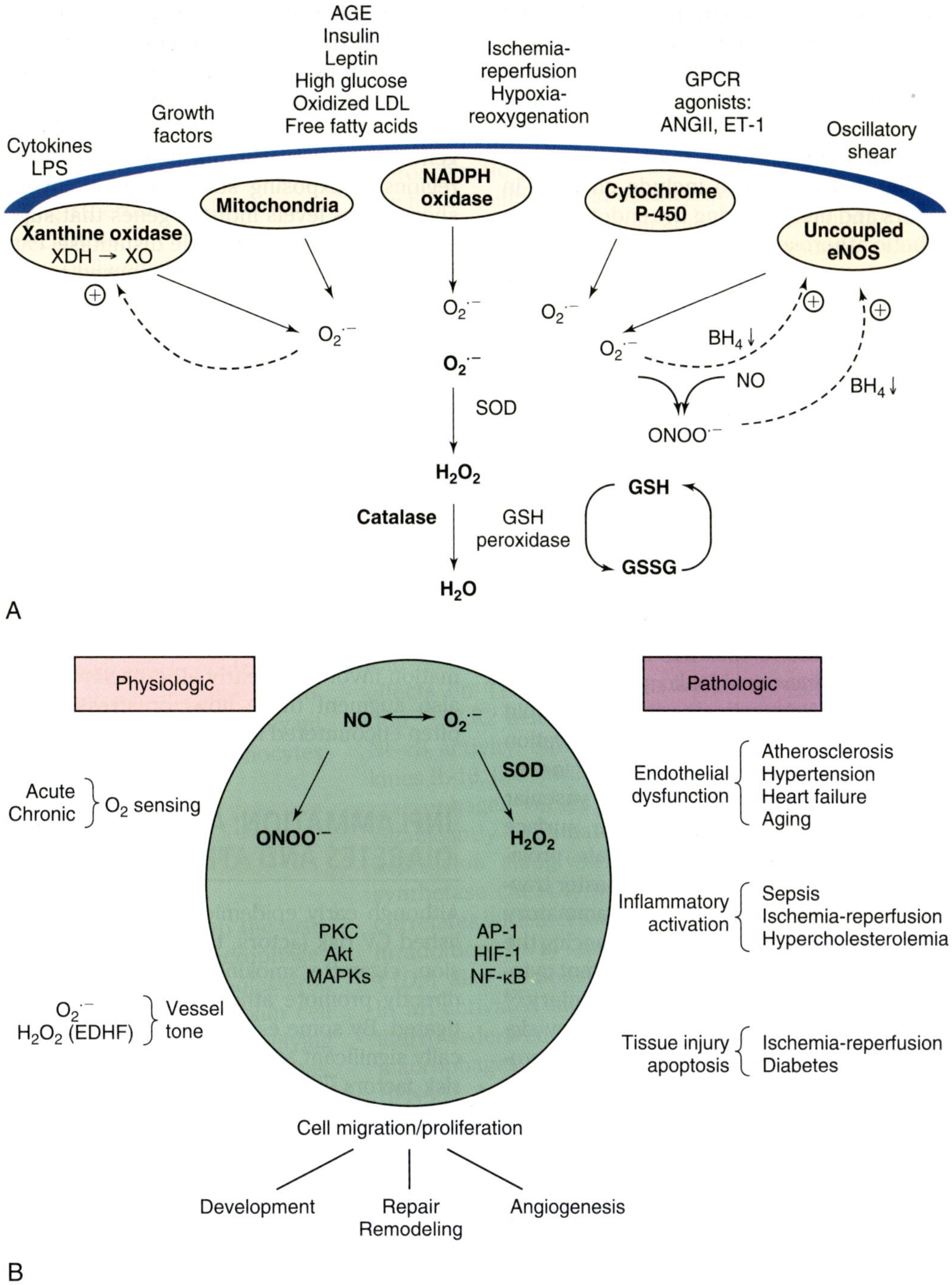

FIG. 7.11 The role of reactive oxygen species in endothelial dysfunction.[242] **A**, Multiple inputs, including proinflammatory cytokines, growth factors, and metabolites, elevated in T2DM, including free fatty acids and glucose, can lead to production of superoxide anion (O_2^-). **B**, Superoxide anion reacts with nitric oxide (NO), reducing NO bioavailability and leading to alterations in vascular tone, endothelial adhesion, angiogenesis, and cell viability. *ANGII*, Angiotensin II; *AP-1*, activator protein 1; *ET-1*, endothelin 1; *GPCR*, g-protein coupled receptor; *GSH*, monomeric glutathione; *GSSG*, glutathione disulfide; *HIF-1*, hypoxia-induced factor-1; *LPS*, lipopolysaccharide; *MAPKs*, mitogen activated protein kinases; *XDH*, xanthine dehydrogenase; *XO*, xanthine oxidase. (From Li JM, Shah AM. Endothelial cell superoxide generation: regulation and relevance for cardiovascular pathophysiology. *Am J Physiol Regul Integr Comp Physiol*. 2004;287:R1014–R1030.)

diabetic macrovascular disease;[253] increased nitrotyrosine levels are detected in diabetic human plasma.[254] Nitrotyrosine levels correlate with EC death while neutralizing peroxynitrite improves endothelial dysfunction in preclinical diabetes models.

Preclinical work has also expanded our perspective on endothelial dysfunction, suggesting the endothelium can also exert effects on metabolic control, like on glucose and FFAs, rather than just reacting to such forces. For example, in mouse models, genetic deletion of PPAR-γ from the endothelium alone alters lipid metabolism, responses to lipid loads, FFA levels, and adiposity, with concomitant changes in diabetes.[255] Other work finds that regulation of insulin receptor adaptor proteins in the endothelium (IRS1 and IRS2) by the Forkhead box proteins (FoxO), a family of DNA binding transcription factors that regulate

in lipoprotein secretion and other basic cellular processes, including mitochondrial function and the unfolded protein response, all with direct relevance to diabetes and atherosclerosis.[296] ER stress in diabetes and diabetic atherosclerosis has been linked to changes in apoptosis, inflammation, hepatic dysfunction, among other settings, offering another way in the complex intersection among cardio-metabolic issues can be further considered and understood.[297]

Lymphocytes in Diabetic Vascular Disease

Both B and T lymphocytes are implicated in atherogenesis in both the absence and presence of diabetes. By immunohistochemistry, most lymphocytes in atherosclerotic plaque are $CD4^+$ cells, which can differentiate along Th1 or Th2 lineages, as directed by cytokines produced by other lymphocytes, ECs, and macrophages. Disruption of the Th1 lineage reduces atherosclerosis in murine models of disease.[298] The role of Th2 cells continues to be explored and is coming into focus, with reported involvement in T1DM, gestational diabetes, MASLD, and other related conditions.[299,300] Smaller subsets of T cells, including T regulatory cells (Tregs) and Th17 lymphocytes, exert local control on plaque inflammation and expansion. In patients with diabetes, a lymphocytosis has been observed with expansion of a less common, proatherogenic $CD4^+$ CD28 null T lymphocyte; moreover, in acute coronary syndrome patients, this specific lymphocyte population's frequency was 12.7% in T2DM versus 3.8% without T2DM, a pattern also independently associated with glycosylated hemoglobin.[301] Increased visceral fat is associated with a loss of local Treg cells,[302] one of many connections between T cells, inflammation, obesity, and CV disease.[303]

Vascular Smooth Muscle Cells

During atherosclerosis, VSMCs proliferate in the media and also migrate from the media to the subintimal space, thus enlarging the neointimal lesion, processes also reported as being part of diabetes and its associated CV complications.[304] VSMC reactivity is increased in isolated human arteries exposed to norepinephrine or phenylephrine, an effect that correlates with reduced subplasmalemmal Ca^{2+}, which helps control K^+ channels and VSMC relaxation.[305] VSMCs grown under high-glucose conditions proliferate, migrate, undergo hypertrophy, and produce ECM more than VSMCs grown in low-glucose media.[306,307] Aortic VSMCs isolated from db/db mice—an established model of aggressive T2DM—manifest increased proinflammatory gene expression (e.g., MCP-1 and IL-6), while other preclinical evidence points to enhanced VSMC responsiveness to stimuli like platelet-derived growth factor.[308,309] These observations, together with other data, suggest that the diabetic environment, including AGEs, "preactivates" VSMCs and thus promotes pathogenic responses involving VSMCs.[310]

Inflammation as a Therapeutic Target in Diabetic Atherosclerosis?

Although cell biology and animal models have provided key scientific insights into atherogenesis, ongoing and extensive efforts have aimed at translating these findings to human disease. The identification of stable, circulating biomarkers of inflammation has allowed consideration of inflammation as an independent CV risk factors and targeting inflammation to decrease atherosclerotic complications, including in diabetes.

PPARs—the family of ligand activated transcription factors/nuclear receptors known to control gene expression in energy balance and metabolism—were also established as being expressed and active in vascular and inflammatory cells, in addition to their role in metabolic tissues and organs.[136] The PPAR family consists of PPAR-α, PPAR-γ, and PPAR-β/δ, with each of these isotypes having unique profiles. The subsequent unfolding of the PPAR data and efforts to use PPAR agonists to improve CV outcomes in diabetes and dyslipidemia provides an example of the challenges in extending scientific findings to clinical benefit.[311] While scientific and therapeutic efforts in diabetic atherosclerosis may have moved on from PPARs, as driven by clinical issues, this obfuscates the clear, important role of PPARs in biology and what unfolded in clinical trials.

Thiazolidinediones (rosiglitazone, pioglitazone) are potent insulin sensitizers that exert their effects by activating PPAR-γ, whereas fibrates lower hypertriglyceridemia and increase HDL by activating PPAR-α. Interestingly, these agents and their effects were identified even before PPARs were identified or well understood. The subsequent extensive evidence for PPAR action in vascular and inflammatory cells, including repressing inflammatory and proatherosclerotic gene expression in ECs, VSMCs, and macrophages, drive interest in these agents for treating diabetic atherosclerosis and diabetes associated dyslipidemia.[312–315] Treating hypercholesterolemic mice with PPAR-α and PPAR-γ activating drugs in vivo also suppressed lesion formation in different models with and without diabetes.[316] PPAR effects correlated with alterations in macrophage foam cell formation in vitro. While PPAR-δ was shown to be involved in these processes, no PPAR-δ agonist ever reached clinical approval.[317] In contrast, considerable evidence argued that both PPAR-γ and PPAR-α activating agents exerted anti-atherosclerotic effects,[318] including early data in humans, like PPAR-γ drugs reducing biomarkers like hsCRP and decreasing surrogate endpoints like carotid intimamedia thickness while fibrates had early positive trials.[319] Despite these prospects, PPAR activators yielded mixed results in translation to humans for different reasons, as discussed elsewhere.

Briefly, for PPAR-γ, a meta-analysis of smaller studies raised concerns about a possible increase in CV events with rosiglitazone.[320] A prospective, placebo-controlled study with pioglitazone—PROACTIVE (Prospective Pioglitazone Clinical Trial in Macrovascular Events)—did demonstrate a 20% reduction in the secondary endpoint of MACE in patients with diabetes but with a potentially flawed primary combined endpoint, which incorporated multiple outcomes, including the notoriously refractory outcome of improving peripheral vascular disease.[321] If in fact the more traditional MACE outcome had been the primary endpoint in PROACTIVE, the field may have unfolded differently. Importantly, pioglitazone did not increase adverse events in this study as had been suggested for rosiglitazone, one of several lines of evidence that establishes how PPAR agonists can have quite distinct transcriptional and functional effects, perhaps as a result of the especially large ligand-binding domain present in PPARs. For example, rosiglitazone does not lower triglycerides while pioglitazone does, perhaps through activity on PPAR-α.[322] In contrast to PRoACTIVE, in the IRIS (Insulin Resistance Intervention after Stroke), pioglitazone decreased stroke as well as MIs,[323,324] in line with the prior preclinical data. Despite this, multiple issues limited the clinical use of PPAR-γ, including ongoing concerns about CV safety for rosiglitazone,[325] fluid retention that could cause issues for patients with heart failure, questions about other untoward side effects like bone fractures and bladder cancer, and weight gain.[326] Interesting, PPAR-γ agonists can cause weight gain, which appears primarily subcutaneous, while also decreasing hsCRP, supporting different adipose depots as having different effects on inflammation.

Similarly, PPAR-α agonists also had a complicated story despite promising science. Fibrates as PPAR-α activating agents that decrease triglycerides and increased HDL, reduced CV events with gemfibrozil, in the Veterans Administration-HDL Intervention Trial ("VA-HIT").[327] Subsequent studies had less definitive evidence for primary endpoint benefit with fibrates, including fenofibrate in diabetes[328] and in combination with statins in patients with T2DM.[329] In these studies, the subgroup of patients with higher TG and lower HDL levels seemed most likely to benefit.[329] However, subsequent data with the PPAR-α agonist pemafibrate failed to show a major adverse CV event benefit in PROMINENT, despite being performed in patients with higher TG levels.[330] A substudy analysis of PROMINENT did suggest a benefit in PAD in patients with diabetes.[331] Omega-3 fatty acids are also considered to be PPAR-α activating agents, in keeping with their effects on lowering triglycerides, again raising the prospect that the benefit of icosapent ethyl seen in REDUCE-IT may have involved PPAR-α activation.[332] The basis for other omega-3 fatty acid trials not showing CV benefit is not clear but may align with the complexity of PPAR biology.

While PPARs are clearly key transcriptional regulators positioned at the intersection of metabolism, inflammation, and atherosclerosis, a distinction exists between any biologic target and the therapeutic agent(s) aimed at that target. While subsequent efforts to develop other PPAR modulators, including ones that would subtract adverse effects or have greater effectiveness, have generally failed, other endogenous mechanisms shown to generate natural PPAR agonists are associated with decreased atherosclerotic risk, such as genetic variants with increased LPL action and apoC3 loss of action.[333]

In contrast to the complexities of PPAR therapeutics, HMG-CoA reductase inhibitors or statins have consistently demonstrated decreased CV risk in patients with diabetes, as also discussed elsewhere.[334,335] Mechanistically, statin benefits involve lowering the LDL-C, with other pleiotropic effects also suggested, including antiinflammatory action. Statins lowered circulating hsCRP levels as compared to a placebo, as seen in randomized, prospective primary and secondary CVD outcomes trials. In the Pravastatin or Atorvastatin Evaluation and Infection Therapy—Thrombolysis in Myocardial Infarction 22 (PROVE IT–TIMI 22) trial, the subjects benefiting the most from high-dose atorvastatin therapy after acute coronary syndrome events were patients who achieved both an LDL-C level below 70 mg/dL and an hsCRP level below 2.0 mg/L.[272] In JUPITER (Justification for the Use of Statins in Prevention: An Intervention Trial Evaluating Rosuvastatin), 17,802 individuals without known CVD and average LDL-C levels (<130 mg/dL, median 108 mg/dL) but hsCRP levels of 2 mg/L or higher were randomized to either a placebo or rosuvastatin 20 mg/day.[336] The study was terminated after only 3 years when the interim analysis revealed a 44% reduction in the primary CV endpoint for those on rosuvastatin, who had significant reductions in hsCRP (37%). Those patients on rosuvastatin also had a major reduction in LDL-C (50%), precluding a definitive conclusion about a specific, causal antiinflammatory effect being the basis for the CV benefit. Preclinical studies continue to suggest various mechanisms through which statins may decrease inflammation independent of LDL lowering, including changes in modification of proteins, induction of other targets such as the kruppel-like factor (KLF) transcription factors, and changes in mRNA stability, as reported for eNOS.[337]

Given that statins decrease both hsCRP and LDL, thus confounding the issue, consideration was given to other therapies that might decrease inflammation without altering LDL, both as proof-of-concept and as an additional potential therapeutic strategy, as relevant to diabetes. The Nod-like receptor protein 3 (NLRP3) inflammasome is a signaling pathway that generates the active form of IL-1β, which is strongly implicated in atherosclerosis and thrombosis, including NLRP3 activation by intracellular cholesterol crystals.[338] The Cardiovascular Risk Reduction Trial (CANTOS; ClinicalTrials.gov identifier NCT013278) was a randomized, double-blind, placebo-controlled, event-driven trial testing if canakinumab, a human IL-1β neutralizing monoclonal antibody, reduces recurrent MI, stroke, and CVD death versus a placebo in patients at least 30 days after MI and who had hsCRP levels of 2 mg/L or higher. In CANTOS, the primary outcome (CV death, MI, or stroke), occurred in 4.11/100 person-years of the 50 mg group versus 3.86/100 person-years of the 150 mg group ($P = 0.02$ for the canakinumab 150 mg group vs. placebo [other doses nonsignificant]).[339] These benefits were seen despite no change in LDL-C, offering proof-of-concept that directly modulating inflammation can reduce CV events. While canakinumab is not being pursued for a CV indication, other direct modulators of inflammation are under investigation, including antibodies to IL-6, now in clinical CV outcome trials.[340]

Other evidence regarding inflammation in CV risk derives from studies using agents for treating rheumatologic conditions. The Cardiovascular Inflammation Reduction Trial (CIRT; NCT01594333), sponsored by the National Institutes of Health, was a multicenter, placebo-controlled trial in subjects with stable CAD on standard care *and* metabolic syndrome or T2DM (n = 7000) randomized to low-dose methotrexate (15–20 mg weekly) with folate supplementation.[341] Methotrexate, which lowers hsCRP without affecting lipid levels, had seven nonrandomized observational studies of patients with rheumatoid arthritis or psoriatic arthritis that suggested significant CV event reduction among those taking low-dose methotrexate. In CIRT, enrolled subjects, which excluded those with chronic inflammatory conditions (e.g., lupus, rheumatoid arthritis, or inflammatory bowel disease), low-dose methotrexate did not reduce CV events versus a placebo among patients with established CAD and either diabetes or metabolic syndrome or both.[342] Importantly, levels of IL-1β, IL-6, and hsCRP were not decreased in the trial while those receiving methotrexate had increased side effects, including transaminitis, leucopenia, anemia, and infections.

In contrast to methotrexate, more positive data on modulating inflammation has been seen with colchicine, an oral tubulin binding and polymerization inhibitory agent that accumulates in neutrophils, exerting antiinflammatory effects on these and other relevant cells, including ECs and macrophages.[343] Aside from studies in pericarditis, atrial fibrillation, and postcardiac surgery, colchicine was reported to reduce atherosclerotic complications in the open label LoDoCo pilot study (ACS, out-of-hospital cardiac arrest, or noncardioembolic ischemic stroke, 5.3% vs. 16%; $P < 0.001$) and LoDoCo2, a multicenter, double-blind, placebo-controlled randomized trial in stable CAD patients.[344] The 5522 patients who tolerated colchicine were randomized and after 29 months (median), colchicine reduced the primary composite CV outcome (CV death, MI, ischemic stroke, or ischemia-driven coronary revascularization) by 31% (6.8% vs. 9.6%; $P < 0.001$) as compared to a placebo. In LoDoCo2, among the 18.2% with baseline T2DM, similar benefits were seen (HR, primary endpoint 0.87 [0.61–1.25] in T2DM, 0.64 [0.51–0.80] without diabetes, *P* interaction = 0.14). Interestingly, the incidence of new-onset T2DM was less in the colchicine group, although not significant (1.5% colchicine group, 2.2% in placebo group, $P = 0.10$). Although various caveats exist, LoDoCo2 supported inflammation as a potential therapeutic target, with relevance to diabetes.

The large, double-blind, placebo-controlled Colchicine Cardiovascular Outcomes Trial (COLCOT) investigated low-dose colchicine in patients within 30 days after MI.[345] After 23 months, colchicine decreased the primary composite endpoint (CV death, resuscitated cardiac arrest, MI, stroke, or urgent hospitalization for angina requiring coronary revascularization) by 23% (HR, 0.77; 95% CI, 0.61–0.96; $P = 0.02$). Colchicine was in general well tolerated with minimal adverse events, aside from a small increase in nonfatal pneumonia hospitalization in those on colchicine. Of note, enrollment in COLCOT was not based on any specific inflammatory marker entry criteria. COLCOT enrolled 959 patients with T2DM, who benefited similarly to those without diabetes, with a primary endpoint event of 8.7% in the colchicine group and 13.1% in the placebo group (HR 0.65; 95% CI, 0.44–0.96; $P = 0.03$) although with more nausea (2.7% vs. 0.8%, $P = 0.03$, and pneumonia, 2.4% vs. 0.4%, $P = 0.008$). More recently, the CLEAR SYNERGY (OASIS 9) reported results in a 2 × 2 randomized controlled trial of low-dose colchicine 0.5 mg daily versus a placebo and spironolactone 25 mg daily versus a placebo in 7062 post-MI participants (mean age 60.5 years; 20% female) treated within 72 hours of the index percutaneous coronary intervention.[346] In this trial, which included 18% of patients with diabetes, colchicine showed no benefit, contrasting with the COLCOT and LoDoCo2 results, which had enrolled different patient populations.

A NEW ERA IN MANAGING CV RISK IN DIABETES: MECHANISTIC INSIGHTS FROM SGLT2I AND GLP-1 RA TRIALS

One explanation raised for the prior conundrum of why treating hyperglycemia and diabetes did not decrease CV events pointed to the specific glucose-lowering agents employed, whether through their specific mechanisms of action or possible adverse effects that might offset CV benefits. As discussed in detail elsewhere, more recent landmark trials with SGLT2is and GLP-1 RAs demonstrating significant reductions in major adverse CV events represent true therapeutic breakthroughs, opening up a new era in managing CV disease in diabetes.[347] The SGLT2i and GLP-1 RA benefits on CV events, CKD, and heart failure are now integrated into current guidelines for managing diabetes as well as other conditions, which also aligns with the increased emphasis on the spectrum of the Cardiovascular-Kidney-Metabolic (CKM) Syndrome.[348,349] As relevant to the discussions in this chapter, the CV benefits with GLP-1 RAs and SGLT2is provide an opportunity to return to and further explore mechanisms at work with these agents as a way of better understanding the pathogenesis of diabetes-associated CVD and why these agents worked to reduce complications. Although these breakthrough therapies warrant the focused consideration provided in separate chapters, it is noteworthy how often data for both SGLT2is and GLP-1 RAs connect directly to the specific mechanisms discussed here,[350,351] with this data providing a basis for understanding and informing future studies into how SGLT2is and GLP-1 RAs modify diabetes-associated CV pathogenesis.

SUMMARY

Diabetes is a disease with a complex pathogenesis that arises over time; involves multiple different inputs; and that is manifest in many distinct, overlapping components. The complexities of this picture are evident in the efforts to deconvolute the nature of the vascular biology of diabetic atherosclerosis—the factors that drive the disorder, determine outcomes, and offer opportunities for improving outcomes. These efforts are informed by the pathologic studies of diabetic atherosclerosis to inputs like AGEs/RAGEs specifically related to diabetes to the many established CV risk factors commonly encountered in diabetes. Understanding the molecular basis of the intersection of diabetes and atherosclerosis remains challenging, given issues shared between these two common diseases: long subclinical phases, the presence of multiple confounding variables, shared mechanistic underpinnings, and cellular players and biologic mechanisms that also overlap. All these issues and clinical experience frame a fundamental question: To what extent is diabetic atherosclerosis distinct from atherosclerosis in the absence of diabetes or is diabetic atherosclerosis simply nondiabetic atherosclerosis accelerated in the context of hyperglycemia, diabetes, and its associated issues? Despite intense efforts and major progress, this question remains incompletely resolved. Clearly the mechanisms and issues considered here are important in diabetic atherosclerosis independent of whether specific to diabetes or not. Despite these challenges, the major advances seen with SGLT2is and GLP-1 RAs provide strong support for the future prospects of enhancing insight into why diabetic atherosclerosis and its complications occur, can be treated, and prevented.

REFERENCES

1. Eckel RH, Bornfeldt KE, Goldberg IJ. Cardiovascular disease in diabetes, beyond glucose. Cell Metab. 2021;33:1519–1545. https://doi.org/10.1016/j.cmet.2021.07.001.
2. Libby P, Plutzky J. Diabetic macrovascular disease: the glucose paradox? Circulation. 2002;106:2760–2763. https://doi.org/10.1161/01.cir.0000037282.92395.ae.
3. Manrique-Acevedo C, Hirsch IB, Eckel RH. Prevention of cardiovascular disease in type 1 diabetes. N Engl J Med. 2024;390:1207–1217. https://doi.org/10.1056/NEJMra2311526.
4. Sattar N, Presslie C, Rutter MK, McGuire DK. Cardiovascular and kidney risks in individuals with type 2 diabetes: contemporary understanding with greater emphasis on excess adiposity. Diabetes Care. 2024;47:531–543. https://doi.org/10.2337/dci23-0041.
5. Tomic D, Shaw JE, Magliano DJ. The burden and risks of emerging complications of diabetes mellitus. Nat Rev Endocrinol. 2022;18:525–539. https://doi.org/10.1038/s41574-022-00690-7.
6. Sattar N, McMurray J, Boren J, et al. Twenty years of cardiovascular complications and risk factors in patients with type 2 diabetes: a nationwide Swedish cohort study. Circulation. 2023;147:1872–1886. https://doi.org/10.1161/CIRCULATIONAHA.122.063374.
7. Wong ND, Sattar N. Cardiovascular risk in diabetes mellitus: epidemiology, assessment and prevention. Nat Rev Cardiol. 2023;20:685–695. https://doi.org/10.1038/s41569-023-00877-z.
8. Neglia D, Caselli C, Maffei E, et al. Rapid plaque progression is independently associated with hyperglycemia and low HDL cholesterol in patients with stable coronary artery disease: a PARADIGM study. *Circ Cardiovasc Imaging.* 2024;17:e016481. https://doi.org/10.1161/CIRCIMAGING.123.016481.
9. Yahagi K, Kolodgie FD, Lutter C, et al. Pathology of human coronary and carotid artery atherosclerosis and vascular calcification in diabetes mellitus. *Arterioscler Thromb Vasc Biol.* 2017;37:191–204. https://doi.org/10.1161/ATVBAHA.116.306256.
10. Kawai K, Kawakami R, Finn AV, Virmani R. Differences in stable and unstable atherosclerotic plaque. *Arterioscler Thromb Vasc Biol.* 2024;44:1474–1484. https://doi.org/10.1161/ATVBAHA.124.319396.
11. Moreno PR, Murcia AM, Palacios IF, et al. Coronary composition and macrophage infiltration in atherectomy specimens from patients with diabetes mellitus. *Circulation.* 2000;102:2180–2184. https://doi.org/10.1161/01.cir.102.18.2180.
12. Cipollone F, Iezzi A, Fazia M, et al. The receptor RAGE as a progression factor amplifying arachidonate-dependent inflammatory and proteolytic response in human atherosclerotic plaques: role of glycemic control. *Circulation.* 2003;108:1070–1077. https://doi.org/10.1161/01.CIR.0000086014.80477.0D.
13. Bull Rasmussen IK, Skriver-Moeller AC, Ripa RS, et al. Increased subclinical coronary artery pathology in type 2 diabetes with albuminuria. *Diabetes.* 2024;73:490–496. https://doi.org/10.2337/db23-0529.
14. Cuccurullo C, Iezzi A, Fazia ML, et al. Suppression of RAGE as a basis of simvastatin-dependent plaque stabilization in type 2 diabetes. *Arterioscler Thromb Vasc Biol.* 2006;26:2716–2723. https://doi.org/10.1161/01.ATV.0000249630.02085.12.
15. Burke AP, Kolodgie FD, Zieske A, et al. Morphologic findings of coronary atherosclerotic plaques in diabetics: a postmortem study. *Arterioscler Thromb Vasc Biol.* 2004;24:1266–1271. https://doi.org/10.1161/01.ATV.0000131783.74034.97.
16. Levin L, Tomer Y. The etiology of autoimmune diabetes and thyroiditis: evidence for common genetic susceptibility. *Autoimmun Rev.* 2003;2:377–386. https://doi.org/10.1016/s1568-9972(03)00080-6.
17. Burke AP, Kolodgie FD, Farb A, et al. Healed plaque ruptures and sudden coronary death: evidence that subclinical rupture has a role in plaque progression. *Circulation.* 2001;103:934–940. https://doi.org/10.1161/01.cir.103.7.934.
18. van Brussel BL, Plokker HW, Voors AA, et al. Multivariate risk factor analysis of clinical outcome 15 years after venous coronary artery bypass graft surgery. *Eur Heart J.* 1995;16:1200–1206. https://doi.org/10.1093/oxfordjournals.eurheartj.a061076.
19. Takazawa K, Hosoda Y, Yamamoto T, Kawasaki S, Sasaguri S. Coronary artery bypass grafting. Late result of actual 10-years follow-up in 376 patients. *Jpn J Thorac Cardiovasc Surg.* 1999;47:110–115. https://doi.org/10.1007/BF03217953.
20. Wang R, Serruys PW, Gao C, et al. Ten-year all-cause death after percutaneous or surgical revascularization in diabetic patients with complex coronary artery disease. *Eur Heart J.* 2021;43:56–67. https://doi.org/10.1093/eurheartj/ehab441.
21. Tam DY, Dharma C, Rocha R, et al. Long-term survival after surgical or percutaneous revascularization in patients with diabetes and multivessel coronary disease. *J Am Coll Cardiol.* 2020;76:1153–1164. https://doi.org/10.1016/j.jacc.2020.06.052.
22. Kolodgie FD, Gold HK, Burke AP, et al. Intraplaque hemorrhage and progression of coronary atheroma. *N Engl J Med.* 2003;349:2316–2325. https://doi.org/10.1056/NEJMoa035655.
23. Moreno PR, Fuster V. New aspects in the pathogenesis of diabetic atherothrombosis. *J Am Coll Cardiol.* 2004;44:2293–2300. https://doi.org/10.1016/j.jacc.2004.07.060.
24. Purushothaman KR, Purushothaman M, Muntner P, et al. Inflammation, neovascularization and intra-plaque hemorrhage are associated with increased reparative collagen content: implication for plaque progression in diabetic atherosclerosis. *Vasc Med.* 2011;16:103–108. https://doi.org/10.1177/1358863X11402249.
25. Stuijfzand WJ, van Rosendael AR, Lin FY, et al. Stress myocardial perfusion imaging vs coronary computed tomographic angiography for diagnosis of invasive vessel-specific coronary physiology: predictive modeling results from the computed tomographic evaluation of atherosclerotic determinants of myocardial ischemia (CREDENCE) trial. *JAMA Cardiol.* 2020;5:1338–1348. https://doi.org/10.1001/jamacardio.2020.3409.
26. Jonas RA, Crabtree TR, Jennings RS, et al. Diabetes, atherosclerosis, and stenosis by AI. *Diabetes Care.* 2023;46:416–424. https://doi.org/10.2337/dc21-1663.
27. Maffei E, Seitun S, Nieman K, et al. Assessment of coronary artery disease and calcified coronary plaque burden by computed tomography in patients with and without diabetes mellitus. *Eur Radiol.* 2011;21:944–953. https://doi.org/10.1007/s00330-010-1996-z.
28. Kato K, Yonetsu T, Kim SJ, et al. Comparison of nonculprit coronary plaque characteristics between patients with and without diabetes: a 3-vessel optical coherence tomography study. *JACC Cardiovasc Interv.* 2012;5:1150–1158. https://doi.org/10.1016/j.jcin.2012.06.019.
29. Patel KV, Budoff MJ, Valero-Elizondo J, et al. Coronary atherosclerosis across the glycemic spectrum among asymptomatic adults: the Miami Heart Study at Baptist Health South Florida. *Circ Cardiovasc Imaging.* 2023;16:e015314. https://doi.org/10.1161/CIRCIMAGING.123.015314.
30. Gyldenkerne C, Maeng M, Kjoller-Hansen L, et al. Coronary artery lesion lipid content and plaque burden in diabetic and nondiabetic patients: PROSPECT II. *Circulation.* 2023;147:469–481. https://doi.org/10.1161/CIRCULATIONAHA.122.061983.
31. Diabetes Control and Complications Trial (DCCT): results of feasibility study. The DCCT Research Group. *Diabetes Care.* 1987;10:1–19. https://doi.org/10.2337/diacare.10.1.1.
32. Nathan DM, et al. Diabetes Control and Complications Trial Research Group. The effect of intensive treatment of diabetes on the development and progression of long-term complications in insulin-dependent diabetes mellitus. *N Engl J Med.* 1993;329:977–986. https://doi.org/10.1056/NEJM199309303291401.
33. Nathan DM, Cleary PA, Backlund JY, et al. Diabetes Control and Complications Trial/Epidemiology of Diabetes Interventions and Complications (DCCT/EDIC) Study Research Group. Intensive diabetes treatment and cardiovascular disease in patients with type 1 diabetes. *N Engl J Med.* 2005;353:2643–2653. https://doi.org/10.1056/NEJMoa052187.
34. Nathan DM, Lachin J, Cleary P, et al. Intensive diabetes therapy and carotid intima-media thickness in type 1 diabetes mellitus. *N Engl J Med.* 2003;348:2294–2303. https://doi.org/10.1056/NEJMoa022314.
35. Intensive blood-glucose control with sulphonylureas or insulin compared with conventional treatment and risk of complications in patients with type 2 diabetes (UKPDS 33). UK Prospective Diabetes Study (UKPDS) Group. *Lancet.* 1998;352:837–853.
36. Holman RR, Paul SK, Bethel MA, Matthews DR, Neil HA. 10-year follow-up of intensive glucose control in type 2 diabetes. *N Engl J Med.* 2008;359:1577–1589. https://doi.org/10.1056/NEJMoa0806470.
37. Gerstein HC, Miller ME, et al. ACCORD Study Group. Long-term effects of intensive glucose lowering on cardiovascular outcomes. *N Engl J Med.* 2011;364:818–828. https://doi.org/10.1056/NEJMoa1006524.
38. Patel A, MacMahon S, et al. ADVANCE Collaborative Group. Intensive blood glucose control and vascular outcomes in patients with type 2 diabetes. *N Engl J Med.* 2008;358:2560–2572. https://doi.org/10.1056/NEJMoa0802987.
39. Duckworth W, Abraira C, Moritz T, et al. Glucose control and vascular complications in veterans with type 2 diabetes. *N Engl J Med.* 2009;360:129–139. https://doi.org/10.1056/NEJMoa0808431.
40. Ramasamy R. Aldose reductase: a novel target for cardioprotective interventions. *Curr Drug Targets.* 2003;4:625–632. https://doi.org/10.2174/1389450033490768.
41. Vedantham S, Ananthakrishnan R, Schmidt AM, Ramasamy R. Aldose reductase, oxidative stress and diabetic cardiovascular complications. *Cardiovasc Hematol Agents Med Chem.* 2012;10:234–240. https://doi.org/10.2174/187152512802651097.
42. Vikramadithyan RK, Hu Y, Noh HL, et al. Human aldose reductase expression accelerates diabetic atherosclerosis in transgenic mice. *J Clin Invest.* 2005;115:2434–2443. https://doi.org/10.1172/JCI24819.
43. Vedantham S, Noh H, Ananthakrishnan R, et al. Human aldose reductase expression accelerates atherosclerosis in diabetic apolipoprotein E-/- mice. *Arterioscler Thromb Vasc Biol.* 2011;31:1805–1813. https://doi.org/10.1161/ATVBAHA.111.226902.

44. Srivastava S, Vladykovskaya E, Barski OA, et al. Aldose reductase protects against early atherosclerotic lesion formation in apolipoprotein E-null mice. *Circ Res.* 2009;105:793–802. https://doi.org/10.1161/CIRCRESAHA.109.200568.
45. Johnson BF, Nesto RW, Pfeifer MA, et al. Cardiac abnormalities in diabetic patients with neuropathy: effects of aldose reductase inhibitor administration. *Diabetes Care.* 2004;27:448–454. https://doi.org/10.2337/diacare.27.2.448.
46. Hothersall JS, Muirhead RP, Taylaur CE, Jones RH. Anti-oxidant status in an in vitro model for hyperglycaemic lens cataract formation: competition for available nicotinamide adenine dinucleotide phosphate between glutathione reduction and the polyol pathway. *Biochem Int.* 1992;27:945–952.
47. Robinson KA, Weinstein ML, Lindenmayer GE, Buse MG. Effects of diabetes and hyperglycemia on the hexosamine synthesis pathway in rat muscle and liver. *Diabetes.* 1995;44:1438–1446. https://doi.org/10.2337/diab.44.12.1438.
48. Du XL, Edelstein D, Rossetti L, et al. Hyperglycemia-induced mitochondrial superoxide overproduction activates the hexosamine pathway and induces plasminogen activator inhibitor-1 expression by increasing Sp1 glycosylation. *Proc Natl Acad Sci U S A.* 2000;97:12222–12226. https://doi.org/10.1073/pnas.97.22.12222.
49. Gabriely I, Yang XM, Cases JA, Ma XH, Rossetti L, Barzilai N. Hyperglycemia induces PAI-1 gene expression in adipose tissue by activation of the hexosamine biosynthetic pathway. *Atherosclerosis.* 2002;160:115–122. https://doi.org/10.1016/s0021-9150(01)00574-3.
50. Du XL, Edelstein D, Dimmeler S, Ju Q, Sui C, Brownlee M. Hyperglycemia inhibits endothelial nitric oxide synthase activity by posttranslational modification at the Akt site. *J Clin Invest.* 2001;108:1341–1348. https://doi.org/10.1172/JCI11235.
51. Hoffman JM, Ishizuka T, Farese RV. Interrelated effects of insulin and glucose on diacylglycerol-protein kinase-C signalling in rat adipocytes and solei muscle in vitro and in vivo in diabetic rats. *Endocrinology.* 1991;128:2937–2948. https://doi.org/10.1210/endo-128-6-2937.
52. Idris I, Gray S, Donnelly R. Protein kinase C activation: isozyme-specific effects on metabolism and cardiovascular complications in diabetes. *Diabetologia.* 2001;44:659–673. https://doi.org/10.1007/s001250051675.
53. Geraldes P, King GL. Activation of protein kinase C isoforms and its impact on diabetic complications. *Circ Res.* 2010;106:1319–1331. https://doi.org/10.1161/CIRCRESAHA.110.217117.
54. Harja E, Chang JS, Lu Y, et al. Mice deficient in PKCbeta and apolipoprotein E display decreased atherosclerosis. *FASEB J.* 2009;23:1081–1091. https://doi.org/10.1096/fj.08-120345.
55. Leitges M, Mayr M, Braun U, et al. Exacerbated vein graft arteriosclerosis in protein kinase Cdelta-null mice. *J Clin Invest.* 2001;108:1505–1512. https://doi.org/10.1172/JCI12902.
56. Mamputu JC, Renier G. Advanced glycation end-products increase monocyte adhesion to retinal endothelial cells through vascular endothelial growth factor-induced ICAM-1 expression: inhibitory effect of antioxidants. *J Leukoc Biol.* 2004;75:1062–1069. https://doi.org/10.1189/jlb.0603265.
57. Devaraj S, Hirany SV, Burk RF, Jialal I. Divergence between LDL oxidative susceptibility and urinary F(2)-isoprostanes as measures of oxidative stress in type 2 diabetes. *Clin Chem.* 2001;47:1974–1979.
58. Wakabayashi Y, Usui Y, Shibauchi Y, Uchino H, Goto H. Increased levels of 8-hydroxydeoxyguanosine in the vitreous of patients with diabetic retinopathy. *Diabetes Res Clin Pract.* 2010;89:e59–61. https://doi.org/10.1016/j.diabres.2010.05.032.
59. Yi X, Xu L, Hiller S, Kim HS, Maeda N. Reduced alpha-lipoic acid synthase gene expression exacerbates atherosclerosis in diabetic apolipoprotein E-deficient mice. *Atherosclerosis.* 2012;223:137–143. https://doi.org/10.1016/j.atherosclerosis.2012.04.025.
60. Yusuf S, Dagenais G, Pogue J, Bosch J, Sleight P. Heart Outcomes Prevention Evaluation Study Investigators. Vitamin E supplementation and cardiovascular events in high-risk patients. *N Engl J Med.* 2000;342:154–160. https://doi.org/10.1056/NEJM200001203420302.
61. Levy Y, Blum S, Levy AP. Antioxidants in the prevention of atherosclerosis: the importance of proper patient selection. *Clin Nutr.* 2009;28:581–582. https://doi.org/10.1016/j.clnu.2009.04.012.
62. Nishikawa T, Edelstein D, Du XL, et al. Normalizing mitochondrial superoxide production blocks three pathways of hyperglycaemic damage. *Nature.* 2000;404:787–790. https://doi.org/10.1038/35008121.
63. Giacco F, Brownlee M. Oxidative stress and diabetic complications. *Circ Res.* 2010;107:1058–1070. https://doi.org/10.1161/CIRCRESAHA.110.223545.
64. Hammes HP, Du X, Edelstein D, et al. Benfotiamine blocks three major pathways of hyperglycemic damage and prevents experimental diabetic retinopathy. *Nat Med.* 2003;9:294–299. https://doi.org/10.1038/nm834.
65. Sedeek M, Montezano AC, Hebert RL, et al. Oxidative stress, Nox isoforms and complications of diabetes—potential targets for novel therapies. *J Cardiovasc Transl Res.* 2012;5:509–518. https://doi.org/10.1007/s12265-012-9387-2.
66. Touyz RM, Briones AM, Sedeek M, Burger D, Montezano AC. NOX isoforms and reactive oxygen species in vascular health. *Mol Interv.* 2011;11:27–35. https://doi.org/10.1124/mi.11.1.5.
67. Wautier MP, Chappey O, Corda S, Stern DM, Schmidt AM, Wautier JL. Activation of NADPH oxidase by AGE links oxidant stress to altered gene expression via RAGE. *Am J Physiol Endocrinol Metab.* 2001;280:E685–694. https://doi.org/10.1152/ajpendo.2001.280.5.E685.
68. Barry-Lane PA, Patterson C, van der Merwe M, et al. p47phox is required for atherosclerotic lesion progression in ApoE(-/-) mice. *J Clin Invest.* 2001;108:1513–1522. https://doi.org/10.1172/JCI11927.
69. Sheehan AL, Carrell S, Johnson B, Stanic B, Banfi B, Miller Jr. FJ. Role for Nox1 NADPH oxidase in atherosclerosis. *Atherosclerosis.* 2011;216:321–326. https://doi.org/10.1016/j.atherosclerosis.2011.02.028.
70. Judkins CP, Diep H, Broughton BR, et al. Direct evidence of a role for Nox2 in superoxide production, reduced nitric oxide bioavailability, and early atherosclerotic plaque formation in ApoE-/- mice. *Am J Physiol Heart Circ Physiol.* 2010;298:H24–32. https://doi.org/10.1152/ajpheart.00799.2009.
71. Lewis P, Stefanovic N, Pete J, et al. Lack of the antioxidant enzyme glutathione peroxidase-1 accelerates atherosclerosis in diabetic apolipoprotein E-deficient mice. *Circulation.* 2007;115:2178–2187. https://doi.org/10.1161/CIRCULATIONAHA.106.664250.
72. Perrotta I, Sciangula A, Perrotta E, Donato G, Cassese M. Ultrastructural analysis and electron microscopic localization of Nox4 in healthy and atherosclerotic human aorta. *Ultrastruct Pathol.* 2011;35:1–6. https://doi.org/10.3109/01913123.2010.510261.
73. Rivera J, Sobey CG, Walduck AK, Drummond GR. Nox isoforms in vascular pathophysiology: insights from transgenic and knockout mouse models. *Redox Rep.* 2010;15:50–63. https://doi.org/10.1179/174329210X12650506623401.
74. Wells-Knecht KJ, Zyzak DV, Litchfield JE, Thorpe SR, Baynes JW. Mechanism of autoxidative glycosylation: identification of glyoxal and arabinose as intermediates in the autoxidative modification of proteins by glucose. *Biochemistry.* 1995;34:3702–3709. https://doi.org/10.1021/bi00011a027.
75. Schalkwijk CG, Miyata T. Early- and advanced non-enzymatic glycation in diabetic vascular complications: the search for therapeutics. *Amino Acids.* 2012;42:1193–1204. https://doi.org/10.1007/s00726-010-0779-9.
76. Farboud B, Aotaki-Keen A, Miyata T, Hjelmeland LM, Handa JT. Development of a polyclonal antibody with broad epitope specificity for advanced glycation endproducts and localization of these epitopes in Bruch's membrane of the aging eye. *Mol Vis.* 1999;5:11.
77. Chang JS, Wendt T, Qu W, et al. Oxygen deprivation triggers upregulation of early growth response-1 by the receptor for advanced glycation end products. *Circ Res.* 2008;102:905–913. https://doi.org/10.1161/CIRCRESAHA.107.165308.
78. Friedlander MA, Witko-Sarsat V, Nguyen AT, et al. The advanced glycation endproduct pentosidine and monocyte activation in uremia. *Clin Nephrol.* 1996;45:379–382.
79. Anderson MM, Requena JR, Crowley JR, Thorpe SR, Heinecke JW. The myeloperoxidase system of human phagocytes generates Nepsilon-(carboxymethyl)lysine on proteins: a mechanism for producing advanced glycation end products at sites of inflammation. *J Clin Invest.* 1999;104:103–113. https://doi.org/10.1172/JCI3042.
80. Negrean M, Stirban A, Stratmann B, et al. Effects of low- and high-advanced glycation endproduct meals on macro- and microvascular endothelial function and oxidative stress in patients with type 2 diabetes mellitus. *Am J Clin Nutr.* 2007;85:1236–1243. https://doi.org/10.1093/ajcn/85.5.1236.
81. Gursinsky T, Ruhs S, Friess U, et al. Air pollution-associated fly ash particles induce fibrotic mechanisms in primary fibroblasts. *Biol Chem.* 2006;387:1411–1420. https://doi.org/10.1515/BC.2006.177.
82. McCann VJ, Davis RE, Welborn TA, Constable IJ, Beale DG. Glyoxalase phenotypes in patients with diabetes mellitus. *Aust N Z J Med.* 1981;11:380–382. https://doi.org/10.1111/j.1445-5994.1981.tb03516.x.
83. Reiniger N, Lau K, McCalla D, et al. Deletion of the receptor for advanced glycation end products reduces glomerulosclerosis and preserves renal function in the diabetic OVE26 mouse. *Diabetes.* 2010;59:2043–2054. https://doi.org/10.2337/db09-1766.
84. Schlondorff D. Cellular mechanisms of lipid injury in the glomerulus. *Am J Kidney Dis.* 1993;22:72–82. https://doi.org/10.1016/s0272-6386(12)70171-3.
85. Harja E, Bu DX, Hudson BI, et al. Vascular and inflammatory stresses mediate atherosclerosis via RAGE and its ligands in apoE-/- mice. *J Clin Invest.* 2008;118:183–194. https://doi.org/10.1172/JCI32703.
86. Boyd-White J, Williams Jr. JC. Effect of cross-linking on matrix permeability. A model for AGE-modified basement membranes. *Diabetes.* 1996;45:348–353. https://doi.org/10.2337/diab.45.3.348.
87. Stitt AW, Li YM, Gardiner TA, Bucala R, Archer DB, Vlassara H. Advanced glycation end products (AGEs) co-localize with AGE receptors in the retinal vasculature of diabetic and of AGE-infused rats. *Am J Pathol.* 1997;150:523–531.
88. Ohgami N, Nagai R, Ikemoto M, et al. Cd36, a member of the class b scavenger receptor family, as a receptor for advanced glycation end products. *J Biol Chem.* 2001;276:3195–3202. https://doi.org/10.1074/jbc.M006545200.
89. Araki N, Higashi T, Mori T, et al. Macrophage scavenger receptor mediates the endocytic uptake and degradation of advanced glycation end products of the Maillard reaction. *Eur J Biochem.* 1995;230:408–415. https://doi.org/10.1111/j.1432-1033.1995.0408h.x.
90. Yan SF, Ramasamy R, Naka Y, Schmidt AM. Glycation, inflammation, and RAGE: a scaffold for the macrovascular complications of diabetes and beyond. *Circ Res.* 2003;93:1159–1169. https://doi.org/10.1161/01.RES.0000103862.26506.3D.
91. Neeper M, Schmidt AM, Brett J, et al. Cloning and expression of a cell surface receptor for advanced glycosylation end products of proteins. *J Biol Chem.* 1992;267:14998–15004.
92. Koch M, Chitayat S, Dattilo BM, et al. Structural basis for ligand recognition and activation of RAGE. *Structure.* 2010;18:1342–1352. https://doi.org/10.1016/j.str.2010.05.017.

93. Yatime L, Andersen GR. Structural insights into the oligomerization mode of the human receptor for advanced glycation end-products. *FEBS J*. 2013;280:6556–6568. https://doi.org/10.1111/febs.12556.
94. Hofmann MA, Drury S, Fu C, et al. RAGE mediates a novel proinflammatory axis: a central cell surface receptor for S100/calgranulin polypeptides. *Cell*. 1999;97:889–901. https://doi.org/10.1016/s0092-8674(00)80801-6.
95. Leclerc E, Fritz G, Vetter SW, Heizmann CW. Binding of S100 proteins to RAGE: an update. *Biochim Biophys Acta*. 2009;1793:993–1007. https://doi.org/10.1016/j.bbamcr.2008.11.016.
96. Hofmann Bowman MA, Schmidt AM. S100/calgranulins EN-RAGEing the blood vessels: implications for inflammatory responses and atherosclerosis. *Am J Cardiovasc Dis*. 2011;1:92–100.
97. Taguchi A, Blood DC, del Toro G, et al. Blockade of RAGE-amphoterin signalling suppresses tumour growth and metastases. *Nature*. 2000;405:354–360. https://doi.org/10.1038/35012626.
98. Rauvala H, Rouhiainen A. Physiological and pathophysiological outcomes of the interactions of HMGB1 with cell surface receptors. *Biochim Biophys Acta*. 2010;1799:164–170. https://doi.org/10.1016/j.bbagrm.2009.11.012.
99. Kang R, Tang D, Schapiro NE, et al. The receptor for advanced glycation end products (RAGE) sustains autophagy and limits apoptosis, promoting pancreatic tumor cell survival. *Cell Death Differ*. 2010;17:666–676. https://doi.org/10.1038/cdd.2009.149.
100. Yan SD, Chen X, Fu J, et al. RAGE and amyloid-beta peptide neurotoxicity in Alzheimer's disease. *Nature*. 1996;382:685–691. https://doi.org/10.1038/382685a0.
101. Ma W, Rai V, Hudson BI, Song F, Schmidt AM, Barile GR. RAGE binds C1q and enhances C1q-mediated phagocytosis. *Cell Immunol*. 2012;274:72–82. https://doi.org/10.1016/j.cellimm.2012.02.001.
102. Rai V, Toure F, Chitayat S, et al. Lysophosphatidic acid targets vascular and oncogenic pathways via RAGE signaling. *J Exp Med*. 2012;209:2339–2350. https://doi.org/10.1084/jem.20120873.
103. Li J, Schmidt AM. Characterization and functional analysis of the promoter of RAGE, the receptor for advanced glycation end products. *J Biol Chem*. 1997;272:16498–16506. https://doi.org/10.1074/jbc.272.26.16498.
104. Goldin A, Beckman JA, Schmidt AM, Creager MA. Advanced glycation end products: sparking the development of diabetic vascular injury. *Circulation*. 2006;114:597–605. https://doi.org/10.1161/CIRCULATIONAHA.106.621854.
105. Park L, Raman KG, Lee KJ, et al. Suppression of accelerated diabetic atherosclerosis by the soluble receptor for advanced glycation endproducts. *Nat Med*. 1998;4:1025–1031. https://doi.org/10.1038/2012.
106. Bucciarelli LG, Wendt T, Qu W, et al. RAGE blockade stabilizes established atherosclerosis in diabetic apolipoprotein E-null mice. *Circulation*. 2002;106:2827–2835. https://doi.org/10.1161/01.cir.0000039325.03698.36.
107. Wendt T, Harja E, Bucciarelli L, et al. RAGE modulates vascular inflammation and atherosclerosis in a murine model of type 2 diabetes. *Atherosclerosis*. 2006;185:70–77. https://doi.org/10.1016/j.atherosclerosis.2005.06.013.
108. Soro-Paavonen A, Watson AM, Li J, et al. Receptor for advanced glycation end products (RAGE) deficiency attenuates the development of atherosclerosis in diabetes. *Diabetes*. 2008;57:2461–2469. https://doi.org/10.2337/db07-1808.
109. Ramasamy R, Shekhtman A, Schmidt AM. RAGE/DIAPH1 axis and cardiometabolic disease: from nascent discoveries to therapeutic potential. *Arterioscler Thromb Vasc Biol*. 2024;44:1497–1501. https://doi.org/10.1161/ATVBAHA.124.320142.
110. DeWard AD, Eisenmann KM, Matheson SF, Alberts AS. The role of formins in human disease. *Biochim Biophys Acta*. 2010;1803:226–233. https://doi.org/10.1016/j.bbamcr.2009.11.006.
111. Toure F, Fritz G, Li Q, et al. Formin mDia1 mediates vascular remodeling via integration of oxidative and signal transduction pathways. *Circ Res*. 2012;110:1279–1293. https://doi.org/10.1161/CIRCRESAHA.111.262519.
112. Engelen L, Ferreira I, Gaens KH, et al. The association between the -374T/A polymorphism of the receptor for advanced glycation endproducts gene and blood pressure and arterial stiffness is modified by glucose metabolism status: the Hoorn and CoDAM studies. *J Hypertens*. 2010;28:285–293. https://doi.org/10.1097/HJH.0b013e3283330931.
113. Senatus L, Egana-Gorrono L, Lopez-Diez R, et al. DIAPH1 mediates progression of atherosclerosis and regulates hepatic lipid metabolism in mice. *Commun Biol*. 2023;6:280. https://doi.org/10.1038/s42003-023-04643-2.
114. Katakami N, Matsuhisa M, Kaneto H, et al. Serum endogenous secretory RAGE level is an independent risk factor for the progression of carotid atherosclerosis in type 1 diabetes. *Atherosclerosis*. 2009;204:288–292. https://doi.org/10.1016/j.atherosclerosis.2008.08.026.
115. Yang SJ, Kim S, Hwang SY, et al. Association between sRAGE, esRAGE levels and vascular inflammation: analysis with (18)F-fluorodeoxyglucose positron emission tomography. *Atherosclerosis*. 2012;220:402–406. https://doi.org/10.1016/j.atherosclerosis.2011.11.008.
116. Gaede P, Vedel P, Larsen N, Jensen GV, Parving HH, Pedersen O. Multifactorial intervention and cardiovascular disease in patients with type 2 diabetes. *N Engl J Med*. 2003;348:383–393. https://doi.org/10.1056/NEJMoa021778.
117. Gaede P, Lund-Andersen H, Parving HH, Pedersen O. Effect of a multifactorial intervention on mortality in type 2 diabetes. *N Engl J Med*. 2008; 358:580–591. https://doi.org/10.1056/NEJMoa0706245.
118. Mooradian AD. Dyslipidemia in type 2 diabetes mellitus. *Nat Clin Pract Endocrinol Metab*. 2009;5:150–159. https://doi.org/10.1038/ncpendmet1066.
119. Neeland IJ, Turer AT, Ayers CR, et al. Dysfunctional adiposity and the risk of prediabetes and type 2 diabetes in obese adults. *JAMA*. 2012;308:1150–1159. https://doi.org/10.1001/2012.jama.11132.
120. Adiels M, Olofsson SO, Taskinen MR, Boren J. Overproduction of very low-density lipoproteins is the hallmark of the dyslipidemia in the metabolic syndrome. *Arterioscler Thromb Vasc Biol*. 2008;28:1225–1236. https://doi.org/10.1161/ATVBAHA.107.160192.
121. Teno S, Uto Y, Nagashima H, et al. Association of postprandial hypertriglyceridemia and carotid intima-media thickness in patients with type 2 diabetes. *Diabetes Care*. 2000;23:1401–1406. https://doi.org/10.2337/diacare.23.9.1401.
122. Bansal S, Buring JE, Rifai N, Mora S, Sacks FM, Ridker PM. Fasting compared with nonfasting triglycerides and risk of cardiovascular events in women. *JAMA*. 2007;298:309–316. https://doi.org/10.1001/jama.298.3.309.
123. Pang J, Chan DC, Barrett PH, Watts GF. Postprandial dyslipidaemia and diabetes: mechanistic and therapeutic aspects. *Curr Opin Lipidol*. 2012;23:303–309. https://doi.org/10.1097/MOL.0b013e328354c790.
124. White KT, Moorthy MV, Akinkuolie AO, et al. Identifying an optimal cutpoint for the diagnosis of hypertriglyceridemia in the Nonfasting State. *Clin Chem*. 2015;61:1156–1163. https://doi.org/10.1373/clinchem.2015.241752.
125. Basu D, Goldberg IJ. Regulation of lipoprotein lipase-mediated lipolysis of triglycerides. *Curr Opin Lipidol*. 2020;31:154–160. https://doi.org/10.1097/MOL.0000000000000676.
126. Shang R, Rodrigues B. Lipoprotein lipase as a target for obesity/diabetes related cardiovascular disease. *J Pharm Pharm Sci*. 2024;27:13199. https://doi.org/10.3389/jpps.2024.13199.
127. Ziouzenkova O, Perrey S, Asatryan L, et al. Lipolysis of triglyceride-rich lipoproteins generates PPAR ligands: evidence for an antiinflammatory role for lipoprotein lipase. *Proc Natl Acad Sci U S A*. 2003;100:2730–2735. https://doi.org/10.1073/pnas.0538015100.
128. Augustus A, Yagyu H, Haemmerle G, et al. Cardiac-specific knock-out of lipoprotein lipase alters plasma lipoprotein triglyceride metabolism and cardiac gene expression. *J Biol Chem*. 2004;279:25050–25057. https://doi.org/10.1074/jbc.M401028200.
129. Chawla A, Lee CH, Barak Y, et al. PPARdelta is a very low-density lipoprotein sensor in macrophages. *Proc Natl Acad Sci U S A*. 2003;100:1268–1273. https://doi.org/10.1073/pnas.0337331100.
130. Plutzky J. The PPAR-RXR transcriptional complex in the vasculature: energy in the balance. *Circ Res*. 2011;108:1002–1016. https://doi.org/10.1161/CIRCRESAHA.110.226860.
131. Chakravarthy MV, Lodhi IJ, Yin L, et al. Identification of a physiologically relevant endogenous ligand for PPARalpha in liver. *Cell*. 2009;138:476–488. https://doi.org/10.1016/j.cell.2009.05.036.
132. Haemmerle G, Moustafa T, Woelkart G, et al. ATGL-mediated fat catabolism regulates cardiac mitochondrial function via PPAR-alpha and PGC-1. *Nat Med*. 2011;17:1076–1085. https://doi.org/10.1038/nm.2439.
133. Zheng C, Azcutia V, Aikawa E, et al. Statins suppress apolipoprotein CIII-induced vascular endothelial cell activation and monocyte adhesion. *Eur Heart J*. 2013;34:615–624. https://doi.org/10.1093/eurheartj/ehs271.
134. de la Parra Soto LG, Gutierrez-Uribe JA, Sharma A, Ramirez-Jimenez AK. Is Apo-CIII the new cardiovascular target? An analysis of its current clinical and dietetic therapies. *Nutr Metab Cardiovasc Dis*. 2022;32:295–308. https://doi.org/10.1016/j.numecd.2021.09.035.
135. Kim NH, Kim SG. Fibrates revisited: potential role in cardiovascular risk reduction. *Diabetes Metab J*. 2020;44:213–221. https://doi.org/10.4093/dmj.2020.0001.
136. Brown JD, Plutzky J. Peroxisome proliferator-activated receptors as transcriptional nodal points and therapeutic targets. *Circulation*. 2007;115:518–533. https://doi.org/10.1161/CIRCULATIONAHA.104.475673.
137. Okopien B, Buldak L, Boldys A. Benefits and risks of the treatment with fibrates—a comprehensive summary. *Expert Rev Clin Pharmacol*. 2018;11:1099–1112. https://doi.org/10.1080/17512433.2018.1537780.
138. Rip J, Nierman MC, Ross CJ, et al. Lipoprotein lipase S447X: a naturally occurring gain-of-function mutation. *Arterioscler Thromb Vasc Biol*. 2006;26:1236–1245. https://doi.org/10.1161/01.ATV.0000219283.10832.43.
139. Hsu CC, Kanter JE, Kothari V, Bornfeldt KE. Quartet of APOCs and the different roles they play in diabetes. *Arterioscler Thromb Vasc Biol*. 2023;43:1124–1133. https://doi.org/10.1161/ATVBAHA.122.318290.
140. Ain Q, Cevc M, Marusic T, et al. Genetic and clinical characteristics of patients with lipoprotein lipase deficiency from Slovenia and Pakistan: case series and systematic literature review. *Front Endocrinol (Lausanne)*. 2024;15:1387419. https://doi.org/10.3389/fendo.2024.1387419.
141. Jo SH, Han SH, Kim SH, Eckel RH, Koh KK. Cardiovascular effects of omega-3 fatty acids: hope or hype? *Atherosclerosis*. 2021;322:15–23. https://doi.org/10.1016/j.atherosclerosis.2021.02.014.
142. Bhat S, Sarkar S, Zaffar D, Dandona P, Kalyani RR. Omega-3 fatty acids in cardiovascular disease and diabetes: a review of recent evidence. *Curr Cardiol Rep*. 2023;25:51–65. https://doi.org/10.1007/s11886-022-01831-0.
143. Doi T, Langsted A, Nordestgaard BG. A possible explanation for the contrasting results of REDUCE-IT vs. STRENGTH: cohort study mimicking trial designs. *Eur Heart J*. 2021;42:4807–4817. https://doi.org/10.1093/eurheartj/ehab555.
144. Taskinen MR, Packard CJ, Boren J. Emerging evidence that ApoC-III inhibitors provide novel options to reduce the residual CVD. *Curr Atheroscler Rep*. 2019;21:27. https://doi.org/10.1007/s11883-019-0791-9.
145. Bergmark BA, Marston NA, Prohaska TA, et al. Olezarsen for hypertriglyceridemia in patients at high cardiovascular risk. *N Engl J Med*. 2024;390:1770–1780. https://doi.org/10.1056/NEJMoa2402309.
146. Asztalos BF, Demissie S, Cupples LA, et al. LpA-I, LpA-I:A-II HDL and CHD-risk: the Framingham Offspring Study and the Veterans Affairs HDL Intervention

Trial. *Atherosclerosis*. 2006;188:59–67. https://doi.org/10.1016/j.atherosclerosis.2005.10.018.
147. Badellino KO, Wolfe ML, Reilly MP, Rader DJ. Endothelial lipase concentrations are increased in metabolic syndrome and associated with coronary atherosclerosis. *PLoS Med*. 2006;3:e22. https://doi.org/10.1371/journal.pmed.0030022.
148. Paradis ME, Badellino KO, Rader DJ, et al. Visceral adiposity and endothelial lipase. *J Clin Endocrinol Metab*. 2006;91:3538–3543. https://doi.org/10.1210/jc.2006-0766.
149. Paradis ME, Badellino KO, Rader DJ, et al. Endothelial lipase is associated with inflammation in humans. *J Lipid Res*. 2006;47:2808–2813. https://doi.org/10.1194/jlr.P600002-JLR200.
150. Badellino KO, Wolfe ML, Reilly MP, Rader DJ. Endothelial lipase is increased in vivo by inflammation in humans. *Circulation*. 2008;117:678–685. https://doi.org/10.1161/CIRCULATIONAHA.107.707349.
151. Kingwell BA, Chapman MJ, Kontush A, Miller NE. HDL-targeted therapies: progress, failures and future. *Nat Rev Drug Discov*. 2014;13:445–464. https://doi.org/10.1038/nrd4279.
152. Ahmed W, Orasanu G, Nehra V, Asatryan L, Rader DJ, Ziouzenkova O, Plutzky J. High-density lipoprotein hydrolysis by endothelial lipase activates PPARalpha: a candidate mechanism for high-density lipoprotein-mediated repression of leukocyte adhesion. *Circ Res*. 2006;98:490–498. https://doi.org/10.1161/01.RES.0000205846.46812.be.
153. Li C, Zhang W, Zhou F, et al. Cholesteryl ester transfer protein inhibitors in the treatment of dyslipidemia: a systematic review and meta-analysis. *PLoS One*. 2013;8:e77049. https://doi.org/10.1371/journal.pone.0077049.
154. Davidson MH, Hsieh A, Kastelein JJP. Cholesteryl ester transfer protein inhibition: a pathway to reducing risk of morbidity and promoting longevity. *Curr Opin Lipidol*. 2024;35:303–309. https://doi.org/10.1097/MOL.0000000000000955.
155. Adiels M, Taskinen MR, Boren J. Fatty liver, insulin resistance, and dyslipidemia. *Curr Diab Rep*. 2008;8:60–64. https://doi.org/10.1007/s11892-008-0011-4.
156. Kaylan KB, Paul S. NAFLD no more: a review of current guidelines in the diagnosis and evaluation of metabolic dysfunction-associated steatotic liver disease (MASLD). *Curr Diab Rep*. 2024;25:5. https://doi.org/10.1007/s11892-024-01558-y.
157. Hernando-Redondo J, Nino OC, Fito M. Atherogenic low-density lipoprotein and cardiovascular risk. *Curr Opin Lipidol*. 2024;36:8–13. https://doi.org/10.1097/MOL.0000000000000963.
158. White-Al Habeeb NMA, Higgins V, Wolska A, Delaney SR, Remaley AT, Beriault DR. The present and future of lipid testing in cardiovascular risk assessment. *Clin Chem*. 2023;69:456–469. https://doi.org/10.1093/clinchem/hvad012.
159. Lichtman AH, Binder CJ, Tsimikas S, Witztum JL. Adaptive immunity in atherogenesis: new insights and therapeutic approaches. *J Clin Invest*. 2013;123:27–36. https://doi.org/10.1172/JCI63108.
160. Suciu CF, Prete M, Ruscitti P, Favoino E, Giacomelli R, Perosa F. Oxidized low density lipoproteins: the bridge between atherosclerosis and autoimmunity. Possible implications in accelerated atherosclerosis and for immune intervention in autoimmune rheumatic disorders. *Autoimmun Rev*. 2018;17:366–375. https://doi.org/10.1016/j.autrev.2017.11.028.
161. Pedreno J, Hurt-Camejo E, Wiklund O, Badimon L, Masana L. Platelet function in patients with familial hypertriglyceridemia: evidence that platelet reactivity is modulated by apolipoprotein E content of very-low-density lipoprotein particles. *Metab Clin Exp*. 2000;49:942–949. https://doi.org/10.1053/meta.2000.6742.
162. Patti G, Cavallari I, Andreotti F, et al. Prevention of atherothrombotic events in patients with diabetes mellitus: from antithrombotic therapies to new-generation glucose-lowering drugs. *Nat Rev Cardiol*. 2019;16:113–130. https://doi.org/10.1038/s41569-018-0080-2.
163. Assert R, Scherk G, Bumbure A, Pirags V, Schatz H, Pfeiffer AF. Regulation of protein kinase C by short term hyperglycaemia in human platelets in vivo and in vitro. *Diabetologia*. 2001;44:188–195. https://doi.org/10.1007/s001250051598.
164. Lemkes BA, Hermanides J, Devries JH, Holleman F, Meijers JC, Hoekstra JB. Hyperglycemia: a prothrombotic factor? *J Thromb Haemost*. 2010;8:1663–1669. https://doi.org/10.1111/j.1538-7836.2010.03910.x.
165. Keating FK, Sobel BE, Schneider DJ. Effects of increased concentrations of glucose on platelet reactivity in healthy subjects and in patients with and without diabetes mellitus. *Am J Cardiol*. 2003;92:1362–1365. https://doi.org/10.1016/j.amjcard.2003.08.033.
166. Yamagishi S, Matsui T, Ueda S, Nakamura K, Imaizumi T. Advanced glycation end products (AGEs) and cardiovascular disease (CVD) in diabetes. *Cardiovasc Hematol Agents Med Chem*. 2007;5:236–240. https://doi.org/10.2174/187152507781058681.
167. Undas A, Wiek I, Stepien E, Zmudka K, Tracz W. Hyperglycemia is associated with enhanced thrombin formation, platelet activation, and fibrin clot resistance to lysis in patients with acute coronary syndrome. *Diabetes Care*. 2008;31:1590–1595. https://doi.org/10.2337/dc08-0282.
168. Yngen M, Ostenson CG, Li N, Hjemdahl P, Wallen NH. Acute hyperglycemia increases soluble P-selectin in male patients with mild diabetes mellitus. *Blood Coagul Fibrinolysis*. 2001;12:109–116. https://doi.org/10.1097/00001721-200103000-00004.
169. Ueno M, Ferreiro JL, Desai B, et al. Cigarette smoking is associated with a dose-response effect in clopidogrel-treated patients with diabetes mellitus and coronary artery disease: results of a pharmacodynamic study. *JACC Cardiovasc Interv*. 2012;5:293–300. https://doi.org/10.1016/j.jcin.2011.09.027.
170. Morel O, Kessler L, Ohlmann P, Bareiss P. Diabetes and the platelet: toward new therapeutic paradigms for diabetic atherothrombosis. *Atherosclerosis*. 2010;212:367–376. https://doi.org/10.1016/j.atherosclerosis.2010.03.019.
171. Tsimerman G, Roguin A, Bachar A, Melamed E, Brenner B, Aharon A. Involvement of microparticles in diabetic vascular complications. *Thromb Haemost*. 2011;106:310–321. https://doi.org/10.1160/TH10-11-0712.
172. Li Y, Woo V, Bose R. Platelet hyperactivity and abnormal Ca(2+) homeostasis in diabetes mellitus. *Am J Physiol Heart Circ Physiol*. 2001;280:H1480–1489. https://doi.org/10.1152/ajpheart.2001.280.4.H1480.
173. Dean WL, Chen D, Brandt PC, Vanaman TC. Regulation of platelet plasma membrane Ca2+-ATPase by cAMP-dependent and tyrosine phosphorylation. *J Biol Chem*. 1997;272:15113–15119. https://doi.org/10.1074/jbc.272.24.15113.
174. Schaeffer G, Wascher TC, Kostner GM, Graier WF. Alterations in platelet Ca2+ signalling in diabetic patients is due to increased formation of superoxide anions and reduced nitric oxide production. *Diabetologia*. 1999;42:167–176. https://doi.org/10.1007/s001250051135.
175. Randriamboavonjy V, Isaak J, Elgheznawy A, et al. Calpain inhibition stabilizes the platelet proteome and reactivity in diabetes. *Blood*. 2012;120:415–423. https://doi.org/10.1182/blood-2011-12-399980.
176. Ferreira IA, Mocking AI, Feijge MA, et al. Platelet inhibition by insulin is absent in type 2 diabetes mellitus. *Arterioscler Thromb Vasc Biol*. 2006;26:417–422. https://doi.org/10.1161/01.ATV.0000199519.37089.a0.
177. Hers I. Insulin-like growth factor-1 potentiates platelet activation via the IRS/PI3Kalpha pathway. *Blood*. 2007;110:4243–4252. https://doi.org/10.1182/blood-2006-10-050633.
178. Anfossi G, Mularoni EM, Burzacca S, et al. Platelet resistance to nitrates in obesity and obese NIDDM, and normal platelet sensitivity to both insulin and nitrates in lean NIDDM. *Diabetes Care*. 1998;21:121–126. https://doi.org/10.2337/diacare.21.1.121.
179. Ferretti G, Rabini RA, Bacchetti T, Vignini A, Salvolini E, Ravaglia F, Curatola G, Mazzanti L. Glycated low density lipoproteins modify platelet properties: a compositional and functional study. *J Clin Endocrinol Metab*. 2002;87:2180–2184. https://doi.org/10.1210/jcem.87.5.8466.
180. Anfossi G, Russo I, Trovati M. Platelet dysfunction in central obesity. *Nutr Metab Cardiovasc Dis*. 2009;19:440–449. https://doi.org/10.1016/j.numecd.2009.01.006.
181. Russo I, Traversa M, Bonomo K, et al. In central obesity, weight loss restores platelet sensitivity to nitric oxide and prostacyclin. *Obesity (Silver Spring)*. 2010;18:788–797. https://doi.org/10.1038/oby.2009.302.
182. Freedman JE. Oxidative stress and platelets. *Arterioscler Thromb Vasc Biol*. 2008;28:s11–16. https://doi.org/10.1161/ATVBAHA.107.159178.
183. Schneider DJ. Factors contributing to increased platelet reactivity in people with diabetes. *Diabetes Care*. 2009;32:525–527. https://doi.org/10.2337/dc08-1865.
184. De Cristofaro R, Rocca B, Vitacolonna E, et al. Lipid and protein oxidation contribute to a prothrombotic state in patients with type 2 diabetes mellitus. *J Thromb Haemost*. 2003;1:250–256. https://doi.org/10.1046/j.1538-7836.2003.00072.x.
185. Lim HS, Blann AD, Lip GY. Soluble CD40 ligand, soluble P-selectin, interleukin-6, and tissue factor in diabetes mellitus: relationships to cardiovascular disease and risk factor intervention. *Circulation*. 2004;109:2524–2528. https://doi.org/10.1161/01.CIR.0000129773.70647.94.
186. Gerrits AJ, Koekman CA, van Haeften TW, Akkerman JW. Platelet tissue factor synthesis in type 2 diabetic patients is resistant to inhibition by insulin. *Diabetes*. 2010;59:1487–1495. https://doi.org/10.2337/db09-1008.
187. Barlovic DP, Soro-Paavonen A, Jandeleit-Dahm KA. RAGE biology, atherosclerosis and diabetes. *Clin Sci (Lond)*. 2011;121:43–55. https://doi.org/10.1042/CS20100501.
188. Heywood DM, Mansfield MW, Grant PJ. Factor VII gene polymorphisms, factor VII:C levels and features of insulin resistance in non-insulin-dependent diabetes mellitus. *Thromb Haemost*. 1996;75:401–406.
189. Meade TW, Ruddock V, Stirling Y, Chakrabarti R, Miller GJ. Fibrinolytic activity, clotting factors, and long-term incidence of ischaemic heart disease in the Northwick Park Heart Study. *Lancet*. 1993;342:1076–1079. https://doi.org/10.1016/0140-6736(93)92062-x.
190. Karatela RA, Sainani GS. Interrelationship between coagulation factor VII and obesity in diabetes mellitus (type 2). *Diabetes Res Clin Pract*. 2009;84:e41–44. https://doi.org/10.1016/j.diabres.2009.02.018.
191. Grant PJ. Diabetes mellitus as a prothrombotic condition. *J Intern Med*. 2007;262:157–172. https://doi.org/10.1111/j.1365-2796.2007.01824.x.
192. Aoki I, Shimoyama K, Aoki N, et al. Platelet-dependent thrombin generation in patients with diabetes mellitus: effects of glycemic control on coagulability in diabetes. *J Am Coll Cardiol*. 1996;27:560–566. https://doi.org/10.1016/0735-1097(95)00518-8.
193. Osende JI, Badimon JJ, Fuster V, et al. Blood thrombogenicity in type 2 diabetes mellitus patients is associated with glycemic control. *J Am Coll Cardiol*. 2001;38:1307–1312. https://doi.org/10.1016/s0735-1097(01)01555-8.
194. Koenig W. Fibrin(ogen) in cardiovascular disease: an update. *Thromb Haemost*. 2003;89:601–609.
195. Le DS, Miles R, Savage PJ, Cornell E, Tracy RP, Knowler WC, Krakoff J. The association of plasma fibrinogen concentration with diabetic microvascular complications in young adults with early-onset of type 2 diabetes. *Diabetes Res Clin Pract*. 2008;82:317–323. https://doi.org/10.1016/j.diabres.2008.08.019.

196. Raynaud E, Perez-Martin A, Brun J, Aissa-Benhaddad A, Fedou C, Mercier J. Relationships between fibrinogen and insulin resistance. *Atherosclerosis*. 2000;150:365–370. https://doi.org/10.1016/s0021-9150(99)00373-1.
197. Barazzoni R, Kiwanuka E, Zanetti M, Cristini M, Vettore M, Tessari P. Insulin acutely increases fibrinogen production in individuals with type 2 diabetes but not in individuals without diabetes. *Diabetes*. 2003;52:1851–1856. https://doi.org/10.2337/diabetes.52.7.1851.
198. Zambon A, Gervois P, Pauletto P, Fruchart JC, Staels B. Modulation of hepatic inflammatory risk markers of cardiovascular diseases by PPAR-alpha activators: clinical and experimental evidence. *Arterioscler Thromb Vasc Biol*. 2006;26:977–986. https://doi.org/10.1161/01.ATV.0000204327.96431.9a.
199. Sobel BE, Schneider DJ. Platelet function, coagulopathy, and impaired fibrinolysis in diabetes. *Cardiol Clin*. 2004;22:511–526. https://doi.org/10.1016/j.ccl.2004.06.009.
200. Hernandez-Espinosa D, Ordonez A, Minano A, Martinez-Martinez I, Vicente V, Corral J. Hyperglycaemia impairs antithrombin secretion: possible contribution to the thrombotic risk of diabetes. *Thromb Res*. 2009;124:483–489. https://doi.org/10.1016/j.thromres.2009.05.020.
201. Falciani M, Gori AM, Fedi S, et al. Elevated tissue factor and tissue factor pathway inhibitor circulating levels in ischaemic heart disease patients. *Thromb Haemost*. 1998;79:495–499.
202. Mitchell CT, Kamineni A, Palmas W, Cushman M. Tissue factor pathway inhibitor, vascular risk factors and subclinical atherosclerosis: the Multi-Ethnic Study of Atherosclerosis. *Atherosclerosis*. 2009;207:277–283. https://doi.org/10.1016/j.atherosclerosis.2009.04.024.
203. Zawadzki C, Susen S, Richard F, et al. Dyslipidemia shifts the tissue factor/tissue factor pathway inhibitor balance toward increased thrombogenicity in atherosclerotic plaques: evidence for a corrective effect of statins. *Atherosclerosis*. 2007;195:e117–125. https://doi.org/10.1016/j.atherosclerosis.2006.10.012.
204. Holroyd EW, Simari RD. Interdependent biological systems, multi-functional molecules: the evolving role of tissue factor pathway inhibitor beyond anti-coagulation. *Thromb Res*. 2010;125(suppl 1):S57–59. https://doi.org/10.1016/j.thromres.2010.01.039.
205. Dahlback B, Villoutreix BO. The anticoagulant protein C pathway. *FEBS Lett*. 2005;579:3310–3316. https://doi.org/10.1016/j.febslet.2005.03.001.
206. Yamaji K, Wang Y, Liu Y, et al. Activated protein C, a natural anticoagulant protein, has antioxidant properties and inhibits lipid peroxidation and advanced glycation end products formation. *Thromb Res*. 2005;115:319–325. https://doi.org/10.1016/j.thromres.2004.09.011.
207. Folsom AR, Ohira T, Yamagishi K, Cushman M. Low protein C and incidence of ischemic stroke and coronary heart disease: the Atherosclerosis Risk in Communities (ARIC) Study. *J Thromb Haemost*. 2009;7:1774–1778. https://doi.org/10.1111/j.1538-7836.2009.03577.x.
208. Matsumoto K, Yano Y, Gabazza EC, et al. Inverse correlation between activated protein C generation and carotid atherosclerosis in type 2 diabetic patients. *Diabet Med*. 2007;24:1322–1328. https://doi.org/10.1111/j.1464-5491.2007.02289.x.
209. Li YH, Shi GY, Wu HL. The role of thrombomodulin in atherosclerosis: from bench to bedside. *Cardiovasc Hematol Agents Med Chem*. 2006;4:183–187. https://doi.org/10.2174/187152506776369953.
210. Karakas M, Baumert J, Herder C, et al. Soluble thrombomodulin in coronary heart disease: lack of an association in the MONICA/KORA case-cohort study. *J Thromb Haemost*. 2011;9:1078–1080. https://doi.org/10.1111/j.1538-7836.2011.04229.x.
211. Salomaa V, Wu KK. Soluble thrombomodulin as predictor of incident coronary heart disease. *Lancet*. 1999;354:1646–1647. https://doi.org/10.1016/S0140-6736(05)77134-8.
212. Thorand B, Baumert J, Herder C, Meisinger C, Koenig W. Soluble thrombomodulin as a predictor of type 2 diabetes: results from the MONICA/KORA Augsburg case-cohort study, 1984–1998. *Diabetologia*. 2007;50:545–548. https://doi.org/10.1007/s00125-006-0568-x.
213. Aso Y, Fujiwara Y, Tayama K, Takanashi K, Inukai T, Takemura Y. Relationship between plasma soluble thrombomodulin levels and insulin resistance syndrome in type 2 diabetes: a comparison with von Willebrand factor. *Exp Clin Endocrinol Diabetes*. 2001;109:210–216. https://doi.org/10.1055/s-2001-15108.
214. Aso Y, Fujiwara Y, Tayama K, Takebayashi K, Inukai T, Takemura Y. Relationship between soluble thrombomodulin in plasma and coagulation or fibrinolysis in type 2 diabetes. *Clin Chim Acta*. 2000;301:135–145. https://doi.org/10.1016/s0009-8981(00)00335-1.
215. Dunn EJ, Ariens RA, Grant PJ. The influence of type 2 diabetes on fibrin structure and function. *Diabetologia*. 2005;48:1198–1206. https://doi.org/10.1007/s00125-005-1742-2.
216. Dunn EJ, Philippou H, Ariens RA, Grant PJ. Molecular mechanisms involved in the resistance of fibrin to clot lysis by plasmin in subjects with type 2 diabetes mellitus. *Diabetologia*. 2006;49:1071–1080. https://doi.org/10.1007/s00125-006-0197-4.
217. Pieters M, Covic N, van der Westhuizen FH, et al. Glycaemic control improves fibrin network characteristics in type 2 diabetes—a purified fibrinogen model. *Thromb Haemost*. 2008;99:691–700. https://doi.org/10.1160/TH07-11-0699.
218. Carter AM, Catto AJ, Grant PJ. Determinants of tPA antigen and associations with coronary artery disease and acute cerebrovascular disease. *Thromb Haemost*. 1998;80:632–636.
219. Hoekstra T, Geleijnse JM, Schouten EG, Kluft C. Plasminogen activator inhibitor-type 1: its plasma determinants and relation with cardiovascular risk. *Thromb Haemost*. 2004;91:861–872. https://doi.org/10.1160/TH03-08-0546.
220. Ajjan R, Grant PJ. Coagulation and atherothrombotic disease. *Atherosclerosis*. 2006;186:240–259. https://doi.org/10.1016/j.atherosclerosis.2005.10.042.
221. Alessi MC, Juhan-Vague I. PAI-1 and the metabolic syndrome: links, causes, and consequences. *Arterioscler Thromb Vasc Biol*. 2006;26:2200–2207. https://doi.org/10.1161/01.ATV.0000242905.41404.68.
222. Festa A, Williams K, Tracy RP, Wagenknecht LE, Haffner SM. Progression of plasminogen activator inhibitor-1 and fibrinogen levels in relation to incident type 2 diabetes. *Circulation*. 2006;113:1753–1759. https://doi.org/10.1161/CIRCULATIONAHA.106.616177.
223. Cefalu WT, Schneider DJ, Carlson HE, et al. Effect of combination glipizide GITS/metformin on fibrinolytic and metabolic parameters in poorly controlled type 2 diabetic subjects. *Diabetes Care*. 2002;25:2123–2128. https://doi.org/10.2337/diacare.25.12.2123.
224. Zabczyk M, Ariens RAS, Undas A. Fibrin clot properties in cardiovascular disease: from basic mechanisms to clinical practice. *Cardiovasc Res*. 2023;119:94–111. https://doi.org/10.1093/cvr/cvad017.
225. Hori Y, Gabazza EC, Yano Y, et al. Insulin resistance is associated with increased circulating level of thrombin-activatable fibrinolysis inhibitor in type 2 diabetic patients. *J Clin Endocrinol Metab*. 2002;87:660–665. https://doi.org/10.1210/jcem.87.2.8214.
226. Yano Y, Kitagawa N, Gabazza EC, et al. Increased plasma thrombin-activatable fibrinolysis inhibitor levels in normotensive type 2 diabetic patients with microalbuminuria. *J Clin Endocrinol Metab*. 2003;88:736–741. https://doi.org/10.1210/jc.2002-020691.
227. Colucci M, D'Aprile AM, Italia A, Gresele P, Morser J, Semeraro N. Thrombin activatable fibrinolysis inhibitor (TAFI) does not inhibit in vitro thrombolysis by pharmacological concentrations of t-PA. *Thromb Haemost*. 2001;85:661–666.
228. Meltzer ME, Doggen CJ, de Groot PG, Rosendaal FR, Lisman T. Plasma levels of fibrinolytic proteins and the risk of myocardial infarction in men. *Blood*. 2010;116:529–536. https://doi.org/10.1182/blood-2010-01-263103.
229. Sakkinen PA, Cushman M, Psaty BM, et al. Relationship of plasmin generation to cardiovascular disease risk factors in elderly men and women. *Arterioscler Thromb Vasc Biol*. 1999;19:499–504. https://doi.org/10.1161/01.atv.19.3.499.
230. Bryk AH, Siudut J, Broniatowska E, et al. Sex-specific alteration to alpha2-antiplasmin incorporation in patients with type 2 diabetes. *Thromb Res*. 2020;185:55–62. https://doi.org/10.1016/j.thromres.2019.09.032.
231. Kanno Y, Hirota M, Matsuo O, Ozaki KI. α2-antiplasmin positively regulates endothelial-to-mesenchymal transition and fibrosis progression in diabetic nephropathy. *Mol Biol Rep*. 2022;49:205–215. https://doi.org/10.1007/s11033-021-06859-z.
232. Guimaraes AH, de Bruijne EL, Lisman T, et al. Hypofibrinolysis is a risk factor for arterial thrombosis at young age. *Br J Haematol*. 2009;145:115–120. https://doi.org/10.1111/j.1365-2141.2008.07568.x.
233. Goldfine AB, Beckman JA, Betensky RA, et al. Family history of diabetes is a major determinant of endothelial function. *J Am Coll Cardiol*. 2006;47:2456–2461. https://doi.org/10.1016/j.jacc.2006.02.045.
234. Moncada S, Higgs A. The L-arginine-nitric oxide pathway. *N Engl J Med*. 1993;329:2002–2012. https://doi.org/10.1056/NEJM199312303292706.
235. Furchgott RF, Zawadzki JV. The obligatory role of endothelial cells in the relaxation of arterial smooth muscle by acetylcholine. *Nature*. 1980;288:373–376. https://doi.org/10.1038/288373a0.
236. Kinlay S, Libby P, Ganz P. Endothelial function and coronary artery disease. *Curr Opin Lipidol*. 2001;12:383–389. https://doi.org/10.1097/00041433-200108000-00003.
237. Adams JA, Uryash A, Lopez JR, Sackner MA. The endothelium as a therapeutic target in diabetes: a narrative review and perspective. *Front Physiol*. 2021;12:638491. https://doi.org/10.3389/fphys.2021.638491.
238. Gerszten RE, Garcia-Zepeda EA, Lim YC, et al. MCP-1 and IL-8 trigger firm adhesion of monocytes to vascular endothelium under flow conditions. *Nature*. 1999;398:718–723. https://doi.org/10.1038/19546.
239. Theodorakopoulou MP, Schoina M, Sarafidis P. Assessment of endothelial and microvascular function in CKD: older and newer techniques, associated risk factors, and relations with outcomes. *Am J Nephrol*. 2020;51:931–949. https://doi.org/10.1159/000512263.
240. Johnstone MT, Creager SJ, Scales KM, Cusco JA, Lee BK, Creager MA. Impaired endothelium-dependent vasodilation in patients with insulin-dependent diabetes mellitus. *Circulation*. 1993;88:2510–2516. https://doi.org/10.1161/01.cir.88.6.2510.
241. Williams SB, Cusco JA, Roddy MA, Johnstone MT, Creager MA. Impaired nitric oxide-mediated vasodilation in patients with non-insulin-dependent diabetes mellitus. *J Am Coll Cardiol*. 1996;27:567–574. https://doi.org/10.1016/0735-1097(95)00522-6.
242. Li JM, Shah AM. Endothelial cell superoxide generation: regulation and relevance for cardiovascular pathophysiology. *Am J Physiol Regul Integr Comp Physiol*. 2004;287:R1014–1030. https://doi.org/10.1152/ajpregu.00124.2004.
243. Takaya T, Hirata K, Yamashita T, et al. A specific role for eNOS-derived reactive oxygen species in atherosclerosis progression. *Arterioscler Thromb Vasc Biol*. 2007;27:1632–1637. https://doi.org/10.1161/ATVBAHA.107.142182.
244. Gallo G, Savoia C. New insights into endothelial dysfunction in cardiometabolic diseases: potential mechanisms and clinical implications. *Int J Mol Sci*. 2024;25:2973. https://doi.org/10.3390/ijms25052973.
245. Steinberg HO, Tarshoby M, Monestel R, et al. Elevated circulating free fatty acid levels impair endothelium-dependent vasodilation. *J Clin Invest*. 1997;100:1230–1239. https://doi.org/10.1172/JCI119636.

246. Griffin ME, Marcucci MJ, Cline GW, et al. Free fatty acid-induced insulin resistance is associated with activation of protein kinase C theta and alterations in the insulin signaling cascade. *Diabetes*. 1999;48:1270–1274. https://doi.org/10.2337/diabetes.48.6.1270.
247. Engin A. Endothelial dysfunction in obesity and therapeutic targets. *Adv Exp Med Biol*. 2024;1460:489–538. https://doi.org/10.1007/978-3-031-63657-8_17.
248. Dickhout JG, Hossain GS, Pozza LM, Zhou J, Lhotak S, Austin RC. Peroxynitrite causes endoplasmic reticulum stress and apoptosis in human vascular endothelium: implications in atherogenesis. *Arterioscler Thromb Vasc Biol*. 2005;25:2623–2629. https://doi.org/10.1161/01.ATV.0000189159.96900.d9.
249. Paixao J, Dinis TC, Almeida LM. Dietary anthocyanins protect endothelial cells against peroxynitrite-induced mitochondrial apoptosis pathway and Bax nuclear translocation: an in vitro approach. *Apoptosis*. 2011;16:976–989. https://doi.org/10.1007/s10495-011-0632-y.
250. Zou MH, Shi C, Cohen RA. High glucose via peroxynitrite causes tyrosine nitration and inactivation of prostacyclin synthase that is associated with thromboxane/prostaglandin H(2) receptor-mediated apoptosis and adhesion molecule expression in cultured human aortic endothelial cells. *Diabetes*. 2002;51:198–203. https://doi.org/10.2337/diabetes.51.1.198.
251. Bauersachs J, Schafer A. Tetrahydrobiopterin and eNOS dimer/monomer ratio—a clue to eNOS uncoupling in diabetes? *Cardiovasc Res*. 2005;65:768–769. https://doi.org/10.1016/j.cardiores.2004.12.011.
252. Kar S, Bhandar B, Kavdia M. Impact of SOD in eNOS uncoupling: a two-edged sword between hydrogen peroxide and peroxynitrite. *Free Radic Res*. 2012;46:1496–1513. https://doi.org/10.3109/10715762.2012.731052.
253. Gow AJ, Farkouh CR, Munson DA, Posencheg MA, Ischiropoulos H. Biological significance of nitric oxide-mediated protein modifications. *Am J Physiol Lung Cell Mol Physiol*. 2004;287:L262–268. https://doi.org/10.1152/ajplung.00295.2003.
254. Ceriello A, Mercuri F, Quagliaro L, et al. Detection of nitrotyrosine in the diabetic plasma: evidence of oxidative stress. *Diabetologia*. 2001;44:834–838. https://doi.org/10.1007/s001250100529.
255. Kanda T, Brown JD, Orasanu G, et al. PPARgamma in the endothelium regulates metabolic responses to high-fat diet in mice. *J Clin Invest*. 2009;119:110–124. https://doi.org/10.1172/JCI36233.
256. Tsuchiya K, Tanaka J, Shuiqing Y, et al. FoxOs integrate pleiotropic actions of insulin in vascular endothelium to protect mice from atherosclerosis. *Cell Metab*. 2012;15:372–381. https://doi.org/10.1016/j.cmet.2012.01.018.
257. Qiang L, Tsuchiya K, Kim-Muller JY, Lin HV, Welch C, Accili D. Increased atherosclerosis and endothelial dysfunction in mice bearing constitutively deacetylated alleles of Foxo1 gene. *J Biol Chem*. 2012;287:13944–13951. https://doi.org/10.1074/jbc.M111.332767.
258. Li H, Cybulsky MI, Gimbrone Jr. MA, Libby P. An atherogenic diet rapidly induces VCAM-1, a cytokine-regulatable mononuclear leukocyte adhesion molecule, in rabbit aortic endothelium. *Arterioscler Thromb*. 1993;13:197–204. https://doi.org/10.1161/01.atv.13.2.197.
259. Cybulsky MI, Gimbrone Jr. MA. Endothelial expression of a mononuclear leukocyte adhesion molecule during atherogenesis. *Science*. 1991;251:788–791. https://doi.org/10.1126/science.1990440.
260. de Lemos JA, Hennekens CH, Ridker PM. Plasma concentration of soluble vascular cell adhesion molecule-1 and subsequent cardiovascular risk. *J Am Coll Cardiol*. 2000;36:423–426. https://doi.org/10.1016/s0735-1097(00)00742-7.
261. Maganto-Garcia E, Tarrio ML, Grabie N, Bu DX, Lichtman AH. Dynamic changes in regulatory T cells are linked to levels of diet-induced hypercholesterolemia. *Circulation*. 2011;124:185–195. https://doi.org/10.1161/CIRCULATIONAHA.110.006411.
262. Hernandez-Mijares A, Rocha M, Rovira-Llopis S, et al. Human leukocyte/endothelial cell interactions and mitochondrial dysfunction in type 2 diabetic patients and their association with silent myocardial ischemia. *Diabetes Care*. 2013;36:1695–1702. https://doi.org/10.2337/dc12-1224.
263. Fukuda D, Pham PT, Sata M. Emerging roles of the innate immune system regulated by DNA sensors in the development of vascular and metabolic diseases. *J Atheroscler Thromb*. 2022;29:297–307. https://doi.org/10.5551/jat.RV17059.
264. Ley K, Laudanna C, Cybulsky MI, Nourshargh S. Getting to the site of inflammation: the leukocyte adhesion cascade updated. *Nat Rev Immunol*. 2007;7:678–689. https://doi.org/10.1038/nri2156.
265. Tabas I. Consequences and therapeutic implications of macrophage apoptosis in atherosclerosis: the importance of lesion stage and phagocytic efficiency. *Arterioscler Thromb Vasc Biol*. 2005;25:2255–2264. https://doi.org/10.1161/01.ATV.0000184783.04864.9f.
266. Farb A, Burke AP, Tang AL, et al. Coronary plaque erosion without rupture into a lipid core. A frequent cause of coronary thrombosis in sudden coronary death. *Circulation*. 1996;93:1354–1363. https://doi.org/10.1161/01.cir.93.7.1354.
267. Libby P, Pasterkamp G, Crea F, Jang IK. Reassessing the mechanisms of acute coronary syndromes. *Circ Res*. 2019;124:150–160. https://doi.org/10.1161/CIRCRESAHA.118.311098.
268. Gimbrone Jr. MA, Topper JN, Nagel T, Anderson KR, Garcia-Cardena G. Endothelial dysfunction, hemodynamic forces, and atherogenesis. *Ann N Y Acad Sci*. 2000;902:230–239. https://doi.org/10.1111/j.1749-6632.2000.tb06318.x. discussion 239-240.
269. Tamargo IA, Baek KI, Kim Y, Park C, Jo H. Flow-induced reprogramming of endothelial cells in atherosclerosis. *Nat Rev Cardiol*. 2023;20:738–753. https://doi.org/10.1038/s41569-023-00883-1.
270. Hajra L, Evans AI, Chen M, Hyduk SJ, Collins T, Cybulsky MI. The NF-kappa B signal transduction pathway in aortic endothelial cells is primed for activation in regions predisposed to atherosclerotic lesion formation. *Proc Natl Acad Sci U S A*. 2000;97:9052–9057. https://doi.org/10.1073/pnas.97.16.9052.
271. Castelli WP. Lipids, risk factors and ischaemic heart disease. *Atherosclerosis*. 1996;124(suppl):S1–9. https://doi.org/10.1016/0021-9150(96)05851-0.
272. Cannon CP, Braunwald E, McCabe CH, et al. Intensive versus moderate lipid lowering with statins after acute coronary syndromes. *N Engl J Med*. 2004;350:1495–1504. https://doi.org/10.1056/NEJMoa040583.
273. Manta E, Thomopoulos C, Kariori M, et al. Revisiting cardiovascular benefits of blood pressure reduction in primary and secondary prevention: focus on targets and residual risk - a systematic review and meta-analysis. *Hypertension*. 2024;81:1076–1086. https://doi.org/10.1161/HYPERTENSIONAHA.123.22610.
274. Ridker PM, Cushman M, Stampfer MJ, Tracy RP, Hennekens CH. Inflammation, aspirin, and the risk of cardiovascular disease in apparently healthy men. *N Engl J Med*. 1997;336:973–979. https://doi.org/10.1056/NEJM199704033361401.
275. Ridker PM, Buring JE, Shih J, Matias M, Hennekens CH. Prospective study of C-reactive protein and the risk of future cardiovascular events among apparently healthy women. *Circulation*. 1998;98:731–733. https://doi.org/10.1161/01.cir.98.8.731.
276. Despres JP. Abdominal obesity and cardiovascular disease: is inflammation the missing link? *Can J Cardiol*. 2012;28:642–652. https://doi.org/10.1016/j.cjca.2012.06.004.
277. d'Aiello A, Filomia S, Brecciaroli M, Sanna T, Pedicino D, Liuzzo G. Targeting inflammatory pathways in atherosclerosis: exploring new opportunities for treatment. *Curr Atheroscl Rep*. 2024;26:707–719. https://doi.org/10.1007/s11883-024-01241-3.
278. Gomes MB, Piccirillo LJ, Nogueira VG, Matos HJ. Acute-phase proteins among patients with type 1 diabetes. *Diabetes Metab*. 2003;29:405–411. https://doi.org/10.1016/s1262-3636(07)70051-4.
279. Schaumberg DA, Glynn RJ, Jenkins AJ, et al. Effect of intensive glycemic control on levels of markers of inflammation in type 1 diabetes mellitus in the diabetes control and complications trial. *Circulation*. 2005;111:2446–2453. https://doi.org/10.1161/01.CIR.0000165064.31505.3B.
280. Davis FM, Gallagher KA. Epigenetic mechanisms in monocytes/macrophages regulate inflammation in cardiometabolic and vascular disease. *Arterioscler Thromb Vasc Biol*. 2019;39:623–634. https://doi.org/10.1161/ATVBAHA.118.312135.
281. Gistera A, Hansson GK. The immunology of atherosclerosis. *Nat Rev Nephrol*. 2017;13:368–380. https://doi.org/10.1038/nrneph.2017.51.
282. Soehnlein O, Libby P. Targeting inflammation in atherosclerosis—from experimental insights to the clinic. *Nat Rev Drug Discov*. 2021;20:589–610. https://doi.org/10.1038/s41573-021-00198-1.
283. Kanter JE, Bornfeldt KE. Inflammation and diabetes-accelerated atherosclerosis: myeloid cell mediators. *Trends Endocrinol Metab*. 2013;24:137–144. https://doi.org/10.1016/j.tem.2012.10.002.
284. Bradshaw EM, Raddassi K, Elyaman W, et al. Monocytes from patients with type 1 diabetes spontaneously secrete proinflammatory cytokines inducing Th17 cells. *J Immunol*. 2009;183:4432–4439. https://doi.org/10.4049/jimmunol.0900576.
285. Wieland EB, Kempen LJ, Donners MM, Biessen EA, Goossens P. Macrophage heterogeneity in atherosclerosis: a matter of context. *Eur J Immunol*. 2024;54:e2350464. https://doi.org/10.1002/eji.202350464.
286. Luo M, Zhao F, Cheng H, Su M, Wang Y. Macrophage polarization: an important role in inflammatory diseases. *Front Immunol*. 2024;15:1352946. https://doi.org/10.3389/fimmu.2024.1352946.
287. Swirski FK, Libby P, Aikawa E, et al. Ly-6Chi monocytes dominate hypercholesterolemia-associated monocytosis and give rise to macrophages in atheromata. *J Clin Invest*. 2007;117:195–205. https://doi.org/10.1172/JCI29950.
288. Schloss MJ, Swirski FK, Nahrendorf M. Modifiable cardiovascular risk, hematopoiesis, and innate immunity. *Circ Res*. 2020;126:1242–1259. https://doi.org/10.1161/CIRCRESAHA.120.315936.
289. Brown AL, Zhu X, Rong S, et al. Omega-3 fatty acids ameliorate atherosclerosis by favorably altering monocyte subsets and limiting monocyte recruitment to aortic lesions. *Arterioscler Thromb Vasc Biol*. 2012;32:2122–2130. https://doi.org/10.1161/ATVBAHA.112.253435.
290. Kanter JE, Kramer F, Barnhart S, et al. Diabetes promotes an inflammatory macrophage phenotype and atherosclerosis through acyl-CoA synthetase 1. *Proc Natl Acad Sci U S A*. 2012;109:E715–724. https://doi.org/10.1073/pnas.1111600109.
291. Jialal I, Kaur H, Devaraj S. Toll-like receptor status in obesity and metabolic syndrome: a translational perspective. *J Clin Endocrinol Metab*. 2014;99:39–48. https://doi.org/10.1210/jc.2013-3092.
292. Devaraj S, Tobias P, Kasinath BS, Ramsamooj R, Afify A, Jialal I. Knockout of toll-like receptor-2 attenuates both the proinflammatory state of diabetes and incipient diabetic nephropathy. *Arterioscler Thromb Vasc Biol*. 2011;31:1796–1804. https://doi.org/10.1161/ATVBAHA.111.228924.
293. Liao X, Sluimer JC, Wang Y, et al. Macrophage autophagy plays a protective role in advanced atherosclerosis. *Cell Metab*. 2012;15:545–553. https://doi.org/10.1016/j.cmet.2012.01.022.
294. Ozcan U, Yilmaz E, Ozcan L, et al. Chemical chaperones reduce ER stress and restore glucose homeostasis in a mouse model of type 2 diabetes. *Science*. 2006;313:1137–1140. https://doi.org/10.1126/science.1128294.
295. Hotamisligil GS. Endoplasmic reticulum stress and atherosclerosis. *Nat Med*. 2010;16:396–399. https://doi.org/10.1038/nm0410-396.

296. Yilmaz E. Endoplasmic reticulum stress and obesity. *Adv Exp Med Biol.* 2024;1460:373–390. https://doi.org/10.1007/978-3-031-63657-8_13.
297. Ren J, Bi Y, Sowers JR, Hetz C, Zhang Y. Endoplasmic reticulum stress and unfolded protein response in cardiovascular diseases. *Nat Rev Cardiol.* 2021;18:499–521. https://doi.org/10.1038/s41569-021-00511-w.
298. Hansson GK, Jonasson L. The discovery of cellular immunity in the atherosclerotic plaque. *Arterioscler Thromb Vasc Biol.* 2009;29:1714–1717. https://doi.org/10.1161/ATVBAHA.108.179713.
299. Desai S, Bhonde R, Sharma H, et al. Th1-Th2 seesaw: an essential aspect in type 1 diabetes. *Curr Diabetes Rev.* 2022;18:e080322201918. https://doi.org/10.2174/1573399818666220308162514.
300. Mendez-Garcia LA, Escobedo G, Baltazar-Perez I, et al. Exploring the Th2 response in obesity and metabolic dysfunction-associated steatotic liver disease (MASLD): a potential modulator of the renin-angiotensin system (RAS) pathway in hypertension development. *Life (Basel).* 2024;14:1080. https://doi.org/10.3390/life14091080.
301. Giubilato S, Liuzzo G, Brugaletta S, et al. Expansion of CD4+CD28null T-lymphocytes in diabetic patients: exploring new pathogenetic mechanisms of increased cardiovascular risk in diabetes mellitus. *Eur Heart J.* 2011;32:1214–1226. https://doi.org/10.1093/eurheartj/ehq499.
302. Deiuliis J, Shah Z, Shah N, et al. Visceral adipose inflammation in obesity is associated with critical alterations in tregulatory cell numbers. *PLoS one.* 2011;6:e16376. https://doi.org/10.1371/journal.pone.0016376.
303. Albany CJ, Trevelin SC, Giganti G, Lombardi G, Scotta C. Getting to the heart of the matter: the role of regulatory T-cells (Tregs) in cardiovascular disease (CVD) and atherosclerosis. *Front Immunol.* 2019;10:2795. https://doi.org/10.3389/fimmu.2019.02795.
304. Montero D, Walther G, Perez-Martin A, Vicente-Salar N, Roche E, Vinet A. Vascular smooth muscle function in type 2 diabetes mellitus: a systematic review and meta-analysis. *Diabetologia.* 2013;56:2122–2133. https://doi.org/10.1007/s00125-013-2974-1.
305. Fleischhacker E, Esenabhalu VE, Spitaler M, et al. Human diabetes is associated with hyperreactivity of vascular smooth muscle cells due to altered subcellular Ca2+ distribution. *Diabetes.* 1999;48:1323–1330. https://doi.org/10.2337/diabetes.48.6.1323.
306. Christopher J, Velarde V, Zhang D, Mayfield D, Mayfield RK, Jaffa AA. Regulation of B(2)-kinin receptors by glucose in vascular smooth muscle cells. *Am J Physiol Heart Circ Physiol.* 2001;280:H1537–1546. https://doi.org/10.1152/ajpheart.2001.280.4.H1537.
307. Sun J, Xu Y, Dai Z, Sun Y. Intermittent high glucose enhances proliferation of vascular smooth muscle cells by upregulating osteopontin. *Mol Cell Endocrinol.* 2009;313:64–69. https://doi.org/10.1016/j.mce.2009.08.019.
308. Li SL, Reddy MA, Cai Q, et al. Enhanced proatherogenic responses in macrophages and vascular smooth muscle cells derived from diabetic db/db mice. *Diabetes.* 2006;55:2611–2619. https://doi.org/10.2337/db06-0164.
309. Reddy MA, Jin W, Villeneuve L, et al. Pro-inflammatory role of microrna-200 in vascular smooth muscle cells from diabetic mice. *Arterioscler Thromb Vasc Biol.* 2012;32:721–729. https://doi.org/10.1161/ATVBAHA.111.241109.
310. Mao L, Yin R, Yang L, Zhao D. Role of advanced glycation end products on vascular smooth muscle cells under diabetic atherosclerosis. *Front Endocrinol (Lausanne).* 2022;13:983723. https://doi.org/10.3389/fendo.2022.983723.
311. Rosenson RS, Wright RS, Farkouh M, Plutzky J. Modulating peroxisome proliferator-activated receptors for therapeutic benefit? Biology, clinical experience, and future prospects. *Am Heart J.* 2012;164:672–680. https://doi.org/10.1016/j.ahj.2012.06.023.
312. Marx N, Schonbeck U, Lazar MA, Libby P, Plutzky J. Peroxisome proliferator-activated receptor gamma activators inhibit gene expression and migration in human vascular smooth muscle cells. *Circ Res.* 1998;83:1097–1103. https://doi.org/10.1161/01.res.83.11.1097.
313. Marx N, Mach F, Sauty A, et al. Peroxisome proliferator-activated receptor-gamma activators inhibit IFN-gamma-induced expression of the T cell-active CXC chemokines IP-10, Mig, and I-TAC in human endothelial cells. *J Immunol.* 2000;164:6503–6508. https://doi.org/10.4049/jimmunol.164.12.6503.
314. Glass CK, Ogawa S. Combinatorial roles of nuclear receptors in inflammation and immunity. *Nat Rev Immunol.* 2006;6:44–55. https://doi.org/10.1038/nri1748.
315. Derosa G, Sahebkar A, Maffioli P. The role of various peroxisome proliferator-activated receptors and their ligands in clinical practice. *J Cell Physiol.* 2018;233:153–161. https://doi.org/10.1002/jcp.25804.
316. Li AC, Binder CJ, Gutierrez A, et al. Differential inhibition of macrophage foam-cell formation and atherosclerosis in mice by PPARalpha, beta/delta, and gamma. *J Clin Invest.* 2004;114:1564–1576. https://doi.org/10.1172/JCI18730.
317. Lee CH, Chawla A, Urbiztondo N, Liao D, Boisvert WA, Evans RM. Curtiss LK. Transcriptional repression of atherogenic inflammation: modulation by PPARdelta. *Science.* 2003;302:453–457. https://doi.org/10.1126/science.1087344.
318. Plutzky J. Medicine. PPARs as therapeutic targets: reverse cardiology? *Science.* 2003;302:406–407. https://doi.org/10.1126/science.1091172.
319. Cariou B, Charbonnel B, Staels B. Thiazolidinediones and PPARγ agonists: time for a reassessment. *Trends Endocrinol Metab.* 2012;23:205–215. https://doi.org/10.1016/j.tem.2012.03.001.
320. Nissen SE, Wolski K. Effect of rosiglitazone on the risk of myocardial infarction and death from cardiovascular causes. *N Engl J Med.* 2007;356:2457–2471. https://doi.org/10.1056/NEJMoa072761.
321. Dormandy JA, Charbonnel B, Eckland DJ, et al. Secondary prevention of macrovascular events in patients with type 2 diabetes in the PROactive Study (PROspective pioglitAzone Clinical Trial In macroVascular Events): a randomised controlled trial. *Lancet.* 2005;366:1279–1289. https://doi.org/10.1016/S0140-6736(05)67528-9.
322. Orasanu G, Ziouzenkova O, Devchand PR, et al. The peroxisome proliferator-activated receptor-gamma agonist pioglitazone represses inflammation in a peroxisome proliferator-activated receptor-alpha-dependent manner in vitro and in vivo in mice. *J Am Coll Cardiol.* 2008;52:869–881. https://doi.org/10.1016/j.jacc.2008.04.055.
323. Young LH, Viscoli CM, Curtis JP, et al. Cardiac outcomes after ischemic stroke or transient ischemic attack: effects of pioglitazone in patients with insulin resistance without diabetes mellitus. *Circulation.* 2017;135:1882–1893. https://doi.org/10.1161/CIRCULATIONAHA.116.024863.
324. Yaghi S, Furie KL, Viscoli CM, et al. Pioglitazone prevents stroke in patients with a recent transient ischemic attack or ischemic stroke: a planned secondary analysis of the IRIS trial (Insulin Resistance Intervention After Stroke). *Circulation.* 2018;137:455–463. https://doi.org/10.1161/CIRCULATIONAHA.117.030458.
325. Graham DJ, Ouellet-Hellstrom R, MaCurdy TE, et al. Risk of acute myocardial infarction, stroke, heart failure, and death in elderly Medicare patients treated with rosiglitazone or pioglitazone. *JAMA.* 2010;304:411–418. https://doi.org/10.1001/jama.2010.920.
326. Lebovitz HE. Thiazolidinediones: the forgotten diabetes medications. *Curr Diab Rep.* 2019;19:151. https://doi.org/10.1007/s11892-019-1270-y.
327. Rubins HB, Robins SJ, Collins D, et al. Gemfibrozil for the secondary prevention of coronary heart disease in men with low levels of high-density lipoprotein cholesterol. Veterans Affairs High-Density Lipoprotein Cholesterol Intervention Trial Study Group. *N Engl J Med.* 1999;341:410–418. https://doi.org/10.1056/NEJM199908053410604.
328. Keech A, Simes RJ, Barter P, et al. Effects of long-term fenofibrate therapy on cardiovascular events in 9795 people with type 2 diabetes mellitus (the FIELD study): randomised controlled trial. *Lancet.* 2005;366:1849–1861. https://doi.org/10.1016/S0140-6736(05)67667-2.
329. Ginsberg HN, Elam MB, et al. ACCORD Study Group Effects of combination lipid therapy in type 2 diabetes mellitus. *N Engl J Med.* 2010;362:1563–1574. https://doi.org/10.1056/NEJMoa1001282.
330. Das Pradhan A, Glynn RJ, Fruchart JC, et al. Triglyceride lowering with pemafibrate to reduce cardiovascular risk. *N Engl J Med.* 2022;387:1923–1934. https://doi.org/10.1056/NEJMoa2210645.
331. Marinho LL, Everett BM, Aday AW, et al. Effect of pemafibrate on diabetic foot ulceration and gangrene: an exploratory analysis from PROMINENT. *J Am Coll Cardiol.* 2024;84:408–410. https://doi.org/10.1016/j.jacc.2024.05.028.
332. Bhatt DL, Steg PG, Miller M, et al. Cardiovascular risk reduction with icosapent ethyl for hypertriglyceridemia. *N Engl J Med.* 2019;380:11–22. https://doi.org/10.1056/NEJMoa1812792.
333. Lotta LA, Stewart ID, Sharp SJ, et al. Association of genetically enhanced lipoprotein lipase-mediated lipolysis and low-density lipoprotein cholesterol-lowering alleles with risk of coronary disease and type 2 diabetes. *JAMA Cardiol.* 2018;3:957–966. https://doi.org/10.1001/jamacardio.2018.2866.
334. Colhoun HM, Betteridge DJ, Durrington PN, et al. Primary prevention of cardiovascular disease with atorvastatin in type 2 diabetes in the Collaborative Atorvastatin Diabetes Study (CARDS): multicentre randomised placebo-controlled trial. *Lancet.* 2004;364:685–696. https://doi.org/10.1016/S0140-6736(04)16895-5.
335. Brugts JJ, Yetgin T, Hoeks SE, et al. The benefits of statins in people without established cardiovascular disease but with cardiovascular risk factors: meta-analysis of randomised controlled trials. *BMJ.* 2009;338:b2376. https://doi.org/10.1136/bmj.b2376.
336. Ridker PM, Danielson E, Fonseca FA, et al. Rosuvastatin to prevent vascular events in men and women with elevated C-reactive protein. *N Engl J Med.* 2008;359:2195–2207. https://doi.org/10.1056/NEJMoa0807646.
337. Oesterle A, Laufs U, Liao JK. Pleiotropic effects of statins on the cardiovascular system. *Circ Res.* 2017;120:229–243. https://doi.org/10.1161/CIRCRESAHA.116.308537.
338. Duewell P, Kono H, Rayner KJ, et al. NLRP3 inflammasomes are required for atherogenesis and activated by cholesterol crystals. *Nature.* 2010;464:1357–1361. https://doi.org/10.1038/nature08938.
339. Ridker PM, Everett BM, Thuren T, et al. Antiinflammatory therapy with canakinumab for atherosclerotic disease. *N Engl J Med.* 2017;377:1119–1131. https://doi.org/10.1056/NEJMoa1707914.
340. Ridker PM, Rane M. Interleukin-6 signaling and anti-interleukin-6 therapeutics in cardiovascular disease. *Circ Res.* 2021;128:1728–1746. https://doi.org/10.1161/CIRCRESAHA.121.319077.
341. Everett BM, Pradhan AD, Solomon DH, et al. Rationale and design of the Cardiovascular Inflammation Reduction Trial: a test of the inflammatory hypothesis of atherothrombosis. *Am Heart J.* 2013;166:199–207. https://doi.org/10.1016/j.ahj.2013.03.018. e115.
342. Ridker PM, Everett BM, Pradhan A, et al. Low-dose methotrexate for the prevention of atherosclerotic events. *N Engl J Med.* 2019;380:752–762. https://doi.org/10.1056/NEJMoa1809798.
343. Deftereos SG, Beerkens FJ, Shah B, et al. Colchicine in cardiovascular disease: in-depth review. *Circulation.* 2022;145:61–78. https://doi.org/10.1161/CIRCULATIONAHA.121.056171.
344. Nidorf SM, Fiolet ATL, Eikelboom JW, et al. The effect of low-dose colchicine in patients with stable coronary artery disease: the LoDoCo2 trial rationale, design, and baseline characteristics. *Am Heart J.* 2019;218:46–56. https://doi.org/10.1016/j.ahj.2019.09.011.
345. Bouabdallaoui N, Tardif JC, Waters DD, et al. Time-to-treatment initiation of colchicine and cardiovascular outcomes after myocardial infarction

in the Colchicine Cardiovascular Outcomes Trial (COLCOT). *Eur Heart J.* 2020;41:4092–4099. https://doi.org/10.1093/eurheartj/ehaa659.

346. Jolly SS, d'Entremont MA, Lee SF, et al. Colchicine in acute myocardial infarction. *N Engl J Med.* 2024;392:633–642. https://doi.org/10.1056/NEJMoa2405922.
347. Jha KK, Adhikari R, Tasdighi E, Osuji N, Rajan T, Blaha MJ. Transitioning to GLP-1 RAs and SGLT2 inhibitors as the first choice for managing cardiometabolic risk in type 2 diabetes. *Curr Atheroscl Rep.* 2022;24:925–937. https://doi.org/10.1007/s11883-022-01066-y.
348. Ndumele CE, Neeland IJ, Tuttle KR, et al. A synopsis of the evidence for the science and clinical management of cardiovascular-kidney-metabolic (CKM) syndrome: a scientific statement from the American Heart Association. *Circulation.* 2023;148:1636–1664. https://doi.org/10.1161/CIR.0000000000001186.
349. American Diabetes Association Professional Practice Committee 10. Cardiovascular disease and risk management: standards of care in diabetes-2024. *Diabetes Care.* 2024;47:S179–S218. https://doi.org/10.2337/dc24-S010.
350. Huang XD, Jiang DS, Feng X, Fang ZM. The benefits of oral glucose-lowering agents: GLP-1 receptor agonists, DPP-4 and SGLT-2 inhibitors on myocardial ischaemia/reperfusion injury. *Eur J Pharmacol.* 2024;976:176698. https://doi.org/10.1016/j.ejphar.2024.176698.
351. Vallon V. State-of-the-art-review: mechanisms of action of SGLT2 inhibitors and clinical implications. *Am J Hypertens.* 2024;37:841–852. https://doi.org/10.1093/ajh/hpae092.

8 Risk Stratification Among Patients With Type 2 Diabetes With or at Risk for Atherosclerotic Cardiovascular Disease

DAVID D. BERG

INTRODUCTION

Type 2 diabetes (T2D) accelerates vascular injury and atherogenesis. Accordingly, T2D is a powerful risk factor for atherosclerotic cardiovascular disease (ASCVD) and its complications, including cardiovascular death, myocardial infarction (MI), and ischemic stroke.[1] However, whereas the aggregate population-level impact of T2D on ASCVD risk is substantial, there is enormous heterogeneity in individual risk of ASCVD among patients with T2D, in part because of their varied clinical characteristics and the diverse pathogenetic mechanisms driving their glucose dysregulation. This variability in risk is seen both in patients with established ASCVD and in those without manifest ASCVD and underscores the importance of effective risk stratification in this population. Refining cardiovascular risk assessment of patients with T2D allows clinicians to appropriately focus the intensity of preventive efforts and allows patients to make informed decisions about managing their own cardiovascular risk.

Multiple tools exist for stratifying risk of ASCVD among patients with T2D, including clinical risk scores, blood-based biomarkers, and cardiovascular imaging studies. In this chapter, we will review the current landscape of instruments used to evaluate ASCVD risk in patients with T2D across the spectrum of primary and secondary prevention. Risk stratification for other types of cardiovascular complications of T2D, including heart failure (see Chapter 15), is covered in other chapters.

TYPE 2 DIABETES AND ATHEROSCLEROTIC CARDIOVASCULAR DISEASE

Epidemiology of Atherosclerotic Cardiovascular Disease Risk in Type 2 Diabetes

Many studies dating back to the 1970s have demonstrated the epidemiologic link between T2D and risk of ASCVD[2] (see also Chapter 6). Although conventional risk factors for ASCVD, including hypertension and dyslipidemia, tend to cluster with T2D, this clustering does not fully account for the excess atherothrombotic risk seen with T2D. In a large meta-analysis of nearly 700,000 individuals from 102 prospective studies, there was an approximate twofold excess in risk of coronary heart disease, stroke, and other vascular diseases conferred by the presence of T2D, independent from other conventional risk factors.[3]

Older studies suggested that these adverse vascular effects resulted in comparable ASCVD risk profiles between diabetic patients without prior MI and nondiabetic patients with prior MI, leading to the notion that T2D should be considered a coronary heart disease risk equivalent.[4] However, with greater attention to the importance of intensive risk factor modification in patients with diabetes,[5] incidence rates of ASCVD-related morbidity and mortality have steadily declined over the last three decades,[6,7] such that T2D alone no longer has the same prognostic significance as a prior MI.[8] Nevertheless, due to the dramatic increase in the prevalence of T2D over that same time period, the overall burden of T2D-related atherothrombotic complications has continued to climb.[6]

Mechanisms of Atherosclerotic Cardiovascular Disease Risk in Type 2 Diabetes

Multiple molecular and cellular mechanisms are responsible for diabetes-associated atherosclerosis[9] (see also Chapters 7 and 19). For example, both hyperglycemia and insulin resistance directly contribute to the formation of advanced glycation end-products and reactive oxygen species (ROS), as well as mitochondrial dysfunction. These processes collectively result in endothelial dysfunction, vascular inflammation, and activation of vascular smooth muscle cells.[10] The dyslipidemia that generally accompanies T2D further accelerates atherogenesis, because oxidized low-density lipoprotein (LDL) particles are deposited in the subendothelial layer of affected portions of the vasculature. Dysfunctional endothelium promotes activation and adhesion of monocytes, which exit the circulation and engulf these oxidized LDL particles, forming lipid-laden foam cells that drive progression of atherosclerotic lesions. Indeed, studies comparing the composition of atherosclerotic plaques in patients with and without T2D have demonstrated that the former contain more lipid-rich atheroma and macrophage infiltration.[11]

Beyond accelerating atherogenesis, diabetes directly promotes atherothrombosis through several mechanisms. For instance, the vascular inflammation that drives atherosclerotic progression also contributes to atherosclerotic plaque instability.[12] In addition, diabetes promotes platelet activation and the release of thrombogenic substances contained within platelet granules.[13] Finally, diabetes increases circulating concentrations of multiple prothrombotic proteins and decreases the concentrations of anticoagulant proteins. Collectively, the prothrombotic milieu that accompanies T2D supports thrombus formation at the site of ruptured atherosclerotic plaques.

The diverse pathophysiological mechanisms by which diabetes contributes to ASCVD underscores the complexity of a disease that paradoxically is defined by a single metabolite—glucose. Mirroring the variable cardiovascular clinical risk profiles of patients with T2D, the pathways driving diabetes-associated atherothrombosis are also highly variable across individuals with T2D. Understanding the basis for this heterogeneity has been and remains an important area of investigation.

HETEROGENEITY OF CARDIOVASCULAR RISK PROFILES IN DIABETES

The varied clinical profiles of patients with diabetes can be characterized through different lenses. The conventional classification system for diabetes is not inherently defined by associations with cardiovascular risk, but rather by the suspected mechanism of dysglycemia.[14] Type 1 diabetes (T1D) results from autoimmune destruction of pancreatic β-cells resulting in absolute insulin deficiency, whereas T2D is a nonautoimmune process characterized by varying degrees of insulin resistance and deficiency (see also Chapters 1 and 5). Other atypical forms of diabetes that do not fit cleanly in the category of T1D or T2D are also part of the current classification system, including some with known genetic causes (e.g., mature-onset diabetes of the young) and some related to diseases of the exocrine pancreas. With deeper understanding of the genetic and metabolomic architecture of different subgroups of patients with diabetes, these categories are continuing to evolve.

Another emerging paradigm for classifying diabetes has been to leverage advances in machine learning techniques to define data-driven metabolic subphenotypes with the goal of expanding our understanding of underlying disease mechanisms and potentially guiding therapeutic approaches. One such effort identified five novel clusters of individuals with adult-onset diabetes using six variables that can be monitored in clinical practice.[15] Interestingly, these clusters not only have distinct clinical features but are associated with varying risk of diabetes-related complications, including coronary heart disease. The heterogeneity in the cardiovascular risk profiles of these clusters highlights the important link between metabolic characteristics and cardiovascular disease manifestations and suggests that this type of framework may eventually be important for precision cardiovascular treatment approaches.

Another more clinically oriented view of the heterogeneous profiles of patients with diabetes is to classify them directly in relation to cardiovascular risk factor control. This concept stems from the evidence-based understanding that multifactorial risk factor management can prevent or delay diabetes-related cardiovascular complications,[5] which has led professional society guidelines to focus not only on glycemic control but also on the management of blood pressure, lipids, and kidney disease risk in this population.[16] In a large cohort study from the Swedish National Diabetes Register that included more than 270,000 individuals with T2D followed for a median of 5.7 years, individuals were categorized by age and according to the presence of five cardiovascular risk factors—elevated glycated hemoglobin (HbA_{1c}), elevated LDL cholesterol, albuminuria, smoking, and elevated blood pressure.[17] When all five of these risk factors were within target ranges, individuals with T2D had only marginal or no excess risk of death, stroke, and MI compared to the general population. However, with each successive increase in the number of risk factors not within the target range, there was a stepwise increase in ASCVD risk. Moreover, age was an important effect modifier of this relationship, such that the incremental cardiovascular risk associated with having poorly controlled risk factors was especially pronounced in younger patients.

Thus, while T2D is a powerful risk factor for ASCVD and its complications, cardiovascular risk is not uniformly elevated in patients with T2D. This increased but varying risk underscores the importance of individualized risk assessment as well as patient-centered considerations when managing cardiovascular risk in patients with diabetes.

PREVENTIVE THERAPIES TO REDUCE CARDIOVASCULAR RISK IN PATIENTS WITH TYPE 2 DIABETES

A broad range of therapeutic strategies, including lifestyle interventions, pharmacologic therapies, and procedural interventions (e.g., coronary artery bypass grafting) have been shown to reduce the risk of cardiovascular complications in patients with T2D (see also Chapters 3, 4, 12, and 13). Over the last decade, the results of multiple large cardiovascular outcomes trials motivated by regulatory directives to demonstrate cardiovascular safety in at-risk populations (see also Chapter 11), have specifically expanded the evidence base supporting the use of certain antihyperglycemic therapies.[18–24] The emergence of these pharmacotherapies, which include sodium-glucose cotransporter-2 inhibitors (SGLT2i) and glucagon-like peptide 1 receptor agonists (GLP-1 RAs), as well as other novel agents, including lipid-lowering therapies[25] and antiplatelet agents,[26–28] have dramatically altered the treatment armamentarium for cardiovascular primary and secondary prevention in T2D.[29]

The full spectrum of therapies used to manage cardiovascular risk in patients with T2D is covered in detail in later chapters. Here, we provide a general overview of these preventive therapies and their effects on ASCVD outcomes to frame the discussion around the value of ASCVD risk stratification.

Glucose-Lowering Medications With Cardiovascular Benefit

Because of its efficacy for lowering glucose and its generally favorable safety profile, metformin has traditionally been viewed as the foundational pharmacologic therapy for patients with T2D. However, while multiple preclinical and clinical studies suggest a potential atheroprotective effect of metformin, there are limited studies directly evaluating the effects of metformin on hard clinical outcomes.[30] In the 10-year posttrial monitoring study of the United Kingdom Prospective Diabetes Study (UKPDS), patients treated with metformin (n = 342) had a significantly lower risk of MI (risk ratio [RR], 0.67; 95% confidence interval [CI], 0.51–0.89) and all-cause mortality (RR, 0.71; 95% CI, 0.59–0.89) compared to those randomized to nonintensive glucose control.[31] Nevertheless, in the larger A Diabetes Outcome Progression Trial (ADOPT), which randomized 4360 patients with newly diagnosed T2D to metformin, glyburide, or rosiglitazone, metformin use did not reduce the risk of cardiovascular events relative to the other agents over a median follow-up of 4 years.[32] Notably, both trials enrolled low-risk populations and thus were limited by low event rates.

Both SGLT2i and GLP-1 RA were also initially introduced as antihyperglycemic agents. SGLT2i lower blood glucose by enhancing urinary glucose excretion, and GLP-1 RAs do so by augmenting glucose-dependent insulin secretion and glucagon suppression. Importantly, the cardiovascular outcomes trials evaluating these agents have demonstrated their powerful cardioprotective properties independent of their glucose-lowering effects, which has shifted the focus of their use towards comprehensive cardiovascular risk reduction.[29,33]

In a meta-analysis of six cardiovascular outcomes trials of four SGLT2i agents enrolling a combined 46,969 patients with T2D, the SGLT2i class was shown to reduce the risk of cardiovascular death by 15% (hazard ratio [HR], 0.85; 95% CI, 0.78–0.93) and of major adverse cardiovascular events (MACE), a composite of cardiovascular death, MI, or ischemic stroke, by 10% (HR, 0.90; 95% CI, 0.85–0.90).[34] Although the pathophysiological mechanisms underlying each component of this composite outcome may be heterogeneous, treatment effects on MACE are generally viewed as modifying ASCVD risk. SGLT2i also robustly reduces the risk of hospitalization for heart failure by 32% (HR, 0.68; 95% CI, 0.61–0.76) and of kidney disease progression by 38% (HR, 0.62; 95% CI, 0.56–0.70).[34]

In a meta-analysis of eight GLP-1 RA trials, comprising 60,080 patients with T2D, the GLP-1 RA class was shown to reduce cardiovascular death by 13% (HR, 0.87; 95% CI, 0.80–0.94) and MACE by 14% (HR, 0.86; 95% CI, 0.80–0.93).[35] Notably, there is clinically important heterogeneity within the GLP-1 RA class. Specifically, semaglutide, dulaglutide, and liraglutide have the most favorable cardiovascular outcomes data,[22–24] and are therefore the agents recommended by current guidelines. Compared to the SGLT2i, the effects of GLP-1 RA on hospitalization for heart failure (HR, 0.89; 95% CI, 0.82–0.98) and kidney disease progression (HR, 0.86; 95% CI, 0.72–1.02) are more modest.[35] However, GLP-1 RA are more effective than SGLT2i for reducing HbA_{1c} and body weight. Thus while the benefits with respect to ASCVD risk reduction are quite similar between the two classes, selection between these agents is often driven by considerations related to their other salutary benefits.

Cardiovascular Risk Factor Management

In addition to using glucose-lowering therapies with known cardiovascular benefits, managing other ASCVD risk factors that tend to cluster with T2D, including hypertension and dyslipidemia, is an important aspect of the multifactorial approach to reducing cardiovascular risk in T2D.[16]

Individual clinical trials testing strategies of intensive blood pressure lowering in patients with T2D have yielded varying results.[36,37] Nevertheless, the totality of the data suggests that targeting lower blood pressures reduces the risk of ASCVD events, with the trade-off of increasing the risk of adverse events related to episodes of hypotension (e.g., syncope). Thus guidelines recommend a blood pressure goal of <130/80 mm Hg in all patients with T2D if this target can be safely attained.

Lowering LDL cholesterol is the cornerstone of ASCVD risk management. In a meta-analysis of 18,686 individuals with T2D from 14 randomized trials of statin therapy followed for a mean of 4.3 years, there was a 13% proportional reduction (rate ratio [RR], 0.87; 99% CI, 0.76–1.00; p = .008) in vascular mortality and a 21% proportional reduction in major vascular events (RR, 0.79; 99% CI, 0.72–0.86; p <0.0001) per mmol/L reduction in LDL cholesterol.[38] Thus statin therapy is recommended for all patients with T2D. For patients with T2D and ASCVD, the addition of ezetimibe or a PCSK9 inhibitor is recommended when an LDL cholesterol goal of <55 mg/dL is not achieved on maximum tolerated statin therapy. The benefit of these therapies with respect to ASCVD risk reduction has been demonstrated in subgroup analyses of patients with T2D enrolled in the pivotal cardiovascular outcomes trials of these agents.[39,40]

TABLE 8.1 Diabetes-Specific Models for ASCVD Risk Prediction in Patients With Type 2 Diabetes

RISK MODEL	PUBLICATION YEAR	DERIVATION COHORT: DATA SOURCE	N	REGIONS SAMPLED	OUTCOME PREDICTED BY RISK MODEL	CLINICAL VARIABLES IN RISK MODEL
Primary Prevention						
UKPDS-Risk Engine (*UKPDS-RE*)	2001	UKDPS	4540	United Kingdom	Fatal and nonfatal CHD or ischemic stroke	Age, gender, ethnicity, diabetes duration, HbA_{1c}, smoking status, atrial fibrillation, SBP, total cholesterol, LDL-C
Advance Risk Model	2011	ADVANCE	7168	Asia, Australia, Europe, Canada	MI, stroke, or vascular death	Age at diagnosis, gender, diabetes duration, pulse pressure, retinopathy, atrial fibrillation, HbA_{1c}, UACR, non-HDL-C, treated hypertension
SCORE2-Diabetes	2023	SCID, CPRD, UK Biobank, ERFC	229,460	Europe, United States	MI, stroke, cardiovascular death	Age, gender, smoking, SBP, total cholesterol, HDL-C, age at diabetes diagnosis, HbA_{1c}, eGFR
Primary and Secondary Prevention						
Diabetes Lifetime-Perspective (*DIAL*) Model	2019	Swedish National Diabetes Register	389,366	Sweden	MI, stroke, vascular death	Age, gender, smoking, SBP, BMI, HbA_{1c}, eGFR, non-HDL-C, UACR, diabetes duration, insulin use, and history of CVD
TIMI Risk Score for Atherothrombosis in Diabetes	2023	SAVOR-TIMI 53, DECLARE-TIMI 58	23,643	Africa, Asia, Australia, Europe, North America, South America	Fatal and nonfatal MI or ischemic stroke	Age, gender, waist circumference (or BMI), HbA_{1c}, insulin use, eGFR, UACR, smoking, SBP, LDL-C, prior CAD, prior MI, PAD, prior ischemic stroke, prior PCI, prior CABG

ADVANCE, Action in Diabetes and Vascular disease: preterax and diamicron-MR controlled evaluation; *CABG*, coronary artery bypass grafting; *CAD*, coronary artery disease; *CHD*, coronary heart disease; *CPRD*, Clinical Practice Research Datalink; *eGFR*, estimated glomerular filtration rate; *ERFC*, Emerging Risk Factors Collaboration; *HbA_{1c}*, glycated hemoglobin; *HDL-C*, high-density lipoprotein-cholesterol; *LDL-C*, low-density lipoprotein-cholesterol; *MI*, myocardial infarction; *PAD*, peripheral artery disease; *PCI*, percutaneous coronary intervention; *SBP*, systolic blood pressure; *SCID*, Scottish Care Information-Diabetes; *UACR*, urine albumin-creatinine ratio; *UKPDS*, United Kingdom Prospective Diabetes Study.

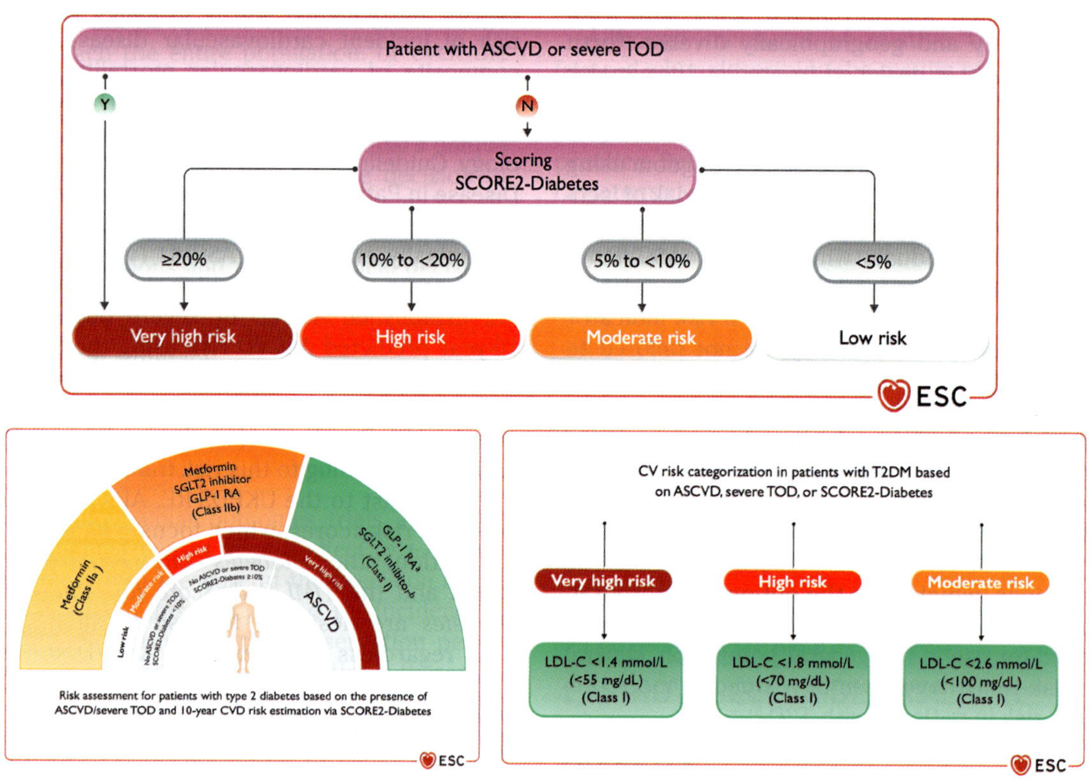

FIG. 8.1 Atherosclerotic cardiovascular disease (*ASCVD*) risk stratification framework in the 2023 European Society of Cardiology (*ESC*) Guidelines for the management of cardiovascular disease in patients with diabetes. *ASCVD*, atherosclerotic cardiovascular disease; *CV*, cardiovascular; *CVD*, cardiovascular disease; *GLP-1 RA*, glucagon-like peptide 1 receptor agonist; *LDL-C*, low-density lipoprotein-cholesterol; *SGLT2*, sodium-glucose cotransporter 2; *T2DM*, type 2 diabetes mellitus; *TOD*, target organ damage. (From *Eur Heart J*. 2023;44(39):4043–4140.)

mass index (BMI), HbA_{1c}, estimated glomerular filtration rate (eGFR), non-HDL cholesterol, albuminuria, diabetes duration, insulin use, and history of CVD.[56] An interactive calculator is available at https://U-Prevent.com/, which combines DIAL model predictions of absolute risk with relative treatment effects from clinical trials to estimate absolute treatment benefit from selected cardiovascular therapies. The TIMI Risk Score for Atherothrombosis in Diabetes was developed and validated in a pooled cohort of 42,181 patients with T2D enrolled in four large cardiovascular outcomes trials.[57] The model predicts risk of fatal and nonfatal MI or ischemic stroke using 16 clinical variables, including 10 variables that apply to all patients with T2D (age, gender, waist circumference [or BMI], HbA_{1c}, insulin use, eGFR, albuminuria, smoking status, SBP, and LDL-C) and 6 variables that reflect the extent of prior atherosclerotic disease in those with known ASCVD (coronary artery disease, prior MI, PAD, prior ischemic stroke, prior percutaneous coronary intervention, and prior coronary artery bypass grafting). The risk model has good discrimination and is well calibrated in patients with and without established ASCVD. It has also been shown to identify strong gradients of absolute treatment benefit from cardiovascular therapies, including SGLT2i and lipid-lowering therapies (PCSK9i). An online calculator is available at https://timibiostat.shinyapps.io/calculators/.

Although beyond the scope of this chapter focused on patients with T2D, several clinical risk scores have been developed for use in patients with T1D, including a model for incident CVD that was developed in the Scottish Care Information-Diabetes register ($n = 27{,}527$) and validated in the Swedish National Diabetes Register ($n = 33{,}183$).[58]

TABLE 8.2 Circulating Protein Biomarkers With Well-Established Associations With ASCVD Risk in Patients With Type 2 Diabetes

BIOMARKER	DESCRIPTION
LDL cholesterol	• Primary atherogenic lipoprotein and the target of most lipid-lowering therapies • Lowering LDL-C has been proven to reduce ASCVD risk
Non-HDL cholesterol	• Includes cholesterol content of all atherogenic lipoproteins, including LDL, IDL, triglyceride-rich lipoproteins (VLDL, chylomicrons, remnants), and lipoprotein (a) • Calculated as the difference between total cholesterol and HDL cholesterol
Apolipoprotein B-100 (*ApoB*)	• Key structural protein component of all atherogenic lipoproteins • There is exactly one apoB molecule on each atherogenic apoB-containing particle • Strongest association with ASCVD risk among lipid biomarkers
C-reactive protein (high-sensitivity assay)	• Biomarker of systemic inflammation • Stronger association with incident ASCVD than recurrent ASCVD
Cardiac troponin (high-sensitivity assay)	• Complex of three regulatory proteins involved in cardiac muscle contraction • Detection in circulation provides direct biochemical evidence of myocardial injury • May provide subclinical indication of cardiac structural abnormality
BNP/NT-proBNP	• Hormone secreted by cardiomyocytes in response to myocardial stretch (hemodynamic stress) • May provide subclinical indication of cardiac structural abnormality

ASCVD, Atherosclerotic cardiovascular disease; *BNP*, B-type natriuretic peptide; *IDL*, intermediate-density lipoproteins; *NT-proBNP*, N-terminal prohormone of B-type natriuretic peptide; *VLDL*, very low-density lipoprotein.

BIOMARKER-BASED ATHEROSCLEROTIC CARDIOVASCULAR DISEASE RISK ASSESSMENT IN PATIENTS WITH TYPE 2 DIABETES

Although most ASCVD risk prediction frameworks used in clinical practice are based primarily on a patient's clinical characteristics, emerging evidence suggests that blood-based biomarkers can help refine ASCVD risk assessment and inform clinical decision making (Table 8.2).

LDL cholesterol is the most important atherogenic lipoprotein in the bloodstream and the target of most lipid-lowering therapies. Nevertheless, other lipid biomarkers, including *non-HDL cholesterol* and *apolipoprotein B-100 (apoB)*, may be superior markers of ASCVD risk. This is because both biomarkers also incorporate other atherogenic lipoprotein subfractions, many of which tend to be particularly elevated in patients with T2D (e.g., triglyceride-rich lipoproteins). Non-HDL cholesterol comprises the cholesterol content of all atherogenic lipoproteins, including LDL, intermediate-density lipoproteins (IDL), triglyceride-rich lipoproteins (very low-density lipoprotein [VLDL], chylomicrons, and their remnants), and lipoprotein (a) [Lp(a)]. It can be easily calculated from a standard lipid panel as total cholesterol minus HDL cholesterol. ApoB is a key structural protein component of each of these atherogenic lipoproteins. Since there is exactly one apoB molecule on each atherogenic apoB-containing particle, measuring apoB enables direct quantification of the total burden of atherogenic particles in the bloodstream. Recent evidence suggests that apoB is the best discriminator of atherothrombotic risk among all lipid parameters,[59] which may suggest that the total number of apoB containing lipoproteins is a more important risk factor for ASCVD than lipid content (cholesterol or triglycerides) or a specific type of lipoprotein.

High-sensitivity C-reactive protein (hsCRP), a biomarker of systemic inflammation, has also been linked to risk of developing T2D and to the risk of incident ASCVD. It has been shown to improve ASCVD risk stratification when added to clinical variables in multiple epidemiologic cohorts, including the Women's Health Study and the Atherosclerosis Risk in Communities (ARIC) study.[60,61] As a result, it has also been incorporated into some general primary prevention risk tools, including the Reynolds Risk Score.[62]

Circulating cardiac-specific biomarkers primarily used in other clinical settings also offer important prognostic information about ASCVD risk in patients with T2D, perhaps by offering insights into subclinical cardiac structural abnormalities. These include the natriuretic peptides (*B-type natriuretic peptide [BNP]* and *N-terminal prohormone of B-type natriuretic peptide [NT-proBNP]*), which are biomarkers of hemodynamic stress most often used in the diagnosis of heart failure,[63] and *cardiac troponin (cTn)*, the canonical biomarker of myocardial injury most often used in the diagnosis of MI.[64]

In a substudy from the BARI 2D (Bypass Angioplasty Revascularization Investigation in Type 2 Diabetes) trial (n = 2,285), which randomized patients with T2D and stable ischemic heart disease to prompt coronary revascularization plus intensive medical therapy or intensive medical therapy alone, cardiac troponin T measured at baseline using a high-sensitivity assay (hsTnT) was a strong, independent predictor of subsequent cardiovascular death, MI, or stroke in models adjusted for cardiovascular risk factors, diabetes severity, electrocardiographic abnormalities, and coronary anatomy (adjusted HR, 1.85; 95% CI, 1.48–2.32).[65]

The associations between cardiac-specific biomarkers and ASCVD risk were also examined in a biomarker substudy (n = 12,310) of the SAVOR (Saxagliptin Assessment of Vascular Outcomes Recorded in Patients with Diabetes Mellitus)-TIMI 53 trial, which enrolled patients with T2D and either established ASCVD or multiple risk factors for ASCVD.[66] In this cohort, elevated levels of hsTnT and NT-proBNP measured at the time of trial enrollment strongly predicted the risk of cardiovascular death, MI, and ischemic stroke during the trial observation period, and these biomarkers significantly improved risk discrimination when added to clinical variables. By contrast, hsCRP was only weakly associated with atherothrombotic outcomes in this analysis, suggesting that this inflammatory biomarker may be less prognostically relevant in patients with clinically manifest ASCVD or with a substantial burden of ASCVD risk factors.[66] In a biomarker substudy (n = 14,565) from the DECLARE (Dapagliflozin Effect on Cardiovascular Events)-TIMI 58 trial, hsTnT and NT-proBNP were again shown to be strongly associated with risk of cardiovascular death, MI, and ischemic stroke in patients with T2D and elevated ASCVD risk. In addition, each of these biomarkers identified patients at particularly high risk of MACE, who had greater absolute reduction in MACE event rates with the SGLT2i dapagliflozin.[67]

Other novel protein biomarkers may provide complementary prognostic information about orthogonal axes of ASCVD risk in patients with T2D. For example, soluble suppression of tumorigenesis-2 (sST2), a biomarker reflecting vascular congestion, tissue inflammation, and fibrosis, and insulin-like growth factor-binding protein 7, a biomarker of cellular senescence, were both shown to predict risk of MACE in patients with T2D enrolled in the CANVAS trial. When these markers were used in combination with hsTnT, discrimination of MACE risk was superior to that of any one biomarker alone, demonstrating the potential value of multimarker ASCVD risk stratification in T2D.[68]

Advances in genomic and proteomic technologies have also motivated interest in using "-omics"-based approaches to refine ASCVD risk stratification. For instance, many common genetic variants associated with ASCVD risk have been identified through genome-wide association studies, and the cumulative genetic risk associated with these genetic variants can be captured in *polygenic risk scores*. Polygenic risk scores for specific forms of ASCVD (e.g., coronary artery disease, ischemic stroke) have been shown to improve discrimination of ASCVD risk when added to clinical variables,[69] and may be particularly helpful when used in younger individuals who have not yet developed ASCVD or ASCVD risk factors.[70] Analogous to large-scale genomic testing, it is now possible to simultaneously measure a very large number of proteins in a single blood sample. Like polygenic risk scores, protein risk scores derived from large-scale proteomics have been shown to improve ASCVD risk stratification compared with clinical variables alone.[71] However, to date, there are limited data on the performance of such genomic and proteomic risk scores, specifically in patients with T2D.

IMAGING-BASED ATHEROSCLEROTIC CARDIOVASCULAR DISEASE RISK ASSESSMENT IN PATIENTS WITH TYPE 2 DIABETES

Cardiovascular imaging studies may help refine ASCVD risk assessment in patients with T2D. Although cardiovascular imaging is most often pursued in the evaluation of clinical symptoms, there has been long-standing interest in using imaging techniques to screen asymptomatic patients with T2D for ASCVD, both because of their increased risk and because the presence of T2D may blunt their appreciation of ischemic pain. Some cardiovascular imaging techniques, such as computed tomography (CT), are based on direct visualization of existing atherosclerosis (i.e., anatomic assessment), whereas other imaging studies assess the functional consequences of clinically significant ASCVD (i.e., myocardial ischemia). Both approaches provide prognostic information about ASCVD risk in patients with T2D, but CT has the strongest evidence base for use in this setting.

Computed Tomography

Electron beam CT and multidetector row CT (MDCT) are noninvasive techniques that enable direct detection of coronary atherosclerosis. Since atherosclerotic plaques result in intimal calcium deposition, CT can be used to visualize and quantify *coronary artery calcification (CAC)* as a measure of coronary atherosclerotic burden. CAC scoring is highly sensitive for coronary atherosclerosis, but it cannot be used to visualize the extent of coronary artery stenosis. To do this, angiographic contrast must be administered and images must be obtained in the coronary arterial phase. This modality, known as *coronary CT angiography (CCTA)*, permits highly accurate detection of obstructive coronary artery disease.

Among asymptomatic individuals with no known coronary artery disease, those with T2D are up to five times more likely to have clinically significant CAC (Agatson score ≥100) as compared to those without T2D.[72] Moreover, in studies of asymptomatic patients with T2D undergoing screening CCTA, approximately one-third have at least one coronary lesion with ≥50% stenosis.[73] On the other hand, approximately one-third of asymptomatic patients with T2D have virtually no detectable coronary calcium (Agatson score <10), demonstrating the substantial phenotypic variability in ASCVD burden among patients with T2D.

Many studies have demonstrated that CAC is a strong, independent predictor of coronary heart disease events with prognostic value that adds to standard clinical risk stratification.[74] Moreover, there is an important interaction between CAC score and T2D, such that each incrementally higher CAC value is associated with a greater increase in ASCVD risk in patients with T2D compared to those without.[75] At the same time, patients with T2D who have no detectable coronary calcium have very low short- and intermediate-term risk of ASCVD events, comparable to that of patients without T2D and a CAC score of 0.[75] However, in observational studies with longer-term follow-up (>10 years), patients with T2D and a CAC score of 0 do appear to have a somewhat higher ASCVD risk than those without T2D and a CAC score of 0, suggesting that the "warranty period" of a CAC score of 0 may be shorter in patients with T2D than it is in patients without T2D. Thus CAC scoring is a powerful tool for ASCVD risk assessment in patients with T2D; however, given the dynamic nature of the atherosclerotic processes driving vascular calcification, serial assessment of CAC may be important for optimal ASCVD risk prediction.

There are limited data comparing the relative prognostic value of CAC scoring versus CCTA. In practice, CCTA is generally used only when a patient either has active ischemic symptoms or when knowledge of the burden and location of obstructive coronary lesions may be important for guiding clinical decision making with respect to revascularization, rather than for initial ASCVD risk stratification.

Stress Testing

Stress testing with radionuclide myocardial perfusion imaging, echocardiography, or magnetic resonance imaging can be used to detect myocardial ischemia. Although stress testing is generally reserved for the evaluation of patients with anginal symptoms, prospective studies of these modalities suggest that approximately 20% of asymptomatic individuals with T2D have silent myocardial ischemia.[76] Furthermore, when stress testing is pursued sequentially after CAC scoring, approximately 50% of asymptomatic patients with T2D and Agatson score ≥100 will have detectable ischemia.[77]

There are limited data on the prognostic significance of detectable ischemia in asymptomatic patients with T2D, but their risk of adverse ASCVD events is comparable to that of symptomatic patients with T2D and detectable ischemia.[78] In addition, normal myocardial perfusion imaging generally reflects low short-term ASCVD risk, though the "warranty period" associated with a normal study is likely shorter than that of a CAC score of 0. Thus it remains uncertain whether stress testing adds clinically important incremental prognostic information beyond CAC scoring. As such, the routine use of stress testing for ASCVD risk stratification in asymptomatic patients with T2D is not recommended by the guidelines.

SUMMARY

T2D is a well-established risk factor for ASCVD, but individual ASCVD risk is highly heterogenous among patients with T2D. Given the varied clinical risk profiles of patients with T2D and the numerous available therapies for cardiovascular prevention, it is important to individualize treatment approaches in this population. ASCVD risk stratification allows clinicians to make well-informed decisions about the risk-benefit calculus of initiating new preventive therapies, and thus to appropriately focus the intensity of preventive efforts. Existing tools used to assess ASCVD risk in patients with T2D include clinical risk scores, blood-based biomarkers, and cardiovascular imaging studies.

REFERENCES

1. Martin SS, Aday AW, Allen NB, et al. Heart disease and stroke statistics: A report of US and global data from the american heart association. *Circulation*. 2025;151(8):e41–e660.
2. Kannel WB, McGee DL. Diabetes and glucose tolerance as risk factors for cardiovascular disease: the Framingham study. *Diabetes Care*. 1979;2(2): 120–126.
3. Sarwar N, Gao P, et al. Emerging Risk Factors Collaboration Diabetes mellitus, fasting blood glucose concentration, and risk of vascular disease: a collaborative meta-analysis of 102 prospective studies. *Lancet*. 2010;375(9733):2215–2222.
4. Haffner SM, Lehto S, Ronnemaa T, Pyorala K, Laakso M. Mortality from coronary heart disease in subjects with type 2 diabetes and in nondiabetic subjects with and without prior myocardial infarction. *N Engl J Med*. 1998;339(4):229–234.
5. Gaede P, Lund-Andersen H, Parving HH, Pedersen O. Effect of a multifactorial intervention on mortality in type 2 diabetes. *N Engl J Med*. 2008;358(6): 580–591.
6. Gregg EW, Li Y, Wang J, et al. Changes in diabetes-related complications in the United States, 1990–2010. *N Engl J Med*. 2014;370(16):1514–1523.
7. Ali MK, Bullard KM, Saaddine JB, Cowie CC, Imperatore G, Gregg EW. Achievement of goals in U.S. diabetes care, 1999–2010. *N Engl J Med*. 2013;368(17):1613–1624.
8. Bulugahapitiya U, Siyambalapitiya S, Sithole J, Idris I. Is diabetes a coronary risk equivalent? Systematic review and meta-analysis. *Diabet Med*. 2009;26(2):142–148.
9. Low Wang CC, Hess CN, Hiatt WR, Goldfine AB. Clinical update: cardiovascular disease in diabetes mellitus: atherosclerotic cardiovascular disease and heart failure in type 2 diabetes mellitus - mechanisms, management, and clinical considerations. *Circulation*. 2016;133(24):2459–2502.
10. Bornfeldt KE. 2013 Russell Ross memorial lecture in vascular biology: cellular and molecular mechanisms of diabetes mellitus-accelerated atherosclerosis. *Arterioscler Thromb Vasc Biol*. 2014;34(4):705–714.
11. Moreno PR, Murcia AM, Palacios IF, et al. Coronary composition and macrophage infiltration in atherectomy specimens from patients with diabetes mellitus. *Circulation*. 2000;102(18):2180–2184.
12. Libby P. Inflammation in atherosclerosis. *Nature*. 2002;420(6917):868–874.
13. Shechter M, Merz CN, Paul-Labrador MJ, Kaul S. Blood glucose and platelet-dependent thrombosis in patients with coronary artery disease. *J Am Coll Cardiol*. 2000;35(2):300–307.
14. American Diabetes Association Professional Practice Committee 2. Diagnosis and classification of diabetes: standards of care in diabetes-2024. *Diabetes Care*. 2023;47(Suppl 1):S20–S42.
15. Ahlqvist E, Storm P, Karajamaki A, et al. Novel subgroups of adult-onset diabetes and their association with outcomes: a data-driven cluster analysis of six variables. *Lancet Diabetes Endocrinol*. 2018;6(5):361–369.
16. American Diabetes Association Professional Practice Committee 10. Cardiovascular disease and risk management: standards of care in diabetes-2024. *Diabetes Care*. 2024;47(Suppl 1):S179–S218.
17. Rawshani A, Rawshani A, Franzen S, et al. Risk factors, mortality, and cardiovascular outcomes in patients with type 2 diabetes. *N Engl J Med*. 2018;379(7):633–644.
18. Zinman B, Wanner C, Lachin JM, et al. Empagliflozin, cardiovascular outcomes, and mortality in type 2 diabetes. *N Engl J Med*. 2015;373(22):2117–2128.
19. Neal B, Perkovic V, Mahaffey KW, et al. Canagliflozin and cardiovascular and renal events in type 2 diabetes. *N Engl J Med*. 2017;377(7):644–657.
20. Wiviott SD, Raz I, Bonaca MP, et al. Dapagliflozin and cardiovascular outcomes in type 2 diabetes. *N Engl J Med*. 2019;380(4):347–357.
21. Cannon CP, Pratley R, Dagogo-Jack S, et al. Cardiovascular outcomes with ertugliflozin in type 2 diabetes. *N Engl J Med*. 2020;383(15):1425–1435.
22. Marso SP, Daniels GH, Brown-Frandsen K, et al. Liraglutide and cardiovascular outcomes in type 2 diabetes. *N Engl J Med*. 2016;375(4):311–322.

23. Marso SP, Bain SC, Consoli A, et al. Semaglutide and cardiovascular outcomes in patients with type 2 diabetes. *N Engl J Med*. 2016;375(19):1834–1844.
24. Gerstein HC, Colhoun HM, Dagenais GR, et al. Dulaglutide and cardiovascular outcomes in type 2 diabetes (REWIND): a double-blind, randomised placebo-controlled trial. *Lancet*. 2019;394(10193):121–130.
25. Sabatine MS, Giugliano RP, Keech AC, et al. Evolocumab and clinical outcomes in patients with cardiovascular disease. *N Engl J Med*. 2017;376(18):1713–1722.
26. Bonaca MP, Bhatt DL, Cohen M, et al. Long-term use of ticagrelor in patients with prior myocardial infarction. *N Engl J Med*. 2015;372(19):1791–1800.
27. Steg PG, Bhatt DL, Simon T, et al. Ticagrelor in patients with stable coronary disease and diabetes. *N Engl J Med*. 2019;381(14):1309–1320.
28. Wiviott SD, Braunwald E, Angiolillo DJ, et al. Greater clinical benefit of more intensive oral antiplatelet therapy with prasugrel in patients with diabetes mellitus in the trial to assess improvement in therapeutic outcomes by optimizing platelet inhibition with prasugrel-Thrombolysis in Myocardial Infarction 38. *Circulation*. 2008;118(16):1626–1636.
29. Davies MJ, Aroda VR, Collins BS, et al. Management of hyperglycemia in type 2 diabetes, 2022. A consensus report by the American Diabetes Association (ADA) and the European Association for the Study of Diabetes (EASD). *Diabetes Care*. 2022;45(11):2753–2786.
30. Goldberg RB, Aroda VR, Bluemke DA, et al. Effect of long-term metformin and lifestyle in the Diabetes Prevention Program and its outcome study on coronary artery calcium. *Circulation*. 2017;136(1):52–64.
31. Holman RR, Paul SK, Bethel MA, Matthews DR, Neil HA. 10-year follow-up of intensive glucose control in type 2 diabetes. *N Engl J Med*. 2008;359(15):1577–1589.
32. Kahn SE, Haffner SM, Heise MA, et al. Glycemic durability of rosiglitazone, metformin, or glyburide monotherapy. *N Engl J Med*. 2006;355(23):2427–2443.
33. Marx N, Federici M, Schutt K, et al. 2023 ESC Guidelines for the management of cardiovascular disease in patients with diabetes. *Eur Heart J*. 2023;44(39):4043–4140.
34. McGuire DK, Shih WJ, Cosentino F, et al. Association of SGLT2 inhibitors with cardiovascular and kidney outcomes in patients with type 2 diabetes: a meta-analysis. *JAMA Cardiol*. 2021;6(2):148–158.
35. Kristensen SL, Rorth R, Jhund PS, et al. Cardiovascular, mortality, and kidney outcomes with GLP-1 receptor agonists in patients with type 2 diabetes: a systematic review and meta-analysis of cardiovascular outcome trials. *Lancet Diabetes Endocrinol*. 2019;7(10):776–785.
36. Cushman WC, Evans GW, et al. ACCORD Study Group Effects of intensive blood-pressure control in type 2 diabetes mellitus. *N Engl J Med*. 2010;362(17):1575–1585.
37. Zhang W, Zhang S, Deng Y, et al. Trial of intensive blood-pressure control in older patients with hypertension. *N Engl J Med*. 2021;385(14):1268–1279.
38. Kearney PM, Blackwell L, et al. Cholesterol Treatment Trialists' (CTT) Collaborators Efficacy of cholesterol-lowering therapy in 18,686 people with diabetes in 14 randomised trials of statins: a meta-analysis. *Lancet*. 2008;371(9607):117–125.
39. Giugliano RP, Cannon CP, Blazing MA, et al. Benefit of adding ezetimibe to statin therapy on cardiovascular outcomes and safety in patients with versus without diabetes mellitus: results from IMPROVE-IT (Improved Reduction of Outcomes: Vytorin Efficacy International Trial). *Circulation*. 2018;137(15):1571–1582.
40. Sabatine MS, Leiter LA, Wiviott SD, et al. Cardiovascular safety and efficacy of the PCSK9 inhibitor evolocumab in patients with and without diabetes and the effect of evolocumab on glycaemia and risk of new-onset diabetes: a prespecified analysis of the FOURIER randomised controlled trial. *Lancet Diabetes Endocrinol*. 2017;5(12):941–950.
41. Bowman L, Mafham M, et al. ASCEND Study Collaborative Group Effects of aspirin for primary prevention in persons with diabetes mellitus. *N Engl J Med*. 2018;379(16):1529–1539.
42. Berg DD, Kolkailah AA, Sarraju A, Kerchberger AM, Eljalby M, McGuire DK. Interpreting absolute and relative risk reduction in the context of recent cardiovascular outcome trials in patients with type 2 diabetes. *Curr Diab Rep*. 2021;21(11):45.
43. Arnett DK, Blumenthal RS, Albert MA, et al. 2019 ACC/AHA Guideline on the primary prevention of cardiovascular disease: executive summary: a report of the American College of Cardiology/American Heart Association Task Force on Clinical Practice Guidelines. *Circulation*. 2019;140(11):e563–e595.
44. Grundy SM, Stone NJ, Bailey AL, et al. 2018 AHA/ACC/AACVPR/AAPA/ABC/ACPM/ADA/AGS/APhA/ASPC/NLA/PCNA Guideline on the management of blood cholesterol: executive summary: a report of the American College of Cardiology/American Heart Association Task Force on Clinical Practice Guidelines. *Circulation*. 2019;139(25):e1046–e1081.
45. Virani SS, Newby LK, Arnold SV, et al. 2023 AHA/ACC/ACCP/ASPC/NLA/PCNA Guideline for the management of patients with chronic coronary disease: a report of the American Heart Association/American College of Cardiology Joint Committee on Clinical Practice Guidelines. *Circulation*. 2023;148(9):e9–e119.
46. Goff Jr. DC, Lloyd-Jones DM, Bennett G, et al. 2013 ACC/AHA Guideline on the assessment of cardiovascular risk: a report of the American College of Cardiology/American Heart Association Task Force on Practice Guidelines. *Circulation*. 2014;129(25 Suppl 2):S49–73.
47. Hippisley-Cox J, Coupland C, Brindle P. Development and validation of QRISK3 risk prediction algorithms to estimate future risk of cardiovascular disease: prospective cohort study. *BMJ*. 2017;357:j2099.
48. Hippisley-Cox J, Coupland CAC, Bafadhel M, et al. Development and validation of a new algorithm for improved cardiovascular risk prediction. *Nat Med*. 2024;30(5):1440–1447.
49. Rana JS, Tabada GH, Solomon MD, et al. Accuracy of the atherosclerotic cardiovascular risk equation in a large contemporary, multiethnic population. *J Am Coll Cardiol*. 2016;67(18):2118–2130.
50. Khan SS, Matsushita K, Sang Y, et al. Development and validation of the American Heart Association's PREVENT Equations. *Circulation*. 2024;149(6):430–449.
51. Stevens RJ, Kothari V, Adler AI, Stratton IM. United Kingdom Prospective Diabetes Study G. The UKPDS risk engine: a model for the risk of coronary heart disease in type II diabetes (UKPDS 56). *Clin Sci (Lond)*. 2001;101(6):671–679.
52. van der Heijden AA, Ortegon MM, Niessen LW, Nijpels G, Dekker JM. Prediction of coronary heart disease risk in a general, pre-diabetic, and diabetic population during 10 years of follow-up: accuracy of the Framingham, SCORE, and UKPDS risk functions: The Hoorn Study. *Diabetes Care*. 2009;32(11):2094–2098.
53. Bannister CA, Poole CD, Jenkins-Jones S, et al. External validation of the UKPDS risk engine in incident type 2 diabetes: a need for new type 2 diabetes-specific risk equations. *Diabetes Care*. 2014;37(2):537–545.
54. Kengne AP, Patel A, Marre M, et al. Contemporary model for cardiovascular risk prediction in people with type 2 diabetes. *Eur J Cardiovasc Prev Rehabil*. 2011;18(3):393–398.
55. Group SC-DW. the ESCCRC. SCORE2-Diabetes: 10-year cardiovascular risk estimation in type 2 diabetes in Europe. *Eur Heart J*. 2023;44(28):2544–2556.
56. Berkelmans GFN, Gudbjornsdottir S, Visseren FLJ, et al. Prediction of individual life-years gained without cardiovascular events from lipid, blood pressure, glucose, and aspirin treatment based on data of more than 500 000 patients with Type 2 diabetes mellitus. *Eur Heart J*. 2019;40(34):2899–2906.
57. Berg DD, Moura FA, Bellavia A, et al. Assessment of atherothrombotic risk in patients with type 2 diabetes mellitus. *J Am Coll Cardiol*. 2023;81(25):2391–2402.
58. McGurnaghan SJ, McKeigue PM, Read SH, et al. Development and validation of a cardiovascular risk prediction model in type 1 diabetes. *Diabetologia*. 2021;64(9):2001–2011.
59. Marston NA, Giugliano RP, Melloni GEM, et al. Association of apolipoprotein b-containing lipoproteins and risk of myocardial infarction in individuals with and without atherosclerosis: distinguishing between particle concentration, type, and content. *JAMA Cardiol*. 2022;7(3):250–256.
60. Ballantyne CM, Hoogeveen RC, Bang H, et al. Lipoprotein-associated phospholipase A2, high-sensitivity C-reactive protein, and risk for incident coronary heart disease in middle-aged men and women in the Atherosclerosis Risk in Communities (ARIC) study. *Circulation*. 2004;109(7):837–842.
61. Pradhan AD, Manson JE, Rossouw JE, et al. Inflammatory biomarkers, hormone replacement therapy, and incident coronary heart disease: prospective analysis from the Women's Health Initiative observational study. *JAMA*. 2002;288(8):980–987.
62. Ridker PM, Paynter NP, Rifai N, Gaziano JM, Cook NR. C-reactive protein and parental history improve global cardiovascular risk prediction: the Reynolds Risk Score for men. *Circulation*. 2008;118(22):2243–2251.
63. Maisel AS, Krishnaswamy P, Nowak RM, et al. Rapid measurement of B-type natriuretic peptide in the emergency diagnosis of heart failure. *N Engl J Med*. 2002;347(3):161–167.
64. Thygesen K, Alpert JS, Jaffe AS, et al. Fourth universal definition of myocardial infarction (2018). *J Am Coll Cardiol*. 2018;72(18):2231–2264.
65. Everett BM, Brooks MM, Vlachos HE, et al. Troponin and cardiac events in stable ischemic heart disease and diabetes. *N Engl J Med*. 2015;373(7):610–620.
66. Scirica BM, Bhatt DL, Braunwald E, et al. Prognostic implications of biomarker assessments in patients with type 2 diabetes at high cardiovascular risk: a secondary analysis of a randomized clinical trial. *JAMA Cardiol*. 2016;1(9):989–998.
67. Zelniker TA, Wiviott SD, Mosenzon O, et al. Association of cardiac biomarkers with major adverse cardiovascular events in high-risk patients with diabetes: a secondary analysis of the DECLARE-TIMI 58 trial. *JAMA Cardiol*. 2023;8(5):503–509.
68. Vaduganathan M, Sattar N, Xu J, et al. Stress cardiac biomarkers, cardiovascular and renal outcomes, and response to canagliflozin. *J Am Coll Cardiol*. 2022;79(5):432–444.
69. Aragam KG, Jiang T, Goel A, et al. Discovery and systematic characterization of risk variants and genes for coronary artery disease in over a million participants. *Nat Genet*. 2022;54(12):1803–1815.
70. Marston NA, Pirruccello JP, Melloni GEM, et al. Predictive utility of a coronary artery disease polygenic risk score in primary prevention. *JAMA Cardiol*. 2023;8(2):130–137.
71. Helgason H, Eiriksdottir T, Ulfarsson MO, et al. Evaluation of large-scale proteomics for prediction of cardiovascular events. *JAMA*. 2023;330(8):725–735.
72. Daga N, Nasir K, Hamirani Y, et al. Prevalence and severity of coronary artery calcium in young persons with diabetes. *J Cardiovasc Comput Tomogr*. 2013;7(4):241–247.
73. Celeng C, Maurovich-Horvat P, Ghoshhajra BB, Merkely B, Leiner T, Takx RA. Prognostic value of coronary computed tomography angiography in patients with diabetes: a meta-analysis. *Diabetes Care*. 2016;39(7):1274–1280.
74. Detrano R, Guerci AD, Carr JJ, et al. Coronary calcium as a predictor of coronary events in four racial or ethnic groups. *N Engl J Med*. 2008;358(13):1336–1345.
75. Raggi P, Shaw LJ, Berman DS, Callister TQ. Prognostic value of coronary artery calcium screening in subjects with and without diabetes. *J Am Coll Cardiol*. 2004;43(9):1663–1669.

76. Wackers FJ, Young LH, Inzucchi SE, et al. Detection of silent myocardial ischemia in asymptomatic diabetic subjects: the DIAD study. *Diabetes Care*. 2004;27(8):1954–1961.
77. Anand DV, Lim E, Hopkins D, et al. Risk stratification in uncomplicated type 2 diabetes: prospective evaluation of the combined use of coronary artery calcium imaging and selective myocardial perfusion scintigraphy. *Eur Heart J*. 2006;27(6):713–721.
78. Zellweger MJ, Hachamovitch R, Kang X, et al. Prognostic relevance of symptoms versus objective evidence of coronary artery disease in diabetic patients. *Eur Heart J*. 2004;25(7):543–550.

9 Epidemiology and Pathophysiology of Heart Failure With Preserved and With Reduced Ejection Fraction in Patients With Type 2 Diabetes

DAVID AGUILAR

KEY POINTS

- Type 2 diabetes mellitus is associated with an approximately twofold increased risk of heart failure, affecting both HFPEF and HFREF
- Heart failure risk increases with longer diabetes duration, poor glycemic control, and comorbidities such as obesity, hypertension, coronary artery disease, and kidney disease
- Subclinical structural and functional cardiac abnormalities, including left ventricular hypertrophy, diastolic dysfunction, and elevated cardiac biomarkers, are common in diabetes and often precede symptomatic heart failure
- A bidirectional relationship exists between diabetes and heart failure, as heart failure itself increases the risk of incident diabetes through mechanisms such as insulin resistance and neurohormonal activation
- The coexistence of diabetes and heart failure is associated with significantly higher morbidity and mortality, including increased risk of hospitalization and cardiovascular death
- Diabetes contributes to heart failure through multiple interrelated mechanisms, including insulin resistance, chronic hyperglycemia, inflammation, oxidative stress, abnormal myocardial metabolism, microvascular dysfunction, and cardiac fibrosis
- Diabetic cardiomyopathy is characterized by concentric left ventricular remodeling, impaired diastolic function, and subclinical systolic dysfunction, often preceding overt reductions in ejection fraction

Multiple observational studies demonstrate that type 2 diabetes mellitus (DM) is associated with increased risk for the development of heart failure (HF). The mechanisms contributing to this greater risk are multifactorial and include the often-accelerated comorbid conditions such as obesity, hypertension, and coronary artery disease (CAD). In addition, diabetes may contribute to cardiac dysfunction through other pathways related to hyperglycemia and glucotoxicity, insulin resistance, inflammation, hyperlipidemia and lipotoxicity, abnormal calcium handling, mitochondrial dysfunction, increased oxidative stress, and abnormalities in autophagy. Importantly, the coexistence of diabetes and HF in a patient is associated with increased morbidity and mortality. Recent trends in the prevalence of type 2 diabetes and HF forecast a growing burden of disease. This chapter reviews the epidemiology and pathophysiology of HF with preserved ejection fraction (HFPEF) and with reduced ejection fraction (HFREF) in patients with type 2 DM.

EPIDEMIOLOGY OF DIABETES AND HEART FAILURE

Association of Diabetes and Incident Heart Failure

Several observational studies have shown that diabetes increases the risk for the development of HF by approximately two- to fourfold.[1–3] In the first 20 years of follow-up in the Framingham Heart Study, diabetes was associated with an almost twofold increased risk of HF in males and a fourfold increased risk in females independent of other risk factors (such as age, systolic blood pressure, tobacco use, cholesterol, and left ventricular [LV] hypertrophy).[4] Multivariable analyses revealed that diabetes had a high population attributable risk for HF in the Framingham Heart Study, accounting for 6% of cases in males and 12% in females. In more recent studies, including a registry of over 3 million people living in Scotland[5] and a meta-analyses of 74 observational studies,[2] the relative risk of incident HF remained approximately twofold higher in

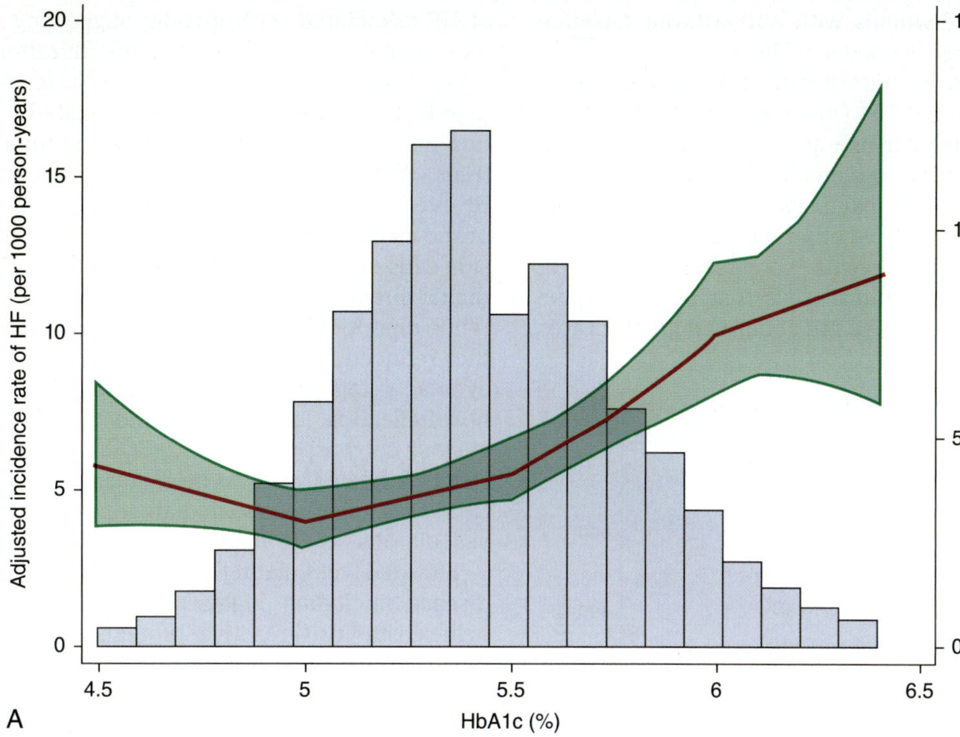

FIG. 9.1 Incident rates of heart failure (*HF*) according to hemoglobin A1c (*HbA1c*). The graph shows incidence-rate (per 1000 person-years) and 95% CI (*shaded area*) of HF with spline terms of A1c (knots at 5.0%, 5.5%, and 6.0%). The histograms represent the frequency distribution of A1C (4.5–6.5%) in the study sample. (From Matsushita K, Blecker S, Pazin-Filho A, et al. The association of hemoglobin a1c with incident heart failure among people without diabetes: the atherosclerosis risk in communities study. *Diabetes*. 2010;59(8):2020–2026.)

people with diabetes compared to those without diabetes.[2,5] The diabetes-associated increased HF risk manifests across different patients populations, including the general population, older people, those with established coronary artery disease, and individuals with kidney disease. The relative risk of HF associated with diabetes may be even in higher in younger adults and in females.[2,3,5]

Diabetes is a risk factor for both HFPEF and HFREF, and studies have shown that the magnitude of risk associated between diabetes and heart failure appears similar for both HF subtype.[2,6] In the Multi-Ethnic Study of Atherosclerosis (MESA), diabetes conferred similar risks for HFPEF (HR, 1.85; 95% CI, 1.57–2.68) and HFREF (HR, 2.02; 95% CI, 1.38–2.97) compared to those without diabetes.[6] Similarly, a meta-analysis of seven studies demonstrated that the risk magnitude associated with diabetes and incident was increased by approximately twofold and was similar for both incident HFPEF or HFREF.[2]

In addition to overt diabetes, epidemiologic studies have demonstrated that milder abnormalities of glucose regulation (below the diagnostic threshold for diabetes) are associated with increased rates of HF. In participants without diabetes or HF at baseline in the Atherosclerosis Risk in Communities (ARIC) study, incident HF rates increased in a stepwise manner with increasing hemoglobin A1c (HbA1c) when compared with the reference group (HbA1c 5.0%–5.4%) (Fig. 9.1).[7] The presence of prediabetes has also been associated with subclinical alterations in cardiac structure and function and greater rates of symptomatic heart failure compared to those with normal glycemia.[8–10] The HF risk observed in individuals with prediabetes is particularly elevated in those with other cardiovascular disease risk factors, such as elevated blood pressure, elevated cholesterol levels, elevated C-reactive protein, or current or former smoking.[8]

Risk Factors for Incident Heart Failure

Risk factors for incident HF in patients with diabetes are similar to those in individuals without diabetes. Studies of individuals with diabetes have shown that risk factors for the development of HF include older age, the presence of ischemic heart disease and CAD, peripheral vascular disease, nephropathy and renal insufficiency, metabolic complications of diabetes, retinopathy, obesity, hypertension, atrial fibrillation, and increased cardiac biomarkers such as high-sensitivity troponin and N-terminal pro-B-type natriuretic peptide (NT-proBNP).[1,5,11] Longer duration of diabetes is associated with echocardiographic abnormalities of left ventricular systolic and diastolic function,[12] and longer duration of diabetes is an important risk factor for HF development.[10,13] In the ARIC study, each 5-year increase in diabetes duration was associated with a 17% relative increase risk of HF, and the incidence HF rate among individuals with a diabetes duration greater than 15 years was at least fourfold higher than those without diabetes (Fig. 9.2).[10] The magnitude of the associations between diabetes duration and incident HF was similar with both HFPEF and HFREF.[10]

Multiple studies have identified that worsened glycemic control is associated with greater risk for the development of HF in individuals with diabetes.[1,13,14] For each 1% increase in HbA1c in individuals with diabetes, the risk of incident HF increases by 8% to 36%.[1] The relationship between HbA1c and incident HF in a community-based study of diabetic individuals with and without baseline coronary heart disease is shown in Fig. 9.3.[14]

Specific glucose-lowering therapies have also been associated with incident HF. Observational studies have demonstrated that insulin use at baseline is associated with increased rates of HF in individuals with diabetes, but it remains unclear whether insulin use is a marker of diabetes duration and severity or whether it directly contributes to increased heart failure events. Long-term follow-up of randomized, controlled clinical trials that have prospectively studied insulin use have not confirmed greater rates of HF associated with insulin, suggesting that insulin is more likely a marker for diabetes duration and severity rather than a contributor to greater rates of HF.[1] Thiazolidinediones (TZDs) have been associated with fluid retention and increased rates of HF in randomized controlled trials. Although the exact mechanisms of the increased HF events with TZDs are not known, the predominant proposed mechanism relates to TZD-associated volume expansion caused by increased renal sodium reabsorption rather than a direct effect on myocardial structure and function.[1] While dipeptidyl peptidase 4 inhibitors have generally neither reduced nor increased major adverse cardiovascular events, saxagliptin has been associated with increased hospitalization for HF compared to a placebo.[15] Sodium glucose cotransporter type-2 (SGLT-2) inhibitors have consistently been shown to be associated with reductions in HF events in patients with diabetes and established cardiovascular disease or high-cardiovascular risk.

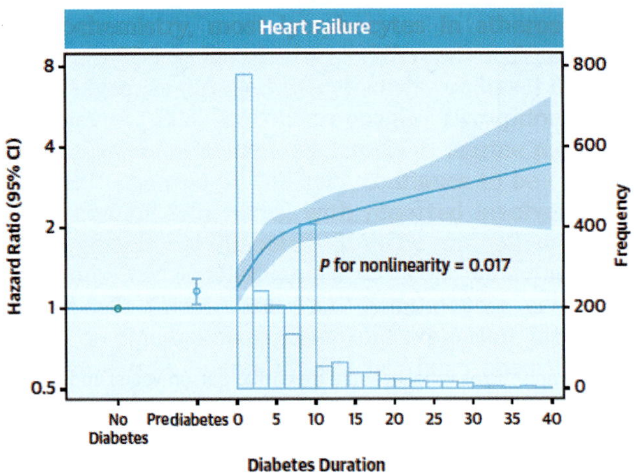

FIG. 9.2 The association of prediabetes, diabetes, and diabetes duration with heart failure (*HF*). The graph shows the hazard ratio and frequency of heart failure among individuals with prediabetes and by diabetes duration. Restricted cubic splines are shown to demonstrate the association of diabetes duration with heart failure. There is a roughly linear relation between diabetes duration and HF risk among individuals with diabetes. From Echouffo-Tcheugui JB, Zhang S, Florido R, et al. Duration of diabetes and incident heart failure: the ARIC (Atherosclerosis Risk in Communities) Study. *JACC Heart Fail*. 2021;9(8):594–603.)

Elevated circulating biomarkers of cardiovascular disease, including high-sensitivity troponin T (hsTnT), high-sensitivity C-reactive protein, and N-terminal pro-B-type natriuretic peptide (NT-proBNP), are also associated with increased risk of incident HF in individuals with diabetes.[16–18] In one study, males and females with a hsTnT level >15 and >10 pg/mL, respectively, had a nearly fourfold increased risk of future HF hospitalization.[17] The adjusted hazard for HF hospitalization in those with elevated levels on NT-proBNP was also nearly fourfold increased.[17]

As expected, rates of incident HF in patients with diabetes vary depending on the duration of diabetes and concomitant HF risk factors present. Several risk scores incorporating multiple factors have been proposed to help identify those with diabetes who have greatest risk for HF. These scores have based on clinical risk factors and cardiac biomarkers. Examples of HF risk scores are demonstrated

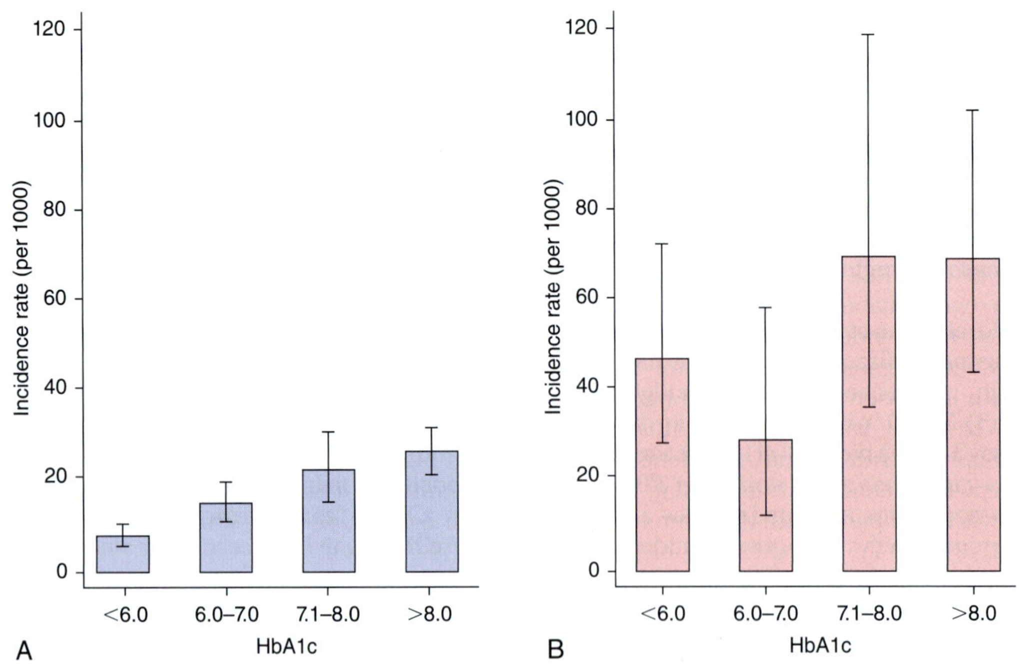

FIG. 9.3 Crude incidence rates (95% CI) of heart failure (*HF*) in participantes with diabetes in the Atherosclerosis Risk in Communities (*ARIC*) study by baseline hemoglobin A1c (*HbA1c*) categories and coronary heart disease (*CHD*) status at baseline (**A**, without CHD; **B**, with CHD). (From Pazin-Filho A, Kottgen A, Bertoni AG, et al. HbA1c as a risk factor for heart failure in persons with diabetes: the Atherosclerosis Risk in Communities (ARIC) study. *Diabetologia*. 2008;51:2197–2204.)

in Table 9.1.[18–20] For instance, the WATCH-DM risk score is a weighted integer scoring system that includes 10 clinical, laboratory, and ECG measures, including weight (BMI), age, hypertension, creatinine, high-density lipoproteiin (HDL) cholesterol, diabetes control (fasting plasma glucose), QRS duration, prior myocardial infarction, and prior coronary artery bypass graft surgery.[20] As demonstrated in Fig. 9.4, those in the highest quintile of WATCH-DM score (score ≥14 points) had a 5-year incidence of HF of 17.4% compared to the lowest quintile score (score ≤7 points) who had a 5-year HF incidence of 1.1%.[20]

TABLE 9.1 **Examples of HF Risk Scores for Individuals With Diabetes**

HEART FAILURE RISK SCORE	VARIABLES INCLUDED IN THE RISK SCORE	C-INDEX
WATCH-DM[20]	Weight (BMI), age, hypertension, creatinine, HDL cholesterol, diabetes control (fasting plasma glucose), QRS duration, myocardial infarction, and coronary artery bypass graft	0.72 (0.69–0.75)
TIMI Risk Score for Heart Failure in Diabetes[19]	Prior HF, history of atrial fibrillation, coronary artery disease, eGFR, urine albumin-to-creatine ratio	0.81 (0.78–0.84)
Pandey et al.[18]	Biomarker based: hs-TnT ≥6 ng/l, NT-proBNP ≥125 pg/ml, hs-CRP ≥3 mg/l, and ECG left ventricular hypertrophy	0.74 (0.68–0.80)

BMI, Body mass index; *ECG*, electrocardiogram; *eGFR*, estimated glomerular filtration rate; *HDL*, high-density lipoprotein cholesterol; *hs-TnT, high-sensitivity cardiac troponin T; hs-CRP*, high-sensitivity C-reactive protein; *TIMI*, thrombolysis in myocardial infarction; *NT-proBNP*, N-terminal pro-B-type natriuretic peptide.

Prevalence of Asymptomatic Left Ventricular Dysfunction Among People With Diabetes

Stage B heart failure (pre-HF) refers to a phase of asymptomatic structural and functional cardiac abnormalities and/or an asymptomatic elevation in cardiac biomarkers (NT-proBNP or high-sensitivity troponin) that is associated with increases in the risk for symptomatic HF.[21] Asymptomatic LV dysfunction and abnormalities of cardiac structure and function are more commonly present in patients with diabetes than in those without diabetes. These abnormalities include LV systolic and diastolic dysfunction and diabetes-associated increases in LV mass, relative wall thickness, and left atrial size. In patients with diabetes in the Framingham Heart Study, the prevalence of asymptomatic LV dysfunction (defined as left ventricular ejection fraction [LVEF] < 50%) was 7%.[22] In a more recent pooled-cohort study of adults older than 40 years (mean age 72 years) without prevalent cardiovascular disease and without LVEF <45%, the prevalence of at least one echocardiographic abnormality consistent with stage B HF (either increased LV mass, increased left atrial (LA) size, or diastolic dysfunction) was 67% (the least restrictive definition), and the prevalence of two or more echocardiographic abnormalities consistent with stage B HF was 20%.[23] In this study, approximately 12% of adults with diabetes had both elevated natriuretic peptide levels and two or more echocardiographic abnormalities (the most restrictive definition for stage B HF) (Fig. 9.5).[23] Importantly, the presence of these imaging and biomarker abnormalities were associated with a stepwise increase in HF risk; the 5-year cumulative incidence of HF among participants with at least one echocardiographic abnormality, at least two echocardiographic abnormalities, and at least

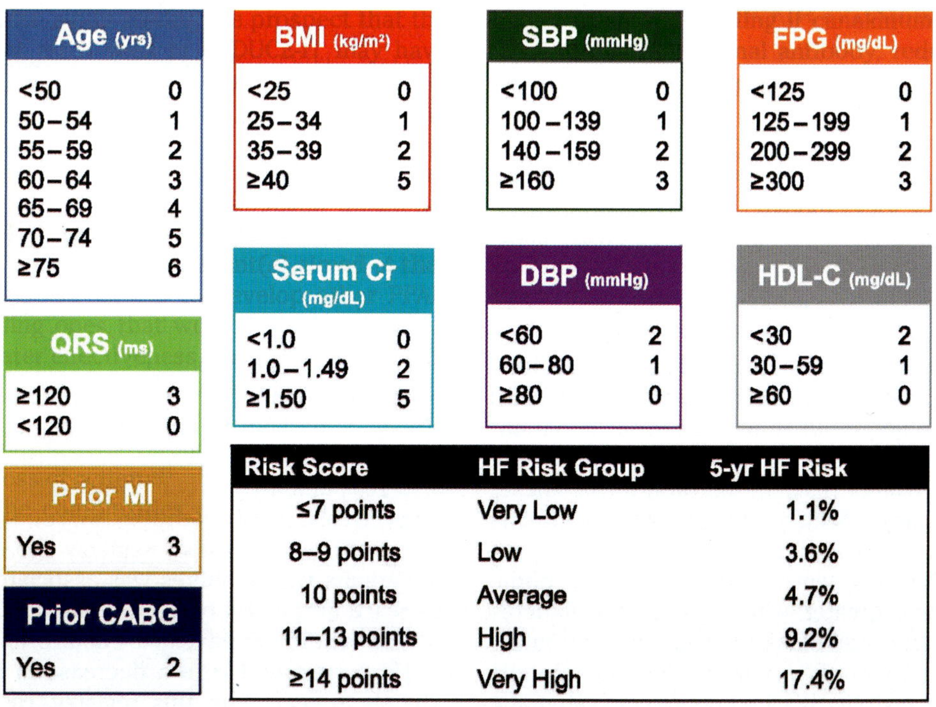

FIG. 9.4 The WATCH-DM scoring variables and 5-year heart failure (*HF*) incidence based on approximate quintiles of WATCH-DM score (very low ≤7, low 8–9, average 10, high 11–13, and very high ≥14). *CABG*, Coronary artery bypass grafting; *CR*, creatinine; *DBP*, diastolic blood pressure; *FPG*, fasting plasma glucose; *HDL-C*, high-density lipoprotein cholesterol; *MI*, myocardial infarction; *SBP*, systolic blood pressure; *yrs*, years. (From Segar MW, et al. Machine learning to predict the risk of incident heart failure hospitalization among patients with diabetes: the WATCH-DM risk score. *Diabetes Care*. 2019;42(12):2298–2306.)

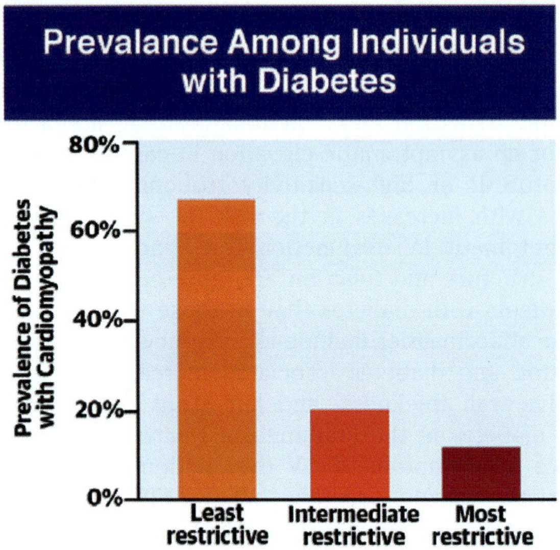

FIG. 9.5 Prevalence of cardiomyopathy in people with diabetes and without known cardiovascular disease in the Atherosclerosis Risk in Communities Study. Among adults with diabetes but without known cardiovascular disease, three separate criteria for asymptomatic cardiomyopathy were assessed. Least restrictive definition was the presence of at least one echocardiographic abnormality (either increased left ventricular mass, increased left atrial size, or diastolic dysfunction); intermediate restrictive included two or more echocardiographic abnormalities; the most restrictive definition included two or more echocardiographic abnormalities plus elevated natriuretic peptide levels. (From Segar MW, et al. Prevalence and prognostic implications of diabetes with cardiomyopathy in community-dwelling adults. *J Am Coll Cardiol.* 2021;78(16):1587–1598.)

two echocardiographic abnormality plus elevated natriuretic peptide was 8.4%, 11.2%, and 12.8%, respectively.[23]

Prevalence of Diabetes Among People With Heart Failure

HF is a growing health and economic burden, in large part due to an aging population. It is estimated that 6 million US adults have HF, and the prevalence is projected to rise to over 8 million adults with HF by 2030.[24] In clinical trials of HF, including both HFREF and HFPEF, the prevalence of diabetes ranges between 20% and 40%. The prevalence of diabetes in clinical HF trial populations varies by age, chronic kidney disease, and coexistence of other cardiovascular conditions. The prevalence of DM appears even higher in patients hospitalized with acute HF, reaching levels greater 40%.[1] There is also significant heterogeneity among different ethnic groups in regards to HF. In patient level data from two large global cohorts, the prevalence of DM was lowest in Whites (29.3%), followed by Japanese/Koreans (34.1%), Blacks (35.9%), Chinese (42.3%), Indians (44.2%), and highest in Malays (51.9%).[25]

Furthermore, the prevalence of diabetes in HF populations may be even greater when systematic diabetes screening occurs and individuals with previously unrecognized diabetes are identified. For example, in a cohort of outpatients with systolic HF who underwent systematic oral glucose tolerance testing, almost 20% of individuals without a prior diagnosis of diabetes were found to have newly diagnosed diabetes.[26]

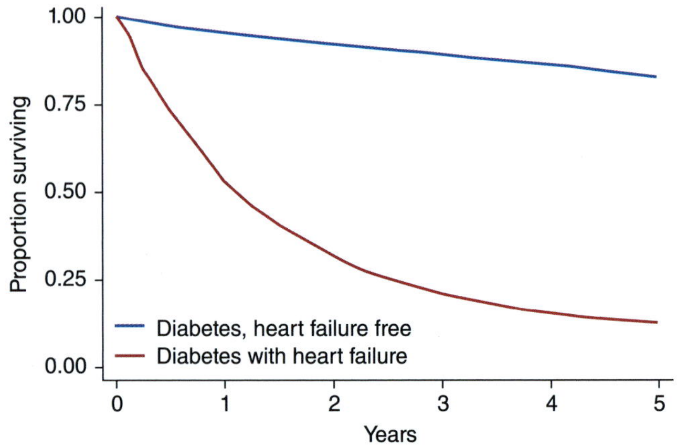

FIG. 9.6 Five-year Kaplan-Meier survival estimates for 115,803 adults aged 65 years or older in fee-for-service Medicare with diabetes by incident heart failure (HF) status. (From Bertoni AG, Hundley WG, Massing MW, et al. Heart failure prevalence, incidence, and mortality in the elderly with diabetes. *Diabetes Care.* 2004;27(3):699–703.)

Incident Diabetes in Patients With Heart Failure

In addition to diabetes contributing to greater HF incidence, evidence suggests that HF itself may be considered an insulin-resistant state with increased risk for incident diabetes.[1,27,28] The potential reasons for this association have not been well established but include potential increased neurohormonal activation promoting both skeletal and myocardial insulin resistance.[28] Increased sympathetic nervous stimulation, renin-angiotensin-aldosterone (RAAS) overactivity, and reduced activity of natriuretic peptides may affect skeletal muscle blood flow, reduce skeletal muscle glucose uptake, and increase systemic and local inflammation and fibrosis.[28] Risk factors for incident diabetes among people with HF include elevated BMI and waist circumference, smoking history, elevated HbA1c or glucose, higher systolic blood pressure, longer duration of HF, diuretic therapy, and higher New York Heart Association functional class.[1] Given bidirectional association, it is not surprising that diabetes and HF frequently coexist.

Diabetes and Adverse Outcomes in Patients With Heart Failure

The development of HF in a person with diabetes is associated with a markedly increased risk of death compared with diabetic individuals who remain free of HF. In a study of individuals 65 years or older, incident HF was associated with markedly reduced survival compared with those diabetic individuals who remained HF free (mortality rate 32.7/100 person-years compared with 3.7/100 person-years, respectively; HR of death 10.6, 95% CI, 10.4–10.9) (Fig. 9.6).[29] In a more recent Danish Registry, the development of HF in patients with diabetes was associated with a threefold increase in the risk of death compared to those with diabetes who did not have heart failure, and the development of HF corresponded to a decrease in lifespan of approximately 1 year. [30] In this registry, HF development was associated with the highest 5-year absolute and relative risk of death and with decrease in lifespan compared to the development of other cardiovascular diagnoses, such as ischemic heart disease, stroke, and peripheral artery disease.[30] These findings underscore the importance of HF prevention in people with diabetes.

Epidemiologic studies and analyses of clinical trials of patients with established HF have shown that patients with diabetes have increased mortality compared with individuals without diabetes.[31] Both CV and non-CV mortality are increased in HF patients with diabetes compared with HF patients without diabetes. In a large meta-analysis of 31 registries and 12 clinical trials, diabetes was associated with a higher risk of all-cause death (HR, 1.28; 95% CI, 1.21–1.35) and cardiovascular death (HR, 1.34; 95% CI, 1.20–1.50).[31] The association with diabetes and increased mortality is seen in both HFREF and HFPEF and appears to be independent of HF etiology.[28] Insulin use has been associated with increased mortality in patients with diabetes and established HF, although, as described earlier, this may be a reflection of diabetes disease severity rather than a direct mediator.

Multiple studies have also demonstrated that patients with diabetes and established HF have greater rates of future HF hospitalization than HF patients without diabetes.[2,31] Individuals with coexistent diabetes and HF have an approximately 35% to 40% increased risk of recurrent HF hospitalization.[2,31] In one meta-analysis, the relative risk of HF hospitalization associated with diabetes appeared to be greater in those with HFPEF (RR, 1.73; 95% CI, 1.32–2.26) compared to HFREF (RR, 1.37; 95% CI, 1.28–1.38).[2] In this meta-analysis, the relative risk of HF hospitalization associated with diabetes was also higher in females than males and in younger individuals compared to older individuals.[2] In survivors of acute myocardial infarction (MI) complicated by LV dysfunction or symptoms of HF, diabetes is also associated with greater rates of subsequent HF hospitalization. The increased rates of HF hospitalization after MI occur despite similar infarct size and LVEF at baseline in patients with and without diabetes and no greater enlargement or reduction in systolic volume over time in patients with diabetes compared with those without diabetes.[32] After MI, patients with diabetes exhibit more pronounced concentric remodeling and demonstrate indications of elevated LV filling pressures, which suggests that diastolic dysfunction could be a key mechanism underlying the heightened risk observed in this patient population.[32]

PATHOPHYSIOLOGY AND MOLECULAR MECHANISMS OF HEART FAILURE IN PATIENTS WITH TYPE 2 DIABETES

The pathways leading to HF in individuals with diabetes are multifaceted and complex, encompassing both ischemic and nonischemic mechanisms (Fig. 9.7). In individuals with diabetes, this complexity is further augmented by the greater presence of coexisting HF risk factors, such as accelerated atherosclerosis, obesity, and hypertension, which contribute to abnormal cardiac remodeling, myocardial stress and injury, leading to cardiac dysfunction and HF. Additionally, the concept of "diabetic cardiomyopathy" describes cardiac structural and functional abnormalities occurring independently of CAD and hypertension. In this condition, chronic dysglycemia, insulin resistance, and hyperinsulinemia induce a cascade of systemic, myocardial, and cellular/molecular derangements, thereby contributing to cardiac dysfunction.[33–37] Systemic processes, such as heightened activity of the renin-angiotensin-aldosterone system and sympathetic nervous system, hyperinsulinemia and hyperglycemia, persistent low-grade inflammation, coexisting hypertension and hyperlipidemia, and autonomic dysfunction, are recognized contributors to the cardiac dysfunction

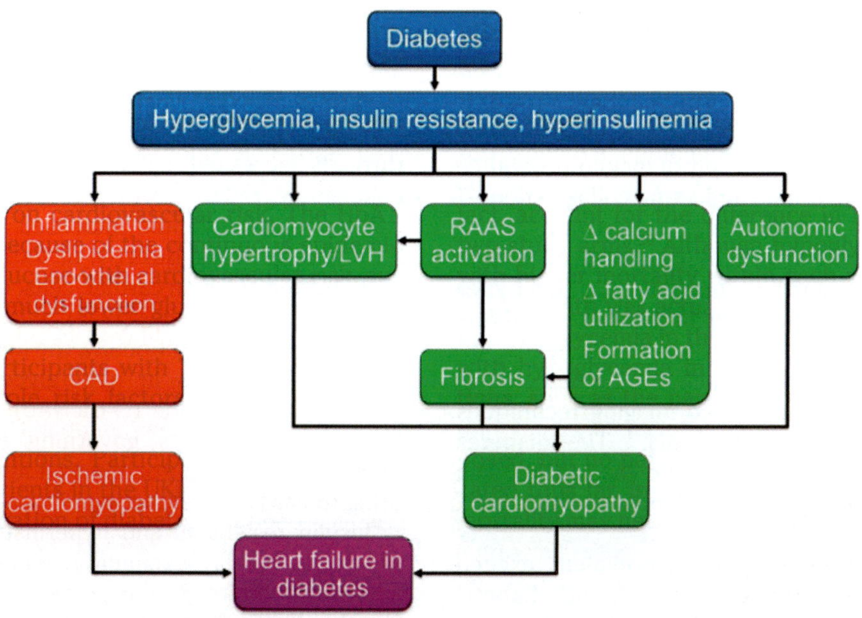

FIG. 9.7 Pathophysiology of diabetes and heart failure. Multiple pathways contributed to the development of heart failure in diabetes. Hyperglycemia, insulin resistance, and hyperinsulinemia can contribute to a variety of adverse effects that can lead to heart failure. *AGES*, Advanced glycation end products; *CAD*, coronary artery disease; *LVH*, left ventricular hypertrophy; *RAAS*, renin-angiotensin-aldosterone system. (Reprinted with permission Circulation. 2022;145:e895-e1032 ©2022 American Heart Association, Inc.)

TABLE 9.2 Diabetic Cardiomyopathy: Hallmark Features

Structural and Morphologic
Near-normal end-diastolic volume
Elevated left ventricular mass relative to chamber volume
Concentric left ventricular remodeling
Myocardial hypertrophy
Myocardial fibrosis
Intramyocardial lipid accumulation
Left atrial enlargement
Functional
Abnormal left ventricular systolic function/contractility
Abnormal left ventricular diastolic function
Reduced left ventricular compliance

associated with diabetes. This intricate network underscores the need for a comprehensive understanding of the diverse pathways involved in diabetes-related heart failure, for effective prevention and management strategies.

Morphologic and Structural Characteristics of Diabetic Cardiomyopathy

Cardiac dysfunction in individuals with diabetes often remains clinically silent, typically going undetected until the disease progresses to more advanced stages. Table 9.2 details various structural and functional impairments characteristic of diabetic cardiomyopathy. Key features of this condition include changes in LV geometry, abnormal diastolic function, and impaired LV systolic function. Myocardial hypertrophy is often considered a hallmark of the cardiomyopathy of diabetes, and there may often be elevated ventricular mass relative to chamber volume (concentric LV remodeling). LV hypertrophy and concentric remodeling often reflect the cumulative effects of cardiac fibrosis, cardiomyocyte hypertrophy, and cardiomyocyte cell death.[34] Myocyte hypertrophy can occur as a result of concomitant hypertension, but it may also occur due to chronic hyperinsulinemia as a result of insulin resistance. Increased extracellular volume, reflecting collagen deposition and fibrosis, also contributes to hypertrophy. Moreover, increased extracellular volume, indicative of collagen deposition and fibrosis, further contributes to this hypertrophy. Cardiac fibrosis is increased in patients with diabetes even in the absence of prior myocardial ischemia, and the increased cardiac fibrosis, which can be detected by certain cardiac magnetic resonance imaging techniques, is associated with adverse prognosis.[34] The diabetes-associated cardiac remodeling and increase in left ventricular mass may be exaggerated in females compared to males.[34]

LV diastolic dysfunction is notably prevalent, exceeding 50% in some studies, among individuals with diabetes and is closely associated with an increased risk of incident heart failure and mortality.[38] Diastolic dysfunction typically precedes systolic abnormalities, marking an early stage in the progression of cardiac dysfunction in diabetes. Key features of diastolic dysfunction include impaired LV relaxation, reduced ventricular compliance, and both structural and functional indications of elevated LV filling pressures. Echocardiographic manifestations of these diastolic impairments include prolonged mitral valve Doppler deceleration time, a decrease in mitral annular early diastolic tissue Doppler velocity (e'), an elevated ratio of early mitral inflow velocity to e' (E/e'), left atrial enlargement, and increased pulmonary artery systolic pressure. Notably, the prevalence of LV diastolic dysfunction in diabetic patients is comparable between males and females.[38]

Sensitive parameters of LV systolic function, such as strain imaging with speckle-tracking echocardiography, can demonstrate reductions in LV systolic function in the presence of preserved ejection fraction. Abnormal global longitudinal strain, sensitive maker of LV systolic dysfunction, can identify systolic dysfunction even while ejection fraction is preserved and is associated with a future risk of HF. With time, LV ejection fraction can fall leading to HFREF.

Mechanisms Contributing to Diabetes-Associated Heart Failure

The pathophysiology of HF associated with diabetes is a complex and multifaceted process, yet to be fully elucidated. It encompasses various interrelated mechanisms, as extensively reviewed in recent literature.[33–37] A few key concepts are described below.

Insulin Resistance and Hyperglycemia

Insulin resistance and hyperglycemia play a key role in the pathophysiology of diabetes-associated HF.[33–37] Chronic hyperglycemia exerts both direct and indirect deleterious effects on cardiomyocytes, cardiac fibroblasts, and endothelial cells. Advance glycation end products (AGEs) are long-lasting proteins or lipid molecules that result from advanced, nonenzymatic glycation of proteins, lipids, and nucleic acid that occur in the setting of chronic hyperglycemia. AGEs can induce cardiovascular dysfunction through increased collagen cross-linking and impaired collagen degradation which contribute to decreased myocardial compliance and increased myocardial and vascular stiffness. AGEs, directly, or indirectly by engaging the receptor for AGEs on cardiac cells, contribute to increased reactive oxygen species (ROS), inflammation, and endothelial dysfunction. Additionally, the hexosamine biosynthetic pathway, enhanced in hyperglycemic states, produces β-N-acetylglucosamine (O-GlcNAc), leading to alterations in critical pathways governing inflammation, calcium homeostasis, and mitochondrial function, further contributing to cardiac dysfunction.[33,34]

Insulin resistance and hyperinsulinemia, characteristic of type 2 DM, play a seminal role in disrupting intracellular signaling and biological processes that lead to cardiac dysfunction.[33–37] For example, insulin resistance and energy surplus activate protein kinase B(Akt) and mammalian target of rapamycin complex 1 and decrease the activation of sirtuin 1 (SIRT-1).[37] These alterations and other alterations in cellular signaling contribute to a spectrum of cardiac abnormalities, including cardiomyocyte hypertrophy, mitochondrial dysfunction and excitation-contraction uncoupling, oxidative stress, aberrant calcium handling, and disruptions in autophagy.[33–37] Insulin resistance also prompts a metabolic shift in cardiomyocytes, increasing fatty acid intake and β-oxidation to sustain ATP production. However, over time, this mechanism becomes insufficient, leading to excessive intracellular lipid accumulation and lipotoxicity.[34,36] Moreover, hyperinsulinemia is implicated in stimulating sodium-hydrogen exchanger isoforms in the heart (NHE1) and kidneys (NHE3), contributing to the complex pathophysiology of diabetes-associated HF.[37] Increased activity of NHE1 in the heart contributes to cardiac hypertrophy and cardiac dysfunction, and increased activity of NHE3 in the kidney can enhance sodium reabsorption in the proximal tubule and has been implicated in the pathogenesis of fluid retention that can contribute to HF.[37]

Oxidative Stress

Oxidative stress, a critical factor in diabetes-associated cardiac dysfunction, represents an imbalance marked by heightened generation of ROS and a diminished capacity for their degradation. These ROS, including superoxide and hydroxyl radicals, are unstable byproducts of cellular respiration and play a pivotal role in diabetic cardiac pathology.[33–35] Excessive ROS generation, coupled with compromised endogenous antioxidant defenses, is central to the development of cardiac complications in diabetes. This oxidative environment triggers a cascade of deleterious effects on the heart, including impaired cardiomyocyte calcium handling and mitochondrial dysfunction.[33–36] Additionally, it induces myocardial inflammation, contributing to structural and functional cardiac alterations, and downregulates cardioprotective physiological signaling pathways.

Myocardial Inflammation

Inflammation, a critical player in the development of HF among diabetic patients, is substantially influenced by the abnormalities associated with insulin resistance, hyperglycemia, and the upregulated renin-angiotensin system.[33–37] Recognized as a fundamental mechanism in both diabetes and its related complications, systemic inflammation contributes significantly to the pathogenesis of diabetic cardiomyopathy. Key inflammatory mediators, including cytokines and chemokines, along with the infiltration of proinflammatory macrophages and lymphocytes, play pivotal roles in this process. A major trigger for cardiac inflammation in this context is the elevation in ROS levels. Additionally, inflammatory factors like tumor necrosis factor (TNF), nuclear factor-kB, and protein kinases such as c-jun N terminal kinase (JNK) and p38 mitogen-activated protein kinase are implicated in the induction of cardiomyocyte hypertrophy and the promotion of cardiac fibrosis.[35,36]

Altered Myocardial Metabolism

Alterations in myocardial glucose and fatty acid metabolism have been identified as contributors to cardiac dysfunction in diabetes.[33–35] Myocardial glucose uptake depends on the presence of glucose transporters (GLUTs). In diabetes, there is reduced insulin-stimulated glucose uptake into the cardiomyocyte due to reduced GLUT4 cardiomyocyte expression and reduced translocation of GLUT4 from the cytoplasm to the cell membrane.[35] GLUT-4 is believed to be required for preservation of cardiac structure and function in response to a pathological process that increases energy demand, such as LV pressure overload.[35]

Circulating levels of free fatty acids and triglycerides are elevated in diabetes due to insulin resistance. In diabetes, there is a notable shift in the heart's substrate utilization, favoring fatty acid oxidation over glucose utilization for energy production.[34] This augmented reliance on fatty acids is partly attributable to increased expression of sarcolemmal transport proteins, especially cluster of differentiation-36 (CD36), on cardiomyocytes. An enhanced CD36 presence on the sarcolemma membrane facilitates greater uptake of long-chain fatty acids, resulting in the accumulation of triglycerides and lipid byproducts within the cardiomyocytes. This accumulation contributes to lipotoxicity, a detrimental condition for cardiac cells.[34–36] Furthermore, the altered substrate utilization pattern, in concert with lipotoxicity, inflammation, and increased ROS, leads to mitochondrial dysfunction. This mitochondrial impairment is a critical factor in the cascade of events that culminates in diabetic cardiac dysfunction.

Impaired Coronary Microvascular Perfusion

Impaired coronary microvascular perfusion associated with diabetes has been implicated in diabetic cardiomyopathy.[33,34,36,37] Diabetes has been associated with impairments in coronary flow reserve, myocardial blood volume and flow, and increased coronary resistance. These perfusion abnormalities are likely multifactorial and include diabetes-associated endothelial dysfunction and abnormal nitric oxide metabolism. Furthermore, the thickening of the vascular basement membrane and increased deposition of extracellular matrix proteins, typical in diabetes, further exacerbate this dysfunction. Epicardial adipose tissue expansion associated with diabetes can also lead to local secretion of proinflammatory cytokines and local inflammatory cell infiltration that can also contribute to coronary microvascular dysfunction.[37] The resultant microvascular impairment limits the adequate delivery of oxygen and nutrients to myocardial tissue, particularly during increased cardiac workload, leading to ischemia and subsequent myocardial injury.

SUMMARY

Multiple studies have demonstrated that diabetes is associated with an increased risk for development of HF in a variety of populations. The relative risk of incident heart failure is approximately twofold higher in people with diabetes compared to those without diabetes, and the relative HF risk associated with diabetes may be even higher in younger people and in females. The magnitude of diabetes-associated risk for HF is similar for both HFREF and

HFPEF. Dysglycemia below the diagnostic threshold of diabetes is also associated with increased HF risk. Importantly, individuals with both diabetes and HF are at increased risk of both morbidity and mortality compared to individuals with either condition alone. Type 2 DM induces a myriad of alterations in cardiac structure and function through mechanisms such as hyperglycemia-induced damage, insulin resistance, altered myocardial metabolism, oxidative stress, inflammation, and microvascular dysfunction. These changes manifest in both HFREF and HFPEF. The epidemiological data underscore a growing prevalence and an intimate association between T2DM and both forms of heart failure, highlighting the significant burden of these comorbid conditions in the population.

REFERENCES

1. Dunlay SM, Givertz MM, Aguilar D, et al. Type 2 diabetes mellitus and heart failure: a scientific statement from the American Heart Association and the Heart Failure Society of America: this statement does not represent an update of the 2017 ACC/AHA/HFSA heart failure guideline update. *Circulation*. 2019;140(7):e294–e324.
2. Kodama S, Fujihara K, Horikawa C, et al. Diabetes mellitus and risk of new-onset and recurrent heart failure: a systematic review and meta-analysis. *ESC Heart Fail*. 2020;7(5):2146–2174.
3. Ohkuma T, Komorita Y, Peters SAE, Woodward M. Diabetes as a risk factor for heart failure in women and men: a systematic review and meta-analysis of 47 cohorts including 12 million individuals. *Diabetologia*. 2019;62(9):1550–1560.
4. Kannel WB, McGee DL. Diabetes and cardiovascular disease. The Framingham study. *JAMA*. 1979;241(19):2035–2038.
5. McAllister DA, Read SH, Kerssens J, et al. Incidence of hospitalization for heart failure and case-fatality among 3.25 million people with and without diabetes mellitus. *Circulation*. 2018;138(24):2774–2786.
6. Echouffo-Tcheugui JB, Ogunmoroti O, Golden SH, et al. Glycemic markers and heart failure subtypes: the multi-ethnic study of atherosclerosis (MESA). *J Card Fail*. 2022;28(11):1593–1603.
7. Matsushita K, Blecker S, Pazin-Filho A, et al. The association of hemoglobin a1c with incident heart failure among people without diabetes: the Atherosclerosis Risk in Communities Study. *Diabetes*. 2010;59(8):2020–2026.
8. Honigberg MC, Zekavat SM, Pirruccello JP, Natarajan P, Vaduganathan M. Cardiovascular and kidney outcomes across the glycemic spectrum: insights from the UK Biobank. *J Am Coll Cardiol*. 2021;78(5):453–464.
9. Skali H, Shah A, Gupta DK, et al. Cardiac structure and function across the glycemic spectrum in elderly men and women free of prevalent heart disease: the Atherosclerosis Risk in the Community Study. *Circ Heart Fail*. 2015;8(3):448–454.
10. Echouffo-Tcheugui JB, Zhang S, Florido R, et al. Duration of diabetes and incident heart failure: the ARIC (Atherosclerosis Risk In Communities) Study. *JACC Heart Fail*. 2021;9(8):594–603.
11. Wamil M, Coleman RL, Adler AI, McMurray JJV, Holman RR. Increased risk of incident heart failure and death is associated with insulin resistance in people with newly diagnosed type 2 diabetes: UKPDS 89. *Diabetes Care*. 2021;44(8):1877–1884.
12. Reis JP, Allen NB, Bancks MP, et al. Duration of diabetes and prediabetes during adulthood and subclinical atherosclerosis and cardiac dysfunction in middle age: the CARDIA Study. *Diabetes Care*. 2018;41(4):731–738.
13. Echouffo-Tcheugui JB, Ndumele CE, Zhang S, et al. Diabetes and progression of heart failure: the Atherosclerosis Risk in Communities (ARIC) Study. *J Am Coll Cardiol*. 2022;79(23):2285–2293.
14. Pazin-Filho A, Kottgen A, Bertoni AG, et al. HbA 1c as a risk factor for heart failure in persons with diabetes: the Atherosclerosis Risk in Communities (ARIC) study. *Diabetologia*. 2008;51(12):2197–2204.
15. Scirica BM, Braunwald E, Raz I, et al. Heart failure, saxagliptin, and diabetes mellitus: observations from the SAVOR-TIMI 53 randomized trial. *Circulation*. 2014;130(18):1579–1588.
16. Berg DD, Wiviott SD, Scirica BM, et al. A biomarker-based score for risk of hospitalization for heart failure in patients with diabetes. *Diabetes Care*. 2021;44(11):2573–2581.
17. Scirica BM, Bhatt DL, Braunwald E, et al. Prognostic implications of biomarker assessments in patients with type 2 diabetes at high cardiovascular risk: a secondary analysis of a randomized clinical trial. *JAMA Cardiol*. 2016;1(9):989–998.
18. Pandey A, Vaduganathan M, Patel KV, et al. Biomarker-based risk prediction of incident heart failure in pre-diabetes and diabetes. *JACC Heart Fail*. 2021;9(3):215–223.
19. Berg DD, Wiviott SD, Scirica BM, et al. Heart failure risk stratification and efficacy of sodium-glucose cotransporter-2 inhibitors in patients with type 2 diabetes mellitus. *Circulation*. 2019;140(19):1569–1577.
20. Segar MW, Vaduganathan M, Patel KV, et al. Machine learning to predict the risk of incident heart failure hospitalization among patients with diabetes: the WATCH-DM risk score. *Diabetes Care*. 2019;42(12):2298–2306.
21. Heidenreich PA, Bozkurt B, Aguilar D, et al. 2022 AHA/ACC/HFSA Guideline for the management of heart failure: a report of the American College of Cardiology/American Heart Association Joint Committee on Clinical Practice Guidelines. *J Am Coll Cardiol*. 2022;79(17):e263–e421.
22. Wang TJ, Evans JC, Benjamin EJ, Levy D, LeRoy EC, Vasan RS. Natural history of asymptomatic left ventricular systolic dysfunction in the community. *Circulation*. 2003;108(8):977–982.
23. Segar MW, Khan MS, Patel KV, et al. Prevalence and prognostic implications of diabetes with cardiomyopathy in community-dwelling adults. *J Am Coll Cardiol*. 2021;78(16):1587–1598.
24. Tsao CW, Aday AW, Almarzooq ZI, et al. Heart disease and stroke statistics-2022 update: a report from the American Heart Association. *Circulation*. 2022;145(8):e153–e639.
25. Cooper LB, Yap J, Tay WT, et al. Multi-ethnic comparisons of diabetes in heart failure with reduced ejection fraction: insights from the HF-ACTION trial and the ASIAN-HF registry. *Eur J Heart Fail*. 2018;20(9):1281–1289.
26. Egstrup M, Schou M, Gustafsson I, Kistorp CN, Hildebrandt PR, Tuxen CD. Oral glucose tolerance testing in an outpatient heart failure clinic reveals a high proportion of undiagnosed diabetic patients with an adverse prognosis. *Eur J Heart Fail*. 2011;13(3):319–326.
27. Pop-Busui R, Januzzi JL, Bruemmer D, et al. Heart failure: an underappreciated complication of diabetes. A consensus report of the American Diabetes Association. *Diabetes Care*. 2022;45(7):1670–1690.
28. Palazzuoli A, Iacoviello M. Diabetes leading to heart failure and heart failure leading to diabetes: epidemiological and clinical evidence. *Heart Fail Rev*. 2023;28(3):585–596.
29. Bertoni AG, Hundley WG, Massing MW, Bonds DE, Burke GL, Goff Jr. DC. Heart failure prevalence, incidence, and mortality in the elderly with diabetes. *Diabetes Care*. 2004;27(3):699–703.
30. Zareini B, Blanche P, D'Souza M, et al. Type 2 diabetes mellitus and impact of heart failure on prognosis compared to other cardiovascular diseases: a nationwide study. *Circ Cardiovasc Qual Outcomes*. 2020;13(7):e006260.
31. Dauriz M, Mantovani A, Bonapace S, et al. Prognostic impact of diabetes on long-term survival outcomes in patients with heart failure: a meta-analysis. *Diabetes Care*. 2017;40(11):1597–1605.
32. Shah AM, Shin SH, Takeuchi M, et al. Left ventricular systolic and diastolic function, remodelling, and clinical outcomes among patients with diabetes following myocardial infarction and the influence of direct renin inhibition with aliskiren. *Eur J Heart Fail*. 2012;14(2):185–192.
33. Marwick TH, Ritchie R, Shaw JE, Kaye D. Implications of underlying mechanisms for the recognition and management of diabetic cardiomyopathy. *J Am Coll Cardiol*. 2018;71(3):339–351.
34. Ritchie RH, Abel ED. Basic mechanisms of diabetic heart disease. *Circ Res*. 2020;126(11):1501–1525.
35. Tan Y, Zhang Z, Zheng C, Wintergerst KA, Keller BB, Cai L. Mechanisms of diabetic cardiomyopathy and potential therapeutic strategies: preclinical and clinical evidence. *Nat Rev Cardiol*. 2020;17(9):585–607.
36. Jia G, Hill MA, Sowers JR. Diabetic cardiomyopathy: an update of mechanisms contributing to this clinical entity. *Circ Res*. 2018;122(4):624–638.
37. Packer M. Differential pathophysiological mechanisms in heart failure with a reduced or preserved ejection fraction in diabetes. *JACC Heart Fail*. 2021;9(8):535–549.
38. Bouthoorn S, Valstar GB, Gohar A, et al. The prevalence of left ventricular diastolic dysfunction and heart failure with preserved ejection fraction in men and women with type 2 diabetes: a systematic review and meta-analysis. *Diab Vasc Dis Res*. 2018;15(6):477–493.

PART III EFFECTS OF ANTIHYPERGLYCEMIC THERAPIES FOR TYPE 2 DIABETES ON CARDIOVASCULAR AND KIDNEY OUTCOMES

10 Effect of Glucose Management on Coronary Heart Disease Risk in Patients With Type 2 Diabetes

KASIA J. LIPSKA AND SILVIO E. INZUCCHI

Coronary heart disease (CHD) is the most common vascular complication of type 2 diabetes (T2D). However, CHD can precede the development of diabetes, and some have suggested that both conditions (CHD and T2D) have common genetic and environmental roots and spring from a "common soil" (Fig. 10.1).[1] Since elevated glucose defines diabetes and since diabetes is a well-recognized risk factor for CHD, strategies that lower glucose should theoretically reduce the risk of CHD events in people with diabetes. In reality, the relationship between glucose-lowering strategies and CHD events is complex: some strategies that lower glucose levels reduce CHD events, but others do not. This suggests that the impact of interventions on patient outcomes cannot be easily predicted from the impact of interventions on glucose or hemoglobin A1c (HbA1c). This chapter describes the epidemiologic relationship between glucose and CHD, reviews clinical trial evidence of the effects of glucose lowering on CHD outcomes (taking into account the types of strategies used to lower glucose levels), discusses the benefits and risks of glucose lowering with specific medications and in specific patient populations, and concludes with implications for clinical practice.

CHANGING EPIDEMIOLOGY OF DIABETES AND CORONARY HEART DISEASE

The general incidence and prevalence of CHD have declined in the United States in the last several decades, and this decline has been accompanied by a decline in CHD-related mortality.[2–4] These trends have been attributed to better cardiovascular risk factor control and treatment during and after acute coronary syndromes over time, primarily with the use of statin medications, blood pressure management, and antiplatelet therapies. In contrast to CHD trends, the prevalence[5] of diabetes has been steadily increasing over time, with the disease now affecting close to a third of older US adults (65 years or older).[6,7] In addition, adults with diabetes are living longer.[8,9] As a result, the burden of CHD attributable to diabetes is increasing.[10] These changes in the epidemiology of diabetes and CHD have important implications. First, strategies that mitigate the risk of CHD in patients with diabetes will be of growing importance because heart disease is increasingly a complication of diabetes. Second, these strategies will be applied to an aging population with a high comorbidity burden and at higher risk for adverse effects of therapy.

EPIDEMIOLOGIC RELATIONSHIP OF GLUCOSE WITH CORONARY HEART DISEASE

Multiple studies have assessed the relationship between various glucose parameters—fasting glucose, 2-hour glucose during an oral glucose tolerance test, or HbA1c levels—and the risk of CHD in populations with and without diabetes. Most of this work suggests a continuous relationship between measures of glycemia and CHD risk,

TABLE 10.1 Major Randomized Controlled Trials in Type 2 Diabetes

	UKPDS	ACCORD	ADVANCE	VADT
Study Participants				
Mean age, years	53	62	66	60
Diabetes duration, years	New	10	8	11.5
Prior macrovascular disease	Excluded[a]	35%	32%	40%
Duration of Study				
Number of years	11	3.5	5	5.6
HbA1c Goal				
Intensive therapy	[b]	<6%	≤6.5%	<6%
Standard therapy	[c]	7%–7.9%	Standard	8%–9%
HbA1c Achieved				
Intensive therapy	7.0%	6.4%	6.4%	6.9%
Standard therapy	7.9%	7.5%	7.0%	8.5%
Severe Hypoglycemia				
Annual events per 100 patients	0.71	4.6	0.56	12.0
Intensive therapy	0.20	1.5	0.30	4.0
Standard therapy	Not reported	<0.001	<0.001	<0.001
P value				
Primary Outcome[d]				
HR (95% CI) for intensive versus standard therapy	**0.88 (0.79–0.99)**	0.90 (0.78–1.04)	0.90 (0.82–0.98)	0.88 (0.74–1.05)
All-Cause Mortality				
HR (95% CI) for intensive versus standard therapy	0.94 (0.80–1.10)	**1.22 (1.01–1.46)**	0.93 (0.83–1.06)	1.07 (0.81–1.42)
Cardiovascular Mortality				
HR (95% CI) for intensive versus standard therapy	0.94 (0.66–1.30)	**1.35 (1.04–1.76)**	0.88 (0.74–1.04)	1.32 (0.81–2.14)

Bolded results represent HR reaching statistical significance, $P < 0.05$.
[a]Excluded myocardial infarction (MI) within 1 year prior, heart failure, angina, or more than one vascular event.
[b]Based on fasting plasma glucose (FPG) < 108 mg/dL.
[c]Based on FPG < 270 mg/dL.
[d]An aggregate endpoint of any diabetes-related endpoint (UKPDS); a composite of nonfatal myocardial infarction, nonfatal stroke, and fatal myocardial infarction and stroke (ACCORD); combined microvascular and macrovascular disease (ADVANCE); and time to occurrence of a composite of major cardiovascular events (VADT).
HR, Hazard ratio; *CI*, confidence interval.
Data from Ismail-Beigi F, Moghissi E, Tiktin M, et al. Individualizing glycemic targets in type 2 diabetes mellitus: implications of recent clinical trials, *Ann Intern Med.* 2011;154:554–559.

endpoint (P = 0.03), which included both macrovascular and microvascular events as well as sudden death or death due to metabolic complications and non-vascular outcomes; not significantly lower for any diabetes-related death (−10%, P = 0.34); and not significantly lower for mortality (−6%, P = 0.44), compared with patients treated with diet only. The reduction in diabetes-related endpoints was driven by a 25% relative risk reduction in microvascular events, with the effect on MI and on stroke neither reaching statistical significance (16% lower, p = 0.052; 11% higher, p = 0.52). A subgroup of UKPDS patients who had overweight or obesity at trial entry (>120% ideal body weight) were randomized either to intensive therapy with metformin (n = 342, median achieved HbA1c 7.4%) or conventional diet therapy (n = 411, median achieved HbA1c 8%).[22] In this subset of patients, any diabetes-related endpoint occurred among 98/341 (29%) patients randomized to metformin versus 160/411 (39%) randomized to conventional therapy (P = 0.002), diabetes-related death occurred among 28/341 (8%) patients randomized to metformin versus 55/411 (13%) randomized to conventional therapy (P = 0.017), and death from any cause occurred among 50/341 (15%) patients randomized to metformin versus 89/411(22%) randomized to conventional therapy (P = 0.011). In addition, MI occurred in 39/341 (11%) of patients randomized to metformin versus 73/411 (18%) randomized to conventional therapy, which represented a significant 39% reduction in MI (P = 0.01) (Fig. 10.3). In summary, the UKPDS trial established that intensive glucose control reduces the risk of microvascular complications in patients with newly diagnosed T2D but suggested that macrovascular benefits may be confined to patients with overweight or obesity treated with metformin therapy.

After the UKPDS trial was completed, study participants and their clinicians were advised to lower levels of blood glucose as much as possible, and patients returned to community or hospital-based diabetes care according to their clinical needs without any attempts to maintain previously randomized therapies. In the 10-year posttrial monitoring study of patients who survived to the end of the UKDPS trial, HbA1c levels were no longer different between the original intensive and conventional arms (approximately 8% at the end of the posttrial monitoring period).[23] In the sulfonylurea-insulin group, relative risk reductions for

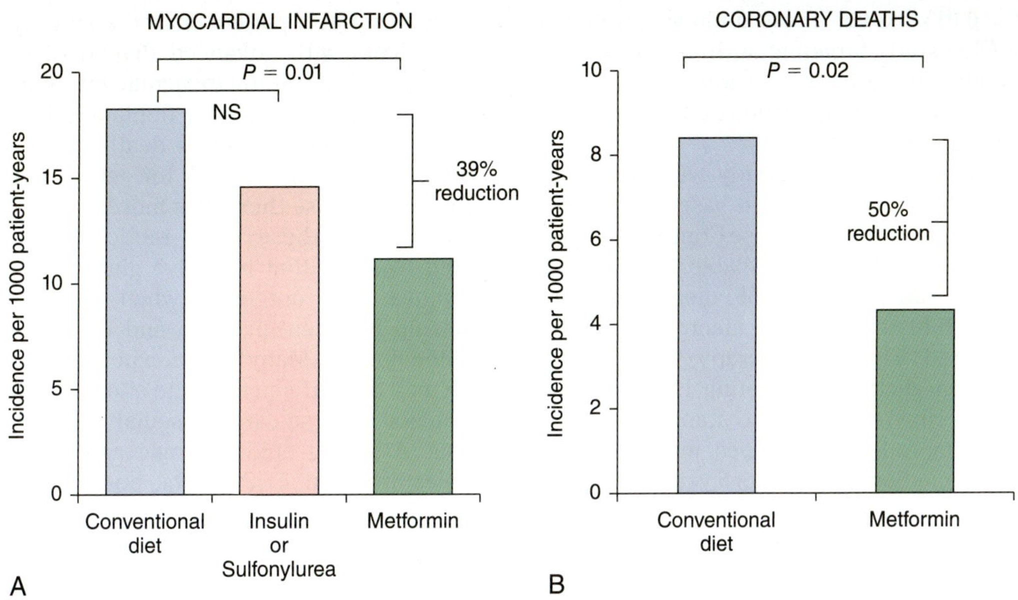

FIG. 10.3 Results of the UKPDS trial with respect to myocardial infarction and coronary deaths. *NS,* Nonsignificant. Data from Effect of intensive blood-glucose control with metformin on complications in overweight patients with type 2 diabetes [UKPDS 34]. UK Prospective Diabetes Study [UKPDS] Group, *Lancet* 1998;352:854.

diabetes-related endpoints persisted, whereas significant risk reductions for MI (15%, $P = 0.010$) and mortality (13%, $P = 0.007$) emerged over time. In the metformin group, relative risk reductions persisted for any diabetes-related endpoint, MI (33%, $P = 0.005$), and mortality (27%, $P = 0.002$). These observations suggest a modest but sustained effect of intensive glucose lowering on cardiovascular events, but only after many years of follow-up. Whether the effect is confined to patients with newly diagnosed T2D or whether it reflects the long period of time required to significantly affect subsequent atherosclerotic outcomes is not entirely clear.

Even before the cardiovascular benefits of intensive glucose therapy emerged in the long-term follow-up of the UKPDS trial, guidelines recommended a target HbA1c level of 7% or less in most patients. This was primarily driven by the expectation of microvascular benefits, albeit with uncertainty over the effects on macrovascular events. To settle the questions about the role of intensive glucose therapy in T2D, three randomized controlled trials were specifically designed to examine the impact of targeting near-normal glycemia on cardiovascular risk. The HbA1c targets were set low because of the continuous epidemiologic relationship of glucose with cardiovascular risk, suggesting that perhaps much lower glucose levels need to be achieved for a significant benefit to emerge. The three trials all recruited participants with T2D who had either a history of or multiple risk factors for cardiovascular disease, thus ensuring adequate event rates to study the effects of the interventions. Participants were therefore quite distinct from patients in the UKPDS trial—they were older, had a longer duration of diabetes, and had a greater comorbidity burden.

The Action to Control Cardiovascular Risk in Diabetes (ACCORD) trial enrolled 10,251 patients (mean age 62, median baseline HbA1c 8.1%, 35% with history of prior cardiovascular event) to intensive glucose therapy (targeting HbA1c <6%, median achieved HbA1c 6.4%) versus conventional therapy (targeting HbA1c 7%–7.9%, median achieved HbA1c 7.5%).[24] This trial was stopped prematurely after a mean follow-up of 3.5 years because of a higher mortality rate in the intensive therapy group compared with the control arm (HR 1.22, $P = 0.04$). The primary endpoint of the trial, major cardiovascular events, was not significantly reduced (HR 0.90, $P = 0.16$), although the rate of nonfatal MI was lower in the intensive therapy group (HR 0.76, $P = 0.004$). To date, analyses have not identified any clear explanation for the higher mortality risk associated with the intensive glucose-lowering strategy. In the intensive therapy group, a median HbA1c level of 6.4% was rapidly achieved and maintained, but subsequent post hoc analyses implicated factors associated with persistently higher HbA1c, rather than low HbA1c, as likely contributors to the higher mortality risk.[25] In addition, rates of serious hypoglycemia requiring medical assistance were threefold higher in the intensive group than during standard therapy (10.5% vs. 3.5%, $P < 0.001$). Subsequent retrospective epidemiologic analyses of ACCORD have suggested, however, that severe hypoglycemia may not, in fact, account for the difference in mortality between the two study arms.[26] Although hypoglycemia was associated with higher mortality within each randomized group, the risk of death was actually lower in participants experiencing hypoglycemia in the intensive arm than in participants with hypoglycemia in the standard arm. Other explanations, such as the particular medication combinations or undetected medication interactions, have also been proposed, but no particular medication class has been implicated thus far. In the end, the explanation for the higher mortality may never be known, but the findings have led to a growing recognition that intensive glucose lowering may be associated with some benefits but also important risks.

Subsequent follow-up of the participants from the ACCORD trial, up to the originally planned 5 years, showed persistently higher mortality rates in the intensive therapy group (HR 1.19, $P = 0.02$), but still lower rates of nonfatal

MI (HR 0.82, P = 0.01).[27] Given these findings, strategies used in the ACCORD study targeting an HbA1c below 6% are not recommended for patients with advanced T2D and established macrovascular complications or multiple risk factors for cardiovascular events.

At the same time the ACCORD study was published, results from the Action in Diabetes and Vascular Disease: Preterax and Diamicron Modified Release Controlled Evaluation (ADVANCE) trial also became available.[28] In this trial, 11,140 patients with T2D (mean age 66, median baseline HbA1c 7.2%, 32% with history of major macrovascular disease) were randomized to intensive therapy (preferentially with the sulfonylurea gliclazide, targeting HbA1c ≤6.5%, with mean achieved HbA1c 6.5%) or to standard therapy (HbA1c goal according to local guidelines, mean achieved HbA1c 7.3%). After a median follow-up of 5 years, there was a reduction in the primary outcome of the study, which was a composite of microvascular and macrovascular events (HR 0.90, P = 0.01), and this was almost entirely driven by effects on intermediate markers of nephropathy. There was no significant effect with respect to major cardiovascular events (HR 0.94, P = 0.32), but also no increase in mortality (HR 0.93, P = 0.28) as was observed in the ACCORD trial. The ADVANCE investigators specifically examined various subgroups at potentially increased risk of death, but none were identified. Overall, the trial findings suggest a modest improvement in markers of microvascular complications with more intensive treatment versus usual care, but no significant benefit gained with respect to CHD endpoints.

One additional trial confirmed the lack of significant benefit of more intensive glucose lowering compared with usual care on major cardiovascular events, the Veterans Affairs Diabetes Trial (VADT). In this study of 1791 US military veterans with T2D (mean age 60, median baseline HbA1c 9.4%, 40% with history of cardiovascular events), participants were randomized to intensive glucose or standard therapy using a combination of agents, with a goal of achieving an absolute reduction in HbA1c of 1.5% in the intensive versus the standard arm. Median HbA1c levels achieved were 6.9% versus 8.4% in the intensive and standard groups, respectively, over a median follow-up of 5.6 years. There was no significant benefit with respect to the primary composite outcome, of cardiovascular events (HR 0.88, P = 0.14), the individual outcome of death from any cause, nor any difference with respect to most microvascular complications (no changes in retinopathy, new neuropathy, or doubling of creatinine, but reduction in some albuminuria-based endpoints). In this study of patients with advanced T2D, other cardiovascular risk factors were well controlled, and differences in HbA1c levels between the two groups were maintained. However, overall, the benefit of decreasing HbA1c from 8.4% to 6.9% was minimal, except in the progression of albuminuria, an intermediate marker with uncertain implications for long-term renal risk.

Multiple meta-analyses have followed the three randomized controlled trials described earlier to determine whether pooling results of existing studies will illuminate our understanding of these relationships (Fig. 10.4). Although these analyses sometimes included studies of different intent (not necessarily glucose-lowering per se) and with variable patient characteristics (newly diagnosed vs. patients with advanced diabetes), they consistently show a modest, although significant, reduction of approximately 15% in the risk for nonfatal MI, but no impact on mortality or cardiovascular death.[29–34] Moreover, all these studies show that the risk for severe hypoglycemia with intensive glucose therapy is more than doubled.

Why have these large randomized controlled trials failed to show that intensive glucose lowering improves cardiovascular outcomes when the epidemiologic relationship between glycemia and cardiovascular events is so convincing? Many of the expectations for reduction in risk may have arisen from the effects of statin medications on major adverse cardiovascular events (MACEs) in early trials. A strong epidemiologic association between LDL cholesterol and CHD exists, and interventional studies show a 23% relative reduction in risk achieved for every 1 mmol/L (38 mg/dL) of LDL cholesterol lowering. Glycemia is a much weaker risk factor for CHD than cholesterol, but the assumption has been that some degree of cardiovascular (CV) risk reduction should result from glucose lowering. However, it is clear that the simple arithmetic (lower the level of a risk factor and cardiovascular events will naturally follow) does not apply in the case of glycemia. There may be a modest reduction in nonfatal MI, but overall disappointing results with respect to mortality and the composite of major cardiovascular events. Several potential explanations can be proposed: significant adverse effects of glucose therapy may counterbalance possible benefits, effects of glucose lowering applied in advanced diabetes may be too late to prevent atherosclerotic events, or the impact of glucose lowering may take a longer time to materialize than the 5 to 7 years assessed in most clinical trials. Regardless of the reasons, currently available therapies tested in these studies do not appear to constitute a "magic bullet" for the increased cardiovascular morbidity of diabetes.

TRIALS OF GLUCOSE-LOWERING INTERVENTIONS IN PREDIABETES AND EARLY DIABETES

Because one potential reason for the lack of benefit of intensive glucose lowering on cardiovascular disease is that it is applied too late to prevent atherosclerosis, it is worthwhile to examine studies that have investigated glucose lowering before diabetes actually develops or very early in the disease course (see also Chapters 3 and 4).

One such study was the Diabetes Prevention Program that randomly assigned 3234 persons without diabetes at high risk for diabetes (with elevated body mass index and fasting and postload glucose values) to intensive lifestyle therapy, metformin monotherapy, or placebo.[35] Lifestyle intervention and metformin both significantly reduced the incidence of subsequent diabetes. In follow-up studies of the trial population, the lifestyle intervention also improved cardiovascular risk factors compared with metformin or placebo treatment, but the number of cardiovascular events was too small (n = 89 at 3 years) to allow any meaningful examination of the differences among

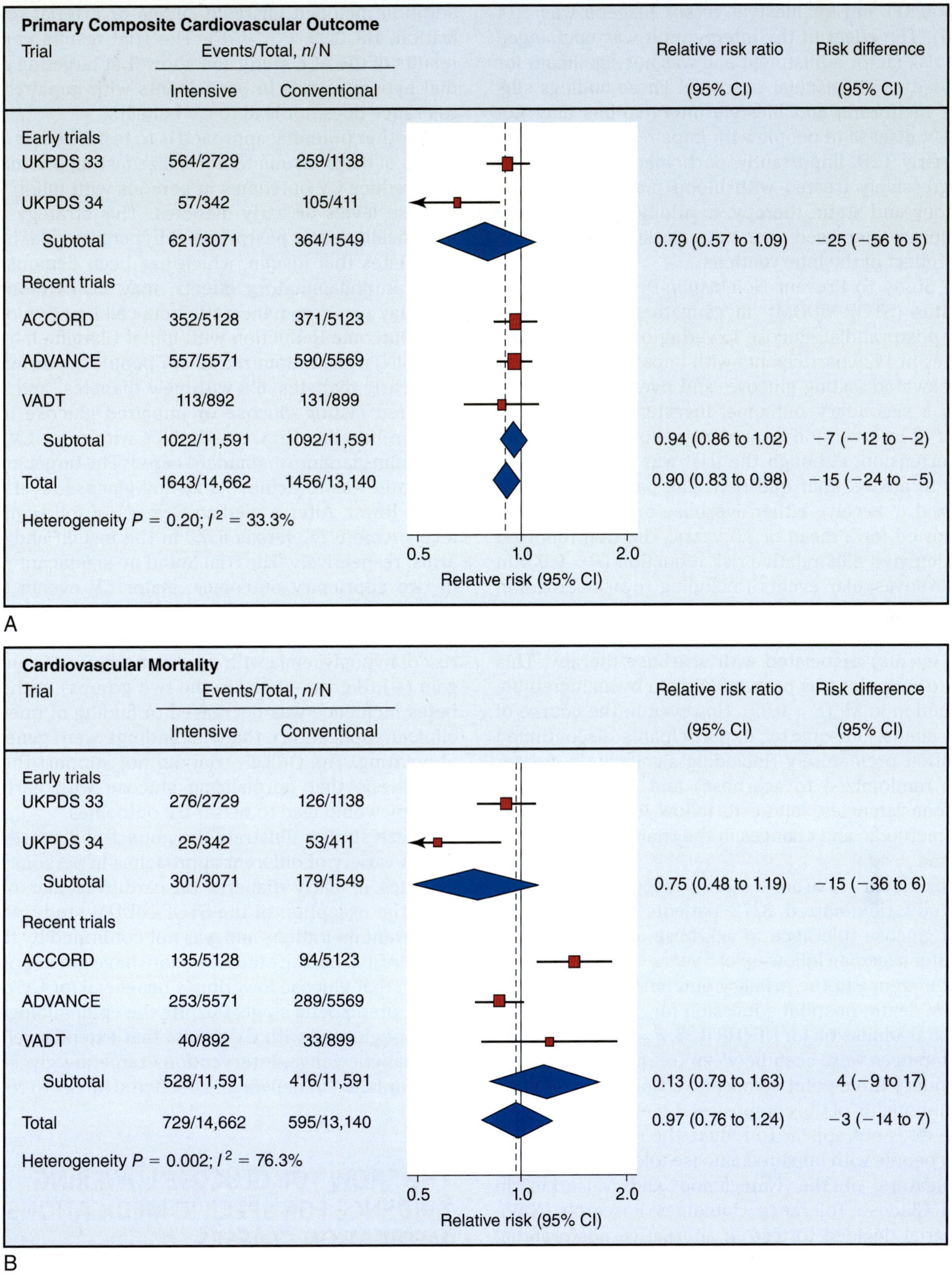

FIG. 10.4 Relative risk and risk differences estimates (per 1000 patients over 5 years of treatment), with 95% confidence intervals (*CIs*), for the main study outcomes in the UKPDS, ACCORD, ADVANCE, and VADT. **A**, Primary composite cardiovascular outcome. **B**, Cardiovascular mortality. From Kelly TN, Bazzano LA, Fonseca VA, et al. Systematic review: glucose control and cardiovascular disease in type 2 diabetes, *Ann Intern Med* 2009;151:394–403.

groups.[36] After 10 years of follow-up of the Diabetes Prevention Program, the cumulative incidence of diabetes was still lowest in the former lifestyle intervention group.[37] Cardiovascular disease risk factors improved in all three treatment groups, but averaged over all follow-up, systolic and diastolic blood pressure and triglyceride levels were lower in the lifestyle than in the other groups (even though the use of antihypertensive medications was less frequent). However, after 21 years of follow-up, neither metformin nor lifestyle intervention reduced major cardiovascular events (nonfatal MI, stroke, or CV death).[38] The hazard ratio for metformin versus placebo was

1.03 ($P = 0.81$) and for lifestyle versus placebo was 1.14 ($P = 0.34$). The effect of the intervention was unchanged after the risk factor adjustment and was not significant for an extended cardiovascular outcome. These findings suggest that metformin and lifestyle interventions may not prevent CV disease in people with impaired glucose tolerance or early T2D. Importantly, participants in the study were aggressively treated with blood pressure–lowering medications and statin therapy; in addition, out-of-study metformin use increased over time, possibly limiting the apparent effect of the interventions.

In the Study to Prevent Non-Insulin-Dependent Diabetes Mellitus (STOP-NIDDM), investigators examined the effect of postprandial glucose lowering on the incidence of diabetes in 1429 participants with impaired glucose tolerance, elevated fasting glucose, and overweight or obesity.[39] As a secondary outcome, investigators examined the effect of intervention on major cardiovascular events and hypertension, although the trial was not adequately powered to answer that question. The participants were randomized to receive either acarbose or a placebo and were followed for a mean of 3.3 years. The trial reported an unanticipated 49% relative risk reduction ($P = 0.03$) in major cardiovascular events (including revascularization procedures, congestive heart failure, and peripheral vascular disease in addition to the conventional major cardiovascular events) associated with acarbose therapy. This composite endpoint was primarily driven by an incredible 91% reduction in MI ($P = 0.02$). However, in the course of the trial, almost one-quarter of participants discontinued participation prematurely (including significantly greater numbers randomized to acarbose) and other concerns about inconsistencies, failure to follow intention-to-treat analysis methods, and changes in the trial endpoints have been raised.

A subsequent Acarbose Cardiovascular Evaluation (ACE) study randomized 3272 patients with CHD and impaired glucose tolerance to acarbose and 3250 to placebo.[40] After a median follow-up of 5 years, there was no significant difference in the primary outcome of nonfatal MI, stroke, CV death, hospital admission for unstable angina, and hospital admission for HF (HR 0.98, $P = 0.73$). No significant differences were seen between treatment groups for the secondary three-point composite CV outcome, or each of the components of the composites. Given these findings, acarbose does not appear to reduce the risk of major CV events in people with impaired glucose tolerance and CHD.

Investigators of the Nateglinide and Valsartan in Impaired Glucose Tolerance Outcomes Research (NAVIGATOR) trial decided to test an alternative postprandial glucose-lowering approach with a short-acting insulin secretagogue, nateglinide, in addition to lifestyle modification. They randomized 9306 persons (mean age 64) with impaired glucose tolerance (baseline HbA1c 5.8%) at high risk for CV disease (24% had a history of CV events) to nateglinide or a placebo and followed participants for a median of 5 years. Nateglinide did not reduce the occurrence of the three coprimary outcomes—incident diabetes (HR 1.07, $P = 0.05$), cardiovascular outcome (death from CV causes, nonfatal MI, nonfatal stroke, or hospitalization for HF, HR 0.94, $P = 0.43$), or the extended CV outcome (which in addition included unstable angina or arterial revascularization, HR 0.93, $P = 0.16$). The trial results confirm the results of the ACE study and show that targeting postprandial hyperglycemia in participants with impaired glucose tolerance does not lead to CV benefits.

Another potential approach is to test whether early provision of basal insulin to normalize fasting plasma glucose may reduce CV outcomes in persons with mildly elevated glucose levels or early diabetes. This strategy does not specifically target postprandial hyperglycemia, but rather postulates that insulin, which has been demonstrated to have antiinflammatory effects, may be cardioprotective and may preserve pancreatic beta-cell function over time. The Outcome Reduction with Initial Glargine Intervention (ORIGIN) trial randomized 12,537 people (mean age 64; 82% with early diabetes, 6% with new diabetes, and 12% with impaired fasting glucose or impaired glucose tolerance; median baseline HbA1c 6.4%; 59% with prior CV disease) to insulin glargine or standard care.[41] The target in the insulin group was to achieve a fasting glucose level of 95 mg/dL or lower. After a median 6 years of follow-up, HbA1c levels were 6.2% versus 6.5% in the insulin and standard arms, respectively. The trial found no significant reduction in two coprimary outcomes: major CV events (HR 1.02, $P = 0.63$) and major CV events plus revascularization and HF (HR 1.04, $P = 0.27$). However, there was an increased risk of hypoglycemia with insulin therapy and some weight gain (+1.6 kg vs. −0.5 kg in the two groups). Although diabetes incidence was decreased (a finding of questionable clinical application), the trial findings were generally disappointing. The ORIGIN trial did not support the original hypothesis that normalizing glucose with early insulin therapy would lead to better CV outcomes.

These studies illustrate the impact of glucose lowering with a variety of different approaches in persons with prediabetes or early diabetes on cardiovascular outcomes. With the exception of the STOP-NIDDM study, which had important limitations and was not confirmed by the subsequent ACE trial, the studies to date have not supported the notion that glucose lowering is beneficial for CV outcomes at the prediabetic stage. Despite the epidemiologic association of glucose with CV events that extends well into the nondiabetic range, interventions targeting glycemia have thus far failed to deliver an effective strategy to reduce this risk.

THE "HOW" OF GLUCOSE LOWERING: EVIDENCE FOR SPECIFIC MEDICATIONS AND MEDICATION CLASSES

Perhaps one of the most important lessons in CV risk reduction in T2D has been the growing recognition that the exact strategy used to reduce glucose may actually matter with respect to outcomes. The early UKPDS experience, albeit based on a small subgroup ($n = 342$) of patients, has given metformin a preferred place in the antihyperglycemic regimen for T2D. In the subsequent glucose-lowering trials (ACCORD, ADVANCE, VADT), combinations of various medications, including insulin, had to be used to lower glucose levels, and there was no particular advantage to one strategy versus another. However, these glucose-lowering trials were not designed to test the effects of specific medications on outcomes.

Interest in the effects of specific antihyperglycemic medications on outcomes was boosted by the publication of a meta-analysis by Nissen and colleagues in 2007 that showed an adverse effect of the thiazolidinedione rosiglitazone on MI risk.[42] In the analysis of 42 trials that was performed, there were 86 MI events in the rosiglitazone group compared with 71 in the comparator arm (including placebo, metformin, sulfonylurea, or insulin), resulting in an odds ratio of 1.43 ($P = 0.03$). Although the methodology and the results of this meta-analysis have been debated, and some have noted no increase in risk associated with rosiglitazone use,[43,44] there is no doubt that the study provided a cautionary tale for glucose lowering. Most important, the study suggested that even though a medication may reduce glucose levels, and thus appear to treat diabetes effectively, it may in fact increase the risk of clinical events that are the target of glucose lowering in the first place. After the rosiglitazone experience, however, the US Food and Drug Administration (FDA) mandated that novel glucose-lowering medications must have data that support their safety with respect to cardiovascular events before they are approved for use in diabetes.[45]

The FDA guidance led to a proliferation of multiple large cardiovascular outcomes trials (CVOTs), which substantially differ in their design from glycemic control trials. CVOTs include participants with established atherosclerotic CV disease, or at high risk for CV events, to ensure accrual of sufficient events in a timely manner. The trials randomize participants to either receive placebo with other diabetes treatments per usual care, or to receive a specific drug being tested with other diabetes treatments as background therapy. Since clinicians are blinded to the intervention, they can adjust participants' glucose-lowering therapies to achieve HbA1c levels according to standards of care. As a result, the study arms differ in the use of the specific study drug but generally achieve similar levels of glycemic control, albeit the active comparator arm is typically associated with reduction in HbA1c levels by ~0.3%.

Although CVOTs were mainly designed to rule out unacceptable cardiovascular risk, many were powered to estimate superiority as well as noninferiority. The results of these trials for SGLT-2 inhibitors and GLP-1 receptor agonists, two classes of antihyperglycemic medications with robustly proven efficacy for cardiovascular and kidney outcomes, are described in detail in Chapters x and y. Below, the evidence for the other antihyperglycemic drug classes including the FDA-mandated CVOTs with DPP-4 inhibitors is summarized (see also Table 10.2).

Metformin[46]

Metformin, which works primarily by reducing hepatic glucose production, effectively reduces HbA1c levels, is weight neutral, and does not lead to hypoglycemia when used as monotherapy. It is also inexpensive, has a favorable safety profile, and may have potential benefit with respect to CV disease, based on the UKPDS substudy.[22] However, despite the many advantages of metformin, the evidence generated from large CVOTs with SGLT2i and GLP1RA has not been matched by large-scale CVOTs with metformin, partly because of its pervasive and entrenched use as first-line therapy in T2D.

As noted above, existing data with respect to CV risk reduction with metformin are relatively sparse. In addition to the UKPDS substudy,[22] only one prior randomized controlled trial was conducted on this subject. In the trial, 390 patients treated with insulin were randomized to receive either metformin or placebo as add-on therapy.[47] The primary endpoint, an aggregate of microvascular and macrovascular outcomes, did not differ between the two groups after 4.3 years of follow-up (HR 0.92, $P = 0.33$), but there was a significant reduction in the secondary endpoint of macrovascular events (HR 0.60, $P = 0.04$). In addition, metformin use was associated with beneficial effects on body weight and insulin requirements.

In observational studies, metformin use (either as monotherapy or in combination with another oral agent) has been associated with reduced mortality,[48–51] CV deaths,[48,51] and CV events.[49,50,52,53] Because metformin is generally the preferred initial agent for diabetes treatment and remains contraindicated in patients with advanced chronic kidney disease, patients who are not treated with this medication in an observational study may differ in important ways from those who are. These analyses either adjusted for potential confounders or matched patient populations for the propensity to be prescribed metformin versus another medication (usually a sulfonylurea). However, these investigations were observational in nature, so unmeasured factors may potentially still have contributed to the differences in outcomes.

Alongside the evidence that supports the safety and effectiveness of metformin, there are data that provide a less reassuring picture. Although the UKPDS substudy showed benefits of metformin in participants with overweight or obesity, the trial also reported an increased death rate in nonoverweight patients who took metformin and a sulfonylurea compared with those who took a sulfonylurea alone (relative risk 1.60, $P = 0.04$).[22] Combined analyses of the two UKPDS studies did not reveal an increased risk for mortality in patients treated with this combination, and the increased mortality in the UKPDS substudy has not been fully explained. In a subsequent meta-analysis of 13 randomized controlled trials involving more than 13,000 patients with T2D, compared with other treatments, metformin therapy had no significant effect on the risk for mortality (relative risk 0.99 with wide 95% confidence intervals that could not exclude a 25% reduction or 31% increase in risk), CV mortality (relative risk 1.05), or rates of MI (relative risk 0.90 with 95% CIs that could not exclude 26% risk reduction or 9% harm).[29] Similar findings were reported in a meta-analysis that specifically examined the effects of metformin with insulin compared with insulin alone in 23 trials with over 2000 participants.[54] The study found that metformin added to insulin did not significantly change mortality risk (relative risk 1.30, with 95% CIs 0.57–2.99) or cardiovascular mortality risk (relative risk 1.70, with 95% CIs 0.35–8.30) but provided little reassurance with regard to each of these endpoints given the wide confidence intervals. Finally, in a

TABLE 10.2 Summary of Cardiovascular Effects Associated With Various Classes of Glucose-Lowering Agents (Excluding SGLT-2 Inhibitors and GLP-1 Receptor Agonists, Which Are Covered Separately)

AGENT	MECHANISM OF ACTION	EXPECTED HBA1C REDUCTION	ADVERSE EFFECTS	CARDIOVASCULAR EFFECTS
Sulfonylureas				
Glyburide (aka glibenclamide) Glipizide Glimepiride Gliclazide Tolbutamide Chlorpropamide	Bind to sulfonylurea receptors on pancreatic islet cells, closing K_{ATP} channels, stimulating insulin release. Relatively long duration of action.	Approximately 1%–2%	Hypoglycemia Weight gain	Hypoglycemia may precipitate ischemia, arrhythmia. Cardiac K_{ATP} channel closure may impair ischemic preconditioning. Observational studies suggest worse CVD outcomes compared with metformin.
Glinides				
Repaglinide Nateglinide	Bind to sulfonylurea receptors on pancreatic islet cells, closing K_{ATP} channels, stimulating insulin release. Relatively short duration of action.	Approximately 1%–2%	Hypoglycemia Weight gain	Hypoglycemia may precipitate ischemia, arrhythmia. Cardiac K_{ATP} channel closure may impair ischemic preconditioning. Few CVD outcome studies exist.
Biguanide				
Metformin	Activates AMP-kinase and reduces hepatic glucose production.	Approximately 1%–2%	Diarrhea, nausea Lactic acidosis Decreases B_{12} levels	May improve CVD outcomes (UKPDS 34). Favorable CVD outcomes in most observational studies. Should not be used in patients with acute or unstable HF because of lactic acidosis risk.
α-Glucosidase Inhibitors				
Voglibose Acarbose Miglitol	Slow gut carbohydrate absorption.	Approximately 0.5%–1.0%	Gas, bloating	Neutral with respect to MACE (ACE Study).
Thiazolidinediones				
Pioglitazone Rosiglitazone	Activate the nuclear receptor PPAR-γ, increasing peripheral insulin sensitivity. Also reduce hepatic glucose production.	Approximately 1%–1.5%	Weight gain Edema, HF Fractures? Bladder cancer (pioglitazone)	Contraindicated in NYHA Class III or IV HF (because of fluid retention); not recommended in Class II HF. Pioglitazone may reduce MI, stroke risk (PROactive, IRIS) but increases HF risk. Rosiglitazone may increase MI risk.
DPP-4 Inhibitors				
Sitagliptin Saxagliptin Linagliptin Vildagliptin Alogliptin	Inhibit degradation of endogenous GLP-1 (and GIP-1), thereby enhancing incretin levels.			Neutral effect on cardiovascular outcomes, but saxagliptin and alogliptin may increase the risk of HF.
Amylin Analog				
Pramlintide	Decreases glucagon secretion and delays gastric emptying.	Approximately 0.4%–0.6%	Nausea, vomiting	Long-term outcomes not known.
Insulins				
Glargine, detemir, degludec NPH Regular Lispro, aspart, glulisine Premixed	Increase insulin supply.	Theoretically limitless	Hypoglycemia Weight gain Edema (at high doses)	Few randomized controlled trials show neutral effects on cardiovascular outcomes, but observational studies suggest higher risk of cardiovascular events and mortality compared with oral antihyperglycemic agents.

Data from Inzucchi and McGuire.

AMP, Adenosine monophosphate; *CVD*, cardiovascular disease; *GFR*, glomerular filtration rate; *GIP-1*, gastric inhibitory polypeptide-1; *GLP-1*, glucagon-like peptide-1; *HF*, heart failure; K_{ATP}, adenosine triphosphate (ATP) sensitive potassium channel; *MACE*, major adverse cardiovascular event; *NYHA*, New York Heart Association; *PPAR-γ*, peroxisome proliferator-activated receptor gamma; *SGLT-2*, sodium-glucose co-transporter 2.

meta-analysis of 301 clinical trials of nine major classes of glucose-lowering medications (metformin, sulfonylureas, thiazolidinediones, meglitinides, alpha-glucosidase inhibitors, DPP-4i, SLGT2i, GLP1RA, and basal insulin), there were no significant differences in associations between any drug class as monotherapy, dual therapy, or triple therapy with the odds of CV or all-cause mortality.[55]

Sulfonylureas

Sulfonylureas, insulin secretagogues, are the oldest oral agent class for treatment of hyperglycemia. Whereas sulfonylureas are effective at glucose lowering, they increase the risk of hypoglycemia, are associated with a modest weight gain, and likely result in less durable effects on glucose control compared with metformin or thiazolidinediones.[56]

Questions about cardiovascular safety of sulfonylureas date back to 1970 when the University Group Diabetes Program (UGDP) trial reported an increased risk for CV death associated with the use of tolbutamide compared with a placebo or insulin.[57] Subsequently the FDA mandated a boxed warning for all sulfonylureas. Sulfonylureas inhibit the adenosine triphosphate (ATP)–dependent potassium channels that are present within cardiomyocytes and coronary vascular endothelial cells, and it has been postulated that the presence of sulfonylureas at the time of an acute coronary event prevents adequate coronary vasodilation and thus may result in a larger area of myocardial damage. However, the risk of CV death noted by the UGDP group was not supported by the subsequent UKPDS study, which showed no difference in CV risk between the use of sulfonylureas (chlorpropamide, glibenclamide, or glipizide) or insulin therapy[21] (but a benefit with the use of metformin, as noted earlier[22]). The large A Diabetes Outcome Prevention Trial (ADOPT) study compared metformin, rosiglitazone, or glyburide therapy with respect to glycemic control, but again found no difference with respect to cardiovascular events (which were not frequent and were collected as adverse events during the trial) across the treatment groups after 4 years of treatment.[56] The ADVANCE study of intensive glucose lowering primarily used gliclazide in its intensive glucose control arm and found no risk associated with this strategy.[28] Finally, the aforementioned meta-analysis found no significant differences in associations between any drug class—including sulfonylureas—as monotherapy, dual therapy, or triple therapy with odds of CV or all-cause mortality.[58]

One CVOT specifically compared linagliptin, a DPP-4 inhibitor, against glimepiride, a sulfonylurea.[58] In this trial, 6042 patients with relatively early T2D and risk factors for or established atherosclerotic CV disease were randomized to these two therapies, and 6033 were treated and included in the analysis. The primary outcome of major CV events occurred in 356 of 3023 participants (11.8%) in the linagliptin group and 362 of 3010 (12.0%) in the glimepiride group (HR, 0.98; $P<.001$ for noninferiority and $P=0.76$ for superiority). Despite a higher risk for hypoglycemia in the glimepiride group, this did not translate into an increase in CV events. Like the meta-analysis above, the trial provides reassuring evidence with respect to the CV safety of sulfonylureas.

Observational studies have, however, mostly suggested harm with sulfonylurea treatment, especially compared with metformin therapy.[48,49,59,60] Whether sulfonylureas are associated with adverse effects or metformin is protective remains debatable. Sulfonylureas are still considered a viable option for second-line therapy in diabetes, primarily based on their effectiveness in lowering glucose and extensive accrued experience with the use of these agents.

Thiazolidinediones

Thiazolidinediones, which lower glucose by activating the nuclear transcription factor peroxisome proliferator-activated receptor gamma (PPAR-γ), are insulin sensitizers. They do not increase the risk of hypoglycemia and may result in more durable blood glucose control than sulfonylureas or metformin.[56] Although these agents improve many intermediate markers of cardiovascular risk (e.g., C-reactive protein and markers of endothelial function), they are associated with substantial weight gain, lower-extremity edema, HF, bone fractures, and possibly bladder cancer risk.

Rosiglitazone, but not pioglitazone, has actually been associated with an increased risk of MI,[42] which led to its restricted use in diabetes. Therefore the two members of the thiazolidinediones class need to be considered separately if their individual risks and benefits are to be understood. It is worth noting that most analyses of the effects of glucose-lowering therapies on clinical outcomes group together medications of the same class and perform class-based comparisons. This practice is based on the assumption that medications in the same class have a similar mode of action and therefore will have a similar effect on clinical outcomes. The experience with rosiglitazone and pioglitazone, both members of the thiazolidinedione class, suggests that individual medications within the same class can affect clinical outcomes in different ways.

As already mentioned, the effect of rosiglitazone on CV events was analyzed in a highly publicized meta-analysis, which showed an increased risk of MI associated with its use.[42] Several other meta-analyses confirmed adverse effects associated with rosiglitazone,[61,62] but not all found harm.[43,44] However, observational studies comparing rosiglitazone with other oral diabetes medications[63] or with pioglitazone[64–66] have consistently shown increased risk of mortality and HF with rosiglitazone use. The only trial specifically designed to evaluate CV outcomes associated with rosiglitazone was the Rosiglitazone Evaluated for Cardiovascular Outcomes in Oral Agent Combination Therapy for Type 2 Diabetes (RECORD) study.[67] RECORD randomized 4447 patients with diabetes with inadequately controlled hyperglycemia treated with metformin or sulfonylurea monotherapy to receive, in addition, a sulfonylurea, metformin, or rosiglitazone. In the final analysis of the trial, there was no difference in the primary endpoint (CV hospitalization or CV death) among the groups, but the event rate was lower than expected and the dropout rate in the trial was high, decreasing the power to detect significant differences in outcomes. Notably, the risk of HF was increased approximately twofold with rosiglitazone.

Finally, in the Bypass Angioplasty Revascularization Investigation 2 Diabetes trial, 2368 patients with T2D and obstructive coronary artery disease were factorially randomized to (1) medical therapy with insulin provision [insulin or sulfonylurea] versus insulin sensitization [metformin or rosiglitazone]); and (2) randomized to medical treatment versus coronary revascularization (a priori determined to be percutaneous coronary intervention [PCI] or coronary artery bypass grafting [CABG]), evaluating the effects on death and major CV events.[68] There was no difference in the rates of death and CV events between patients undergoing revascularization or medical therapy, or between strategies of insulin provision and insulin sensitization. However, in the CABG stratum, the risk of major CV events was significantly lower with revascularization and insulin sensitization (18.7%) compared with insulin sensitization therapy alone (32%, $P = 0.002$). Because rosiglitazone was the primary thiazolidinedione used for insulin sensitization, there did not appear to be harm associated with its use in the setting of this trial. However, the trial was not designed to specifically address rosiglitazone's safety.

Given the weight of the evidence, in 2011 the FDA placed restrictions on the prescription and use of rosiglitazone-containing medications through a Risk Evaluation and Mitigation Strategy.[69] The use of rosiglitazone was limited to patients already successfully treated with this medication, or patients whose blood glucose levels could not be controlled with other antihyperglycemia medicines and who did not wish to use pioglitazone instead. In June 2013, the FDA reviewed readjudicated data from the RECORD trial and concluded that the trial had not found an elevated risk of MI or death associated with rosiglitazone. Therefore in November 2013 the FDA lifted its earlier restrictions on rosiglitazone use. Given the highly publicized debates over the safety of rosiglitazone, this medication is essentially never used even in those countries where it is still available.

In contrast to rosiglitazone, data with pioglitazone are more reassuring with respect to CV outcomes.[60,64–66,70] One trial investigating the effects of pioglitazone on CV outcomes was the Prospective Pioglitazone Clinical Trial in Macrovascular Events (PROactive) study, in which 5238 patients with T2D and established macrovascular disease received pioglitazone or placebo, added to their baseline diabetes therapy.[71] After an average follow-up of 2.9 years, there was a 10% relative risk reduction in the primary endpoint (including all-cause mortality, nonfatal MI, stroke, acute coronary syndrome, revascularization, and above-knee amputation), but this did not reach statistical significance ($P = 0.095$) (Fig. 10.5). The secondary, and more conventional, outcome of major CV events was significantly decreased with pioglitazone (HR 0.84, $P = 0.03$). Concerns have been raised about the late definition of the secondary endpoint after the trial was underway, the large number of secondary endpoints (more than eight), and the increased risk of HF in the intervention group (16% vs. 11.5%), which may have, over time, negatively affected study results.

Two additional trials specifically examined CV outcomes associated with pioglitazone. The Insulin Resistance after Stroke (IRIS) trial included 3876 insulin-resistant patients without diabetes who had a recent ischemic stroke or

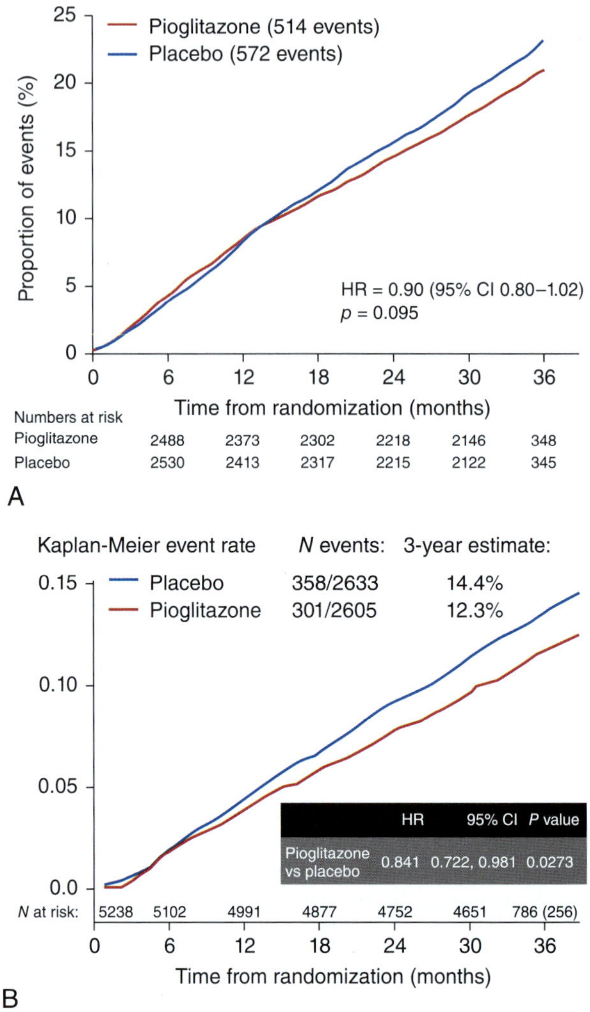

FIG. 10.5 PROactive study. Time to primary composite endpoint (all-cause mortality, nonfatal myocardial infarction, stroke, acute coronary syndrome, revascularization, and above-knee amputation) and time to secondary endpoint (major cardiovascular events).

TIA.[72] These subjects were randomly assigned to receive either pioglitazone or placebo. In the IRIS trial, pioglitazone reduced the combined endpoint of fatal or nonfatal stroke or MI by 24% versus placebo over a median follow-up of 4.8 years (HR, 0.76; 95% CI, 0.62–0.93; $P = 0.007$). However, the use of pioglitazone increased the risk of weight gain, edema, and fracture. In contrast, the Thiazolidinediones Or Sulfonylureas and Cardiovascular Accidents Intervention Trial (TOSCA.IT) randomly assigned 3028 patients with T2D to pioglitazone or to sulfonylureas (mostly glimepiride and gliclazide) in addition to baseline metformin therapy.[73] TOSCA.IT was stopped early on the basis of futility. Only 11% of the study population had established CV disease at baseline and the rate of events in the trial was low at 1.5 per 100 person-years. The primary outcome, which included a composite of nonfatal MI, nonfatal stroke, all-cause mortality, or urgent coronary revascularization did not differ between pioglitazone versus sulfonylurea groups (HR, 0.96; 95% CI, 0.74–1.26; $P = 0.79$). Moderate weight gain, edema, and fractures did not differ between the groups. Whether the differences between the results of IRIS and TOSCA.IT are due to different sample populations with respect to diabetes status and baseline CV risk, or due to the comparison drug (placebo or sulfonylureas) is difficult to parse out.

In summary, the CV benefits of thiazolidinediones are not entirely clear. The association of rosiglitazone with MI, HF, and mortality is concerning, and most guidelines recommend against the use of rosiglitazone for those reasons. The potential benefits of pioglitazone in the PROactive study and IRIS studies must be weighed against the increased risk of HF and fractures. Based on the data and net benefit-risk assessment, European Society of Cardiology guidelines consider the use of pioglitazone to mitigate CV risk in patients with T2D and prevalent CHD as a reasonable option.[74]

Dipeptidyl Peptidase 4 Inhibitors

Dipeptidyl peptidase 4 (DPP-4) inhibitors reduce the activity of the enzyme DPP-4, which deactivates glucose-insulinotropic polypeptide (GIP) and GLP-1. Thus DPP-4 inhibitors raise GIP and GLP-1 levels, but the effects are more modest compared with administration of a GLP-1 receptor agonist. DPP-4 inhibitors modestly lower HbA1c levels, are weight neutral, and do not cause hypoglycemia. Due to infrequent side effects and lack of contraindications with respect to chronic kidney disease, these agents tend to be popular among older patients with T2D.

Data from CVOT demonstrate that DPP-4 inhibitors are neutral with respect to major cardiovascular events, but some trials have shown increased risk of heart failure with the use of certain DPP-4 inhibitors. In the Saxagliptin Assessment of Vascular Outcomes Recorded in Patients with Diabetes Mellitus–Thrombolysis in Myocardial Infarction 53 (SAVOR-TIMI 53) trial, 16,492 patients with T2D who had risk factors or a history of CV events were assigned to receive saxagliptin or placebo in addition to their existing diabetes medication therapy.[75] After a median of 2.1 years, there was no difference in the primary endpoint (MI, ischemic stroke, or CV death) between the two groups (HR, 1.0; 95% CI, 0.89–1.12). However, more patients in the saxagliptin group reported hypoglycemic events (15.3% vs. 11.7%, $P < 0.001$), and, somewhat unexpectedly, more patients on saxagliptin were hospitalized for HF (3.5% vs. 2.8%, $P = 0.007$). In the Examination of Cardiovascular Outcomes with Alogliptin Versus Standard of Care (EXAMINE) trial, 5380 patients with T2D who had had an acute coronary event in the preceding 15 to 90 days were randomly assigned to receive either alogliptin or placebo in addition to an existing antihyperglycemic regimen.[76] Similar to the findings of the SAVOR trial, there was no difference in the primary endpoint (MI, stroke, or CV death) between the two groups (HR, 0.96; upper boundary of the one-sided CI, 1.16). HF hospitalization was not a prespecified endpoint in EXAMINE, but when it was examined in a post hoc fashion (including those events that occurred after a primary endpoint), there were numerically, but not statistically, more events in the alogliptin group (106 vs. 89; HR, 1.19; $P = 0.22$).[77] In another trial (TECOS), 14,671 patients with T2D with established CV disease were randomized to receive either sitagliptin or placebo.[78] The primary outcome of nonfatal MI, nonfatal stroke, hospitalization for unstable angina, or CV death occurred in 839 versus 851 patients in the sitagliptin versus placebo groups (HR, 0.98; $P < 0.001$) for noninferiority. Unlike the EXAMINE and SAVOR trials, HF hospitalization rates did not differ between the groups (HR, 1.00; $P = 0.98$). Finally, in the CARMELINA trial, patients with T2D at high risk for CV disease were randomized to linagliptin versus a placebo.[79] In this trial, the primary composite outcome of nonfatal MI, nonfatal stroke, and CV death occurred in 434 of 3494 patients in the linagliptin group and 420 of 3485 in the placebo group (HR, 1.02; $P = 0.62$). Hospitalization for heart failure occurred in 209 of 3494 patients randomized to linagliptin and in 226 of 3485 patients randomized to a placebo, with no significant difference between the two treatment groups (HR, 0.90; $P = 0.26$).

These trials demonstrate neutral effects of DPP-4 inhibitors with respect to major CV events, which appear consistent across trials and across slightly different definitions of the primary composite outcome. In contrast, the risk of HF admission with the use of DPP-4 inhibitors has not been a consistent finding across trials, suggesting it may not be a class effect, and a causal mechanism remains unclear. The FDA added warnings about the risk of HF hospitalization with alogliptin and saxagliptin, but subsequently expanded the warning to all DPP-4 inhibitors in patients at risk for HF. Certainly, in patients at high risk of HF best available evidence suggests preferential use of sitagliptin or linagliptin over alogliptin or saxagliptin.[80,81]

Insulin

As T2D progresses, beta-cell function declines and the effectiveness of oral agents for glucose control diminishes. However, endogenous insulin secretion is not entirely lost in T2D, and strategies for insulin use can be less complex than those used in the treatment of T1D. The main side effects of insulin use are weight gain and hypoglycemia. Given that insulin has been used in clinical practice for decades and is a naturally occurring peptide hormone, fewer concerns have been previously raised about its CV safety. However, insulin may obviously induce hypoglycemia, which may in turn promote adrenergic discharges and arrhythmia, promotes fluid retention, and may result in hypokalemia (especially when administered intravenously) as a result of potassium shifts from the extracellular to intracellular space.

Concerns about the CV safety of insulin use in T2D have been raised.[82] These concerns are primarily based on observational studies that show an increased risk of mortality, CV mortality, and CV events in patients with diabetes treated with insulin compared with other agents.[18,83–86] In one analysis, data on over 84,000 patients with T2D in the GPRD were used to determine the risk of the primary outcome (first major adverse cardiac event, first cancer, or mortality) associated with five different glucose-lowering regimens (metformin monotherapy, sulfonylurea monotherapy, insulin monotherapy, metformin plus sulfonylurea, and insulin plus metformin).[85] When compared with all other regimens, insulin monotherapy was associated with an increased risk of the primary outcome and all-cause mortality. Another analysis used data on patients initially treated with metformin only who either added on insulin (n = 2948) or sulfonylurea (n = 39,990).[86] In a propensity matched sample, patients whose regimen was intensified with insulin had higher rates of nonfatal CV events (adjusted HR, 1.30; P = 0.009) and all-cause mortality (adjusted HR, 1.44; P = 0.001) compared with those whose regimen was intensified using a sulfonylurea. The observational nature of these studies does not permit conclusions about the causal nature of these associations; the risk of harms may be mediated by insulin itself or by the clinical characteristics of patients who require and are prescribed insulin. Indeed, there were important differences in baseline characteristics among treatment groups; despite adjustment for a variety of variables, residual confounding remains an important limitation.

Although few trials have specifically focused on the effectiveness and safety of insulin for prevention of CV events, several trials have tested the use of insulin during and after an acute MI for secondary prevention of CV disease and mortality. The first Diabetes Mellitus, Insulin Glucose Infusion in Acute Myocardial Infarction (DIGAMI) study showed a significant reduction in mortality (absolute reduction of 11%) associated with the use of insulin-glucose infusion during admission and subcutaneous insulin after hospitalization for glycemic control compared with standard therapy in patients with diabetes.[87] Because it was unclear whether the mortality benefit was the result of inpatient or outpatient glycemic control in DIGAMI, the DIGAMI-2 study tested three different strategies, including combinations of insulin-based inpatient and outpatient glycemic control regimens.[88] However, the study struggled with patient recruitment and did not achieve differences in glycemic control among the three groups. There were no differences in mortality among the three groups. However, in a post hoc analysis of the DIGAMI-2 trial, insulin treatment was actually associated with a higher risk for nonfatal cardiovascular events, but not mortality.[89] In another trial conducted in the setting of acute myocardial infarction (HEART2D), 1115 patients with T2D were randomly assigned to prandial insulin or to basal insulin within 21 days of an acute myocardial event.[90] Interim analysis demonstrated no difference between the two arms with respect to the risk of CV events, and the trial was halted for statistical futility based on the advice of the data safety monitoring board.

The previously described ORIGIN trial provided reassuring evidence on the use of insulin glargine in adults with prediabetes or early diabetes but did not suggest CV benefits.[41] The use of insulin in this trial was associated with a very modest reduction in already low HbA1c levels (6.3% vs. 6.0% in the standard vs. insulin group, respectively) at the end of 2 years, no significant reduction in the cardiovascular endpoints, but increase in weight gain and hypoglycemic events. Moreover, there was no effect of glargine on the incidence of various cancers, a concern raised because of insulin's role in cell growth, differentiation, and proliferation and because of epidemiologic studies pointing to the increased risk of cancer associated with its use.[91,92]

The DEVOTE trial specifically compared different types of insulin with respect to major CV events. In this trial, 7637 patients with T2D were randomized to receive either insulin degludec or insulin glargine.[93] The vast majority of patients in this trial had either established CV disease, chronic kidney disease, or both. However, major CV events did not differ between the two arms (HR, 0.91; $P < 0.001$ for noninferiority), while hypoglycemia was significantly less common with insulin degludec.

Other Agents

Acarbose is an alpha-glucosidase inhibitor that delays gut carbohydrate absorption. Acarbose is infrequently used in the United States because of gastrointestinal side effects. Post hoc analyses of the STOP-NIDDM trial showed a reduction in CV endpoints, but as mentioned earlier, there were problems with the trial design and conduct.[39] The ACE study did not confirm CV benefits of this drug class.[94] Another agent, colesevelam, a bile acid sequestrant, is typically used to lower low-density lipoprotein (LDL) levels, but also modestly reduces glucose. The dopamine agonist bromocriptine reduces glucose levels, but very modestly, and is available in the United States only for antihyperglycemic therapy. A 52-week trial evaluated the short-term overall and CV safety of bromocriptine in T2D.[95] The frequency of serious adverse events was comparable between treatment arms, but fewer patients experienced CV events in the bromocriptine compared with the placebo group (HR, 0.60; 95% CI, 0.35–0.96). Future studies will need to confirm whether bromocriptine is indeed associated with CV risk reduction in the long term.

RISKS ASSOCIATED WITH ANTIHYPERGLYCEMIC MEDICATIONS

If efforts to reduce glucose levels were not associated with any risk, there might be less hesitation to normalize them in patients with diabetes. In reality, the benefits of glucose lowering must be weighed against the burden of treatment and known, as well as potential, risks of therapy. Because data on the impact of various antihyperglycemic agents on long-term clinical outcomes are limited for many of the drug classes, clinical decisions about the type and intensity of glucose lowering must be made with some uncertainty in mind (Fig. 10.6). Data on the known risks associated with antihyperglycemic agents will be reviewed. This information is critical to informed decision making and should be discussed with patients as strategies for treatment are considered.

Hypoglycemia

The pursuit of strict glucose control is frequently hampered by concerns over hypoglycemia. Hypoglycemia requiring third-party assistance is common in the course of T2D therapy and occurs with a frequency of approximately 35 episodes per 100 patient-years among insulin-treated patients.[96] Hypoglycemia occurring during treatment has been associated with several adverse events, including higher mortality,[97,98] higher risk of dementia,[99] falls,[100] fall-related fractures,[101] cardiovascular events,[98,102,103] and poor health-related quality of life.[104,105]

In particular, the relationship between hypoglycemia and subsequent cardiac events warrants attention. There

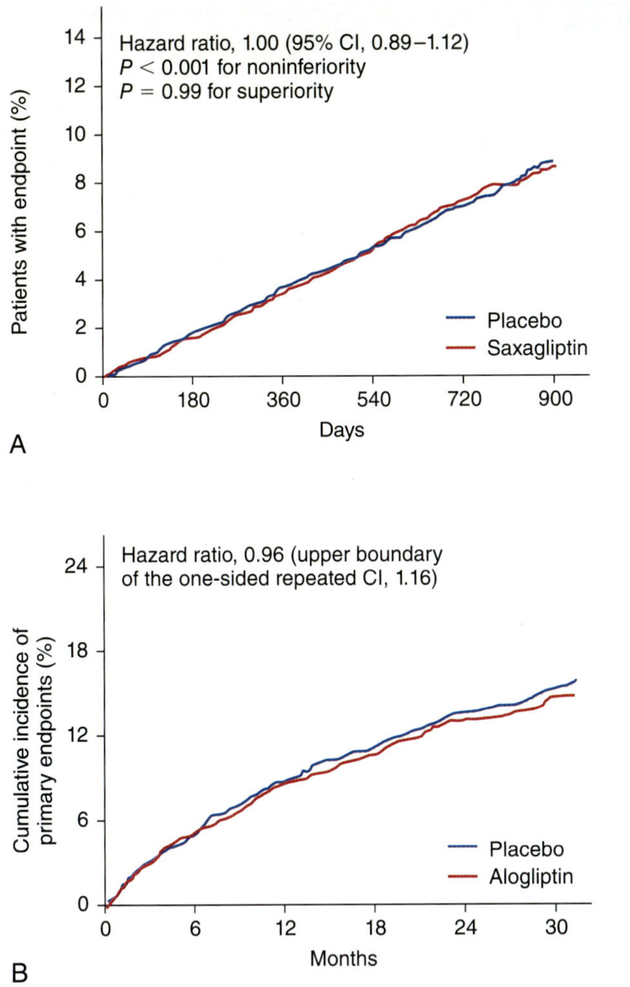

FIG. 10.6 Summary of results from **A**, SAVOR and **B**, EXAMINE trials, in which saxagliptin and alogliptin were compared against placebo with respect to major cardiovascular outcomes (myocardial infarction, stroke, or cardiovascular death). (From White WB, Cannon CP, Heller SR, et al. Alogliptin after acute coronary syndrome in patients with type 2 diabetes. *N Engl J Med.* 2013;369:1327–1335.)

are a number of plausible mechanisms by which acute hypoglycemia may trigger ischemia, arrhythmia, and CV events (Fig. 10.7). Hypoglycemia increases the levels of counterregulatory hormones, such as epinephrine and norepinephrine, which may induce increased cardiac rate and/or contractility, heightening myocardial oxygen consumption, while also precipitating vasoconstriction and platelet aggregation. Acute hypoglycemia in the presence of hypokalemia prolongs cardiac repolarization and increases the QT interval, favoring a proarrhythmic state. One study of patients with T1D and T2D who presented to the hospital with severe hypoglycemia documented frequent hypokalemia, QT prolongation, and severe hypertension during the hypoglycemic events.[106] Although animal studies have verified the effect of hypoglycemia on myocardial ischemic injury,[107] the data in humans are less clear, and debates continue on whether hypoglycemia is a mediator or merely a marker of such adverse outcomes—that is, does the propensity toward hypoglycemia simply identify sicker individuals who have lost the ability to counterregulate?

Clinical trial data consistently show that assignment to an intensive glucose control strategy is associated with a twofold to threefold higher risk of hypoglycemia compared with standard care.[21,24,28,108,109] In trial settings, hypoglycemia requiring third-party assistance occurred with a frequency of 0.6 to 12 events annually per 100 patients in the intensive therapy group and 0.2 to 4 events in the standard therapy group—much less frequently than in the community setting. Although the relationship between intensive therapy and hypoglycemia appears clear, the relationship between achieved levtrol and hypoglycemia is more complex. In the Diabetes Control and Complications Trial of patients with T1D, an inverse relationship between HbA1c level and serious hypoglycemia was noted, with the number of events higher with lower HbA1c.[109] In contrast, however, detailed post hoc analyses of ACCORD participants with T2D showed that patients with poorer glycemic control had a higher risk of hypoglycemia, irrespective of treatment assignment.[110] In fact, a greater drop in HbA1c level during the first 4 months of the trial was not associated with increased hypoglycemia risk. Rather, patients who started out with higher baseline HbA1c levels and were unable to reduce their blood glucose levels appeared to be at the highest risk for this complication. Moreover, participants with persistently elevated HbA1c levels above 7% after initiation of the intensive strategy had a higher mortality risk than those achieving lower glycemic levels (<7%).[25] What is actually mediating the higher risk of hypoglycemia and mortality in this setting is unclear, but the findings suggest that aggressive attempts to intensify treatment in patients who remain hyperglycemic may confer a very high risk for subsequent hypoglycemia.

Other apparent risk factors for hypoglycemia, aside from intensive glucose lowering, include treatment with insulin or sulfonylurea medications,[111] older age,[110] lower health literacy level,[112] longer duration of diabetes,[110] renal impairment,[111] polypharmacy,[113] baseline cognitive impairment,[114] and recent admission to the hospital within 30 days.[113]

Multiple studies have compared the impact of a specific type of insulin and the risk of hypoglycemia. Based on a recent Cochrane review, treatment with glargine and detemir resulted in fewer patients with T2D experiencing hypoglycemia compared with the use of NPH insulin.[115] Treatment with detemir was also associated with a reduced incidence of severe hypoglycemia. However, severe hypoglycemic events were rare and approximately 1 in 100 people treated with detemir instead of NPH were estimated to benefit from its use. In the previously mentioned trial of degludec versus glargine, severe hypoglycemia occurred in 187 patients (4.9%) in the degludec group versus 252 (6.6%) in the glargine group, for an absolute difference of 1.7% (RR, 0.60; $P < 0.001$ for superiority of degludec).[116] Although differences in the risk of hypoglycemia across types of basal insulins have been found, most of these differences are relatively modest. Practically, the choice of insulin preparation is often driven by insurance coverage given its high price. For patients aiming for intensive glycemic control and at high risk for hypoglycemic events, a specific type of basal insulin with a low risk for hypoglycemia may be appropriate (e.g., degludec).[117]

Based on a meta-analysis of 10 trials, there is no clear difference in hypoglycemic events with the use of regular

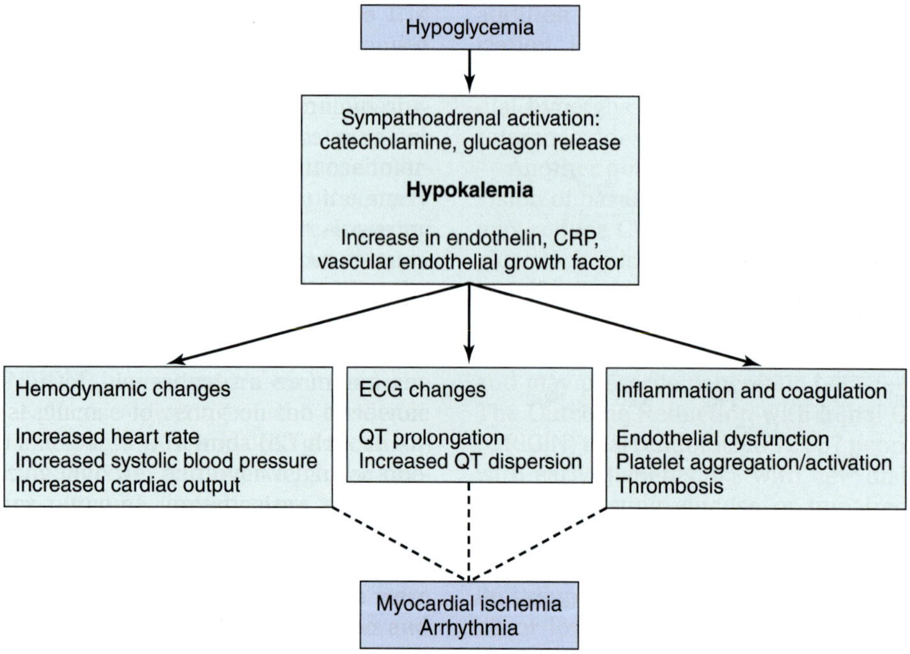

FIG. 10.7 Proposed mechanisms linking hypoglycemia with cardiovascular events. *CRP,* C-reactive protein; *ECG,* electrocardiogram.

insulin versus the use of insulin analogs (lispro, aspart) in patients with T2D.[118] However, there are differences in convenience. Rapid-acting insulin analogs can be injected immediately before meals; in contrast, regular insulin needs to be injected 30 to 45 minutes before meals. Factors such as insurance coverage, convenience, and patient preference may play a key role in the choice of specific therapy.

Other Adverse Effects of Medications

Intensive glucose control usually requires polypharmacy to achieve HbA1c targets, and adverse effects of medications require careful consideration. Even in patients who do not choose tight glycemic targets, multiple medications to lower glucose are often required with increasing duration of the disease, as beta-cell function declines.

The relative importance of various adverse effects of medications may vary from patient to patient. Weight gain is typically associated with the use of insulin, sulfonylureas, and thiazolidinediones. Heart failure, edema, and fractures are associated with the use of thiazolidinediones. Gastrointestinal side effects complicate treatment with metformin, acarbose, and some of the incretin-based therapies. In general, drug reactions increase in frequency with the use of multiple medications. The addition of another medication to lower glucose may also pose a financial burden and significantly increase time and effort required to manage diabetes (including, potentially, capillary blood glucose monitoring).

IMPLICATIONS FOR CLINICAL PRACTICE

What is the effect of glucose management on CHD events in patients with T2D? Based on the available data, intensive glucose lowering appears, at best, to modestly decrease the risk of CHD by approximately 15% when compared with standard glucose strategies. Assuming a 10-year risk of CHD of 17.4% (control arm of UKPDS), the number needed to treat (NNT) ranges on the order of 41 to 46 over 10 years to prevent one CHD event.[119]

How to prioritize glucose lowering within the patient's overall diabetes care plan is also critically important. Statin therapy, smoking cessation, aspirin for appropriate patients, and blood pressure control are the central pillars of CV risk reduction. On a population level, based on UKPDS data, fewer persons would need to be treated with tight blood pressure control (NNT 23) than intensive glucose control (NNT 46) to prevent one MI event.[120] Similarly, LDL-C lowering therapy for patients without (NNT 34 or 35) and with established atherosclerotic CV disease (NNT 13 or 14) appears to be more effective for reducing the risk for CV events than intensive glucose control.[121]

Who is the patient, and what are their goals for care? To help patients make the best decisions about their care, clinicians must consider the clinical characteristics of a patient and the context in which they live to determine how these various factors may influence the relationship between treatment and outcomes. For example, based on existing data, patients with high levels of comorbidity may derive less CV benefit from intensive glucose control,[122] and most guidelines suggest higher glycemic targets for older patients with longer duration of diabetes, established CV disease, and high risk of hypoglycemia. Naturally, these patients are at higher underlying risk of CHD, but they appear to benefit less from tight glycemic control. In contrast, the benefits of aggressive lipid and blood pressure control appear to be greatest based on high underlying CHD risk, although the relative benefits will depend also on competing mortality risk and current medications.[122]

What about types of glucose-lowering therapy? Our understanding of the implications of the specific type of therapy on these outcomes has begun to emerge with the advent of CVOTs. Some glucose-lowering therapies (SGLT2i,

GLP1RA) reduce the risk of major CV events compared with a placebo, and these effects appear to be unrelated to achieved glycemic control levels. Therefore these therapies are specifically endorsed in patients with T2D with either established, or at high/very high risk for, CV disease. Yet, the evidence generated from large CVOTs with SGLT2i and GLP1RA has not been matched by large-scale CVOTs with older agents, including metformin. Based on the evidence on SGLT2i and GLP1RA, the 2023 European Society of Cardiology (ESC) guidelines for the management of CVD in patients with diabetes recommend in patients with T2DM and ASCVD the use SGLT2i and GLP1RA for the reduction of CV risk independent of HbA1c and independent of concomitant glucose-lowering medication.[123] The American Diabetes Association (ADA) and UK NICE guidelines still recommend metformin as a first-line therapy in T2D but endorse SGLT-2i or GLP1RA as additional therapies in patients with CV indications, regardless of glycemic control levels.

As already suggested, central to the decision making about treatment are patient's preferences and goals for care. Patient-centered care needs to begin by eliciting these preferences and goals because understanding them is indispensable for providing care that is responsive to and respectful of patients' needs. A shared decision-making process stresses a partnership between the patient's values and preferences and the physician's knowledge of clinical evidence and judgment. Decisions are highly individualized, based on available evidence, and uncertainty must be acknowledged when it exists. As an example, more intensive glycemic control in a patient already struggling with a complex regimen may lead to an overburdened patient who is unable to cope with their disease. Indeed, somewhat paradoxically, pushing forward with intensive antihyperglycemic therapy may decrease adherence to other more evidence-based therapies. In such a circumstance, it may be reasonable to liberalize glycemic targets to some degree. On the other hand, a patient whose most important goal is prevention of diabetes complications may choose to take on the additional burden of insulin therapy or multiple medications to control blood glucose levels with high intensity.

REFERENCES

1. Stern MP. Diabetes and cardiovascular disease. The "common soil" hypothesis. *Diabetes*. 1995;44:369–374.
2. Roger VL, Go AS, Lloyd-Jones DM, et al. Heart disease and stroke statistics–2012 update: a report from the American Heart Association. *Circulation*. 2012;125:e2–e220.
3. https://pubmed.ncbi.nlm.nih.gov/35078371/
4. https://www.ahajournals.org/doi/epub/10.1161/CIR.0000000000001209
5. Selvin E, Ali MK. Declines in the incidence of diabetes in the U.S.-real progress or artifact? *Diabetes Care*. 2017;40(9):1139–1143. https://doi.org/10.2337/dc16-2442.
6. Cowie CC, Rust KF, Ford ES, et al. Full accounting of diabetes and pre-diabetes in the U.S. population in 1988–1994 and 2005–2006. *Diabetes Care*. 2009;32:287–294.
7. National diabetes fact sheet: general information and national estimates on diabetes in the United States; 2011.
8. Gregg EW, Cheng YJ, Saydah S, et al. Trends in death rates among U.S. adults with and without diabetes between 1997 and 2006: findings from the national health interview survey. *Diabetes Care*. 2012;35:1252–1257.
9. https://pubmed.ncbi.nlm.nih.gov/32632526/
10. Fox CS, Coady S, Sorlie PD, et al. Increasing cardiovascular disease burden due to diabetes mellitus: the Framingham Heart Study. *Circulation*. 2007;115:1544–1550.
11. Coutinho M, Gerstein HC, Wang Y, et al. The relationship between glucose and incident cardiovascular events. A metaregression analysis of published data from 20 studies of 95,783 individuals followed for 12.4 years. *Diabetes Care*. 1999;22:233–240.
12. https://pubmed.ncbi.nlm.nih.gov/21551215/
13. Khaw KT, Wareham N, Bingham S, et al. Association of hemoglobin A1c with cardiovascular disease and mortality in adults: the European Prospective Investigation into Cancer in Norfolk. *Ann Intern Med*. 2004;141:413–420.
14. Selvin E, Steffes MW, Zhu H, et al. Glycated hemoglobin, diabetes, and cardiovascular risk in nondiabetic adults. *N Engl J Med*. 2010;362:800–811.
15. https://www.ahajournals.org/doi/10.1161/JAHA.112.000077
16. Stratton IM, Adler AI, Neil HA, et al. Association of glycaemia with macrovascular and microvascular complications of type 2 diabetes (UKPDS 35): prospective observational study. *Br Med J (Clin Res Ed)*. 2000;321:405–412.
17. Selvin E, Marinopoulos S, Berkenblit G, et al. Meta-analysis: glycosylated hemoglobin and cardiovascular disease in diabetes mellitus. *Ann Intern Med*. 2004;141:421–431.
18. Currie CJ, Peters JR, Tynan A, et al. Survival as a function of HbA(1c) in people with type 2 diabetes: a retrospective cohort study. *Lancet*. 2010;375:481–489.
19. Huang ES, Liu JY, Moffet HH, et al. Glycemic control, complications, and death in older diabetic patients: the diabetes and aging study. *Diabetes Care*. 2011;34:1329–1336.
20. Colayco DC, Niu F, McCombs JS, et al. A1c and cardiovascular outcomes in type 2 diabetes: a nested case-control study. *Diabetes Care*. 2011;34:77–83.
21. Intensive blood-glucose control with sulphonylureas or insulin compared with conventional treatment and risk of complications in patients with type 2 diabetes (UKPDS 33). UK Prospective Diabetes Study (UKPDS) Group. *Lancet*. 1998;352:837–853.
22. Effect of intensive blood-glucose control with metformin on complications in overweight patients with type 2 diabetes (UKPDS 34).. UK Prospective Diabetes Study (UKPDS) Group. *Lancet*. 1998;352:854–865.
23. Holman RR, Paul SK, Bethel MA, et al. 10-year follow-up of intensive glucose control in type 2 diabetes. *N Engl J Med*. 2008;359:1577–1589.
24. Gerstein HC, Miller ME, Byington RP, et al. Effects of intensive glucose lowering in type 2 diabetes. *N Engl J Med*. 2008;358:2545–2559.
25. Riddle MC, Ambrosius WT, Brillon DJ, et al. Epidemiologic relationships between A1C and all-cause mortality during a median 3.4-year follow-up of glycemic treatment in the accord trial. *Diabetes Care*. 2010;33:983–990.
26. Bonds DE, Miller ME, Bergenstal RM, et al. The association between symptomatic, severe hypoglycaemia and mortality in type 2 diabetes: retrospective epidemiological analysis of the accord study. *Br Med J (Clin Res Ed)*. 2010;340:b4909.
27. Gerstein HC, Miller ME, Genuth S, et al. Long-term effects of intensive glucose lowering on cardiovascular outcomes. *N Engl J Med*. 2011;364:818–828.
28. Patel A, MacMahon S, Chalmers J, et al. Intensive blood glucose control and vascular outcomes in patients with type 2 diabetes. *N Engl J Med*. 2008;358:2560–2572.
29. Boussageon R, Supper I, Bejan-Angoulvant T, et al. Reappraisal of metformin efficacy in the treatment of type 2 diabetes: a meta-analysis of randomised controlled trials. *PLoS Med*. 2012;9:e1001204.
30. Hemmingsen B, Lund SS, Gluud C, et al. Intensive glycaemic control for patients with type 2 diabetes: systematic review with meta-analysis and trial sequential analysis of randomised clinical trials. *Br Med J (Clin Res Ed)*. 2011;343:d6898.
31. Kelly TN, Bazzano LA, Fonseca VA, et al. Systematic review: glucose control and cardiovascular disease in type 2 diabetes. *Ann Intern Med*. 2009;151:394–403.
32. Marso SP, Kennedy KF, House JA, et al. The effect of intensive glucose control on all-cause and cardiovascular mortality, myocardial infarction and stroke in persons with type 2 diabetes mellitus: a systematic review and meta-analysis. *Diab Vasc Dis Res*. 2010;7:119–130.
33. Ray KK, Seshasai SR, Wijesuriya S, et al. Effect of intensive control of glucose on cardiovascular outcomes and death in patients with diabetes mellitus: a meta-analysis of randomised controlled trials. *Lancet*. 2009;373:1765–1772.
34. Turnbull FM, Abraira C, Anderson RJ, et al. Intensive glucose control and macrovascular outcomes in type 2 diabetes. *Diabetologia*. 2009;52:2288–2298.
35. Knowler WC, Barrett-Connor E, Fowler SE, et al. Reduction in the incidence of type 2 diabetes with lifestyle intervention or metformin. *N Engl J Med*. 2002;346:393–403.
36. Ratner R, Goldberg R, Haffner S, et al. Impact of intensive lifestyle and metformin therapy on cardiovascular disease risk factors in the diabetes prevention program. *Diabetes Care*. 2005;28:888–894.
37. Knowler WC, Fowler SE, Hamman RF, et al. 10-year follow-up of diabetes incidence and weight loss in the diabetes prevention program outcomes study. *Lancet*. 2009;374:1677–1686.
38. https://pubmed.ncbi.nlm.nih.gov/35603600/
39. Chiasson JL, Josse RG, Gomis R, et al. Acarbose treatment and the risk of cardiovascular disease and hypertension in patients with impaired glucose tolerance: the STOP-NIDDM trial. *JAMA*. 2003;290:486–494.
40. https://pubmed.ncbi.nlm.nih.gov/28917545/
41. ORIGIN Trial Investigators, Gerstein HC, Bosch J, Dagenais GR, et al. Basal insulin and cardiovascular and other outcomes in dysglycemia. *N Engl J Med*. 2012;367:319–328.
42. Nissen SE, Wolski K. Effect of rosiglitazone on the risk of myocardial infarction and death from cardiovascular causes. *N Engl J Med*. 2007;356:2457–2471.

43. Richter B, Bandeira-Echtler E, Bergerhoff K, et al. Rosiglitazone for type 2 diabetes mellitus. *Cochrane Database Syst Rev*. 2007;2007:CD006063.
44. Diamond GA, Bax L, Kaul S. Uncertain effects of rosiglitazone on the risk for myocardial infarction and cardiovascular death. *Ann Intern Med*. 2007;147:578–581.
45. US Department of Health and Human Services, Food and Drug Administration, Center for Drug Evaluation and Research (CDER). Guidance for industry: diabetes mellitus—evaluating cardiovascular risk in new antidiabetic therapies to treat type 2 diabetes; 2008.
46. https://pubmed.ncbi.nlm.nih.gov/35605236/
47. Kooy A, de Jager J, Lehert P, et al. Long-term effects of metformin on metabolism and microvascular and macrovascular disease in patients with type 2 diabetes mellitus. *Arch Intern Med*. 2009;169:616–625.
48. Johnson JA, Majumdar SR, Simpson SH, et al. Decreased mortality associated with the use of metformin compared with sulfonylurea monotherapy in type 2 diabetes. *Diabetes Care*. 2002;25:2244–2248.
49. Tzoulaki I, Molokhia M, Curcin V, et al. Risk of cardiovascular disease and all cause mortality among patients with type 2 diabetes prescribed oral antidiabetes drugs: retrospective cohort study using UK general practice research database. *Br Med J (Clin Res Ed)*. 2009;339:b4731.
50. Roumie CL, Hung AM, Greevy RA, et al. Comparative effectiveness of sulfonylurea and metformin monotherapy on cardiovascular events in type 2 diabetes mellitus: a cohort study. *Ann Intern Med*. 2012;157:601–610.
51. https://pubmed.ncbi.nlm.nih.gov/35032305/
52. McAfee AT, Koro C, Landon J, et al. Coronary heart disease outcomes in patients receiving antidiabetic agents. *Pharmacoepidemiol Drug Saf*. 2007;16:711–725.
53. https://pubmed.ncbi.nlm.nih.gov/35277396/
54. Hemmingsen B, Christensen LL, Wetterslev J, et al. Comparison of metformin and insulin versus insulin alone for type 2 diabetes: systematic review of randomised clinical trials with meta-analyses and trial sequential analyses. *Br Med J (Clin Res Ed)*. 2012;344:e1771.
55. https://jamanetwork.com/journals/jama/fullarticle/2533506
56. Kahn SE, Haffner SM, Heise MA, et al. Glycemic durability of rosiglitazone, metformin, or glyburide monotherapy. *N Engl J Med*. 2006;355:2427–2443.
57. A study of the effects of hypoglycemia agents on vascular complications in patients with adult-onset diabetes. VI. Supplementary report on nonfatal events in patients treated with tolbutamide.. *Diabetes*. 1976;25:1129–1153.
58. https://pubmed.ncbi.nlm.nih.gov/31536101/
59. Simpson SH, Majumdar SR, Tsuyuki RT, et al. Dose-response relation between sulfonylurea drugs and mortality in type 2 diabetes mellitus: a population-based cohort study. *CMAJ*. 2006;174:169–174.
60. Morgan CL, Poole CD, Evans M, et al. What next after metformin? A retrospective evaluation of the outcome of second- line, glucose-lowering therapies in people with type 2 diabetes. *J Clin Endocrinol Metab*. 2012;97:4605–4612.
61. Singh S, Loke YK, Furberg CD. Long-term risk of cardiovascular events with rosiglitazone: a meta-analysis. *JAMA*. 2007;298:1189–1195.
62. Cobitz A, Zambanini A, Sowell M, et al. A retrospective evaluation of congestive heart failure and myocardial ischemia events in 14,237 patients with type 2 diabetes mellitus enrolled in 42 short-term, double-blind, randomized clinical studies with rosiglitazone. *Pharmacoepidemiol Drug Saf*. 2008;17:769–781.
63. Lipscombe LL, Gomes T, Levesque LE, et al. Thiazolidinediones and cardiovascular outcomes in older patients with diabetes. *JAMA*. 2007;298:2634–2643.
64. Winkelmayer WC, Setoguchi S, Levin R, Solomon DH. Comparison of cardiovascular outcomes in elderly patients with diabetes who initiated rosiglitazone vs pioglitazone therapy. *Arch Intern Med*. 2008;168:2368–2375.
65. Juurlink DN, Gomes T, Lipscombe LL, et al. Adverse cardiovascular events during treatment with pioglitazone and rosiglitazone: population based cohort study. *Br Med J (Clin Res Ed)*. 2009;339:b2942.
66. Graham DJ, Ouellet-Hellstrom R, MaCurdy TE, et al. Risk of acute myocardial infarction, stroke, heart failure, and death in elderly medicare patients treated with rosiglitazone or pioglitazone. *JAMA*. 2010;304:411–418.
67. Home PD, Pocock SJ, Beck-Nielsen H, et al. Rosiglitazone evaluated for cardiovascular outcomes in oral agent combination therapy for type 2 diabetes (record): a multicentre, randomised, open-label trial. *Lancet*. 2009;373:2125–2135.
68. Frye RL, August P, Brooks MM, et al. A randomized trial of therapies for type 2 diabetes and coronary artery disease. *N Engl J Med*. 2009;360:2503–2515.
69. FDA drug safety communication: updated risk evaluation and mitigation strategy (REMS) to restrict access to resiglitazone containing medicines including Avandia, Avandamet, and Avandaryl, 2011. http://fda.gov/Drugs/DrugSafety/ucm2555005.htm. Accessed January 09, 2013.
70. Lincoff AM, Wolski K, Nicholls SJ, et al. Pioglitazone and risk of cardiovascular events in patients with type 2 diabetes mellitus: a meta-analysis of randomized trials. *JAMA*. 2007;298:1180–1188.
71. Dormandy JA, Charbonnel B, Eckland DJ, et al. Secondary prevention of macrovascular events in patients with type 2 diabetes in the PROACTIVE study (prospective pioglitazone clinical trial in macrovascular events): a randomised controlled trial. *Lancet*. 2005;366:1279–1289.
72. https://www.nejm.org/doi/full/10.1056/nejmoa1506930
73. https://www.thelancet.com/journals/landia/article/PIIS2213-8587(17)30317-0/fulltext
74. https://academic.oup.com/eurheartj/article/44/39/4043/7238227?login=true#437089057
75. Scirica BM, Bhatt DL, Braunwald E, et al. Saxagliptin and cardiovascular outcomes in patients with type 2 diabetes mellitus. *N Engl J Med*. 2013;369:1317–1326.
76. White WB, Cannon CP, Heller SR, et al. Alogliptin after acute coronary syndrome in patients with type 2 diabetes. *N Engl J Med*. 2013;369:1327–1335.
77. White W.B. Cardiovascular outcomes with alogliptin in patients with type 2 diabetes mellitus and recent acute coronary syndromes. In *49th Annual Meeting of the European Association for the Study of Diabetes (EASD), September 26, 2013*; 2013.
78. https://pubmed.ncbi.nlm.nih.gov/26052984/
79. https://pubmed.ncbi.nlm.nih.gov/30418475/
80. McGuire DK, Van de Werf F, Armstrong PW, Peterson ED and Trial Evaluating Cardiovascular Outcomes With Sitagliptin Study G., et al. Association between sitagliptin use and heart failure hospitalization and related outcomes in type 2 diabetes mellitus: secondary analysis of a randomized clinical trial. *JAMA Cardiol*. 2016;1:126–135.
81. McGuire DK, Alexander JH, Johansen OE, et al. Linagliptin effects on heart failure and related outcomes in individuals with type 2 diabetes mellitus at high cardiovascular and renal risk in CARMELINA. *Circulation*. 2019;139:351–361.
82. Currie CJ, Johnson JA. The safety profile of exogenous insulin in people with type 2 diabetes: justification for concern. *Diabetes Obes Metab*. 2012;14:1–4.
83. Gamble JM, Simpson SH, Eurich DT, et al. Insulin use and increased risk of mortality in type 2 diabetes: a cohort study. *Diabetes Obes Metab*. 2010;12:47–53.
84. Anselmino M, Ohrvik J, Malmberg K, et al. Glucose lowering treatment in patients with coronary artery disease is prognostically important not only in established but also in newly detected diabetes mellitus: a report from the Euro Heart Survey on diabetes and the heart. *Eur Heart J*. 2008;29:177–184.
85. Currie CJ, Poole CD, Evans M, et al. Mortality and other important diabetes-related outcomes with insulin vs other antihyperglycemic therapies in type 2 diabetes. *J Clin Endocrinol Metab*. 2013;98:668–677.
86. https://pubmed.ncbi.nlm.nih.gov/24915260/
87. Malmberg K. Prospective randomised study of intensive insulin treatment on long term survival after acute myocardial infarction in patients with diabetes mellitus. Digami (diabetes mellitus, insulin glucose infusion in acute myocardial infarction) study group. *BMJ*. 1997;314:1512–1515.
88. Malmberg K, Ryden L, Wedel H, et al. Intense metabolic control by means of insulin in patients with diabetes mellitus and acute myocardial infarction (digami 2): effects on mortality and morbidity. *Eur Heart J*. 2005;26:650–661.
89. Mellbin LG, Malmberg K, Norhammar A, et al. Prognostic implications of glucose-lowering treatment in patients with acute myocardial infarction and diabetes: experiences from an extended follow-up of the diabetes mellitus insulin- glucose infusion in acute myocardial infarction (digami) 2 study. *Diabetologia*. 2011;54:1308–1317.
90. https://pubmed.ncbi.nlm.nih.gov/19246588/
91. Currie CJ, Poole CD, Gale EA. The influence of glucose-lowering therapies on cancer risk in type 2 diabetes. *Diabetologia*. 2009;52:1766–1777.
92. Li C, Zhao G, Okoro CA, et al. Prevalence of diagnosed cancer according to duration of diagnosed diabetes and current insulin use among U.S. adults with diagnosed diabetes: findings from the 2009 behavioral risk factor surveillance system. *Diabetes Care*. 2013;36:1569–1576.
93. https://pubmed.ncbi.nlm.nih.gov/28605603/
94. https://pubmed.ncbi.nlm.nih.gov/28917545/
95. Gaziano JM, Cincotta AH, O'Connor CM, et al. Randomized clinical trial of quick-release bromocriptine among patients with type 2 diabetes on overall safety and cardiovascular outcomes. *Diabetes Care*. 2010;33:1503–1508.
96. Donnelly LA, Morris AD, Frier BM, et al. Frequency and predictors of hypoglycaemia in type 1 and insulin-treated type 2 diabetes: a population-based study. *Diabet Med*. 2005;22:749–755.
97. McCoy RG, Van Houten HK, Ziegenfuss JY, et al. Increased mortality of patients with diabetes reporting severe hypoglycemia. *Diabetes Care*. 2012;35:1897–1901.
98. Hsu PF, Sung SH, Cheng HM, et al. Association of clinical symptomatic hypoglycemia with cardiovascular events and total mortality in type 2 diabetes: a nationwide population-based study. *Diabetes Care*. 2013;36:894–900.
99. Whitmer RA, Karter AJ, Yaffe K, et al. Hypoglycemic episodes and risk of dementia in older patients with type 2 diabetes mellitus. *JAMA*. 2009;301:1565–1572.
100. Schwartz AV, Vittinghoff E, Sellmeyer DE, et al. Diabetes-related complications, glycemic control, and falls in older adults. *Diabetes Care*. 2008;31:391–396.
101. Johnston SS, Conner C, Aagren M, et al. Association between hypoglycaemic events and fall-related fractures in medicare-covered patients with type 2 diabetes. *Diabetes Obes Metab*. 2012;14:634–643.
102. Johnston SS, Conner C, Aagren M, et al. Evidence linking hypoglycemic events to an increased risk of acute cardiovascular events in patients with type 2 diabetes. *Diabetes Care*. 2011;34:1164–1170.
103. Desouza C, Salazar H, Cheong B, et al. Association of hypoglycemia and cardiac ischemia: a study based on continuous monitoring. *Diabetes Care*. 2003;26:1485–1489.
104. Laiteerapong N, Karter AJ, Liu JY, et al. Correlates of quality of life in older adults with diabetes: the diabetes & aging study. *Diabetes Care*. 2011;34:1749–1753.
105. Williams SA, Shi L, Brenneman SK, et al. The burden of hypoglycemia on healthcare utilization, costs, and quality of life among type 2 diabetes mellitus patients. *J Diabetes Complications*. 2012;26:399–406.

106. Tsujimoto T, Yamamoto-Honda R, Kajio H, et al. Vital signs, QT prolongation, and newly diagnosed cardiovascular disease during severe hypoglycemia in type 1 and type 2 diabetic patients. *Diabetes Care*. 2014;37: 217–225.
107. Libby P, Maroko PR, Braunwald E. The effect of hypoglycemia on myocardial ischemic injury during acute experimental coronary artery occlusion. *Circulation*. 1975;51:621–626.
108. Duckworth W, Abraira C, Moritz T, et al. Glucose control and vascular complications in veterans with type 2 diabetes. *N Engl J Med*. 2009;360:129–139.
109. The Diabetes Control and Complications Trial Research Group. The effect of intensive treatment of diabetes on the development and progression of long-term complications in insulin-dependent diabetes mellitus. *N Engl J Med*. 1993;329:977–986.
110. Miller ME, Bonds DE, Gerstein HC, et al. The effects of baseline characteristics, glycaemia treatment approach, and glycated haemoglobin concentration on the risk of severe hypoglycaemia: post hoc epidemiological analysis of the accord study. *BMJ*. 2010;340:b5444.
111. Davis TM, Brown SG, Jacobs IG, et al. Determinants of severe hypoglycemia complicating type 2 diabetes: the fremantle diabetes study. *J Clin Endocrinol Metab*. 2010;95:2240–2247.
112. Sarkar U, Karter AJ, Liu JY, et al. Hypoglycemia is more common among type 2 diabetes patients with limited health literacy: the diabetes study of Northern California (distance). *J Gen Intern Med*. 2010;25:962–968.
113. Shorr RI, Ray WA, Daugherty JR, et al. Incidence and risk factors for serious hypoglycemia in older persons using insulin or sulfonylureas. *Arch Intern Med*. 1997;157:1681–1686.
114. Punthakee Z, Miller ME, Launer LJ, et al. Poor cognitive function and risk of severe hypoglycemia in type 2 diabetes: post hoc epidemiologic analysis of the accord trial. *Diabetes Care*. 2012;35:787–793.
115. Semlitsch T, Engler J, Siebenhofer A, Jeitler K, Berghold A, Horvath K. (Ultra-)long-acting insulin analogues versus NPH insulin (human isophane insulin) for adults with type 2 diabetes mellitus. *Cochrane Database Systematic Rev*. 2020;11:CD005613. https://doi.org/10.1002/14651858.CD005613.pub4.
116. https://pubmed.ncbi.nlm.nih.gov/28605603/
117. Standl E, Stevens SR, Armstrong PW, et al. Increased risk of severe hypoglycemic events before and after cardiovascular outcomes in TECOS suggests an at-risk type 2 diabetes frail patient phenotype. *Diabetes Care*. 2018;41:596–603.
118. https://pubmed.ncbi.nlm.nih.gov/30556900/
119. Yudkin JS, Richter B. Intensive glucose control and cardiovascular outcomes. *Lancet*. 2009;374:523–524.
120. Vijan S, Hayward RA. Treatment of hypertension in type 2 diabetes mellitus: blood pressure goals, choice of agents, and setting priorities in diabetes care. *Ann Intern Med*. 2003;138:593–602.
121. Vijan S, Hayward RA. Pharmacologic lipid-lowering therapy in type 2 diabetes mellitus: background paper for the American College of Physicians. *Ann Intern Med*. 2004;140:650–658.
122. Greenfield S, Billimek J, Pellegrini F, et al. Comorbidity affects the relationship between glycemic control and cardiovascular outcomes in diabetes: a cohort study. *Ann Intern Med*. 2009;151:854–860.
123. Marx N, Federici M, et al. 2023 ESC Guidelines for the management of cardiovascular disease in patients with diabetes. *European Heart J*. 2023;44:4043–4140. https://doi.org/10.1093/eurheartj/ehad192.

11 Regulatory Approach to Medications for Type 2 Diabetes: Past, Present, and Future

BRENDAN M. EVERETT, NEHA PAGIDIPATI, AND CECILIA C. LOW WANG

INTRODUCTION

Improved glucose control improves clinical outcomes in all patients with diabetes, including those affected by type 2 diabetes. The surrogate endpoint for glucose control is hemoglobin A1c (A1c), a measure of average glycemia over the preceding few months. The 2008 guidance by the United States (US) Food and Drug Administration (FDA) requiring the assessment of cardiovascular safety of new drugs for diabetes mellitus was issued because of safety concerns surrounding certain glucose-lowering drugs.[1] Subsequent large-scale cardiovascular outcome trials (CVOTs) demonstrated an absence of excess cardiovascular risk with few exceptions. These trials unexpectedly led to the discovery that two new drug classes for glucose-lowering, the sodium-glucose cotransporter-2 inhibitors (SGLT2i) and glucagon-like peptide-1 receptor agonists (GLP1RA), also had significant beneficial effects on cardiovascular disease and kidney disease risk as compared with placebo control, despite minor differences in glycemic control between treatment groups, and in the setting of contemporary background therapy. To understand the regulation of diabetes drugs, this chapter will review the historical context of the 2008 guidance by the US FDA and parallel events in the European Union, the impact of the FDA guidance, the current regulatory environment, and the future.

HISTORY OF REGULATION OF DIABETES DRUGS

Regulatory Standards Prior to 2008

The treatment of diabetes has evolved significantly since the purification of insulin in 1921 leading to awarding of the Nobel Prize in Physiology or Medicine to Frederick G. Banting and John JR MacCleod in 1923. The Diabetes Control and Complications Trial (DCCT), the United Kingdom Prospective Diabetes Study, and subsequent follow-up studies demonstrated conclusively that lowering A1c decreases the risk of diabetes complications in type 1 diabetes (T1D) and type 2 diabetes (T2D), respectively.[2–5] Therefore the goals for diabetes therapy advanced from survival to alleviating symptoms to prevention of complications.

New antihyperglycemic agents were and are based on demonstrating efficacy for A1c-lowering in different treatment scenarios.[1,6] Trial populations before 2008 were generally composed of patients with T2D with relatively short duration of diabetes who were not otherwise at high risk for cardiovascular events. Trial durations were short (less than 6 or at most 12 months' duration). Patients with recent or advanced cardiovascular disease were excluded from trials. The assessment of adverse cardiovascular events was based on adverse event term reporting by investigators. One analysis using a specific custom query of adverse event terms found the numbers of events in these trials to be low, as outlined in Table 11.1, making evaluation of cardiovascular safety problematic.[16,17]

In addition to the low numbers of cardiovascular adverse events in drug development trials was a growing concern regarding potential cardiovascular risk with certain antihyperglycemic agents. For example, tolbutamide, a first-generation sulfonylurea, was found to result in significantly higher cardiovascular mortality in the University Group Diabetes Program.[18,19] Muraglitazar, a dual-peroxisome proliferator-activated receptor (PPAR) agonist, was associated with excess incidence of a composite of death, major adverse cardiovascular events (myocardial infarction, stroke, transient ischemic attack) and congestive heart failure.[20] Finally, a meta-analysis of trials of rosiglitazone, a thiazolidinedione, revealed an increased risk of myocardial infarction and an increased odds ratio for cardiovascular death that just missed statistical significance.[21,22] Although this was later not confirmed by a comprehensive readjudication of the Rosiglitazone Evaluated for Cardiovascular

TABLE 11.1 Cardiovascular Outcomes Data for Selected T2D Drugs Before and After the 2008 FDA Requirement That New Antihyperglycemic Drugs Demonstrate Cardiovascular.

MEDICATION	TRIALS CNDUCTED BEFORE OR AFTER 2008 GUIDANCE	TRIAL PHASE(S) OR TRIAL (YEAR) AND IDENTIFIER	CARDIOVASCULAR SAFETY SIGNALS OR 3-POINT MACE HAZARD RATIO (95%CI)	SUBJECTS, N	MAJOR ADVERSE CARDIOVASCULAR EVENTS, N	OTHER OUTCOMES
DPP4i						
Saxagliptin	Before	Phase 3	Custom MACE SMQ	4607	40	
Saxagliptin	After	SAVOR-TIMI 53 (2013)[9]	1.00 (0.89–1.12)	16,492	1222	HHF 1.27 (1.07–1.51)
Alogliptin	Before	Phase 3	Custom MACE SMQ	4702	18	
Alogliptin	After	EXAMINE (2013)[10]	0.96 (0.80–1.16)	5380	621	HHF 1.19 (0.90–1.58)
Sitagliptin	Before	Phase 3	Cardiac disorders SAEs	2342	12	
Sitagliptin	After	TECOS (2015)[11]	0.98 (0.89–1.08)	14,671	1690	HHF 1.00 (0.83–1.20)
GLP1RA						
Exenatide	Before	Phase 2 and 3	Cardiac disorders SAEs	2371	27	
Exenatide	After	EXSCEL (2017)[12]	0.91 (0.83–1.00)	14,752	1744	
Liraglutide	Before	Phase 3	Custom MACE SMQ	6638	38	
Liraglutide	After	LEADER (2016)[13]	0.87 (0.78–0.97)	9340	1302	
SGLT2i						
Dapagliflozin	Before	Meta-analysis phase II/III data[8]	0.73 (0.46–1.16)	4359	48	
Dapagliflozin	After	DECLARE-TIMI 58 (2018)[14]	0.93 (0.84–1.03)[a]	17,160	1559	Diabetic ketoacidosis 2.18 (1.10–4.30)
Canagliflozin	Before	Meta-analysis phase II/III data[8]	0.95 (0.71–1.26)[a]	6769	132	
Canagliflozin	After	CANVAS program (2017)[15]	0.86 (0.75–0.97)	10,142	1011	Amputation 1.97 (1.41–2.75)

[a]Cardiovascular death, myocardial infarction, nonfatal stroke, or hospitalization for unstable angina.
Safety Trials conducted before the 2008 guidance are displayed in darker green and represent combined phase 2 or 3 approval trials for selected drugs.[7] Also included and displayed in darker green are data from a meta-analysis of phase 2 or 3 data for dapagliflozin and canagliflozin, where the primary aim of the included trials was to demonstrate A1c reduction rather than cardiovascular safety.[8] The trials in the displayed in darker green area are characterized by low numbers of major adverse cardiovascular events, in contrast to the numbers of events collected in trials conducted after the 2008 guidance.
CI, Confidence interval; *CVD*, cardiovascular disease; *DPP4i*, dipeptidyl peptidase-4 inhibitor; *GLP1RA*, glucagon-like peptide-1 receptor agonist; *HHF*, hospitalization for heart failure; *3-point MACE*, major adverse cardiovascular event: myocardial infarction, stroke, or cardiovascular death; *SAE*, serious adverse event; *SGLT2i*, sodium-glucose cotransporter-2 inhibitor; *SMQ*, standardized medical query (of adverse event terms).
Adapted in part from Wang L, et al.[7] with copyright permission from the American Heart Association.

Outcomes and Regulation of Glycemic in Diabetes randomized controlled trial[23] resulting in removal of prescribing restrictions by the FDA,[24] the meta-analysis raised significant concern regarding potential unacceptable cardiovascular risk of a therapy for T2D.

The Action to Control Cardiovascular Risk in Diabetes trial was designed to determine whether normalization of A1c in individuals with T2D would reduce cardiovascular events as compared with standard therapy targeting an A1c of 7% to 7.9%, but the intensive treatment regimen was terminated in 2008, before the scheduled end of the study, because of a finding of increased cardiovascular and all-cause mortality in the intensive therapy arm.[25]

This series of events called into question the adequacy of the regulatory pathway for determining overall clinical benefit of diabetes drugs since it was focused on A1c lowering, and whether development programs were able to detect an unacceptable level of cardiovascular risk in this intended patient population already at higher cardiovascular risk than those without diabetes. The FDA Endocrinologic and Metabolic Drugs Advisory Committee met on July 1 and 2, 2008, to discuss the role of cardiovascular risk assessment during diabetes drug development, and whether a long-term cardiovascular trial should be required of all drugs or biologics for diabetes regardless of the presence or absence of a safety signal during development.[17] The majority of the committee was in favor of recommending more extensive, standardized assessment of cardiovascular risk in the pre- and postmarketing phases, with the goal of ruling out cardiovascular risk, but not necessarily to demonstrate cardiovascular benefit.

In the European Union, new diabetes medications were required to undergo European Medicines Agency (EMA) review starting in 2005, and a guideline for diabetes drug development outlined the criterion for efficacy, which was A1c lowering.[6,26] Just as the rosiglitazone meta-analysis led to concerns about the cardiovascular safety of antihyperglycemic medications in the United States, similar concerns were identified in Europe.[21,22]

The 2008 FDA Guidance

In December 2008 the FDA released the Guidance for Industry: *Diabetes Mellitus–Evaluating Cardiovascular Risk in New Antidiabetic Therapies to Treat Type 2 Diabetes* and focused on "excluding an unacceptable increase in cardiovascular risk for all new therapies to improve glycemic control in patients with T2D regardless of the presence or absence of a signal for cardiovascular risk in the development program."[1] The safety signals prompting the FDA guidance also led to concerns in Europe, and eventually to new requirements for the assessment of cardiovascular safety of new diabetes medications for the European market.[22,27] While cardiovascular outcome trials were not required for approval of new antihyperglycemic medications in Europe, they could be mandated prior to approval. Because companies often develop medications for both the American and European markets in tandem, the evidence generated in trials conducted to comply with the 2008 FDA Guidance described below was often used in drug applications to the EMA.[6]

Specific Recommendations From the FDA Guidance Included

- Establishment of an independent cardiovascular endpoints committee for prospective adjudication of cardiovascular mortality, myocardial infarction, and stroke in phase 2 and 3 clinical trials. Other outcomes felt to be acceptable included hospitalization for acute coronary syndrome and urgent revascularization procedures.
- Inclusion of patients at higher risk for cardiovascular events in phase 2 and phase 3 trials to obtain sufficient outcomes to allow for a meaningful estimate of risk.
- Trial designs that allow for meta-analysis, lasting more than 3 to 6 months and at a minimum of 2 years to evaluate longer-term cardiovascular risk.
- Exclusion of 1.8 from the upper bound of the two-sided 95% confidence interval for the estimated risk ratio for major adverse cardiovascular events prior to approval.
- Exclusion of 1.3 from the upper bound of the two-sided 95% confidence interval for the estimated risk ratio for major adverse cardiovascular events after approval, to conclude that there is no unacceptable increase in cardiovascular risk.

In terms of trial design, these recommendations for demonstrating absence of increased risk required that for an event rate of 3% per year, 122 events and 4067 patient-years would be needed to achieve 90% power to exclude a risk ratio of 1.8 for major adverse cardiovascular events. To exclude a risk ratio of 1.3 for major adverse cardiovascular events with 90% power, 611 events and 20,367 patient-years would be needed.[17] In the years following the release of the 2008 Guidance, more than 20 large-scale CVOTs of diabetes drugs have been conducted (Fig. 11.1). Most of these trials reported that newly approved antihyperglycemic therapies were not associated with an increased risk of major adverse cardiovascular events, and a few demonstrated evidence of cardiovascular benefit. As anticipated, the larger, longer trials required to meet this regulatory standard meant a substantial increase in the number of randomized patients enrolled, and major adverse cardiovascular events ascertained during the trials, providing far more robust signals of cardiovascular safety (and in some cases, efficacy), and offering insight into other nonatherosclerotic cardiovascular disease (ASCVD) risks and benefits. Table 11.1 provides a contrast of the numbers of patients and cardiovascular events ascertained for select dipeptidyl peptidase-4 inhibitor (DPP4i), GLP1RA, and SGLT2i registration trials with and without major adverse cardiovascular events as the trial outcome.

LESSONS LEARNED IN THE 2008 FDA GUIDANCE FOR INDUSTRY ERA

Since the advent of the 2008 FDA guidance for the pharmaceutical industry on assessing cardiovascular safety for antihyperglycemic agents, more than 20 CVOTs conducted in patients with T2D have been completed, with many more underway as of 2024 (Fig. 11.1).[28] These trials have expanded our understanding of the cardiovascular, kidney, and metabolic effects of various classes of antihyperglycemic agents, many of which might never have come to light without the 2008 FDA guidance. Importantly, however, the evolution of these trials has added greatly to our understanding of how to conduct conclusive, efficient, and impactful trials that assess both cardiovascular safety and other important clinical outcomes. Below, we outline some of the learnings gained in trial design and conduct since the 2008 FDA guidance.

CLASSES OF DRUGS ASSESSED

First, we will briefly review the various drug classes that have been evaluated for cardiovascular safety under the 2008 FDA guidance. A table summarizing key aspects of the study design is presented in Table 11.2. The initial CVOTs assessed the cardiovascular effects of DPP4i, with each of the tested drugs showing noninferiority with respect to major adverse cardiovascular events (MACE) compared with a placebo or active comparator.[9–11,35,36] Of note, the SAVOR-TIMI 53 trial did show an increased rate of heart failure hospitalization with saxagliptin compared with a placebo,[9] but this effect was not seen with the other DPP4i agents. Seven CVOTs have evaluated the cardiovascular impact of SGLT2i solely among patients with T2D; all of these have not only confirmed cardiovascular safety but have also mostly shown significant benefit in various outcomes, including heart failure hospitalization and progression of kidney disease.[15,30,37–41] Subsequent studies in populations both with and without T2D have shown the benefits of empagliflozin and dapagliflozin in heart failure with reduced ejection fraction,[46,47] heart failure with preserved ejection fraction,[48,49] and chronic kidney disease.[50,51]

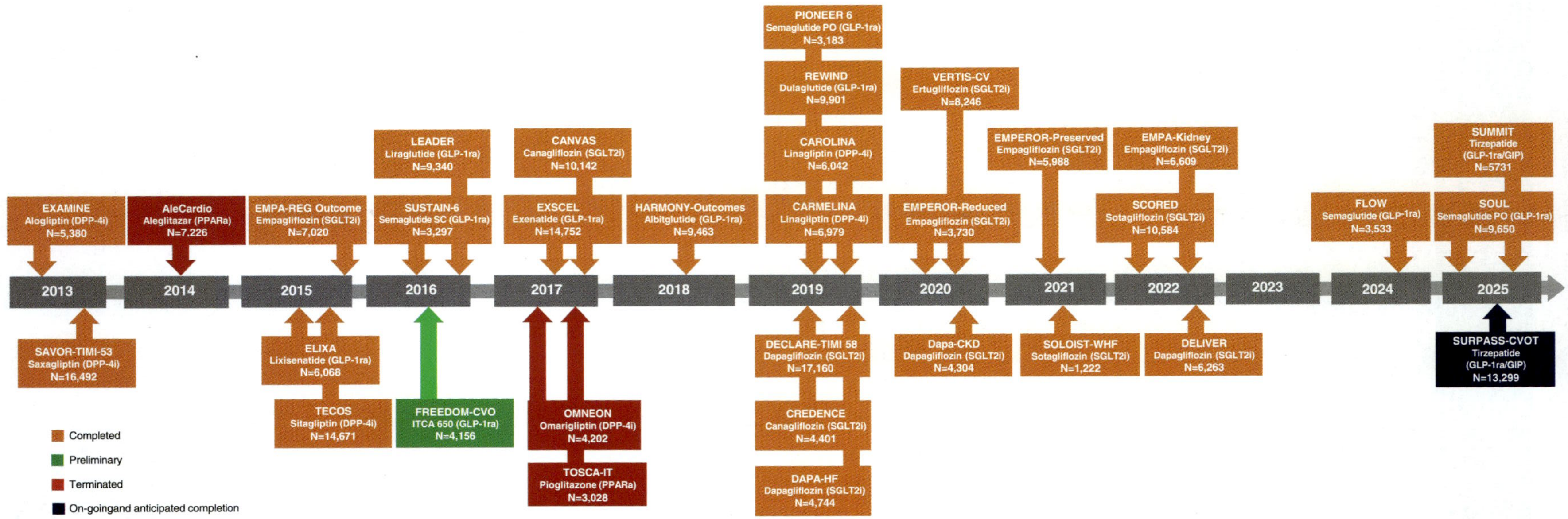

FIG. 11.1 Timeline of cardiovascular and kidney outcome trials since the 2008 US Food and Drug Administration guidance. *AleCardio*, Aleglitazar to Reduce CV Events in Patients with ACS and Diabetes; *CANVAS*, Canagliflozin Cardiovascular Assessment Study; *CARMELINA*, Cardiovascular and Renal Microvascular Outcome Study with Linagliptin; *CAROLINA*, Cardiovascular Outcome Study of Linagliptin Versus Glimepiride in Patients with Type 2 Diabetes; *CREDENCE*, Canagliflozin and Renal Events in Diabetes with Established Nephropathy Clinical Evaluation; *DAPA-CKD*, Dapagliflozin and Prevention of Adverse Outcomes in Chronic Kidney Disease; *DAPA-HF*, Dapagliflozin and Prevention of Adverse Outcomes in Heart Failure; *DECLARE-TIMI 58*, Dapagliflozin Effect on Cardiovascular Events–Thrombolysis in Myocardial Infarction 58; *DELIVER*, Dapagliflozin Evaluation to Improve the Lives of Patients with Preserved Ejection Fraction Heart Failure; *DPP-4*, dipeptidyl peptidase-4; *ELIXA*, Evaluation of Lixisenatide in Acute Coronary Syndrome; *EMPA-REG OUTCOME*, BI 10773 (Empagliflozin) Cardiovascular Outcome Event Trial in Type 2 Diabetes Mellitus Patients; *EMPEROR-Preserved*, Empagliflozin Outcome Trial in Patients with Chronic Heart Failure with Preserved Ejection Fraction; *EMPEROR-Reduced*, Empagliflozin Outcome Trial in Patients with Chronic Heart Failure with Reduced Ejection Fraction; *EXAMINE*, Examination of Cardiovascular Outcomes with Alogliptin Versus Standard of Care; *EXSCEL*, Exenatide Study of Cardiovascular Event Lowering; *FLOW*, Effect of Semaglutide Versus Placebo on the Progression of Renal Impairment in Subjects with Type 2 Diabetes and Chronic Kidney Disease; *FREEDOM-CVO*, Study to Evaluate Cardiovascular Outcomes with ITCA 650 in Patients Treated with Standard of Care for Type 2 Diabetes; *GLP-1RA*, glucagon-like peptide 1 receptor agonist; *LEADER*, Liraglutide Effect and Action in Diabetes: Evaluation of Cardiovascular Outcome Results; *OMNEON*, Study to Assess Cardiovascular Outcomes Following Treatment with Omarigliptin (MK-3102) in Participants with Type 2 Diabetes Mellitus; *PIONEER-6*, A Trial Investigating the Cardiovascular Safety of Oral Semaglutide in Subjects with Type 2 Diabetes; *PPAR*, peroxisome proliferator-activated receptor agonist; *REWIND*, Researching Cardiovascular Events with a Weekly Incretin in Diabetes; *SAVOR-TIMI 53*, Saxagliptin Assessment of Vascular Outcomes Recorded in Patients with Diabetes–Thrombolysis in Myocardial Infarction 53; *SCORED*, Effect of Sotagliflozin on Cardiovascular and Renal Events in Patients with Type 2 Diabetes and Moderate Renal Impairment Who Are at Cardiovascular Risk; *SGLT2*, sodium-glucose cotransporter-2; *SOLOIST-WHF*, Effect of Sotagliflozin on Cardiovascular Events in Patients with Type 2 Diabetes Post Worsening Heart Failure; *SOUL*, Semaglutide Cardiovascular Outcomes Trial in Patients with Type 2 Diabetes; *SUMMIT*, Study of Tirzepatide in Participants with Heart Failure with Preserved Ejection Fraction and Obesity; *SURPASS-CVOT*, The Effect of Tirzepatide Versus Dulaglutide on Major Adverse Cardiovascular Events in Patients with Type 2 Diabetes; *SUSTAIN-6*, Trial to Evaluate Cardiovascular and Other Long-term Outcomes with Semaglutide in Subjects with Type 2 Diabetes; *TECOS*, Trial Evaluating Cardiovascular Outcomes with Sitagliptin; *TOSCA-IT*, Thiazolidinediones or Sulfonylureas Cardiovascular Accidents Intervention Trial; and *VERTIS-CV*, Cardiovascular Outcomes Following Ertugliflozin Treatment in Type 2 Diabetes Mellitus Participants with Vascular Disease.

TABLE 11.2 Study Design Aspects of CVOTs in patients with T2D since 2008 FDA Guidance. All trials are placebo-controlled except CAROLINA, which used glimepiride as an active comparator; SURPASS, which uses dulaglutide as an active comparator; and PRECIDENTD, which is a comparative effectiveness study of active GLP-1RA versus active SGLT2i.

TRIAL	DRUG	N	STUDY POPULATION	PRIMARY OUTCOME	MEDIAN FOLLOW-UP (Y)	HR (95% CI) FOR THE PRIMARY ENDPOINT	UNIQUE ASPECTS
EXAMINE[10]	Alogliptin	5380	T2D, ACS 15-90 days before randomization	3p MACE	1.5	0.96 (≤1.16)	Post-ACS population
SAVOR-TIMI 53[9]	Saxagliptin	16,492	T2D, HRPP (21%) or ASCVD (79%)	3p MACE	2.1	1.00 (0.89–1.12)	Only CVOT to show increased HF hospitalization
ELIXA[29]	Lixisenatide	6068	T2D, ACS 0-180 d before screening	4p MACE	2.1	1.02 (0.89–1.17)	Post-ACS population
EMPA-REG Outcomes[30]	Empagliflozin	7020	T2D, ASCVD (99%)	3p MACE	3.1	0.86 (0.74–0.99)	
TECOS[11]	Sitagliptin	14,671	T2D, ASCVD (100%)	4p MACE	3.0	0.98 (0.88-1.09)	
LEADER[13]	Liraglutide	9340	T2D, ASCVD (including CKD or HF) (81%) or HRPP (19%)	3p MACE	3.8	0.87 (0.78–0.97)	
SUSTAIN-6[31]	Injectable Semaglutide	3297	T2D, ASCVD (including CKD or HF) (83%) or HRPP (17%)	3p MACE	2.1	0.74 (0.58–0.95)	
EXSCEL[12]	Exenatide	14,752	T2D, HRPP (27%) or ASCVD (73%)	3p MACE	3.2	0.91 (0.83–1.00)	
CANVAS Program[15]	Canagliflozin	10,142	T2D, HRPP (34%) or ASCVD (66%)	3p MACE	3.6	0.86 (0.75–0.97)	Integrated data from 2 trials
HARMONY Outcomes[32]	Albiglutide	9463	T2D, ASCVD (100%)	3p MACE	1.6	0.78 (0.68–0.90)	
PIONEER-6[33]	Oral Semaglutide	3183	T2D, [ASCVD or CKD (85%)] or HRPP (15%)	3p MACE	1.3	0.79 (0.57–1.11)	
REWIND[34]	Dulaglutide	9901	T2D, HRPP (69%) or ASCVD (31%)	3p MACE	5.4	0.88 (0.79–0.99)	Largest HRPP population in a CVOT
CARMELINA[35]	Linagliptin	6979	T2D, [ASCVD and albuminuria] or CKD	3p-MACE	2.2	1.02 (0.89–1.17)	
CAROLINA[36]	Linagliptin	6033	T2D, HRPP (58%) or ASCVD (42%)	3p MACE	6.3	0.98 (0.84–1.14)	Only CVOT with active comparator
DECLARE TIMI-58[37]	Dapagliflozin	17,160	T2D, HRPP (59%) or ASCVD (41%)	Co-primaries: 3pMACE; CV death or HF hospitalization	4.2	0.93 (0.84–1.03)	
CREDENCE[38]	Canagliflozin	4401	T2D, CKD, and albuminuria	ESKD, doubling of serum Cr, or kidney or CV death	2.6	0.80 (0.67–0.95)	Terminated early due to benefit
VERTIS-CV[39]	Ertugliflozin	8246	T2D, ASCVD (100%)	3p MACE	3.5	0.97 (0.85–1.11)	
SOLOIST-WHF[40]	Sotagliflozin	1222	T2D, hospitalized for worsening HF	Total CV deaths, HF hospitalization, and HF urgent visits	0.75	0.67 (0.52–0.85)	SGLT1 and SGLT2 inhibitor; trial terminated early due to loss of funding
SCORED[41]	Sotagliflozin	10,584	T2D, CKD, and RFs	Total CV deaths, HF hospitalization, and HF urgent visits	1.3	0.74 (0.63–0.88)	SGLT1 and SGLT2 inhibitor; primary outcome changed during the trial; trial terminated early due to loss of funding
AMPLITUDE-O[42]	Efpeglenatide	4076	T2D, ASCVD (90%) or CKD (32%) or both (22%)	3p MACE	1.8	0.73 (0.58–0.92)	Randomization was stratified by use of SGLT2i

Continued

TABLE 11.2 Study Design Aspects of CVOTs in patients with T2D since 2008 FDA Guidance. All trials are placebo-controlled except CAROLINA, which used glimepiride as an active comparator; SURPASS, which uses dulaglutide as an active comparator; and PRECIDENTD, which is a comparative effectiveness study of active GLP-1RA versus active SGLT2i.**—cont'd**

TRIAL	DRUG	N	STUDY POPULATION	PRIMARY OUTCOME	MEDIAN FOLLOW-UP (Y)	HR (95% CI) FOR THE PRIMARY ENDPOINT	UNIQUE ASPECTS
FLOW[43]	Semaglutide	3533	T2D, CKD	Major kidney events, kidney or CV death	3.4	0.76 (0.66–0.88)	First trial of GLP-1RA with kidney disease as primary outcome
SURPASS CVOT (NCT04255433)[44]	Tirzepatide	13,299	T2D, ASCVD and BMI ≥25 kg/m²	3p MACE	ongoing	ongoing	First trial of a dual GIP/GLP1RA. Estimated completion: 6/2025
PRECIDENTD (NCT05390892)[45]	GLP-1RA vs. SGLT2 inhibitor	Goal 6000	T2D, ASCVD (70%) or high ASCVD risk	Total CV and kidney events or death	Enrolling now	Enrolling now	Only current comparative effectiveness trial of GLP-1RA vs. SGLT2i

ACS, Acute coronary syndrome; *ASCVD*, atherosclerotic cardiovascular disease; *CI*, confidence interval; *CKD*, chronic kidney disease; *Cr*, creatinine; *CVOT*, cardiovascular outcome trial; *ESKD*, end stage kidney disease; *GIP*, glucose-dependent insulinotropic polypeptide; *GLP-1RA*, glucagon-like peptide 1 receptor agonist; *HF*, heart failure; *HR*, hazard ratio; *HRPP*, high risk primary prevention; *SGLT*, sodium glucose cotransporter; *N*, number of subjects; *RF*, risk factor for ASCVD; *T2D*, type 2 diabetes mellitus; *y*, years; *3p MACE*, 3 point major adverse cardiovascular event (myocardial infarction, stroke, cardiovascular death); *4p MACE*, 4 point major adverse cardiovascular event (myocardial infarction, stroke, hospitalization for unstable angina, cardiovascular death).

Sotagliflozin, a combined sodium-glucose cotransporter 1 (SGLT1) and sodium-glucose cotransporter 2 (SGLT2) inhibitor, has demonstrated efficacy in preventing recurrent heart failure[40] and kidney disease progression[41] in patients with T2D. Eight published CVOTs with GLP1RA in patients with T2D have shown cardiovascular safety and a few (liraglutide, semaglutide, dulaglutide) have also demonstrated reduction in risk of MACE and kidney outcomes.[12,13,29,31–33,42,43,52] CVOTs were terminated due to safety or business concerns for the following agents: thiazolidinediones,[53] aleglitazar,[54] fasiglifam,[55] omarigliptin,[56] and taspoglutide.[57] Ongoing CVOTs are assessing additional drug classes including dual GLP1 receptor/glucose-dependent insulinotropic polypeptide (GIP) agonists (NCT04255433).

Patient Populations

Several of the initial CVOTs after the 2008 FDA guidance focused exclusively on patients with known ASCVD in order to both satisfy the guidance requirement to demonstrate cardiovascular safety in individuals at high cardiovascular risk, and to ensure enough events to complete the trial.[9–11,29,30,32,36,39] However, as time progressed and the wide-ranging impact of some of the agents became more apparent, additional trial populations within T2D were included. Several trials have included high-risk primary prevention patients in varying proportions of the overall trial population,[12,13,15,31,33–37,42] though no trials to date have included only primary prevention patients. Additionally, four trials of SGLT2i have focused on patients with chronic kidney disease (CKD): two in those with T2D only[38,41] and two in the broader population of CKD.[50,58] With clear heart failure benefit seen in the early SGLT2i trials,[30,37] subsequent trials enrolled patients with heart failure with reduced ejection fraction[46,47] and with preserved ejection fraction,[49,59,60] regardless of T2D status. The beneficial effects of GLP-1RA on ASCVD have also been extended to patients who have obesity but do not have T2D.[61] Thus since the FDA guidance was first issued, the patient populations evaluated in CVOTs have broadened considerably to include many severe comorbidities associated with T2D beyond ASCVD or high risk for ASCVD, such as heart failure or kidney disease, and the evidence base has expanded to support the use of SGLT2i and GLP-1RA use for those same conditions in patients without T2D.[47,48,61]

Comparator Groups

The vast majority of CVOTs conducted under the 2008 FDA guidance utilized a placebo control arm as the comparator group. The CAROLINA trial, which compared linagliptin and glimepiride, and SURPASS-CVOT, which is comparing tirzepatide to dulaglutide, have utilized an active comparator arm (though glimepiride has no known cardiovascular benefit).[36,44] All other trials have tested the agent of interest compared with placebo on the background of standard of care diabetes agents. However, as the efficacy of various SGLT2i and GLP1RA agents has become apparent, the background standard of care therapy has changed over time. For example, in the EMPA-REG OUTCOME trial (empagliflozin), published in 2015, 3% of patients in the placebo arm were on GLP1RA.[30] In comparison, by the end of the VERTIS-CV trial (ertugliflozin) in 2020, 5.6% of patients in the placebo arm were on GLP1RA.[39] More strikingly, in the 2016 LEADER trial (liraglutide), 2.8% of the placebo arm was initiated on SGLT2i during the trial,[13] whereas in the more recent AMPLITUDE-O trial (efpeglenitide), 21.2% of patients in the placebo arm were on SGLT2i by the end of the study in 2021.[42] As agents with proven cardiovascular (CV) benefit are increasingly used as background therapy, the bar to prove noninferiority from a CV perspective is anticipated to rise. Indeed, the ongoing SURPASS CVOT for tirzepatide, a dual GIP/GLP21RA, uses the active comparator dulaglutide, a GLP-1RA with established cardiovascular benefit.[34,44]

Outcomes Assessed

The 2008 FDA guidance specifically mandated that all antihyperglycemic agents be assessed for impact on CV mortality, myocardial infarction, and stroke[1]. Additional outcomes that were considered "optional" included hospitalization for acute coronary syndrome and urgent revascularization procedures. Thus the majority of the CVOTs that were conducted early after the guidance was published utilized 3-point MACE (CV death, nonfatal MI, or nonfatal stroke) as the primary outcome. Once the heart failure and kidney benefits of empagliflozin became apparent,[30,62] however, a shift towards expanded outcomes began to take place. For example, the DECLARE-TIMI 58 trial of dapagliflozin among patients with T2D had completed enrollment and was ongoing at the time the EMPA-REG Outcomes trial was published, and the trial executive committee elected to add a second primary efficacy endpoint of CV death or heart failure hospitalization in addition to the prior primary efficacy endpoint of 3-point MACE.[37] DECLARE-TIMI 58 demonstrated that dapagliflozin was superior to placebo for reducing the CV death/heart failure hospitalization outcome but not the MACE outcome. Subsequent trials have utilized kidney disease progression and hospitalization for heart failure as components of the primary outcome, highlighting the trend towards tailoring the trial design to the expected benefit of specific agents, rather than focusing solely on demonstrating ASCVD safety.

MOVING FORWARD: 2020 REVISED FDA GUIDANCE FOR INDUSTRY

In October 2018 the FDA convened a meeting of the Endocrinologic and Metabolic Drugs Advisory Committee to discuss the 2008 Guidance. The FDA asked the committee to vote on the question of whether *all* new antihyperglycemic medications for T2D should need to demonstrate cardiovascular safety (i.e., an absence of unacceptable increase in CV risk) regardless of presence or absence of a signal for CV risk in the development program. A number of other key questions were raised, such as whether the current atherothrombotic endpoint (3-point or 4-point MACE) was appropriate, and to what extent it should be expanded to consider a broader array of cardiovascular and noncardiovascular outcomes such as kidney disease, heart failure, and atrial fibrillation.

The FDA used the feedback provided in that 2018 Advisory Committee meeting to shape a new 2020 draft guidance document.[63] This document includes a number of key modifications to the 2008 guidance, including a broader perspective on safety. The 2020 guidance eliminates the two-step approach of requiring manufacturers to demonstrate ASCVD safety events by excluding an upper bound of the 95% confidence interval of 1.8 prior to bringing a drug to market. The guidance also eliminates the requirement for a large, phase 4 cardiovascular safety or efficacy trial to exclude an increased risk of ASCVD events by excluding an upper bound of the 95% confidence interval of 1.3. Instead, the FDA suggests that manufacturers conduct trials in patients of sufficient CV risk to capture meaningful numbers of cardiovascular events. In this way the FDA hopes to be able to exclude an increased risk for a number of outcomes including major CV events and can mandate further trials focused on safety if there are concerns. The draft guidance specifies a number of different aspects of a drug development program, including the size and duration of the trials required, as well as specific requirements for the types of comorbidities that must be present in those trials[63]:

- At least 4000 patient-years of exposure to the new drug in phase 3 clinical trials.
- At least 1500 patients exposed to the new drug for at least 1 year.
- At least 500 patients exposed to the new drug for at least 2 years.
- At least 500 patients with stage 3/4 chronic kidney disease exposed to the new drug.
- At least 600 patients with established CV disease (e.g., previous myocardial infarction, documented coronary artery disease, previous stroke, peripheral vascular disease) exposed to the new drug.
- At least 600 patients older than 65 years of age exposed to the new drug.

Furthermore, the FDA notes that CV safety remains an important concern for patients with diabetes and recommends that rigorous methods be used to ascertain and adjudicate CV events. They also note that a minimum number of adverse events is required in order to detect a risk signal and recommend independent adjudication of noncardiovascular risks as well. Then, if a concern is identified, the FDA can require more rigorous studies to specifically address that safety concern. While the 2008 guidance was focused almost exclusively on CV safety, one important effect of conducting large CVOTs was to increase the number of patients with significant burden of illness who were exposed to the novel medications for years, instead of weeks or months. In addition to testing CV safety, the increase in the patient-years of exposure allowed the detection of important noncardiovascular adverse effects, including allergic reactions to taspoglutide, upper gastrointestinal bleeding with aleglitazar, liver abnormalities with fasiglifam, and others.[54,55,57] The FDA writes that the updated guidance allows subsequent trials to focus on a broader assessment of premarket safety, to include both CV and noncardiovascular adverse effects.[63,64] Bexagliflozin, an SGLT2i, is the first antihyperglycemic agent for T2D approved after the updated FDA draft guidance was released in 2020. While the phase 3 cardiovascular safety trial for bexagliflozin was complete as of July 2024,[65] it has not yet been published except in abstract[66] or meta-analysis form.[67]

REAL-WORLD EVIDENCE AND THE ASSESSMENT OF SAFETY AND EFFICACY

There is broad interest in using real-world evidence (RWE) to assess drug safety and efficacy. RWE comes from routine health data collected in the usual care of patients. The interest in novel approaches is driven in part by the escalating cost of large, randomized pivotal trials and an appreciation for the limitations of the randomized trial to produce generalizable knowledge adequate to assess effectiveness and safety in broad populations with a range of comorbidities. RWEs can use randomized or nonrandomized study designs and typically use routine health data (e.g., data collected from billing codes or from the electronic health record) for follow-up and outcome ascertainment. The 21st Century Cures Act was passed by the US Congress in 2016 and was "designed to help accelerate medical product development and bring new innovations and advances to patients who need them faster and more efficiently." It directed the FDA to develop RWE approaches for the assessment of new drugs, and a number of studies have tried to address the ways in which RWE may offer valid assessments of drug efficacy and safety.[68,69]

Real-World Evidence for Safety

While randomized trials provide critical safety information, most do not provide the patient-years of drug exposure needed to detect events that occur only very rarely or only after sustained exposure. The FDA has long used the Sentinel System to monitor the safety of approved drugs. Sources of data for the Sentinel System include the Center for Medicare and Medicaid Services (CMS) and the Veterans Health Administration (VA), among others. The Sentinel Initiative seeks to expand data sources to include electronic health records, medical claims data, and other sources.[69] Using observational and uncontrolled RWE to assess short- and long-term safety, and to capture unexpected or rare events, has been an area of sustained interest and effort by the FDA. As a result, there is a significant history and experience with using RWE to assess the safety of new drugs.

Real-World Evidence for Efficacy

The issue of using RWE to support a claim of efficacy is more uncertain. As noted above, the efficacy for new antihyperglycemic agents is defined by the FDA as demonstrating evidence of A1c lowering in different treatment scenarios. As noted earlier in this chapter, A1c lowering is a clinically relevant and FDA-accepted surrogate endpoint for the efficacy of antihyperglycemic medications, although the FDA released draft guidance regarding other glycemic efficacy endpoints for clinical trials of antidiabetic and biological products in May 2023 including postprandial glucose and continuous glucose monitoring-based metrics.[70] Because A1c is a continuous measure, and generally shows clinically important change within 3 to 6 months, smaller, shorter, traditional randomized trials will likely continue to be the preferred approach for demonstrating the effect of a new drug on this endpoint. However, multiple drugs from the SGLT2i and GLP1RA classes now have labeling indications for the prevention of major adverse cardiovascular and kidney outcomes. Thus manufacturers, investigators, clinicians, and patients are less likely to adopt new therapies simply for their effects to lower A1c without similarly robust evidence of cardiovascular, kidney, or other benefits in patients with T2D. Manufacturers and others involved in drug development may have an interest in demonstrating broader efficacy and may turn to large, extended-duration, cost-efficient trials using RWE to provide support for those claims.

However, whether RWE can conclusively demonstrate efficacy at a level of evidence required for registration of a new drug with major cardiovascular, kidney, or other effects is far less certain. While FDA guidance on the use of RWE does not require a randomization step in study design,[68] and some advocates for the use of RWE argue that randomization is not necessary to achieve valid results, the potential for residual confounding to alter the size and even the direction of the observed effect of a new drug is substantial and could lead to imprecise or incorrect estimates of the drug's benefit or risk.

One group of investigators has directly addressed the question of whether an observational approach with careful adjustment for baseline confounders can produce results that are similar in direction and magnitude to the results of RCTs in the cardiovascular and diabetes space. In the RCT DUPLICATE initiative, Franklin and colleagues sought to emulate the results from 10 randomized controlled trials which evaluated the cardiovascular outcomes of antihyperglycemic or antiplatelet medications.[71] The trials of antihyperglycemic medications that the investigators tried to emulate were the LEADER,[13] DECLARE-TIMI 58,[14] EMPA-REG OUTCOME,[30] CANVAS,[15] CARMELINA,[35] TECOS,[11] SAVOR-TIMI 53,[9] and CAROLINA[36] trials. The investigators used insurance claims data to emulate inclusion and exclusion criteria, primary outcomes, and comparator populations. They created propensity scores to balance measured and unmeasured confounders. For the diabetes trials, agreement was high except for those that compared a DPP4i with a placebo (CARMELINA, TECOS, SAVOR-TIMI 53). The choice of a comparator for these studies was particularly challenging. While agreement between these trials and the RWE was good, the authors note that they were unable to emulate a placebo, and thus had to choose an active comparator, such as a sulfonylurea. This challenge fundamentally alters the study question. Another important consideration is that randomized trials are analyzed with an intention to treat principle, while RWE such as the RCT DUPLICATE study uses on-treatment analyses, which raises a number of other important analytic and interpretation issues and potential for bias.[71,72]

Pragmatic trials, which include a randomization step but then use real-world data for follow-up, are another hybrid approach for demonstrating efficacy with RWE. Pragmatic trial design includes trials that are incorporated into routine clinical practice and use either electronic health record data or registry data to ascertain clinical outcomes. Recently, this approach has been used in the ADAPTABLE trial, a pragmatic trial of two different doses of aspirin in patients with ASCVD,[73] and in the VALIDATE-SWEDEHEART trial,[74] a comparative effectiveness trial of bivalirudin versus heparin in patients with myocardial infarction. These trials are based on the well-tested assumption that ascertainment of outcomes are well captured in real-world data.[75,76] While this may be true for outcomes like myocardial infarction, stroke, or death, other outcomes, such as peripheral artery disease, are not captured well in electronic health records, with low concordance between traditionally ascertained and adjudicated events when compared with those events collected through billing data.[76] Thus the role of RWE in demonstrating efficacy will rely heavily on how well the outcome of interest can be ascertained from routine health data. Furthermore, other aspects of study design, such as the presence or absence of double-blind treatment allocation, can lead to important differences in adherence, outcome ascertainment, and outcome validity in RWE studies designed to assess the efficacy of a new therapy.[73]

CONCLUSIONS

Regulatory requirements for the approval of new antihyperglycemic medications have evolved substantially over the past 14 or more years. Concern for the cardiovascular safety of antihyperglycemic medications led the FDA in 2008 to require large cardiovascular outcome trials to demonstrate the cardiovascular safety of new antihyperglycemic medications. Similar, though somewhat less stringent, requirements were adopted by the EMA. The trials that were conducted to comply with this guidance were instrumental in identifying drugs from the SGLT2i and GLP1RA classes as important new therapies with novel beneficial cardiovascular and kidney effects for patients with T2D. The FDA revised its guidance in 2020 and no longer requires dedicated cardiovascular outcome trials. The ongoing challenge and expense of conducting large clinical trials, as well as language in the 21st Century Cures Act, have prompted the FDA to consider the roles of RWE in the assessment of both safety and efficacy of new drugs. The dramatic shift in regulation of antihyperglycemic drugs with the 2008 FDA guidance transformed the field of diabetes care and beyond, catalyzing the understanding of paradigm-shifting beneficial effects of SGLT2i and GLP1RA in high-risk patients with and without diabetes. As the regulatory environment for antihyperglycemic medications continues to evolve, the hope is that optimal use of RWE and novel trial design will facilitate the development and testing of safe therapies with important benefits to improve health and quality of life for patients with diabetes.

REFERENCES

1. U.S. Food And Drug Administration. Food and Drug Administration. Diabetes Mellitus—Evaluating Cardiovascular Risk in New Antidiabetic Therapies to Treat Type 2 Diabetes. U.S. Department of Health and Human Services Food and Drug Administration Center for Drug Evaluation and Research (CDER). 2008. https://www.fda.gov/media/71297/download.
2. Diabetes Control and Complications Research Group, Nathan DM, Genuth S, Lachin J, et al. The effect of intensive treatment of diabetes on the development and progression of long-term complications in insulin-dependent diabetes mellitus. *N Engl J Med.* 1993;329:977–986. https://doi.org/10.1056/NEJM199309303291401.
3. UK Prospective Study Group. Intensive blood-glucose control with sulphonylureas or insulin compared with conventional treatment and risk of complications in patients with type 2 diabetes (UKPDS 33). UK Prospective Diabetes Study (UKPDS) Group. *Lancet.* 1998;352:837–853.
4. The Diabetes Control and Complications Trial/Epidemiology of Diabetes Interventions and Complications (DCCT/EDIC) Study Research Group, Nathan DM, Cleary PA, Backlund JY, et al. Intensive diabetes treatment and cardiovascular disease in patients with type 1 diabetes. *N Engl J Med.* 2005;353:2643–2653. https://doi.org/10.1056/NEJMoa052187.
5. Holman RR, Paul SK, Bethel MA, Matthews DR, Neil HAW. 10-year follow-up of intensive glucose control in type 2 diabetes. *N Engl J Med.* 2008;359:1577–1589. https://doi.org/10.1056/NEJMoa0806470.
6. Blind E, Janssen H, Dunder K, de Graeff PA. The European Medicines Agency's approval of new medicines for type 2 diabetes. *Diabetes Obes Metab.* 2018;20:2059–2063. https://doi.org/10.1111/dom.13349.
7. Low Wang CC, Everett BM, Burman KD, Wilson PWF. Cardiovascular Safety Trials for All New Diabetes Mellitus Drugs? *Circulation.* 2019;139:1741–1743. https://doi.org/10.1161/CIRCULATIONAHA.118.038771.
8. Vasilakou D, Karagiannis T, Athanasiadou E, et al. Sodium-glucose cotransporter 2 inhibitors for type 2 diabetes: a systematic review and meta-analysis. *Ann Intern Med.* 2013;159:262–274. https://doi.org/10.7326/0003-4819-159-4-201308200-00007.
9. Scirica BM, Bhatt DL, Braunwald E, et al. Saxagliptin and cardiovascular outcomes in patients with type 2 diabetes mellitus. *N Engl J Med.* 2013;369:1317–1326. https://doi.org/10.1056/NEJMoa1307684.
10. White WB, Cannon CP, Heller SR, et al. Alogliptin after acute coronary syndrome in patients with type 2 diabetes. *N Engl J Med.* 2013;369:1327–1335. https://doi.org/10.1056/NEJMoa1305889.
11. Green JB, Bethel MA, Armstrong PW, et al. Effect of sitagliptin on cardiovascular outcomes in type 2 diabetes. *N Engl J Med.* 2015;373:232–242. https://doi.org/10.1056/NEJMoa1501352.
12. Holman RR, Bethel MA, Mentz RJ, et al. Effects of once-weekly exenatide on cardiovascular outcomes in type 2 diabetes. *N Engl J Med.* 2017;377:1228–1239. https://doi.org/10.1056/NEJMoa1612917.
13. Marso SP, Daniels GH, Brown-Frandsen K, et al. Liraglutide and cardiovascular outcomes in type 2 diabetes. *N Engl J Med.* 2016;375:311–322. https://doi.org/10.1056/NEJMoa1603827.
14. Wiviott SD, Raz I, Bonaca MP, et al. Dapagliflozin and cardiovascular outcomes in type 2 diabetes. *N Engl J Med.* 2018;380:347–357. https://doi.org/10.1056/NEJMoa1812389.
15. Neal B, Perkovic V, Mahaffey KW, et al. Canagliflozin and cardiovascular and renal events in type 2 diabetes. *N Engl J Med.* 2017;377:644–657. https://doi.org/10.1056/NEJMoa1611925.
16. U.S. Food And Drug Administration. FDA Background Document: Endocrinologic and Metabolic Drugs Advisory Committee Meeting October 24-25, 2018. https://www.fda.gov/media/121272/download.
17. Chong W. Endocrinologic and Metabolic Drugs Advisory Committee Meeting October 24-25, 2018 Introductory Remarks. 2018. https://www.fda.gov/media/121276/download.
18. Meinert CL, Knatterud GL, Prout TE, Klimt CR. A study of the effects of hypoglycemic agents on vascular complications in patients with adult-onset diabetes. II. Mortality results. *Diabetes.* 1970;19:Suppl:789–830.
19. A study of the effects of hypoglycemia agents on vascular complications in patients with adult-onset diabetes. VI. Supplementary report on nonfatal events in patients treated with tolbutamide. *Diabetes.* 1976;25:1129–1153. https://doi.org/10.2337/diab.25.12.1129.
20. Nissen SE, Wolski K, Topol EJ. Effect of muraglitazar on death and major adverse cardiovascular events in patients with type 2 diabetes mellitus. *JAMA.* 2005;294:2581–2586. https://doi.org/10.1001/jama.294.20.joc50147.
21. Nissen SE, Wolski K. Effect of rosiglitazone on the risk of myocardial infarction and death from cardiovascular causes. *N Engl J Med.* 2007;356:2457–2471. https://doi.org/10.1056/NEJMoa072761.
22. European Medicines Agency. Concept paper on the need for revision of the note for guidance on clinical investigation of medicinal products in the treatment of diabetes mellitus. 2008. https://www.ema.europa.eu/en/documents/scientific-guideline/concept-paper-need-revision-note-guidance-clinical-investigation-medicinal-products-treatment_en-2.pdf.
23. U.S. Food And Drug Administration. FDA Briefing Document: Readjudication of the Rosiglitazone Evaluated for Cardiovascular Outcomes and Regulation of Glycemia in Diabetes Trial (RECORD). Joint Meeting of the Endocrinologic and Metabolic Drugs Advisory Committee and the Drug Safety and Risk Management Advisory Committee. 2013. http://wayback.archive-it.org/7993/20161024135214/http://www.fda.gov/downloads/AdvisoryCommittees/CommitteesMeetingMaterials/Drugs/EndocrinologicandMetabolicDrugsAdvisoryCommittee/UCM354859.pdf.
24. U.S. Food And Drug Administration. FDA Drug Safety Communication: FDA requires removal of some prescribing and dispensing restrictions for rosiglitazone-containing diabetes medicines. 2013.
25. Action to Control Cardiovascular Risk in Diabetes Study Group, Gerstein HC, Miller ME, Byington RP, et al. Effects of intensive glucose lowering in type 2 diabetes. *N Engl J Med.* 2008;358:2545–2559. https://doi.org/10.1056/NEJMoa0802743. NEJMoa0802743 [pii].
26. European Medicines Agency. Guideline on clinical investigation of medicinal products in the treatment or prevention of diabetes mellitus. 2012. https://www.ema.europa.eu/en/documents/scientific-guideline/guideline-clinical-investigation-medicinal-products-treatment-prevention-diabetes-mellitus-revision_en.pdf.
27. European Medicines Agency. Reflection paper on assessment of cardiovascular safety profile of medicinal products. 2016. https://www.ema.europa.eu/en/documents/scientific-guideline/reflection-paper-assessment-cardiovascular-safety-profile-medicinal-products_en.pdf.
28. Sharma A, Pagidipati NJ, Califf RM, et al. Impact of regulatory guidance on evaluating cardiovascular risk of new glucose-lowering therapies to treat type 2 diabetes mellitus: lessons learned and future directions. *Circulation.* 2020;141:843–862. https://doi.org/10.1161/CIRCULATIONAHA.119.041022.
29. Pfeffer MA, Claggett B, Diaz R, et al. Lixisenatide in patients with type 2 diabetes and acute coronary syndrome. *N Engl J Med.* 2015;373:2247–2257. https://doi.org/10.1056/NEJMoa1509225.

30. Zinman B, Wanner C, Lachin JM, et al. Empagliflozin, Cardiovascular outcomes, and mortality in type 2 diabetes. *N Engl J Med*. 2015;373:2117–2128. https://doi.org/10.1056/NEJMoa1504720.
31. Marso SP, Bain SC, Consoli A, et al. Semaglutide and cardiovascular outcomes in patients with type 2 diabetes. *N Engl J Med*. 2016;375:1834–1844. https://doi.org/10.1056/NEJMoa1607141.
32. Hernandez AF, Green JB, Janmohamed S, et al. Albiglutide and cardiovascular outcomes in patients with type 2 diabetes and cardiovascular disease (Harmony Outcomes): a double-blind, randomised placebo-controlled trial. *Lancet*. 2018;392:1519–1529. https://doi.org/10.1016/S0140-6736(18)32261-X.
33. Husain M, Birkenfeld AL, Donsmark M, et al. Oral semaglutide and cardiovascular outcomes in patients with type 2 diabetes. *N Engl J Med*. 2019;381:841–851. https://doi.org/10.1056/NEJMoa1901118.
34. Gerstein HC, Colhoun HM, Dagenais GR, et al. Dulaglutide and cardiovascular outcomes in type 2 diabetes (REWIND): a double-blind, randomised placebo-controlled trial. *Lancet*. 2019;394:121–130. https://doi.org/10.1016/S0140-6736(19)31149-3.
35. Rosenstock J, Perkovic V, Johansen OE, et al. Effect of linagliptin vs placebo on major cardiovascular events in adults with type 2 diabetes and high cardiovascular and renal risk: the CARMELINA Randomized Clinical Trial. *JAMA*. 2019;321:69–79. https://doi.org/10.1001/jama.2018.18269.
36. Rosenstock J, Kahn SE, Johansen OE, et al. Effect of linagliptin vs glimepiride on major adverse cardiovascular outcomes in patients with type 2 diabetes: the CAROLINA randomized clinical trial. *JAMA*. 2019;322:1155–1166. https://doi.org/10.1001/jama.2019.13772.
37. Wiviott SD, Raz I, Bonaca MP, et al. Dapagliflozin and cardiovascular outcomes in type 2 diabetes. *N Engl J Med*. 2019;380:347–357. https://doi.org/10.1056/NEJMoa1812389.
38. Perkovic V, Jardine MJ, Neal B, et al. Canagliflozin and renal outcomes in type 2 diabetes and nephropathy. *N Engl J Med*. 2019;380:2295–2306. https://doi.org/10.1056/NEJMoa1811744.
39. Cannon CP, Pratley R, Dagogo-Jack S, et al. Cardiovascular outcomes with ertugliflozin in type 2 diabetes. *N Engl J Med*. 2020;383:1425–1435. https://doi.org/10.1056/NEJMoa2004967.
40. Bhatt DL, Szarek M, Steg PG, et al. Sotagliflozin in patients with diabetes and recent worsening heart failure. *N Engl J Med*. 2021;384:117–128. https://doi.org/10.1056/NEJMoa2030183.
41. Bhatt DL, Szarek M, Pitt B, et al. Sotagliflozin in patients with diabetes and chronic kidney disease. *N Engl J Med*. 2021;384:129–139. https://doi.org/10.1056/NEJMoa2030186.
42. Gerstein HC, Sattar N, Rosenstock J, et al. Cardiovascular and renal outcomes with efpeglenatide in type 2 diabetes. *N Engl J Med*. 2021;385:896–907. https://doi.org/10.1056/NEJMoa2108269.
43. Perkovic V, Tuttle KR, Rossing P, et al. Effects of semaglutide on chronic kidney disease in patients with type 2 diabetes. *N Engl J Med*. 2024. https://doi.org/10.1056/NEJMoa2403347.
44. Nicholls SJ, Bhatt DL, Buse JB, et al. Comparison of tirzepatide and dulaglutide on major adverse cardiovascular events in participants with type 2 diabetes and atherosclerotic cardiovascular disease: SURPASS-CVOT design and baseline characteristics. *Am Heart J*. 2024;267:1–11. https://doi.org/10.1016/j.ahj.2023.09.007.
45. Everett B.M., R.J. G., Wexler D.J. PREvention of CardIovascular and DiabEtic kidNey Disease in Type 2 Diabetes (PRECIDENTD) (NCT05390892). 2024. https://clinicaltrials.gov/study/NCT05390892?term=PRECIDENTD&rank=1.
46. Packer M, Anker SD, Butler J, et al. Cardiovascular and renal outcomes with empagliflozin in heart failure. *N Engl J Med*. 2020;383:1413–1424. https://doi.org/10.1056/NEJMoa2022190.
47. McMurray JJV, Solomon SD, Inzucchi SE, et al. Dapagliflozin in patients with heart failure and reduced ejection fraction. *N Engl J Med*. 2019;381:1995–2008. https://doi.org/10.1056/NEJMoa1911303.
48. Solomon SD, McMurray JJV, Claggett B, et al. Dapagliflozin in heart failure with mildly reduced or preserved ejection fraction. *N Engl J Med*. 2022;387:1089–1098. https://doi.org/10.1056/NEJMoa2206286.
49. Anker SD, Butler J, Filippatos G, et al. Empagliflozin in heart failure with a preserved ejection fraction. *N Engl J Med*. 2021;385:1451–1461. https://doi.org/10.1056/NEJMoa2107038.
50. Heerspink HJL, Stefansson BV, Correa-Rotter R, et al. Dapagliflozin in patients with chronic kidney disease. *N Engl J Med*. 2020;383:1436–1446. https://doi.org/10.1056/NEJMoa2024816.
51. The Empa-Kidney Collaborative Group, Herrington WG, Staplin N, Wanner C, et al. Empagliflozin in patients with chronic kidney disease. *N Engl J Med*. 2023;388:117–127. https://doi.org/10.1056/NEJMoa2204233.
52. Gerstein HC, Colhoun HM, Dagenais GR, et al. Design and baseline characteristics of participants in the Researching cardiovascular Events with a Weekly INcretin in Diabetes (REWIND) trial on the cardiovascular effects of dulaglutide. *Diabetes Obes Metab*. 2018;20:42–49. https://doi.org/10.1111/dom.13028.
53. Punthakee Z, Bosch J, Dagenais G, et al. Design, history and results of the Thiazolidinedione Intervention with vitamin D Evaluation (TIDE) randomised controlled trial. *Diabetologia*. 2012;55:36–45. https://doi.org/10.1007/s00125-011-2357-4.
54. Lincoff AM, Tardif JC, Schwartz GG, et al. Effect of aleglitazar on cardiovascular outcomes after acute coronary syndrome in patients with type 2 diabetes mellitus: the AleCardio randomized clinical trial. *JAMA*. 2014;311:1515–1525. https://doi.org/10.1001/jama.2014.3321.
55. Menon V, Lincoff AM, Nicholls SJ, et al. Fasiglifam-induced liver injury in patients with type 2 diabetes: results of a randomized controlled cardiovascular outcomes safety trial. *Diabetes Care*. 2018;41:2603–2609. https://doi.org/10.2337/dc18-0755.
56. Gantz I, Chen M, Suryawanshi S, et al. A randomized, placebo-controlled study of the cardiovascular safety of the once-weekly DPP-4 inhibitor omarigliptin in patients with type 2 diabetes mellitus. *Cardiovasc Diabetol*. 2017;16:112. https://doi.org/10.1186/s12933-017-0593-8.
57. Rosenstock J, Balas B, Charbonnel B, Group TeS., et al. The fate of taspoglutide, a weekly GLP-1 receptor agonist, versus twice-daily exenatide for type 2 diabetes: the T-emerge 2 trial. *Diabetes Care*. 2013;36:498–504. https://doi.org/10.2337/dc12-0709.
58. Herrington WG, Preiss D, Haynes R, et al. The potential for improving cardio-renal outcomes by sodium-glucose co-transporter-2 inhibition in people with chronic kidney disease: a rationale for the EMPA-KIDNEY study. *Clin Kidney J*. 2018;11:749–761. https://doi.org/10.1093/ckj/sfy090.
59. Solomon SD, de Boer RA, DeMets D, et al. Dapagliflozin in heart failure with preserved and mildly reduced ejection fraction: rationale and design of the DELIVER trial. *Eur J Heart Fail*. 2021;23:1217–1225. https://doi.org/10.1002/ejhf.2249.
60. Kosiborod MN, Abildstrom SZ, Borlaug BA, et al. Semaglutide in patients with heart failure with preserved ejection fraction and obesity. *N Engl J Med*. 2023;389:1069–1084. https://doi.org/10.1056/NEJMoa2306963.
61. Lincoff AM, Brown-Frandsen K, Colhoun HM, et al. Semaglutide and cardiovascular outcomes in obesity without diabetes. *N Engl J Med*. 2023 https://doi.org/10.1056/NEJMoa2307563.
62. Wanner C, Inzucchi SE, Lachin JM, et al. Empagliflozin and progression of kidney disease in type 2 diabetes. *N Engl J Med*. 2016;375:323–334. https://doi.org/10.1056/NEJMoa1515920.
63. U.S. Food and Drug Administration. Type 2 Diabetes: Evaluating the Safety of New Drugs for Improving Glycemic Control. 2020. https://www.fda.gov/media/135936/download.
64. Chong WH, Yanoff LB, Andraca-Carrera E, Thanh Hai M. Assessing the safety of glucose-lowering drugs - a new focus for the FDA. *N Engl J Med*. 2020;383:1199–1202. https://doi.org/10.1056/NEJMp2004889.
65. Theracos. Bexagliflozin Efficacy and Safety Trial (BEST) (NCT02558296). 2024. https://clinicaltrials.gov/study/NCT02558296?term=bexagliflozin&rank=2.
66. McMurray JJV, Freeman MW, Massaro J, et al. The Bexagliflozin Efficacy and Safety Trial (BEST): a randomized, double-blind, placebo-controlled, phase IIII, clinical trial. *Diabetes*. 2020;69:32.
67. McMurray JJV, Solomon SD, Lock JP, et al. Meta-analysis of risk of major adverse cardiovascular events in adults with type 2 diabetes treated with bexagliflozin. *Diabetes Obes Metab*. 2024;26:971–979. https://doi.org/10.1111/dom.15394.
68. U.S. Food And Drug Administration. Real-World Data: Assessing Electronic Health Records and Medical Claims Data To Support Regulatory Decision-Making for Drug and Biological Products. 2021. https://www.fda.gov/media/152503/download.
69. U.S. Food And Drug Administration. Framework for FDA's Real-World Evidence Program. 2021. https://www.fda.gov/media/120060/download
70. U.S. Food And Drug Administration. Diabetes Mellitus: Efficacy Endpoints for Clinical Trials Investigating Antidiabetic Drugs and Biological Products Guidance for Industry. U.S. Department of Health and Human Services Food and Drug Administration Center for Drug Evaluation and Research (CDER). 2023. https://www.fda.gov/media/168475/download.
71. Franklin JM, Patorno E, Desai RJ, et al. Emulating randomized clinical trials with nonrandomized real-world evidence studies: first results from the RCT DUPLICATE initiative. *Circulation*. 2021;143:1002–1013. https://doi.org/10.1161/CIRCULATIONAHA.120.051718.
72. Hernan MA, Hernandez-Diaz S. Beyond the intention-to-treat in comparative effectiveness research. *Clin Trials*. 2012;9:48–55. https://doi.org/10.1177/1740774511420743.
73. Jones WS, Mulder H, Wruck LM, et al. Comparative effectiveness of aspirin dosing in cardiovascular disease. *N Engl J Med*. 2021;384:1981–1990. https://doi.org/10.1056/NEJMoa2102137.
74. Erlinge D, Omerovic E, Frobert O, et al. Bivalirudin versus heparin monotherapy in myocardial infarction. *N Engl J Med*. 2017;377:1132–1142. https://doi.org/10.1056/NEJMoa1706443.
75. Strom JB, Faridi KF, Butala NM, et al. Use of administrative claims to assess outcomes and treatment effect in randomized clinical trials for transcatheter aortic valve replacement: findings from the EXTEND study. *Circulation*. 2020;142:203–213. https://doi.org/10.1161/CIRCULATIONAHA.120.046159.
76. Rodrigues C, Odutayo A, Patel S, et al. Accuracy of cardiovascular trial outcome ascertainment and treatment effect estimates from routine health data: a systematic review and meta-analysis. *Circ Cardiovasc Qual Outcomes*. 2021;14:e007903. https://doi.org/10.1161/CIRCOUTCOMES.120.007903.

12 Cardiovascular and Kidney Effects of Sodium Glucose Cotransporter Inhibitors

SILVIO E. INZUCCHI AND MIKHAIL KOSIBOROD

OVERVIEW OF MECHANISM OF ACTION

The sodium-glucose cotransporter (SGLT)-2 inhibitors are glucose-lowering agents initially approved for use in patients with type 2 diabetes. They exert their antihyperglycemic effects through the induction of glucosuria. The precise mechanism involves the blockade of a transporter in the proximal nephron that is responsible for about 90% of the reclamation of glucose from the early glomerular filtrate. As a result, the urinary glucose excretion threshold is reduced from the normal of approximately 180 mg/dL (the threshold in those with type 2 diabetes is actually higher in 230–240 mg/dL) down to less than 70 mg/dL.[1] Urinary glucose losses average approximately 70 to 80 g/day, with calorie losses of about 300 kcal/day.[1] Modest urinary sodium losses also occur, at least early in the treatment course.

Currently available SGLT2 inhibitors for use in patients with type 2 diabetes in the United States and Europe include canagliflozin, empagliflozin, dapagliflozin, and ertugliflozin. In Japan, other available members of the class include luseogliflozin, tofogliflozin, and ipragliflozin. In India, remogliflozin is also available. An SGLT1/SGLT2 inhibitor, sotagliflozin, is also available in Europe.

Some SGLT2 inhibitors also carry indications for use in heart failure and/or in chronic kidney disease, irrespective of diabetes status.

ANTIHYPERGLYCEMIC EFFECTS

Meta-analyses of glycemic control studies involving SGLT2 inhibitors have demonstrated mean reductions in HbA1c on the order of 0.6% to 0 7%, more when baseline values are higher (as is common with all glucose lowering medications.)[2] This drug category was initially approved for use as monotherapy or in conjunction with other glucose-lowering agents in patients with type 2 diabetes. Most commonly, this has included metformin, but these agents are also effective when combined with a variety of other agents with additive effects, including insulin. Due to their mechanism of action which does not involve the stimulation of insulin secretion, hypoglycemia rates are not increased when used in monotherapy or in conjunction with other diabetes medications that did not themselves induce hypoglycemia.[1,2] Of course, if used in combination with sulfonylureas or insulin, particularly those already under tight glycemic control, hypoglycemia may ensue, which would necessitate reduction in the doses of the agents with which the SGLT2 inhibitor is being paired.

NONGLYCEMIC EFFECTS

Modest reductions in body weight (approximately 2 kg) and blood pressure (approximately 4/2 mm Hg) occur.[1,2] Interestingly, despite ongoing calorie losses through the urine, weight loss plateaus are likely the result of increased calorie intake. Urine albumin:creatinine ratios are also reduced.[1] Other studies have found small reductions in liver fat.[3] The rest of this chapter reviews the important cardiorenal benefits of this class of medication.

CARDIOVASCULAR OUTCOMES

SGLT inhibitors have now been convincingly demonstrated to provide substantial cardiovascular benefits in multiple randomized controlled trials of various patient populations, including participants with type 2 diabetes, the first group that was extensively evaluated with these agents, as well as those who have heart failure with reduced, mildly reduced, and preserved ejection fraction (HFrEF, HFmrEF, and HFpEF) and those with chronic kidney disease (CKD), regardless of diabetes status.

Cardiovascular Outcomes in Dedicated CVOTs of Participants With Type 2 Diabetes

EMPA-REG OUTCOME

EMPA-REG Outcome[4] was the first large-scale randomized controlled trial of an SGLT2 inhibitor to demonstrate cardiovascular benefits of this class. It was designed in accordance the PREVAILING United States (US) Food and Drug Administration (FDA) Guidance to Industry concerning evaluation of the cardiovascular safety of new antihyperglycaemic therapies for type 2 diabetes.[5]

In total, 7020 participants with type 2 diabetes and established atherosclerotic cardiovascular disease (ASCVD) were randomized to either empagliflozin (10 or 25 mg) or a placebo once daily. The primary endpoint in this event-driven trial was a composite of 3-point MACE (major adverse cardiovascular events) defined as time to first nonfatal myocardial infraction (MI), stroke, or death from cardiovascular causes. The key secondary outcome was a 4-point MACE (which also included hospitalization for unstable angina). Both the primary and key secondary endpoints were tested for noninferiority first, and then for superiority (if noninferiority was met) in a hierarchical fashion. Cardiovascular death, all-cause death, and hospitalizations for heart failure were exploratory endpoints.

The primary outcome occurred less frequently in participants randomized to empagliflozin (490 of 4687 [10.5%]) than a placebo (282 of 2333 [12.1%]) (hazard ratio [HR], 0.86; 95% confidence interval [CI], 0.74– 0.99; $P < 0.001$ for noninferiority and $P = .04$ for superiority). The key secondary outcome occurred in 599 of 4687 patients (12.8%) with empagliflozin and 333 of 2333 patients (14.3%) with a placebo (HR, 0.89; 95% CI, 0.78–1.01; $P < 0.001$ for noninferiority and $P = .08$ for superiority). The reduction in the primary endpoint of 3-point MACE was driven predominantly by the lower incidence of cardiovascular (CV) death (HR, 0.62; 95% CI, 0.49–0.77; $P < 0.001$), with no significant difference in the risk of nonfatal MI (4.8% of participants in the empagliflozin group and 5.4% in the placebo group) or stroke (3.5% of participants in the empagliflozin group and 3.0% in the placebo group). The effects of empagliflozin versus placebo were also consistent across the prespecified subgroups of interest.

In addition, empagliflozin also reduced the risk of death from any cause (HR, 0.68; 95% CI, 0.57–0.82, $P < 0.001$), and hospitalization for heart failure (HR, 0.65; 95% CI, 0.50–0.85; $P = .002$).

Overall, empagliflozin was well tolerated, and the proportions of participants who experienced adverse events, serious adverse events, and adverse events leading to the discontinuation of the study medication were similar in the empagliflozin and placebo groups.

In subsequent secondary analyses, the favorable effects of empagliflozin on CV death occurred early, with the first statistically significant benefit seen at 59 days postrandomization.[6] The first statistically significant benefit for heart failure hospitalizations was seen at 17 days postrandomization.

CANVAS PROGRAM

The CANVAS Program consisted of two sister trials, CANVAS and CANVAS-R, which collectively randomized 10,142 participants (4330 in CANVAS and 5812 in CANVAS-R) with type 2 diabetes and either established ASCVD or at high risk for ASCVD to either canagliflozin 100 mg (in CANVAS-R with optional up-titration to 300 mg) or placebo once daily.[7] The primary endpoint was 3-point MACE (time to first event of cardiovascular causes, nonfatal MI, or nonfatal stroke). The primary endpoint was tested for noninferiority first and then for superiority (if noninferiority was met) in a hierarchical fashion. Secondary endpoints (tested hierarchically) included all-cause death, CV death, progression of albuminuria, and the composite of CV death and hospitalization for heart failure. Hospitalization for heart failure was an exploratory endpoint.

The primary outcome occurred less frequently among participants randomized to canagliflozin than a placebo (HR, 0.86; 95% CI, 0.75–0.97; $P < 0.001$ for noninferiority; $P = .02$ for superiority), with consistent findings observed across multiple demographic and clinical subgroups. Although the point estimates for the secondary endpoints of all-cause and CV death favored canagliflozin, they were not statistically significant (for all-cause death, HR, 0.87; 95% CI, 0.74–1.01; for CV death, HR, 0.87; 95% CI, 0.72–1.06). It was the same case for the individual endpoints of nonfatal MI and nonfatal stroke. The results for the composite endpoint of CV death or hospitalization for heart failure (HF), and hospitalization for HF alone were considered to be exploratory, but canagliflozin reduced the risk of these outcomes (HR, 0.78; 95% CI, 0.67–0.91; and HR, 0.67; 95% CI, 0.52–0.87, respectively).

Overall, canagliflozin was well tolerated, with fewer serious adverse events than placebo (HR, 0.93; 95% CI, 0.87–1.00). However, there was a higher risk of lower limb amputation with canagliflozin than a placebo (HR, 1.97; 95% CI, 1.41–2.75), a signal that was not seen in subsequent trials of canagliflozin or in trials of other SGLT inhibitors.

DECLARE

DECLARE was the largest of the SGLT2 inhibitor safety cardiovascular outcome trial (CVOTs), and randomly assigned 17,160 patients with type 2 diabetes and either established ASCVD (~40%) or multiple risk factors for ASCVD (~60%) to dapagliflozin 10 mg or a placebo daily.[8] This event-driven trial had one primary safety endpoint of 3-point MACE (time to first event of CV death, nonfatal MI, or nonfatal stroke), tested for noninferiority. There were also two dual primary efficacy endpoints: 3-point MACE and a composite of CV death or hospitalization for HF. Secondary endpoints included a renal composite (≥40% decrease in estimated glomerular filtration rate to <60 mL per minute per 1.73 m^2, end-stage renal disease, or death from renal or CV causes) and death from any cause.

In the analysis of the primary safety endpoint (3-point MACE), dapagliflozin was noninferior to a placebo (upper boundary of the 95% CI, <1.3; $P < 0.001$). In the analyses of the dual primary efficacy endpoints, dapagliflozin did not reduce 3-point MACE (HR, 0.93; 95% CI, 0.84–1.03; $P = .17$), but did lower the risk of CV death or hospitalization for HF (HR, 0.83; 95% CI, 0.73–0.95; $P = .005$), which was driven by a lower rate of hospitalizations for HF (HR, 0.73; 95% CI, 0.61–0.88), with no between-group difference in CV death (HR, 0.98; 95% CI, 0.82–1.17). No significant reductions were seen with dapagliflozin versus placebo in nonfatal MI, nonfatal stroke, or all-cause death (HR, 0.93; 95% CI, 0.82–1.04). The beneficial effects of dapagliflozin on CV death or hospitalization for HF were consistent across multiple subgroups, including among patients with established ASCVD and those with multiple ASCVD risk factors (*P* value for interaction was .99).

Similar to other CVOTs of SGLT2 inhibitors, dapagliflozin was well tolerated, with fewer serious adverse events than a placebo. There were more genital mycotic infections observed with dapagliflozin versus a placebo. Although diabetic ketoacidosis occurred rarely, more dapagliflozin than placebo-treated patients experienced such events (0.3% vs. 0.1%; HR, 2.18; 95% CI, 1.10–4.30; $P = .02$).

VERTIS-CV

In the VERTIS-CV trial, a total of 8246 participants with type 2 diabetes and established ASCVD were randomly assigned to either ertugliflozin (at the dose of 5 or 15 mg) or a placebo daily.[9] The primary safety endpoint in this event-driven trial was a composite of 3-point MACE (time to first nonfatal MI, stroke, or death from CV causes). Secondary efficacy endpoints, tested hierarchically, included a composite of CV death or hospitalization for HF; CV death; and a composite of death from renal causes, renal replacement therapy, or doubling of the serum creatinine level.

Ertugliflozin was noninferior as compared with a placebo for the primary safety endpoint; 11.9% of participants in the ertugliflozin group and 11.9% in the placebo group experienced a composite of 3-point MACE (HR, 0.97; 95% CI, 0.85–1.11; $P < 0.001$ for noninferiority). There were no between-group differences in any of the confirmatory secondary endpoints, including occurrence of CV death or hospitalization for HF (HR, 0.88; 95% CI, 0.75–1.03; $P = .11$ for superiority, or CV death (HR, 0.92; 95% CI, 0.77–1.11). The rates of hospitalizations for HF were lower with ertugliflozin than a placebo (HR, 0.70; 95% CI, 0.54–0.90), although this endpoint was not tested hierarchically and therefore is considered exploratory.

The incidence of serious adverse events and all adverse events were similar between ertugliflozin and placebo, although more urinary tract infections and genital mycotic infections were observed in the ertugliflozin- versus placebo-treated participants.

SCORED

SCORED was the cardiovascular outcome trial of sotagliflozin, which offers both SGLT1 and SGLT2 inhibition.[10] Unlike other CVOTs of SGLT2 inhibitors, it was designed to primarily test superiority (rather than noninferiority) of sotagliflozin versus placebo.

The event-driven trial randomly assigned 10,584 participants with type 2 diabetes and CKD, as well as ASCVD risk factors to either sotagliflozin (200 mg, up-titrated to 400 mg) or a placebo daily. The primary endpoint (revised during the trial) was the composite of the total number of CV deaths, and HF events (hospitalizations or urgent visits for HF). The final secondary endpoints (following the protocol amendment) included the total number of HF events; CV death; total number of CV deaths, hospitalizations for HF, nonfatal MI, and nonfatal stroke; the total number of CV deaths, and expanded definition of HF events; time to first kidney endpoint (sustained decrease of at least 50% in the eGFR, long-term dialysis, renal transplantation, or a sustained eGFR of less than 15 mL per minute per 1.73 m^2); all-cause deaths; and the total number of CV deaths, nonfatal MIs, and nonfatal strokes.

The trial ended early owing to loss of funding. This resulted in the protocol amendment, which included the change in the primary and secondary endpoints (as listed above); in addition, planned adjudication of endpoints was not completed, and investigator-reported events were used instead for all efficacy analyses.

Sotagliflozin reduced the risk of the primary efficacy endpoint (total number of CV deaths and HF events) by 26% (HR, 0.74; 95% CI, 0.63–0.88; $P < 0.001$). Sotagliflozin also reduced the risk of total HF events (HR, 0.67; 95% CI, 0.55–0.82; $P < 0.001$). There was no significant between-group difference in CV death (HR, 0.90; 95% CI, 0.73–1.12) or all-cause death (HR, 0.99; 95% CI, 0.83–1.18). Although considered exploratory, the analyses of time to first CV death or HF event (HR, 0.77; 95% CI, 0.66–0.91), and time to first event of 3-point MACE (HR, 0.84; 95% CI, 0.72–0.99) were favorable for sotagliflozin versus a placebo. Interestingly, and in contrast to the trials of pure SGLT2 inhibitors, the exploratory endpoints of time to first MI and time to first stroke were also favorable for sotagliflozin versus a placebo, potentially reflecting its different mechanism of action (which also includes SGLT1 inhibition).

Overall, sotagliflozin was well tolerated, with similar rates of adverse events and serious adverse events as compared with placebo. The rates of diarrhea (likely as a result of SGLT1 inhibition), genital mycotic infections, diabetic ketoacidosis (which occurred rarely), and volume depletion were higher with sotagliflozin than placebo.

META-ANALYSES

A number of meta-analyses of SGLT2 inhibitor CVOTs among participants with type 2 diabetes have been conducted, including by several trialist groups.[11] These studies have confirmed, using very large sample[12] sizes, that SGLT inhibitors modestly reduce the risk of ASCVD events, such as 3-point MACE (by ~10%), with a much larger (>20%) reduction in the risk of CV death or HF hospitalizations, and a very large, more than 30%, reduction in HF hospitalizations (Fig. 12.1).

Dedicated Outcome Trials of Participants With Heart Failure

The initial data from EMPA-REG OUTCOME and other CVOTs in participants with type 2 diabetes generated enthusiasm for testing SGLT inhibitors in dedicated outcome trials among patients with established HF (both heart failure with reduced ejection fraction (HFrEF) and heart failure with preserved ejection fraction (HFmrEF/HFpEF)).

DAPA-HF

DAPA-HF was the first trial to report the effects of SGLT2 inhibitors in patients with established HFrEF.[13] In this multicenter, randomized, international, event-driven trial, 4744 participants with symptomatic HFrEF (left ventricular ejection fraction of 40% or less) and elevated natriuretic

A Effects of Sodium-Glucose Cotransporter 2 Inhibitors on Major Adverse Cardiovascular Events–Composite of Myocardial Infarction, Stroke, or Cardiovascular Death

A Overall MACEs

	Treatment		Placebo			
	No./total No.	Rate/1000 patient-years	No./total No.	Rate/1000 patient-years	Hazard ratio (95% CI)	Weight, %
EMPA-REG OUTCOME	490/4687	37.4	282/2333	43.9	0.86 (0.74–0.99)	15.72
CANVAS program	NA/5795	26.9	NA/4347	31.5	0.86 (0.75–0.97)	20.12
DECLARE-TIMI 58	756/8582	22.6	803/8578	24.2	0.93 (0.84–1.03)	32.02
CREDENCE	217/2202	38.7	269/2199	48.7	0.80 (0.67–0.95)	10.92
VERTIS CV	735/5499	40.0	368/2747	40.3	0.99 (0.88–1.12)	21.23
Fixed-effects model (Q = 5.22; df = 4; P = .27; I^2 = 23.4%)					0.90 (0.85–0.95)	

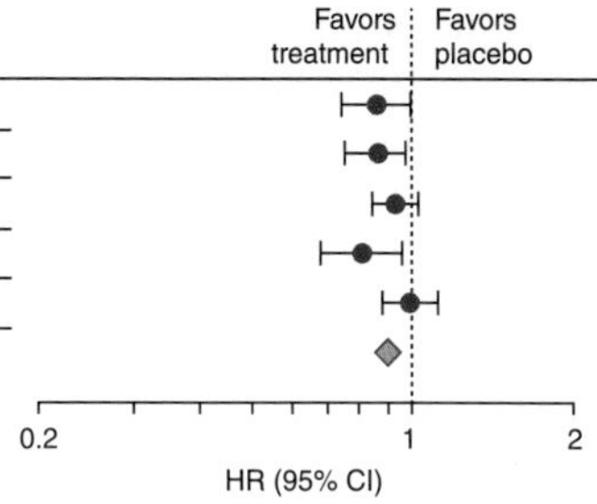

B Effects of Sodium-Glucose Cotransporter 2 Inhibitors on Cardiovascular Death

A Overall CV death

	Treatment		Placebo			
	No./total No.	Rate/1000 patient-years	No./total No.	Rate/1000 patient-years	Hazard ratio (95% CI)	Weight, %
EMPA-REG OUTCOME	172/4687	12.4	137/2333	20.2	0.62 (0.49–0.77)	15.61
CANVAS program	NA/5795	11.6	NA/4347	12.8	0.87 (0.72–1.06)	21.32
DECLARE-TIMI 58	245/8582	7.0	249/8578	7.1	0.98 (0.82–1.17)	25.24
CREDENCE	110/2202	19.0	140/2199	24.4	0.78 (0.61–1.00)	13.05
VERTIS CV	341/5499	17.6	184/2747	19.0	0.92 (0.77–1.10)	24.77
Fixed-effects model (Q = 11.22; df = 4; P = .02; I^2 = 64.3%)					0.85 (0.78–0.93)	

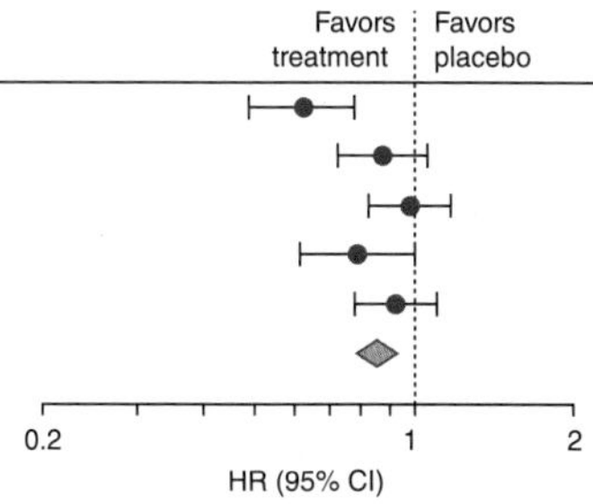

C Effects of Sodium-Glucose Cotransporter 2 Inhibitors on Hospitalisation for heart failure

A Overall HHF

	Treatment		Placebo			
	No./total No.	Rate/1000 patient-years	No./total No.	Rate/1000 patient-years	Hazard ratio (95% CI)	Weight, %
EMPA-REG OUTCOME	126/4687	9.4	95/2333	14.5	0.652 (0.50–0.85)	16.09
CANVAS program	NA/5795	5.5	NA/4347	8.7	0.67 (0.52–0.87)	17.10
DECLARE-TIMI 58	212/8582	6.2	286/8578	8.5	0.73 (0.61–0.88)	33.72
CREDENCE	89/2202	15.7	141/2199	25.3	0.61 (0.47–0.80)	16.01
VERTIS CV	139/5499	7.3	99/2747	10.5	0.70 (0.54–0.90)	17.08
Fixed-effects model (Q = 1.39; df = 4; P = .85; I^2 = 0.0%)					0.68 (0.61–0.76)	

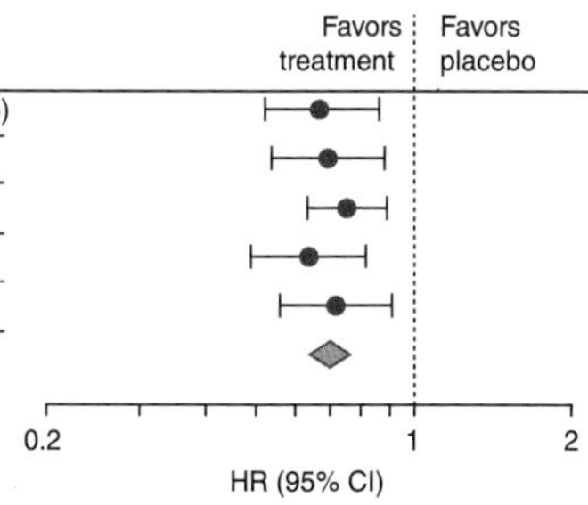

FIG. 12.1 Effects of SGLT2 inhibitors on MACE (A), CV mortality (B), and hospitalization for heart failure (C). *CI*, Confidence interval; *CV*, cardiovascular; *MACE*, major adverse cardiovascular events; *SGLT2*, sodium-glucose cotransporter-2. Cumulative data from five large CV outcomes trials involving SGLT2 inhibitors in high-risk people with type 2 diabetes (EMPA-REG OUTCOME [empagliflozin], CANVAS program [canagliflozin], DECLARE-TIMI 58 [dapagliflozin], CREDENCE [canagliflozin], and VERTIS CV [ertugliflozin]). The overall relative risk reductions were 10% for MACE, 15% for CV mortality, and a more robust 32% for HF. There was a significant variability across the trials for the first two outcomes but greater consistency for the HF outcome. From McGuire DK, et al. Association of SGLT2 inhibitors with cardiovascular and kidney outcomes in patients with type 2 diabetes: a meta-analysis, *JAMA Cardiol*. 2021;6(2):148–158.

peptides were assigned to dapagliflozin 10 mg or a placebo daily. The primary endpoint was a composite of time to first CV death or worsening HF event (hospitalizations or urgent visit due to HF).

Dapagliflozin significantly reduced the risk of the primary efficacy endpoint, which occurred in 16.3% of participants in the dapagliflozin group and 21.2% in the placebo group (HR, 0.74, 95% CI, 0.65–0.85; $P < 0.001$). Importantly, dapagliflozin significantly improved each of the components of the primary composite endpoint, including worsening HF events (HR, 0.70; 95% CI, 0.59–0.83) and CV death (HR, 0.82; 95% CI, 0.69–0.98). Dapagliflozin also reduced all-cause death (HR, 0.83; 95% CI, 0.71–0.97). The benefits of dapagliflozin were consistent across multiple subgroups, including among patients both with and without diabetes. Dapagliflozin also significantly improved HF-related symptoms as measured by the Kansas City Cardiomyopathy Questionnaire[14]–Total Symptom Score (KCCQ-TSS). Dapagliflozin was well tolerated, with fewer serious adverse events than placebo.

Subsequent secondary analyses demonstrated that the benefits of dapagliflozin emerged within 2 weeks of randomization,[15] were highly consistent regardless of baseline guideline-directed medical therapy for HFrEF,[16] and regardless of baseline HbA1c.[16] In addition, dapagliflozin also significantly reduced the risk of sudden death and serious ventricular arrhythmias.[17]

EMPEROR-REDUCED

In the EMPEROR-REDUCED, an international, multicenter, event-driven trial,[18] a total of 3730 participants with symptomatic HFrEF (left ventricular ejection fraction of 40% or less) and elevated natriuretic peptides were randomized to either empagliflozin 10 mg or a placebo daily. The primary endpoint was time to first event of CV death or hospitalization for HF.

The results were overall consistent with those of DAPA-HF. Empagliflozin significantly reduced the risk of the primary efficacy endpoint (19.4% participants in the empagliflozin group versus 24.7% in the placebo group; HR, 0.75; 95% CI, 0.65–0.86; $P < 0.001$); this was consistent across multiple subgroups, including patients with and without diabetes. Empagliflozin also reduced the total number of HF (HR, 0.70; 95% CI, 0.58–0.85; $P < 0.001$). The point estimates for CV death and all-cause death were favorable for empagliflozin versus placebo, but did not reach statistical significance. Empagliflozin also had a favorable effect on the kansas city cardiomyopathy questionnaire (KCCQ), and was well tolerated.

Subsequent meta-analysis of the DAPA-HF and EMPEROR-REDUCED trials confirmed large benefits of SGLT2 inhibitors on CV death or hospitalizations for HF, as well as CV death and all-cause mortality, independent of diabetes status.[19]

EMPEROR-PRESERVED

EMPEROR-PRESERVED was the first large, international multicenter, event-driven trial to test the effects of SGLT2 inhibitors in patients with HFmrEF and HFpEF, a group that now represents the majority of patients with HF but until recently had no disease-modifying treatments available.

In the EMPEROR-PRESERVED trial,[20] 5988 participants with symptomatic HFmrEF/HFpEF (ejection fraction higher than 40%) and elevated natriuretic peptides were randomized to empagliflozin 10 mg or placebo daily. The primary endpoint was the same as in EMPEROR-REDUCED, time to first CV death or hospitalization for HF.

Fewer empagliflozin- versus placebo-treated participants experienced the primary endpoint (13.8% vs 17.1%, HR, 0.79; 95% CI, 0.69–0.90; $P < 0.001$). This was driven predominantly by lower risk of HF hospitalizations (HR, 0.71; 95% CI, 0.60–0.83), with no significant reduction in CV death (HR, 0.91; 95% CI, 0.76–1.09), or all-cause death (HR; 1.00, 95% CI, 0.87–1.15). Similar to the SGLT2 inhibitor trials in patients with HFrEF, the effects were consistent in participants with and without diabetes. Subsequent analyses demonstrated that the effects of empagliflozin on the primary endpoint occurred early, with the first statistically significant benefit observed at 18 days postrandomization.[21] Empagliflozin was well tolerated, with fewer serious adverse events than with a placebo.

DELIVER

DELIVER was the largest trial of SGLT2 inhibitors in patients with HFmrEF/HFpEF. Overall, 6263 participants with symptomatic HFmrEF/HFpEF (left ventricular ejection fraction of greater than 40%) and elevated natriuretic peptides were randomized to dapagliflozin 10 mg or a placebo daily.[22] The primary endpoint was the same as in DAPA-HF: time to first event of CV death or worsening HF (hospitalization or urgent visit due to HF).

Fewer patients experienced the primary endpoint with dapagliflozin than placebo (16.4% vs 19.5%, HR, 0.82; 95% CI, 0.73–0.92; $P < 0.001$). This was driven predominantly by fewer events of worsening HF with dapagliflozin versus placebo (HR, 0.79; 95% CI, 0.69–0.91), with no significant reduction in CV death (HR, 0.88; 95% CI, 0.74–1.05). There was no significant reduction in all-cause death (HR, 0.94; 95% CI, 0.83–1.07). Dapagliflozin improved HF-related symptoms as measured by KCCQ-TSS,[23] and was well tolerated.

The benefits of dapagliflozin on the primary efficacy endpoint were consistent across multiple subgroups, including those with mildly reduced, preserved and completely normal ejection fraction, those with and without diabetes, participants randomized in the hospital versus ambulatory setting, and participants who had HF with improved ejection fraction (who were excluded from most other HFmrEF/HFpEF trials).

Subsequent meta-analysis of the EMPEROR-PRESERVED and DELIVER trials confirmed large benefits of SGLT2 inhibitors on reducing the risk of CV death and HF hospitalizations, driven primarily by the large reduction in HF hospitalizations (30% relative risk reduction), with a modest beneficial effect on CV death (12% relative risk reduction)[24] (Fig. 12.2).[24]

Pooled analyses both from the DAPA-HF/DELIVER and the EMPEROR Program demonstrated that the beneficial effects of dapagliflozin and empagliflozin are consistent across the entire range of left ventricular ejection fraction.[25]

SOLOIST-WHF

SOLOIST was the HF outcome trial of sotagliflozin, which offers both SGLT1 and SGLT2 inhibition.[26] Unlike other HF outcome trials, it focused on participants with type 2 diabetes, and those either hospitalized or within few days of discharge after an episode of worsening HF; it also included participants with HF regardless of left ventricular ejection fraction. The primary endpoint (following a protocol amendment) was the total number of CV deaths and hospitalizations and urgent visits for HF. A total of 1222 participants were randomized to sotagliflozin 200 mg (titrated to 400 mg) or a placebo daily

The trial ended early owing to loss of funding. This resulted in the protocol amendment, which included the change in the primary and secondary endpoints (as listed above); in addition, planned adjudication of endpoints was not completed and investigator-reported events were used instead for all efficacy analyses.

Sotagliflozin significantly reduced the risk of the primary endpoint as compared with a placebo (HR, 0.67; 95%

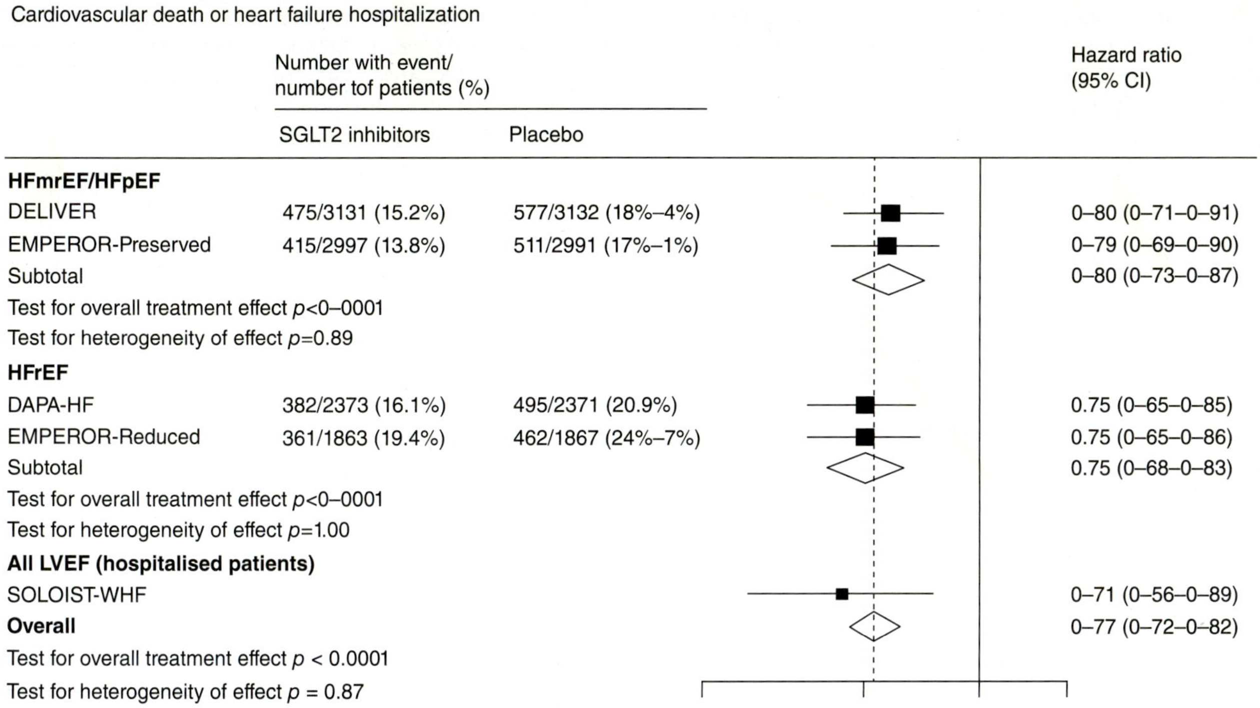

FIG. 12.2 Effects of SGLT2 inhibitors on CV mortality or hospitalization for heart failure from four dedicated HF trials using the SGLT2 inhibitors, dapagliflozin or empagliflozin. *CI*, Confidence interval; *CV*, cardiovascular; *SGLT2*, sodium-glucose cotransporter-2. Cumulative data from five large heart failure (*HF*) outcomes trials involving SGLT inhibitors in people with HF. The HF with reduced ejection fraction (HFrEF; ≤40%) trials were DAPA-HF (dapagliflozin) and EMPEROR-Reduced (empagliflozin). The HF with preserved ejection fraction (HFpEF; ≥50%) trials also included those with mildly reduced ejection fraction (HFmrEF; 41%–49%) and were EMPEROR-Preserved (empagliflozin) and DELIVER (dapagliflozin). One study, SOLOIST, enrolled hospitalized HF patients, not distinguishing by ejection fraction and tested the effects of a combined SGLT-1 and SGLT-2 inhibitor, sotagliflozin. The overall relative risk reduction in the primary outcomes from these trials (CV mortality or HF hospitalization) was 25% for the two HFrEF trials, 20% for the two HFpEF/HFmrEF trials, and 23% overall, with notable consistency across the five studies. From Vaduganathan M, Docherty KF, Claggett BL, et al. SGLT-2 inhibitors in patients with heart failure: a comprehensive meta-analysis of five randomised controlled trials. *Lancet*. 2022;400(10354):757–767. Erratum in *Lancet*. 2023;401(10371):104.

CI, 0.52–0.85; $P < 0.001$). This was driven predominantly by a large reduction in HF events, with no significant difference in CV death. The benefits of sotagliflozin were consistent across multiple subgroups, including across the range of left ventricular ejection fraction.

EMPULSE

In the EMPULSE multicenter, international trial,[27] 530 patients hospitalized with acute HF (regardless of ejection fraction, both with de novo or worsening of chronic HF) were randomized to empagliflozin 10 mg or placebo daily. The primary endpoint was "total clinical benefit," defined as a hierarchical composite of death from any cause, number of HF events and time to first HF event, or a 5-point or greater difference in change from baseline in the KCCQ-TSS at 90 days, assessed with a win ratio.

Empagliflozin resulted in more participants experiencing the clinical benefit versus placebo (win ratio 1.36; 95% CI, 1.09–1.68; $P = .0054$). This benefit was consistent across both acute de novo and decompensated chronic HF, and regardless of ejection fraction. Importantly, empagliflozin was well tolerated in this acute setting, with fewer serious adverse events than a placebo (32.3% vs. 43.6%, respectively).

TRIALS OF SGLT2 INHIBITORS FOCUSING ON HF-RELATED SYMPTOMS AND FUNCTION

Several dedicated multicenter, randomized controlled trials focused on the outcomes of HF-related symptoms and function. In the DEFINE-HF (HFrEF) and PRESERVED-HF (HFmrEF and HFpEF) trials which enrolled participants across multiple centers in the United States, dapagliflozin was demonstrated to significantly improve HF-related health status as measured by KCCQ. Dapagliflozin also significantly improved 6-minute walking distance in patients with HFmrEF/HFpEF, but not those with HFrEF.

The DETERMINE trial showed improved HF-related health status in participants with HFrEF, but not HFpEF with dapagliflozin versus placebo, whereas the EMPERIAL trials of empagliflozin did not demonstrate significant improvements in KCCQ in participants with either HFrEF or HFpEF. Neither trial program showed significant improvements with SGLT2 inhibitors versus a placebo in the 6-minute walking distance. The likely explanation between these results versus more favorable effects of dapagliflozin in the DEFINE-HF and PRESERVED-HF trials is the considerably greater burden of HF symptoms and physical limitations at baseline in these latter studies.[28–31]

Cardiovascular Effects of SGLT2 Inhibitors in Kidney Outcome Trials

Several kidney outcome trials of SGLT2 inhibitors (which are described below) demonstrated substantial CV benefits of these agents in participants with CKD. In the CREDENCE trial,[32] participants in the canagliflozin group experienced a lower risk of CV death or hospitalization for HF (HR, 0.69; 95% CI, 0.57–0.83; $P < 0.001$), CV death, myocardial infarction, or stroke (HR, 0.80; 95% CI, 0.67–0.95; P = .01), and hospitalization for HF (HR, 0.61; 95% CI, 0.47–0.80; P < 0.001), in addition to favorable effects on CV death (HR, 0.78; 95% CI, 0.61–1.00).

In the DAPA-CKD trial,[33] dapagliflozin significantly reduced the risk of CV death or hospitalization for HF (HR, 0.71; 95% CI, 0.55–0.92; P = .009), as well as total mortality (HR, 0.69; 95% CI, 0.53–0.88; P = .004).

In the EMPA-KIDNEY trial,[34] although the point estimates for the composite of CV deaths or hospitalizations for HF were favorable for empagliflozin versus placebo, these effects were not statistically significant (HR, 0.84; 95% CI, 0.67–1.07; P = .15).

Mechanistic Insights

The mechanisms behind the cardiovascular benefits of SGLT inhibitors remain a subject of debate. Multiple mechanistic trials have been completed, which collectively demonstrated the favorable effects of these agents on reducing filling pressures, improving diuretic efficiency, and having benefits on left ventricular remodeling.[35–37]

KIDNEY OUTCOMES

In early studies with SGLT2 inhibitors, an interesting 20% to 40% reduction in urinary albumin:creatinine ratio was observed.[1] This, in addition, to the drugs' glucose and blood pressure lowering effects, stimulated interest in these agents as possibly nephroprotective medication. As initially demonstrated in cardiovascular outcome trials, SGLT2 inhibitors were shown to reduce progression of CKD in patients with type 2 diabetes at high CV risk. Subsequently, because this effect appeared to have little to do with SGLT2 inhibitors' glycemic lowering properties, this benefit has been extended to patients with heart failure and, most recently, to patients with CKD, irrespective of diabetes status.

Kidney Outcomes in Cardiovascular Outcome Trials

EMPA-REG OUTCOME

The first trial to demonstrate a clear beneficial effect on adverse renal outcomes was EMPA-REG OUTCOME.[38] As noted previously, this trial randomized 7020 patients with type 2 diabetes and established CV disease and estimated glomerular filtration rate (eGFR) of at least 30 mL/min/1.73 m^2 to the SGLT2 inhibitor empagliflozin or a placebo. It was designed, per regulatory mandate, as a CV outcome trial, primarily to assess long-term CV safety of the medication. The primary outcome and related secondary CV outcomes have already been described. Incident or worsening nephropathy and incident albuminuria were the prespecified renal outcomes. The former was defined as a progression to persistent macroalbuminuria, the doubling of the serum creatinine concentration (with an estimated glomerular filtration rate [eGFR] <45 mL/min/1.73 kg/m^2) of body surface area; the initiation of renal replacement therapy (dialysis, transplantation); or death from renal disease.[39] Relevant baseline characteristics included a mean age of 63 years, 28% were females, and mean eGFR 72 mL/min/1.73 kg/m^2; 24% of participants had an eGFR <60 mL/min/1.73 kg/m^2; and 33% had urine albumin:creatinine ratio ≥30 mg/g. Over a mean follow-up of 3.1 years, the main renal outcome occurred in 12.7% of the empagliflozin group versus 18.8% in the placebo group (HR, 0.61; 95% CI, 0.53, 0.70; P < 0.001), yielding a 39% relative risk reduction. As for individual components of the renal composite outcome, risk of the progression to macroalbuminuria was reduced by 38% (11.2% vs. 16.2%), the risk of doubling of serum creatinine was decreased by 44% (1.5% vs. 2.6%; P < 0.001) and the risk of initiating renal replacement therapy was 55% lower (0.3% vs. 0.6%; P = .04), all in favor of empagliflozin. Although the number of events was relatively small, the investigators also reported significant reductions with empagliflozin on the "harder" kidney outcome of doubling of serum creatinine, initiation of renal replacement therapy, or renal death (i.e., removing macroalbuminuria from the composite; HR, 0.54; 95% CI, 0.40, 0.75; P < 0.001).

These results were consistent across a variety of prespecified subgroups including age, sex, race/ethnicity, baseline eGFR (<45, 45–<60, 60–<90, and ≥90 mL/min/1.73 kg/m^2), baseline albuminuria status (<30, ≥30 mg/g Cr), and prevalent use of renin-angiotensin system blockers like ACE inhibitors or ARBs. The investigators also reported an initial "dip" in eGFR in the active therapy group with subsequent stabilization versus a slow reduction over time in the placebo patients. By the end of the trial, eGFR was actually lower in the placebo than in the empagliflozin group.

There have been multiple follow-up studies focusing on the kidney from this key trial. For example, the cardiovascular benefits from empagliflozin (reductions in MACE, CV death, and HF hospitalization) were similar in those with or without baseline CKD.[40] Further exploration into the initial eGFR "dip" has also been conducted.[41,42] Risk factors for a larger initial dip included diuretic use and more advanced CKD (i.e., higher kidney disease: improving global outcomes (KDIGO) risk category) at baseline.[41] Both the beneficial CV and kidney effects and safety parameters with empagliflozin were consistent across subgroups based on these predictive factors, suggesting that the initial decrease in eGFR is not a clinical concern. In a post hoc analysis, the short-term reduction in urinary albumin-to-creatinine ratio was actually found to be significantly associated with a decreased risk of CV and renal outcomes, so it may portend ultimate benefit.[43] Finally, as has been shown with the SGLT2 inhibitor's CV benefits, the impact on kidney outcomes appeared to be independent of the drug's effects to lower HbA1c.[44]

CANVAS

The positive effects of SGLT2 inhibitors on the kidney were subsequently confirmed by the CANVAS program, which combined data from two trials: CANVAS and CANVAS-R.[45] The former enrolled patients with type 2 diabetes and either CV disease (about two-thirds) or at high CV risk (about one-third). In all 10,142 were enrolled and followed for a mean of 3.5 years. The primary CV outcome has been discussed earlier. A secondary renal outcome was the composite of a sustained 40% reduction in eGFR, renal replacement therapy, or death due to renal causes. The mean age of participants in the trial was 63.3 years, with a mean duration of diabetes of 13.5 years, and 36% were females. At baseline, the mean eGFR was 77 mL/min/1.73 kg/m^2 and 30% had at least microalbuminuria. The risk for the renal outcome was reduced by 40% with canagliflozin versus a placebo (5.54 vs. 9.01 events per 1000 patient-years; HR, 0.60; 95% CI, 0.47–0.77). Regression of albuminuria was more likely to occur in the canagliflozin group (HR, 1.70; 95% CI, 1.51–1.91). As with EMPA-REG OUTCOME, subgroup analyses in CANVAS also found no significant heterogeneity of the canagliflozin kidney benefit across multiple baseline features, including eGFR and albuminuric category.

DECLARE

In DECLARE, the SGLT2i dapagliflozin was studied in a somewhat lower-risk population of patients comprising a total of 17,160 individuals with type 2 diabetes, in which about 60% did not have any known underlying atherosclerotic cardiovascular disease.[46] Follow-up in DECLARE was 4.2 years, longer than in either of the other two trials. A prespecified renal outcome consisted of at least 40% in eGFR to <60 mL/min/1.73 kg/m^2, end-stage renal disease (defined as dialysis or kidney transplantation), or confirmed sustained eGFR <15 mL/min/1.73 kg/m^{2}or renal death. At baseline, the mean age was 64 years, duration of diabetes 10.5 years, with 37% females, and mean eGFR higher than in the prior two studies at 85 mL/min/1.73 kg/m. The renal outcome occurred in 3.7% in the dapagliflozin group and in 7.0% in the placebo group, yielding a 46% relative reduction (HR, 0.53; 95% CI, 0.43, 0.66; $P < 0.0001$).[47] The risk of end-stage renal disease or renal death was reduced by 59% in the dapagliflozin group (0.1% vs. 0·3% with a placebo; HR, 0.41; 95% CI, 0.20, 0.82; $P = .012$). As with both EMPA-REG OUTCOME and CANVAS, the kidney benefit was shared across multiple baseline risk groups.

The generally healthier population and higher mean eGFR in DECLARE allowed the investigators to determine if dapagliflozin could prevent new CKD from developing. Those in the lowest KDIGO risk group randomized to dapagliflozin indeed experienced a 46% reduction in their risk of developing the kidney-specific outcome (HR, 0.54; 95% CI, 0.38, 0.77) versus a placebo.[48] Moreover, those participants with baseline eGFR >60 mL/min/1.73 kg/m^2 randomized to the dapagliflozin group were at 44% reduced risk for a >57% decline in eGFR (HR, 0.52; 95% CI, 0.30, 0.91).

VERTIS CV

The VERTIS CV trial, testing the CV safety/efficacy of ertugliflozin proved neutral for major adverse CV events. The prespecified renal outcome (doubling of serum creatinine, renal dialysis or kidney transplantations, or renal death) was nonsignificantly reduced by active therapy (HR, 0.81; 95% CI, 0.63, 1.04).[49] In a reanalysis of the data, however, using the more standard 40% reduction in eGFR in lieu of doubling in creatinine, the data appeared more similar to other SGLT2 inhibitor trials, however (6.0 vs. 9.0 events per 1000 patient-years; HR, 0.66; 95% CI, 0.50, 0.88).[50]

SCORED[51]

As noted, sotagliflozin is a SGLT1/2 inhibitor, with a blockade of SGLT1, mainly expressed in the gut, dampening intestinal glucose absorption. In the SCORED trial, 10,584 patients with type 2 diabetes, eGFR 25 to 60 mL/min/1.73 kg/m^2, and at high CV risk were randomized to sotagliflozin or a placebo and followed for a median of 16 months. The results of the primary outcome (composite of total CV deaths and HF hospitalizations or urgent visits) are described above. The main renal outcome incorporated a sustained decrease of at least 50% in eGFR, or to <15 mL/min/1.73 kg/m^2, or renal dialysis, kidney transplantation. This is numerically reduced from 0.7 to 0.5 events per 100 patient-years, but the HR of 0.71 did not reach statistical significance (95% CI, 0.46, 1.08), likely owing to short duration of follow-up.

META-ANALYSES

Several meta-analyses of the kidney effects of SGLT2 inhibitors in CV outcome trials have been published.[52–54] In the most comprehensive to date, McGuire et al.[54] reported a pooled estimate HR of 0.621 (95% CI, 0.56, 0.70; I^2 49.7%) for progression of CKD (Fig. 12.3). There was also no

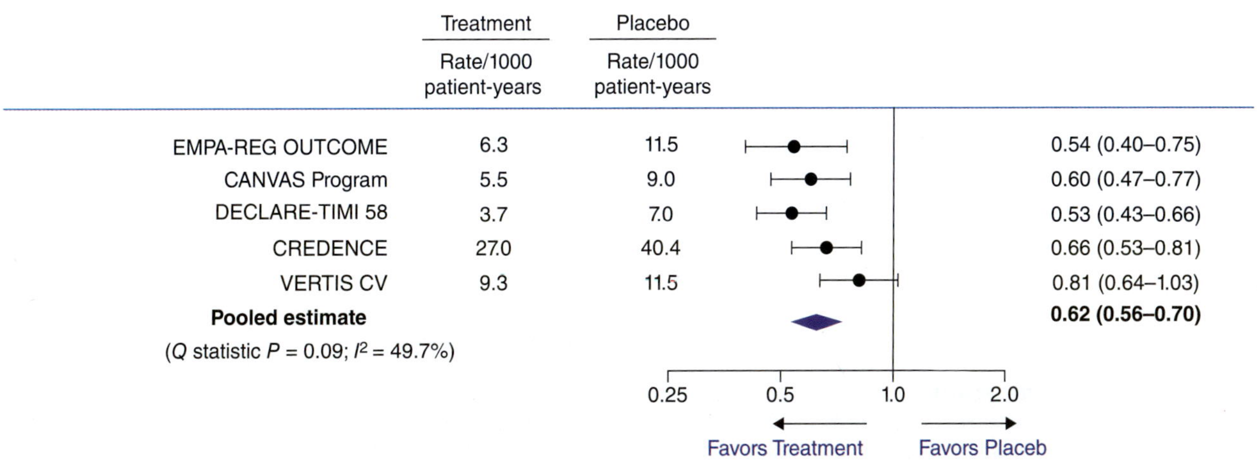

FIG. 12.3 SGLT2 inhibitor meta-analysis from diabetes cardiovascular outcome trials. *CV*, cardiovascular; *SGLT2*, sodium-glucose cotransporter-2. The pooled risk estimate of time to first renal composite outcome from these five SGLT2 inhibitor trials in individuals with type 2 diabetes was significantly reduced by 38% SGLT2 inhibitors versus a placebo. From McGuire DK, Shih WJ, Cosentino F, et al. Association of SGLT2 inhibitors with cardiovascular and kidney outcomes in patients with type 2 diabetes: a meta-analysis. *JAMA Cardiol*. 2021;6(2):148–158.

heterogeneity based on baseline presence (HR, 0.64) or absence (HF, 0.60) of atherosclerotic CV disease.

Kidney Outcome Trials

CREDENCE

CREDENCE was the first dedicated renal outcome trial involving an SGLT2 inhibitor, in this case, canagliflozin.[55] The trial randomized 4401 individuals with eGFR of 30 to <90 mL/min/1.73 m² and macroalbuminuria already on a renin-angiotensin blockade to canagliflozin or placebo. The primary outcome was a renal composite comprised of end-stage kidney disease, a doubling of serum creatinine, or renal or CV death. The trial was actually stopped prematurely due to overwhelming efficacy after a mean follow-up of 2.6 years. Relevant baseline characteristics included a mean age of 63 years, 34% were females, and the mean eGFR was 56 mL/min/1.73 kg/m², and a median urinary albumin-to-creatinine ratio of 927 mg/g. The relative risk of the primary renal composite outcome was decreased by 30% in the canagliflozin group (HR, 0.70; 95% CI, 0.59–0.82; $P = .00001$). The relative risk of a secondary outcome that excluded renal death was cut by 34% (HR, 0.66; 95% CI, 0.53–0.81; $P < 0.001$); for end-stage kidney disease alone, the relative risk reduction (RRR) was 32% (HR, 0.68; 95% CI, 0.54–0.86; $P = .002$). This trial garnered canagliflozin a specific indication in the US FDA to prevent the progression of diabetic kidney disease in those with type 2 diabetes and established renal impairment. Serious adverse events occurred at a similar frequency between the two therapies.

DAPA-CKD

DAPA-CKD was the first SGLT2 inhibitor renal outcome trial enrolling patients both with or without diabetes.[56] It randomized 4304 patients with an eGFR between 25 and 75 mL/min/1.73 m² and urinary albumin-to-creatinine ratio of at least 200 mg/g to dapagliflozin or a placebo. Here, the primary composite outcome was a decline of at least 50% in eGFR, end-stage kidney disease, or renal or CV death. This trial was also stopped early due to efficacy, after a median of 2.4 years. Important baseline characteristics include a mean age of 62 years, with 33% of participants being female. The mean eGFR was 43 mL/min/1.73 kg/m², with nearly 90% having GFR <60 mL/min/1.73 kg/m² and nearly 60% being below 45 mL/min/1.73 kg/m². The median urinary albumin-to-creatinine ratio was 949 mg/g. About two-thirds of the patients had a prior diagnosis of type 2 diabetes. The risk of the primary outcome was reduced by 39% in the dapagliflozin arm (HR, 0.61; 95% CI, 0.51–0.72; $P < 0.001$) (Fig. 12.4). For the renal-specific secondary outcome (primary less CV death), the risk reduction was 44% (HR, 0.56; 95% CI, 0.45–0.68; $P < 0.001$). A HF secondary outcome (HF hospitalization and CV death) was reduced by 29% (HR, 0.71; 95% CI, 0.55–0.92; $P = .009$) and all-cause mortality by 31% (HR, 0.69; 95% CI, 0.53–0.88; $P = .004$). Patients with or without type 2 diabetes responded similarly to dapagliflozin (type 2 diabetes: HR, 0.64; 95% CI, 0.52, 0.79); no diabetes: HR, 0.50; 95% CI, 0.35, 0.72). There was also no heterogeneity in the response across multiple other subgroups including age, sex, race, and ethnicity, nor by the degree of renal impairment or albuminuria. After DAPA-CKD, the canagliflozin prescribing label was expanded by the US FDA to include the prevention of the progression of established CKD, regardless of the presence of type 2 diabetes. The rates of serious adverse events were similar in the two treatment groups.

EMPA-KIDNEY

EMPA-KIDNEY was the primary renal outcome trial involving empagliflozin, and the largest to date involving an

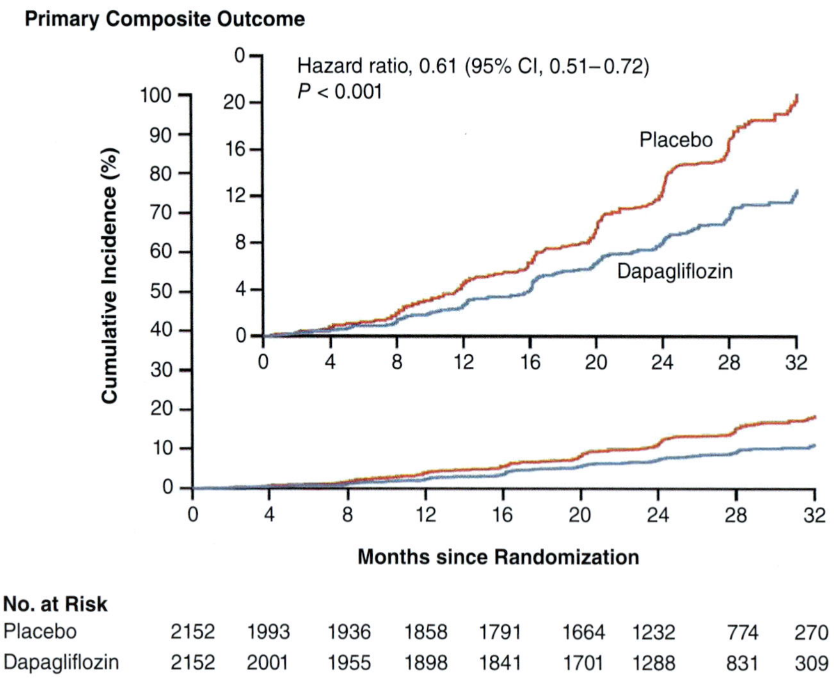

FIG. 12.4 Primary outcome result from the DAPA-CKD trial. *CI*, Confidence interval. The risk for the composite outcome of a sustained decline in the eGFR of at least 50%, end-stage kidney disease, or death from renal or cardiovascular causes was reduced by the SGLT2 inhibitor dapagliflozin. From Heerspink HJL, Stefánsson BV, Correa-Rotter R, et al.; DAPA-CKD Trial Committees and Investigators. Dapagliflozin in patients with chronic kidney disease. *N Engl J Med.* 2020;383(15):1436–1446.

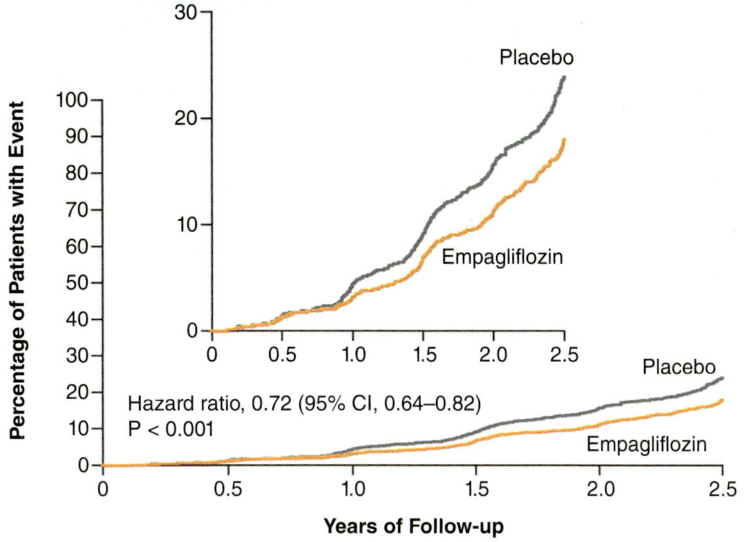

No. at Risk						
Placebo	3305	3250	3129	2243	1496	592
Empagliflozin	3304	3252	3163	2275	1538	624

FIG. 12.5 Primary outcome result from the EMPA-Kidney trial. *CI*, Confidence interval. The risk for the composite outcome of a sustained decline in the eGFR of at least 50%, end-stage kidney disease, or death from renal or cardiovascular causes was reduced by the SGLT2 inhibitor empagliflozin. From EMPA-KIDNEY Collaborative Group, Herrington WG, Staplin N, Wanner C, et al. Empagliflozin in patients with chronic kidney disease. *N Engl J Med*. 2023;388:117–127.

SGLT2 inhibitor.[57] The trial was similar to DAPA-CKD, the main exception being that the enrollment criteria allow for eGFR down to 20 in patients who were not albuminuric; 6609 patients were randomized to empagliflozin or a placebo and followed for a median of 2.0 years. The primary outcome was sustained reduction in eGFR of at least 40% or to less than 10 mL/min/1.73 kg/m^2, or renal or CV death. The primary outcome occurred in 13.1% of patients assigned to empagliflozin and 16.9% of those assigned to a placebo, for a 28% relative risk reduction (HR, 0.72; 95% CI, 0.64, 0.82, $P < 0.001$) (Fig. 12.5). Cardiovascular and all-cause mortality were not reduced by empagliflozin, however. As with DAPA-CKD, the results were similar in those with or without diabetes and across multiple other subgroups, including those describing the degree of renal dysfunction and albuminuria. Serious adverse event rates were similar between the two treatment arms.

Kidney Outcomes in Heart Failure Trials

The HF benefits of SGLT2 inhibitors in dedicated HF trials have been described previously. Given the frequent coexistence of CKD in HF, their relationship is of extreme clinical importance. As a result, renal events and kidney function were also assessed as exploratory outcomes in these trials.

In DAPA-HF, involving 4744 patients with reduced (<40%) ejection fraction HF, 41% of participants had eGFR <60 mL/min/1.73 kg/m^2 and the effects of dapagliflozin on the primary outcome were similar in those with eGFR above or below this threshold.[58] The composite renal outcome of a sustained decline eGFR of at least 50%, end-stage renal disease, or renal death was numerically reduced by dapagliflozin (HR, 0.71; 95% CI, 0.44, 1.16) but the results did not achieve statistical significance. The annual rates of eGFR decline after the first 2 weeks of the trial were less in those randomized to dapagliflozin than to a placebo (−1.09 vs. −2.85 mL/min/1.73 kg/m^2 [$P < 0.001$]), with no heterogeneity by diabetes status.

In DELIVER, involving 6263 patients with HF and left ventricular ejection fraction ≥40%, 49% of patients had eGFR <60 mL/min/1.73 kg/m^2.[59] Here, too, the benefits of dapagliflozin on HF outcomes were not modified by a baseline kidney function. Incidence rates for the renal composite outcome (identical to that in DAPA-HF) were not affected by treatment assignment (HR, 1.08; 95% CI, 0.79–1.49). However, the annual decline in eGFR from baseline was attenuated with dapagliflozin (difference vs. placebo, 0.5 mL/min/1.73 kg/m^2 [95% CI, 0.1–0.9]; $P = .01$), with a larger difference when calculated beyond month 1, after the eGFR dip: difference versus placebo: 1.4 mL/min/1.73 kg/m^2 (95% CI, 1.0–1.8).

In the EMPEROR trials, the HF benefits of empagliflozin in both reduced and preserved HF were experienced similarly across the eGFR spectrum.[60,61] Also, in EMPEROR-Reduced ($N = 3730$), less major adverse renal events (dialysis or transplantation or profound, sustained decrease in eGFR occurred in the empagliflozin group (1.6% vs. 3.1%; HR, 0.50; 95% CI, 0.32, 0.77).[56] Interestingly, the same pattern was not seen in the EMPEROR-Preserved trial ($N = 5958$). The annual decline in eGFR decline versus a placebo also appeared to be reduced to a greater extent in EMPEROR-Reduced than in EMPEROR-Preserved (adjusted mean difference, 1.77 [95% CI, 0.80, 2.74] vs. 0.94 [95% CI, 0.60, 1.27]).[62]

Mechanisms

The precise mechanisms underlying the SGLT2 inhibitors' renoprotective effect are not well understood. There are experimental data to suggest that these agents, by blocking proximal tubular sodium reabsorption, increase the amount of sodium reaching the macula densa. This, in turn, normalizes tubule-glomerular feedback and decreases glomerular flow by increasing afferent arteriolar tone.[63] In this fashion progressive glomerular barotrauma is attenuated. This theory is similar to the effects of a renin-angiotensin system blockade, although in that circumstance, glomerular hypertension is decreased by an increase in vascular tone of the efferent arteriole. Importantly, the presence of a baseline angiotensin converting enzyme (ACE) inhibition or angiotensin II receptor blockade (ARB) does not at all abrogate the benefits of SGLT2 inhibition, so these mediation categories are felt to be complementary. Other data, however, do not support this theory.[64] Additional proposed mechanisms include reductions in tubular hypoxia, inflammation, and/or oxidative stress and alternative fuel utilization.[35–69] Ongoing mechanistic studies will hopefully elucidate the underlying mediators of the renal benefits of this drug category.

Guidelines

The international KDIGO guidelines[70] endorse SGLT2 inhibitors be used as part of the treatment program for any individual with type 2 diabetes and CKD, down to an eGFR of 25 mL/min/1.73 kg/m^2. Based on specific renal outcome trials involving the CKD population, this recommendation now also applies to patients with renal dysfunction who do not have diabetes.[71] International diabetes guidelines[68] also recommend choosing an SGLT2 inhibitor as part of the antihyperglycemic therapy regimen in anyone with type 2 diabetes and CKD, so long as there is sufficient glomerular filtration, typically defined as above 30 mL/min/1.73 kg/m^2.[72]

SAFETY

The main side effects from SGLT2 inhibitors are genitourinary in nature, in keeping with their mechanism of action.[1,3,66] Patients described increased urination, particularly early in the treatment course. Increased rates of genital yeast infections, especially in females, are reported. Urinary tract infections, while a conceivable risk, appear not to be a significant concern, however. Cases of Fournier's gangrene have also been reported; these are rare events and it remains unknown if the SGLT2 inhibitor was actually the cause. A small decrease in eGFR is seen in most patients but should be of little concern, given that it is reversible and the drugs, if anything, reduce the chronic decline in renal function. Euglycemic diabetic ketoacidosis can occur, particularly in patients with type 1 diabetes, in whom these agents are not approved in most countries and should generally not be used.[68] In dedicated HF and CKD trials, the SGLT2 inhibitors have been shown to have a serious adverse event profile indistinguishable from a placebo and are surprisingly well tolerated in these generally sicker groups of patients. DKA can occur in type 2 diabetes but it is a rare event. Patients who are acutely ill or undergoing surgical procedures, in whom calorie intake may be curtailed, should temporarily hold this medication until their status is back to the baseline and are consuming their usual diet.

SUMMARY

The SGLT2 inhibitors are newer glucose-lowering medications widely used in type 2 diabetes. They were found to have surprising benefits in both CV and kidney outcomes in initial CVOTs involving patients with type 2 diabetes at high CV risk. Their main benefits are improvements in HF and renal outcomes, effects which have now been clearly demonstrated in patient populations beyond diabetes, including those with HF (with either reduced and preserved ejection fractions) and CKD.

REFERENCES

1. Fonseca-Correa JI, Correa-Rotter R. Sodium-glucose cotransporter 2 inhibitors mechanisms of action: a review. *Front Med (Lausanne)*. 2021;8:777861. https://doi.org/10.3389/fmed.2021.777861.
2. Vasilakou D, Karagiannis T, Athanasiadou E, et al. Sodium-glucose cotransporter 2 inhibitors for type 2 diabetes: a systematic review and meta-analysis. *Ann Intern Med*. 2013;159(4):262–274.
3. Scheen AJ. Beneficial effects of SGLT2 inhibitors on fatty liver in type 2 diabetes: a common comorbidity associated with severe complications. *Diabetes Metab*. 2019;45(3):213–223.
4. Zinman B, Wanner C, Lachin JM, et al. EMPA-REG OUTCOME Investigators Empagliflozin, cardiovascular outcomes, and mortality in type 2 diabetes. *N Engl J Med*. 2015;373(22):2117–2128. https://doi.org/10.1056/NEJMoa1504720. Epub 2015 Sep 17. PMID: 26378978.
5. Draft Guidance for Industry on Diabetes Mellitus: Developing Drugs and Therapeutic Biologics for Treatment and Prevention (A Notice by the Food and Drug Administration on 03/03/2008). https://www.federalregister.gov/documents/2008/03/03/E8-3974/draft-guidance-for-industry-on-diabetes-mellitus-developing-drugs-and-therapeutic-biologics-for.
6. Verma S, Leiter LA, Zinman B, et al. Time to cardiovascular benefits of empagliflozin: a post hoc observation from the EMPA-REG OUTCOME trial. *ESC Heart Fail*. 2021;8(4):2603–2607. https://doi.org/10.1002/ehf2.13374. Epub 2021 Jun 16. PMID: 34132492; PMCID: PMC8318423.
7. Neal B, Perkovic V, Mahaffey KW, et al. CANVAS Program Collaborative Group Canagliflozin and cardiovascular and renal events in type 2 diabetes. *N Engl J Med*. 2017;377(7):644–657. https://doi.org/10.1056/NEJMoa1611925. Epub 2017 Jun 12. PMID: 28605608.
8. Wiviott SD, Raz I, Bonaca MP, et al. DECLARE–TIMI 58 Investigators Dapagliflozin and cardiovascular outcomes in type 2 diabetes. *N Engl J Med*. 2019;380(4):347–357. https://doi.org/10.1056/NEJMoa1812389. Epub 2018 Nov 10. PMID: 30415602.
9. Cannon CP, Pratley R, Dagogo-Jack S, et al. VERTIS CV Investigators Cardiovascular outcomes with ertugliflozin in type 2 diabetes. *N Engl J Med*. 2020;383(15):1425–1435. https://doi.org/10.1056/NEJMoa2004967. Epub 2020 Sep 23. PMID: 32966714.
10. Bhatt DL, Szarek M, Pitt B, et al. SCORED Investigators. Sotagliflozin in patients with diabetes and chronic kidney disease. *N Engl J Med*. 2021;384(2):129–139. https://doi.org/10.1056/NEJMoa2030186. Epub 2020 Nov 16. PMID: 33200891.
11. Zelniker TA, Wiviott SD, Raz I, et al. SGLT2 inhibitors for primary and secondary prevention of cardiovascular and renal outcomes in type 2 diabetes: a systematic review and meta-analysis of cardiovascular outcome trials. *Lancet*. 2019;393(10166):31–39. https://doi.org/10.1016/S0140-6736(18)32590-X. Epub 2018 Nov 10. Erratum in: Lancet. 2019 Jan 5;393(10166):30. doi: 10.1016/S0140-6736(18)33206-9. PMID: 30424892.
12. McGuire DK, Shih WJ, Cosentino F, et al. Association of SGLT2 inhibitors with cardiovascular and kidney outcomes in patients with type 2 diabetes: a meta-analysis. *JAMA Cardiol*. 2021;6(2):148–158. https://doi.org/10.1001/jamacardio.2020.4511. PMID: 33031522; PMCID: PMC7542529.
13. McMurray JJV, Solomon SD, Inzucchi SE, et al. DAPA-HF Trial Committees and Investigators. Dapagliflozin in patients with heart failure and reduced ejection fraction. *N Engl J Med*. 2019;381(21):1995–2008. https://doi.org/10.1056/NEJMoa1911303. Epub 2019 Sep 19. PMID: 31535829.
14. Kosiborod MN, Jhund PS, Docherty KF, et al. Effects of dapagliflozin on symptoms, function, and quality of life in patients with heart failure and reduced ejection fraction: results from the DAPA-HF trial. *Circulation*. 2020;141(2):90–99. https://doi.org/10.1161/CIRCULATIONAHA.119.044138. Epub 2019 Nov 17. PMID: 31736335; PMCID: PMC6964869.
15. Berg DD, Jhund PS, Docherty KF, et al. Time to clinical benefit of dapagliflozin and significance of prior heart failure hospitalization in patients with heart failure with reduced ejection fraction. *JAMA Cardiol*. 2021;6(5):499–507. https://doi.org/10.1001/jamacardio.2020.7585. PMID: 33595593; PMCID: PMC7890451.
16. Docherty KF, Jhund PS, Inzucchi SE, et al. Effects of dapagliflozin in DAPA-HF according to background heart failure therapy. *Eur Heart J*. 2020;41(25):2379–2392. https://doi.org/10.1093/eurheartj/ehaa183. PMID: 32221582; PMCID: PMC7327533.
17. Curtain JP, Docherty KF, Jhund PS, et al. Effect of dapagliflozin on ventricular arrhythmias, resuscitated cardiac arrest, or sudden death in DAPA-HF. *Eur*

Heart J. 2021;42(36):3727–3738. https://doi.org/10.1093/eurheartj/ehab560. PMID: 34448003; PMCID: PMC8455345.

18. Packer M, Anker SD, Butler J, et al. EMPEROR-Reduced Trial Investigators. Cardiovascular and renal outcomes with empagliflozin in heart failure. *N Engl J Med.* 2020;383(15):1413–1424. https://doi.org/10.1056/NEJMoa2022190. Epub 2020 Aug 28. PMID: 32865377.
19. Zannad F, Ferreira JP, Pocock SJ, et al. SGLT2 inhibitors in patients with heart failure with reduced ejection fraction: a meta-analysis of the EMPEROR-Reduced and DAPA-HF trials. *Lancet.* 2020;396(10254):819–829. https://doi.org/10.1016/S0140-6736(20)31824-9. Epub 2020 Aug 30. PMID: 32877652.
20. Anker SD, Butler J, Filippatos G, et al. EMPEROR-Preserved Trial Investigators. Empagliflozin in heart failure with a preserved ejection fraction. *N Engl J Med.* 2021;385(16):1451–1461. https://doi.org/10.1056/NEJMoa2107038. Epub 2021 Aug 27. PMID: 34449189.
21. Butler J, Siddiqi TJ, Filippatos G, Ferreira JP, Pocock SJ, Zannad F, Anker SD. Early benefit with empagliflozin in heart failure with preserved ejection fraction: insights from the EMPEROR-Preserved trial. *Eur J Heart Fail.* 2022;24(2):245–248. https://doi.org/10.1002/ejhf.2420. Epub 2022 Jan 18. PMID: 34989083.
22. Solomon SD, McMurray JJV, Claggett B, et al. DELIVER Trial Committees and Investigators. Dapagliflozin in heart failure with mildly reduced or preserved ejection fraction. *N Engl J Med.* 2022;387(12):1089–1098. https://doi.org/10.1056/NEJMoa2206286. Epub 2022 Aug 27. PMID: 36027570.
23. Kosiborod MN, Bhatt AS, Claggett BL, et al. Effect of Dapagliflozin on health status in patients with preserved or mildly reduced ejection fraction. *J Am Coll Cardiol.* 2023;81(5):460–473. https://doi.org/10.1016/j.jacc.2022.11.006. Epub 2022 Dec 14. PMID: 36526515.
24. Vaduganathan M, Docherty KF, Claggett BL, et al. SGLT-2 inhibitors in patients with heart failure: a comprehensive meta-analysis of five randomised controlled trials. *Lancet.* 2022;400(10354):757–767. https://doi.org/10.1016/S0140-6736(22)01429-5. Epub 2022 Aug 27. Erratum in: Lancet. 2023 Jan 14;401(10371):104. doi: 10.1016/S0140-6736(23)00018-1. PMID: 36041474.
25. Jhund PS, Kondo T, Butt JH, et al. Dapagliflozin across the range of ejection fraction in patients with heart failure: a patient-level, pooled meta-analysis of DAPA-HF and DELIVER. *Nat Med.* 2022;28(9):1956–1964. https://doi.org/10.1038/s41591-022-01971-4. Epub 2022 Aug 27. PMID: 36030328; PMCID: PMC9499855.
26. Bhatt DL, Szarek M, Steg PG, et al. SOLOIST-WHF Trial Investigators Sotagliflozin in patients with diabetes and recent worsening heart failure. *N Engl J Med.* 2021;384(2):117–128. https://doi.org/10.1056/NEJMoa2030183. Epub 2020 Nov 16. PMID: 33200892.
27. Voors AA, Angermann CE, Teerlink JR, et al. The SGLT2 inhibitor empagliflozin in patients hospitalized for acute heart failure: a multinational randomized trial. *Nat Med.* 2022;28(3):568–574. https://doi.org/10.1038/s41591-021-01659-1. Epub 2022 Feb 28. PMID: 35228754; PMCID: PMC8938265.
28. Abraham WT, Lindenfeld J, Ponikowski P, et al. Effect of empagliflozin on exercise ability and symptoms in heart failure patients with reduced and preserved ejection fraction, with and without type 2 diabetes. *Eur Heart J.* 2021;42(6):700–710. https://doi.org/10.1093/eurheartj/ehaa943. PMID: 33351892.
29. McMurray JJV, Docherty KF, de Boer RA, et al. Effect of dapagliflozin versus placebo on symptoms and 6-minute walk distance in patients with heart failure: the DETERMINE randomized clinical trials. *Circulation.* 2024;149(11):825–838. https://doi.org/10.1161/CIRCULATIONAHA.123.065061. Epub 2023 Dec 7. PMID: 38059368.
30. Nassif ME, Windsor SL, Tang F, et al. Dapagliflozin effects on biomarkers, symptoms, and functional status in patients with heart failure with reduced ejection fraction: the DEFINE-HF trial. *Circulation.* 2019;140(18):1463–1476. https://doi.org/10.1161/CIRCULATIONAHA.119.042929. Epub 2019 Sep 16. PMID: 31524498.
31. Nassif ME, Windsor SL, Borlaug BA, et al. The SGLT2 inhibitor dapagliflozin in heart failure with preserved ejection fraction: a multicenter randomized trial. *Nat Med.* 2021;27(11):1954–1960. https://doi.org/10.1038/s41591-021-01536-x. Epub 2021 Oct 28. PMID: 34711976; PMCID: PMC8604725.
32. Perkovic V, Jardine MJ, Neal B, et al. CREDENCE Trial Investigators. Canagliflozin and renal outcomes in type 2 diabetes and nephropathy. *N Engl J Med.* 2019;380(24):2295–2306. https://doi.org/10.1056/NEJMoa1811744. Epub 2019 Apr 14. PMID: 30990260.
33. Heerspink HJL, Stefánsson BV, Correa-Rotter R, et al. DAPA-CKD Trial Committees and Investigators Dapagliflozin in Patients with Chronic Kidney Disease. *N Engl J Med.* 2020;383(15):1436–1446. https://doi.org/10.1056/NEJMoa2024816. Epub 2020 Sep 24. PMID: 32970396.
34. Herrington WG, Staplin N, Wanner C, et al. The EMPA-KIDNEY Collaborative Group Empagliflozin in patients with chronic kidney disease. *N Engl J Med.* 2023;388(2):117–127. https://doi.org/10.1056/NEJMoa2204233. Epub 2022 Nov 4. PMID: 36331190; PMCID: PMC7614055.
35. Nassif ME, Qintar M, Windsor SL, et al. Empagliflozin effects on pulmonary artery pressure in patients with heart failure: results from the EMBRACE-HF trial. *Circulation.* 2021;143(17):1673–1686. https://doi.org/10.1161/CIRCULATIONAHA.120.052503. Epub 2021 Feb 8. PMID: 33550815.
36. Griffin M, Rao VS, Ivey-Miranda J, et al. Empagliflozin in heart failure: diuretic and cardiorenal effects. *Circulation.* 2020;142(11):1028–1039. https://doi.org/10.1161/CIRCULATIONAHA.120.045691. Epub 2020 May 15. PMID: 32410463; PMCID: PMC7521417.
37. Verma S, Mazer CD, Yan AT, et al. Effect of empagliflozin on left ventricular mass in patients with type 2 diabetes mellitus and coronary artery disease: the EMPA-HEART CardioLink-6 randomized clinical trial. *Circulation.* 2019;140(21):1693–1702. https://doi.org/10.1161/CIRCULATIONAHA.119.042375. Epub 2019 Aug 22. PMID: 31434508.
38. Zinman B, Wanner C, Lachin JM, et al. EMPA-REG OUTCOME Investigators. Empagliflozin, cardiovascular outcomes, and mortality in type 2 diabetes. *N Engl J Med.* 2015;373(22):2117–2128.
39. Wanner C, Inzucchi SE, Lachin JM, et al. EMPA-REG OUTCOME Investigators. Empagliflozin and progression of kidney disease in type 2 diabetes. *N Engl J Med.* 2016;375(4):323–334.
40. Wanner C, Lachin JM, Inzucchi SE, et al. EMPA-REG OUTCOME Investigators. Empagliflozin and clinical outcomes in patients with type 2 diabetes mellitus, established cardiovascular disease, and chronic kidney disease. *Circulation.* 2018;137(2):119–129.
41. Kraus BJ, Weir MR, Bakris GL, et al. Characterization and implications of the initial estimated glomerular filtration rate 'dip' upon sodium-glucose cotransporter-2 inhibition with empagliflozin in the EMPA-REG OUTCOME trial. *Kidney Int.* 2021;99(3):750–762.
42. Wanner C, Heerspink HJL, Zinman B, et al. EMPA-REG OUTCOME Investigators. Empagliflozin and kidney function decline in patients with type 2 diabetes: a slope analysis from the EMPA-REG OUTCOME trial. *J Am Soc Nephrol.* 2018;29(11):2755–2769.
43. Waijer SW, Xie D, Inzucchi SE, et al. Short-term changes in albuminuria and risk of cardiovascular and renal outcomes in type 2 diabetes mellitus: a post hoc analysis of the EMPA-REG OUTCOME trial. *J Am Heart Assoc.* 2020;9(18):e016976.
44. Cooper ME, Inzucchi SE, Zinman B, et al. Glucose control and the effect of empagliflozin on kidney outcomes in type 2 diabetes: an analysis from the EMPA-REG OUTCOME trial. *Am J Kidney Dis.* 2019;74(5):713–715.
45. Neal B, Perkovic V, Mahaffey KW, et al. CANVAS Program Collaborative Group Canagliflozin and cardiovascular and renal events in type 2 diabetes. *N Engl J Med.* 2017;377(7):644–657.
46. Wiviott SD, Raz I, Bonaca MP, et al. DECLARE–TIMI 58 Investigators Dapagliflozin and cardiovascular outcomes in type 2 diabetes. *N Engl J Med.* 2019;380(4):347–357.
47. Mosenzon O, Wiviott SD, Cahn A, et al. Effects of dapagliflozin on development and progression of kidney disease in patients with type 2 diabetes: an analysis from the DECLARE-TIMI 58 randomised trial. *Lancet Diabetes Endocrinol.* 2019;7(8):606–617.
48. Mosenzon O, Raz I, Wiviott SD, et al. Dapagliflozin and prevention of kidney disease among patients with type 2 diabetes: post hoc analyses from the DECLARE-TIME 58 trial. *Diabetes Care.* 2022;45(10):2350–2359.
49. Cannon CP, Pratley R, Dagogo-Jack S, et al. VERTIS CV Investigators Cardiovascular outcomes with ertugliflozin in type 2 diabetes. *N Engl J Med.* 2020;383(15):1425–1435.
50. Cherney DZI, Charbonnel B, Cosentino F, et al. VERTIS CV Investigators Effects of ertugliflozin on kidney composite outcomes, renal function and albuminuria in patients with type 2 diabetes mellitus: an analysis from the randomised VERTIS CV trial. *Diabetologia.* 2021;64(6):1256–1267.
51. Bhatt DL, Szarek M, Pitt B, et al. SCORED Investigators Sotagliflozin in patients with diabetes and chronic kidney disease. *N Engl J Med.* 2021;384(2):129–139.
52. Cherney DZI, Dagogo-Jack S, McGuire DK, et al. VERTIS CV Investigators Kidney outcomes using a sustained ≥40% decline in eGFR: a meta-analysis of SGLT2 inhibitor trials. *Clin Cardiol.* 2021;44(8):1139–1143.
53. Giugliano D, Longo M, Caruso P, Maiorino MI, Bellastella G, Esposito K. Sodium-glucose co-transporter-2 inhibitors for the prevention of cardiorenal outcomes in type 2 diabetes: an updated meta-analysis. *Diabetes Obes Metab.* 2021;23(7):1672–1676.
54. McGuire DK, Shih WJ, Cosentino F, et al. Association of SGLT2 inhibitors with cardiovascular and kidney outcomes in patients with type 2 diabetes: a meta-analysis. *JAMA Cardiol.* 2021;6(2):148–158.
55. Perkovic V, Jardine MJ, Neal B, et al. CREDENCE Trial Investigators Canagliflozin and renal outcomes in type 2 diabetes and nephropathy. *N Engl J Med.* 2019;380(24):2295–2306.
56. Heerspink HJL, Stefánsson BV, Correa-Rotter R, et al. DAPA-CKD Trial Committees and Investigators Dapagliflozin in patients with chronic kidney disease. *N Engl J Med.* 2020;383(15):1436–1446.
57. EMPA-KIDNEY Collaborative Group, et al. Herrington WG, Staplin N, Wanner C, et al. Empagliflozin in patients with chronic kidney disease. *N Engl J Med.* 2022 https://doi.org/10.1056/NEJMoa2204233.
58. McMurray JJV, Solomon SD, Inzucchi SE, et al. DAPA-HF Trial Committees and Investigators Dapagliflozin in patients with heart failure and reduced ejection fraction. *N Engl J Med.* 2019;381(21):1995–2008.
59. Solomon SD, McMurray JJV, Claggett B, et al. DELIVER Trial Committees and Investigators Dapagliflozin in heart failure with mildly reduced or Preserved Ejection Fraction. *N Engl J Med.* 2022;387(12):1089–1098.
60. Packer M, Anker SD, Butler J, et al. EMPEROR-Reduced Trial Investigators Cardiovascular and renal outcomes with empagliflozin in feart failure. *N Engl J Med.* 2020;383(15):1413–1424.
61. Anker SD, Butler J, Filippatos G, et al. EMPEROR-Preserved Trial Investigators Empagliflozin in heart failure with preserved ejection fraction. *N Engl J Med.* 2022;385(16):1451–1461.
62. Packer M, Butler J, Zannad F, et al. EMPEROR Study Group Empagliflozin and major renal outcomes in heart failure. *N Engl J Med.* 2021;385(16):1531–1533.
63. Cherney DZ, Perkins BA, Soleymanlou N, et al. Renal hemodynamic effect of sodium-glucose cotransporter 2 inhibition in patients with type 1 diabetes mellitus. *Circulation.* 2014;129(5):587–597.

64. van Bommel EJM, Muskiet MHA, van Baar MJB, et al. The renal hemodynamic effects of the SGLT2 inhibitor dapagliflozin are caused by post-glomerular vasodilatation rather than pre-glomerular vasoconstriction in metformin-treated patients with type 2 diabetes in the randomized, double-blind RED trial. *Kidney Int.* 2020;97(1):202–212.
65. Heerspink HJ, Perkins BA, Fitchett DH, Husain M, Cherney DZ. Sodium glucose cotransporter 2 inhibitors in the treatment of diabetes mellitus: cardiovascular and kidney effects, potential mechanisms, and clinical applications. *Circulation.* 2016;134(10):752–772.
66. Christopher S. Wilcox Antihypertensive and renal mechanisms of SGLT2 (sodium-glucose linked transporter 2) inhibitors. *Hypertension.* 2020;75: 894–901.
67. Tuttle KR, Brosius 3rd FC, Cavender MA, et al. SGLT2 Inhibition for CKD and cardiovascular disease in type 2 diabetes: report of a scientific workshop sponsored by the National Kidney Foundation. *Am J Kidney Dis.* 2021;77(1):94–109.
68. Sen T, Hiddo J.L.Heerspink HJL. A kidney perspective on the mechanism of action of sodium glucose co-transporter 2 inhibitors. *Cell Metabolism.* 2021;33(4):732–739.
69. Lupsa BC, Inzucchi SE. Ketones: the double-edge sword of SGLT2 inhibitors? *Diabetologia.* 2022 (in press).
70. *KDIGO 2022 Clinical Practice Guideline for Diabetes Management in Chronic Kidney Disease.* https://kdigo.org/guidelines/diabetes-ckd/.
71. *KDIGO 2022 Clinical Practice Guideline for CKD Evaluation and Management.* https://www.guidelinecentral.com/guideline/25092/.
72. American Diabetes Association Professional Practice Committee/ Pharmacologic Approaches to Glycemic Treatment Standards of Medical Care in Diabetes—2022. *Diabetes Care.* 2022;45(Suppl 1):S125–S143.

13 Cardiovascular and Kidney Effects of Glucagon-Like Peptide 1 Receptor Agonists

NAVEED AMJID SATTAR

KEY POINTS

- GLP-1RAs lower MACE by around 14% to 15% overall with broadly consistent benefits across its constituents' outcomes, including CV death.
- Three drugs in the class—liraglutide, semaglutide, and dulaglutide—are available for use and approved by regulatory agents for protection against CV outcomes.
- Most preparations are injectable and given once weekly, but once daily oral semaglutide is also available.
- GLP-1RAs lower glucose, weight, and blood pressure and improve lipids but do not increase hypoglycemia rates.
- On the basis of available evidence, relevant guidelines recommend the use of either GLP-1RA or SGLT2i in people with diabetes and existing cardiovascular disease.
- GLP-1RAs may be prioritized in those with much higher BMIs or post stroke or where atherosclerotic disease dominates.
- GLP-1RAs are also recommended in people with diabetes but without existing cardiovascular disease based either on high measured cardiovascular risk or imaging evidence of atherosclerotic disease.
- Present limited trial data suggest GLP-1RAs improve MACE and other outcomes beyond SGLT2i, a finding that fits with distinct mechanisms of action of these two classes of drugs.
- GLP-1RAs also robustly reduce important kidney outcomes with an impact for kidney guidelines, marking them as additional treatment pillars for preventing CKD.
- Semaglutide at higher doses and tirzepatide have clear symptomatic benefits in patients with heart failure and preserved ejection fraction, with preliminary evidence for harder outcome benefits in such patients.
- Finally, higher-dose semaglutide lowered MACE in people with high BMI and established cardiovascular disease but no diabetes, widening indications to beyond diabetes. Other drugs that also lower weight more, such as the GLP-1RA-GIP agonist, tirzepatide, and several others, are being tested in outcome trials that will report in next 1 to 5 years.

BACKGROUND

Glucagon-like peptide (GLP)-1 is a small peptide hormone released from gastrointestinal L-cells after food intake. It binds to the GLP-1 receptor (GLP-1R), leading to an incretin effect that enhances glucose-dependent insulin secretion from pancreatic beta cells and promotes inhibition of glucagon release from pancreatic alpha cells. It also leads to a slowing of gastric emptying. The result of such actions is a reduction in fasting blood glucose and improved postprandial glucose metabolism. By stimulating GLP-1R in the brain, GLP-1 also induces satiety and, this action together with slowing gastric emptying, leads to weight loss.

GLP-1R agonists (GLP-1RAs) have been developed as novel antidiabetic agents that replicate the actions of incretin hormone GLP-1. Initially, exenatide (exendin-4) was developed. It is a GLP-1 mimetic found in the saliva of the gila monster with 53% sequence homology with human GLP-1. This peptide has been shown to be a full agonist of the GLP-1R. Subsequently, other GLP-1RAs were developed based on human GLP-1, such as liraglutide, semaglutide, and dulaglutide. The vast majority are delivered by subcutaneous injection, but recent technology has allowed the development of an orally available GLP-1 RA with the coformulation of semaglutide and the absorption enhancer Sodium *N*-(8-[2-hydroxybenzoyl] Amino) Caprylate (SNAC). Other oral nonpeptide GLP-1 RAs are in development and could come to the market within 1–2 years.

All GLP-1RAs improve glucose levels, variably lower body weight, lower blood pressure, and improve lipids.[1]

They do, however, increase the heart rate by one to three beats per minute. Up to 2021, several cardiovascular outcome trials had been reported in people with diabetes with different GLP-1RAs.[2–9] The first to report was the LEADER trial[4] and the last, AMPLITUDE-O.[2] The characteristics of all eight trials are given in Table 13.1, adapted from a 2022 meta-analysis of all eight trials.[10] Since then, the FLOW[11] and SELECT[12] trials have reported out expanding data. A more recent meta-analysis (2024)[13] including such data has recently reported with a focus on kidney outcomes and included patients with and without diabetes. The key findings from all the available evidence from both a cardiovascular and kidney perspective are summarized below.

CARDIOVASCULAR OUTCOME TRIALS OF GLP-1RA IN TYPE 2 DIABETES AND RELEVANT META-ANALYSES

Baseline Characteristics of Populations Studied in Outcome the First Eight Outcome Trials

Of all the eight trials included in the 2022 meta-analysis, ELIXA was unusual as it enrolled patients with a recent acute coronary syndrome; all other trials included patients with stable cardiovascular disease, cardiovascular risk factors, or both. All trials, except ELIXA, had 3-point MACE as the primary endpoint; in ELIXA the primary endpoint was an expanded 4-point composite, including hospitalization for unstable angina. The mean age at baseline ranged from 60 years in ELIXA to 66 years in PIONEER 6 and REWIND. The proportion of patients with established cardiovascular disease at baseline ranged from 100% in ELIXA and Harmony Outcomes to 31% of those in REWIND (Table 13.1). Kidney function was similar across trials (median/mean estimated glomerular filtration rate ranged from 72–80 mL/min per 1.73 m^2), whereas mean HbA1c was lowest in REWIND and ELIXA (7.2% and 7.7%, respectively) and highest in AMPLITUDE-O at 8.9%. REWIND had the lowest proportional use of insulin at baseline (24% compared with 39%–63% in remaining trials). The median length of follow-up ranged from 1.3 years in PIONEER 6 to 5.4 years in REWIND.

MACE Outcomes and Specific Drugs Approved for CV Prevention

In the pooled analysis, treatment with a GLP-1 receptor agonist led to a 14% relative risk reduction in 3-point MACE (Fig. 13.1) with moderate heterogeneity. The following trials showed superiority for MACE: LEADER (liraglutide), SUSTAIN-6 (semaglutide), HARMONY Outcomes (albiglutide), REWIND (dulaglutide), and AMPLITUDE-0 (efpeglenatide). Of these, albiglutide and efpeglenatide are not available for use in practice but the other three agents are now licensed for CV protection, widely available and increasingly used for this purpose.

EXPANDING EVIDENCE BASE: NEW TRIALS IN CHRONIC KIDNEY DISEASE AND IN PATIENTS WITH ASCVD BUT WITHOUT TYPE 2 DIABETES

Two important trials have been reported in the last 2 years, widening the evidence base for GLP-1RAs. Below is a brief description of these trials followed by a new meta-analysis incorporating these new data.

FLOW Trial

The FLOW trial tested the efficacy of 1 mg semaglutide versus placebo in 3533 people living with T2 diabetes and chronic kidney disease (CKD).[11] The primary outcome was major kidney disease events, a composite of the onset of kidney failure (dialysis, transplantation, or an eGFR of <15 mL/min/1.73 m^2), at least a 50% reduction in the eGFR from baseline, or death from kidney-related or CV causes. It was stopped early at 3.4 years mean follow-up for overwhelming efficacy with a 24% reduction in the primary endpoint in the placebo group (Fig. 13.2). The results were similar for a composite of the kidney-specific components of the primary outcome. Further, death from CV causes (by 29%), MACE (by 18%), and all-cause mortality (by 20%) were all significantly reduced with semaglutide relative to a placebo. Serious adverse events were reported in a lower percentage of participants in the semaglutide group than in the placebo group (49.6% vs. 53.8%).[11]

SELECT Trial

The SELECT trial tested the impact of 2.4 mg semaglutide versus a placebo on MACE outcomes in 17,604 patients 45 years of age or older who had preexisting CV disease and a body mass index (the weight in kilograms divided by the square of the height in meters) of 27 or greater but no history of diabetes.[12] The mean duration of follow-up was nearly 40 months and the mean weight loss of 8.51% with semaglutide relative to a placebo. The primary MACE outcome was reduced by 20% in those allocated to semaglutide relative to a placebo with nominal reductions in incident HF outcomes and all-cause mortality (Fig. 13.3). Around 1 in 6 patients discontinued semaglutide versus 1 in 12 for a placebo during the trial, and notably serious adverse events were less in the semaglutide group at 33.4% versus 36.4% with a placebo.[12] SELECT was the first outcome trial of GLP-1RA outside of type 2 diabetes and it was also the first randomized trial of an agent approved for weight loss to show cardiovascular benefit. Consequently, it is a seminal trial with results set to influence all future relevant guidelines in the cardiometabolic space.

NEW META-ANALYSIS OF GLP-1RA OUTCOMES TRIALS INCORPORATING FLOW AND SELECT FROM A CV PERSPECTIVE

A 2024 meta-analysis included 11 GLP-1RA trials (including SELECT and FLOW) and so was able to add important new

TABLE 13.1 Baseline Characteristics and Use of Glucose-Lowering Agents Across Trials

	ELIXA (N = 6068)	LEADER (*N* = 9340)	SUSTAIN-6 (*N* = 3297)	EXSCEL (*N* = 14,752)	HARMONY OUTCOMES (*N* = 9463)	REWIND (*N* = 9903)	PIONEER 6 (*N* = 3183)	AMPLITUDE-O (*N* = 4076)
Drug	Lixisenatide	Liraglutide	Semaglutide	Exenatide	Albiglutide	Dulaglutide	Semaglutide	Efpeglenatide
Year reported								
Structural basis	Exendin-4	Human GLP-1	Human GLP-1	Exendin-4	Human GLP-1	Human GLP-1	Human GLP-1	Exendin-4
Administration route	Subcutaneous	Subcutaneous	Subcutaneous	Subcutaneous	Subcutaneous	Subcutaneous	Oral	Subcutaneous
Dose	20 µg/day	1.8 mg/day	0.5 or 1 mg/week	2 mg/week	30 or 50 mg/week	1.5 mg/week	14 mg/day	4 or 6 mg/day
Age, mean, years	60 ± 10	64 ± 7	65 ± 7	62 ± 9	64 ± 7	66 ± 7	66 ± 7	65 ± 8
Female gender, no. (%)	1861 (31%)	3337 (36%)	1295 (39%)	5603 (38%)	2894 (31%)	4589 (46%)	1007 (32%)	1344 (33%)
BMI (kg/m^2)	30.1 ± 5.6	32.5 ± 6.3	32.8 ± 6.2	32.7 ± 6.4	32.3 ± 5.9	32.3 ± 5.7	32.3 ± 6.5	32.7 ± 6.2
Caucasian	4576 (75%)	7238 (78%)	2736 (83%)	11,175 (76%)	6583 (70%)	7498 (76%)	2300 (72%)	3534 (87%)
Diabetes duration, years	9.2 ± 8.2	12.8 ± 8.0	13.9 ± 8.1	13.1 ± 8.3	14.2 ± 8.8	10.6 ± 7.2	14.9 ± 8.5	15.4 ± 8.8
HbA_{1c} (%)	7.7 ± 1.3	8.7 ± 1.6	8.7 ± 1.5	8.1 ± 1.0	8.7 ± 1.5	7.3 ± 1.1	8.2 ± 1.6	8.9 ± 1.5
Established CVD	6068 (100%)	7598 (81%)	2735 (83%)	11,175 (76%)	6678 (71%)	3114 (31%)	2692 (85%)	3650 (90%)
History of heart failure	1358 (22%)	1667 (18%)	777 (24%)	2389 (16%)	1922 (20%)	852 (9%)	388 (12%)	737 (18%)
Systolic blood pressure (mmHg)	129 ± 17	136 ± 18	136 ± 17	135 ± 17	135 ± 17	137 ± 17	136 ± 18	135 ± 16
eGFR (mL/min per 1.73 m^2)*	78 ± 21	80 (NR)	80 (61–92)	77 (61–92)	79 ± 25	75 ± 24	74 ± 21	72 ± 22
Glucose-Lowering Drugs Used (%)								
Insulin	2374 (39%)	4159 (45%)	1913 (58%)	6838 (46%)	5597 (59%)	2398 (24%)	1943 (61%)	2560 (63%)
Biguanide	4021 (66%)	7136 (76%)	2414 (73%)	11,295 (77%)	7970 (84%)	8016 (81%)	2437 (77%)	2985 (73%)
Sulfonylurea	2004 (33%)	4721 (51%)	1410 (43%)	5401 (37%)	2725 (29%)	5644 (57%)	1007 (32%)	1036 (25%)
Thiazolidinedione	95 (2%)	573 (6%)	76 (2%)	579 (4%)	194 (2%)	168 (2%)	NR	NR
DPP-4 inhibitor	NR	6 (<1%)	5 (<1%)	2203 (15%)	1437 (15%)	88 (1%)	0	0
SGLT2 inhibitor	NR	NR	5 (<1%)	77 (1%)	575 (6%)	12 (0%)	301 (10%)	618 (15%)

Risk of MACE in 2021 meta–analysis with eight CVOTs

Total	GLP–1 receptor agonist *n/N* (%)	Placebo n/ (%)	Hazard ratio (95% CI)	NNT (95% CI)	*P* value
Three–component MACE					
ELIXA	400/3034 (13%)	392/3034 (13%)	1.02 (0.89, 1.17)		0.776
LEADER	608/4668 (13%)	694/4672 (15%)	0.87 (0.78, 0.97)		0.01
SUSTAIN–6	108/1648 (7%)	146/1649 (9%)	0.74 (0.58, 0.95)		0.016
EXSCEL	839/7356 (11%)	905/7396 (12%)	0.91 (0.83, 1.00)		0.061
Harmony Outcomes	338/4731 (7%)	428/4732 (9%)	0.78 (0.68, 0.90)		0.0006
REWIND	594/4949 (12%)	663/4952 (13%)	0.88 (0.79, 0.99)		0.026
PIONEER 6	61/1591 (4%)	76/1592 (5%)	0.79 (0.57, 1.11)		0.17
AMPLITUDE–O	189/2717 (7%)	125/1359 (9%)	0.73 (0.58, 0.92)		0.0069
Subtotal (*I*–squared = 44.5%, *p* = 0.082)			0.86 (0.80, 0.93)	65 (45–130)	<0.001

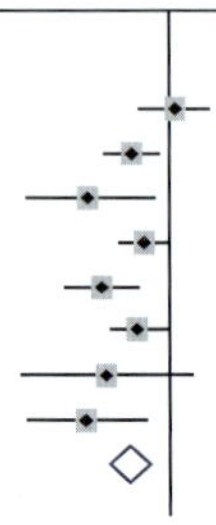

FIG. 13.1 Risk of MACE. Three-component MACE consisted of cardiovascular death, myocardial infarction, and stroke. NNTs are calculated over a weighted average median follow-up of 3.0 years. *P* values for superiority. *CVOTs*, Cardiovascular outcome trials; *CI*, confidence interval; *GLP-1*, glucagon-like peptide-1; *MACE*, major adverse cardiovascular events; *NNT*, number needed to treat. Taken from Sattar N, Lee MMY, Kristensen SL, et al. Cardiovascular, mortality, and kidney outcomes with GLP-1 receptor agonists in patients with type 2 diabetes: a systematic review and meta-analysis of randomised trials. *Lancet Diabetes Endocrinol.* 2021;9(10):653–662. https://doi:10.1016/S2213-8587(21)00203-5.

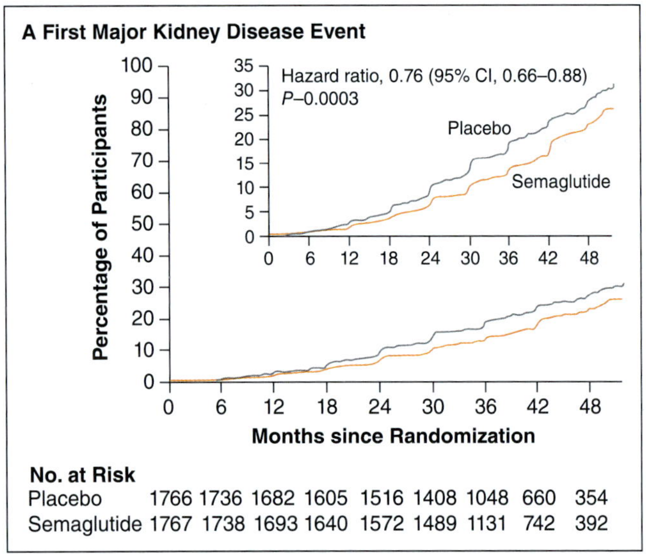

FIG. 13.2 Primary outcome plot from FLOW. Cumulative incidence plot of the primary outcome, major kidney disease events (a composite of the onset of kidney failure [dialysis, transplantation, or an estimated glomerular filtration rate (eGFR) of < 15 mL per minute per 1.73 m^2 of body-surface area], ≥50% reduction in eGFR from baseline, or death from kidney-related or cardiovascular causes). *CI*, Confidence interval. Taken from Perkovic V, Tuttle KR, Rossing P, et al.; FLOW Trial Committees and Investigators. Effects of semaglutide on chronic kidney disease in patients with type 2 diabetes. *N Engl J Med.* 2024;391(2):109–121. https://doi:10.1056/NEJMoa2403347. Epub 2024 May 24. PMID: 38785209.

data to determine impact of this class of drugs on CKD outcomes and in patients without type 2 diabetes.

Broadly, as with the prior 2022 meta-analysis, MACE with GLP-1RAs was reduced by 14% (moderate heterogeneity) relative to a placebo, with all-cause death reduced by 13% (no heterogeneity) (Fig. 13.4). Reductions in MI and stroke were also broadly similar at 13% and 12%, respectively. More importantly, the results suggest broadly consistent benefits of GLP-1RAs on differing atherosclerotic outcomes in patients with or without type 2 diabetes with no evidence of heterogeneity by diabetes status.[13]

SPECIFIC POINTS OF RELEVANCE TO PRACTICE FROM META-ANALYSES

Heterogeneity by Key Baseline Characteristics

In this 2024 meta-analysis,[13] the key demographics were examined for evidence of heterogeneity for the primary MACE outcome. Notably, there were no significant interactions by major criteria examined, including gender, age (<65 vs. ≥65), BMI (<30 vs. ≥0), evidence of prior CVD (yes vs. no), or eGFR (<60 vs. ≥60). For prior CVD, the HR for efficacy was 0.84 for those with CVD and 0.96 for those without CVD but with a *P* = 0.13 for interaction. Of note, the REWIND trial, which included a large (68.5%) proportion of people without prior CVD, showed near identical benefits of dulaglutide in people with and without (but at high risk of) prior CVD.[8]

Key Safety Outcomes of Interest

This 2024 meta-analysis[13] also captured adverse events of interest. Fig. 13.5 shows these results and while there were clearly more people stopping GLP-1RA for adverse events, no imbalance was noted for total serious adverse events, nor for incident cancers, including pancreatic cancer, and nor for acute pancreatitis. There was also no excess risk for retinopathy, whereas the numbers of medullary thyroid cancers were very small in active and placebo groups. These results are therefore reassuring.

Benefits on Top of SGLT2i

Three outcome trials (Amplitude-O, Harmony Outcomes, and FLOW) included enough patients to allow researchers to test whether the benefits of GLP-1RAs were consistent, whether patients were already taking SGLT2 inhibitors.[15] In these three trials, GLP-1 receptor agonists reduced the risk of MACE events by 21% (hazard ratio [HR], 0.79 [95% CI,

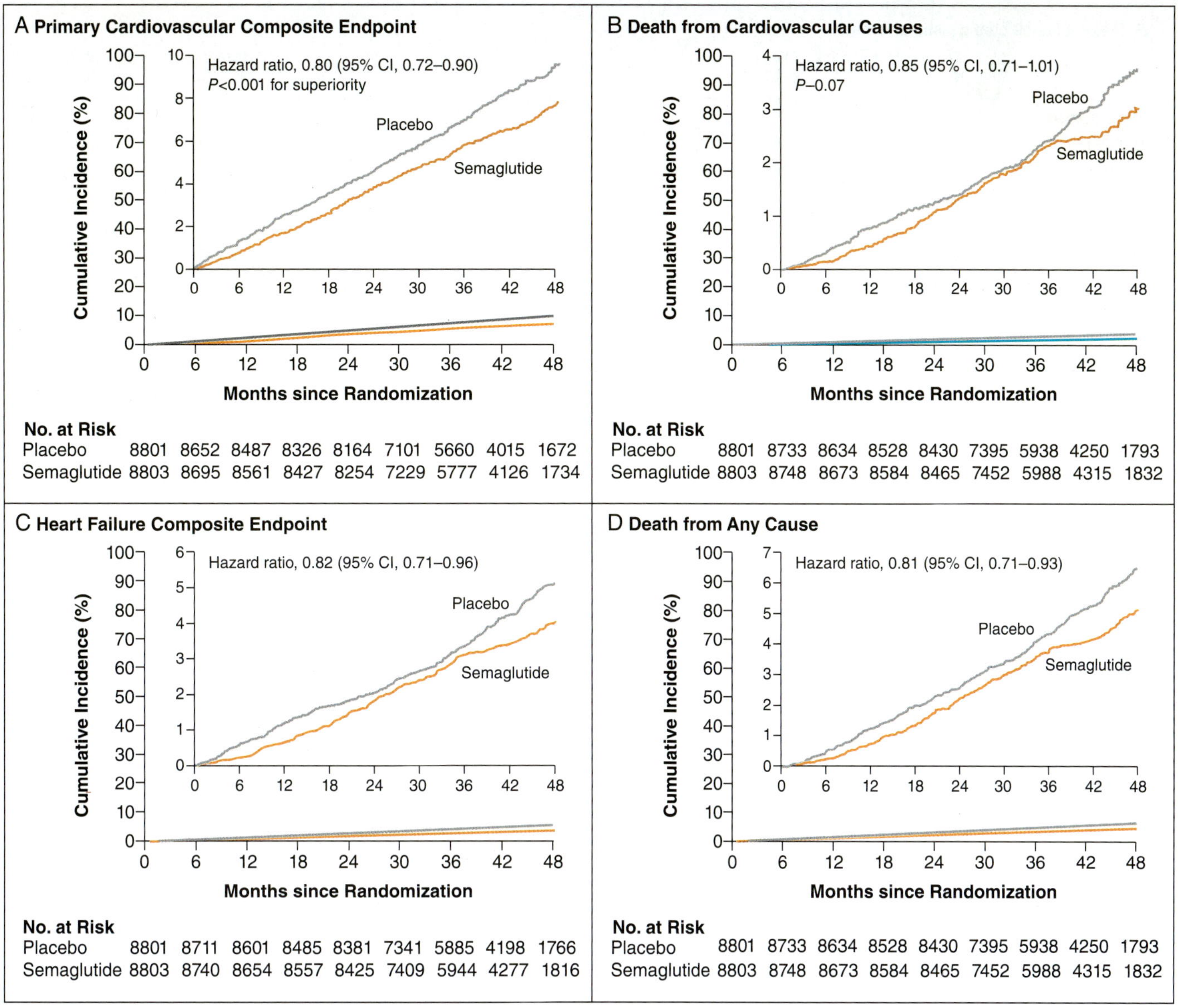

FIG. 13.3 Time-to-first-event analysis for primary and confirmatory secondary efficacy end points from the SELECT trial. Panel **(A)** shows the cumulative incidence of the primary cardiovascular composite endpoint (death from cardiovascular causes, nonfatal myocardial infarction, or nonfatal stroke). Panel **(B)** shows the cumulative incidence of the first confirmatory secondary endpoint (death from cardiovascular causes). Panel **(C)** shows the cumulative incidence of the second confirmatory secondary end point (heart failure composite endpoint: death from cardiovascular causes or hospitalization or an urgent medical visit for heart failure). Panel **(D)** shows the cumulative incidence of the third confirmatory secondary endpoint (death from any cause). The definitions of all endpoints are provided in the Supplementary Appendix. Cumulative incidence was estimated with the use of the Aalen-Johansen method with accounting for competing risk,[14] and hazard ratios were estimated with the Cox proportional hazards regression model. Because the between-group difference in death from cardiovascular causes did not meet the required *P* value for hierarchical testing, results for the two subsequent endpoints in the testing hierarchy are reported as point estimates and 95% confidence intervals. The widths of these confidence intervals have not been adjusted for multiplicity and therefore should not be used to infer definitive treatment effects for these secondary endpoints. The insets show the same data on an enlarged *y* axis. The *x* axis is truncated at 48 months because of the limited number of patients in the trial after 48 months. *CI*, Confidence interval. From Lincoff AM, Brown-Frandsen K, Colhoun HM, Deanfield J, Emerson SS, Esbjerg S, Hardt-Lindberg S, Hovingh GK, Kahn SE, Kushner RF, Lingvay I, Oral TK, Michelsen MM, Plutzky J, Tornøe CW, Ryan DH; SELECT Trial Investigators. Semaglutide and Cardiovascular Outcomes in Obesity without Diabetes. *N Engl J Med*. 2023 Dec 14;389(24): 2221–2232. https://doi.org/10.1056/NEJMoa2307563. Epub 2023 Nov 11. PMID: 37952131.

0.71–0.87]), with consistent effects in those receiving and not receiving SGLT2 inhibitors at baseline (HR, 0.77 [95% CI, 0.54–1.09] and HR, 0.79 [95% CI, 0.71–0.87], respectively; *P*-heterogeneity = 0.78). These results are reassuring and suggest additive benefits of these two classes of drugs in combination at least for MACE benefits and potentially other additive benefits for other outcomes.

SOUL Trial

More recently, oral Semaglutide has been shown in the SOUL trial to lower cardiovascular events by 14% (95% CI: 45%–23%) in people with diabetes and prior cardiovascular events.[16] A subsequent meta-analysis confirmed that the athersoclerotic cardiovascular benefits were similar for injectable versus oral GLP-1RAs.[17]

BENEFITS OF INCRETIN-BASED WEIGHT LOSS DRUGS IN PEOPLE LIVING WITH HFpEF

Recognition of the importance of obesity to the development and progression of heart failure with preserved ejection fraction has led to three randomized trials of weight loss

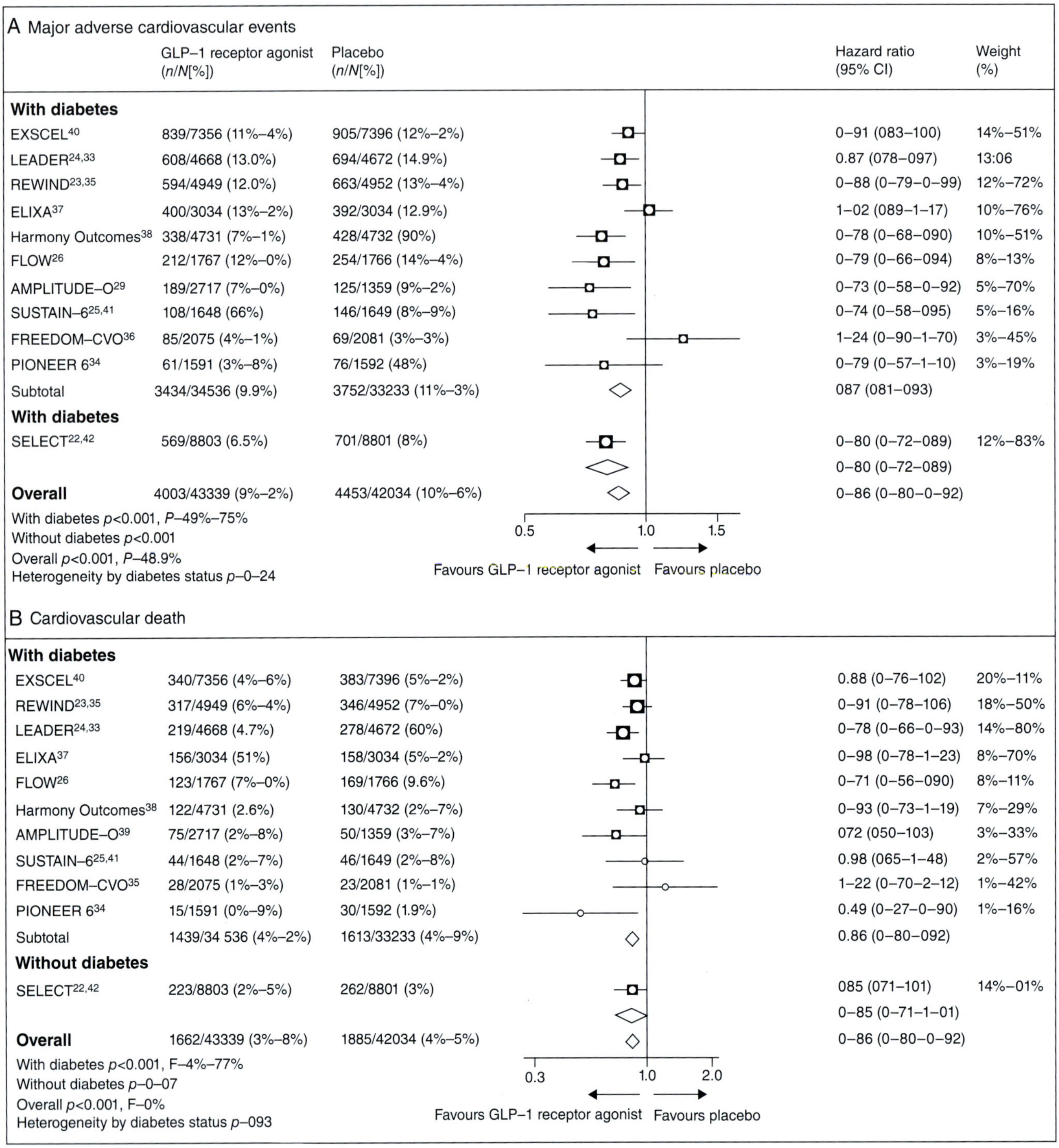

FIG. 13.4 **Individual and pooled estimates for cardiovascular outcomes from 2024 meta-analysis of GLP-1RA cardiovascular or kidney outcome trials in diabetes and nondiabetes.** Trials are sorted by weight. **(A)** Major adverse cardiovascular events outcomes. (**B**) Cardiovascular death. Taken from Badve SV, Bilal A, Lee MMY, et al. Effects of GLP-1 receptor agonists on kidney and cardiovascular disease outcomes: a meta-analysis of randomised controlled trials. *Lancet Diabetes Endocrinol*. 2025;13(1):15–28. https://doi:10.1016/S2213-8587(24)00271-7. Epub 2024 Nov 25. PMID: 39608381.

agents. Two of these trials were conducted with higher-dose semaglutide in patients with high BMI but with and without diabetes,[18,19] whereas the third trial was conducted with tirzepatide.[20] Briefly, the results show these drugs help such patients lose considerable weight, with parallel, substantial improvements in KCCQ, well in excess of KCCQ improvements seen with SGLT2i. The findings also showed improvement in 6-minute walk tests, in CRP levels, variably in NT proBNP levels, and in cardiac remodeling.[18,19,21]

Overall, while the extent to which these findings are related to the weight loss from these drugs versus their direct effects on cardiac tissue continues to be debated, these new results as well as preliminary evidence for their benefits on harder outcomes, will rapidly influence relevant guidelines. A recent viewpoint, however, concluded that drug-induced weight loss was likely the primary reason for symptomatic benefits in HFpEF.[22] Clearly, improving patient symptoms and quality of life is vitally important in the context of HF.

	Trials (*n*)	GLP–1 receptor agonist (*n*)	Placebo (*n*/*N* [%])	Hazard ratio (95% CI)	*P*(%)
Total serious adverse events	9	11286/35644 (31%–7%)	11731/35680 (32%–9%)	0–95 (0–90–1–01)	88%–5%
Discontinuation due to adverse event	9	4494/35329 (12.7%)	3127/33996 (9%–2%)	1–51 (1–18–1–94)	96%–3%
Cancers	10	1884/41235 (4%–6%)	1838/39910 (46%)	1–01 (0–95–1–07)	0%
Pancreatic cancer	9	63/32739 (0%–2%)	56/31413 (0%–2%)	1–04 (0–63–1–71)	30%–5%
Medullary thyroid cancer	8	4/30665 (<0%–1%)	2/29343 (<0%–01%)	1–63 (0–38–7–03)	0%
Acute pancreatitis	11	138/43309 (0%–3%)	104/41980 (0%–3%)	1–02 (0–78–1–33)	10.8%
Severe hypoglycaemia	11	943/43309 (2%–5%)	949/41980 (2%–3%)	0–95 (080–1–12)	57%–4%
Retinopathy	10	1107/34506 (3%–2%)	1059/33196 (3%–2%)	1–04 (0–92–1–18)	39.9%

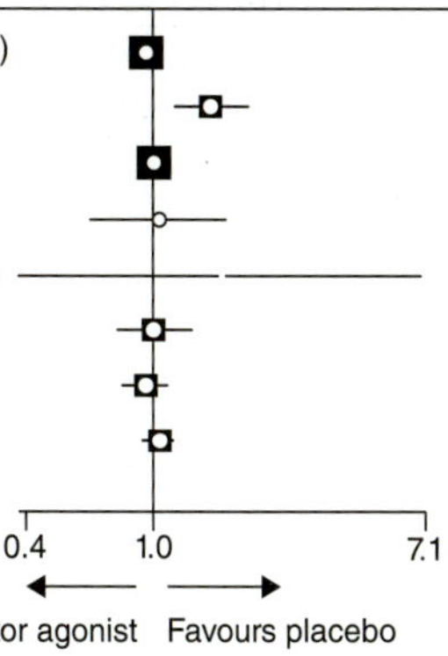

FIG. 13.5 Pooled estimates for adverse events from 2024 meta-analysis. (Taken from Badve SV, Bilal A, Lee MMY, et al. Effects of GLP-1 receptor agonists on kidney and cardiovascular disease outcomes: a meta-analysis of randomised controlled trials. *Lancet Diabetes Endocrinol.* 2025;13(1):15–28.) https://doi:10.1016/S2213-8587(24)00271-7. Epub 2024 Nov 25. PMID: 39608381.

TABLE 13.2 Selected Ongoing Trial in the GLP-1RA (or GLP-1RA-GIP) Class of Particular Interest

TRIAL NAME	STUDY POPULATION	INTERVENTION	PRIMARY OUTCOME	ANTICIPATED STUDY COMPLETION DATE
SURPASS CVOT (a study of tirzepatide compared with dulaglutide on major cardiovascular events in participants with type 2 diabetes); unique identifier: NCT04255433	***N*** = 12,500; key inclusion criteria: adults age ≥ 45 years; BMI ≥ 25 kg/m^2; type 2 diabetes; established CVD	Tirzepatide weekly subcutaneous injection versus dulaglutide weekly subcutaneous injection	Time to first occurrence of composite endpoint of cardiovascular death, nonfatal myocardial infarction, or nonfatal stroke	Q3/4 2025

DIABETES AND CARDIOLOGY GUIDELINES RECOMMENDATIONS ON GLP-1RAS IN PEOPLE WITH EXISTING DISEASE OR AT ELEVATED CARDIOVASCULAR RISK

Given GLP-1RAs lower CV outcomes in people with type 2 diabetes, and do so independently of baseline HbA1c, their use is now recommended (alongside SGLT2i) in patients with diabetes and ASCVD, irrespective of glucose control. These two classes of drugs are considered disease modifying and the evidence base for their cardiovascular benefits is robust, elevating their use beyond all other agents proven to lower glucose. The 2022 updated ADA/EASD guidelines[23] and the 2023 ESC-led guidelines[24] recommend their use, regardless of metformin use at baseline in those with ASCVD or evidence of target organ damage or multiple risk factors.

In people with high BMI and ASCVD but without T2D, the findings of SELECT have led the FDA to approve their use for prevention of cardiovascular disease in this population,[25] making them the first class of weight loss agents to achieve this approval. Notably, different countries or health authorities will continue to make individualized treatment decisions, taking into consideration costs, accessibility, and benefits of GLP-1RAs.

ONGOING CARDIOVASCULAR OUTCOME TRIAL OF CLINICAL RELEVANCE

SURPASS-CVOT[26] is comparing the effect of high-dose (15 mg) tirzepatide, associated with average weight losses of > 10% in people with diabetes, versus dulaglutide (limited weight loss) in patients living with diabetes and established CV disease (Table 13.2). Notably, dulaglutide has already been shown to lower CV outcomes in the REWIND trial.[8] There is preliminary evidence that tirzepatide is at least safe with respect to CV outcomes in a meta-analysis of phase 3 trial data[27] (Fig. 13.6), but its longer-term CV impact is eagerly awaited as this is the first GLP-1RA-GIP drug to be tested for CV outcomes, as well as being the first diabetes head-to-head trial of incretin-based agents. Furthermore, the contribution of greater sustained weight loss on CV outcomes in context of diabetes, a disease that is primary caused by excess adiposity is, yet, unknown but will be of interest given this is likely one of the main differences in effect between the two agents. This trial will report in 2025.

KIDNEY OUTCOMES WITH GLP-1RA—UPDATED META-ANALYSIS

With the addition of FLOW and SELECT,[11,12] Badve et al.[13] updated the kidney outcomes data across the class in their

	All tirzepatide $N = 4,887$ n (n/100 person-years")	All comparator $N = 2,328$ n (n/100 person-years")	Hazard ratio (95% CI)	P value
Composite MACE-4	72 (1.35)	70 (1.61)	0.80 (0.57, 1.11)	0.183
Death due to cardiovascular cause[b]	25 (0.46)	22 (0.43)	0.90 (0.50, 1.61)	
Myocardial infarction	30 (0.56)	30 (0.71)	0.76 (0.45, 1.28)	
Stroke	15 (0.27)	15 (0.35)	0.81 (0.39, 1.68)	
Hospitalization for unstable angina	5 (0.09)	9 (0.20)	0.46 (0.15, 1.41)	
Composite MACE-3[c]	67 (1.25)	62 (1.42)	0.83 (0.58, 1.18)	0.306
Composite MACE-3 or hospitalization for heart failure	74 (1.39)	71 (1.71)	0.78 (0.56, 1.08)	0.137
Hospitalization for heart failure	10 (0.19)	9 (0.29)	0.67 (0.26, 1.70)	
All-cause death	41 (0.76)	39 (0.86)	0.80 (0.51, 1.25)	

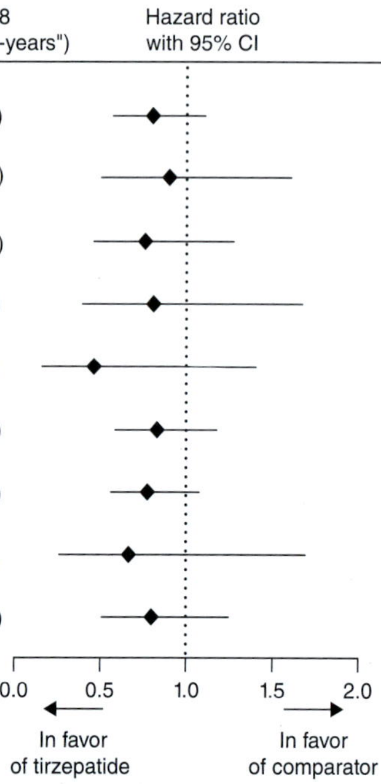

FIG. 13.6 Tirzepatide cardiovascular event risk assessment: a prespecified meta-analysis. Primary and secondary cardiovascular outcomes confirmed by central-blinded adjudication. Data are point estimates of HR (illustrated by the diamond symbol) and range of two-sided 95% CI of the HR. Strata size adjusted estimate. Strata are defined as trial-level cardiovascular risk (SURPASS-4 forms one stratum, and all other trials form one stratum). Death due to cardiovascular causes includes adjudication-confirmed deaths due to cardiovascular or undetermined cause. cMACE-3 includes deaths due to cardiovascular or undetermined causes, MIs, and strokes. Note: *P* values were based on the Wald chi-square test. *n*, number of participants in the specified category. *CI*, Confidence interval; *MACE*, major adverse cardiovascular events. Taken from: Sattar N, McGuire DK, Pavo I, et al. Tirzepatide cardiovascular event risk assessment: a pre-specified meta-analysis. *Nat Med*. 2022;28(3):591–598. https://doi:10.1038/s41591-022-01707-4.

2024 meta-analysis. The results showed that the GLP-1RA class lowered a compositive kidney outcome (Fig. 13.7 for more details) by 19% (95% CI, 8%–28%), with minimal heterogeneity. For worsening of kidney function, the reduction in risk with GLP-1RAs was 22% (9%–32%) but with modest heterogeneity. In this meta-analysis, while the results for the one trial in those without diabetes—SELECT—were directionally concordant so that there was no heterogeneity by diabetes, such reductions were not nominally significant. The authors reported that their comprehensive meta-analysis provided high-quality and predominantly high-certainty evidence for the benefits of GLP-1RAs for clinically important kidney disease outcomes.[13]

GUIDELINE CONSIDERATIONS IN CHRONIC KIDNEY DISEASE

The 2020 KDIGO guidelines[14] firmly placed SGLT2i and metformin as first-line therapy after lifestyle interventions for patients with diabetes and CKD, with the caveats of eGFR criteria. If additional drug therapy was then required for glycemic control, the guidelines recommended GLP-1RA be the preferred next therapy in view of evidence of CV benefits from trials, and no need for dose adjustments for the commonly used drugs, dulaglutide, liraglutide, and semaglutide, currently used in clinical practice in patients with type 2 diabetes (Table 13.3). The recent FLOW data[11] allied to the recent Badve et al. meta-analysis[13] will push GLP-1RA as one of the key treatment pillars in the treatment of CKD in diabetes, with further evidence needed for their use outside of diabetes.

OTHER CONSIDERATIONS IN THE USE OF GLP-1RA

Side Effects/Safety

Gastrointestinal complaints are the most common side effects: nausea (25%–60%), vomiting (5%–15%), and diarrhea. However, nausea and vomiting are often transient in most patients leading to discontinuation in 5% to 15% of participants in clinical trials. Escalating doses more slowly is increasingly used to mitigate such side effects.

The risk of hypoglycemia with GLP-1RA is minimal unless these drugs are used in combination with insulin or sulfonylureas. These latter two classes should be stopped or their doses reduced when starting these patients on a GLP-1RA. Such decisions are influenced depending on the patient's baseline HbA1C. For example, it may be helpful to reduce the dose of concomitant insulin (e.g., basal insulin) by 10% to 20% if the HbA1c is below 8% (Table 13.4). Given that Dipeptidyl peptidase 4 (DPP4-IV) also acts via GLP-1, these agents should be discontinued when starting GLP-1RA.

There are rare cases of gallbladder disease, such a cholelithiasis in GLP-1RA–treated patients. Of note, large CVOTs with extensive follow-up of these agents have not seen an increase in pancreatitis, which is reassuring on prior concerns about these agents.[9] Even so, patients should be

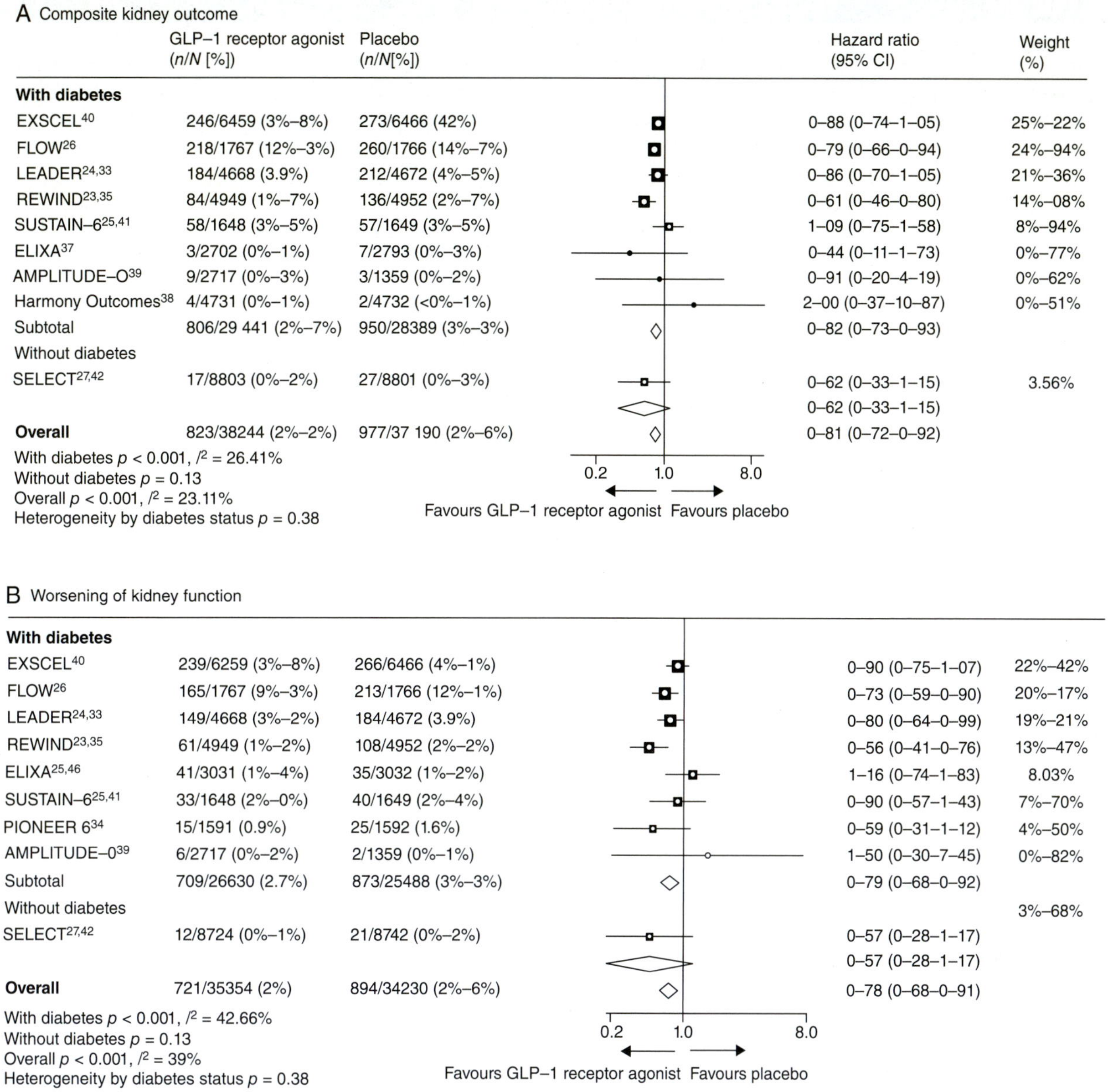

FIG. 13.7 Individual and pooled estimates for kidney outcomes. Trials are sorted by weight. **(A)** Composite kidney outcome. In the FLOW, LEADER, REWIND, SUSTAIN-6, SELECT, and AMPLITUDE-O trials, this outcome was a sustained reduction in eGFR by 50% or more, kidney failure (persistent eGFR < 15 mL/min per 1.73 m^2 or initiation of kidney replacement therapy), or death due to kidney failure. In the EXSCEL trial, this outcome was a sustained reduction in eGFR by 40% or more, kidney failure (persistent eGFR < 15 mL/min per 1.73 m^2 or initiation of kidney replacement therapy), or death due to kidney failure. In the ELIXA and Harmony Outcomes trials, this outcome was kidney replacement therapy. **(B)** Worsening of kidney function. In the FLOW, LEADER, REWIND, SUSTAIN-6, PIONEER 6, SELECT, and AMPLITUDE-O trials, this outcome was a sustained decline in eGFR by 50% or more. In the EXSCEL trial, this outcome was a sustained decline in eGFR by 40% or more. In the ELIXA trial, this outcome was a doubling of serum creatinine. Taken from Badve SV, Bilal A, Lee MMY, et al. Effects of GLP-1 receptor agonists on kidney and cardiovascular disease outcomes: a meta-analysis of randomised controlled trials. *Lancet Diabetes Endocrinol*. 2025;13(1):15–28. https://doi:10.1016/S2213-8587(24)00271-7. Epub 2024 Nov 25. PMID: 39608381.

TABLE 13.3 Dosing for Available GLP-1 RA and Dose Modification for Chronic Kidney Disease (*CKD*)

GLP-1RA	DOSE	CKD ADJUSTMENT
Dulaglutide	0.75 mg and 1.5 mg once weekly	No dosage adjustmentUse with eGFR > 15 mL/min per 1.73 m^2
Liraglutide	0.6 mg, 1.2 mg, and 1.8 mg once daily	No dosage adjustment Limited data for severe CKD
Semaglutide (injection)	0.5 mg and 1 mg once weekly	No dosage adjustment Limited data for severe CKD
Semaglutide (oral)	3 mg, 7 mg, or 14 mg daily	No dosage adjustment Limited data for severe CKD

CrCl, creatinine clearance; *eGFR*, estimated glomerular filtration rate; *GLP-1RA*, glucagon-like peptide-1 receptor agonist.

TABLE 13.4 Practical Recommendations and Patient Counseling

POTENTIAL CONCERNS	PRACTICAL RECOMMENDATION
Concomitant glucose-lowering medication	Stop dipeptidyl peptidase (DPP-IV) inhibitors Depending on HbA1C: stop or reduce (~25%) insulin dose or sulfonylurea to reduce risk of hypoglycemia
GI side effects (nausea, vomiting)	Start with low dose and uptitrate slowly Consider symptomatic therapy (e.g., proton pump inhibitor) for short period of time Counsel patients on: • side effects only transient; • small meals; • eat slowly; • stop before feeling full; and to • avoid fatty, spicy, and strong flavored foods
Injectable therapy	Use small needle (≤32 gauge) Fear of injection: consider oral available GLP-1RA (semaglutide)
Laboratory controls	Kidney function: not necessary Pancreatic enzymes: – only if patient is symptomatic; – levels increase on average by ~20% (no increased risk of acute pancreatitis in studies) Liver enzymes: not necessary

counseled to report severe or persisting abdominal pain and GLP-1RA should not be presently recommended in patients with a history of pancreatitis. In addition, injection-site pruritus and erythema are also common, most notably with the longer-acting medications in this class. In contrast to other antihyperglycemic drugs such as metformin or SGLT2 inhibitors, there are no special sick-day rules to follow for GLP-1 RA. However, recent concerns about delayed gastric emptying prior to surgery means some mitigation is followed in the preoperative period.[28]

Contraindications

GLP-1RAs are contraindicated in pregnancy and breastfeeding and, as such, contraception is recommended in females of childbearing age. Patients with severe gastrointestinal diseases, such as gastroparesis and inflammatory bowel disease, should also not be prescribed GLP-1RA due to their effects of slowed gastric emptying and potential exacerbation of disease. GLP-1RAs are also not recommended in patients with a personal or family history significant for multiple endocrine neoplasia 2A, multiple endocrine neoplasia 2B, or medullary thyroid cancer.

CONCLUSIONS

GLP-1RA is a class of drugs proven to lower cardiovascular outcomes and recommended as potential first-line agents in patients with diabetes and established cardiovascular disease. As they also lower weight, blood pressure, and improve glucose levels, they offer multiple benefits to such patients. Higher doses or new formulations that yield even greater weight loss may offer even greater benefits in patients with diabetes and those without, including improved quality of life and better impacts on a range of other chronic diseases such as sleep apnea, liver outcomes, and osteoarthritis. More recently, these drugs have been shown to robustly slow CKD damage, with notable data for semaglutide. Higher-dose semaglutide has also now shown CV benefits in those without diabetes but with established CVD and higher BMI, leading to the widening of its indication. Similarly, both semaglutide and tirzepatide have shown clinical benefit in patients with HFpEF, linked in large part to greater weight loss. Accordingly, the GLP-1RA class and related medicines are revolutionizing medical care in cardiometabolic and kidney disease.

REFERENCES

1. Dalsgaard NB, Vilsbøll T, Knop FK. Effects of glucagon-like peptide-1 receptor agonists on cardiovascular risk factors: A narrative review of head-to-head comparisons. *Diabetes Obes Metab.* 2018;20(3):508–519. https://doi.org/10.1111/dom.13128.
2. Gerstein HC, Sattar N, Rosenstock J, et al. Cardiovascular and renal outcomes with efpeglenatide in type 2 diabetes. *N Engl J Med.* 2021;385(10):896–907. https://doi.org/10.1056/nejmoa2108269.
3. Pfeffer MA, Claggett B, Diaz R, et al. Lixisenatide in patients with type 2 diabetes and acute coronary syndrome. *N Engl J Med.* 2015;373(23):2247–2257. https://doi.org/10.1056/NEJMoa1509225.
4. Marso SP, Daniels GH, Brown-Frandsen K, et al. Liraglutide and cardiovascular outcomes in type 2 diabetes. *N Engl J Med.* 2016;375(4):311–322. https://doi.org/10.1056/NEJMoa1603827.
5. Marso SP, Bain SC, Consoli A, et al. Semaglutide and cardiovascular outcomes in patients with type 2 diabetes. *N Engl J Med.* 2016;375(19):1834–1844. https://doi.org/10.1056/nejmoa1607141.
6. Hernandez AF, Green JB, Janmohamed S, et al. Albiglutide and cardiovascular outcomes in patients with type 2 diabetes and cardiovascular disease (Harmony Outcomes): a double-blind, randomised placebo-controlled trial. *Lancet.* 2018;392(10157):1519–1529. https://doi.org/10.1016/S0140-6736(18)32261-X.
7. Holman RR, Bethel MA, Mentz RJ, et al. Effects of once-weekly exenatide on cardiovascular outcomes in type 2 diabetes. *N Engl J Med.* 2017;377(13):1228–1239. https://doi.org/10.1056/NEJMoa1612917.
8. Gerstein HC, Colhoun HM, Dagenais GR, et al. Dulaglutide and cardiovascular outcomes in type 2 diabetes (REWIND): a double-blind, randomised placebo-controlled trial. *Lancet.* 2019;394(10193):121–130. https://doi.org/10.1016/S0140-6736(19)31149-3.
9. Husain M, Birkenfeld AL, Donsmark M, et al. Oral semaglutide and cardiovascular outcomes in patients with type 2 diabetes. *N Engl J Med.* 2019;381(9):841–851. https://doi.org/10.1056/NEJMoa1901118.
10. Sattar N, Lee MMY, Kristensen SL, et al. Cardiovascular, mortality, and kidney outcomes with GLP-1 receptor agonists in patients with type 2 diabetes: a systematic review and meta-analysis of randomised trials. *Lancet Diabetes Endocrinol.* 2021;9(10):653–662. https://doi.org/10.1016/S2213-8587(21)00203-5.
11. Perkovic V, Tuttle KR, Rossing P, et al. Effects of semaglutide on chronic kidney disease in patients with type 2 diabetes. *N Engl J Med.* 2024;391(2):109–121. https://doi.org/10.1056/NEJMoa2403347.
12. Lincoff AM, Brown-Frandsen K, Colhoun HM, et al. Semaglutide and cardiovascular outcomes in obesity without diabetes. *N Engl J Med.* 2023;389(24):2221–2232. https://doi.org/10.1056/NEJMoa2307563.
13. Badve SV, Bilal A, Lee MMY, et al. Effects of GLP-1 receptor agonists on kidney and cardiovascular disease outcomes: a meta-analysis of randomised controlled trials. *Lancet Diabetes Endocrinol.* 2025;13(1):15–28. https://doi.org/10.1016/S2213-8587(24)00271-7.
14. Kidney Disease: Improving Global Outcomes (KDIGO) Diabetes Work Group. KDIGO 2020 clinical practice guideline for diabetes management in chronic

kidney disease. *Kidney Int.* 2020;98(4):S1–S115. https://doi.org/10.1016/j.kint.2020.06.019.

15. Neuen BL, Fletcher RA, Heath L, et al. Cardiovascular, kidney, and safety outcomes with GLP-1 receptor agonists alone and in combination with SGLT2 inhibitors in type 2 diabetes: a systematic review and meta-analysis. *Circulation.* 2024;150(22):1781–1790. https://doi.org/10.1161/CIRCULATIONAHA.124.071689.
16. McGuire DK, Marx N, Mulvagh SL, et al. Oral semaglutide and cardiovascular outcomes in high-risk type 2 diabetes. *N Engl J Med.* 2025;392(20):2001–2012.
17. Lee MMY, Sattar N, Pop-Busui R, et al. Cardiovascular and kidney outcomes and mortality with long-acting injectable and oral glucagon-like peptide 1 receptor agonists in individuals with type 2 diabetes: A systematic review and meta-analysis of Randomized Trials. *Diabetes Care.* 2025;48(5):846–859.
18. Kosiborod MN, Abildstrøm SZ, Borlaug BA, et al. Semaglutide in patients with heart failure with preserved ejection fraction and obesity. *N Engl J Med.* 2023;389(12):1069–1084. https://doi.org/10.1056/NEJMoa2306963.
19. Kosiborod MN, Petrie MC, Borlaug BA, et al. Semaglutide in patients with obesity-related heart failure and type 2 diabetes. *N Engl J Med.* 2024;390(15):1394–1407. https://doi.org/10.1056/NEJMoa2313917.
20. Packer M, Zile MR, Kramer CM, et al. Tirzepatide for heart failure with preserved ejection fraction and obesity. *N Engl J Med.* 92(5):427-437. doi:10.1056/NEJMoa2410027.
21. Borlaug BA, Zile MR, Kramer CM, et al. Effects of tirzepatide on circulatory overload and end-organ damage in heart failure with preserved ejection fraction and obesity: a secondary analysis of the SUMMIT trial. *Nat Med.* 2025;31(2):544–551. https://doi.org/10.1038/s41591-024-03374-z.
22. Sattar N, Lee MMY. Estimating direct tissue effects versus weight loss effects of incretin-based drugs for obesity on various chronic conditions. *Lancet Diabetes Endocrinol.* 2025;13(4):347–354.
23. Davies MJ, Aroda VR, Collins BS, et al. Management of hyperglycaemia in type 2 diabetes, 2022. A consensus report by the American Diabetes Association (ADA) and the European Association for the Study of Diabetes (EASD). *Diabetologia.* 2022;65(12):1925–1966. https://doi.org/10.1007/s00125-022-05787-2.
24. Marx N, Federici M, Schütt K, et al. 2023 ESC Guidelines for the management of cardiovascular disease in patients with diabetes. *Eur Heart J.* 2023;44(39):4043–4140. https://doi.org/10.1093/eurheartj/ehad192.
25. U.S. Food and Drug Administration (FDA). FDA Approves First Treatment to Reduce Risk of Serious Heart Problems Specifically in Adults with Obesity or Overweight. 2024. https://www.fda.gov/news-events/press-announcements/fda-approves-first-treatment-reduce-risk-serious-heart-problems-specifically-adults-obesity-or.
26. A Study of Tirzepatide (LY3298176) Compared With Dulaglutide on Major Cardiovascular Events in Participants With Type 2 Diabetes. https://clinicaltrials.gov/ct2/show/NCT04255433.
27. Sattar N, McGuire DK, Pavo I, et al. Tirzepatide cardiovascular event risk assessment: a pre-specified meta-analysis. *Nat Med.* 2022;28(3):591–598. https://doi.org/10.1038/s41591-022-01707-4.
28. Gariani K, Putzu A. Glucagon-like peptide-1 receptor agonists in the perioperative period. *Eur J Anaesthesiol.* 2024;41(3):245–246. https://doi.org/10.1097/JA.0000000000001914.

14 Antihyperglycemic Medications With Proven Cardiovascular Safety

JENNIFER B. GREEN

CARDIOVASCULAR EFFECTS OF ANTIHYPERGLYCEMIC AGENTS USED IN TYPE 2 DIABETES

Clinical research in type 2 diabetes was historically focused upon interventions designed to achieve ever-tighter degrees of glycemic control. One of the most important lessons in cardiovascular risk reduction in type 2 diabetes has been the growing recognition that the specific medications used to reduce glucose, rather than the degree of glucose lowering itself, are likely the most effective means of reducing the risk of cardiovascular complications.

Of course, not all medications developed to manage hyperglycemia have a reassuring safety profile. As an example, the biguanide phenformin was removed from the US market in the 1970s given its association with high rates of lactic acidosis.[1] Interest in the effects of specific antihyperglycemic medications on outcomes was boosted by the rapid development of new drug classes to treat an ever-expanding population of people with type 2 diabetes. Uncertainty regarding the cardiovascular effects of these newer agents was highlighted by the publication of a meta-analysis by Nissen and colleagues in 2007 that suggested an increase in risk of myocardial infarction (MI) with the use of thiazolidinedione (TZD) rosiglitazone.[2] In the analysis of 42 trials that was performed, there were 86 MI events in the rosiglitazone group compared with 71 in the comparator arm (including placebo, metformin, sulfonylurea, or insulin), resulting in an increased odds ratio of 1.43 ($P = .03$). Although the methodology and results of this meta-analysis have been debated, and some have noted no increase in risk associated with rosiglitazone use,[3,4] the study was a cautionary tale in the selection of agents for glucose lowering. Most importantly, the study suggested that even though a medication may effectively reduce glucose levels, it may in fact increase the risk of important cardiovascular events that were the rationale for glucose lowering in the first place. After the rosiglitazone experience, the US Food and Drug Administration (FDA) mandated that glucose-lowering medications must have data to support their cardiovascular safety before they are approved for clinical use in type 2 diabetes.[5] Fortunately, there is now available over a decade of robust data from subsequent dedicated cardiovascular outcomes trials that permit selection of agents to specifically reduce the risks of cardiovascular morbidity and mortality in patients with type 2 diabetes with some agents, and demonstrating cardiovascular safety with others. This chapter will review the available evidence for the major classes of antihyperglycemic therapy that have been demonstrated to be safe, or have a neutral effect, in cardiovascular outcomes trials.

Metformin

Metformin, which lowers glucose by reducing hepatic glucose production and increasing intestinal glucose uptake, has long been the recommended first-line agent in the treatment of type 2 diabetes.[6] Metformin effectively reduces glycated hemoglobin (HbA1c) levels, may promote modest weight loss, and does not lead to hypoglycemia when used as monotherapy. It is also inexpensive and has a generally favorable safety profile. Metformin may also reduce the risk of long-term cardiovascular events when given as first-line therapy to patients with new-onset type 2 diabetes.[7]

The United Kingdom Prospective Diabetes Study (UKPDS) was an early landmark trial in type 2 diabetes that investigated the effect of intensive glucose lowering on microvascular and macrovascular outcomes. The trial was begun in 1977 and the results were published in 1998. In this trial, 3867 patients with newly diagnosed type 2 diabetes (median age 54) were randomized to intensive treatment with sulfonylureas (chlorpropamide, glibenclamide [glyburide in the United States], or glipizide) or with insulin, versus conventional therapy with diet alone.[8] A subgroup of UKPDS patients who were overweight (>120% ideal body weight) were randomized either to intensive therapy with metformin ($n = 342$, median HbA1c 7.4%) or conventional diet therapy ($n = 411$, median HbA1c 8%).[7] In the overall trial, tighter glycemic control (median HbA1c level 7% in the intensive group vs. 7.9% in the conventional group) reduced the risk for a broad, diabetes-related endpoint by 12% ($P = .03$) over 10 years of follow-up.

This reduction in risk was primarily driven by a 25% risk reduction in microvascular events; no reduction in the risk of mortality was found, and a numeric reduction in the risk of MI did not reach statistical significance (−16%, $P = .052$). Further, an unfavorable point estimate for stroke with intensive therapy was identified but the increase was not statistically significant (RR [relative risk], 1.14; 95% CI [confidence interval], 0.70–1.84). However, in the metformin-treated subset of patients, intensive management with metformin was associated with a 32% reduction in any diabetes-related endpoint ($P = .002$) and a 36% reduction in mortality ($P = .011$) that exceeded the reductions in risk seen with sulfonylurea or insulin therapy.[7] In summary, the UKPDS trial established that intensive glucose control reduces the risk of microvascular complications in patients with newly diagnosed type 2 diabetes, but also suggested that only overweight patients treated with metformin therapy will derive significant macrovascular benefits within the first 10 years of treatment.

After the UKPDS trial was completed, study participants and their clinicians were advised to pursue appropriate glycemic control, and patients were returned to community or hospital-based diabetes care according to their clinical needs without any attempts to maintain previously randomized therapies. In the 10-year posttrial monitoring study of patients who survived to the end of the UKDPS trial, HbA1c levels were no longer different between the original intensive and conventional arms (approximately 8% at the end of the posttrial monitoring period).[9] In the sulfonylurea-insulin group, RR reductions for diabetes-related endpoints persisted, whereas significant risk reductions for MI (15%, $P = .010$) and mortality (13%, $P = .007$) emerged over time. In the metformin group, RR reductions were shown for any diabetes-related endpoint, MI (33%, $P = .005$), and mortality (27%, $P = .002$). These observations suggest a modest but sustained effect of intensive glucose lowering on cardiovascular events, but only after many years of follow-up.

Despite the many advantages of metformin, data with respect to cardiovascular risk reduction with metformin are not entirely consistent. In addition to the UKPDS substudy,[7] only one prior randomized controlled trial was conducted on this subject. In the trial, 390 patients treated with insulin were randomized to receive either metformin or a placebo as add-on therapy.[10] The primary endpoint, an aggregate of microvascular and macrovascular outcomes, did not differ between the two groups after 4.3 years of follow-up (HR [hazard ratio], 0.92; $P = .33$), but there was a significant reduction in the secondary endpoint of macrovascular events (HR, 0.60; $P = .04$). In addition, metformin use was associated with beneficial effects on body weight and insulin requirements.

In observational studies, metformin use (either as monotherapy or in combination with another oral agent) has been associated with reduced mortality,[11–13] cardiovascular deaths,[11] and cardiovascular events.[12–14] Because metformin is generally the preferred initial agent for diabetes treatment and remains contraindicated in patients with advanced chronic kidney disease, patients who are not treated with this medication in an observational study may differ in important ways from those who are. These analyses either adjusted for potential confounders or matched patient populations for the propensity to be prescribed metformin versus another medication (usually a sulfonylurea). However, these investigations were observational in nature, so unmeasured factors may potentially still have contributed to the differences in outcomes.

Alongside the evidence that supports the safety and effectiveness of metformin, there are data that provide a less reassuring picture. Although the UKPDS substudy showed benefits of metformin in overweight participants, the trial also reported an increased death rate in nonoverweight patients who took metformin and a sulfonylurea compared with those who took a sulfonylurea alone (RR, 1.60, $P = .04$).[7] Combined analysis of the two UKPDS studies did not reveal an increased risk for mortality in patients treated with this combination, and the increased mortality in the UKPDS substudy has not been fully explained. In a subsequent meta-analysis of 13 randomized controlled trials involving more than 13,000 patients with type 2 diabetes, compared with other treatments, metformin therapy had no significant effect on the risk for mortality (RR 0.99 with wide 95% CIs that could not exclude a 25% reduction or 31% increase in risk), cardiovascular mortality (RR, 1.05), or rates of MI (RR 0.90 with 95% CIs that could not exclude 26% risk reduction or 9% harm).[15] Similar findings were reported in a meta-analysis that specifically examined the effects of metformin with insulin compared with insulin alone in 23 trials with over 2000 participants.[16] The study found that metformin added to insulin did not significantly change mortality risk (RR, 1.30, with 95% CI, 0.57–2.99) or cardiovascular mortality risk (RR, 1.70, with 95% CI, 0.35–8.30) but provided little reassurance with regard to each of these endpoints given the wide CIs.

Interestingly, analyses of observational studies including approximately 34,500 patients with heart failure (HF) and type 2 diabetes suggest a benefit to the use of metformin for glycemic control compared with older antihyperglycemic therapy. Patients with HF receiving metformin ($n = 6624$) had a 20% lower adjusted death rate compared with other antihyperglycemic medications (primarily sulfonylureas): 23% versus 37%; pooled adjusted HR, 0.80; 95% CI, 0.74–0.87 with no increase in risk of lactic acidosis.[17,18] This suggests that among the older classes of antihyperglycemic medications, metformin represents a safer choice than sulfonylureas for patients with type 2 diabetes and HF.

EFFECTS OF METFORMIN IN PREDIABETES

Additional studies have been conducted to determine if metformin therapy might provide a greater degree of cardiovascular protection when initiated earlier in the course of development of type 2 diabetes. One such study was the Diabetes Prevention Program (DPP) that randomly assigned 3234 persons without but at high risk for diabetes (with elevated body mass index and fasting and postload glucose values) to intensive lifestyle therapy, metformin monotherapy, or a placebo.[19] Lifestyle intervention and metformin both significantly reduced the incidence of subsequent type 2 diabetes. In follow-up studies of the trial population, the lifestyle intervention also improved cardiovascular risk factors compared with metformin or a placebo treatment, but the number of cardiovascular events was too small (*n* = 89 at 3 years) to allow any meaningful examination of the differences among groups.[20] After 10 years of follow-up of the DPP, the cumulative incidence of diabetes was still lowest in the former lifestyle intervention group.[21] Cardiovascular disease risk factors improved in all three treatment groups, but averaged over all follow-up, systolic and diastolic blood pressure and triglyceride levels were lower in the lifestyle than in the other groups (even though the use of antihypertensive medications was less frequent). However, the number of clinical events remained too small to determine the effect of diabetes prevention strategies on actual cardiovascular events. Most recently, assessment of DPP outcomes at a median 21 years of follow-up has identified no reduction in rates of major cardiovascular events or all-cause, cancer, or cardiovascular mortality with either lifestyle modification or metformin therapy.[22,23]

Sulfonylureas and Other Insulin Secretagogues

Sulfonylureas, the most commonly prescribed insulin secretagogues, are the oldest oral agent class for treatment of hyperglycemia. Whereas sulfonylureas are effective at glucose lowering, they increase the risk of hypoglycemia, are associated with a modest weight gain, and may provide less durable glycemic control compared with other antihyperglycemic classes.[24]

Hypoglycemia, which commonly occurs during treatment with sulfonylureas, other insulin secretagogues, and insulin, has been associated with adverse events in patients with diabetes including increased mortality, higher risk of dementia, falls, fall-related fractures, cardiovascular events, and poor health-related quality of life.[25–33] The relationship between hypoglycemia and cardiovascular events has been of particular clinical concern. There are a number of plausible mechanisms through which acute hypoglycemia may trigger ischemia, arrhythmia, and cardiovascular events. Hypoglycemia increases levels of counterregulatory hormones, such as epinephrine and norepinephrine, which may induce increased cardiac rate and/or contractility, heightening myocardial oxygen consumption, while also precipitating vasoconstriction and platelet aggregation. Acute hypoglycemia in the presence of hypokalemia prolongs cardiac repolarization and increases the QT interval, favoring a proarrhythmic state. One study of patients with type 1 and type 2 diabetes who presented to the hospital with severe hypoglycemia documented frequent hypokalemia, QT prolongation, and severe hypertension during the hypoglycemic events.[34]

Although animal studies have verified the effect of hypoglycemia on myocardial ischemic injury,[35] the data in humans are less clear, and debates continue on whether hypoglycemia is a mediator or merely a marker of such adverse outcomes—that is, the propensity toward hypoglycemia may simply identify sicker individuals who have lost the ability to counterregulate. Other risk factors for hypoglycemia include intensive glucose lowering, older age, lower health literacy level, longer duration of diabetes, renal impairment, polypharmacy, baseline cognitive impairment, and recent admission to the hospital within 30 days.[36–40] Notably, analyses of cardiovascular outcomes trials data have suggested that the relationship between severe hypoglycemia and cardiovascular events may be bidirectional, and each type of event indicative of a common at-risk type 2 diabetes frail patient phenotype.[41]

Questions about the cardiovascular safety of sulfonylureas date back to 1970 when the University Group Diabetes Program (UGDP) trial reported an increased risk of cardiovascular death associated with the use of tolbutamide compared with a placebo or insulin.[42] Subsequently, the FDA mandated a boxed warning to that effect for all sulfonylureas that remains in every sulfonylurea label to this day. Sulfonylureas inhibit the adenosine triphosphate–dependent potassium channels that are present within cardiomyocytes and coronary vascular endothelial cells, and it has been postulated that the presence of sulfonylureas at the time of an acute coronary event prevent adequate coronary vasodilation and thus may result in a larger area of myocardial damage. However, the risk of cardiovascular death noted by the UGDP group was not supported by the subsequent UKPDS study, which showed no difference in cardiovascular risk between the use of sulfonylureas (chlorpropamide, glibenclamide [aka glyburide], or glipizide) or insulin therapy[8] (but a benefit with the use of metformin, as noted earlier[7]). The large A Diabetes Outcome Prevention Trial (ADOPT) compared the glycemic effectiveness of metformin, rosiglitazone, or glyburide therapy, but again identified no between-group difference with respect to cardiovascular events (which were not frequent and were collected as adverse events during the trial) after 4 years of treatment.[24]

The Action in Diabetes and Vascular Disease: Preterax and Diamicron Modified Release Controlled Evaluation (ADVANCE) trial assessed the effects of intensive glucose lowering in patients with type 2 diabetes at high cardiovascular risk, preferentially using the sulfonylurea gliclazide in its intensive glucose control strategy.[43] In ADVANCE, 11,140 patients with type 2 diabetes (mean age 66, median baseline HbA1c 7.2%, 32% with history of major macrovascular disease) were randomized to intensive therapy (primarily with the sulfonylurea gliclazide, targeting HbA1c ≤6.5%, with mean achieved HbA1c 6.5%) or to standard therapy (HbA1c goal according to local guidelines, mean achieved HbA1c 7.3%). After a median follow-up of 5 years, there was a reduction in the risk of the primary outcome of the study, which was a composite of microvascular and macrovascular events (HR, 0.90; *P* = .01); the reduction in risk was almost entirely attributable to effects on intermediate markers of nephropathy. There was no significant between-group difference with respect to the risk of major cardiovascular events (HR, 0.94; *P* = .32) in ADVANCE, and no increase in mortality (HR, 0.93; *P* = .28).

Most recently, the cardiovascular effects of sulfonylurea therapy have been assessed in the Cardiovascular Outcome Study of Linagliptin versus Glimepiride in Type 2 Diabetes (CAROLINA), which assessed the cardiovascular impact of treatment with the dipeptidyl-peptidase 4 inhibitor linagliptin to the sulfonylurea glimepiride in 6033 patients with type 2 diabetes and established or multiple risk factors for atherosclerotic cardiovascular disease.[44]

At a median 6.3 years of follow-up, the treatment groups had similar rates of the primary composite outcome (cardiovascular death, nonfatal MI, or nonfatal stroke); 11.8% with linagliptin versus 12.0% with glimepiride. The upper limit of the 95.47% CI of the HR was 1.14, which met prespecified criteria for noninferiority. The CAROLINA findings indirectly support the cardiovascular safety of glimepiride therapy, as linagliptin itself did not increase the risk of major adverse cardiovascular events compared with a placebo in the Cardiovascular and Renal Microvascular Outcome Study with Linagliptin (CARMELINA).[45]

Insulin Secretagogues in Prediabetes

The Nateglinide and Valsartan in Impaired Glucose Tolerance Outcomes Research (NAVIGATOR) trial assessed the impact of postprandial glucose-lowering with a short-acting insulin secretagogue, nateglinide, in addition to lifestyle modification, in patients with impaired glucose tolerance.[46] The trial randomized 9306 persons (mean age 64) with baseline HbA1c 5.8% and high risk for cardiovascular disease (24% had a prior history of cardiovascular events) to nateglinide or placebo. Over a median 5 years of follow-up, nateglinide did not reduce the occurrence of the three coprimary outcomes—incident diabetes (HR, 1.07; $P = .05$), cardiovascular outcomes (death from cardiovascular causes, nonfatal MI, nonfatal stroke, or hospitalization for HF; HR, 0.94; $P = .43$), or the extended cardiovascular outcome (which in addition included unstable angina or arterial revascularization; HR, 0.93; $P = .16$). Thus use of an insulin secretagogue cannot be recommended in patients with prediabetes to reduce the risks of either diabetes or cardiovascular events.

Insulins

As type 2 diabetes progresses, beta-cell function declines and the effectiveness of oral agents in maintaining glucose control diminishes. However, endogenous insulin secretion is not entirely lost in type 2 diabetes, and strategies for insulin use can be less complex than those used in the treatment of type 1 diabetes. The main side effects of insulin use are weight gain and hypoglycemia. As insulin has been used in clinical practice for decades and is a naturally occurring peptide hormone, fewer concerns have been previously raised about the cardiovascular safety of such therapy. However, insulin may obviously induce hypoglycemia, which may in turn promote adrenergic discharges and arrhythmia, promotes fluid retention, and may result in hypokalemia (especially when administered intravenously) as a result of potassium shifts from the extracellular to intracellular space.

Concerns about the cardiovascular safety of insulin use in type 2 diabetes have been raised, primarily based on observational studies showing an increased risk of overall and cardiovascular mortality, and cardiovascular events in patients treated with insulin compared with other antihyperglycemic agents.[47–51] In one such analysis, data from over 84,000 patients with type 2 diabetes in the UK General Practice Research Database were used to determine the risk of the primary outcome (first major adverse cardiac event, first cancer, or mortality) associated with five different glucose-lowering regimens (metformin monotherapy, sulfonylurea monotherapy, insulin monotherapy, metformin plus sulfonylurea, and insulin plus metformin).[51] When compared with all other regimens, insulin monotherapy was associated with an increased risk of the primary outcome and all-cause mortality. The observational nature of the study does not permit conclusions about the causal nature of these associations; the risk of harms may be mediated by insulin itself or by the clinical characteristics of patients who require and are prescribed insulin. Indeed, there were important differences in baseline characteristics among treatment groups; despite adjustment for a variety of variables, residual confounding remains an important limitation.

Although few trials have specifically focused on the effectiveness and safety of insulin for prevention of cardiovascular events, several trials have tested the use of insulin during and after an acute MI for secondary prevention of cardiovascular events and mortality. The first Diabetes Mellitus, Insulin Glucose Infusion in Acute Myocardial Infarction (DIGAMI) study showed significant reduction in mortality (absolute reduction of 11%) associated with the use of insulin-glucose infusion during admission and subcutaneous insulin for glycemic control after hospitalization for acute MI compared with standard therapy in patients with diabetes.[52] Because it was unclear whether the mortality benefit was the result of inpatient or outpatient glycemic control in DIGAMI, the DIGAMI-2 study tested three different strategies, including combinations of insulin-based inpatient and outpatient glycemic control regimens.[53] However, the study struggled with patient recruitment and did not achieve differences in glycemic control among the three groups. There were no differences in mortality among the three groups. However, in the post hoc analysis of the DIGAMI-2 trial, insulin treatment was actually associated with an increased risk for nonfatal cardiovascular events, but not mortality.[54] Therefore, although insulin treatment is a particularly effective means of achieving glycemic control, it cannot be recommended as an intervention to reduce cardiovascular risk in the setting of an acute coronary event.

Cardiovascular outcomes with the use of two different, long-acting basal insulin analogues were compared in the Trial Comparing the Cardiovascular Safety of Insulin Degludec versus Insulin Glargine in Patients with Type 2 Diabetes at High Risk of Cardiovascular Events (DEVOTE).[55] DEVOTE enrolled 7637 patients with long-standing type 2 diabetes, 82.5% of whom also had cardiovascular and/or kidney disease, who were then randomly assigned to once-daily treatment with either the newer insulin analogue degludec or insulin glargine. At 24 months of follow-up, severe hypoglycemia was significantly less frequent in the degludec-treated group. However, rates of the primary outcome of death from cardiovascular causes, nonfatal MI, or nonfatal stroke were similar: 8.5% in the degludec group and 9.3% in the glargine group (HR, 0.91; 95% CI, 0.78–1.06; $P < .001$ for noninferiority). Despite an association noted between severe hypoglycemia and subsequent HF hospitalization (HHF), there were no between-group differences in rates of hospitalization for HF.[56] As DEVOTE assessed the cardiovascular effects of two different types of insulin, the trial findings are not useful in comparing the safety of insulin to other, noninsulin antihyperglycemic therapy.

EFFECTS OF INSULIN IN PREDIABETES AND EARLY DIABETES

Early provision of basal insulin to normalize fasting plasma glucose has been assessed as a strategy to reduce cardiovascular outcomes in persons with mildly elevated glucose levels or early diabetes. The Outcome Reduction with Initial Glargine Intervention (ORIGIN) trial randomized 12,537 people (mean age 64; 82% with early diabetes, 6% with new diabetes, and 12% with impaired fasting glucose or impaired glucose tolerance; median baseline HbA1c 6.4%; 59% with prior cardiovascular disease) to treatment with insulin glargine or standard care.[57] The target in the insulin-treated group was to achieve a fasting glucose level of 95 mg/dL or lower. After a median 6 years of follow-up, HbA1c levels were 6.2% versus 6.5% in the insulin and standard arms, respectively. The trial found no significant reduction in two coprimary outcomes, major cardiovascular events (HR, 1.02; $P = .63$) and major cardiovascular events plus revascularization and HF (HR, 1.04; $P = .27$) with early insulin initiation. However, there was an increased risk of hypoglycemia with insulin therapy and some weight gain (+1.6 vs. −0.5 kg in the two groups). Although the incidence of type 2 diabetes was decreased in the insulin group (a finding of questionable clinical application), the trial findings were generally disappointing. The ORIGIN trial did not support the original hypothesis that normalizing glucose with early insulin therapy would lead to better cardiovascular outcomes, but also did not identify an increase in cardiovascular risk with insulin treatment.

Incretin-Based Therapies

Medications that lower glucose through effect on the incretin system have been relatively recently introduced into the type 2 diabetes pharmacopeia. These agents either mimic the effects of or increase the circulating concentrations of the endogenous incretin hormone glucagon-like peptide 1 (GLP-1), which include stimulation of pancreatic insulin secretion in a glucose-dependent fashion, suppression of pancreatic glucagon output, slowed gastric emptying, and decreases in appetite through central mechanisms.[58] The oral dipeptidyl peptidase 4 (DPP-4) inhibitors slow the metabolism and inactivation of endogenously produced GLP-1, resulting in modest decreases in HbA1c with little impact on body weight.[59] The main advantages of the GLP-1 receptor agonists (GLP-1RAs), which most closely mimic the effects of endogenous GLP-1, are their potency in both weight loss and glucose lowering.[58,59] A potentially limiting side effect of GLP-1RA therapy may be nausea and vomiting, particularly early in the course of treatment and with dose uptitration, and both classes have been associated with an increased risk of pancreatitis and/or biliary disease. Typically, neither of these incretin-based classes causes hypoglycemia as monotherapy as their hypoglycemic effects are glucose dependent.[59]

Dipeptidyl Peptidase 4 Inhibitors

DPP-4 inhibitors (DPP4i), newer oral agents that have been studied in numerous large outcomes trials to date, appear to neither increase nor decrease the risk of major adverse cardiovascular events compared with placebo. These trials include assessment of the cardiovascular safety of saxagliptin in the Saxagliptin Assessment of Vascular Outcomes Recorded in Patients with Diabetes Mellitus–Thrombolysis in Myocardial Infarction 53 (SAVOR-TIMI 53)[60]; alogliptin in the Examination of Cardiovascular Outcomes with Alogliptin versus Standard of Care (EXAMINE)[61]; sitagliptin in the Trial Evaluating Cardiovascular Outcomes with Sitagliptin (TECOS)[62]; and linagliptin in CARMELINA and the previously described CAROLINA trial.[44,45] The inclusion criteria, patient populations, study interventions, and primary outcomes of these trials are summarized in Table 14.1. In all of the trials other than CAROLINA, the effects of DPP4i therapy have been compared with placebo in the context of otherwise usual care.

Unexpectedly, a significantly increased risk of hospitalization for HF was noted with saxagliptin treatment in the SAVOR-TIMI 53 trial.[60] In that trial, 16,492 patients with type 2 diabetes who had risk factors or a history of cardiovascular events were assigned to receive saxagliptin or placebo in addition to their existing diabetes medication regimen. After a median of 2.1 years, there was no difference in the primary endpoint (MI, ischemic stroke, or cardiovascular death) between the two groups (HR, 1.0; 95% CI, 0.89–1.12). However, more saxagliptin-treated patients were hospitalized for HF (3.5% vs. 2.8%; HR, 1.27 [1.07–1.51]; $P = .007$) compared with those assigned to placebo. This increase in HF risk has not been clearly explained; however, participants at greatest risk for saxagliptin-associated HF were those with elevated levels of natriuretic peptides, prior HF, or chronic kidney disease.[63] In the EXAMINE trial, there were also numerically, but not statistically, more HHF events in the alogliptin group compared with a placebo (106 vs. 89; HR, 1.19; $P = .22$).[61] As the SAVOR-TIMI findings have not been replicated in other DPP4i cardiovascular outcomes trials, it is unclear whether this increase in HHF risk represents a true within-class difference or is perhaps due to play of chance. Notably, the more robust, prospectively planned HF analyses of TECOS, CAROLINA, and CARMELINA outcomes demonstrated no increase in risk of HHF with use of sitagliptin or linagliptin in those trials.[64,65] A recent meta-analysis including data from 182 DPP4i trials identified no significant increase in risk of incident HF for the class, with the exception of saxagliptin.[66] However, the saxagliptin effects were primarily attributable to the SAVOR-TIMI 53 findings and the analyses were limited by inconsistent outcome adjudication across trials.

GLUCAGON-LIKE PEPTIDE 1 RECEPTOR AGONISTS

Numerous cardiovascular outcomes trials of GLP-1RAs have been completed, with results suggesting within-class heterogeneity of effects. Clear evidence of cardiovascular benefit has been found in the outcomes trials of the GLP-1RA liraglutide, the injected formulation of semaglutide, albiglutide, and dulaglutide (see also Chapters 12 and 13). Although several of the GLP-1RA agents that

TABLE 14.1 Cardiovascular Outcomes Trials of DPP-4 Inhibitors

	SAVOR-TIMI 53[60] (N = 16,492)	EXAMINE[61] (N = 5380)	TECOS[62] (N = 14,671)	CARMELINA[45] (N = 6979)	CAROLINA[44] (N = 6042)
Intervention	Saxagliptin/placebo	Alogliptin/placebo	Sitagliptin/placebo	Linagliptin/placebo	Linagliptin/glimepiride
Main inclusion criteria	Type 2 diabetes and history of or multiple risk factors for CVD	Type 2 diabetes and ACS within 15–90 days before randomization	Type 2 diabetes and preexisting CVD	Type 2 diabetes and high CV and renal risk	Type 2 diabetes and high CV risk
A1c inclusion criteria (%)	≥6.5	6.5–11.0	6.5–8.0	6.5–10.0	6.5–8.5
Age (years) [a]	65.1	61.0	65.4	65.8	64.0
Race (% White)	75.2	72.7	67.9	80.2	73.0
Sex (% male)	66.9	67.9	70.7	62.9	60.0
Diabetes duration (years)[a]	10.3	7.1	11.6	14.7	6.2
Median follow-up (years)	2.1	1.5	3.0	2.2	6.3
Statin use (%)	78	91	80	71.8	64.1
Metformin use (%)	70	66	82	54.8	82.5
Prior CVD/CHF (%)	78/13	100/28	74/18	57/26.8	34.5/4.5
Mean baseline A1c (%)	8.0	8.0	7.2	7.9	7.2
Mean difference in A1c between groups at end of treatment (%)	−0.3[d]	−0.3[d]	−0.3[d]	−0.36[d]	0
Year started/reported	2010/2013	2009/2013	2008/2015	2013/2018	2010/2019
Primary outcome[b]	3-point MACE 1.00 (0.89–1.12)	3-point MACE 0.96 (95% UL ≤1.16)	4-point MACE 0.98 (0.89–1.08)	3-point MACE 1.02 (0.89–1.17)	3-point MACE 0.98 (0.84–1.14)
Key secondary outcome[b]	Expanded MACE 1.02 (0.94–1.11)	4-point MACE 0.95 (95% UL ≤1.14)	3-point MACE 0.99 (0.89–1.10)	Kidney composite (ESRD, sustained ≥40% decrease in eGFR, or renal death) 1.04 (0.89–1.22)	4-point MACE 0.99 (0.86–1.14)
Cardiovascular death[b]	1.03 (0.87–1.22)	0.85 (0.66–1.10)	1.03 (0.89–1.19)	0.96 (0.81–1.14)	1.00 (0.81–1.24)
MI[b]	0.95 (0.80–1.12)	1.08 (0.88–1.33)	0.95 (0.81–1.11)	1.12 (0.90–1.40)	1.03 (0.82–1.29)
Stroke[b]	1.11 (0.88–1.39)	0.91 (0.55–1.50)	0.97 (0.79–1.19)	0.91 (0.67–1.23)	0.86 (0.66–1.12)
HF hospitalization[b]	1.27 (1.07–1.51)	1.19 (0.90–1.58)	1.00 (0.83–1.20)	0.90 (0.74–1.08)	1.21 (0.92–1.59)
Unstable angina hospitalization[b]	1.19 (0.89–1.60)	0.90 (0.60–1.37)	0.90 (0.70–1.16)	0.87 (0.57–1.31)	1.07 (0.74–1.54)
All-cause mortality[b]	1.11 (0.96–1.27)	0.88 (0.71–1.09)	1.01 (0.90–1.14)	0.98 (0.84–1.13)	0.91 (0.78–1.06)
Worsening nephropathy[b,c]	1.08 (0.88–1.32)	—	—	Kidney composite (see above)	—

[a]Age was reported as means in all trials except EXAMINE, which reported medians; diabetes duration was reported as means in all trials except SAVOR-TIMI 53 and EXAMINE, which reported medians.
[b]Outcomes reported as hazard ratio (95% CI).
[c]Worsening nephropathy is defined as doubling of creatinine level, initiation of dialysis, renal transplantation, or creatinine > 6.0 mg/dL (530 mmol/L) in SAVOR-TIMI 53. Worsening nephropathy was a prespecified exploratory adjudicated outcome in SAVOR-TIMI 53.
[d]Significant difference in A1c between groups (*P* < .05).
—, Not assessed/reported; *ACS*, acute coronary syndrome; *CHF*, congestive heart failure; *CV*, cardiovascular; *CVD*, cardiovascular disease; *DPP-4*, dipeptidyl peptidase 4; *eGFR*, estimated glomerular filtration rate; *ESRD*, end-stage renal disease; *HF*, heart failure; *MACE*, major adverse cardiac event; *MI*, myocardial infarction; *UL*, upper limit.
Reproduced/amended from ADA SOC 2024, Section 10; Adapted from American Diabetes Association Professional Practice Committee. 10. Cardiovascular disease and risk management: standards of medical care in diabetes-2024. *Diabetes Care*. 2024;47(Suppl 1):S179–S218.

have undergone cardiovascular outcomes assessments were not found to significantly reduce risk, those agents (including lixisenatide and once-weekly exenatide) did not increase the risk of cardiovascular events compared with aplacebo. Details of the lixisenatide and exenatide once-weekly outcomes trials are summarized in Table 14.2.

The Evaluation of Lixisenatide in Acute Coronary Syndrome (ELIXA) trial assessed the cardiovascular impact of treatment with the once-daily GLP-1RA lixisenatide in patients with type 2 diabetes who had had a recent acute coronary event.[67] In ELIXA, 6068 patients with type 2 diabetes and recent hospitalization for MI or unstable angina were randomized to receive lixisenatide or a placebo and followed for a median of 2.1 years. Lixisenatide did not significantly reduce the risk of cardiovascular events, but was found noninferior to a placebo with respect to the primary outcome of cardiovascular death, MI, stroke, or hospitalization for unstable angina (HR, 1.2; 95% CI, 0.89–1.17; $P_{\text{noninferiority}} < .001$).

The Exenatide Study of Cardiovascular Event Lowering (EXSCEL) trial of 14,752 patients with type 2 diabetes and established or high risk for atherosclerotic cardiovascular

TABLE 14.2 GLP-1/Dual Incretin Receptor Agonists With Cardiovascular Safety

	ELIXA [67] (N = 6068)	EXSCEL [68] (N = 14,752)	PIONEER-6 [69] (N = 3183)	TIRZEPATIDE META-ANALYSIS [70] (N = 7215)
Intervention	Lixisenatide/placebo	Exenatide QW/placebo	Semaglutide oral/placebo	Tirzepatide/active or placebo comparators
Main inclusion criteria	Type 2 diabetes and history of ACS (180 days)	Type 2 diabetes with or without preexisting CVD	Type 2 diabetes and high CV risk (age of ≥50 years with established CVD or CKD, or age of ≥60 years with CV risk factors only)	Varied across trials
A1c inclusion criteria (%)	5.5–11.0	6.5–10.0	None	Varied
Age (years)[a]	60.3	62	66	58.8
Race (% White)	75.2	75.8	72.3	73.4
Sex (% male)	69.3	62	68.4	56.7
Diabetes duration (years)[a]	9.3	12	14.9	6.83
Median follow-up (years)	2.1	3.2	1.3	0.85 (all trials at least 26 weeks in duration)
Statin use (%)	93	74	85.2 (all lipid-lowering)	—
Metformin use (%)	66	77	77.4	—
Prior CVD/CHF (%)	100/22	73.1/16.2	84.7/12.2	34.9
Mean baseline A1c (%)	7.7	8.0	8.2	8.29
Mean difference in A1c between groups at end of treatment (%)	−0.3[c]	−0.53[c]	−0.7	—
Year started/reported	2010/15	2010/17	2017/19	n/a
Primary outcome[b]	4-point MACE 1.02 (0.89–1.17)	3-point MACE 0.91 (0.83–1.00)	3-point MACE 0.79 (0.57–1.11)	4-point MACE 0.80 (0.57–1.11)
Key secondary outcome[b]	Expanded MACE (0.90–1.11)	Individual components of MACE (see below)	Expanded MACE or HF hospitalization 0.82 (0.61–1.10)	3-point MACE 0.83 (0.58–1.18); MACE-3 or HF 0.78 (0.56–1.08)
Cardiovascular death[b]	0.98 (0.78–1.22)	0.88 (0.76–1.02)	0.49 (0.27–0.92)	0.90 (0.50–1.61)
MI[b]	1.03 (0.87–1.22)	0.97 (0.85–1.10)	1.18 (0.73–1.90)	0.76 (0.45–1.28)
Stroke[b]	1.12 (0.79–1.58)	0.85 (0.70–1.03)	0.74 (0.35–1.57)	—
HF hospitalization[b]	0.96 (0.75–1.23)	0.94 (0.78–1.13)	0.86 (0.48–1.55)	—
Unstable angina hospitalization[b]	1.11 (0.47–2.62)	1.05 (0.94–1.18)	1.56 (0.60–4.01)	0.46 (0.15–1.41)
All-cause mortality[b]	0.94 (0.78–1.13)	0.86 (0.77–0.97)	0.51 (0.31–0.84)	—

[a]Age was reported as means in all trials; diabetes duration was reported as means in all trials except EXSCEL, which reported medians.
[b]Outcomes reported as hazard ratio (95% CI).
[c]Significant difference in A1c between groups ($P < .05$).
—, Not assessed/reported; *ACS*, acute coronary syndrome; *ASCVD*, atherosclerotic cardiovascular disease; *CHF*, congestive heart failure; *CKD*, chronic kidney disease; *CV*, cardiovascular; *CVD*, cardiovascular disease; *GLP-1*, glucagon-like peptide 1; *HF*, heart failure; *MACE*, major adverse cardiac event; *MI*, myocardial infarction.
Reproduced/amended from ADA SOC 2024, Section 10; Adapted from American Diabetes Association Professional Practice Committee. 10. Cardiovascular disease and risk management: standards of medical care in diabetes-2024. *Diabetes Care*. 2024;47(Suppl 1):S179–S218.

disease similarly found that treatment with the once-weekly formulation of the GLP-1RA exenatide did not significantly reduce the risk of major adverse cardiovascular events compared with placebo over a median 3.2 years of follow-up.[68] The primary endpoint of cardiovascular death, MI, or stroke occurred in 11.4% of patients in the exenatide group and 12.2% in the placebo group, which confirmed the noninferiority of exenatide treatment (HR, 0.91; 95% CI, 0.83–1.00; $P_{noninferiority} < .001$).

Dedicated cardiovascular outcomes trials of additional incretin-based therapies, including the oral formulation of semaglutide and the new dual-incretin receptor agonist tirzepatide, are ongoing.[70,71] Analyses of cardiovascular events occurring in premarketing studies of both agents have excluded a significant increase in risk associated with the drugs, thus permitting approval of the agents for clinical use in type 2 diabetes management. These findings are also summarized in Table 14.2.

Thiazolidinediones

TZDs, which lower glucose by activating the nuclear transcription factor peroxisome proliferator–activated receptor gamma, are insulin sensitizers. They do not increase the risk of hypoglycemia and may result in more durable blood glucose control than sulfonylureas or metformin.[24]

Although these agents improve many intermediate markers of cardiovascular risk (e.g., C-reactive protein and markers of endothelial function), they are associated with substantial weight gain; volume expansion with lower-extremity edema; and an increased risk of HF, bone fractures, and possibly bladder cancer risk.

ROSIGLITAZONE

Rosiglitazone, but not pioglitazone, was associated with an increased risk of MI in a now-controversial meta-analysis.[2] These findings initially led to a regulatory restriction in the use of rosiglitazone, which even after resolution has likely permanently limited the use of rosiglitazone in clinical practice. The only trial specifically designed to evaluate cardiovascular outcomes associated with rosiglitazone treatment has been the Rosiglitazone Evaluated for Cardiovascular Outcomes in Oral Agent Combination Therapy for Type 2 Diabetes (RECORD) study.[72] RECORD randomized 4447 patients with diabetes with inadequately controlled hyperglycemia treated with metformin or sulfonylurea monotherapy to receive, in addition, a sulfonylurea, metformin, or rosiglitazone. In the final analysis of the trial, there was no difference in the primary endpoint (cardiovascular hospitalization or cardiovascular death) among the groups, but the event rate was lower than expected and the dropout rate in the trial was high, decreasing the power to detect significant differences in outcomes. Notably, the risk of HF was increased approximately twofold with rosiglitazone. In June 2013 the FDA reviewed readjudicated data from the RECORD trial and confirmed that the trial had not found an elevated risk of MI or death associated with rosiglitazone: the regulatory restrictions to rosiglitazone use were subsequently removed.

Of note, in the Bypass Angioplasty Revascularization Investigation 2 Diabetes (BARI 2D) trial, 2368 patients with type 2 diabetes and obstructive coronary artery disease were factorially randomized to (a) medical therapy with insulin provision (insulin or sulfonylurea) versus insulin sensitization (metformin or rosiglitazone); and also (b) randomized to medical treatment versus coronary revascularization (a priori determined to be percutaneous coronary intervention or coronary artery bypass grafting) for management of coronary disease.[73] In BARI 2D, at over 5 years of follow-up, there was no difference in the rates of death and cardiovascular events between patients undergoing revascularization or medical therapy, or between the strategies of insulin provision and insulin sensitization. However, in the coronary intervention stratum, the risk of major cardiovascular events was significantly lower with CABG revascularization plus insulin sensitization (18.7%) compared with insulin sensitization therapy alone (32%, $P = .002$). There did not appear to be harm associated with use of rosiglitazone in the setting of this trial; however, the trial was not designed to specifically address the cardiovascular safety of rosiglitazone.

PIOGLITAZONE

In contrast to rosiglitazone, outcomes data available for the TZD pioglitazone appear to be more consistently reassuring, other than the increased risk of HF that is universal to the class.[74–78] The largest completed trial investigating effects of pioglitazone on cardiovascular outcomes was the Prospective Pioglitazone Clinical Trial in Macrovascular Events (PROactive) study, in which 5238 patients with type 2 diabetes and established macrovascular disease received pioglitazone or a placebo added to their baseline diabetes therapy.[79] After an average follow-up of 2.9 years, there was a 10% RR reduction in the primary endpoint (including all-cause mortality, nonfatal MI, stroke, acute coronary syndrome, revascularization, and above-knee amputation), which did not reach statistical significance ($P = .095$). The secondary, and more conventional, outcome of major cardiovascular events was significantly decreased with pioglitazone (HR, 0.84; $P = .03$). Concerns have been raised about the late definition and inclusion of the secondary endpoint after the trial was underway, the large number of secondary endpoints (more than eight) assessed, and the increased risk of any HF event in the pioglitazone group (11% vs. 8%, $P < .0001$), which may have, over time, impacted the study results and their clinical translation.

In the Thiazolidinediones Or Sulfonylureas Cardiovascular Accidents Intervention Trial (TOSCA.IT) study, the incidence of cardiovascular events was similar with the addition of unblinded pioglitazone versus sulfonylurea added to the care of older Italian patients with type 2 diabetes inadequately controlled on metformin monotherapy; the trial was halted for futility at a median follow-up of 57.3 months.[80] Additional meta-analyses have suggested either no effect of pioglitazone therapy on non-HF cardiovascular events, or perhaps a benefit restricted to patients with type 2 diabetes and established atherosclerotic cardiovascular disease.[81,82]

PIOGLITAZONE IN PATIENTS WITH INSULIN RESISTANCE

The Insulin Resistance Intervention after Stroke (IRIS) trial assessed whether pioglitazone would reduce rates of stroke and MI in patients with insulin resistance and recent ischemic stroke or TIA.[83] In IRIS, 3876 such patients were randomly assigned to pioglitazone or a placebo and followed for a median duration of 4.8 years. In the pioglitazone group, 9.0% of participants experienced the primary outcome of a stroke or MI compared with 11.8% in the placebo group (HR, 0.76; 95% CI, 0.62–0.93; $P = .007$). The rate of progression to diabetes was also significantly lower in the pioglitazone-treated group. Of note, pioglitazone-treated patients had more edema and weight gain than those receiving a placebo, but not higher rates of HF. The risk of HF may have been mitigated by the exclusion of patients with HF from enrollment, and safety algorithms that prompted pioglitazone dose reduction in patients with excess edema and/or weight gain.

In summary, the cardiovascular effects of TZDs in patients with type 2 diabetes or prediabetes appear mixed. The potential benefits of TZD therapy in reducing the risks of major adverse cardiovascular events must be weighed against the known increased risk of HF. The risk/benefit ratio with TZD treatment may be most significant in patients at intrinsically higher HF risk. Individuals with long-standing, complicated type 2 diabetes with comorbidities such as coronary and kidney disease will likely derive greater overall benefit from the use of other classes of antihyperglycemic agents.

Other Agents

ACARBOSE

Acarbose is an alpha-glucosidase inhibitor that delays intestinal carbohydrate absorption: the agent is infrequently used in the United States due to gastrointestinal side effects. In the Study to Prevent Non–Insulin-Dependent Diabetes Mellitus (STOP-NIDDM), investigators examined the effect of postprandial glucose lowering with acarbose on the incidence of diabetes in 1429 participants with impaired glucose tolerance, elevated fasting glucose, and overweight or obesity.[84] As a secondary outcome, investigators specifically examined the effect of the study intervention on major cardiovascular events, although the trial was not adequately powered to answer that question. The participants were randomized to receive either acarbose or placebo and were followed for a mean of 3.3 years. In the course of the trial, almost one-quarter of participants discontinued participation prematurely (including significantly greater numbers randomized to acarbose). Moreover, concerns about inconsistencies, failure to follow intention-to-treat analysis, and changes in the trial endpoints have been raised. Nevertheless, the trial reported an unanticipated 49% RR reduction ($P = .03$) in major cardiovascular events (including revascularization procedures, congestive HF, and peripheral vascular disease in addition to the conventional major cardiovascular events) associated with acarbose therapy. This composite endpoint was primarily driven by a marked 91% reduction in MI ($P = .02$).

The Acarbose Cardiovascular Evaluation (ACE) study has subsequently tested the impact of acarbose on cardiovascular outcomes in 6522 Chinese patients with impaired glucose tolerance and established cardiovascular disease or acute coronary syndromes. In ACE, no reduction in cardiovascular events was found with acarbose treatment compared with a placebo over a median 5 years of follow-up, but acarbose did reduce progression to type 2 diabetes.[85] Given the lack of consistently demonstrated outcomes benefit, acarbose cannot be recommended to reduce the risk of cardiovascular events in patients with prediabetes. However, there is no evidence of increased cardiovascular risk when the medication is used to reduce the risk of progression to frank type 2 diabetes.

QUICK-RELEASE BROMOCRIPTINE

The dopamine agonist bromocriptine very modestly reduces glucose levels and is available in the United States for antihyperglycemic therapy. A 52-week trial enrolling 3095 patients with type 2 diabetes evaluated the short-term overall and cardiovascular safety of quick-release bromocriptine compared with a placebo.[86] The frequency of serious adverse events was comparable between treatment arms, and fewer bromocriptine-treated patients experienced the composite outcome of MI, stroke, coronary revascularization, and hospitalization for angina or congestive HF than the placebo group (HR, 0.60; 95% CI, 0.35–0.96). This agent is not widely used for diabetes management.

PLACE OF THERAPIES IN GUIDELINES

Current guidelines for the care of patients with type 2 diabetes recommend preferential use of agents with demonstrated cardiovascular and kidney outcomes benefits in those at highest risk.[87,88] However, there remains a clear role and need for antihyperglycemic agents with demonstrated cardiovascular safety in diabetes management. A summary of the glycemic efficacy and side effect profile of these medications is provided in Table 14.3.[89] The natural history of type 2 diabetes suggests that most affected patients will require gradual intensification of medical therapy, and indeed ultimately require insulin therapy, to meet their individually appropriate glycemic goals. Thus an appropriate regimen of care for the high-risk patient with diabetes may include combinations of cardiovascular-beneficial and cardiovascular-neutral medications to meet a wide array of individual metabolic and outcomes goals. Demonstrated safe medications are also reasonable therapeutic options for lower-risk patients with type 2 diabetes, and may provide a means of achieving glycemic and weight-related goals with lower costs than those associated with newer classes of medications. In particular, the use of combinations of classes of known cardiovascular-safe drugs, which also pose little to no risk of hypoglycemia, may permit many patients with diabetes to achieve excellent glycemic control more safely than has been historically possible. This is particularly important for patients in whom hypoglycemia would be particularly hazardous, and for patients with recently diagnosed diabetes who are likely to benefit most from rapidly achieved and sustained intensive glycemic control.

TABLE 14.3 Other Characteristics of Glucose-Lowering Medications With Proven Cardiovascular Safety

MEDICATION (ROUTE OF ADMINISTRATION)	GLUCOSE-LOWERING EFFICACY	HYPOGLYCEMIA RISK	WEIGHT EFFECTS	KIDNEY EFFECTS		CLINICAL CONSIDERATIONS AND ADVERSE EFFECTS
				PROGRESSION OF CKD	DOSING/USE CONSIDERATIONS[a]	
Metformin (oral)	High	No	Neutral (or modest weight loss)	Neutral	Contraindicated with eGFR <30 mL/min/1.73 m^2	GI side effects: mitigate with slow dose titration, extended-release formulations, and administration with food. Potential for vitamin B_{12} deficiency: monitor and replete as appropriate.

TABLE 14.3 Other Characteristics of Glucose-Lowering Medications With Proven Cardiovascular Safety—cont'd

MEDICATION (ROUTE OF ADMINISTRATION)	GLUCOSE-LOWERING EFFICACY	HYPOGLYCEMIA RISK	WEIGHT EFFECTS	KIDNEY EFFECTS		CLINICAL CONSIDERATIONS AND ADVERSE EFFECTS
				PROGRESSION OF CKD	DOSING/USE CONSIDERATIONS[a]	
GLP-1RAs (SQ; semaglutide also available in oral formulation)	High to very high	No	Loss (intermediate to very high)	Benefit for kidney end points in CVOTs, driven by albuminuria outcomes: dulaglutide, liraglutide, semaglutide (SQ) Demonstrated benefit for progression of CKD for semaglutide (SQ)	See labels of individual agents for dosage considerations for kidney function. No dose adjustment for dulaglutide, liraglutide, or semaglutide. Monitor kidney function when initiating or escalating doses in individuals with kidney impairment reporting severe adverse GI reactions.	Thyroid C-cell tumors identified in rodents; human relevance not determined. Ileus: risk level is not well established; provide guidance on discontinuation prior to surgical procedures. Pancreatitis: acute pancreatitis has been reported, but causality has not been established. Do not initiate if at high risk for pancreatitis, and discontinue if pancreatitis is suspected. Biliary disease: evaluate for gallbladder disease if cholelithiasis or cholecystitis is suspected; avoid use in at-risk individuals. Diabetic retinopathy: close monitoring of retinopathy in those at high risk (older individuals and those with longer duration of T2D [≥10 years]). Impact on drug absorption: orally administered drug absorption may be impaired during dose titration (including of oral contraceptives). GI side effects: counsel on potential for GI side effects; provide guidance on dietary modifications to mitigate GI side effects (reduction in meal size, mindful eating practices [e.g., stop eating once full], decreasing intake of high-fat or spicy foods); consider slower dose titration for those experiencing GI challenges. Not recommended for individuals with gastroparesis.
Dual GIP and GLP-1RA (SQ)	Very high	No	Loss (very high)	Under investigation	See labels of individual agents for dosage considerations for kidney function. No dose adjustment. Monitor kidney function when initiating or escalating doses in individuals with kidney impairment reporting severe adverse GI reactions.	
DPP-4 inhibitors (oral)	Intermediate	No	Neutral	Neutral	Dose adjustment required based on kidney function (sitagliptin, saxagliptin, alogliptin). No dose adjustment required for linagliptin.	Pancreatitis has been reported, but causality has not been established. Discontinue if pancreatitis is suspected. Postmarketing concerns about joint pain (consider discontinuing if debilitating and other treatment options are feasible) and bullous pemphigoid (discontinue if suspected).

(Continued)

TABLE 14.3 Other Characteristics of Glucose-Lowering Medications With Proven Cardiovascular Safety—cont'd

MEDICATION (ROUTE OF ADMINISTRATION)	GLUCOSE-LOWERING EFFICACY	HYPOGLYCEMIA RISK	WEIGHT EFFECTS	KIDNEY EFFECTS: PROGRESSION OF CKD	KIDNEY EFFECTS: DOSING/USE CONSIDERATIONS[a]	CLINICAL CONSIDERATIONS AND ADVERSE EFFECTS
Pioglitazone (oral)	High	No	Gain	Neutral	No dose adjustment required. May not be recommended in kidney impairment due to potential for fluid retention.	Risk of volume expansion and HF. Do not initiate therapy in patients with established New York Heart Association (NYHA) Class III or IV HF. Risk of bone fractures. Bladder cancer: do not use in individuals with active bladder cancer, and use caution in those with prior history of bladder cancer.
Sulfonylureas (2nd generation) (oral)	High	Yes	Gain	Neutral	Glyburide: generally not recommended in CKD. Glipizide and glimepiride: initiate conservatively to avoid hypoglycemia.	FDA Special Warning on increased risk of CV mortality based on studies of an older sulfonylurea (tolbutamide); glimepiride shown to be CV safe (see text). Use with caution in individuals at risk for hypoglycemia, particularly if in combination with insulin.
Insulin (human) (SQ; regular insulin also available as inhaled formulation) Insulin (analogs) (SQ)	High to very high	Yes	Gain	Neutral	Lower insulin doses required with a decrease in eGFR; titrate per clinical response.	Injection site reactions. Higher risk of hypoglycemia with human insulin (NPH or premixed formulations) vs. analogs. Risk of hypoglycemia and duration of activity increases with the severity of impaired kidney function. Refer to device-specific instructions for insulins compatible with different delivery systems (i.e., pumps, connected insulin pens, insulin patches).

[a]For agent-specific dosing recommendations, please refer to manufacturers' prescribing information.
CKD, Chronic kidney disease; *CV*, cardiovascular; *DPP-4*, dipeptidyl peptidase 4; *eGFR*, estimated glomerular filtration rate; *FDA*, US Food and Drug Administration; *GI*, gastrointestinal; *GIP*, glucose-dependent insulinotropic polypeptide; *GLP-1RA*, glucagon-like peptide 1 receptor agonist; *HF*, heart failure; *SQ*, subcutaneous; *T2D*, type 2 diabetes.
Reproduced/amended from American Diabetes Association Professional Practice Committee. Pharmacologic approaches to glycemic treatment: standards of care in diabetes—2025. *Diabetes Care.* 2025;48(Suppl. 1):S181–S206.

REFERENCES

1. Misbin Robert I. The phantom of lactic acidosis due to metformin in patients with diabetes. *Diabetes Care.* 2004;27(7):1791–1793.
2. Nissen SE, Wolski K. Effect of rosiglitazone on the risk of myocardial infarction and death from cardiovascular causes. *N Engl J Med.* 2007;356: 2457–2471.
3. Richter B, Bandeira-Echtler E, Bergerhoff K, et al. Rosiglitazone for type 2 diabetes mellitus. *Cochrane Database Syst Rev.* 2007:CD006063.
4. Diamond GA, Bax L, Kaul S. Uncertain effects of rosiglitazone on the risk for myocardial infarction and cardiovascular death. *Ann Intern Med.* 2007;147: 578–581.
5. US Department of Health and Human Services, Food and Drug Administration Center for Drug Evaluation and Research (CDER), guidance for industry; diabetes mellitus—evaluating cardiovascular risk in new antidiabetic therapies to treat type 2 diabetes, 2008.
6. Sansome DJ, Xie C, Veedfald S, Horowitz M, Rayner CK, Wu T. Mechanism of glucose-lowering by metformin in type 2 diabetes: role of bile acids. *Diabetes Obes Metab.* 2020;22(2):141–148. https://doi.org/10.1111/dom.13869. Epub 2019 Oct 7. PMID: 31468642.
7. UK Prospective Diabetes Study (UKPDS) Group. Effect of intensive blood-glucose control with metformin on complications in overweight patients with type 2 diabetes (UKPDS 34). *Lancet.* 1998;352:854–865.
8. UK Prospective Diabetes Study (UKPDS) Group. Intensive blood-glucose control with sulphonylureas or insulin compared with conventional treatment and risk of complications in patients with type 2 diabetes (UKPDS 33). *Lancet.* 1998;352:837–853.
9. Holman RR, Paul SK, Bethel MA, et al. 10-year follow-up of intensive glucose control in type 2 diabetes. *N Engl J Med.* 2008;359:1577–1589.
10. Kooy A, de Jager J, Lehert P, et al. Long-term effects of metformin on metabolism and microvascular and macrovascular disease in patients with type 2 diabetes mellitus. *Arch Intern Med.* 2009;169:616–625.
11. Johnson JA, Majumdar SR, Simpson SH, et al. Decreased mortality associated with the use of metformin compared with sulfonylurea monotherapy in type 2 diabetes. *Diabetes Care.* 2002;25:2244–2248.
12. Tzoulaki I, Molokhia M, Curcin V, et al. Risk of cardiovascular disease and all cause mortality among patients with type 2 diabetes prescribed oral antidiabetes drugs: retrospective cohort study using UK general practice research database. *Br Med J (Clin Res Ed).* 2009;339:b4731.
13. Roumie CL, Hung AM, Greevy RA, et al. Comparative effectiveness of sulfonylurea and metformin monotherapy on cardiovascular events in type 2 diabetes mellitus: a cohort study. *Ann Intern Med.* 2012;157:601–610.
14. McAfee AT, Koro C, Landon J, et al. Coronary heart disease outcomes in patients receiving antidiabetic agents. *Pharmacoepidemiol Drug Saf.* 2007;16: 711–725.

15. Boussageon R, Supper I, Bejan-Angoulvant T, et al. Reappraisal of metformin efficacy in the treatment of type 2 diabetes: a meta-analysis of randomised controlled trials. *PLoS Med*. 2012;9:e1001204.
16. Hemmingsen B, Christensen LL, Wetterslev J, et al. Comparison of metformin and insulin versus insulin alone for type 2 diabetes: systematic review of randomised clinical trials with meta-analyses and trial sequential analyses. *Br Med J (Clin Res Ed)*. 2012;344:e1771.
17. Eurich DT, Majumdar SR, McAlister FA, Tsuyuki RT, Johnson JA. Improved clinical outcomes associated with metformin in patients with diabetes and heart failure. *Diabetes Care*. 2005;28:2345–2351. 74.
18. Eurich DT, Weir DL, Majumdar SR, et al. Comparative safety and effectiveness of metformin in patients with diabetes mellitus and heart failure: systematic review of observational studies involving 34,000 patients. *Circ Heart Fail*. 2013;6:395–402. https://doi.org/10.1161/CIRCHEARTFAILURE.112.000162.
19. Knowler WC, Barrett-Connor E, Fowler SE, et al. Reduction in the incidence of type 2 diabetes with lifestyle intervention or metformin. *N Engl J Med*. 2002;346:393–403.
20. Ratner R, Goldberg R, Haffner S, et al. Impact of intensive lifestyle and metformin therapy on cardiovascular disease risk factors in the diabetes prevention program. *Diabetes Care*. 2005;28:888–894.
21. Knowler WC, Fowler SE, Hamman RF, et al. 10-year follow-up of diabetes incidence and weight loss in the diabetes prevention program outcomes study. *Lancet*. 2009;374:1677–1686.
22. Lee CG, Heckman-Stoddard B, Dabelea D, et al. Diabetes Prevention Program Research Group: Effect of metformin and lifestyle interventions on mortality in the diabetes prevention program and diabetes prevention program outcomes study. *Diabetes Care*. 2021;44(12):2775–2782. https://doi.org/10.2337/dc21-1046. Epub 2021 Oct 25. PMID: 34697033; PMCID: PMC8669534.
23. Goldberg RB, Orchard TJ, Crandall JP, et al. Diabetes Prevention Program Research Group*. Effects of long-term metformin and lifestyle interventions on cardiovascular events in the diabetes prevention program and its outcome study. *Circulation*. 2022;145(22):1632–1641. https://doi.org/10.1161/CIRCULATIONAHA.121.056756. Epub 2022 May 23. PMID: 35603600; PMCID: PMC9179081.
24. Kahn SE, Haffner SM, Heise MA, et al. Glycemic durability of rosiglitazone, metformin, or glyburide monotherapy. *N Engl J Med*. 2006;355:2427–2443.
25. McCoy RG, Van Houten HK, Ziegenfuss JY, et al. Increased mortality of patients with diabetes reporting severe hypoglycemia. *Diabetes Care*. 2012;35:1897–1901.
26. Hsu PF, Sung SH, Cheng HM, et al. Association of clinical symptomatic hypoglycemia with cardiovascular events and total mortality in type 2 diabetes mellitus: a nationwide population-based study. *Diabetes Care*. 2012
27. Whitmer RA, Karter AJ, Yaffe K, et al. Hypoglycemic episodes and risk of dementia in older patients with type 2 diabetes mellitus. *JAMA*. 2009;301:1565–1572.
28. Schwartz AV, Vittinghoff E, Sellmeyer DE, et al. Diabetes-related complications, glycemic control, and falls in older adults. *Diabetes Care*. 2008;31:391–396.
29. Johnston SS, Conner C, Aagren M, et al. Association between hypoglycaemic events and fall-related fractures in Medicare-covered patients with type 2 diabetes. *Diabetes Obes Metab*. 2012;14:634–643.
30. Johnston SS, Conner C, Aagren M, et al. Evidence linking hypoglycemic events to an increased risk of acute cardiovascular events in patients with type 2 diabetes. *Diabetes Care*. 2011;34:1164–1170.
31. Desouza C, Salazar H, Cheong B, et al. Association of hypoglycemia and cardiac ischemia: a study based on continuous monitoring. *Diabetes Care*. 2003;26:1485–1489.
32. Laiteerapong N, Karter AJ, Liu JY, et al. Correlates of quality of life in older adults with diabetes: the diabetes & aging study. *Diabetes Care*. 2011;34:1749–1753.
33. Williams SA, Shi L, Brenneman SK, et al. The burden of hypoglycemia on healthcare utilization, costs, and quality of life among type 2 diabetes mellitus patients. *J Diabetes Complications*. 2012;26:399–406.
34. Tsujimoto T, Yamamoto-Honda R, Kajio H, et al. Vital signs, QT prolongation, and newly diagnosed cardiovascular disease during severe hypoglycemia in type 1 and type 2 diabetic patients. *Diabetes Care*. 2013.
35. Libby P, Maroko PR, Braunwald E. The effect of hypoglycemia on myocardial ischemic injury during acute experimental coronary artery occlusion. *Circulation*. 1975;51:621–626.
36. Miller ME, Bonds DE, Gerstein HC, et al. The effects of baseline characteristics, glycaemia treatment approach, and glycated haemoglobin concentration on the risk of severe hypoglycaemia: post hoc epidemiological analysis of the accord study. *BMJ*. 2010;340:b5444.
37. Davis TM, Brown SG, Jacobs IG, et al. Determinants of severe hypoglycemia complicating type 2 diabetes: the fremantle diabetes study. *J Clin Endocrinol Metab*. 2010;95:2240–2247.
38. Sarkar U, Karter AJ, Liu JY, et al. Hypoglycemia is more common among type 2 diabetes patients with limited health literacy: the diabetes study of Northern California (distance). *J Gen Intern Med*. 2010;25:962–968.
39. Shorr RI, Ray WA, Daugherty JR, et al. Incidence and risk factors for serious hypoglycemia in older persons using insulin or sulfonylureas. *Arch Intern Med*. 1997;157:1681–1686.
40. Punthakee Z, Miller ME, Launer LJ, et al. Poor cognitive function and risk of severe hypoglycemia in type 2 diabetes: post hoc epidemiologic analysis of the accord trial. *Diabetes Care*. 2012;35:787–793.
41. Standl E, Stevens SR, Armstrong PW, et al. TECOS Study Group. Increased risk of severe hypoglycemic events before and after cardiovascular outcomes in TECOS suggests an at-risk type 2 diabetes frail patient phenotype. *Diabetes Care*. 2018;41(3):596–603. https://doi.org/10.2337/dc17-1778. Epub 2018 Jan 8. PMID: 29311155.
42. A study of the effects of hypoglycemia agents on vascular complications in patients with adult-onset diabetes. Vi. Supplementary report on nonfatal events in patients treated with tolbutamide. *Diabetes*. 1976;25:1129–1153.
43. Patel A, MacMahon S, Chalmers J, et al. Intensive blood glucose control and vascular outcomes in patients with type 2 diabetes. *N Engl J Med*. 2008;358:2560–2572.
44. Rosenstock J, Kahn SE, Johansen OE, et al. CAROLINA Investigators. Effect of linagliptin vs glimepiride on major adverse cardiovascular outcomes in patients with type 2 diabetes: the CAROLINA randomized clinical trial. *JAMA*. 2019;322(12):1155–1166. https://doi.org/10.1001/jama.2019.13772. Erratum in: JAMA. 2019 Dec 3;322(21):2138. PMID: 31536101; PMCID: PMC6763993.
45. Rosenstock J, Perkovic V, Johansen OE, et al. CARMELINA Investigators. Effect of linagliptin vs placebo on major cardiovascular events in adults with type 2 diabetes and high cardiovascular and renal risk: the CARMELINA randomized clinical trial. *JAMA*. 2019;321(1):69–79. https://doi.org/10.1001/jama.2018.18269. PMID: 30418475; PMCID: PMC6583576.
46. NAVIGATOR Study Group, Holman RR, Haffner SM, McMurray JJ, et al. Effect of nateglinide on the incidence of diabetes and cardiovascular events. *N Engl J Med*. 2010;362(16):1463–1476. https://doi.org/10.1056/NEJMoa1001122. Epub 2010 Mar 14. Erratum in: N Engl J Med. 2010 May 6;362(18):1748. PMID: 20228402.
47. Currie CJ, Peters JR, Tynan A, et al. Survival as a function of HbA(1c) in people with type 2 diabetes: a retrospective cohort study. *Lancet*. 2010;375:481–489.
48. Currie CJ, Johnson JA. The safety profile of exogenous insulin in people with type 2 diabetes: justification for concern. *Diabetes Obes Metab*. 2012;14:1–4.
49. Gamble JM, Simpson SH, Eurich DT, et al. Insulin use and increased risk of mortality in type 2 diabetes: a cohort study. *Diabetes Obes Metab*. 2010;12:47–53.
50. Anselmino M, Ohrvik J, Malmberg K, et al. Glucose lowering treatment in patients with coronary artery disease is prognostically important not only in established but also in newly detected diabetes mellitus: a report from the Euro Heart Survey on diabetes and the heart. *Eur Heart J*. 2008;29:177–184.
51. Currie CJ, Poole CD, Evans M, et al. Mortality and other important diabetes-related outcomes with insulin vs other antihyperglycemic therapies in type 2 diabetes. *J Clin Endocrinol Metab*. 2013
52. Malmberg K. Prospective randomised study of intensive insulin treatment on long term survival after acute myocardial infarction in patients with diabetes mellitus. DIGAMI (diabetes mellitus, insulin glucose infusion in acute myocardial infarction) study group. *BMJ*. 1997;314:1512–1515.
53. Malmberg K, Ryden L, Wedel H, et al. Intense metabolic control by means of insulin in patients with diabetes mellitus and acute myocardial infarction (DIGAMI 2): effects on mortality and morbidity. *Eur Heart J*. 2005;26:650–661.
54. Mellbin LG, Malmberg K, Norhammar A, et al. Prognostic implications of glucose-lowering treatment in patients with acute myocardial infarction and diabetes: experiences from an extended follow-up of the diabetes mellitus insulin- glucose infusion in acute myocardial infarction (DIGAMI) 2 study. *Diabetologia*. 2011;54:1308–1317.
55. Marso SP, McGuire DK, Zinman B, et al. DEVOTE Study Group. Efficacy and safety of degludec versus glargine in type 2 diabetes. *N Engl J Med*. 2017;377(8):723–732. https://doi.org/10.1056/NEJMoa1615692. Epub 2017 Jun 12. PMID: 28605603; PMCID: PMC5731244.
56. Pratley RE, Husain M, Lingvay I, et al. DEVOTE Study Group. Heart failure with insulin degludec versus glargine U100 in patients with type 2 diabetes at high risk of cardiovascular disease: DEVOTE 14. *Cardiovasc Diabetol*. 2019;18(1):156. https://doi.org/10.1186/s12933-019-0960-8. PMID: 31729990; PMCID: PMC6858747.
57. ORIGIN Trial Investigators, Gerstein HC, Bosch J, Dagenais GR, et al. Basal insulin and cardiovascular and other outcomes in dysglycemia. *N Engl J Med*. 2012;367:319–328.
58. Tan Q, Akindehin SE, Orsso CE, et al. Recent advances in incretin-based pharmacotherapies for the treatment of obesity and diabetes. *Front Endocrinol (Lausanne)*. 2022;13:838410. https://doi.org/10.3389/fendo.2022.838410. PMID: 35299971; PMCID: PMC8921987.
59. Nauck MA, Meier JJ, Cavender MA, Abd El Aziz M, Drucker DJ. Cardiovascular actions and clinical outcomes with glucagon-like peptide-1 receptor agonists and dipeptidyl peptidase-4 inhibitors. *Circulation*. 2017;136(9):849–870. https://doi.org/10.1161/CIRCULATIONAHA.117.028136. PMID: 28847797.
60. Scirica BM, Bhatt DL, Braunwald E, et al. Saxagliptin and cardiovascular outcomes in patients with type 2 diabetes mellitus. *N Engl J Med*. 2013;369:1317–1326.
61. White WB, Cannon CP, Heller SR, et al. EXAMINE Investigators. Alogliptin after acute coronary syndrome in patients with type 2 diabetes. *N Engl J Med*. 2013;369(14):1327–1335. https://doi.org/10.1056/NEJMoa1305889. Epub 2013 Sep 2. PMID: 23992602.
62. Green JB, Bethel MA, Armstrong PW, et al. TECOS Study Group. Effect of sitagliptin on cardiovascular outcomes in type 2 diabetes. *N Engl J Med*. 2015;373(3):232–242. https://doi.org/10.1056/NEJMoa1501352. Epub 2015 Jun 8. Erratum in: N Engl J Med. 2015 Aug 6;373(6):586. PMID: 26052984.
63. Scirica BM, Braunwald E, Raz I. SAVOR-TIMI 53 Steering Committee and Investigators. Heart failure, saxagliptin, and diabetes mellitus: observations from the SAVOR-TIMI 53 randomized trial. *Circulation*. 2015;132(15):e198. https://doi.org/10.1161/CIR.0000000000000330. Erratum for: Circulation. 2014 Oct 28;130(18):1579-88. PMID: 26459088.

64. McGuire DK, Van de Werf F, Armstrong PW, et al. Association between sitagliptin use and heart failure hospitalization and related outcomes in type 2 diabetes mellitus: secondary analysis of a randomized clinical trial. *JAMA Cardiol*. 2016;1(2):126–135.
65. McGuire DK, Alexander JH, Johansen OE, et al. Linagliptin effects on heart failure and related outcomes in individuals with type 2 diabetes mellitus at high cardiovascular and renal risk in CARMELINA. *Circulation*. 2019;139 (3):351–361.
66. Mannucci E, Nreu B, Montereggi C, et al. SID-AMD joint panel for Italian Guidelines on Treatment of Type 2 Diabetes. Cardiovascular events and all-cause mortality in patients with type 2 diabetes treated with dipeptidyl peptidase-4 inhibitors: an extensive meta-analysis of randomized controlled trials. *Nutr Metab Cardiovasc Dis*. 2021;31(10):2745–2755. https://doi.org/10.1016/j.numecd.2021.06.002. Epub 2021 Jul 5. PMID: 34364771.
67. Pfeffer MA, Claggett B, Diaz R, et al. ELIXA Investigators. Lixisenatide in patients with type 2 diabetes and acute coronary syndrome. *N Engl J Med*. 2015;373(23):2247–2257. https://doi.org/10.1056/NEJMoa1509225. PMID: 26630143.
68. Holman RR, Bethel MA, Mentz RJ, et al. EXSCEL Study Group. Effects of once-weekly exenatide on cardiovascular outcomes in type 2 diabetes. *N Engl J Med*. 2017;377(13):1228–1239. https://doi.org/10.1056/NEJMoa1612917. Epub 2017 Sep 14. PMID: 28910237.
69. Husain M, Birkenfeld AL, Donsmark M, et al. PIONEER 6 Investigators. Oral semaglutide and cardiovascular outcomes in patients with type 2 diabetes. *N Engl J Med*. 2019;381(9):841–851. https://doi.org/10.1056/NEJMoa1901118. Epub 2019 Jun 11. PMID: 31185157.
70. A study of tirzepatide (LY3298176) compared with dulaglutide on major cardiovascular events in participants with type 2 diabetes (SURPASS-CVOT) https://clinicaltrials.gov/ct2/show/NCT04255433.
71. A heart disease study of semaglutide in patients with type 2 diabetes (SOUL). https://clinicaltrials.gov/ct2/show/NCT03914326.
72. Home PD, Pocock SJ, Beck-Nielsen H, et al. Rosiglitazone evaluated for cardiovascular outcomes in oral agent combination therapy for type 2 diabetes (record): a multicentre, randomised, open-label trial. *Lancet*. 2009;373:2125–2135.
73. Frye RL, August P, Brooks MM, et al. A randomized trial of therapies for type 2 diabetes and coronary artery disease. *N Engl J Med*. 2009;360:2503–2515.
74. Morgan CL, Poole CD, Evans M, et al. What next after metformin? A retrospective evaluation of the outcome of second-line, glucose-lowering therapies in people with type 2 diabetes. *J Clin Endocrinol Metab*. 2012;97:4605–4612.
75. Winkelmayer WC, Setoguchi S, Levin R, Solomon DH. Comparison of cardiovascular outcomes in elderly patients with diabetes who initiated rosiglitazone vs pioglitazone therapy. *Arch Intern Med*. 2008;168:2368–2375.
76. Juurlink DN, Gomes T, Lipscombe LL, et al. Adverse cardiovascular events during treatment with pioglitazone and rosiglitazone: population based cohort study. *Br Med J (Clin Res Ed)*. 2009;339:b2942.
77. Graham DJ, Ouellet-Hellstrom R, MaCurdy TE, et al. Risk of acute myocardial infarction, stroke, heart failure, and death in elderly Medicare patients treated with rosiglitazone or pioglitazone. *JAMA*. 2010;304:411–418.
78. Lincoff AM, Wolski K, Nicholls SJ, et al. Pioglitazone and risk of cardiovascular events in patients with type 2 diabetes mellitus: a meta-analysis of randomized trials. *JAMA*. 2007;298:1180–1188.
79. Dormandy JA, Charbonnel B, Eckland DJ, et al. Secondary prevention of macrovascular events in patients with type 2 diabetes in the PRoACTIVE study (prospective pioglitazone clinical trial in macrovascular events): a randomised controlled trial. *Lancet*. 2005;366:1279–1289.
80. Vaccaro O, Masulli M, Nicolucci A, et al. Thiazolidinediones Or Sulfonylureas Cardiovascular Accidents Intervention Trial (TOSCA.IT) study group; Italian Diabetes Society. Effects on the incidence of cardiovascular events of the addition of pioglitazone versus sulfonylureas in patients with type 2 diabetes inadequately controlled with metformin (TOSCA.IT): a randomised, multicentre trial. *Lancet Diabetes Endocrinol*. 2017;5(11):887–897. https://doi.org/10.1016/S2213-8587(17)30317-0. Epub 2017 Sep 13. Erratum in: Lancet Diabetes Endocrinol. 2017 Nov;5(11):e7. PMID: 28917544.
81. Mannucci E, Giaccari A, Gallo M, et al. SID-AMD joint panel for Italian Guidelines on Treatment of Type 2 Diabetes. Effects of pioglitazone on cardiovascular events and all-cause mortality in patients with type 2 diabetes: a meta-analysis of randomized controlled trials. *Nutr Metab Cardiovasc Dis*. 2022;32(3):529–536. https://doi.org/10.1016/j.numecd.2021.12.006. Epub 2021 Dec 10. PMID: 35144855.
82. Zhou Y, Huang Y, Ji X, Wang X, Shen L, Wang Y. Pioglitazone for the primary and secondary prevention of cardiovascular and renal outcomes in patients with or at high risk of type 2 diabetes mellitus: a meta-analysis. *J Clin Endocrinol Metab*. 2020;105(5):dgz252. https://doi.org/10.1210/clinem/dgz252. PMID: 31822895.
83. Kernan WN, Viscoli CM, Furie KL, et al. IRIS Trial Investigators. Pioglitazone after ischemic stroke or transient ischemic attack. *N Engl J Med*. 2016;374(14):1321–1331. https://doi.org/10.1056/NEJMoa1506930. Epub 2016 Feb 17. PMID: 26886418; PMCID: PMC4887756.
84. Chiasson JL, Josse RG, Gomis R, et al. Acarbose treatment and the risk of cardiovascular disease and hypertension in patients with impaired glucose tolerance: the STOP-NIDDM trial. *JAMA*. 2003;290:486–494.
85. Holman RR, Coleman RL, Chan JCN, et al. ACE Study Group. Effects of acarbose on cardiovascular and diabetes outcomes in patients with coronary heart disease and impaired glucose tolerance (ACE): a randomised, double-blind, placebo-controlled trial. *Lancet Diabetes Endocrinol*. 2017; 5(11):877–886. https://doi.org/10.1016/S2213-8587(17)30309-1. Epub 2017 Sep 13. Erratum in: Lancet Diabetes Endocrinol. 2017 Nov;5(11):e7. Erratum in: Lancet Diabetes Endocrinol. 2019 May;7(5):e5. PMID: 28917545.
86. Gaziano JM, Cincotta AH, O'Connor CM, et al. Randomized clinical trial of quick-release bromocriptine among patients with type 2 diabetes on overall safety and cardiovascular outcomes. *Diabetes Care*. 2010;33:1503–1508.
87. American Diabetes Association Professional Practice Committee Draznin B, Aroda VR, Bakris G. 9. Pharmacologic approaches to glycemic treatment: standards of medical care in diabetes-2022. *Diabetes Care*. 2022;45 (Suppl 1):S125–S143. https://doi.org/10.2337/dc22-S009. PMID: 34964831.
88. American Diabetes Association Professional Practice Committee. 10. Cardiovascular disease and risk management: standards of medical care in diabetes-2024. *Diabetes Care*. 2024;47(Suppl 1):S179–S218. https://doi.org/10.2337/dc22-S010.
89. American Diabetes Association Professional Practice Committee. 9. Pharmacologic approaches to glycemic treatment: standards of care in diabetes—2025. *Diabetes Care*. 2025;48(Supp 1):S181–S206. https://doi.org/10.2337/dc25-S009.

15 Prevention of Heart Failure in People With Diabetes

AMBARISH PANDEY AND ADRIAN F. HERNANDEZ

INTRODUCTION

Chronic heart failure (HF) is increasing in prevalence affecting over 6.9 million patients in the United States, and it is estimated that over 20 million individuals have HF globally.[1–3] An aging population, improved survival after myocardial infarction, and a rising burden of cardio-kidney-metabolic conditions such as hypertension, chronic kidney disease, and diabetes in developing economies have all contributed to the increased disease burden worldwide.[4] Furthermore, while optimal control of traditional risk factors in patients with diabetes has been shown to reduce the risk of atherothrombotic adverse events, the risk of HF persists.[5] Although studies show progress in evidence-based treatment for HF with systolic dysfunction, it often remains a progressive condition and is associated with high mortality risk.[3] These treatments are often instituted late in the disease course when patients are symptomatic with significant LV dysfunction, and its impact on overall survival may be modest on a population basis. Given the irreversible nature of late-stage HF syndromes, prevention and early detection of HF should be a priority. Broadly, the prevention of HF is targeted at risk stratification and the implementation of effective therapeutic approaches to lower the risk of HF. These approaches range from lifestyle modification to intensive management of coexisting cardiovascular risk factors and, more recently, the implementation of novel, effective therapies such as Sodium-Glucose Transport Protein 2/1 inhibitors (SGLT2/1-i) and Glucagon-like peptide-1 receptor agonists (GLP-1RA) for the prevention of HF.

Diabetes has long been associated with an increased risk of incident HF[6–9] (see also Chapter 23). Longitudinal epidemiological studies, such as the Framingham Heart Study, have shown that diabetes increases the lifetime risk of developing symptomatic HF by 2.4-fold in men and a 5.0-fold increase in women, independent of coexisting hypertension or coronary artery disease.[8,10,11] The increased risk of HF associated with diabetes is comparable for the two HF subtypes—HF with reduced ejection fraction and HF with preserved ejection fraction.[12] In addition to diabetes, dysglycemia and higher hemoglobin A1c levels, even below the threshold for diabetes, are associated with incrementally greater risk for HF.[13–16] Therefore patients with dysglycemia represent a critical target population for risk stratification and prevention of HF. Considering the high burden of HF in patients with diabetes and associated worse outcomes, HF prevention should be taken equally as preventing other atherosclerotic cardiovascular complications in patients with diabetes. This is particularly relevant as the burden of ischemic heart disease has declined by up to two-thirds in the past two decades, while the decline in HF hospitalization rates has been more gradual and plateaued in the past decade.[17] In this chapter, we address the strategies and challenges of preventing and screening for HF among patients with diabetes, including consideration of diabetes management in patients at risk of developing HF.

STRATEGIES FOR PREVENTION OF HEART FAILURE

The fundamental principle of effective preventive strategies is to reliably detect individuals either at risk of developing a disease or exhibit evidence of pathological processes capable of causing progression to a clinical disease state. Effective interventions should reduce the risk of progression to disease, significantly delay the clinical onset, or alter the trajectory of disease progression. In addition, the condition targeted by preventive strategies should carry significant morbidity and mortality risks that must be balanced against the resources required and potential risks associated with the screening process or any preemptive treatment. To achieve these goals, a thorough understanding of the prevalence and natural history of the risk factors and the disease state is crucial.

IDENTIFYING PRECURSORS OF SYMPTOMATIC HEART FAILURE

HF is a progressive disorder. Despite the heterogeneity of HF etiology, structural or ventricular dysfunction begins in individuals with risk factors contributing to insults to or persistent stress on the myocardium, which may remain asymptomatic in many individuals. The resultant maladaptive changes in the ventricular geometry (remodeling), hypertrophy, stiffness, and neurohormonal activation culminate in a failing heart with patients experiencing dyspnea, congestion, and decreased exercise tolerance, requiring repeated hospitalizations and having increased mortality risk. Recognizing the importance of prevention in addressing the rising prevalence of HF, international professional guidelines and scientific statements have highlighted the need for aggressive risk modification among individuals at risk of developing HF. The American College of Cardiology and the American Heart Association introduced an HF classification based on stages of risk, development, and progression of HF.[18] This ranges from individuals with risk factors associated with increased risk of developing clinical HF without evidence of structural heart disease (Stage A), patients with structural heart disease but without overt clinical symptoms (Stage B), clinical HF syndromes with either current or past HF symptoms (Stage C), or end-stage refractory HF (Stage D) (Fig. 15.1). By incorporating those who are at increased risk for HF but do not exhibit HF symptoms (Stages A and B) but are nevertheless at significant risk of progressing to irreversible cardiac dysfunction, the American College of Cardiology/American Heart Association (ACC/AHA) classification highlighted the need to target these "pre-HF" patients for preventive measures to alter the natural history progression.

Stage A HF: Among patients with diabetes, coexisting risk factors for HF such as hyperglycemia, hypertension, hyperlipidemia, and obesity increase the risk of developing subsequent ventricular dysfunction. These risk factors are highly prevalent among patients with diabetes, are often suboptimally controlled, and represent an important clustering of modifiable cardiometabolic risk factors to consider for population-targeted intensive risk factor intervention for HF prevention (Fig. 15.2). From population studies, the prevalence of Stage A HF among individuals aged 45 years or older is approximately 20%.[20] The underlying assumption is that aggressively treating these modifiable risk factors underpinning the hazard of HF could mitigate the risk of progression to overt ventricular dysfunction. However, recent studies have questioned this paradigm and highlighted the need for novel approaches to HF prevention. These approaches may include more targeted lifestyle modifications and pharmacological therapies such as SGLT2i that may lower the risk of HF in diabetes.

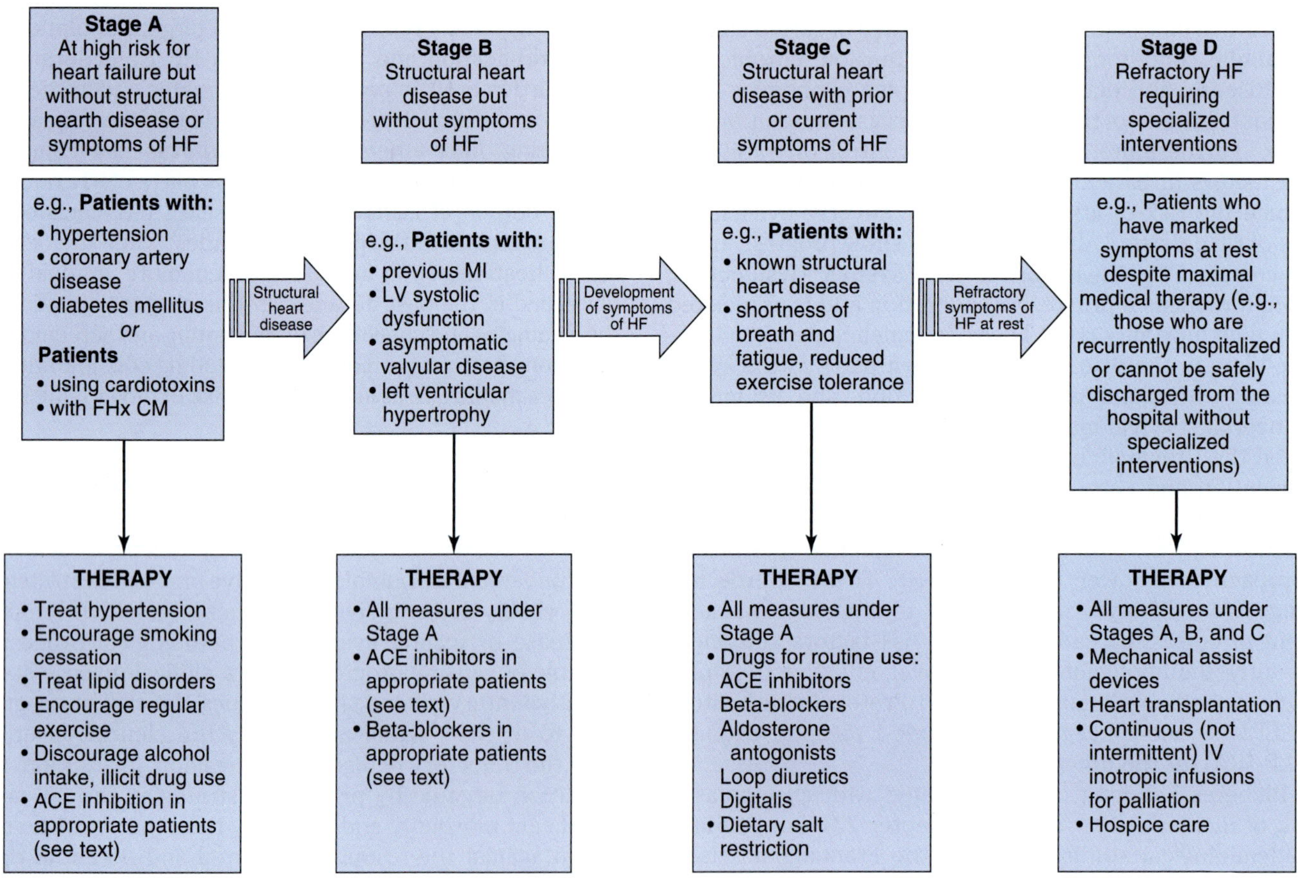

FIG. 15.1 ACC/AHA stages of HF evolution and recommended therapy. *FHx CM*, Family history of cardiomyopathy; *HF*, heart failure; *MI*, myocardial infarction; *LV*, left ventricular; *IV*, intravenous. From Sharon A Hunt et.al., ACC/AHA guidelines for the evaluation and management of chronic heart failure in the adult: executive summary: A report of the american college of cardiology/american heart association task force on practice guidelines (committee to revise the 1995 guidelines for the evaluation and management of heart failure) developed in collaboration with the international society for heart and lung transplantation endorsed by the heart failure society of america. *J Am Coll Cardiol*. 2001;38(7):2101–2113.

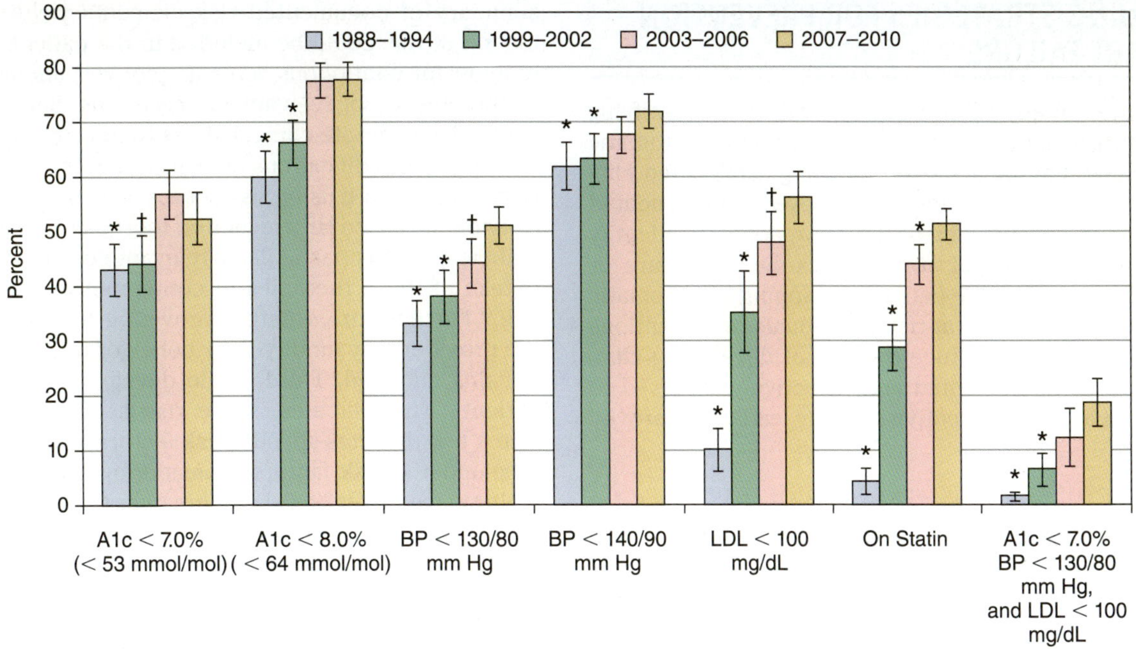

FIG. 15.2 Prevalence of meeting ABC goals among adults aged ≥20 years with diagnosed diabetes, NHANES 1988–2010. Estimates are age and gender standardized to the 2007–2010 NHANES population with diabetes. **P* < 0.01, estimates are compared with those of 2007–2010. †*P* < 0.05, estimates are compared with those of 2007–2010. From Stark Casagrande S, et al. The prevalence of meeting A1C, blood pressure, and LDL goals among people with diabetes. *Diabetes Care* 2013;1988–2010.

Stage B HF: Stage B HF refers to structural and functional cardiac abnormalities without overt clinical manifestations of HF, based predominantly on cardiac imaging results. For practical purposes, it has been narrowly defined as previous myocardial infarction (MI) with regional dysfunction or scar, LV hypertrophy (LVH), LV systolic dysfunction (LVSD; or reduced ejection fraction), or structural valve disease. Based on data from cross-sectional population studies, stage B HF is estimated to affect approximately 1/3 of the population ≥45 years of age.[20] Depending on the age of the population studied and the HF threshold chosen to characterize abnormal LV function, the prevalence of asymptomatic LVSD in predominantly middle-aged and older adults ranges between 2% and 10%, with higher rates reported among men and the older adults.[20–29] Asymptomatic LVSD is associated with a significantly increased risk of clinical HF, particularly HF with reduced ejection fraction, and death.[22,31] In the Framingham cohort, 26% of participants with asymptomatic LVSD progressed to symptomatic HF during the 5-year follow-up, representing an approximately fivefold increased risk compared with subjects with normal LV function.[22] This was associated with a 60% higher mortality risk, but more importantly, over half of the deaths occurred before symptomatic HF developed.[22] Although most studies examining the risk of Stage B HF progressing to symptomatic HF have predominantly included older white individuals, in a large cohort of white and Black young adults (18–30 years old at baseline), the presence of asymptomatic LVSD was a strong predictor of incident HF (greater than 30 times the rate compared with individuals with normal EF) before the age of 50 years, independent of other clinical risk factors, including blood pressure.[32] Given the irrefutable evidence suggesting asymptomatic LV dysfunction as a precursor to symptomatic HF, particularly HF with reduced ejection fraction, and its associated risk of mortality, targeting these high-risk individuals with aggressive preventive measures may meaningfully modify the trajectory of the disease progression into symptomatic HF.

More recently, studies have also focused on identifying diabetic cardiomyopathy. This subclinical Stage B HF phenotype precedes the development of clinical HF in the absence of ischemic heart disease or LV systolic dysfunction.[33] The diabetic cardiomyopathy phenotype is considered an intermediate stage in the development of HF with preserved ejection fraction (HFpEF), and its prevalence varies from 67% to 11.7%, based on the definition used. In a recent pooled analysis from three community-based cohorts, the prevalence of diabetic cardiomyopathy was 67% when defined by any echocardiographic abnormality (LVH or diastolic dysfunction) and 16% when defined by the presence of two out of three echocardiographic abnormalities and elevated natriuretic peptide levels. Diabetic cardiomyopathy was associated with a significantly higher risk of HF, even without other cardiometabolic risk factors such as hypertension and obesity. These findings suggest that diabetic cardiomyopathy may identify a unique subclinical or Stage B HF phenotype that may benefit from effective screening approaches for early identification and efficient implementation of preventive interventions.[33] This is also an important subset of high-risk patients to target for clinical trials of early pharmacological intervention for systolic and diastolic dysfunction. To this end, recent trials have evaluated the role of established and novel cardiometabolic therapies in preventing HF among those with diabetic cardiomyopathy. Specifically, the ARISE-HF trial evaluated the efficacy of an aldose reductase inhibitor in patients with diabetic cardiomyopathy and demonstrate no significant effect of the therapy on changes in peak exercise oxygen uptake or HF symptoms.[34]

SCREENING STRATEGIES FOR PREVENTION OF HEART FAILURE

The first step of any HF preventive strategy is identifying the patient population at risk of developing symptomatic HF. Screening may be achieved by using established clinical risk markers, as mentioned above, complemented by biomarker and imaging-based approaches to identify patients with subclinical abnormal cardiac structure or function on a progressive path of developing symptomatic HF. By identifying these at-risk individuals, interventions aimed to modify and reduce the risk of developing clinical HF may be implemented and objectively assessed to determine if a given preventive strategy leads to improved outcomes.

SCREENING WITH CLINICAL RISK FACTORS

As described, several well-established clinical risk factors, including the diagnosis of DM, increase the risk of HF and should be used by clinicians to identify high-risk individuals who will benefit from aggressive risk factor modification and primary prevention. The advantages of this strategy are the broad availability and generalized feasibility to clinicians, even in areas of limited healthcare resources. Nevertheless, despite the well-documented association of individual risk factors for HF, quantifying the magnitude of risk for a particular patient with multiple risk markers may be challenging. Validated HF risk scores for community-dwelling individuals, such as those derived from the Framingham Heart Study, the Health Aging and Body Composition (ABC) study, and the pooled cohorts (PCP-HF risk score), can identify individuals with an increased risk of developing HF.[35–38] Although these risk scores are not specific for patients with diabetes, the presence of diabetes or elevated fasting blood glucose has been consistently found to be independent predictors for incident HF. More recently, novel risk scores have been developed to predict HF risk among patients with diabetes.[39] One such risk score, the WATCH-DM score, has been developed and validated to predict the risk of new-onset HF among patients with diabetes. Similarly, the Thrombolysis in Myocardial Infarction-HF (TIMI-HF) risk score was recently developed and validated in patients with diabetes to predict the risk of HF hospitalization among diabetes patients with or without prevalent HF.[40] These risk scores use readily available clinical risk factors to identify individuals at the highest risk of HF and can be implemented in electronic medical records for risk stratification.

Several limitations exist concerning using risk prediction scores based on clinical risk factors as a screening strategy. First, while easy to use, their integration with the routine clinical workflow for real-world implementation remains untested. Therefore there remains an unmet need to effectively translate risk prediction model results into a clinical tool to further advance efforts in the prevention of HF through aggressive management of these risk factors. One potential direction is to capitalize on the evolution of integrated health systems and the increasing use of electronic health data, whereby an automated analysis and summary of documented risk elements yielding an estimation of risk could be included in the patient care fields to allow for continuous screening for risk and assessment of the efficacy of relevant interventions. Such a process could also generate clinical alerts to inform screening and therapeutic modifications (see also Chapter 31). Second, it remains unclear if using risk scores may modify the uptake of evidence-based HF prevention therapies in patients with diabetes. This is particularly relevant considering the low uptake of these therapies in contemporary clinical practice.[41] Furthermore, whether providing risk information to the provider may modify their behavior in clinical settings remains untested. Third, while developed in a cohort of patients with diabetes, these risk scores only incorporate a few diabetes-specific risk factors and do not utilize time-updated risk factors. Considering the availability of multiple measures of risk factors over time, novel risk prediction models that use time-updated covariates may have better risk prediction abilities. Finally, these risk scores do not include cardiac biomarkers of myocardial injury or stress, which are well-established predictors of HF risk in patients with and without diabetes.[42,43]

ROLE OF CARDIAC BIOMARKERS IN HEART FAILURE RISK PREDICTION AND SCREENING

In theory, biomarkers are biological variables that can provide information about the presence, severity, and prognosis of a condition of interest. In practice, the term biomarker in HF is limited to circulating serum and plasma analytes that reflect various aspects of the pathophysiology of HF beyond routine hematology and biochemistry panels. To be clinically useful, a particular biomarker must be shown to provide additional information that may alter clinical decision-making or guide interventions, above and beyond careful clinical assessment.

Natriuretic peptides: Circulating levels of biologically active brain natriuretic peptide (BNP) and its biologically inert precursor N-terminal peptide (NT-ProBNP) are elevated in response to high ventricular filling pressure and have been well established as important diagnostic and prognostic biomarkers among patients with signs and symptoms of overt HF. The success observed demonstrating their value in the clinical context of symptomatic HF has prompted interest in evaluating these biomarkers as screening tools for HF risk. In population studies and cohorts with Stage A/B HF, the addition of either NT-ProBNP or BNP measurements helps refine the predictive capability of traditional clinical risk factors in predicting risk for incident HF hospitalization and mortality, especially in patients with diabetes.[37,44–46] Furthermore, population studies that included cardiac imaging, a high clinical risk score, and an elevated BNP or NT-ProBNP had the ideal predictive characteristics to detect subclinical LVSD, LV hypertrophy, and diastolic dysfunction.[47,48] Whether the improved risk prediction and stratification may alter management strategies and improve patient outcomes remains uncertain. Data suggest that a refined HF risk assessment using NT-ProBNP and clinical risk factors in conjunction with multifaceted collaborative clinical care may reduce the incidence of clinical HF. The St Vincent's Screening to Prevent Heart Failure (STOP-HF) study was designed as a pragmatic, prospective randomized trial to examine the efficacy of a screening program using BNP and collaborative care in an at-risk population in reducing newly diagnosed HF and the prevalence of Stage B HF. The study found that patients randomized to the intervention arm (BNP screening and collaborative care) had a lower incidence of LV dysfunction with or without overt HF (odds ratio [OR], 0.55; 95% CI, 0.37–0.82; $P = 0.003$). This may be mediated by better-coordinated care, increased emphasis on adherence to guideline-recommended treatments and healthy lifestyle behaviors, a higher rate of screening echocardiography, and significantly more prescriptions of renin-angiotensin-aldosterone system (RAAS)-based therapy. Nevertheless, the proportion of patients with diabetes in the study was relatively low (less than 20%). Furthermore, the event rate in the STOP-HF study was relatively low, and whether the lower rate of HF diagnosis will indeed translate to improved clinical outcomes long term compared with standard care practice remains to be determined.

Cardiac troponin: Cardiac troponins are key sarcomeric proteins responsible for the contractile function of cardiac myocytes. Detectable circulating levels, a marker of myocyte necrosis, have long been used in the diagnosis and prognostication of acute coronary syndromes,[49–52] myocarditis,[53] and HF.[54–56] The specificity of cardiac troponin as a biomarker for myocardial necrosis underpins its demonstrated adjunctive utility when added to clinical risk factors for risk stratifying apparent healthy individuals to discriminate those at the highest risk of developing HF.[57–60] Moreover, newer generations of cardiac troponin assays with markedly improved detection sensitivity have resulted in much larger proportions of cohorts tested having detectable levels, allowing analysis of their association with subclinical cardiovascular pathology and subsequent cardiovascular risk across the spectrum of circulating concentrations. For example, in the multiethnic, population-based Dallas Heart Study, detectable levels of high sensitivity troponin T (hs-cTnT; lower detection limit 0.003 ng/mL) were associated with increased LV hypertrophy and LV end-diastolic volume (LVEDV) and modestly reduced LV ejection fraction identified by cardiac magnetic resonance imaging.[57] Higher levels of hs-cTnT were also associated with increased risk of subsequent all-cause mortality from 1.9% (95% CI, 1.5%–2.6%) to 28.4% (95% CI, 21.0%–37.8%) across incrementally higher quartiles of hs-cTnT levels ($P < 0.001$) during a median follow-up of 6.4 years.[57] A separate population-based study focused on older individuals (65 years or older) showed higher baseline hs-cTnT levels, and changes in cTnT levels were significantly associated with incident HF and cardiovascular death[60] (Fig. 15.3). Although the overall predictive value of troponins is independent of the presence of diabetes, the magnitude of the incremental value of troponins in predicting incident HF among patients with diabetes is less defined.[61]

As different biomarkers may reflect specific and different pathophysiological pathways contributing to myocardial damage, incorporating multiple such biomarkers in risk prediction models may further improve risk prediction

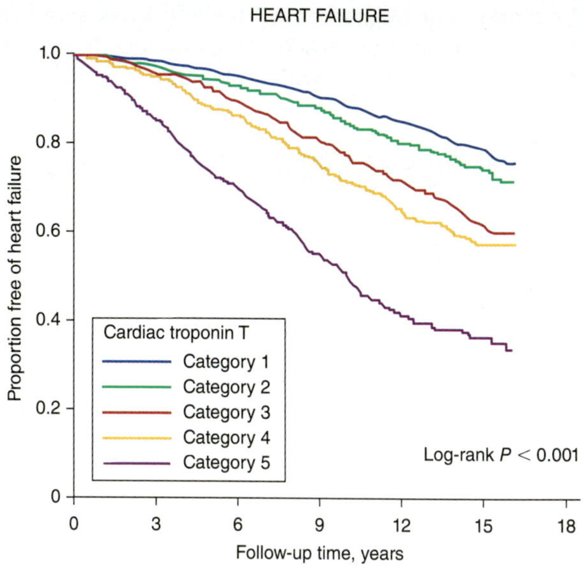

No. at risk							
Category 1	1427	1380	1281	1131	956	763	461
Category 2	697	658	586	508	401	291	169
Category 3	700	642	550	435	333	231	131
Category 4	697	628	505	377	272	176	99
Category 5	700	532	357	213	119	77	36

FIG. 15.3 Association of serial measures of cardiac troponin T using a sensitive assay with incident heart failure and cardiovascular mortality in older adults. Categories of cardiac troponin T concentrations were divided into category 1 (<3.00 pg/mL), category 2 (3.00–5.44 pg/mL), category 3 (5.45–8.16 pg/mL), category 4 (8.17–12.94 pg/mL), and category 5 (>12.94 pg/mL). From deFilippi CR, et al. Association of serial measures of cardiac troponin T using a sensitive assay with incident heart failure and cardiovascular mortality in older adults. *JAMA*. 2010;304(22):2494–2502.

beyond that obtained using individual biomarker predictors.[62–64] Before such strategies can easily be incorporated into practice, more data on the cost-effectiveness and the impact of biomarker-based screening strategies on clinical outcomes will be needed.

Multimarker approach to risk prediction: Studies have evaluated a multimarker approach to predict HF risk among individuals with type 2 DM. The presence of elevated cardiac biomarkers of hs-TnT or NT-ProBNP with LV hypertrophy, a phenotype referred to as malignant LV hypertrophy, identifies a very high-risk subgroup for HF.[65–67] In a pooled analysis from multiple community-based cohort studies, an integer-based biomarker score was developed combining hs-TnT, natriuretic peptides, CRP, and LV hypertrophy.[68] The abnormal elevation in two or more biomarkers identified high-risk individuals with an elevated risk of HF on follow-up. Furthermore, the performance of the biomarker-based risk score was comparable to that of clinical risk factors. More recently, in the CANVAS trial in persons with type 2 DM, a panel of three biomarkers, hs-TnT, sST2, and IGFBP-7, also identified individuals with an elevated risk of adverse CV outcomes, including HF.[69] Furthermore, recent studies have also demonstrated the usefulness of combining biomarkers with clinical risk scores to optimize risk prediction performance.[70,71] Specifically, the addition of biomarker testing, specifically natriuretic peptides, to individuals with low/intermediate risk based on clinical risk scores has been shown to improve risk prediction performance.[70,71] Future studies are needed to determine whether such approaches to risk prediction combining multiple biomarkers or biomarkers with clinical risk scores may be feasible and effective in allocating evidence-based therapies to high-risk individuals with type 2 DM.

STRATEGIES FOR RISK MODIFICATION

The goal of the primary prevention of HF in patients with diabetes is to minimize adverse cardiac remodeling by reducing the risk of myocardial necrosis or stressors. This can be achieved by directly addressing prevalent risk factors among patients with diabetes, such as coronary heart disease, hypertension, dyslipidemia, and obesity. Specific pharmacological agents indicated for other diabetes micro- and macrovascular complications might offer a parallel reduction in the risk of incident HF, in addition to their primary indications. Direct evidence on the efficacy of HF preventive measures are now emerging for SGLT2i and GLP-1RA. Besides these therapies, most of other recommendations are based on either (1) observational data on associations of certain risk factors with the risk of HF or (2) secondary endpoints of randomized controlled trials where incident HF has been inconsistently measured and often lacks adequate statistical power to detect true efficacy. Lastly, special considerations on the diabetes treatment regimens among patients at risk of developing HF are warranted and will be briefly reviewed here.

OPTIMAL MANAGEMENT OF CARDIOVASCULAR RISK FACTORS TO MITIGATE HEART FAILURE RISK IN DIABETES MELLITUS

The conventional approach to preventing HF in diabetes focused on aggressive modification of traditional HF risk factors such as ischemic heart disease, hypertension, and glycemic control. Recently, there have been advances in the preventive approach to HF, with studies evaluating the role of aggressive lifestyle intervention, weight loss surgeries, and specific pharmacotherapies for HF prevention.

Ischemic heart disease: In addition to the initial ischemic insult caused by an episode of acute MI, patients with diabetes are at risk of recurrent ischemic events, which may lead to HF. Therapies aimed at reducing post-MI adverse remodeling and future MIs will likely lead to a lower risk of HF development.

The RAAS is activated immediately post-MI. Angiotensin II plays a key role in the early remodeling of the infarct area and mediates fibrosis via aldosterone and fibrotic pathways such as transforming growth factor β (TGF-β), connective tissue growth factor, and tissue inhibitor of matrix metalloproteinase (MMP) 1. One of the first studies to demonstrate the cardiac protection effect of angiotensin-converting enzymes (ACE) inhibitors in post-MI patients with LVSD was the SAVE (the Survival and Ventricular Enlargement) trial.[72] This study showed that long-term administration of captopril among post-MI patients with LV ejection fraction (LVEF) < 40% was associated with a significant reduction in all-cause mortality, risk of recurrent MI, and incidence of severe HF (relative risk reduction of 34%).[72] In a subgroup analysis, the point estimate of risk reduction among patients with diabetes was consistent with the main study. However, due to the relatively smaller sample size and the lack of statistical power, the treatment difference within the diabetes subset was not statistically significant.[72,73] This finding was confirmed by the SOLVD (Studies of Left Ventricular Dysfunction) prevention trial, which enrolled 4228 patients with an LVEF of less than 35%, of whom 83% had an MI more than 30 days from entry. The study showed that treatment with enalapril (up to 20 mg once per day) significantly reduced the incidence of progression to overt HF and the rate of related hospitalizations.[74] In the echocardiography substudy of the SOLVD-prevention trial, enalapril was associated with less LV dilatation and hypertrophy in patients with Stage B HF.[75] Similarly, subgroup analysis of the SOLVD-prevention study showed that the presence of diabetes was associated with an adverse prognosis. However, the treatment effect of enalapril and its impact on incident HF was similar across the patient's risk profile, including the history of diabetes.[76] In congruence with other studies, the TRACE study showed that treatment with trandolopril in the subset of enrolled patients with diabetes (237/1749 patients; 14%) was associated with a lower risk of progression to severe HF (RR, 0.38; 95% CI, 0.21–0.67), but no significant reduction of this endpoint was seen in the nondiabetic group.[77] Similarly, in the GISSI-3 trial, treatment with lisinopril versus a placebo was evaluated in patients with acute MI, and the magnitude of relative risk reduction for all-cause mortality at 6 weeks favoring lisinopril was greatest in the subset of patients with versus without diabetes (Fig. 15.4).[78] In contrast, treatment with lisinopril versus a placebo was not statistically different in either subgroup stratified by diabetes status for the combined endpoint of mortality and LV dysfunction morbidity [defined as (1) clinical HF, (2) asymptomatic LVEF of ≤35%, or (3) LVEF > 35% but with ≥45% injured myocardial segments evaluated by 2D echocardiography] with diabetes: 21.6% versus 24.5% (OR, 0.85; 95% CI, 0.71–1.01); and without diabetes: 14.3% versus 15.5% (OR, 0.91; 95% CI, 0.83–1.00) (Fig. 15.5). The apparent paradox compared to the primary endpoint of mortality could be explained by the lower mortality during the acute phase in patients treated with lisinopril, which consequently leads to a remnant burden of morbidity for post-MI LVSD among survivors.

Hypertension: Hypertension often coexists with diabetes and visceral adiposity and represents a major risk factor for both macro- and microvascular complications, including an increased risk of incident HF among patients with diabetes (see also Chapter 18). Untreated hypertension accelerates the progression of atherosclerosis, and chronic pressure overload leads to maladaptive LV hypertrophy, diastolic dysfunction, subendocardial ischemia due to impaired microvascular perfusion, and in some cases LV systolic dysfunction ensues. As such, appropriate hypertension management is a key treatment goal in improving the overall clinical outcomes of patients with diabetes and specifically preventing progression to HF.

The United Kingdom Prospective Diabetes Study Group (UKPDS) compared more intensive blood pressure control (<150/85 mm Hg) with lesser control of blood pressure

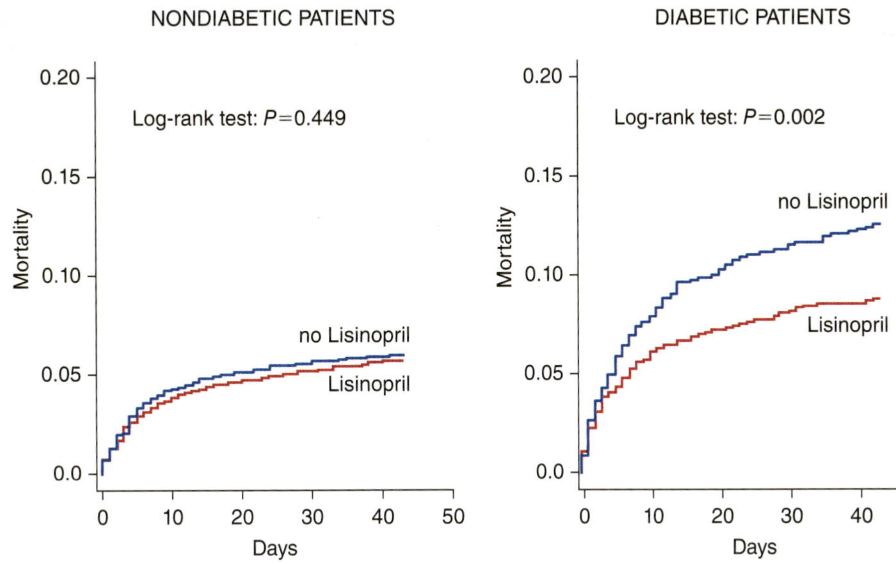

FIG. 15.4 Differential effects of lisinopril compared to placebo on all-cause mortality in patients with or without diabetes mellitus. From Zuanetti G, et al. Effect of the ACE inhibitor lisinopril on mortality in diabetic patients with acute myocardial infarction: data from the GISSI-3 study. *Circulation*. 1997;96(12):4239–4245.

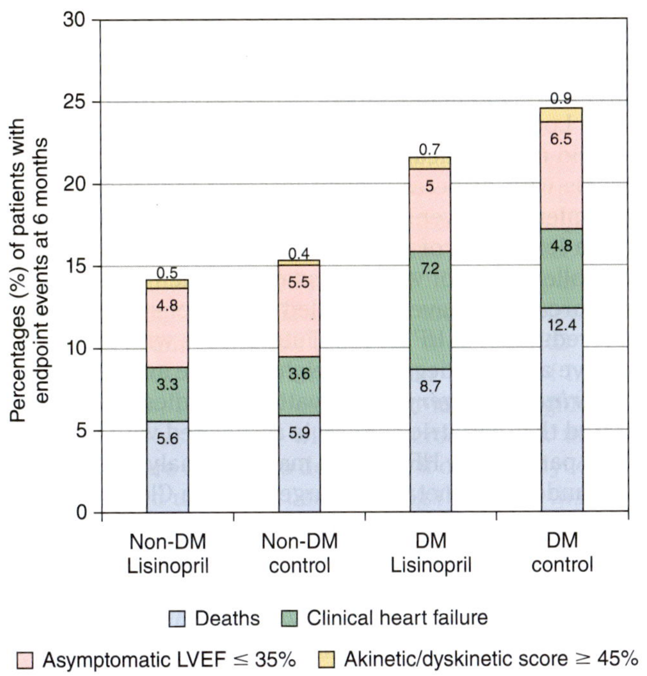

FIG. 15.5 Effect of the ACE inhibitor lisinopril on mortality and secondary endpoints in diabetic (DM) and nondiabetic (Non-DM) patients with acute myocardial infarction at 6 months follow-up. Data from Zuanetti G, et al. Effect of the ACE inhibitor lisinopril on mortality in diabetic patients with acute myocardial infarction: data from the GISSI-3 study. *Circulation*. 1997;96(12):4239–4245.

(<180/105 mm Hg) in 1148 patients with newly diagnosed type 2 diabetes and hypertension.[79] Over a median follow-up period of approximately 10 years, more intensive blood pressure (BP) control decreased the risk of developing HF (hazard ratio 0.44; 95% CI 0.2–0.94, $P = 0.0043$).

Despite the benefits associated with the treatment of hypertension among patients with diabetes, the ideal target BP remains debatable. In the ACCORD-Blood pressure trial, intensive control of BP (systolic BP < 120 mm Hg) was not associated with a lower risk of HF compared with standard control (systolic BP < 140 mm Hg) in patients with diabetes and high cardiovascular risk.[80] In an individual-level metanalysis of 24,444 patients with diabetes, intensive BP lowering was associated with a lower risk of all-cause death, MI, and stroke, but not HF.[81] More recently, in the CHINA trial that included patients with and without diabetes, intensive BP control was associated with a significant reduction in risk of MACE and HF in the overall cohort with comparable treatment effects across the diabetes strata.[82] Similarly, in the recently published BPROAD (Intensive Blood Pressure Control in Patients with Type-2 Diabetes) trial of 12,821 participants with type 2 DM intensive BP control (vs. standard control: target systolic BP < 120 mm Hg systolic vs. <140 mm Hg) was associated with clinically meaningful 19% reduction in the risk of composite endpint of nonfatal stroke, nonfatal-MI, HF hospitalization, or cardiovascular death (HR 0.79; 95% CI, 0.69–0.90, $P < 0.001$).[83] The American Diabetes Association and ACC/AHA recommend a risk-based approach to BP reduction in patients with diabetes.[84] For individuals with a 10-year estimated ASCVD risk of <15%, a blood pressure target of <140/90 mm Hg is recommended.[84] In contrast, for individuals with diabetes and prevalent cardiovascular disease or a 10-year estimated risk of atherosclerotic cardiovascular disease ≥15%, the recommended BP target is <130/90.

The role of specific anti-HTN therapies in preventing HF among individuals with type 2 DM has been studied previously. The UKPDS demonstrated that captopril and atenolol were comparably efficacious in reducing the risk of HF and other diabetes-related complications. The role of angiotensin receptor blocker (ARB), losartan, in reducing the risk of incident HF hospitalization among patients with diabetes was reported from analyses of the patients with diabetes enrolled in two randomized trials: (i) the LIFE (Losartan Intervention For Endpoint reduction in hypertension) trial enrolling patients with hypertension and LV hypertrophy[85,86] and (ii) the RENAAL (Reduction of Endpoints in NIDDM with the Angiotensin II Antagonist Losartan) trial of patients with diabetic nephropathy.[85,87] Although the RENAAL trial enrolled patients with

outcome trial of pioglitazone, the PROspective pioglitAzone Clinical Trial In macroVascular Events (PROACTIVE) study, which enrolled patients with a long duration of diabetes and prevalent cardiovascular disease. In this high-risk population, edema was observed in 27.4% of pioglitazone-treated patients compared with 15.9% of the placebo-treated patients ($P < 0.001$).[140,141] Similar trends were also observed with rosiglitazone, with edema observed in 4.8% of patients treated with rosiglitazone alone compared with 1.3% on a placebo in randomized trials with rosiglitazone.[30] A higher incidence of edema has been observed with rosiglitazone use in combination with metformin or sulfonylurea (3%–4%) than with either comparator drug alone (1.1%–2.2%).[30] Similarly, concomitant use of insulin was associated with higher rates of edema, with 13.1% and 16.2% rosiglitazone 4 or 8 mg per day, respectively, compared with 4.7% in those taking insulin alone.[142]

Pioglitazone and rosiglitazone also increase the risk of HF, as has been observed in patients with diabetes participating in major outcome trials designed to assess the cardiovascular safety of TZDs. In the PROACTIVE trial, a significantly higher proportion of patients in the pioglitazone versus placebo arm had an HF event (11% vs. 8%; $P < 0.0001$). Of these HF events, more pioglitazone than placebo patients (5.7% vs. 4.1%) had serious HF, defined by a requirement for hospitalization or prolonged hospital stay; was fatal or life threatening; or resulted in persistent, significant disability or incapacity ($P = 0.007$). It is important to highlight that HF events were not prespecified endpoints in the PROACTIVE study but were detected as part of standard adverse event reporting. Subsequently, the HF risk was confirmed through adjudication of these safety events.[143] Similarly, in the RECORD study, rosiglitazone use was associated with an increased risk of HF hospitalization.[144] HF-related hospitalization or mortality occurred in 61 people in the rosiglitazone group and 29 in the active control group (HR, 2.10; 1.35–3.27; risk difference per 1000 person-years 2.6; 1.1–4.1) (Fig. 15.7).

The mechanistic and causal relationship between TZDs and incident HF remains unclear. However, it is generally accepted that this is predominantly mediated by the effect of TZDs on increased fluid retention; hence, unmasking underlying LV dysfunction (either diastolic or systolic), rather than direct cardiotoxicity. Nonetheless, clinicians should not discount the clinical significance of such events, as patients who developed HF events experienced high mortality rates (approximately 30%) during the follow-up period.[145]

Earlier observations and findings from the PROACTIVE and RECORD trials support the recommendations from the AHA and American Diabetes Association advising clinicians to assess individual patient's risks prior to commencing TZDs (see Table 15.1) and to discontinue TZDs use in patients with symptomatic HF.[30] More importantly, the experiences from TZDs highlighted the pitfall of relying on intermediate markers, such as HbA1c, in assessing the clinical effectiveness of glucose-lowering agents in the risk of macrovascular complications.

Dipeptidyl peptidase (DPP)-4 inhibitors: DPP-4 inhibitors (saxagliptin, sitagliptin, linagliptin, alogliptin, and vildagliptin) potentiate endogenous action of glucagon-like peptide (GLP)-1 by inhibiting its enzymatic degradation by DPP-4. Once-daily tablets with low risk for hypoglycemia, DPP-4 inhibitors are increasingly used for glycemic control and have generally been considered safe regarding cardiovascular risk based on the absence of adverse cardiovascular signals from Phase I–IIIa trials.

The Saxagliptin Assessment of Vascular Outcomes Recorded in Patients with Diabetes Mellitus (SAVOR) TIMI 53 trial enrolled over 16,000 patients with type 2 DM with or at increased risk of cardiovascular disease complications, evaluating randomized blinded treatment with

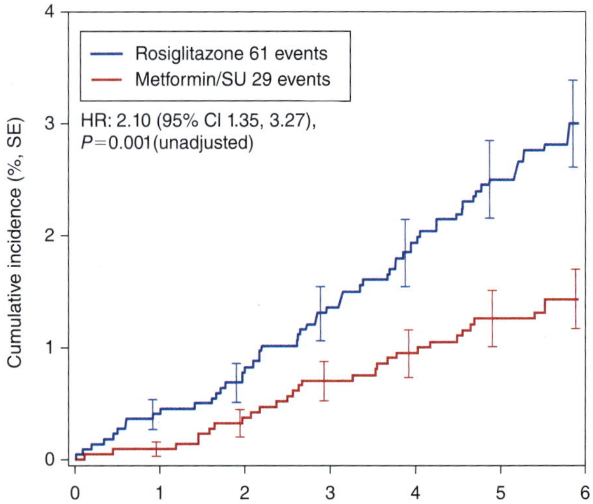

FIG. 15.7 Kaplan–Meier plots of time to heart failure (fatal or nonfatal) in the RECORD study (intent-to-treat analysis). *HR*, hazard ratio; *CI*, confidence interval; *SE*, Standard error. From Komajda M, et al. Heart failure events with rosiglitazone in type 2 diabetes: data from the RECORD clinical trial. *Eur Heart J*. 2010;317:824–831.

TABLE 15.1 Risk Factors Associated With Increased Risk of Heart Failure in Diabetic Patients Treated With Thiazolidinediones (*TZDs*)

RISK FACTORS FOR HEART FAILURE IN PATIENTS TREATED WITH TZDS
History of heart failure (either systolic or diastolic)
History of prior myocardial infarction or symptomatic coronary artery disease
Hypertension
Left ventricular hypertrophy
Significant aortic or mitral valve heart disease
Advanced age (>70 years)
Long-standing diabetes (>10 years)
Preexisting edema or current treatment with loop diuretics
Development of edema or weight gain on TZD therapy
Insulin coadministration
Chronic renal failure (creatinine > 2.0 mg/dL)

From Nesto RW, et al. Thiazolidinedione use, fluid retention, and congestive heart failure: a consensus statement from the American Heart Association and American Diabetes Association. *Circulation*. 2003;108(23):2941–2948.

saxagliptin versus a placebo with a primary efficacy and safety outcome the composite of cardiovascular death, MI, and stroke. Over a median follow-up of 2.1 years, there was no benefit and no harm detected for the primary major adverse cardiovascular event endpoint, meeting the regulatory threshold to exclude an upper 95% noninferiority confidence limit (HR, 1.00; 95% CI, 0.89–1.12). In the present context, a safety signal of increased risk for adjudicated HF hospitalization, a predefined component of the secondary efficacy endpoint, was observed with saxagliptin (3.5% vs. 2.8%; HR, 1.27, 95% CI, 1.07–1.51; $P = 0.007$).[146] This was an unexpected finding given prior observations of favorable myocardial effects of DPP-4 inhibitors in various HF experimental models.[147–151] The Examination of Cardiovascular Outcomes with Alogliptin versus Standard of Care (EXAMINE) trial evaluated the effects of alogliptin versus a placebo in 5380 patients with type 2 diabetes and a recent acute coronary syndrome event, and similar to SAVOR, demonstrated noninferiority with regard to the same three-point MACE primary outcomes (HR, 0.96; 95% UCL, 1.16) over a median follow-up of 18 months.[152] In preliminary post hoc analyses (unpublished), a numerical increase in hospitalized HF events was observed in the alogliptin group, though this difference did not achieve statistical significance (3.9% vs. 3.3%; HR, 1.19; 95% CI, 0.89–1.58). No systematic assessment of cardiac structure or function was performed in either of these two clinical trials and the mechanism underlying the potential increased risk of HF with DPP-4 is not clear. Moreover, the TECOS and CAREMELINA trials were prospective cardiovascular outcomes trials to evaluate the safety of sitagliptin and linagliptin, respectively, and robustly excluded an increased risk of HF with the use of these DPP-4 inhibitors.[153,154]

Insulin: The relationship between insulin use and the risk of incident HF is unclear. Mechanistically, acute insulin administration is associated with fluid retention, potentially mediated by increased renal sodium retention caused by insulin,[155] and may theoretically contribute to overt HF among at-risk patients. Furthermore, chronic insulin administration is associated with weight gain and obesity, a known risk factor for incident HF. However, data from prospective randomized trials are largely lacking, except for the Outcome Reduction with an Initial Glargine Intervention (ORIGIN) trial that assessed the cardiovascular effects of insulin glargine versus usual care in patients with early diabetes or prediabetic impaired glucose metabolism. ORIGIN randomized individuals older than 50 years with prediabetes or diabetes and cardiovascular risk factors to receive insulin glargine or standard care. HF hospitalization was a prespecified component of the secondary composite endpoint. At a median follow-up of 6.2 years (interquartile range, 5.8–6.7), there was no statistical difference in the risk of HF hospitalization between the study groups (HR, 0.90; 95% CI, 0.77–1.05; $P = 0.16$).[156] Moreover, in the Trial Comparing Cardiovascular Safety of Insulin Degludec versus Insulin Glargine in Patients With Type 2 Diabetes at High Risk of Cardiovascular Events (DEVOTE), the ultra-long-acting insulin degludac was noninferior to insulin glargine and did not increase the risk for HF hospitalization (HR, 0.88; 95% CI, 0.72–1.08; $P = 0.23$).[157,158]

CHALLENGES IN PREVENTION OF HEART FAILURE AND FUTURE DIRECTIONS

Preventing HF is a public health priority, and creating strategies to detect and treat patients at risk for HF will be critical. Recognition of major risk factors such as diabetes is important. However, much work remains to be done to implement the best strategies to identify patients to prevent them from progressing to Stage B (asymptomatic with left ventricular dysfunction) or Stage C/D (symptomatic HF). Moving forward, prevention strategies in the population with diabetes will likely require multidimensional efforts, including managing hyperglycemia, effective implementation of lifestyle interventions to promote exercise and weight loss, treatment of other cardiometabolic conditions that tend to cluster with DM, and use of therapies such as SGLT-2 inhibitors and GLP-1 agonists that meaningfully reduce the risk of major adverse cardiovascular events. Furthermore, as newer effective treatments emerge for modifying cardiovascular disease risk in DM, there is also a need for developing effective implementation strategies to promote the utilization of these therapies in optimal combinations in the real world.

REFERENCES

1. Martin SS, et al. Heart disease and stroke statistics: A report of US and Global Data From the American Heart Association. *Circulation.* 2025;151(8): e41–e660.
2. Bozkurt B, et al. Heart failure epidemiology and outcomes statistics: A report of the heart failure society of america. *J Card Fail.* 2023;29(10): 1412–1451.
3. Savarese G, et al. Cardiovasc Res. 2023;118(17):3272–3287.
4. Ostrominski JW, et al. Prevalence and overlap of cardiac, renal, and metabolic conditions in US Adults, 1999–2020. *JAMA Cardiol.* 2023;8(11):1050–1060.
5. Rawshani A, et al. Risk factors, mortality, and cardiovascular outcomes in patients with type 2 diabetes. *N Engl J Med.* 2018;379(7):633–644.
6. Gottdiener JS, et al. Predictors of congestive heart failure in the elderly: the Cardiovascular Health Study. *J Am Coll Cardiol.* 2000;35(6):1628–1637.
7. He J, et al. Risk factors for congestive heart failure in US men and women: NHANES I epidemiologic follow-up study. *Arch Intern Med.* 2001;161(7):996–1002.
8. Kannel WB, Hjortland M, Castelli WP. Role of diabetes in congestive heart failure: the Framingham study. *Am J Cardiol.* 1974;34(1):29–34.
9. Khera R, et al. Temporal trends in heart failure incidence among medicare beneficiaries across risk factor strata, 2011 to 2016. *JAMA Network Open.* 2020;3(10): e2022190-e2022190.
10. Ho JE, et al. Predicting heart failure with preserved and reduced ejection fraction: the International Collaboration on Heart Failure Subtypes. *Circ Heart Fail.* 2016;9(6).
11. Pandey A, et al. Sex and race differences in lifetime risk of heart failure with preserved ejection fraction and heart failure with reduced ejection fraction. *Circulation.* 2018;137(17):1814–1823.
12. Honigberg Michael C, et al. Cardiovascular and kidney outcomes across the glycemic spectrum. *J. Am. Coll. Cardiol.* 2021;78(5):453–464.
13. Nichols GA, et al. The incidence of congestive heart failure in type 2 diabetes: an update. *Diabetes Care.* 2004;27(8):1879–1884.
14. Stratton IM, et al. Association of glycaemia with macrovascular and microvascular complications of type 2 diabetes (UKPDS 35): prospective observational study. *Bmj.* 2000;321(7258):405–412.
15. Iribarren C, et al. Glycemic control and heart failure among adult patients with diabetes. *Circulation.* 2001;103(22):2668–2673.
16. Vaur L, et al. Development of congestive heart failure in type 2 diabetic patients with microalbuminuria or proteinuria: observations from the DIABHYCAR (type 2 DIABetes, Hypertension, CArdiovascular Events and Ramipril) study. *Diabetes Care.* 2003;26(3):855–860.
17. Honigberg MC, et al. Trends in hospitalizations for heart failure and ischemic heart disease among US adults with diabetes. *JAMA Cardiol.* 2021;6(3):354–357.
18. Hunt SA, et al. ACC/AHA guidelines for the evaluation and management of chronic heart failure in the adult: executive summary. A Report of the American College of Cardiology/American Heart Association Task Force on Practice Guidelines (Committee to revise the 1995 Guidelines for the Evaluation and Management of Heart Failure). *Circulation.* 2001;104(24):2996–3007.
19. Stark Casagrande S, et al. The prevalence of meeting A1C, blood pressure, and LDL goals among people with diabetes, 1988–2010. *Diabetes Care.* 2013.

20. Ammar KA, et al. Prevalence and prognostic significance of heart failure stages: application of the American College of Cardiology/American Heart Association heart failure staging criteria in the community. *Circulation*. 2007;115(12):1563–1570.
21. Abhayaratna WP, et al. Prevalence of heart failure and systolic ventricular dysfunction in older Australians: the Canberra Heart Study. *Med J Aust*. 2006;184(4):151–154.
22. Wang TJ, et al. Natural history of asymptomatic left ventricular systolic dysfunction in the community. *Circulation*. 2003;108(8):977–982.
23. Redfield MM, et al. Burden of systolic and diastolic ventricular dysfunction in the community: appreciating the scope of the heart failure epidemic. *JAMA*. 2003;289(2):194–202.
24. Devereux RB, et al. A population-based assessment of left ventricular systolic dysfunction in middle-aged and older adults: the Strong Heart Study. *Am Heart J*. 2001;141(3):439–446.
25. Davies M, et al. Prevalence of left-ventricular systolic dysfunction and heart failure in the Echocardiographic Heart of England Screening study: a population based study. *Lancet*. 2001;358(9280):439–444.
26. Mosterd A, et al. Prevalence of heart failure and left ventricular dysfunction in the general population; The Rotterdam Study. *Eur Heart J*. 1999;20(6):447–455.
27. Schunkert H, et al. Left-ventricular dysfunction. *Lancet*. 1998;351(9099):372.
28. McDonagh TA, et al. Symptomatic and asymptomatic left-ventricular systolic dysfunction in an urban population. *Lancet*. 1997;350(9081):829–833.
29. Gardin JM, et al. Sex, age, and disease affect echocardiographic left ventricular mass and systolic function in the free-living elderly. The Cardiovascular Health Study. *Circulation*. 1995;91(6):1739–1748.
30. Nesto RW, et al. Thiazolidinedione use, fluid retention, and congestive heart failure: a consensus statement from the American Heart Association and American Diabetes Association. October 7, 2003. *Circulation*. 2003;108(23):2941–2948.
31. Lam CSP, et al. Cardiac dysfunction and noncardiac dysfunction as precursors of heart failure with reduced and preserved ejection fraction in the community. *Circulation*. 2011;124(1):24–30.
32. Bibbins-Domingo K, et al. Racial differences in incident heart failure among young adults. *N Engl J Med*. 2009;360(12):1179–1190.
33. Segar Matthew W, et al. Prevalence and prognostic implications of diabetes with cardiomyopathy in community-dwelling adults. *Journal of the American College of Cardiology*. 2021;78(16):1587–1598.
34. Januzzi Jr. JL, et al. Randomized trial of a selective aldose reductase inhibitor in patients with diabetic cardiomyopathy. *J Am Coll Cardiol*. 2024;84(2):137–148.
35. Kannel WB, et al. Profile for estimating risk of heart failure. *Arch Intern Med*. 1999;159(11):1197–1204.
36. Butler J, et al. Incident heart failure prediction in the elderly: the health ABC heart failure score. *Circ Heart Fail*. 2008;1(2):125–133.
37. Kalogeropoulos A, et al. Validation of the health ABC heart failure model for incident heart failure risk prediction: the Cardiovascular Health Study. *Circ Heart Fail*. 2010;3(4):495–502.
38. Khan SS, et al. 10-Year risk equations for incident heart failure in the general population. *J Am Coll Cardiol*. 2019;73(19):2388–2397.
39. Segar MW, et al. Machine learning to predict the risk of incident heart failure hospitalization among patients with diabetes: the WATCH-DM risk score. *Diabetes Care*. 2019;42(12):2298–2306.
40. Berg DD, et al. Heart failure risk stratification and efficacy of sodium-glucose cotransporter-2 inhibitors in patients with type 2 diabetes mellitus. *Circulation*. 2019;140(19):1569–1577.
41. Vaduganathan M, et al. Prescriber patterns of SGLT2i after expansions of U.S. Food and Drug Administration labeling. *J Am Coll Cardiol*. 2018;72(25):3370–3372.
42. McEvoy JW, et al. Six-year change in high-sensitivity cardiac troponin T and risk of subsequent coronary heart disease, heart failure, and death. *JAMA Cardiol*. 2016;1(5):519–528.
43. Pandey A, et al. Incorporation of biomarkers into risk assessment for allocation of antihypertensive medication according to the 2017 ACC/AHA high blood pressure guideline. *Circulation*. 2019;140(25):2076–2088.
44. McKie PM, et al. The prognostic value of N-terminal pro-B-type natriuretic peptide for death and cardiovascular events in healthy normal and stage A/B heart failure subjects. *J Am Coll Cardiol*. 2010;55(19):2140–2147.
45. Onodera M, et al. Plasma B-type natriuretic peptide is useful for cardiovascular risk assessment in community-based diabetes subjects: comparison with albuminuria. *Int Heart J*. 2012;53(3):176–181.
46. Wang TJ, et al. Plasma natriuretic peptide levels and the risk of cardiovascular events and death. *N Engl J Med*. 2004;350(7):655–663.
47. Gupta S, et al. Risk scores versus natriuretic peptides for identifying prevalent stage B heart failure. *Am Heart J*. 2011;161(5):923–930. e2.
48. McGrady M, et al. N-terminal B-type natriuretic peptide and the association with left ventricular diastolic function in a population at high risk of incident heart failure: results of the SCReening Evaluationof the Evolution of New-Heart Failure Study (SCREEN-HF). *Eur J Heart Fail*. 2013;15(5):573–580.
49. Thygesen K, et al. Third universal definition of myocardial infarction. *J Am Coll Cardiol*. 2012;60(16):1581–1598.
50. Reichlin T, et al. Early diagnosis of myocardial infarction with sensitive cardiac troponin assays. *N Engl J Med*. 2009;361(9):858–867.
51. Keller T, et al. Sensitive troponin I assay in early diagnosis of acute myocardial infarction. *N Engl J Med*. 2009;361(9):868–877.
52. Newby LK, et al. Frequency and clinical implications of discordant creatine kinase-MB and troponin measurements in acute coronary syndromes. *J Am Coll Cardiol*. 2006;47(2):312–318.
53. Lauer B, et al. Cardiac troponin T in patients with clinically suspected myocarditis. *J Am Coll Cardiol*. 1997;30(5):1354–1359.
54. Peacock WFt, et al. Cardiac troponin and outcome in acute heart failure. *N Engl J Med*. 2008;358(20):2117–2126.
55. Del Carlo CH, et al. Serial measure of cardiac troponin T levels for prediction of clinical events in decompensated heart failure. *J Card Fail*. 2004;10(1):43–48.
56. Latini R, et al. Prognostic value of very low plasma concentrations of troponin T in patients with stable chronic heart failure. *Circulation*. 2007;116(11):1242–1249.
57. de Lemos JA, et al. Association of troponin T detected with a highly sensitive assay and cardiac structure and mortality risk in the general population. *JAMA*. 2010;304(22):2503–2512.
58. Saunders JT, et al. Cardiac troponin T measured by a highly sensitive assay predicts coronary heart disease, heart failure, and mortality in the Atherosclerosis Risk in Communities Study. *Circulation*. 2011;123(13):1367–1376.
59. Sundstrom J, et al. Cardiac troponin-I and risk of heart failure: a community-based cohort study. *Eur Heart J*. 2009;30(7):773–781.
60. deFilippi CR, et al. Association of serial measures of cardiac troponin T using a sensitive assay with incident heart failure and cardiovascular mortality in older adults. *JAMA*. 2010;304(22):2494–2502.
61. Hallen J, et al. Determinants and prognostic implications of cardiac troponin T measured by a sensitive assay in type 2 diabetes mellitus. *Cardiovasc Diabetol*. 2010;9:52.
62. Velagaleti RS, et al. Multimarker approach for the prediction of heart failure incidence in the community. *Circulation*. 2010;122(17):1700–1706.
63. Nambi V, et al. Troponin T and N-terminal pro-B-type natriuretic peptide: a biomarker approach to predict heart failure risk–the atherosclerosis risk in communities study. *Clin Chem*. 2013;59(12):1802–1810.
64. de Antonio M, et al. Combined use of high-sensitivity cardiac troponin T and N-terminal pro-B type natriuretic peptide improves measurements of performance over established mortality risk factors in chronic heart failure. *Am Heart J*. 2012;163(5):821–828.
65. Pandey A, et al. Association of cardiac injury and malignant left ventricular hypertrophy with risk of heart failure in African Americans: The Jackson Heart Study. *JAMA Cardiol*. 2019;4(1):51–58.
66. Neeland IJ, et al. Biomarkers of chronic cardiac injury and hemodynamic stress identify a malignant phenotype of left ventricular hypertrophy in the general population. *J Am Coll Cardiol*. 2013;61(2):187–195.
67. Seliger SL, et al. Older adults, "malignant" left ventricular hypertrophy, and associated cardiac-specific biomarker phenotypes to identify the differential risk of new-onset reduced versus preserved ejection fraction heart failure: CHS (Cardiovascular Health Study). *JACC Heart Fail*. 2015;3(6):445–455.
68. Pandey A, et al. Biomarker-based risk prediction of incident heart failure in pre-diabetes and diabetes. *JACC Heart Fail*. 2021;9(3):215–223.
69. Vaduganathan M, et al. Stress cardiac biomarkers, cardiovascular and renal outcomes, and response to canagliflozin. *J Am College Cardiol*. 2022;79(5):432–444.
70. Patel KV, et al. Optimal screening for predicting and preventing the risk of heart failure among adults with diabetes without atherosclerotic cardiovascular disease: A pooled cohort analysis. *Circulation*. 2024;149(4):293–304.
71. Segar MW, et al. Incorporation of natriuretic peptides with clinical risk scores to predict heart failure among individuals with dysglycaemia. *Eur J Heart Fail*. 2022;24(1):169–180.
72. Pfeffer MA, et al. Effect of captopril on progressive ventricular dilatation after anterior myocardial infarction. *N Engl J Med*. 1988;319(2):80–86.
73. Moye LA, et al. Uniformity of captopril benefit in the SAVE Study: subgroup analysis. Survival and Ventricular Enlargement Study. *Eur Heart J*. 1994;15(Suppl B):2–8; discussion 26-30.
74. Effect of enalapril on mortality. and the development of heart failure in asymptomatic patients with reduced left ventricular ejection fractions. The SOLVD Investigattors. *N Engl J Med*. 1992;327(10):685–691.
75. Greenberg B, et al. Effects of long-term enalapril therapy on cardiac structure and function in patients with left ventricular dysfunction. Results of the SOLVD echocardiography substudy. *Circulation*. 1995;91(10):2573–2581.
76. Parker AB, Yusuf S, Naylor CD. The relevance of subgroup-specific treatment effects: the Studies Of Left Ventricular Dysfunction (SOLVD) revisited. *Am Heart J*. 2002;144(6):941–947.
77. Gustafsson I, et al. Effect of the angiotensin-converting enzyme inhibitor trandolapril on mortality and morbidity in diabetic patients with left ventricular dysfunction after acute myocardial infarction. Trace Study Group. *J Am Coll Cardiol*. 1999;34(1):83–89.
78. Zuanetti G, et al. Effect of the ACE inhibitor lisinopril on mortality in diabetic patients with acute myocardial infarction: data from the GISSI-3 study. *Circulation*. 1997;96(12):4239–4245.
79. UK Prospective Diabetes Study Group Tight blood pressure control and risk of macrovascular and microvascular complications in type 2 diabetes: UKPDS 38.. *BMJ*. 1998;317(7160):703–713.
80. ACCORD Study Group et al. Effects of intensive blood-pressure control in type 2 diabetes mellitus. *N Engl J Med*. 2010;362(17):1575–1585.
81. Wang J, et al. Effects of intensive blood pressure lowering on mortality and cardiovascular and renal outcomes in type 2 diabetic patients: a meta-analysis. *PLoS One*. 2019;14(4):e0215362.
82. Zhang W, et al. Trial of intensive blood-pressure control in older patients with hypertension. *N Engl J Med*. 2021;385(14):1268–1279.
83. Bi Y, et al. Intensive blood-pressure control in patients with type 2 diabetes. *N Engl J Med*. 2025 Mar 27;392(12):1155–1167.

84. American Diabetes Association 10. Cardiovascular disease and risk management: standards of medical care in diabetes—2019. *Diabetes Care.* 2018;42(Suppl 1):S103–S123.
85. Carr AA, et al. Hospitalizations for new heart failure among subjects with diabetes mellitus in the RENAAL and LIFE studies. *Am J Cardiol.* 2005;96(11):1530–1536.
86. Dahlof B, et al. Cardiovascular morbidity and mortality in the Losartan Intervention For Endpoint reduction in hypertension study (LIFE): a randomised trial against atenolol. *Lancet.* 2002;359(9311):995–1003.
87. Brenner BM, et al. Effects of losartan on renal and cardiovascular outcomes in patients with type 2 diabetes and nephropathy. *N Engl J Med.* 2001;345(12):861–869.
88. ALLHAT Officers and Coordinators for the ALLHAT Collaborative Research Group Major Outcomes in high-risk hypertensive patients randomized to angiotensin-converting enzyme inhibitor or calcium channel blocker vs diuretic: The Antihypertensive and Lipid-Lowering Treatment to Prevent Heart Attack Trial (ALLHAT). *JAMA.* 2002;288(23):2981–2997.
89. Pandey A, et al. Dose–response relationship between physical activity and risk of heart failure. *Circulation.* 2015;132(19):1786–1794.
90. Florido R, et al. Physical activity and incident heart failure in high-risk subgroups: the ARIC study. *J Am Heart Assoc.* 2020;9(10):e014885.
91. Jung I, et al. Changes in patterns of physical activity and risk of heart failure in newly diagnosed diabetes mellitus patients. *Diabetes Metabol J.* 2022;46(2):327–336.
92. Pandey A, et al. Relationship between physical activity, body mass index, and risk of heart failure. *J Am Coll Cardiol.* 2017;69(9):1129–1142.
93. Pandey A, et al. Association of intensive lifestyle intervention, fitness, and body mass index with risk of heart failure in overweight or obese adults with type 2 diabetes mellitus. *Circulation.* 2020;141(16):1295–1306.
94. Patel KV, et al. Association of baseline and longitudinal changes in body composition measures with risk of heart failure and myocardial infarction in type 2 diabetes: findings from the look AHEAD trial. *Circulation.* 2020;142(25):2420–2430.
95. Pandey A, et al. Association of intensive lifestyle intervention, fitness, and body mass index with risk of heart failure in overweight or obese adults with type 2 diabetes mellitus: an analysis from the look AHEAD trial. *Circulation.* 2020;141(16):1295–1306.
96. Patel KV, et al. Association of baseline and longitudinal changes in body composition measures with risk of heart failure and myocardial infarction in type 2 diabetes. *Circulation.* 2020;142(25):2420–2430.
97. Patel KV, et al. Diabetes status modifies the association between different measures of obesity and heart failure risk among older adults: a pooled analysis of community-based NHLBI cohorts. *Circulation.* 2022;145(4):268–278.
98. Marso SP, et al. Liraglutide and cardiovascular outcomes in type 2 diabetes. *N Engl J Med.* 2016;375(4):311–322.
99. Bohula EA, et al. Cardiovascular safety of lorcaserin in overweight or obese patients. *N Engl J Med.* 2018;379(12):1107–1117.
100. Aminian A, et al. Association of metabolic surgery with major adverse cardiovascular outcomes in patients with type 2 diabetes and obesity. *JAMA.* 2019;322(13):1271–1282.
101. Sundstrom J, et al. Weight loss and heart failure: a nationwide study of gastric bypass surgery versus intensive lifestyle treatment. *Circulation.* 2017;135(17):1577–1585.
102. Lewis KH, et al. Risk of incident cardiovascular events following Roux en Y gastric bypass versus sleeve gastrectomy: a claims-based retrospective cohort study. *Ann Surg.* 2024
103. Wolff Sagy Y, et al. Effectiveness of bariatric metabolic surgery versus glucagon-like peptide-1 receptor agonists for prevention of congestive heart failure. *Nat Med.* 2024;30(8):2337–2342.
104. American Diabetes A. Standards of medical care in diabetes–2014. *Diabetes Care.* 2014;37(Suppl 1):S14–S80.
105. Hennekens CH, et al. Academic perspectives on the United States Food and Drug Administration's guidance for industry on diabetes mellitus. *Contemp Clin Trials.* 2010;31(5):411–413.
106. Drucker DJ, Goldfine AB. Cardiovascular safety and diabetes drug development. *Lancet.* 2011;377(9770):977–979.
107. Yancy CW, et al. 2013 ACCF/AHA guideline for the management of heart failure: executive summary: a report of the American College of Cardiology Foundation/American Heart Association Task Force on practice guidelines. *Circulation.* 2013;128(16):1810–1852.
108. Authors/Task Force M, et al. ESC Guidelines on diabetes, pre-diabetes, and cardiovascular diseases developed in collaboration with the EASD: the Task Force on diabetes, pre-diabetes, and cardiovascular diseases of the European Society of Cardiology (ESC) and developed in collaboration with the European Association for the Study of Diabetes (EASD). *Eur Heart J.* 2013;34(39):3035–3087.
109. UK Prospective Diabetes Study (UKPDS) Group Intensive blood-glucose control with sulphonylureas or insulin compared with conventional treatment and risk of complications in patients with type 2 diabetes (UKPDS 33). *Lancet.* 1998;352(9131):837–853.
110. Action to Control Cardiovascular Risk in Diabetes Study Effects of intensive glucose lowering in type 2 diabetes. *N Engl J Med.* 2008;358(24):2545–2559.
111. Group AC, et al. Intensive blood glucose control and vascular outcomes in patients with type 2 diabetes. *N Engl J Med.* 2008;358(24):2560–2572.
112. Duckworth W, et al. Glucose control and vascular complications in veterans with type 2 diabetes. *N Engl J Med.* 2009;360(2):129–139.
113. Turnbull FM, et al. Intensive glucose control and macrovascular outcomes in type 2 diabetes. *Diabetologia.* 2009;52(11):2288–2298.
114. Segar MW, et al. Association of long-term change and variability in glycemia with risk of incident heart failure among patients with type 2 diabetes: a secondary analysis of the ACCORD Trial. *Diabetes Care.* 2020;43(8):1920–1928.
115. Zinman B, et al. Empagliflozin, cardiovascular outcomes, and mortality in type 2 diabetes. *N Engl J Med.* 2015;373(22):2117–2128.
116. Neal B, et al. Canagliflozin and cardiovascular and renal events in type 2 diabetes. *N Engl J Med.* 2017;377(7):644–657.
117. Wiviott SD, et al. Dapagliflozin and cardiovascular outcomes in type 2 diabetes. *N Engl J Med.* 2019;380(4):347–357.
118. Bhatt DL, et al. Sotagliflozin in Patients with diabetes and chronic kidney disease. *N Engl J Med.* 2021;384(2):129–139.
119. Cannon CP, et al. Cardiovascular outcomes with ertugliflozin in type 2 diabetes. *N Engl J Med.* 2020;383(15):1425–1435.
120. McGuire DK, et al. Association of SGLT2 Inhibitors with cardiovascular and kidney outcomes in patients with type 2 diabetes: a meta-analysis. *JAMA Cardiol.* 2021;6(2):148–158.
121. Inzucchi SE, et al. How does empagliflozin reduce cardiovascular mortality? Insights from a mediation analysis of the EMPA-REG OUTCOME Trial. *Diabetes Care.* 2017;41(2):356–363.
122. Li J, et al. Mediators of the effects of canagliflozin on heart failure in patients with type 2 diabetes. *JACC: Heart Failure.* 2020;8(1):57–66.
123. Segar MW et al. Mediators of ertugliflozin effects on heart failure and kidney outcomes among patients with type 2 diabetes. *Diabetes Obes Metab.* 2022;24(9):1829-1839.
124. ElSayed NA, et al. 10. Cardiovascular disease and risk management: standards of care in diabetes-2023. *Diabetes Care.* 2023;46(Suppl 1):S158–S190.
125. Marx N, et al. 2023 ESC Guidelines for the management of cardiovascular disease in patients with diabetes. *Eur Heart J.* 2023;44(39):4043–4140.
126. Heidenreich PA, et al. 2022 AHA/ACC/HFSA guideline for the management of heart failure: a report of the American College of Cardiology/American Heart Association Joint Committee on Clinical Practice Guidelines. *J Am Coll Cardiol.* 2022;79(17):e263–e421.
127. Sattar N, et al. Cardiovascular, mortality, and kidney outcomes with GLP-1 receptor agonists in patients with type 2 diabetes: a systematic review and meta-analysis of randomised trials. *Lancet Diabetes Endocrinol.* 2021;9(10):653–662.
128. Hernandez AF, et al. Albiglutide and cardiovascular outcomes in patients with type 2 diabetes and cardiovascular disease (Harmony Outcomes): a double-blind, randomised placebo-controlled trial. *Lancet.* 2018;392(10157):1519–1529.
129. Gerstein HC, et al. Cardiovascular and renal outcomes with efpeglenatide in type 2 diabetes. *N Engl J Med.* 2021;385(10):896–907.
130. Jorsal A, et al. Effect of liraglutide, a glucagon-like peptide-1 analogue, on left ventricular function in stable chronic heart failure patients with and without diabetes (LIVE)-a multicentre, double-blind, randomised, placebo-controlled trial. *Eur J Heart Fail.* 2017;19(1):69–77.
131. Margulies KB, et al. Effects of liraglutide on clinical stability among patients with advanced heart failure and reduced ejection fraction: a randomized clinical trial. *JAMA.* 2016;316(5):500–508.
132. Lepore JJ, et al. Effects of the novel long-acting GLP-1 agonist, albiglutide, on cardiac function, cardiac metabolism, and exercise capacity in patients with chronic heart failure and reduced ejection fraction. *JACC Heart Fail.* 2016;4(7):559–566.
133. Yki-Jarvinen H. Thiazolidinediones. *N Engl J Med.* 2004;351(11):1106–1118.
134. Masoudi FA, et al. Thiazolidinediones, metformin, and outcomes in older patients with diabetes and heart failure: an observational study. *Circulation.* 2005;111(5):583–590.
135. Dargie HJ, et al. A randomized, placebo-controlled trial assessing the effects of rosiglitazone on echocardiographic function and cardiac status in type 2 diabetic patients with New York Heart Association Functional Class I or II Heart Failure. *J Am Coll Cardiol.* 2007;49(16):1696–1704.
136. Delea TE, et al. Use of thiazolidinediones and risk of heart failure in people with type 2 diabetes: a retrospective cohort study. *Diabetes Care.* 2003;26(11):2983–2989.
137. Singh S, Loke YK, Furberg CD. Thiazolidinediones and heart failure: a teleo-analysis. *Diabetes Care.* 2007;30(8):2148–2153.
138. Lago RM, Singh PP, Nesto RW. Congestive heart failure and cardiovascular death in patients with prediabetes and type 2 diabetes given thiazolidinediones: a meta-analysis of randomised clinical trials. *Lancet.* 2007;370(9593):1129–1136.
139. Home PD, et al. Rosiglitazone evaluated for cardiovascular outcomes in oral agent combination therapy for type 2 diabetes (RECORD): a multicentre, randomised, open-label trial. *Lancet.* 2009;373(9681):2125–2135.
140. Holman RR, et al. PROactive study. *Lancet.* 2006;367(9504):25–26. author reply 26-7.
141. Erdmann E, et al. Pioglitazone use and heart failure in patients with type 2 diabetes and preexisting cardiovascular disease: data from the PROactive study (PROactive 08). *Diabetes Care.* 2007;30(11):2773–2778.
142. Raskin P, et al. A randomized trial of rosiglitazone therapy in patients with inadequately controlled insulin-treated type 2 diabetes. *Diabetes Care.* 2001;24(7):1226–1232.
143. Ryden L, Thrainsdottir I, Swedberg K. Adjudication of serious heart failure in patients from PROactive. *Lancet.* 2007;369(9557):189–190.
144. Komajda M, et al. Heart failure events with rosiglitazone in type 2 diabetes: data from the RECORD clinical trial. *Eur Heart J.* 2010;31(7):824–831.
145. Lincoff AM, et al. Pioglitazone and risk of cardiovascular events in patients with type 2 diabetes mellitus: a meta-analysis of randomized trials. *JAMA.* 2007;298(10):1180–1188.

146. Scirica BM, et al. Saxagliptin and cardiovascular outcomes in patients with type 2 diabetes mellitus. *N Engl J Med.* 2013;369(14):1317–1326.
147. Gomez N, et al. Dipeptidyl peptidase IV inhibition improves cardiorenal function in overpacing-induced heart failure. *Eur J Heart Fail.* 2012;14(1):14–21.
148. Shigeta T, et al. Dipeptidyl peptidase-4 modulates left ventricular dysfunction in chronic heart failure via angiogenesis-dependent and -independent actions. *Circulation.* 2012;126(15):1838–1851.
149. Lourenco P, et al. Dipeptidyl peptidase IV and mortality after an acute heart failure episode. *J Cardiovasc Pharmacol.* 2013;62(2):138–142.
150. Scheen AJ. Cardiovascular effects of gliptins. *Nat Rev Cardiol.* 2013;10(2):73–84.
151. Takahashi A, et al. Dipeptidyl-peptidase IV inhibition improves pathophysiology of heart failure and increases survival rate in pressure-overloaded mice. *Am J Physiol Heart Circ Physiol.* 2013;304(10):H1361–H1369.
152. White WB, et al. Alogliptin after acute coronary syndrome in patients with type 2 diabetes. *N Engl J Med.* 2013;369(14):1327–1335.
153. McGuire DK, et al. Association between sitagliptin use and heart failure hospitalization and related outcomes in type 2 diabetes mellitus: secondary analysis of a randomized clinical trial. *JAMA Cardiol.* 2016;1(2):126–135.
154. McGuire DK, et al. Linagliptin effects on heart failure and related outcomes in individuals with type 2 diabetes mellitus at high cardiovascular and renal risk in CARMELINA. *Circulation.* 2019;139(3):351–361.
155. DeFronzo RA, et al. The effect of insulin on renal handling of sodium, potassium, calcium, and phosphate in man. *J Clin Invest.* 1975;55(4):845–855.
156. Investigators OT, et al. Basal insulin and cardiovascular and other outcomes in dysglycemia. *N Engl J Med.* 2012;367(4):319–328.
157. Pratley RE, et al. Heart failure with insulin degludec versus glargine U100 in patients with type 2 diabetes at high risk of cardiovascular disease: DEVOTE 14. *Cardiovasc Diabetol.* 2019;18(1):156.
158. Marso SP, et al. Efficacy and safety of degludec versus glargine in type 2 diabetes. *N Engl J Med.* 2017;377(8):723–732.

16 Treatment of Patients With Reduced and With Preserved Ejection Fraction Heart Failure in Patients With Type 2 Diabetes

KATHARINA MARX-SCHÜTT

DEFINITION

Heart failure (HF) is not a singular pathological condition but rather a clinical syndrome characterized by current or prior symptoms and/or signs resulting from structural and/or functional cardiac abnormalities. This diagnosis is supported by elevated natriuretic peptides and/or objective evidence of cardiogenic pulmonary or systemic congestion through diagnostic modalities like imaging or invasive hemodynamic measurements.[1]

HF is one of the most common initial manifestations of cardiovascular disease (CVD) in individuals with type 2 diabetes mellitus (T2DM), presenting as HF with preserved ejection fraction (HFpEF), mildly reduced ejection fraction (HFmrEF), or reduced ejection fraction (HFrEF)[1] (Table 16.1).

Symptoms include, for example, breathlessness, ankle swelling, and fatigue. Signs may not be present at an early stage or in patients receiving diuretics.

Major causes of HF in diabetes include ischemic heart disease (IHD), hypertension, direct or indirect effects of hyperglycemia, as well as obesity-related factors affecting the myocardium.[2,3] IHD often presents as accelerated, severe, diffuse coronary atherosclerosis and/or symptomatically silent coronary artery disease (CAD) that are all associated with higher risk of myocardial infarction (MI) and ischemic myocardial dysfunction. Observational data also indicate that lower-extremity artery disease, prolonged duration of diabetes, aging, increased body mass index (BMI), and chronic kidney disease (CKD) are associated with HF in patients with diabetes. Pathophysiological mechanisms may contribute to myocardial dysfunction even in the absence of IHD or hypertension.[4] The concept of diabetic cardiomyopathy has been debated for decades. A recent consensus document introduced the term diabetic myocardial disorder, which is defined as systolic and/or diastolic myocardial dysfunction in the presence of diabetes, also stating that diabetes is rarely exclusively responsible for myocardial dysfunction but usually acts in association with obesity, arterial hypertension, chronic kidney disease, and/or coronary artery disease, causing additive myocardial impairment.[5]

EPIDEMIOLOGY AND SCREENING

Diabetes significantly increases the risk for HF.[6] Studies consistently show that individuals with versus without diabetes face a two- to fourfold higher risk.[7–9] The prevalence of chronic HF rises steadily with age among both patients with and without diabetes. Patients with T2DM develop chronic HF more frequently and earlier than their counterparts without T2DM—e.g., one study reported an incident rate ratio of 1.1 for those under 45 years, decreasing to 1.8 for those aged 75 to 84 years, highlighting higher absolute risks among older adults without diabetes. Data from 679,072 individuals with T2DM from the Swedish National Diabetes Register and 2,643,800 matched controls demonstrate that among individuals with T2DM, incidence rates for HF per 10,000 person-years in 2001 and 2019 were 98.3 (95% CI, 89.4–112.0) and 75.9 (95% CI, 74.4–77.5). The incidence for HF plateaued around 2013, a trend that then persisted[10] (Fig. 16.1).

Mortality and hospitalization for HF are clinically meaningful endpoints with respect to the prognosis of patients with HF and as such used in clinical and epidemiological studies. Patients with diabetes exhibit a significantly higher risk for these endpoints compared with patients with HF without diabetes. As such, various population-based studies demonstrate higher mortality in patients with diabetes and HF. The Danish Investigations of Arrhythmia and Mortality on Dofetilide (DIAMOND) study examined in 5499 patients hospitalized because of congestive HF the mortality rate depending on the presence of diabetes. This study could show that 31% of all patients with HF and diabetes died within 1 and 50% after 3 years, suggesting a markedly increased mortality in patients with diabetes and HF[11].

TABLE 16.1 Heart Failure Phenotypes According to Ejection Fraction Distribution

HF	HFPEF	HFMREF	HFREF
Phenotype			
Criterion 1	Symptoms and/or Signs[a]	Symptoms and/or signs[a]	Symptoms and/or signs[a]
Criterion 2	LVEF ≥ 50%	LVEF 41%–49%	LVEF ≤ 40%
Criterion 3	Objective evidence of cardiac structural and/or functional abnormalities consistent with the presence of LV diastolic dysfunction or raised filling pressures, including raised natriuretic peptides	None	None

[a]Symptoms include, for example, breathlessness, ankle swelling, and fatigue. Signs may not be present at an early stage or in patients receiving diuretics.
HF, Heart failure; *HFmrEF*, heart failure with mildly reduced ejection fraction; *HFpEF*, heart failure with preserved ejection fraction; *HFrEF*, heart failure with reduced ejection fraction; *LV*, left ventricular; *LVEF*, left ventricular ejection fraction.
From McDonagh TA, Metra M, Adamo M, et al. 2021 ESC Guidelines for the diagnosis and treatment of acute and chronic heart failure: Developed by the Task Force for the diagnosis and treatment of acute and chronic heart failure of the European Society of Cardiology (ESC) With the special contribution of the Heart Failure Association (HFA) of the ESC. *Eur Heart J*. 2021;42(36):3599-3726. https://doi.org/10.1093/eurheartj/ehab368.

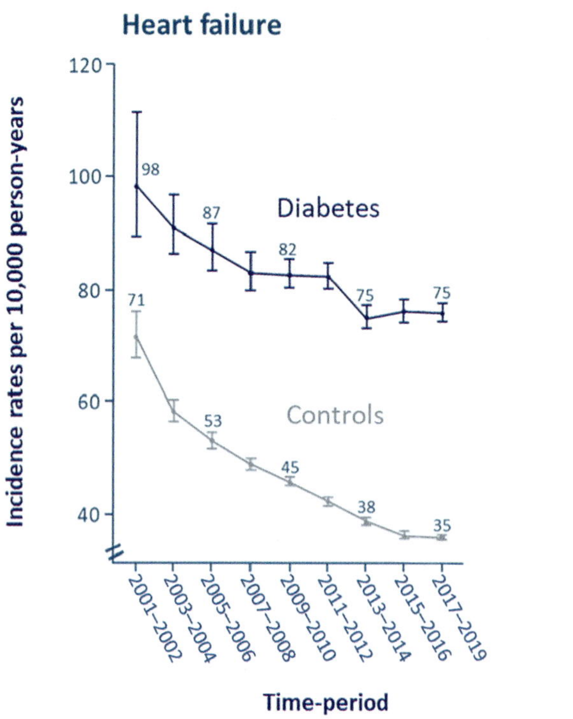

FIG. 16.1 Age- and sex-standardized incidence rates for heart failure (*HF*) among individuals with type 2 diabetes mellitus (*T2DM*) compared with controls from the general population. Adapted from Sattar N, McMurray J, Borén J, et al. Twenty years of cardiovascular complications and risk factors in patients with type 2 diabetes: a nationwide Swedish cohort study. *Circulation*. 2023;147(25):1872–1886. https://doi.10.1161/circulationaha.122.063374. (In eng).

Additional data on the prognosis of diabetes and established HF came from the large HF trials the survival and ventricular enlargement study (SAVE), the VALsartan In Acute myocardial iNfarcTion trial (VALIANT), and Candesartan in heart failure-assessment of reduction in mortality and morbidity (CHARM). All of these studies confirmed a higher mortality risk in patients with diabetes. For example, data from the CHARM trial suggest that 40% of all patients with diabetes reached the CV endpoint of CV death or rehospitalization for HF within 3 years. Among these patients, those with reduced left-ventricular ejection fraction exhibited the highest risk followed by patients with diabetes and preserved ejection fraction. The risk of patients without diabetes both with preserved and reduced ejection fraction was significantly lower compared with persons with diabetes. A similar trend has been shown for the overall mortality.[12] Such data underscore that patients with diabetes and HF exhibit a worse prognosis and that the risk for hospitalization of HF or CV death ranges from 12% to 15% within 1 year.

Screening for Heart Failure in Patients With Diabetes

As outlined above, patients with diabetes are at increased risk of HF (stage A HF), but not every patient will develop HF (stages B to D). Therefore the 2023 European Society of Cardiology (ESC) guidelines on the management of CV disease in patients with diabetes recommends a regular, systematic survey for HF symptoms (including breathlessness, dyspnea on exertion, orthopnea, paroxysmal nocturnal dyspnea, fatigue, tiredness, increased time to recover following exercise) or signs (peripheral edema, weight gain, rales, hepatojugular reflux, third heart sound, or laterally displaced apical impulse).[13] If one or more signs or symptoms are present, measurement of natriuretic peptides is recommended, if available. While values below the following cutoffs make the diagnosis unlikely, it should be considered that concentrations can be disproportionately low in patients with obesity and women and disproportionally high in patients with advanced CKD, advanced age, and atrial fibrillation (AF):

- B-type natriuretic peptide (BNP) < 35 pg/mL (AF threshold < 105 pg/mL)
- NT-ProBNP < 125 pg/mL (AF threshold < 365 pg/mL)

In all patients with suspected HF, the following diagnostic tests should be performed:

- ECG to detect abnormalities such as AF, signs of LV hypertrophy, Q waves, or widened QRS, each of which may be a sign of HF.
- Echocardiography to assess cardiac function including LV function, chamber size, LV hypertrophy, regional wall motion abnormalities (that may suggest CAD), right ventricular function, estimated pulmonary pressure, valvular function, and markers of diastolic dysfunction.
- Chest X-ray to investigate other causes of dyspnea (e.g., pulmonary disease). In addition, it may give supportive evidence of HF (e.g., cardiomegaly, pulmonary congestion, pleural effusion).
- Routine blood tests, including a full blood count, urea, creatinine, electrolytes, thyroid and liver function tests, lipid profile, and iron status (ferritin and transferrin

saturation), are recommended to help distinguish HF from other conditions, provide prognostic insights, and guide treatment decisions. If there is suspicion of a specific condition, such as amyloidosis, additional diagnostic tests should be considered.

In addition to traditional screening using signs and symptoms of HF, different risk scores have been developed. To estimate the risk of HF in outpatients with T2DM mellitus (T2DM), the WATCH-DM risk score was created.[14] This score incorporates factors like BMI, age, hypertension, creatinine levels, HDL-C, fasting plasma glucose, QRS duration, history of myocardial infarction (MI), and coronary artery bypass grafting. Each 1-point increase in this score correlates with a 24% higher likelihood of developing HF within 5 years. Additionally, a risk score based on biomarkers—such as high-sensitivity cardiac troponin T (≥6 ng/L), NT-ProBNP (≥125 pg/mL), high-sensitivity C-reactive protein (≥3 mg/L), and left ventricular hypertrophy seen on ECG—was shown to effectively predict the 5- and 10-year HF risk in patients with diabetes. Patients with a score of 3 or higher were at the highest risk of HF over a 5-year period.[15] After reviewing clinical evidence, the Heart Failure Association of the European Society of Cardiology (ESC) concluded that additional biomarker testing is not currently recommended.[16]

TREATMENT OF HEART FAILURE IN DIABETES

Treatment recommendations for patients with HF are different for patients with HFrEF, HFmrEF, and HFpEF.

Treatment of Heart Failure With Reduced Ejection Fraction

Treatment of HFrEF encompasses therapeutic lifestyle modifications, as well as pharmacological and device therapies with confirmed benefits in RCTs, in which ~30% to 40% of patients had diabetes. Treatment effects of medications and devices for HFrEF have been consistently demonstrated to not differ in patients with versus without diabetes. Importantly, while the RR reductions are consistently similar for those with and without diabetes, given the higher absolute clinical risk associated with diabetes, the ARR in patients with diabetes is typically higher, yielding a lower NNT for benefit among patients with diabetes.

The cornerstone of treatment for HFrEF is pharmacotherapy alongside lifestyle interventions, which should be implemented before considering device therapy (Fig. 16.2).

Recent HF guidelines recommend starting quadruple therapy at the same time: angiotensin receptor-neprilysin inhibitor [ARNI]/ACE-I, MRA, beta-blocker, SGLT2 inhibitor.[1] These four foundational treatments should be initiated within the first 4 weeks from diagnosis,[13] as many of the benefits are seen within 30 days of starting treatment, and adding new medications yields greater benefits than uptitrating existing medications, as shown in the STRONG-HF trial.[17] The sequence of therapy initiation should be based on the individual patient phenotype, taking into account BP, heart rhythm, and heart rate, as well as kidney function and risk of hyperkalemia. While SGLT2 inhibitors have the same starting and target dose, ARNI/ACEi/ARB, beta-blockers, and MRAs should be started at low dose and uptitrated to the maximum tolerated dose. In the following, the specific characteristics for HFrEF treatment in patients with diabetes are presented.

ANGIOTENSIN RECEPTOR-NEPRILYSIN INHIBITORS AND ANGIOTENSIN-CONVERTING ENZYME INHIBITORS

The ARNI sacubitril/valsartan has shown superior efficacy compared with enalapril in reducing CV death and HF hospitalization in patients with HFrEF, with or without diabetes.[18] Patients were uptitrated to sacubitril/valsartan 97/103 mg twice daily within 2 to 4 weeks.[18] The beneficial effect of sacubitril/valsartan over enalapril was consistent for patients with and without diabetes and across the spectrum of baseline HbA1c. Angiotensin-converting enzyme inhibitors (ACE-I) were the first class of medications shown to reduce mortality and morbidity and improve symptoms in patients with HFrEF.[19] There is no difference in efficacy between patients with and without diabetes.[20–22] As renin–angiotensin–aldosterone system (RAAS) inhibitors increase the risk of hyperkalemia and may acutely alter kidney function, routine surveillance of serum creatinine and potassium levels is advised.[23,24] However, misinterpretation of eGFR changes as injury as opposed to understanding that it is due to favorable hemodynamic effects at the glomerular level often leads to inappropriate discontinuation of these disease-modifying agents, which should be avoided.[23–25]

SODIUM-GLUCOSE COTRANSPORTER-2 INHIBITORS

Two randomized placebo-controlled trials have investigated the effect of an SGLT2 inhibitor compared with placebo added to optimal medical therapy (OMT) in patients with HFrEF with and without diabetes. The DAPA-HF (Dapagliflozin and Prevention of Adverse Outcomes in HF) trial included patients if they were in New York Heart Association (NYHA) class II–IV, an LVEF ≤40% despite OMT, and had elevated NT-ProBNP (in sinus rhythm ≥600 pg/mL, in atrial fibrillation ≥900 mg/mL, or ≥400 pg/mL if they had been hospitalized for HF within the previous 12 months). Patients with T1DM or an eGFR < 30 mL/min/1.73 m^2 were excluded. Therapy with dapagliflozin 10 mg once daily versus a placebo reduced the risk for the primary outcome, a composite of worsening HF (hospitalization or an urgent visit resulting in intravenous therapy for HF) or CV death, by 26% (HR, 0.74; 95% CI, 0.65–0.85). In addition, dapagliflozin reduced all-cause mortality (HR, 0.83; 95% CI, 0.71–0.97) and improved symptoms, physical function, and quality of life in patients with HFrEF.[26,27] All of the clinical benefits observed were independent of baseline diabetes status and background glucose-lowering therapy and consistent across the spectrum of HbA1c.[26,28]

The EMPEROR-Reduced (Empagliflozin Outcome Trial in Patients with Chronic Heart Failure with Reduced Ejection Fraction) trial evaluated empagliflozin versus a placebo and included patients with HFrEF with and without diabetes, with NYHA class II–IV, and LVEF ≤40% despite OMT; an eGFR ≥ 20 mL/min/1.73 m^2; and an elevated NT-ProBNP (ejection fraction [EF] ≤30% or EF ≤40% and HF hospitalization within 12 months, NT-ProBNP ≥600 pg/mL; EF 31%–35%, NT-ProBNP ≥1000 pg/mL; EF 36%–40%, NT-ProBNP ≥2500 pg/mL). Empagliflozin reduced the risk for

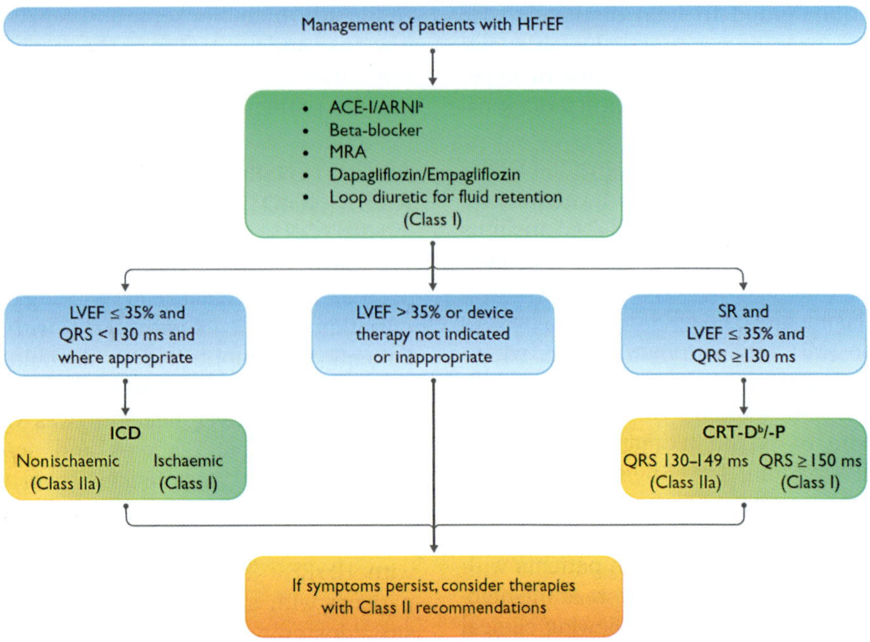

FIG. 16.2 Therapeutic algorithm for patients with HF with reduced ejection fraction based on the 2021 ESC Guidelines for the diagnosis and treatment of acute and chronic HF.[1] *ACE-I*, Angiotensin-converting enzyme inhibitor; *ARNI*, angiotensin receptor-neprilysin inhibitor; *CRT-D*, cardiac resynchronization therapy with defibrillator; *CRT-P*, cardiac resynchronization therapy with pacemaker; *ICD*, implantable cardioverter-defibrillator; *HFrEF*, HF with reduced ejection fraction; *MRA*, mineralocorticoid receptor antagonist; *QRS*, Q, R, and S waves (on a 12-lead electrocardiogram); *SR*, sinus rhythm. [a]As a replacement for ACE-I. [b]Where appropriate. Class I, green; Class IIa, yellow.

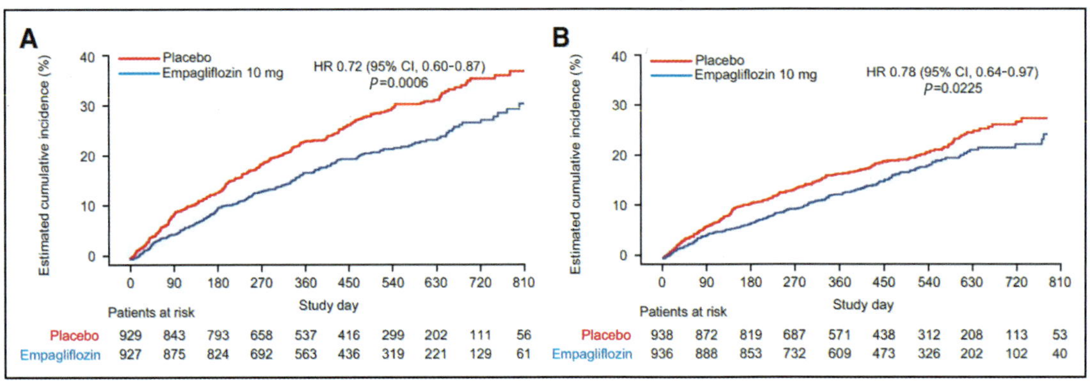

FIG. 16.3 Effect of empagliflozin on the primary endpoint in EMPEROR-Reduced (Empagliflozin Outcome Trial in Patients With Chronic HF With Reduced Ejection Fraction). Time to first event of either cardiovascular death or HF hospitalization in (A) patients with diabetes and (B) patients without diabetes. *CI*, Confidence interval; *HR*, hazard ratio.[30]

the primary outcome, a composite of CV death and HF hospitalization, by 25% versus a placebo (HR, 0.75; 95% CI, 0.65–0.86).[29] The effect of empagliflozin on the primary outcome was consistent across patients with and without diabetes at baseline[30] (Fig. 16.3).

Treatment with empagliflozin also improved quality of life.[31] A meta-analysis of the DAPA-HF and EMPEROR-Reduced trials showed a consistent reduction in HF hospitalization or CV death and all-cause mortality by SGLT2-inhibitor treatment without significant heterogeneity between trials. The combined SGLT1 and -2 inhibitor sotagliflozin was investigated in patients with T2DM who were recently hospitalized for worsening HF, irrespective of their LVEF (SOLOIST-WHF trial). Patients with an eGFR < 30 mL/min/1.73 m^2 were excluded. Sotagliflozin significantly reduced the risk for the composite primary outcome (CV death, HF hospitalization, or urgent visit for HF) by 33% compared with a placebo (HR, 0.67; 95% CI, 0.52–0.85). The treatment effect was consistent across the spectrum of LVEF.[32] Thus the SGLT inhibitors dapagliflozin, empagliflozin, and sotagliflozin are recommended, in addition to OMT (with an ARNI/ACEi/ARB, beta-blocker, and MRA), in patients with HFrEF and diabetes to reduce CV death and HF hospitalization. Three studies have investigated whether SGLT2 inhibitors can be safely started in patients hospitalized for acute HF. The EMPA-RESPONSE-AHF trial randomized 80 patients with acute HF with (approximately one-third) and without diabetes to either empagliflozin or placebo for 30 days. Treatment with empagliflozin did not affect visual analog scale dyspnea, diuretic response, NT-ProBNP levels, and length of hospital stay but was safe, increased urinary output, and reduced a combined endpoint of worsening HF, rehospitalization for HF, or death at 60 days.[33] In the SOLOIST-WHF trial mentioned above, 1222 patients with T2DM were randomized to sotagliflozin or placebo with a median follow-up of

9 months (trial stopped prematurely due to loss of sponsor support). Sotagliflozin therapy, initiated before or shortly after discharge, resulted in significantly fewer deaths from CV causes and hospitalizations and urgent visits for HF than a placebo, with no increase in acute kidney injury.[34] The EMPULSE trial randomized 530 hospitalized patients with and without diabetes with a primary diagnosis of acute de novo or decompensated HF, regardless of LVEF when clinically stable, to receive either empagliflozin or a placebo. More patients treated with empagliflozin had a clinical benefit (win ratio, 1.36; 95% CI, 1.09–1.68) compared with a placebo. This effect was consistent for acute de novo and decompensated chronic HF and was observed regardless of LVEF or the presence of diabetes.[35] In these trials, very few cases of euglycemic diabetic ketoacidosis were reported; still, physicians treating patients with diabetes with SGLT2 inhibitors in this setting should be aware of this rare but potentially serious complication.

MINERALOCORTICOID ANTAGONISTS

In large CVOTs, the MRAs spironolactone or eplerenone have shown to reduce death and HF hospitalization in patients with HFrEF, with consistent results in patients with or without diabetes.[36,37] Eplerenone is more specific for blocking aldosterone and, therefore, causes less gynecomastia. Caution should be exercised when using MRAs in patients with impaired kidney function and in those with serum potassium concentration >5.0 mmol/L.

BETA-BLOCKERS

No dedicated trials have specifically assessed the impact of beta-blockers on HF-related outcomes in patients with HF with HFrEF who also have diabetes. However, posthoc analyses from various studies indicate that beta-blockers provide comparable benefits for HF in patients with HFrEF, with or without diabetes by reducing all-cause death and hospitalization for HF in patients with HFrEF.[38–41] Treatment benefits strongly support using beta-blockers with proven efficacy in patients with HFrEF and diabetes.

DIURETICS

Although there is insufficient evidence regarding the efficacy of thiazide or loop diuretics in reducing CV outcomes in HF patients, these diuretics are effective in preventing and treating symptoms and signs of fluid congestion with no known differentiation in efficacy or recommendation for use by diabetes status.[42]

ANGIOTENSIN-II RECEPTOR BLOCKERS

The place of angiotensin-II receptor blockers (ARBs) in managing HFrEF has changed over the last few years. They are now recommended for patients who cannot tolerate either ARNI or ACE-I due to serious side effects. ARBs have similar treatment effects in patients with HFrEF with or without diabetes.[43–45]

IVABRADINE

Ivabradine slows the heart rate by inhibiting the If channel in the sinus node and is therefore only effective in patients with sinus rhythm. Ivabradine reduced the combined endpoint of CV death or HF hospitalization irrespective of diabetes status.[46]

HYDRALAZINE AND ISOSORBIDE DINITRATE

There is no evidence to support the use of this fixed-dose combination therapy in all patients with HFrEF but rather limited to self-identified Black patients as per product labeling. An RCT conducted in self-identified Black patients with HFrEF showed that adding the combination of hydralazine and isosorbide dinitrate to conventional therapy (ACE-I, beta-blocker, MRA) reduced mortality and HF hospitalization in patients with HFrEF in NYHA class III–IV.[47] The beneficial effects were consistent in patients with or without diabetes.[48]

DIGOXIN

Digoxin may reduce the risk of HF hospitalization in patients with HFrEF treated with ACE-Is, irrespective of diabetes status.[49]

DEVICE THERAPY

Device therapies (implantable cardioverter defibrillator [ICD], cardiac resynchronization therapy [CRT], and CRT with an implantable defibrillator [CRT-D]) have similar efficacies and risks in patients with HFrEF with or without diabetes.[50–53] These therapies should be considered according to treatment guidelines in the HFrEF population. Briefly, an ICD is recommended in patients who have recovered from a ventricular arrhythmia causing hemodynamic instability and who are expected to survive for more than 1 year with good functional status in the absence of reversible causes or unless the ventricular arrhythmia occurred within 48 hours after MI, to reduce the risk of sudden death and all-cause mortality. In primary prevention, an ICD is recommend to reduce the risk of sudden cardiac death and all-cause mortality in patients with symptomatic HFrEF (NYHA class II–III) and LVEF ≤35% despite ≥3 months of optimal medical therapy, provided they are expected to survive more than 1 year with good functional status. ICD implantation is not recommended within 40 days after MI and in patients with NYHA class IV with severe symptoms refractory to pharmacological therapy unless they are candidates for CRT, left ventricular assist device, or heart transplantation. CRT is recommended for symptomatic patients with HF in sinus rhythm with a QRS duration ≥130 ms and left or right (less evidence with lower class of recommendation) bundle branch block morphology (and LVEF ≤35% despite optimal medical therapy to improve symptoms and reduce mortality). In addition, CRT rather than RV pacing is recommended for patients with HFrEF, regardless of NYHA class or QRS width, who have an indication for ventricular pacing for high-degree AV block. In contrast, a CRT is not recommended in patients with a QRS duration <130 ms who do not have an indication for pacing due to high-degree AV block.[1] Heart transplantation could be considered in end-stage HF, but a large, prospective study of transplanted patients indicated a decreased likelihood of 10-year survival in those with diabetes.[54]

Treatment of Heart Failure With Mildly Reduced Ejection Fraction and Heart Failure With Preserved Ejection Fraction

Until 2016, HF phenotypes were defined as those with HF with preserved EF (HFpEF) and those with reduced

LVEF (typically considered as < 40%; HF with reduced EF [HFrEF]). This classification was revised in 2016, and patients with an LVEF in the range of 40% to 49% were defined as HFmrEF.[55] Since many trials were conducted before this revised definition was used, results are often based on patient populations with an EF > 40% not separating HFmrEF from HFpEF. Retrospective analyses from RCTs in both HF with HFrEF and HFpEF suggest that patients with an LVEF between 40% and 50% may benefit from similar therapies as those with an LVEF ≤40%. However, no definitive RCT has yet evaluated therapies exclusively for patients with HFmrEF or HFpEF.

Over the past decade, several large RCTs have failed to achieve statistical significance regarding their primary outcomes in patients with HFpEF. These include PEP-CHF (perindopril), CHARM-Preserved (candesartan), I-PRESERVE (irbesartan), TOPCAT (spironolactone), the DIG Ancillary Trial (digoxin), and PARAGON-HF (sacubitril/valsartan).[56–61] Although the PARAGON-HF trial, which involved patients with an ejection fraction (EF) of ≥45%, did not meet its primary endpoint overall, it revealed a significant EF-by-treatment interaction. Specifically, sacubitril/valsartan reduced the likelihood of the primary composite outcome—CV death and total HF hospitalization—by 22% among participants with LVEF at or below the median of 57%.[57]

SGLT2 INHIBITORS

The strongest evidence to date for the treatment of HFpEF comes from trials involving SGLT2 inhibitors. The EMPEROR-Preserved trial included patients classified as NYHA class II to IV, with an LVEF > 40% and elevated NT-ProBNP levels (> 300 pg/mL in sinus rhythm; >900 pg/mL in atrial fibrillation). Patients with an estimated glomerular filtration rate (eGFR) < 20 mL/min/1.73 m^2 were excluded. Compared with a placebo, empagliflozin reduced the risk of the primary outcome—a composite of cardiovascular death or hospitalization for HF—by 21%, largely due to a 29% lower risk of hospitalization for HF. This effect was independent of diabetes status, and baseline HbA1c levels did not influence outcomes.[30]

Similarly, the DELIVER trial involved 6263 patients who were also classified as NYHA class II–IV and had an LVEF > 40%, elevated NT-ProBNP levels (> 300 pg/mL in sinus rhythm; > 600 pg/mL in atrial fibrillation), and an eGFR ≥25 mL/min/1.73 m^2. Dapagliflozin reduced the primary outcome—a composite of worsening HF or CV death—by 18%, primarily driven by a decrease in hospitalizations for HF. This effect was also independent of diabetes status.[62] A meta-analysis encompassing data from both DELIVER and EMPEROR-Preserved indicated that SGLT2 inhibitors significantly lowered the composite outcome of CV death and first hospitalization for HF compared with a placebo (HR, 0.80; 95% CI, 0.73–0.87). Consistent reductions were observed for both components: CV death (HR, 0.88; 95% CI, 0.77–1.00) and first hospitalization for HF (HR, 0.74; 95% CI, 0.67–0.83).[63] The treatment effects on this primary outcome did not vary between different LVEF subgroups and among patients with or without diabetes.[62,64]

The combined SGLT1 and SGLT2 inhibitor sotagliflozin was studied in patients with T2DM who had recently been hospitalized due to worsening HF, regardless of their LVEF status; notably, 20.9% had an LVEF ≥50%. Sotagliflozin led to a reduction in the risk of the primary composite outcome—CV death, HF hospitalization, and urgent visits for HF—by 33%, demonstrating consistent effects across various baseline LVEFs.[34]

DIURETICS

As is standard practice in other forms of HF, diuretics should be used to manage congestion.

SEMAGLUTIDE

The GLP-1 receptor agonist semaglutide has been tested in patients with HF and preserved ejection fraction in the STEP-HFpEF DM trial. In this trial, 616 participants with obesity-related HF (BMI ≥30 kg/m^2) and T2DM and HFpEF (LVEF ≥45%) were randomized to a placebo or the once-weekly GLP-1 receptor agonist semaglutide (2.4 mg for 52 weeks). Primary outcomes were the change from baseline in the Kansas City Cardiomyopathy Questionnaire Clinical Summary Score (KCCQ-CSS) and the change in body weight. The mean change in KCCQ-CSS was 13.7 points with semaglutide and 6.6 points with a placebo (estimated difference, 7.3 points; 95% CI, 4.1–10.4; $P < 0.001$), and the mean percentage change in body weight was −9.8% with semaglutide and −3.4% with a placebo ($P < 0.01$) (Fig. 16.4). In addition, the confirmatory secondary endpoint of difference in change in 6-minute walk distance was 14.3 m in favor of semaglutide. In addition, semaglutide led to a significantly greater reduction in hsCRP. This trial demonstrates that among patients with obesity-related HFpEF and T2DM, treatment with semaglutide significantly reduced HF-related symptoms and physical limitations in addition to a greater weight loss compared with a placebo after 1 year.[65] Data on the improvement of the prognosis of these patients are currently lacking.

A similar trial has been conducted in patients with obesity-related HF without diabetes (STEP-HFpEF).[66] A pooled analysis of both trials demonstrated that semaglutide treatment improved HF-related symptoms and physical limitations across subgroups who were versus were not treated with diuretics.[67,68] Moreover, an additional analysis of these pooled trials reported that participants with a higher baseline NT-ProBNP had a similar degree of weight loss but experienced larger reduction in HF-related symptoms and physical limitations with semaglutide compared with those with NT-ProBNP.[69]

NONSTEROIDAL MRA FINERENONE

Additional data on HF endpoints in patients with T2DM can be derived from clinical trials with the nonsteroidal mineralocorticoid receptor antagonist finerenone. Two dedicated cardiovascular outcome trials in patients with T2DM and chronic kidney disease (FIGARO DKD[70] and FIDELIO DKD[71]) assessed the effect of finerenone on CV outcomes. The predefined analysis of both trials, FIDELITY, demonstrated that finerenone in combination with optimal RAAS-inhibition in patients with T2DM and CKD but without HFrEF reduced the combined CV outcomes of CV death, nonfatal MI, nonfatal stroke, or HF hospitalization significantly by 14% compared with a placebo.[70] This effect was mainly driven by a reduction in HF hospitalization

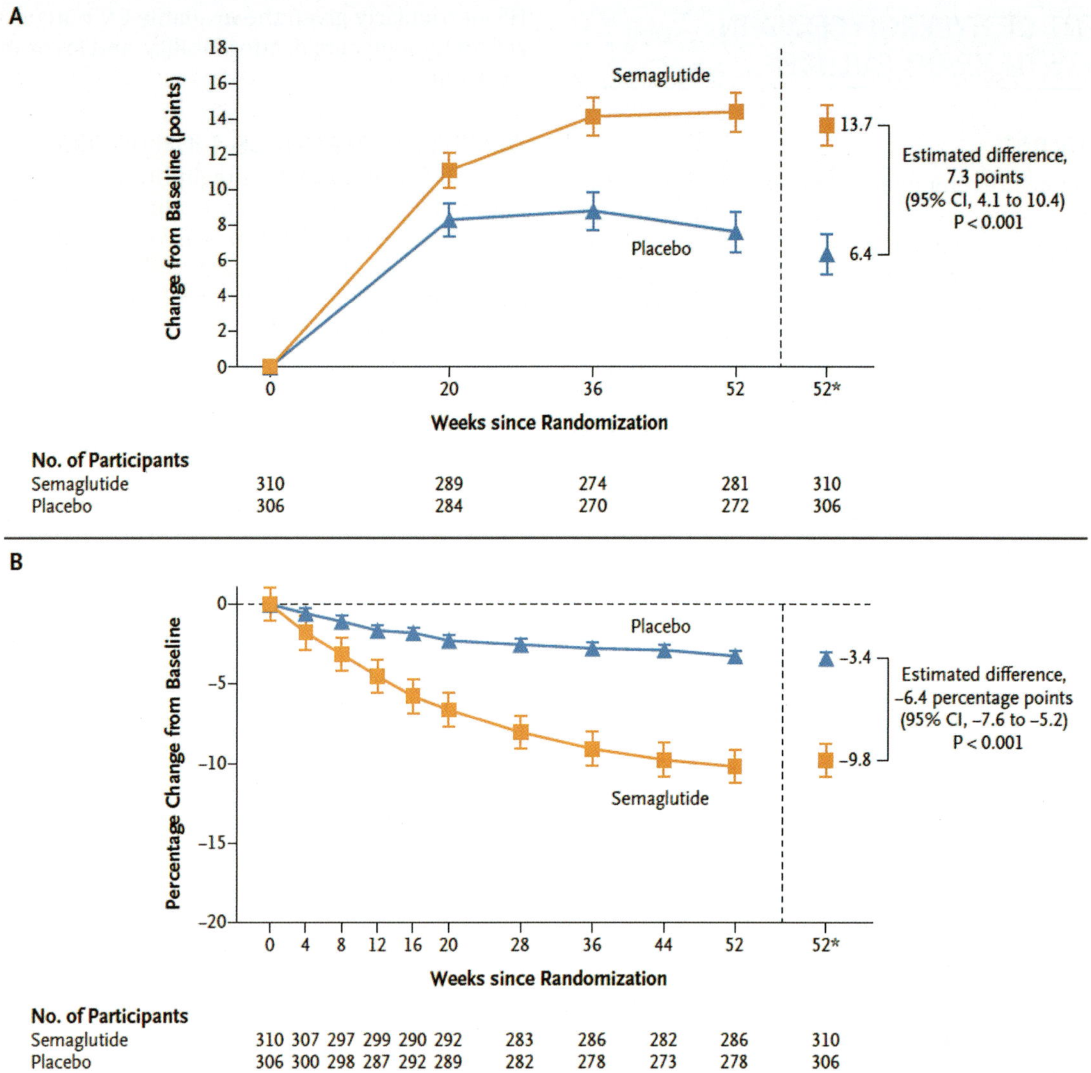

FIG. 16.4 Change from baseline to week 52 in the dual primary endpoints. (A) Change in KCCQ-CSS and (B) change in body weight. Shown are the observed (i.e., as-measured) mean changes from baseline in the Kansas City in the STEP-HFpEF DM trial Cardiomyopathy Questionnaire clinical summary score (KCCQ-CSS; scores range from 0 to 100, with higher scores indicating fewer symptoms and physical limitations) and percentage changes in body weight. I bars indicate the standard error, and the numbers below the graphs are the numbers of participants contributing to the mean (with variations in participants attending certain trial visits). The data at week 52* are the estimated mean changes from baseline to week 52 based on analysis of covariance (*ANCOVA*) and an imputation approach for missing data.[65]

even though patients with HFrEF were excluded. The beneficial effect of finerenone on HF-related outcomes was not modified by baseline eGFR and/or UACR or the presence of HF at baseline. Overall, the prevalence of a history of HF in this patient population was 7.7%, suggesting that finerenone may be effective in the prevention of new-onset HF in T2DM and CKD.

The FINEARTS-HF (Finerenone in HF with Mildly Reduced or Preserved Ejection Fraction) trial assessed the effect of finerenone in patients with HF and mildly reduced or preserved ejection fraction. This trial enrolled patients with HF and a left ventricular ejection fraction of 40% or greater, with or without diabetes; 6001 patients were randomized to finerenone or a placebo, and the primary combined endpoint was CV death or total HF events (hospitalization/urgent visits). Though this trial was not a dedicated diabetes trial, about 40% of all patients had a medical history of T2DM. Overall, treatment with finerenone over a median follow-up of 32 months led a significant reduction of the primary endpoint with a rate ratio of 0.84 (95% CI, 0.74–0.95; $P = 0.07$). This effect was mainly driven by the reduction of the total number of worsening HF events with a relative risk reduction of 18% that was significant. There was a trend toward a reduction of cardiovascular death (HR, 0.93), which did not reach statistical significance. Of note, statistical significance for the primary endpoint was observed within 1 month of therapeutic initiation, a benefit that was sustained until the final follow-up.[72] The beneficial effect of finerenone was comparable in patients with or without diabetes, suggesting that finerenone treatment is effective in reducing HF-related endpoints in patients with T2DM and HF with an ejection fraction of 40 or above.[73] Of note, finerenone was associated with an increased risk of hyperkalemia. These findings were consistent across prespecified subgroups, including across LVEF[74] and in those on SGLT-2 inhibitors.[75]

TREATMENT OF HYPERGLYCEMIA IN PATIENTS WITH HEART FAILURE

Glycemic Targets

Current guidelines recommend individualizing HbA1c targets according to comorbidities, diabetes duration, and life expectancy. In general, an HbA1c < 7% is recommended in patients with a longer life expectancy, while a less stringent glucose control should be applied in those with comorbidities and a shorter life expectancy (e.g., target 7.5%–8%). In any case, hypoglycemic episodes should be avoided. Hypoglycemia is linked to an elevated risk of vascular events, which has led to recent consensus recommendations for limiting hypoglycemic exposure to less than 1% (i.e., less than 15 minutes per day) in individuals at high CV risk. However, the causal relationship between hypoglycemia and adverse outcomes is not always straightforward, as low glucose levels may also indicate underlying health issues[13] (Fig. 16.5).

Glucose-Lowering Agents

METFORMIN

Metformin is considered safe for use at all stages of HF in patients with preserved or stable, moderately reduced kidney function (i.e., eGFR > 30 mL/min/1.73 m^2). Observational studies suggest that it is associated with a lower risk of death and HF hospitalization compared with insulin and sulfonylureas.[76,77] However, dedicated randomized controlled CVOTs evaluating the safety and efficacy of metformin have yet to be conducted. Thus caution regarding metformin use in HF was lifted in 2006 based on data indicating no increased risk of lactic acidosis and potential clinical benefits. Current evidence supports the consideration of metformin for individuals with stable and compensated HF, particularly given the available CV outcomes data, low risk of hypoglycemia, affordability, and favorable tolerability profile.

DIPEPTIDYL PEPTIDASE-4 INHIBITORS

Four DPP-4 inhibitors—sitagliptin, saxagliptin, alogliptin, and linagliptin—have been evaluated in dedicated placebo-controlled CV safety trials involving patients with T2DM who are either at high risk for ASCVD or already diagnosed. Saxagliptin was found to significantly increase the risk of HF hospitalization and is therefore not recommended for patients with diabetes who have or are at increased risk for HF.[78] Alogliptin showed a nonsignificant trend toward an increase in HF hospitalizations.[79] In contrast, sitagliptin[80] and linagliptin[81] demonstrated a neutral effect on HF outcomes. Vildagliptin has not been tested in a CVOT; however, it did not significantly affect LVEF but was associated with an increase in LV volumes in a small study.[82] So if DPP-4 inhibitors are to be used, to avoid HF risk, priority should be given to sitagliptin or linagliptin.

SODIUM-GLUCOSE COTRANSPORTER-2 INHIBITORS

SGLT2 inhibitors have been investigated in different populations with diabetes, ranging from patients with ASCVD or multiple ASCVD risk factors to patients recently hospitalized for worsening HF, with increasing absolute risk reductions for HF-related outcomes as patient risk increases.

As outlined above, in dedicated HF trials, dapagliflozin and empagliflozin reduced CV death and HF hospitalization in patients with HFrEF with or without diabetes, and sotagliflozin reduced CV death and HF hospitalization in patients with T2DM and recent hospitalization for HF of any etiology.[26,29,34] Moreover, empagliflozin and dapagliflozin reduced the risk of CV death or HF hospitalization in patients with HFmrEF or HFpEF.[30,62] While the EMPA-REG OUTCOME (empagliflozin) and VERTIS CV (ertugliflozin)

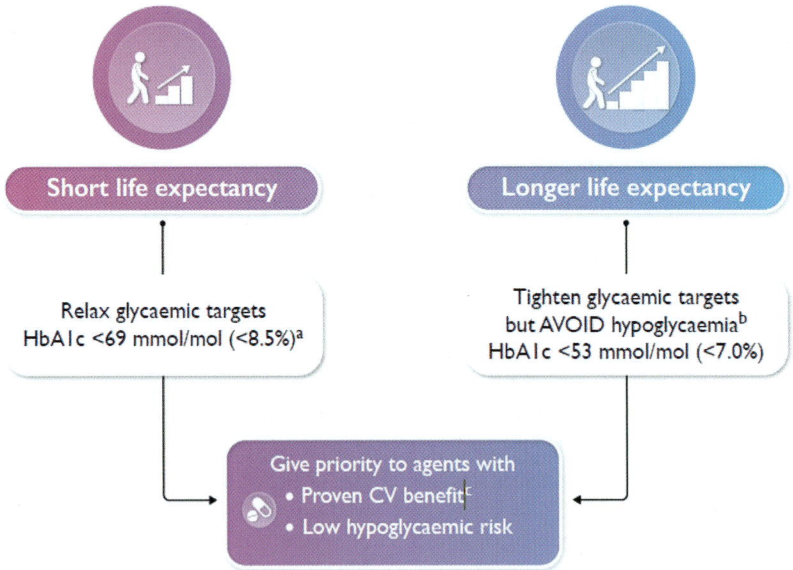

FIG. 16.5 Simple guide to glycemic targets in patients with T2DM and cardiovascular disease. *CV*, Cardiovascular; *GLP-1 RA*, glucagon-like peptide-1 receptor agonist; *HbA1c*, glycated hemoglobin; *s.c.*, subcutaneous; *SGLT2*, sodium-glucose cotransporter-2. [a]Adjust target in the presence of hyperglycemic symptoms (polyuria and polydipsia). [b]Hypoglycemia is usually a concern only in those on a sulphonylurea and/or insulin. [c]SGLT2 inhibitors (empagliflozin, canagliflozin, dapagliflozin, sotagliflozin) or GLP-1 RAs (liraglutide, semaglutide s.c., dulaglutide, efpeglenatide). From Marx N, Federici M, Schütt K, et al. 2023 ESC Guidelines for the management of cardiovascular disease in patients with diabetes. *Eur Heart J*. 2023;44(39):4043–4140.

trials investigated patients with T2DM and established ASCVD risk, the CANVAS Trials Program (canagliflozin) and DECLARE-TIMI 58 trial (dapagliflozin) included patients with established ASCVD or multiple ASCVD risk factors. In all of these placebo-controlled CVOTs of SGLT2 inhibitors, only a small proportion of patients had a baseline history of HF. Empagliflozin reduced the risk of HF hospitalization by 35% in patients with and without previous HF.[83] Canagliflozin also significantly reduced the risk of HF hospitalization by 33%.[84] Dapagliflozin significantly reduced the combined endpoint of CV death and HF hospitalization, a result driven mainly by lower rates of HF hospitalization.[85] This effect was independent of preexisting HF.[86] Ertugliflozin did not reduce the combined endpoint of CV death and HF hospitalization, although there was a significant reduction in HF hospitalization and repeated hospitalizations.[87,88] In addition, four trials investigated the effect of SGLT2 inhibitors in patients with T2DM with moderate or worsening CKD (CREDENCE [canagliflozin] and SCORED [sotagliflozin]) with and without diabetes (DAPA-CKD [dapagliflozin] and EMPA-KIDNEY [empagliflozin]). In these patients at high risk for HF, a consistent risk reduction of CV death or HF hospitalization was observed, ranging from 23% to 31%.[32,84,89,90] A meta-analysis of six outcome trials of four SGLT2 inhibitors in patients with T2DM (EMPA-REG OUTCOME, CANVAS Program [two trials], DECLARE-TIMI, CREDENCE, VERTIS CV) demonstrated a 32% reduction in HF hospitalization, with no heterogeneity between trials; the effect on HF hospitalization was independent of ASCVD.[91]

GLUCAGON-LIKE PEPTIDE-1 RECEPTOR AGONISTS

Eight CVOTs have been conducted with GLP-1RAs in patients with T2DM, revealing a prevalence of established HF ranging from 9% to 24%. Most GLP-1RAs demonstrated a neutral effect on the risk of HF hospitalization in placebo-controlled RCTs assessing the CV safety of glucose-lowering medications in patients with T2DM, even though these agents increased their heart rate by 3 to 5 beats per minute. Additionally, a meta-analysis encompassing eight trials with a total of 60,080 patients found that GLP-1RAs reduced HF hospitalization compared with a placebo.[92] The AMPLITUDE-O trial, which compared efpeglenatide to a placebo, showed a nominally significant reduction in hospitalizations for HF. This trial featured stratified randomization based on baseline or anticipated use of SGLT2 inhibitors and reported the highest prevalence (15.2%) of SGLT2 inhibitor use among GLP-1RA studies. An exploratory analysis from AMPLITUDE-O suggested that the efficacy and safety of efpeglenatide were independent of concurrent SGLT2 inhibitor use concerning HF hospitalization.[93]

Two small RCTs have specifically evaluated GLP-1RAs in patients with HF with HFrEF. The LIVE trial randomly assigned 241 patients with chronic, stable HFrEF—both with and without diabetes—to receive either liraglutide or placebo. After 24 weeks, there were no changes observed in LVEF, quality of life, or functional class; however, serious adverse cardiac events were more prevalent in the liraglutide group (12 events [10%] vs. 3 events [3%] for placebo; $P = 0.04$).[94] The FIGHT trial (Functional Impact of GLP-1 for HF Treatment) involved randomly assigning 300 patients—with and without diabetes—who had HFrEF and a recent hospitalization for HF to either liraglutide or a placebo. After 180 days of treatment, there was no significant difference between groups regarding the primary outcome measures: time to death, time to rehospitalization for HF, and average proportional change in NT-ProBNP levels from baseline to day 180. Furthermore, there was a nonsignificant difference in rehospitalizations for HF between groups (63 [41%] in the liraglutide group vs. 50 [34%] in the placebo group; HR, 1.30; 95% CI, 0.89–1.88; $P = 0.17$).[95]

Additional data on HF outcomes in patients with T2DM are available from the FLOW trial. The FLOW trial was the first dedicated kidney outcome study, enrolling 3534 adults with CKD.[96] Semaglutide resulted in a 24% reduction in the incidence of the primary kidney composite endpoint, which included kidney failure, a sustained 50% decline in eGFR, or CV or kidney death (HR, 0.76; 95% CI, 0.66–0.88). Additionally, an 18% relative risk reduction in 3P-MACE—comprising CV death, MI, or stroke—was observed (HR, 0.82; 95% CI, 0.68–0.98). These CV risk reductions were consistent with findings from the SELECT trial involving a non-CKD cohort at high CV risk, where a 20% reduction in 3P-MACE was reported.[97]

Secondary analyses of the FLOW trial also indicated that semaglutide reduced the risk of HF events or CV death by 17%, regardless of baseline HF history, and showed no treatment heterogeneity across subgroups classified by KDIGO risk.[98] Furthermore, the use of SGLT2 inhibitors alongside semaglutide was relatively low in the FLOW trial (15.6%), and secondary subset analyses demonstrated that concomitant SGLT2 inhibitor use did not significantly affect treatment outcomes on kidney and CV composite endpoints.[99]

Secondary analyses from the SELECT trial, assessing the effect of semaglutide versus a placebo in 17,604 patients with a BMI $\geq 27\,kg/m^2$ and ASCVD but no diabetes, suggest that treatment with semaglutide reduced MACE and composite HF endpoints in those with ($n = 4286$) and without clinical HF ($n = 13{,}314$), regardless of HF subtype.[100]

Overall, based on the totality of current evidence, GLP-1RAs are safe and potentially beneficial in patients with T2DM and HF.

INSULIN

In patients with T2DM and advanced HF, the use of insulin is independently linked to a significantly worse prognosis. Two basal insulins have been formally evaluated in dedicated CVOTs.

In the ORIGIN trial, 12,537 participants (mean age 63.5 years) at high CV risk, including those with impaired fasting glucose, impaired glucose tolerance, or T2DM, were randomized to receive insulin glargine titrated to achieve a fasting blood glucose level of $\leq 95\,mg/dL$ ($\leq 5.3\,mmol/L$) or standard care. After a median follow-up of 6.2 years, insulin glargine showed a neutral effect on HF hospitalizations.[101] The DEVOTE trial was a double-blind study comparing ultra-long-acting, once-daily insulin degludec with insulin glargine U100 and included 7637 patients with T2DM who had established ASCVD or were at high ASCVD risk. Treatment with insulin degludec did not result in any significant difference in HF hospitalization rates compared with insulin glargine; however, prior HF was independently associated with a higher risk of future HF hospitalization.[102]

THIAZOLIDINEDIONES

Thiazolidinediones increased the risk of HF hospitalization in several trials and are not recommended in patients with diabetes and symptomatic HF.[103]

SULFONYLUREAS

Data regarding the effects of sulfonylureas on HF are inconsistent. Two retrospective cohort studies involving 111,971 patients with diabetes suggest an adverse safety profile, indicating a 20% to 60% higher mortality rate and a 20% to 30% higher risk of HF compared with metformin.[104,105] However, trials such as UKPDS, NAVIGATOR (Nateglinide And Valsartan in Impaired Glucose Tolerance Outcomes Research), and ADOPT (A diabetes outcome progression trial) did not show any increased signals for HF.[106–108] Additionally, data from the CAROLINA trial, which compared linagliptin—shown not to increase the risk of HF hospitalization versus a placebo in the CARMELINA trial—with glimepiride indicated no elevated risk of HF hospitalization associated with this sulfonylurea.[109,110]

GUIDELINE RECOMMENDATIONS

The 2023 guidelines for the management of CV disease in patients with diabetes give a class I recommendation for the treatment with an SGLT2 inhibitor (empagliflozin, dapagliflozin, sotagliflozin) to reduce HF-related outcomes (HF hospitalization or CV death) in all patients with T2DM and HF, irrespective of ejection fraction (HFpEF, HFmrEF, HFrEF). Treatment should be initiated independent of HbA1c and independent of concomitant glucose-lowering medications. If additional glucose control is needed, other glucose-lowering agents with neutral effects on HF in CVOTs should be considered. This includes GLP-1RAs, the DPP-4 inhibitors sitagliptin and linagliptin, and metformin, as well as insulin glargine and insulin degludec, all of which have a class IIa recommendation for additional glucose control in these patients. In contrast, pioglitazone and the DPP-4 inhibitor saxagliptin are not recommended because these agents demonstrated an increased risk of HF hospitalization in CVOTs. Fig. 16.6 summarizes the current ESC recommendations for the use of glucose-lowering medications in patients with HF and T2DM.[13]

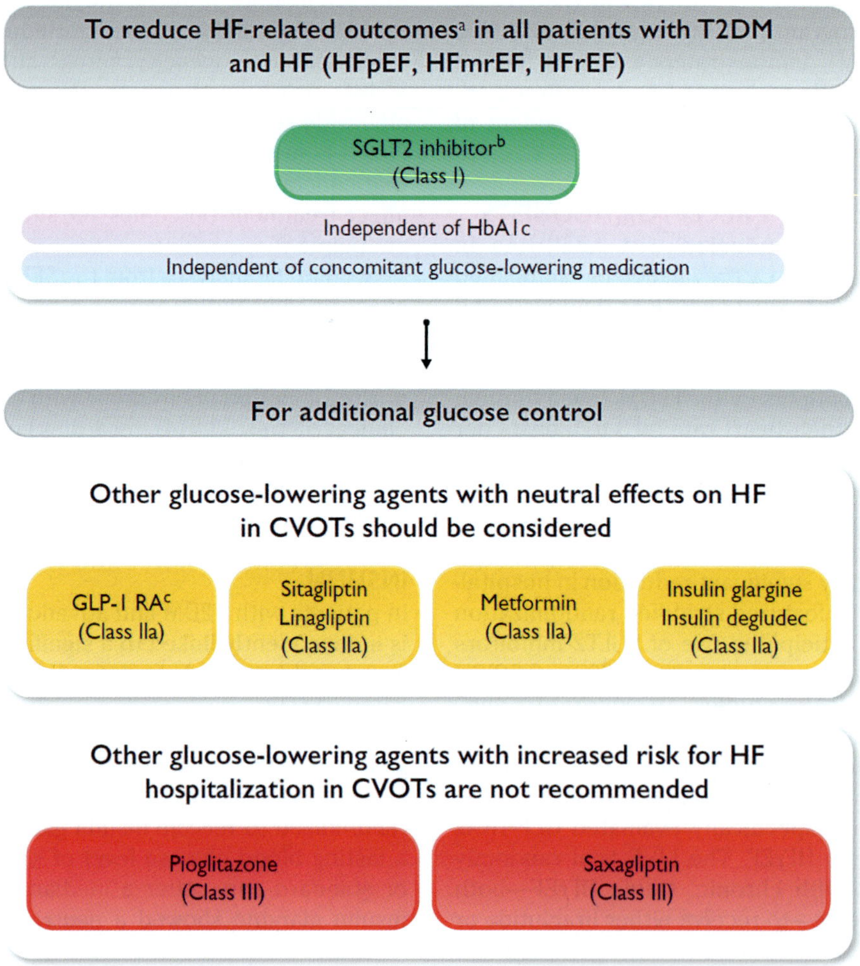

FIG. 16.6 Glucose-lowering treatment of patients with HF and T2DM. *CVOT*, Cardiovascular outcomes trial; *DPP-4*, dipeptidyl peptidase-4; *GLP-1RA*, glucagon-like peptide-1 receptor agonist; *Hb1Ac*, glycated hemoglobin; *HF*, heart failure; *HFmrEF*, HF with mildly reduced ejection fraction; *HFpEF*, HF with preserved ejection fraction; *HFrEF*, HF with reduced ejection fraction; *SGLT2*, sodium-glucose cotransporter-2; *T2DM*, type 2 diabetes mellitus. [a]This includes HF hospitalization or CV death. [b]Empagliflozin, dapagliflozin, or sotagliflozin in patients with HFrEF, empagliflozin, or dapagliflozin in patients with HFpEF and HFmrEF. [c]Preferred in patients with atherosclerotic cardiovascular disease and if weight reduction is needed; do not combine with DPP-4 inhibitors. From Marx N, Federici M, Schütt K, et al. 2023 ESC Guidelines for the management of cardiovascular disease in patients with diabetes. *Eur Heart J*. 2023;44(39):4043–4140. https://doi.10.1093/eurheartj/ehad192. (In eng).

SUMMARY

Patients with T2DM exhibit an increased risk to develop HF, and the presence of both comorbidities has a major impact on the prognosis. According to current guideline recommendations, a systematic survey of HF symptoms and/or signs of HF is recommended at each clinical encounter on all patients with diabetes. If HF is suspected, it is recommended to measure BNP/NT-ProBNP. Based on the data from large CV outcomes trials, including but not exclusively performed in patients with diabetes, treatment strategies and clinical decision-making should be based on the presence of HFrEF, HFmrEF, or HFpEF. In general, therapies proven effective for HF treatment in the general population are effective in persons with diabetes and HF. When HF is diagnosed in patients with T2DM, glucose-lowering medication should be reevaluated given that some agents like pioglitazone or saxagliptin increase the risk of HF hospitalization.

REFERENCES

1. McDonagh TA, Metra M, Adamo M, et al. 2021 ESC Guidelines for the diagnosis and treatment of acute and chronic heart failure: developed by the task force for the diagnosis and treatment of acute and chronic heart failure of the European Society of Cardiology (ESC) with the special contribution of the Heart Failure Association (HFA) of the ESC. Eur Heart J. 2021;42(36):3599–3726. https://doi.org/10.1093/eurheartj/ehab368.
2. Seferović PM, Paulus WJ. Clinical diabetic cardiomyopathy: a two-faced disease with restrictive and dilated phenotypes. Eur Heart J. 2015;36(27):1718–1727. https://doi.org/10.1093/eurheartj/ehv134.
3. Sattar N, McGuire DK. Pathways to cardiorenal complications in type 2 diabetes mellitus: a need to rethink. Circulation. 2018;138(1):7–9. https://doi.org/10.1161/CIRCULATIONAHA.118.035083.
4. Maack C, Lehrke M, Backs J, et al. Heart failure and diabetes: metabolic alterations and therapeutic interventions: a state-of-the-art review from the Translational Research Committee of the Heart Failure Association–European Society of Cardiology. Eur Heart J. 2018;39(48):4243–4254. https://doi.org/10.1093/eurheartj/ehy596.
5. Seferović PM, Paulus WJ, Rosano G, et al. Diabetic myocardial disorder. A clinical consensus statement of the Heart Failure Association of the ESC and the ESC Working Group on Myocardial & Pericardial Diseases. Eur J Heart Fail. 2024 https://doi.org/10.1002/ejhf.3347. (In eng).
6. Thrainsdottir IS, Aspelund T, Thorgeirsson G, et al. The association between glucose abnormalities and heart failure in the population-based Reykjavik study. Diabetes Care. 2005;28(3):612–616. http://www.ncbi.nlm.nih.gov/pubmed/15735197.
7. Nichols GA, Gullion CM, Koro CE, Ephross SA, Brown JB. The incidence of congestive heart failure in type 2 diabetes: an update. Diabetes Care. 2004;27(8):1879–1884. http://www.ncbi.nlm.nih.gov/pubmed/15277411.
8. Kannel WB, McGee DL. Diabetes and cardiovascular disease. The Framingham study. *JAMA*. 1979;241(19):2035–2038. (In eng). http://www.ncbi.nlm.nih.gov/pubmed/430798.
9. van Melle JP, Bot M, de Jonge P, de Boer RA, van Veldhuisen DJ, Whooley MA. Diabetes, glycemic control, and new-onset heart failure in patients with stable coronary artery disease: data from the heart and soul study. *Diabetes Care*. 2010;33(9):2084–2089. https://doi.org/10.2337/dc10-0286. (In eng).
10. Sattar N, McMurray J, Borén J, et al. Twenty years of cardiovascular complications and risk factors in patients with type 2 diabetes: a Nationwide Swedish Cohort Study. *Circulation*. 2023;147(25):1872–1886. https://doi.org/10.1161/circulationaha.122.063374. (In eng).
11. Gustafsson I, Brendorp B, Seibaek M, et al. Influence of diabetes and diabetes-gender interaction on the risk of death in patients hospitalized with congestive heart failure. *J Am Coll Cardiol*. 2004;43(5):771–777. https://doi.org/10.1016/j.jacc.2003.11.024.
12. MacDonald MR, Petrie MC, Varyani F, et al. Impact of diabetes on outcomes in patients with low and preserved ejection fraction heart failure: an analysis of the Candesartan in Heart failure: Assessment of Reduction in Mortality and morbidity (CHARM) programme. *Eur Heart J*. 2008;29(11):1377–1385. http://www.ncbi.nlm.nih.gov/entrez/query.fcgi?cmd=Retrieve&db=PubMed&dopt=Citation&list_uids=18413309.
13. Marx N, Federici M, Schütt K, et al. 2023 ESC Guidelines for the management of cardiovascular disease in patients with diabetes. *Eur Heart J*. 2023;44(39):4043–4140. https://doi.org/10.1093/eurheartj/ehad192. (In eng).
14. Segar MW, Vaduganathan M, Patel KV, et al. Machine learning to predict the risk of incident heart failure hospitalization among patients with diabetes: the WATCH-DM risk score. *Diabetes Care*. 2019;42(12):2298–2306. https://doi.org/10.2337/dc19-0587.
15. Pandey A, Vaduganathan M, Patel KV, et al. Biomarker-based risk prediction of incident heart failure in pre-diabetes and diabetes. *Heart Fail*. 2021;9(3):215–223. https://doi.org/10.1016/j.jchf.2020.10.013.
16. Seferović P, Farmakis D, Bayes-Genis A, et al. Biomarkers for the prediction of heart failure and cardiovascular events in patients with type 2 diabetes: a position statement from the Heart Failure Association of the European Society of Cardiology. *Eur J heart Fail*. 2022;24(7):1162–1170. https://doi.org/10.1002/ejhf.2575.
17. Mebazaa A, Davison B, Chioncel O, et al. Safety, tolerability and efficacy of up-titration of guideline-directed medical therapies for acute heart failure (STRONG-HF): a multinational, open-label, randomised, trial. *Lancet*. 2022;400(10367):1938–1952. https://doi.org/10.1016/S0140-6736(22)02076-1.
18. McMurray JJ, Packer M, Desai AS, et al. Angiotensin–neprilysin inhibition versus enalapril in heart failure. *N Engl J Med*. 2014;371:993–1004. https://doi.org/10.1056/NEJMoa1409077.
19. Garg R, Yusuf S. Overview of randomized trials of angiotensin-converting enzyme inhibitors on mortality and morbidity in patients with heart failure. Collaborative Group on ACE Inhibitor Trials. *JAMA*. 1995;273(18):1450–1456. (In eng).
20. Gustafsson I, Torp-Pedersen C, Køber L, Gustafsson F, Hildebrandt P, Group TS. Effect of the angiotensin-converting enzyme inhibitor trandolapril on mortality and morbidity in diabetic patients with left ventricular dysfunction after acute myocardial infarction. *J Am Coll Cardiology*. 1999;34(1):83–89. https://doi.org/10.1016/S0735-1097(99)00146-1.
21. Moye L, Pfeffer M, Wun C, et al. Uniformity of captopril benefit in the SAVE study: subgroup analysis. *Eur Heart J*. 1994;15(Suppl_B):2–8. https://doi.org/10.1093/eurheartj/15.suppl_B.2.
22. Shekelle PG, Rich MW, Morton SC, et al. Efficacy of angiotensin-converting enzyme inhibitors and beta-blockers in the management of left ventricular systolic dysfunction according to race, gender, and diabetic status: a meta-analysis of major clinical trials. *J Am Coll Cardiology*. 2003;41(9):1529–1538. https://doi.org/10.1016/S0735-1097(03)00262-6.
23. Vijayakumar S, Butler J, Bakris GL. Barriers to guideline mandated renin–angiotensin inhibitor use: focus on hyperkalaemia. *Eur Heart J Suppl*. 2019;21(Supplement_A):A20–A27. https://doi.org/10.1093/eurheartj/suy030.
24. Beldhuis IE, Streng KW, Ter Maaten JM, et al. Renin-angiotensin system inhibition, worsening renal function, and outcome in heart failure patients with reduced and preserved ejection fraction: a meta-analysis of published study data. *Circ Heart Fail*. 2017;10(2):e003588. https://doi.org/10.1161/CIRCHEARTFAILURE.116.003588.
25. Mullens W, Damman K, Testani JM, et al. Evaluation of kidney function throughout the heart failure trajectory–a position statement from the Heart Failure Association of the European Society of Cardiology. *Eur J Heart Fail*. 2020;22(4):584–603. https://doi.org/10.1002/ejhf.1697.
26. McMurray JJ, Solomon SD, Inzucchi SE, et al. Dapagliflozin in patients with heart failure and reduced ejection fraction. *N Engl J Med*. 2019;381(21):1995–2008. https://doi.org/10.1056/NEJMoa1911303.
27. Kosiborod MN, Jhund PS, Docherty KF, et al. Effects of dapagliflozin on symptoms, function, and quality of life in patients with heart failure and reduced ejection fraction: results from the DAPA-HF trial. *Circulation*. 2020;141(2):90–99. https://doi.org/10.1161/CIRCULATIONAHA.119.044138.
28. Docherty KF, Jhund PS, Bengtsson O, et al. Effect of dapagliflozin in DAPA-HF according to background glucose-lowering therapy. *Diabetes Care*. 2020;43(11):2878–2881. https://doi.org/10.2337/dc20-1402.
29. Packer M, Anker SD, Butler J, et al. Cardiovascular and renal outcomes with empagliflozin in heart failure. *N Engl J Med*. 2020;383(15):1413–1424. https://doi.org/10.1056/NEJMoa2022190.
30. Anker SD, Butler J, Filippatos G, et al. Empagliflozin in heart failure with a preserved ejection fraction. *N Engl J Med*. 2021;385(16):1451–1461. https://doi.org/10.1056/NEJMoa2107038. (In eng).
31. Butler J, Anker SD, Filippatos G, et al. Empagliflozin and health-related quality of life outcomes in patients with heart failure with reduced ejection fraction: the EMPEROR-Reduced trial. *Eur Heart J*. 2021;42(13):1203–1212. https://doi.org/10.1093/eurheartj/ehaa1007.
32. Bhatt DL, Szarek M, Pitt B, et al. Sotagliflozin in patients with diabetes and chronic kidney disease. *N Engl J Med*. 2021;384(2):129–139. https://doi.org/10.1056/NEJMoa2030186. (In eng).
33. Damman K, Beusekamp JC, Boorsma EM, et al. Randomized, double-blind, placebo-controlled, multicentre pilot study on the effects of empagliflozin on clinical outcomes in patients with acute decompensated heart failure (EMPA-RESPONSE-AHF). *Eur J Heart Fail*. 2020;22(4):713–722. https://doi.org/10.1002/ejhf.1713.
34. Bhatt DL, Szarek M, Steg PG, et al. Sotagliflozin in patients with diabetes and recent worsening heart failure. *N Engl J Med*. 2021;384(2):117–128. https://doi.org/10.1056/NEJMoa2030183.
35. Voors AA, Angermann CE, Teerlink JR, et al. The SGLT2 inhibitor empagliflozin in patients hospitalized for acute heart failure: a multinational randomized trial. *Nat Med*. 2022;28(3):568–574. https://doi.org/10.1038/s41591-021-01659-1.
36. Pitt B, Zannad F, Remme WJ, et al. Randomized Aldactone Evaluation Study Investigators The effect of spironolactone on morbidity and mortality in patients with severe heart failure. *N Engl J Med*. 1999;341(10):709–717. https://doi.org/10.1056/nejm199909023411001. (In eng).

37. Swedberg K, Zannad F, McMurray JJ, et al. Eplerenone and atrial fibrillation in mild systolic heart failure: results from the EMPHASIS-HF (Eplerenone in Mild Patients Hospitalization and Survival Study in Heart Failure) study. *J Am Coll Cardiology*. 2012;59(18):1598–1603. https://doi.org/10.1016/j.jacc.2011.11.063.
38. Bobbio M, Ferrua S, Opasich C, et al. Survival and hospitalization in heart failure patients with or without diabetes treated with β-blockers. *J Card Fail*. 2003;9(3):192–202. https://doi.org/10.1054/jcaf.2003.31.
39. Deedwania PC, Giles TD, Klibaner M, et al. Efficacy, safety and tolerability of metoprolol CR/XL in patients with diabetes and chronic heart failure: experiences from MERIT-HF. *Am heart J*. 2005;149(1):159–167. https://doi.org/10.1016/j.ahj.2004.05.056.
40. Erdmann E, Philippe L, Patricia V, Hermann W. Results from post-hoc analyses of the CIBIS II trial: effect of bisoprolol in high-risk patient groups with chronic heart failure. *Eur J Heart Fail*. 2001;3(4):469–479. https://doi.org/10.1016/S1388-9842(01)00174-X.
41. Packer M, Fowler MB, Roecker EB, et al. Effect of carvedilol on the morbidity of patients with severe chronic heart failure: results of the carvedilol prospective randomized cumulative survival (COPERNICUS) study. *Circulation*. 2002;106(17):2194–2199. https://doi.org/10.1161/01.CIR.0000035653.72855.BF.
42. Faris R, Flather M, Purcell H, Henein M, Poole-Wilson P, Coats A. Current evidence supporting the role of diuretics in heart failure: a meta analysis of randomised controlled trials. *Int J cardiology*. 2002;82(2):149–158. https://doi.org/10.1016/S0167-5273(01)00600-3.
43. Granger CB, McMurray JJ, Yusuf S, et al. Effects of candesartan in patients with chronic heart failure and reduced left-ventricular systolic function intolerant to angiotensin-converting-enzyme inhibitors: the CHARM-Alternative trial. *Lancet*. 2003;362(9386):772–776. http://www.ncbi.nlm.nih.gov/entrez/query.fcgi?cmd=Retrieve&db=PubMed&dopt=Citation&list_uids=13678870.
44. Konstam MA, Neaton JD, Dickstein K, et al. Effects of high-dose versus low-dose losartan on clinical outcomes in patients with heart failure (HEAAL study): a randomised, double-blind trial. *Lancet*. 2009;374(9704):1840–1848. https://doi.org/10.1016/S0140-6736(09)61913-9.
45. Maggioni AP, Anand I, Gottlieb SO, Latini R, Tognoni G, Cohn JN, Val-HeFT Investigators. Effects of valsartan on morbidity and mortality in patients with heart failure not receiving angiotensin-converting enzyme inhibitors. *J Am Coll Cardiology*. 2002;40(8):1414–1421. https://doi.org/10.1016/S0735-1097(02)02304-5.
46. Komajda M, Tavazzi L, Francq BG, et al. Efficacy and safety of ivabradine in patients with chronic systolic heart failure and diabetes: an analysis from the SHIFT trial. *Eur J heart Fail*. 2015;17(12):1294–1301. https://doi.org/10.1002/ejhf.347.
47. Taylor AL, Ziesche S, Yancy C, et al. Combination of isosorbide dinitrate and hydralazine in blacks with heart failure. *N Engl J Med*. 2004;351(20):2049–2057. https://doi.org/10.1056/NEJMoa042934.
48. Taylor AL, Ziesche S, Yancy CW, et al. Early and sustained benefit on event-free survival and heart failure hospitalization from fixed-dose combination of isosorbide dinitrate/hydralazine: consistency across subgroups in the African-American Heart Failure Trial. *Circulation*. 2007;115(13):1747–1753. https://doi.org/10.1161/CIRCULATIONAHA.106.644013.
49. Abdul-Rahim AH, MacIsaac RL, Jhund PS, Petrie MC, Lees KR, McMurray JJ, VICCTA-Heart Failure Collaborators. Efficacy and safety of digoxin in patients with heart failure and reduced ejection fraction according to diabetes status: An analysis of the Digitalis Investigation Group (DIG) trial. *Int J Cardiology*. 2016;209:310–316. https://doi.org/10.1016/j.ijcard.2016.02.074.
50. Bristow MR, Saxon LA, Boehmer J, et al. Cardiac-resynchronization therapy with or without an implantable defibrillator in advanced chronic heart failure. *N Engl J Med*. 2004;350(21):2140–2150. https://doi.org/10.1056/NEJMoa032423.
51. Ghali JK, Boehmer J, Feldman AM, et al. Influence of diabetes on cardiac resynchronization therapy with or without defibrillator in patients with advanced heart failure. *J Card Fail*. 2007;13(9):769–773. https://doi.org/10.1016/j.cardfail.2007.06.723.
52. Køber L, Thune JJ, Nielsen JC, et al. Defibrillator implantation in patients with nonischemic systolic heart failure. *N Engl J Med*. 2016;375(13):1221–1230. https://doi.org/10.1056/NEJMoa1608029.
53. Rørth R, Thune JJ, Nielsen JC, et al. The effect of implantable cardioverter-defibrillator in patients with diabetes and non-ischaemic systolic heart failure. *Europace*. 2019;21(8):1203–1210. https://doi.org/10.1093/europace/euz114.
54. Kilic A, Weiss ES, George TJ, Arnaoutakis GJ, Yuh DD, Shah AS, Conte JV. What predicts long-term survival after heart transplantation? An analysis of 9,400 ten-year survivors. *Ann Thorac Surg*. 2012;93(3):699–704. https://doi.org/10.1016/j.athoracsur.2011.09.037.
55. Ponikowski P, Voors AA, Anker SD, et al. 2016 ESC Guidelines for the diagnosis and treatment of acute and chronic heart failure: the task force for the diagnosis and treatment of acute and chronic heart failure of the European Society of Cardiology (ESC). Developed with the special contribution of the Heart Failure Association (HFA) of the ESC. *Eur J Heart Fail*. 2016;18(8):891–975. https://doi.org/10.1002/ejhf.592.
56. Yusuf S, Pfeffer MA, Swedberg K, et al. Effects of candesartan in patients with chronic heart failure and preserved left-ventricular ejection fraction: the CHARM-Preserved Trial. *Lancet*. 2003;362(9386):777–781. http://www.ncbi.nlm.nih.gov/entrez/query.fcgi?cmd=Retrieve&db=PubMed&dopt=Citation&list_uids=13678871.
57. Solomon SD, McMurray JJ, Anand IS, et al. Angiotensin–neprilysin inhibition in heart failure with preserved ejection fraction. *N Engl J Med*. 2019;381(17):1609–1620. https://doi.org/10.1056/NEJMoa1908655.
58. Pitt B, Pfeffer MA, Assmann SF, et al. Spironolactone for heart failure with preserved ejection fraction. *N Engl J Med*. 2014;370:1383–1392. https://doi.org/10.1056/NEJMoa1313731.
59. Cleland JG, Tendera M, Adamus J, et al. Perindopril for elderly people with chronic heart failure: the PEP-CHF study. The PEP investigators. *Eur J Heart Fail*. 1999;1(3):211–217. https://doi.org/10.1016/s1388-9842(99)00039-2. (In eng).
60. Massie BM, Carson PE, McMurray JJ, et al. Irbesartan in patients with heart failure and preserved ejection fraction. *N Engl J Med*. 2008;359(23):2456–2467. https://doi.org/10.1056/NEJMoa0805450.
61. Ahmed A, Rich MW, Fleg JL, et al. Effects of digoxin on morbidity and mortality in diastolic heart failure: the ancillary digitalis investigation group trial. *Circulation*. 2006;114(5):397–403. https://doi.org/10.1161/CIRCULATIONAHA.106.628347.
62. Solomon SD, McMurray JJ, Claggett B, et al. Dapagliflozin in heart failure with mildly reduced or preserved ejection fraction. *N Engl J Med*. 2022;387(12):1089–1098. https://doi.org/10.1056/NEJMoa2206286.
63. Vaduganathan M, Docherty KF, Claggett BL, et al. SGLT-2 inhibitors in patients with heart failure: a comprehensive meta-analysis of five randomised controlled trials. *Lancet*. 2022;400(10354):757–767. https://doi.org/10.1016/S0140-6736(22)01429-5.
64. Filippatos G, Butler J, Farmakis D, et al. Empagliflozin for heart failure with preserved left ventricular ejection fraction with and without diabetes. *Circulation*. 2022;146:676–686. https://doi.org/10.1161/CIRCULATIONAHA.122.059785.
65. Kosiborod MN, Petrie MC, Borlaug BA, et al. Semaglutide in patients with obesity-related heart failure and type 2 diabetes. *N Engl J Med*. 2024; 390(15):1394–1407. https://doi.org/10.1056/NEJMoa2313917. (In eng).
66. Kosiborod MN, Abildstrøm SZ, Borlaug BA, et al. Semaglutide in patients with heart failure with preserved ejection fraction and obesity. *N Engl J Med*. 2023;389(12):1069–1084. https://doi.org/10.1056/NEJMoa2306963. (In eng).
67. Butler J, Shah SJ, Petrie MC, et al. Semaglutide versus placebo in people with obesity-related heart failure with preserved ejection fraction: a pooled analysis of the STEP-HFpEF and STEP-HFpEF DM randomised trials. *Lancet*. 2024;403(10437):1635–1648. https://doi.org/10.1016/s0140-6736(24)00469-0. (In eng).
68. Shah SJ, Sharma K, Borlaug BA, et al. Semaglutide and diuretic use in obesity-related heart failure with preserved ejection fraction: a pooled analysis of the STEP-HFpEF and STEP-HFpEF-DM trials. *Eur Heart J*. 2024;45(35):3254–3269. https://doi.org/10.1093/eurheartj/ehae322. (In eng).
69. Petrie MC, Borlaug BA, Butler J, et al. Semaglutide and NT-proBNP in obesity-related HFpEF: insights from the STEP-HfpEF program. *J Am Coll Cardiol*. 2024;84(1):27–40. https://doi.org/10.1016/j.jacc.2024.04.022. (In eng).
70. Pitt B, Filippatos G, Agarwal R, et al. Cardiovascular events with finerenone in kidney disease and type 2 diabetes. *N Engl J Med*. 2021;385(24):2252–2263. https://doi.org/10.1056/NEJMoa2110956.
71. Bakris GL, Agarwal R, Anker SD, et al. Effect of finerenone on chronic kidney disease outcomes in type 2 diabetes. *N Engl J Med*. 2020;383(23):2219–2229. https://doi.org/10.1056/NEJMoa2025845. (In eng).
72. Vaduganathan M, Claggett BL, Desai AS, et al. Time to significant benefit of finerenone in patients with heart failure. *J Am Coll Cardiol*. 2024. https://doi.org/10.1016/j.jacc.2024.09.018. (In eng).
73. Solomon SD, McMurray JJV, Vaduganathan M, et al. Finerenone in heart failure with mildly reduced or preserved ejection fraction. *N Engl J Med*. 2024 https://doi.org/10.1056/NEJMoa2407107. (In eng).
74. Docherty KF, Henderson AD, Jhund PS, et al. Efficacy and safety of finerenone across the ejection fraction spectrum in heart failure with mildly reduced and preserved ejection fraction: a prespecified analysis of the FINEARTS-HF trial. *Circulation*. 2024. https://doi.org/10.1161/circulationaha.124.072011. (In eng).
75. Vaduganathan M, Claggett BL, Kulac IJ, et al. Effects of the non-steroidal MRA finerenone with and without concomitant SGLT2 inhibitor use in heart failure. *Circulation*. 2024. https://doi.org/10.1161/circulationaha.124.072055. (In eng).
76. Eurich DT, Majumdar SR, McAlister FA, Tsuyuki RT, Johnson JA. Improved clinical outcomes associated with metformin in patients with diabetes and heart failure. *Diabetes Care*. 2005;28(10):2345–2351. https://doi.org/10.2337/diacare.28.10.2345.
77. Masoudi FA, Inzucchi SE, Wang Y, Havranek EP, Foody JM, Krumholz HM. Thiazolidinediones, metformin, and outcomes in older patients with diabetes and heart failure: an observational study. *Circulation*. 2005;111(5):583–590. http://www.ncbi.nlm.nih.gov/entrez/query.fcgi?cmd=Retrieve&db=PubMed&dopt=Citation&list_uids=15699279.
78. Scirica BM, Bhatt DL, Braunwald E, et al. Saxagliptin and cardiovascular outcomes in patients with type 2 diabetes mellitus. *N Engl J Med*. 2013;369(14):1317–1326. https://doi.org/10.1056/NEJMoa1307684. (In eng).
79. White WB, Cannon CP, Heller SR, et al. Alogliptin after acute coronary syndrome in patients with type 2 diabetes. *N Engl j Med*. 2013;369:1327–1335. https://doi.org/10.1056/NEJMoa1305889.
80. Green JB, Bethel MA, Armstrong PW, et al. Effect of sitagliptin on cardiovascular outcomes in type 2 diabetes. *N Engl J Med*. 2015;373(3):232–242. https://doi.org/10.1056/NEJMoa1501352.

81. McGuire DK, Alexander JH, Johansen OE, et al. Linagliptin effects on heart failure and related outcomes in individuals with type 2 diabetes mellitus at high cardiovascular and renal risk in CARMELINA. *Circulation*. 2018. https://doi.org/10.1161/circulationaha.118.038352. (In eng).
82. McMurray JJ, Ponikowski P, Bolli GB, et al. Effects of vildagliptin on ventricular function in patients with type 2 diabetes mellitus and heart failure: a randomized placebo-controlled trial. *JACC: Heart Fail*. 2018;6(1):8–17. https://doi.org/10.1016/j.jchf.2017.08.004.
83. Zinman B, Wanner C, Lachin JM, et al. Empagliflozin, cardiovascular outcomes, and mortality in type 2 diabetes. *N Engl J Med*. 2015;373(22). https://doi.org/10.1056/NEJMoa1504720.
84. Neal B, Perkovic V, Mahaffey KW, et al. Canagliflozin and cardiovascular and renal events in type 2 diabetes. *N Engl J Med*. 2017. https://doi.org/10.1056/NEJMoa1611925. (In eng).
85. Wiviott SD, Raz I, Bonaca MP, et al. Dapagliflozin and cardiovascular outcomes in type 2 diabetes. *N Engl J Med*. 2018. https://doi.org/10.1056/NEJMoa1812389. (In eng).
86. Kato ET, Silverman MG, Mosenzon O, et al. Effect of dapagliflozin on heart failure and mortality in type 2 diabetes mellitus. *Circulation*. 2019;139(22):2528–2536. https://doi.org/10.1161/CIRCULATIONAHA.119.040130.
87. Cannon CP, Pratley R, Dagogo-Jack S, et al. Cardiovascular outcomes with ertugliflozin in type 2 diabetes. *N Engl J Med*. 2020;383(15):1425–1435. https://doi.org/10.1056/NEJMoa2004967. (In eng).
88. Cosentino F, Cannon CP, Cherney DZ, et al. Efficacy of ertugliflozin on heart failure–related events in patients with type 2 diabetes mellitus and established atherosclerotic cardiovascular disease: results of the VERTIS CV Trial. *Circulation*. 2020;142(23):2205–2215. https://doi.org/10.1161/CIRCULATIONAHA.120.050255.
89. Heerspink HJL, Stefánsson BV, Correa-Rotter R, et al. Dapagliflozin in patients with chronic kidney disease. *N Engl J Med*. 2020;383(15):1436–1446. https://doi.org/10.1056/NEJMoa2024816. (In eng).
90. Herrington WG, Staplin N, Wanner C, et al. Empagliflozin in patients with chronic kidney disease. *N Engl J Med*. 2022. https://doi.org/10.1056/NEJMoa2204233. (In eng).
91. McGuire DK, Shih WJ, Cosentino F, et al. Association of SGLT2 inhibitors with cardiovascular and kidney outcomes in patients with type 2 diabetes: a meta-analysis. *JAMA Cardiol*. 2021;6(2):148–158. https://doi.org/10.1001/jamacardio.2020.4511. (In eng).
92. Sattar N, Lee MMY, Kristensen SL, et al. Cardiovascular, mortality, and kidney outcomes with GLP-1 receptor agonists in patients with type 2 diabetes: a systematic review and meta-analysis of randomised trials. *Lancet Diabetes Endocrinol*. 2021;9(10):653–662. https://doi.org/10.1016/s2213-8587(21)00203-5. (In eng).
93. Gerstein HC, Sattar N, Rosenstock J, et al. Cardiovascular and renal outcomes with efpeglenatide in type 2 diabetes. *N Engl J Med*. 2021;385(10):896–907. https://doi.org/10.1056/NEJMoa2108269. (In eng).
94. Jorsal A, Kistorp C, Holmager P, et al. Effect of liraglutide, a glucagon-like peptide-1 analogue, on left ventricular function in stable chronic heart failure patients with and without diabetes (LIVE)—a multicentre, double-blind, randomised, placebo-controlled trial. *Eur J heart Fail*. 2017;19(1):69–77. https://doi.org/10.1002/ejhf.657.
95. Margulies KB, Hernandez AF, Redfield MM, et al. Effects of liraglutide on clinical stability among patients with advanced heart failure and reduced ejection fraction: a randomized clinical trial. *JAMA*. 2016;316(5):500–508. https://doi.org/10.1001/jama.2016.10260. (Clinical Trial, Phase II Multicenter Study Randomized Controlled Trial Research Support, N.I.H., Extramural) (In Eng).
96. Perkovic V, Tuttle KR, Rossing P, et al. Effects of semaglutide on chronic kidney disease in patients with type 2 diabetes. *N Engl J Med*. 2024;391(2):109–121. https://doi.org/10.1056/NEJMoa2403347. (In eng).
97. Lincoff AM, Brown-Frandsen K, Colhoun HM, et al. Semaglutide and cardiovascular outcomes in obesity without diabetes. *N Engl J Med*. 2023;389(24):2221–2232. https://doi.org/10.1056/NEJMoa2307563. (In eng).
98. Pratley RE, Tuttle KR, Rossing P, et al. Effects of semaglutide on heart failure outcomes in diabetes and chronic kidney disease in the FLOW trial. *J Am Coll Cardiol*. 2024. https://doi.org/10.1016/j.jacc.2024.08.004. (In eng).
99. Mann JFE, Rossing P, Bakris G, et al. Effects of semaglutide with and without concomitant SGLT2 inhibitor use in participants with type 2 diabetes and chronic kidney disease in the FLOW trial. *Nat Med*. 2024. https://doi.org/10.1038/s41591-024-03133-0. (In eng).
100. Deanfield J, Verma S, Scirica BM, et al. Semaglutide and cardiovascular outcomes in patients with obesity and prevalent heart failure: a prespecified analysis of the SELECT trial. *Lancet*. 2024;404(10454):773–786. https://doi.org/10.1016/s0140-6736(24)01498-3. (In eng).
101. Gerstein HC, Bosch J, Dagenais GR, et al. Basal insulin and cardiovascular and other outcomes in dysglycemia. *N Engl J Med*. 2012;367(4):319–328. https://doi.org/10.1056/NEJMoa1203858. (In eng).
102. Pratley RE, Husain M, Lingvay I, et al. Heart failure with insulin degludec versus glargine U100 in patients with type 2 diabetes at high risk of cardiovascular disease: DEVOTE 14. *Cardiovas Diabetol*. 2019;18(1):156. https://doi.org/10.1186/s12933-019-0960-8.
103. Erdmann E, Charbonnel B, Wilcox RG, et al. Pioglitazone use and heart failure in patients with type 2 diabetes and preexisting cardiovascular disease: data from the PROactive study (PROactive 08). *Diabetes Care*. 2007;30(11):2773–2778. http://www.ncbi.nlm.nih.gov/entrez/query.fcgi?cmd=Retrieve&db=PubMed&dopt=Citation&list_uids=17666462.
104. Pantalone KM, Kattan MW, Yu C, et al. The risk of developing coronary artery disease or congestive heart failure, and overall mortality, in type 2 diabetic patients receiving rosiglitazone, pioglitazone, metformin, or sulfonylureas: a retrospective analysis. *Acta Diabetol*. 2009;46(2):145–154. https://doi.org/10.1007/s00592-008-0090-3.
105. Tzoulaki I, Molokhia M, Curcin V, et al. Risk of cardiovascular disease and all cause mortality among patients with type 2 diabetes prescribed oral antidiabetes drugs: retrospective cohort study using UK general practice research database. *BMJ*. 2009;339:b4731. https://doi.org/10.1136/bmj.b4731.
106. Holman RR, Haffner SM, McMurray JJ, et al. Effect of nateglinide on the incidence of diabetes and cardiovascular events. *N Engl J Med*. 2010;362(16):1463–1476. https://doi.org/10.1056/NEJMoa1001122. (In eng).
107. Uk P. Intensive blood-glucose control with sulfonureas or insulin compared with conventional treatment and risk of complications in patients with type II diabetes. *Lancet*. 1998;352:837–853.
108. Viberti G, Kahn SE, Greene DA, et al. A Diabetes Outcome Progression Trial (ADOPT) An international multicenter study of the comparative efficacy of rosiglitazone, glyburide, and metformin in recently diagnosed type 2 diabetes. *Diabetes care*. 2002;25(10):1737–1743. https://doi.org/10.2337/diacare.25.10.1737.
109. Rosenstock J, Kahn SE, Johansen OE, et al. Effect of linagliptin vs glimepiride on major adverse cardiovascular outcomes in patients with type 2 diabetes: the CAROLINA randomized clinical trial. *JAMA*. 2019. https://doi.org/10.1001/jama.2019.13772. (In eng).
110. Rosenstock J, Perkovic V, Johansen OE, et al. Effect of linagliptin vs placebo on major cardiovascular events in adults with type 2 diabetes and high cardiovascular and renal risk: the CARMELINA randomized clinical trial. *JAMA*. 2019;321(1):69–79. https://doi.org/10.1001/jama.2018.18269.

PART IV MANAGEMENT OF CORONARY HEART DISEASE RISK, CHRONIC AND ACUTE CORONARY SYNDROMES IN PATIENTS WITH TYPE 2 DIABETES

17 Effect of Lifestyle Interventions on Coronary Heart Disease Risk in Patients With Type 2 Diabetes

BARRY A. FRANKLIN, WENDY M. MILLER, AND MICHAEL R. BRENNAN

In the United States and worldwide, the prevalence of high cholesterol, hypertension, and cigarette smoking together with age-adjusted cardiovascular (CV) deaths have declined over the last several decades.[1] On the other hand, the prevalence of type 2 diabetes mellitus (T2DM) has risen steadily, largely because of an epidemic of obesity and adiposity and our increasingly inactive lifestyle.[2] These trends will likely mitigate further reductions in CV mortality and even reverse the decline in CV disease (CVD) incidence.[3]

Using 2010 as the baseline, the estimated direct and indirect costs of CVD are expected to triple by the year 2030, making this a critical medical and societal issue.[4,5] These sobering projections and other data[6,7] suggest that effective preventive strategies are needed if we are to limit the growing burden of CVD. The current reactive-based health care model, in which patients are seen when they become ill, typically during outpatient visits or hospitalizations, often fails to proactively improve health, because so many health outcomes are explained by individual behaviors and the lifestyle choices people make on a daily basis.[6,8]

Unfortunately, many patients as well as individuals in the medical community continue to rely on costly cardioprotective medications and/or coronary revascularization procedures as a first-line strategy to stabilize or favorably modify established risk factors and the course of coronary heart disease (CHD). However, these therapies do not address the foundational causes of the problem, that is, the most proximal risk factors for CHD, including poor dietary practices, overweight and obesity, physical inactivity, and cigarette smoking, as shown in Fig. 17.1.[3] Unhealthy lifestyle habits strongly influence not only conventional risk factors (e.g., blood pressure, lipid and lipoprotein levels, glucose-insulin homeostasis, adiposity) but also novel or emerging risk factors such as endothelial dysfunction, inflammation (e.g., C-reactive protein), thrombosis and coagulation, arrhythmias, and other disease modulators (e.g., psychosocial stressors),[3] even among users of lipid-lowering and antihypertensive medications.[9] Collectively, these data suggest it is time to change our emphasis from disease management to disease prevention, focusing on the foundational causes of CVD by reengineering prevention into the US health care system.[7]

This chapter emphasizes the role of lifestyle interventions in the prevention and treatment of atherosclerotic CVD (ASCVD) in patients with diabetes mellitus (DM), with specific reference to weight management and energy balance, dietary intake and cardiometabolic risk, smoking cessation, exercise and physical activity (PA), cardiorespiratory fitness (CRF), and research-based psychosocial interventions (e.g., readiness to change, motivational interviewing, counseling strategies) to support cardioprotective lifestyle changes in this at-risk patient subset.

WEIGHT MANAGEMENT AND ENERGY BALANCE

Obesity is an independent risk factor for hypertension, dyslipidemia, and CVD, increasing the risk of CV events and mortality in patients with DM.[10] More than 80% of cases of DM can be attributed to obesity. Weight loss in

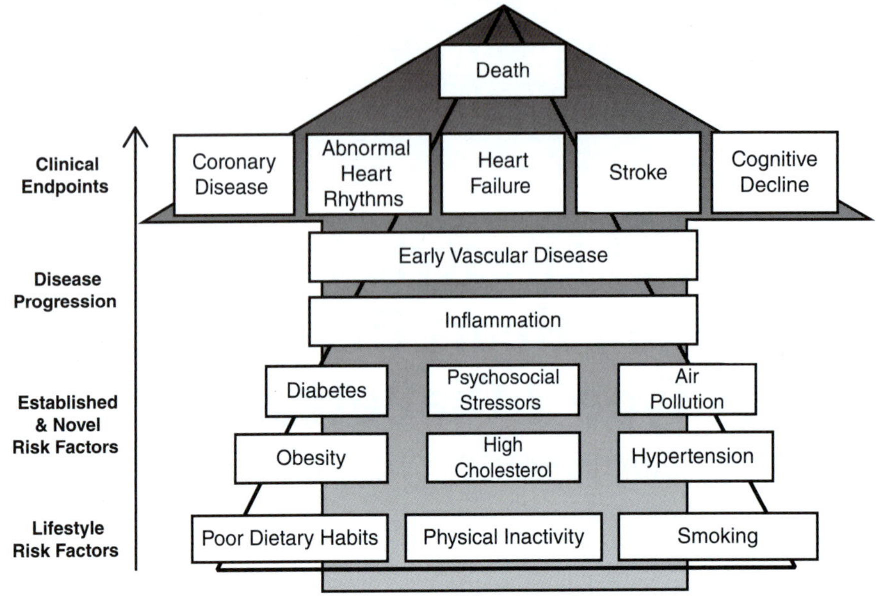

FIG. 17.1 Unhealthy lifestyle habits lead to coronary heart disease risk factors, the progression of atherosclerotic cardiovascular disease, and ultimately adverse clinical outcomes. Thus the first-line strategy to prevent coronary heart disease (or recurrent cardiac events) is to favorably modify poor lifestyle habits or practices, including suboptimal dietary habits, physical inactivity, overweight/obesity, and cigarette smoking. Modified from Mozaffarian D, Wilson PW, Kannel WB. Beyond established and novel risk factors: lifestyle risk factors for cardiovascular disease. *Circulation*. 2008;117(23):3031–3038.

TABLE 17.1 Determining Prescribed Calorie Content

PRESCRIBED CALORIE CONTENT (KCAL/DAY)	CURRENT TOTAL BODY WEIGHT (LB)
1000–1200	150–199
1200–1500	200–249
1500–1800	250–299
1800–2000	300–349
2000	300 or higher

individuals with overweight or obesity and DM is associated with clinical improvement in CV risk factors, including improvements in glycemia, dyslipidemia, and blood pressure. Substantial weight loss can lead to remission of DM, which is defined as maintaining a glycosylated hemoglobin (HbA1c) <6.5% without blood glucose–lowering pharmacotherapy. Therefore weight management is a crucial component of DM treatment and CVD prevention.

Weight loss occurs when energy intake is lower than energy expenditure. An energy deficit of 500 to 1000 kcal/day (3500–7000 kcal/week) usually results in a weight loss of 1 to 2 lb/week. Rate of weight loss can vary, however, depending on genetic factors, age, fidgeting, amount of lean body mass, and habitual PA. Older individuals tend to lose weight more slowly than younger persons due to a decline in metabolic rate of ~2% each decade.[11] Most overweight or obese adults will lose weight if they comply with a diet of 1200 to 1500 kcal/day for females or 1200 to 1600 kcal/day for males. Adjusting the daily calorie content based on baseline body weight is a more individualized and likely more effective approach (Table 17.1).[12]

Expert guidelines recommend an initial weight loss goal of 5% to 10% of body weight within 6 months.[13] Clinical improvements in triglycerides, blood glucose, and HbA1c typically occur with a 3% to 5% body weight loss. Additional body weight loss of >10% can lead to further clinical improvement, including reductions in blood pressure; improvement in low-density lipoprotein cholesterol (LDL-C) and high-density lipoprotein cholesterol (HDL-C); reduction in the need for medications to control blood pressure, blood glucose, and lipids; as well as potential remission of DM.[14]

Investigators have attempted to define the dietary macronutrient composition that is optimal for weight reduction, improvement in cardiometabolic risk factors, and long-term weight maintenance in individuals who are overweight or obese, as well as patients with DM. Overall, it appears that lower-carbohydrate diets (<40% of total calories) may result in short-term weight loss, improvement in hypertriglyceridemia, and possibly improvement in insulin resistance and HbA1c. At 1 to 2 years, however, the degree of weight loss and improvement in cardiometabolic risk factors is similar to that seen with low-fat or high-protein diets.[15] The true long-term impact of differing macronutrient composition dietary intake is not known, however, as many participants have difficulty maintaining their assigned macronutrient composition after 6 to 12 months. Accordingly, the optimal macronutrient composition varies for different individuals with regard to long-term compliance; thus dietary guidance should be individualized. The American Diabetes Association (ADA) 2023 Standards of Medical Care in Diabetes advises that the diet choice should be based on the patient's health status and preferences, including a determination of food availability and other cultural circumstances that could affect dietary patterns.[16] Nevertheless, even without considering macronutrient composition, dietary modifications that result in a net reduction of daily caloric intake below energy expenditure should promote weight reduction.

Comprehensive lifestyle interventions to support dietary changes, PA, and behavior strategies are recommended per expert guidelines and the ADA.[13,16] These interventions are in person, high intensity, and are provided in individual or group sessions by trained interventionists, such as dietitians, psychologists, and exercise specialists. The ADA 2023 Standards of Medical Care recommends ≥16 sessions over 6 months. High-intensity comprehensive lifestyle interventions have been shown to be the most effective behavioral treatment for weight loss. The required components include prescribing a moderately reduced-calorie diet, regular PA, and the implementation of behavioral strategies to facilitate adherence to diet and activity recommendations. The average weight loss in a 6-month period with frequent in-person treatment is 8 kg, which approximates 5% to 10% of initial body weight. Long-term (>1 year) maintenance programs that are comprehensive and provide at least monthly contact with trained interventionists are advised after achieving a marked weight loss. Ongoing monitoring of weight at least weekly is recommended as well as other self-monitoring strategies, such as tracking food intake and daily steps. To prevent weight regain, ≥150 to 200 min of brisk walking per week is recommended.[13]

Per the ADA society recommendations and as shown in the Action for Health in Diabetes (Look AHEAD) trial, meal replacement diet plans can be a beneficial approach for weight management but should be prescribed by trained practitioners with close patient monitoring.[13,17] The Look AHEAD trial that randomized persons with T2DM and with body mass index (BMI) ≥25 kg/m^2 to intensive lifestyle intervention versus usual care demonstrated the feasibility of long-term weight loss in patients with DM via an intensive lifestyle intervention that included a meal replacement diet plan. At 8 years, the average weight loss was 4.7%.[17,18]

Dietary Intake and Cardiometabolic Risk

Nutrition therapy that targets optimizing glucose levels, blood pressure, and lipid profiles in individuals with DM is associated with a lower risk of CVD, CHD, and stroke.[19] The ADA advises replacement of saturated fat with unsaturated fats, especially polyunsaturated fat. This has been associated with significant reductions in both total cholesterol and LDL-C. Additionally, replacement of saturated fat with monounsaturated fat from plant sources, such as olive oil and nuts, is associated with lower CVD risk. Replacing saturated fat with carbohydrate is not advised; although this reduces total cholesterol and LDL-C, it also significantly increases triglycerides and reduces HDL-C. Replacing foods high in carbohydrate with foods lower in carbohydrate and higher in fat may improve glucose, triglyceride, and HDL-C levels. However, the replacement of carbohydrate with fat should be with unsaturated fat.

Individuals with DM should consume <2300 mg/day of sodium, which has been shown to have beneficial effects on blood pressure. A serving of fish, particularly fatty fish such as salmon, mackerel, or rainbow trout, at least two times per week is recommended. Fatty fish contains long-chain omega-3 fatty acids eicosapentaenoic acid and docosahexaenoic acid, which have beneficial effects on lipoproteins and have been associated with prevention of ASCVD. Individuals following a vegetarian or vegan eating plan are encouraged to consume omega-3 α-linoleic acid, which is found in plant foods such as flax, walnuts, and soy, and may provide some CVD benefits. Other dietary recommendations for CVD risk reduction include consuming 8 to 10 servings per day of fruits and vegetables, 2 to 3 servings per day of low-fat dairy products, and limiting alcohol consumption to ≤2 servings per day for males and no more than 1 serving per day for females (Box 17.1).[19]

The Mediterranean diet, which is inclusive of the above dietary recommendations, includes consumption of whole grains; legumes; fruits; vegetables; nuts; fish and olive oil; wine in moderation; and a low intake of meat, dairy products, processed foods, and sweets.[20] This diet has been shown in numerous prospective clinical trials to have beneficial effects on CV health. Additionally, the Mediterranean diet has been shown to have a favorable impact on the CV risk factor profile of individuals with DM.[20]

Smoking Abstinence

Cigarette smoking in people with DM heightens the risk of CVD, premature death, microvascular complications, and worsens glycemic control when compared with those who do not smoke.[21] Quitting smoking has been shown to reduce the risk of CVD to that of someone who has never smoked in ~10 to 15 years, with the greatest decline of CVD risk within the first 5 years of quitting.[22]

BOX 17.1 Dietary Habits Associated with Cardioprotective Benefits

- Consume:
  - Fish and shellfish[a] (≥2 servings per week)
  - White poultry without skin and occasional lean meat (e.g., bison)[a]
  - Intact and minimally processed whole grains (e.g., quinoa and brown rice)
  - Fruits
  - Vegetables
  - Nuts and legumes (e.g., black beans and pinto beans)
  - Nonfat dairy products, plain yogurt, fortified soy milk
  - Most vegetable oils (e.g., olive, canola, and soybean oil)
  - Egg whites
  - Foods rich in soluble fiber (e.g., beans, oats, barley, yams, and oatmeal)
  - Consume 20–30 g of fiber daily
- Limit or avoid:
  - Saturated fat to <7% of total calories
  - Cheese and other dairy products
  - Egg yolks
  - Refined grains
  - Processed meats (e.g., hot dogs, bacon, and bologna)
  - Fried foods (e.g., chicken)
  - Sugars, sweetened beverages, and diet sodas
  - Grain-based desserts and bakery goods
  - Fats, oils, or foods with partially hydrogenated vegetable oils, and shortening
  - Tropical oils (coconut and palm kernel oil)
  - Salt (≤2300 mg/day [ADA guidelines] or <1500 mg/day for adults with high blood pressure or at risk for high blood pressure [AHA guidelines])
  - Alcohol[b]

[a]The portion should be no greater than the size of the individual's palm.
[b]For adults who drink alcohol, moderate consumption (≤2 drinks/day for males and ≤1 drink/day for females), ideally with meals.
ADA, American Diabetes Association; *AHA*, American Heart Association.

The ADA recommends including smoking cessation counseling and other forms of treatment as routine components of care for patients with DM who smoke. Assessment of smoking should be completed with every patient and those who smoke should be counseled on quitting. Results from numerous large randomized clinical trials have demonstrated the efficacy and cost-effectiveness of brief counseling in smoking cessation in reducing tobacco use.[23] Patients should also be advised not to use electronic nicotine delivery systems, commonly known as e-cigarettes or "vaping," or heated tobacco products. There are no rigorous studies that have demonstrated that noncombustible tobacco products are a healthier alternative to smoking or that e-cigarettes can facilitate smoking cessation.

Pharmacologic therapy can assist with smoking cessation and has been shown to be effective in people with DM. For motivated patients, the addition of pharmacologic therapy to counseling is more effective than either treatment alone. Pharmacological therapies, including bupropion and nicotine replacement therapy, can lessen the symptoms of nicotine withdrawal during smoking cessation. Behavioral support programs have also been shown to be effective for smoking cessation. A clinician's referral and recommendation to participate in a behavioral support program for smoking cessation is more effective than simply providing information about these resources. There is strong evidence that combining pharmacotherapy with behavioral interventions is the most effective way to help smokers sustain abstinence.[23] Community-based behavioral support resources for smoking cessation are listed in Table 17.2.[23]

EXERCISE AND PHYSICAL ACTIVITY IN THE TREATMENT OF TYPE 2 DIABETES MELLITUS

There is a pathophysiologic cascade by which physical inactivity predisposes to a cluster of cardiometabolic diseases, including DM. The associated metabolic perturbations reduce the somatic capacity to burn fuel, resulting in hyperinsulinemia, insulin resistance, hypertriglyceridemia, and ultimately increased CV risk. On the other hand, regular moderate-to-vigorous leisure-time PA, structured aerobic exercise, or both, can often reverse these adverse sequelae. A significant increase in PA and daily energy expenditure also improves insulin action in obesity, with or without a concomitant reduction in body weight and fat stores.[24] This is an important (and often overlooked) salutary effect, suggesting that PA is as efficacious in preventing insulin resistance as losing body weight.

TABLE 17.2 **Behavioral Support Resources for Smoking Cessation**

RESOURCE	SERVICES PROVIDED
Telephone Quitline 1-800-QUIT-NOW (1-800-784-8669)	• Counseling by telephone from a trained interventionist • Support provided via a series of scheduled telephone calls before and after quit date • Text messaging and web coaching support are available with some quitlines
Smokefree.gov (National Cancer Institute website)	• Smokefree TXT (text messaging program) • QuitGuide (mobile phone app) • Web-based information about quitting resources
Becomeanex.org (Truth Initiative)	• Web-based support program • Includes support from experts as well as online community to help smokers quit

From Rajat S. Barua et al. 2018 ACC expert consensus decision pathway on tobacco cessation treatment: a report of the American College of Cardiology Task Force on clinical expert consensus documents. *J Am Coll Cardiol.* 2018;72(25): 3332–3365.

Several recent randomized controlled trials in patients with DM have investigated the effects of moderate-to-vigorous aerobic exercise and resistance training on CRF, modifiable CV risk factors, and arterial stiffness, with specific reference to changes in body weight and fat stores.[25–27] Compared with the control group and/or counseling alone, supervised exercise produced significant improvements in CRF, upper and lower body strength, HbA1c, systolic and diastolic blood pressure, total serum cholesterol, HDL-C and LDL-C, BMI, waist circumference, insulin resistance, inflammation (high-sensitivity C-reactive protein), leptin, and CHD risk scores, independent of body weight losses. Structured exercise durations >150 min/week were associated with greater HbA1c declines than those of ≤150 min/week (0.89% and 0.36% reductions, respectively).[28] Results from another systematic review and meta-analysis revealed that combined aerobic exercise and resistance training, as well as aerobic exercise alone, were related to statistically significant declines in HbA1c, triglyceride levels, waist circumference, and systolic blood pressure among individuals with DM.[29] In contrast, the meta-analysis found little support for the benefits of resistance training alone on CV risk factors, including changes in HbA1c or resting systolic blood pressure, in patients with DM. Others, however, have reported that resistance training alone is associated with reductions in HbA1c as compared with a control group of patients with DM.[28]

Compared with individuals with overweight or obesity, those with a normal weight at the time of DM diagnosis have higher mortality rates, even after adjustment for potential confounding variables.[30] Because these data extend the "obesity paradox" to patients with DM, other potential modulators of survival, including body composition, fat distribution, regular PA, and CRF, beyond the measurement of BMI, may help the medical community clarify the relationships among obesity, morbidity, and mortality in adults with DM.[31]

Numerous investigations and systematic reviews have examined the relationships among habitual PA, CRF, DM, BMI, and mortality. The risk for all-cause and/or CV mortality is lower among overweight and obese individuals with good aerobic fitness than in individuals with normal BMI and low fitness.[32,33] This finding has also been reported in a study of African American and White veterans with DM, in whom the obesity paradox was observed along with an independent association between poor exercise capacity and mortality within BMI categories.[34] Others have reported that higher levels of CRF are associated with a substantially lower health risk for a given level of visceral and subcutaneous fat,[35] and that increased PA and/or CRF is inversely associated with all-cause and CV mortality in persons with DM.[31,36–38] Collectively, these data and other reports[39,40] strongly support the role of structured exercise, regular moderate-to-vigorous PA, or both, in interventions designed to prevent and treat DM, regardless of the patient's BMI.

Walking: "Exercise is Medicine" for Patients With Diabetes Mellitus

Epidemiologic studies and clinical trials have consistently demonstrated the survival benefits of regular exercise, especially walking, in the prevention and treatment of DM. In epidemiologic studies, brisk walking for ≥30 min/day has been associated with a 30% to 40% lower risk of developing DM in females.[41] Two clinical trials demonstrated that regular walking or other moderate exercise in conjunction with dietary changes and modest weight losses resulted in a 58% lower risk for the development of DM in overweight patients with impaired fasting glucose, as compared with usual-care control groups.[42,43] In the Diabetes Prevention Program, drug therapy with metformin reduced the risk by only 31%.[43]

In a nationally representative sample (n = 2896) of Americans with DM aged ≥18 years, regular walking was associated with significantly lower risk for all-cause and CV mortality, up to 39% and 54% for walking at least 2 h/week and 3 to 4 h/week, respectively.[44] The inverse association held in multivariable analyses after potential confounding variables (e.g., risk factors, BMI, comorbid conditions) were controlled for. Compared with inactive individuals, the mortality rates were lowest for those who walked 3 to 4 h/week, and for those who reported that their walking involved moderate increases in heart rate and breathing.[44] In the Nurses' Health Study, in which patients with CVD or cancer at screening were excluded, moderate and vigorous levels of PA were associated with lower rates of overall CV events among females with diabetes aged 30 to 55 years.[45] Similarly, the Aerobics Center Longitudinal Study reported that males with DM who had a low CRF level and were physically inactive had higher mortality rates during follow-up than did their counterparts who were active and fit.[36] The clinical and public health implications of these data are enormous, because the survival benefits of moderate-to-vigorous-intensity PA, often achieved by brisk walking alone, may be even greater than those achieved by contemporary pharmacologic therapies to manage DM.[46]

Cardioprotective Effects of Regular Exercise

An inverse association between CRF and the incidence of chronic disease has been established by large, well-designed epidemiologic studies. The findings indicate that these associations are observed at relatively moderate levels of PA or structured exercise and increase in a graded fashion across increasing levels of PA, associated with a significant survival advantage.[47] A systematic review and meta-analysis of 33 PA studies including 883,372 participants reported pooled estimates of 35% and 33% lower risk for CV and all-cause mortality, respectively, among the most physically active cohorts.[48] More recently, researchers estimated the influence of five low-risk lifestyle factors, including ≥30 min/day of moderate-to-vigorous PA, on premature mortality and life expectancy in the US population.[49] During the follow-up period, which extended up to 34 years for some participants, the most physically active cohorts of males and females demonstrated 7- to 8-year gains in life expectancy from age 50 years.

Regular moderate-to-vigorous PA, increased CRF, or both can decrease the risk of initial or recurrent CV events, presumably from multiple mechanisms, including antiatherosclerotic, antiischemic, antiarrhythmic, antithrombotic, and improved psychologic effects (Fig. 17.2). Specific antiischemic effects of regular exercise include reducing the rate-pressure product and associated myocardial oxygen demands at rest and at any given submaximal workload. Decreased vulnerability to threatening ventricular arrhythmias and increased resistance to

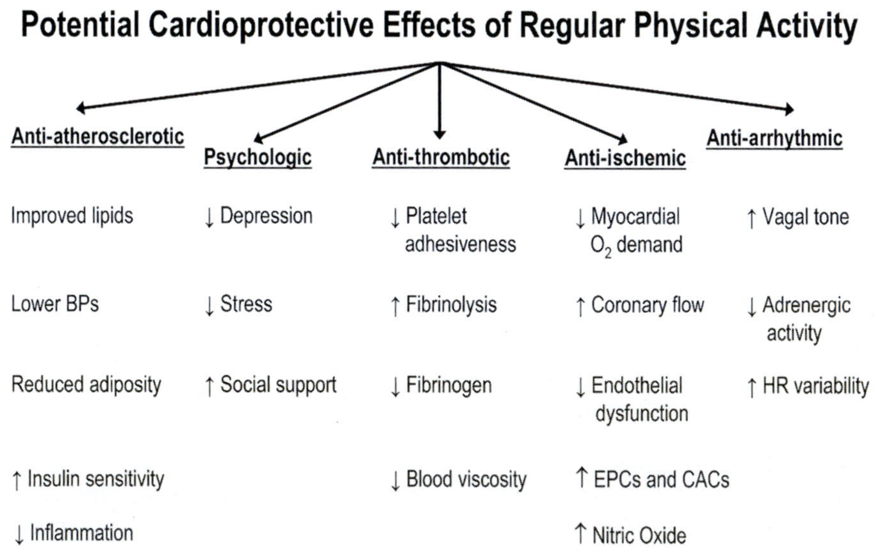

FIG. 17.2 A structured endurance exercise program, increased lifestyle physical activity, or both are sufficient to maintain and enhance cardiorespiratory fitness, which favorably affects multiple atherosclerotic cardiovascular risk factors in patients with diabetes. *BP*, Blood pressure; *CACs*, cultured angiogenic cells; *EPCs*, endothelial progenitor cells; *HR*, heart rate; O_2, oxygen; ↑, increased; ↓, decreased.

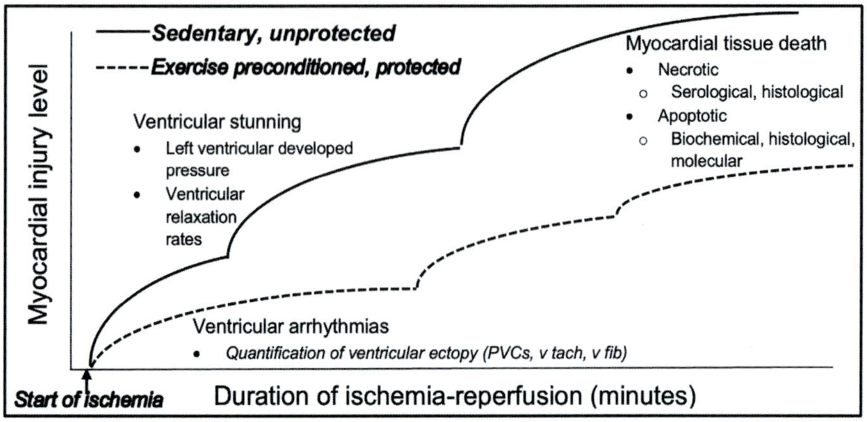

FIG. 17.3 Exercise ischemic preconditioning prevents myocellular injury and death in multiple animal models. Ischemia-reperfusion injury is a time-dependent pathology, as shown conceptually above by the appearance of ventricular ectopy on the ECG, and later by declines in ventricular pump function. Unremitting ischemia is invariably marked by cardiomyocyte death due to necrotic and apoptotic processes. Exercise preconditioning lessens the magnitude of all facets of ischemia-reperfusion injury (*dashed line*). Protection afforded by exercise is due to the upregulation of multiple cellular mechanisms. Importantly, the mechanisms of biochemical cardioprotection against MI are unique to each phase of injury; for example, the factors preventing ventricular ectopy can be different than the other factors which prevent ventricular pump dysfunction. *ECG*, Electrocardiogram; *MI*, myocardial infarction; *MRI*, magnetic resonance imaging; *PVCs*, premature ventricular contractions.

ventricular fibrillation have also been postulated to reflect exercise-related adaptations in autonomic control, including reduced sympathetic drive and increased vagal tone, as well as increasing the period of diastole as a result of decreased resting heart rate, during which coronary perfusion predominates.

Exercise preconditioning. This phenomenon provides an underappreciated independent and additive mechanism for protecting the heart against acute myocardial infarction.[50] First described decades ago in animal studies, subsequent clinical investigations confirm that exercise preconditions the human heart.[51] The benefits of exercise preconditioning are attributed to a host of endogenous biochemical factors activated within hours to days following the first bout of PA so that an ischemic-resistance phenotype is conferred, and appears to be continuously activated in those who remain regularly engaged in exercise (Fig. 17.3).[50] Accordingly, the phenomenon is distinct from other established exercise-induced adaptations, such as those described in Fig. 17.2. Most importantly, the immediate benefits of exercise preconditioning can be conferred in males or females, young or old, who engage in even brief bouts of PA that achieve a minimum threshold of 50% $\dot{V}O_2$ max.[50]

Increasing scientific evidence also suggests that aerobic exercise training improves blood rheology in individuals with and without CHD. Endurance exercise has been shown to improve hemostatic/fibrinolytic parameters, with decreases in plasma fibrinogen levels, platelet aggregability, and hematocrit standardized blood viscosity and increases in fibrinolysis.[52] Finally, well-designed studies now highlight the value of regular aerobic exercise in reducing chronic stress, anxiety, and depression.[53]

Collectively, these data and related reports suggest that regular moderate-to-vigorous PA and higher levels of CRF are associated with a reduced risk of developing hypertension, DM, atrial fibrillation, chronic kidney disease, and major adverse CV events, including heart failure, MI, coronary artery bypass surgery, and death.[47] This inverse association of lower incidence of DM has also been noted against the diabetogenic effects of statins. Accordingly, it appears that the risk of DM incidence in dyslipidemic patients treated with statins may be significantly attenuated by achieving moderate levels of CRF.[54]

PHYSICAL ACTIVITY, EXERCISE PROGRAMMING, AND PRESCRIPTION

In many patients with DM, adequate glycemic control can often be achieved by dietary changes, regular PA, structured exercise, and weight reduction. The exercise program should generally follow contemporary guidelines for the treatment of excessive body weight and fat stores,[55] and other risk factors associated with this common metabolic condition. Overall, individuals with DM have an increased risk of morbidity and mortality from CVD as compared with their age- and sex-matched counterparts without this comorbidity. Accordingly, a physical examination and a careful preliminary CV assessment, including peak or symptom-limited exercise testing, with estimated or directly measured peak oxygen consumption ($\dot{V}O_2$ peak), should be considered before beginning an exercise training program. $\dot{V}O_2$ peak is generally expressed as mL O_2/min/kg or as metabolic equivalents (METs), where 1 MET = 3.5 mL O_2/min/kg. Both the American Health Association (AHA)[56] and the American College of Sports Medicine (ACSM) guidelines for exercise testing and prescription[57] recommend that peak or symptom-limited exercise testing be considered before initiation of exercise training in individuals with known or suspected CVD, including patients with DM.[58]

Type of Exercise

Aerobic (or endurance) exercise has been the most frequently studied mode of physical conditioning, and the resultant increases in CRF in patients with DM have been consistently associated with improvements in modifiable CV risk factors, independent of weight loss.[27] The most effective exercises for the endurance phase use large muscle groups, are maintained continuously through the exercise session, and are rhythmic in nature, such as walking, jogging, elliptical training, stationary or outdoor cycling, swimming, rowing, stair climbing, and combined arm-leg ergometry. Other exercise modalities commonly used in structured exercise training programs for patients with DM include calisthenics, particularly those involving sustained total-body movement, recreational activities (e.g., golf, doubles tennis, pickleball), and resistance training.[59] The last is a particularly important option, because traditional aerobic-conditioning regimens often fail to accommodate participants who require improved muscle strength or endurance to perform occupational or leisure-time activities. Moreover, studies have now shown that muscular strength is inversely associated with all-cause mortality, independent of CRF levels.[60]

Because of the high prevalence of underlying ischemic heart disease, and the heightened risk for exertion-related CV events and orthopedic injuries, adoption of a moderate intensity (e.g., walking), rather than a vigorous PA program (e.g., jogging, running), may be more appropriate for patients with diabetes, especially those who are middle-aged and older.[46] Due to lack of data and observation hours in varied populations with known or occult CVD, including patients with DM, it is currently premature to conclude that high-intensity interval training is a safe and superior exercise intervention compared with moderate-intensity continuous training.[61] Walking has several advantages over other forms of exercise during the initial phase of a physical conditioning program, including inherent neuromuscular limitations on the speed of walking (and therefore the rate of energy expenditure).

Rule of 2 and 3 miles per hour (mph). Because most patients with diabetes, many of whom are overweight or obese, prefer to walk at moderate intensities, it is helpful to recognize that walking on level ground at 2 and 3 mph approximates 2 and 3 METs, respectively. For patients who prefer the slower walking pace (2 mph; 3.2 km/h), each 3.5% increase in treadmill grade adds ~1 MET to the gross energy cost. Therefore patients who desire to walk at a 2-mph pace, but require a 4-MET workload for training, would be advised to add 7.0% grade to this speed. For patients who can negotiate the faster walking speed (3 mph; 4.8 km/h), each 2.5% increase in treadmill grade adds an additional 1 MET to the gross energy expenditure. Accordingly, a workload of 3 mph, 7.5% grade, would approximate an aerobic requirement of 6 METs. Use of this practical rule can be helpful to clinicians in prescribing level or graded treadmill walking workloads for their patients with DM.[62]

RESISTANCE TRAINING

Resistance training, also know as strength or weight training, improves musculoskeletal function through the progressive overload principle. The intensity and volume of exercise can be manipulated by varying the weight load, the number of repetitions and sets completed, the rest interval between sets and exercises, or combinations thereof. Although muscular strength and endurance can be developed by static and dynamic exercises, the latter are generally recommended because they best simulate activities of daily living. Options for strength training include: body weight exercises; machines; free weights; "digital weight" resistance systems; body bars; kettlebells; spring devices; elastic bands; weighted balls; weighted clubs; eccentric, concentric, and isometric exercises; ballistic movements; unilateral and bilateral exercises; and strength training straps.

Although resistance exercise has generally been considered to be less effective in preventing and treating DM, some suggest that it provides independent and additive benefits to an aerobic exercise program for virtually the entire cluster of associated CV factors.[63] For example, numerous studies show that resistance training improves insulin sensitivity; significantly decreases HbA1c and blood pressure in adults with diabetes and with hypertension, respectively; and reduces body fat stores and visceral adipose tissue in both males and females. In addition, the maintenance or enhancement of lean body mass from chronic resistance training is associated with a modest increase in basal metabolic rate, which over time may facilitate greater reductions in body weight than can be achieved with increased aerobic PA and/or structured exercise. Weight training–induced attenuation of the hemodynamic response to lifting fixed loads over time, using a percentage of *baseline* maximal voluntary contraction or perceived exertion, has also been reported in older males and patients with CVD.[64,65] This may decrease cardiac demands during daily activities such as carrying packages or lifting moderate to heavy objects.[59] In the absence of contraindications, patients with DM should be encouraged to participate in resistance training.[66]

Although the traditional weight-training prescription has involved performing each exercise three times (e.g., three sets of 10–15 repetitions per set), it appears that one set provides similar improvements in muscular strength, endurance, and hypertrophy, at least for the novice exerciser.[67,68] Consequently, single-set programs performed at least two times a week are recommended rather than multiset programs because they are highly effective, less time consuming, and less likely to cause musculoskeletal injury or soreness. Such regimens should include 8 to 10 different exercises involving the trunk and upper and lower extremities at loads that permit 8 to 15 repetitions per set. At least 60 min of resistance training should be completed each week (e.g., two 30-min sessions).

LIFESTYLE PHYSICAL ACTIVITY

Lifestyle PA involves bodily movement produced by the contraction of muscles that increase aerobic requirements or energy expenditure. In contrast, structured exercise is PA/planned exercise that is performed with an underlying purpose or goal. Despite contemporary exercise guidelines and the Surgeon General's report,[69] the traditional model for getting people to be more physically active (i.e., a regimented or structured exercise program) has been only marginally effective. Randomized clinical trials have shown that a lifestyle approach to PA among previously sedentary adults has similar effects on CRF, body composition, and coronary risk factors as a structured exercise program.[70,71] These findings have important implications for public health, suggesting an alternative approach for sedentary people who are not ready to integrate a formal exercise commitment into their daily schedule.[72] The skyrocketing prevalence of overweight and obesity and related sequelae (e.g., DM, metabolic syndrome) suggests the need for "real-world" interventions designed to circumvent and attenuate barriers to achieving an adequate daily energy expenditure.[73] Accordingly, physicians and allied health professionals should counsel patients to integrate multiple short bouts of PA into their day.[74,75] Nonexercise activity thermogenesis—the spontaneous physical activities of daily living (e.g., fidgeting while sitting, standing while reading, moving the lower extremities while working at the computer)—represents another source of energy expenditure for many people.[76] Standing also elevates lipoprotein lipase, an enzyme that improves fat metabolism while reducing insulin resistance.[77,78] Thus energy expenditure during nonexercise time may be as critical for preventative health as structured exercise time. Pedometers can be helpful in this regard, as can programs that use them (e.g., America on the Move) to enhance awareness of PA by progressively increasing daily step totals. According to one systematic review, pedometer users significantly increased their PA by an average of 2491 steps per day more than their control counterparts.[79] Although 10,000 steps/day has been the traditional recommendation to improve health, few data are available to support this recommendation. The CARDIA study of 2100 Black and White males and females (aged 38–50 years), with a mean follow-up of 10.8 years, reported that participants taking 7000 or more steps/day, compared with those taking fewer than 7000 steps/day, had a 50% to 70% lower risk of mortality.[80] These findings suggest a viable alternative to a moderate-to-vigorous PA regimen to increase life expectancy.

The Activity Pyramid (Fig. 17.4) has also been suggested as a model to combat America's increasingly hypokinetic environment.[81] This schematic presents a tiered set of weekly goals to promote improved CRF and health, building on a base that emphasizes the importance of accumulating at least 30 min of moderate-intensity activity on 5 or more days per week.

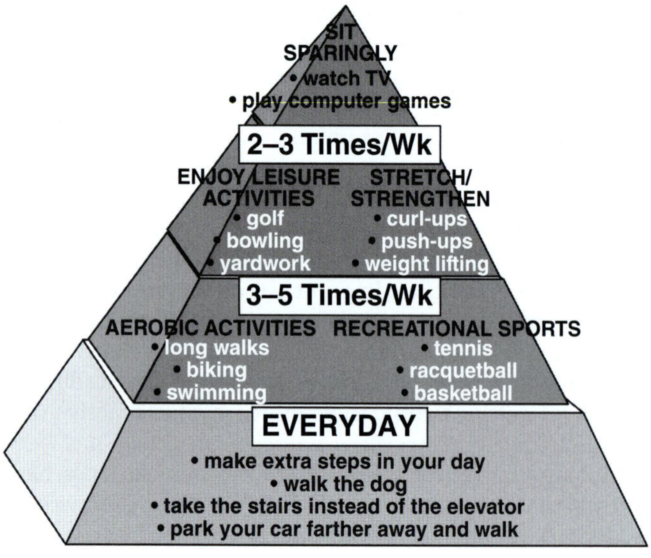

FIG. 17.4 The Activity Pyramid, analogous to the US Department of Agriculture (USDA) Food Guide Pyramid, has been suggested as a model to facilitate public and patient education for adoption of a progressively more active lifestyle.

INTENSITY AND DURATION

There is some controversy regarding the most appropriate exercise intensity and duration that are needed to optimally physically condition patients with the insulin resistance syndrome.[82] Different risk factors associated with this condition may respond more favorably to different exercise frequency, intensity, and duration. For example, a randomized, controlled trial of previously inactive, overweight males and females with abnormal lipoprotein profiles compared the effectiveness of three different exercise regimens versus controls: high-amount, high-intensity exercise; low-amount, high-intensity exercise; and low-amount, moderate-intensity exercise.[83] Although all exercise groups demonstrated improved responses on a variety of lipid and lipoprotein variables as compared with the control group, the most beneficial changes were noted in the high-amount, high-intensity exercise regimen. Because DM has been associated with increased body weight and fat stores, a sedentary lifestyle, and a low level of CRF, the initial exercise training intensity should approximate at least 40% of the peak $\dot{V}O_2$, or heart rate reserve or 55% of the maximal heart rate. In the absence of data from an individual standard exercise test or a cardiopulmonary exercise test to volitional fatigue, this approximates a rating of perceived exertion (6–20 category scale)[84] of 11 (fairly light) to 13 (somewhat hard), for a minimum accumulated duration of 30 min/day.[85] Over time, in the absence of adverse signs and symptoms, the exercise intensity should be gradually increased, generally corresponding to a rating of perceived exertion up to 15 (somewhat hard to hard), to further improve CRF, based on age-, sex-, and good fitness-adjusted target intensities for training (Fig. 17.5).[86]

The exercise intensity recommendation can be achieved with a combination of moderate and vigorous PA, which approximates 40% to 59% and 60% to 84% of peak $\dot{V}O_2$ or heart rate reserve, respectively. The ACSM/AHA recommends that most adults engage in moderate-intensity exercise training for at least 30 min/day on at least 5 days of the week for a total of more than 150 min/week, or vigorous exercise training for at least 20 min/day on at least 3 days of the week for a total of more than 75 min/week,[87] or a combination of moderate- and vigorous-intensity exercise to achieve a total energy expenditure of >500 to 1000 MET/min/week or more.[88]

FREQUENCY

The frequency of exercise is an important consideration when structured exercise and/or increased lifestyle PA are used to treat the abnormalities associated with DM, especially insulin sensitivity and glucose use. Although even twice-weekly exercise sessions may favorably influence glycemic control, patients with DM should exercise at least 3 days each week with no more than 2 consecutive days without training,[85] because increases in insulin sensitivity decline markedly by 48 h after exercise.[89] Nevertheless, more frequent exercise (i.e., at least 5 days/week) may serve to maximize both the acute glucose-lowering effect and the effect on CV risk reduction.[85]

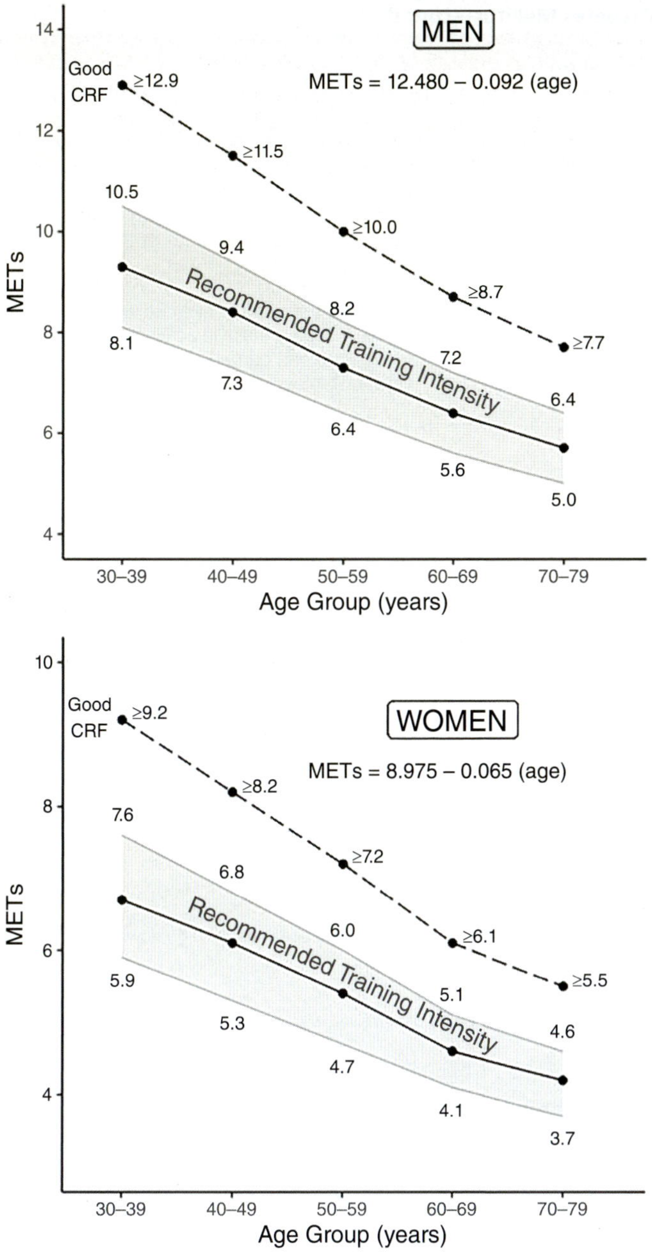

FIG. 17.5 Age- and sex-adjusted "good" levels of cardiorespiratory fitness *(CRF)* for males and females and the recommended training intensity (60%–80% $\dot{V}O_2R$, expressed as metabolic equivalents [*METs*]) to achieve these fitness levels. Regression equations signify 70% $\dot{V}O_2R$.

A summary of exercise prescription and PA guidelines for patients with DM is shown in Table 17.3, with specific reference to the type of exercise; major goals and objectives; and the recommended intensity, frequency, and duration. It should be emphasized, however, that if these recommended levels of exercise are deemed by the patient to be unrealistic or excessive, the patient should be counseled to achieve more moderate exercise dosages or intensities, because the primary beneficiaries are individuals with and without CVD who are in the least fit, least active subgroup (bottom 20%).[90,91]

The Structured Exercise Session: Special Considerations for Exercisers with Diabetes

Structured exercise training sessions should include a preliminary aerobic warm-up (approximately 10 min), a conditioning phase (≥20 min of vigorous-intensity or ≥30 min of moderate-intensity exercise), a cool-down (5–10 min), and ideally an optional recreational game. Stretching (5–10 min) may be incorporated before or after the conditioning or endurance exercise phase. The warm-up facilitates the transition from rest to the conditioning phase by stretching postural muscles and increasing blood flow. A gradual warm-up may also reduce the likelihood of exercise-induced ischemic responses, which can occur with sudden strenuous exertion.[92] A walking cool-down enhances venous return during recovery, decreasing the possibility of hypotension and related sequelae, and ameliorates the potential, deleterious effects of the postexercise rise in plasma catecholamines.[93] In addition, it facilitates more rapid removal of lactic acid than stationary recovery.

For patients with DM with adequate blood glucose control or those who are mildly hyperglycemic, regular PA acutely decreases blood glucose levels and, in some patients with DM treated with insulin, actually reduces insulin requirements. This is because of the insulin-like effect of aerobic exercise. However, PA can also result in a hypoglycemic state that is the most common problem experienced by exercising patients with diabetes treated with insulin or, to a lesser extent, oral hypoglycemic drugs. Recommendations and precautionary measures to reduce the potential for exercise-related complications in patients with DM have been previously described.[16,21,57]

TABLE 17.3 Exercise Recommendations for Patients with Type 2 Diabetes Mellitus

TYPE OF EXERCISE[a]	MAJOR GOALS AND OBJECTIVES	INTENSITY, FREQUENCY, DURATION
Aerobic (large muscle activities)—for example, walking, jogging, stationary or outdoor cycling, swimming	Increase $\dot{V}o_2$ peak; ADLs	40%–84% $\dot{V}o_2R$[b] or HRR; 55%–89% HR max; RPE 11–16 (6–20 scale)
	Improve glycemic control and coronary risk factors	No more than 2 consecutive days without exercising; four to five sessions per week (or more) may be needed to reduce body weight and fat stores
	Decrease rate-pressure product during submaximal exercise	≥150 or ≥75 min/week for moderate-intensity or vigorous-intensity exercise, respectively; ≥20 min per session

(Continued)

TABLE 17.3 Exercise Recommendations for Patients with Type 2 Diabetes Mellitus—cont'd

TYPE OF EXERCISE[a]	MAJOR GOALS AND OBJECTIVES	INTENSITY, FREQUENCY, DURATION
	Induce other cardioprotective benefits (e.g., enhanced nitric oxide vasodilator function, improved vascular reactivity, altered vascular structure, increased resistance to ventricular tachycardia and fibrillation)	For moderate-intensity activity (≤59% $\dot{V}o_2R$ or HRR and/or ≤69% HR max and/or RPE ≤13), multiple shorter periods of exercise (10- to 15-min exercise bouts) accumulated throughout the day may elicit similar (or even greater) reductions in body weight and fat stores than a single bout of the same duration
		Complement structured exercise with an increase in daily lifestyle activities (walking breaks at work, gardening, household activities); move more, sit less
Resistance training (multijoint exercises, large muscle groups, progressive)	Increase muscle strength and endurance	8–10 different exercises that work major muscle groups; weight loads gradually increased over time
	Increase ability to perform leisure and occupational activities and ADLs	≥2 times/week
	Decrease the rate-pressure product at any given resistance (e.g., during lifting or carrying objects)	Moderate-to-vigorous intensity; one to four sets of 8–10 reps at a weight that cannot be lifted more than 8–10 times,[c] or 12–15 reps at a weight that cannot be lifted more than 12–15 times (for patients with known CHD), with 1- to 2-min rest periods between sets
	Assist in the maintenance of basal metabolic rate by maintaining or increasing lean body mass over time	
Flexibility and stretching (upper and lower body ROM activities)	Improve balance and agility	Static stretches: hold for 10–30 s
	Decrease risk of musculoskeletal and orthopedic injury	2–3 days/week

[a]Aerobic exercise should be preceded by a warm-up (approximately 10 min) and followed by a cool-down (5–10 min) at a reduced exercise intensity (e.g., slow walking). Stretching (5–10 min) may be incorporated before or after the endurance exercise phase.
[b]$\dot{V}o_2$ reserve formula = ($\dot{V}o_2$ peak − $\dot{V}o_2$ rest) × 40%–84% intensity + $\dot{V}o_2$ rest, where $\dot{V}o_2$ values are expressed in METs.
[c]Approximates 70%–84% of one repetition maximum.
ADLs, Activities of daily living; *HR max*, maximal heart rate; *HRR*, heart rate reserve; *ROM*, range of motion; *RPE*, rating of perceived exertion (6–20 scale); $\dot{V}o_2R$, $\dot{V}o_2$ reserve; *CHD*, coronary heart disease.

Exercise at approximately the same time each day is a good practice to take advantage of the glucose-lowering effect of PA by timing the session at ~1 h after a meal. Inject insulin in body areas where muscles are not actively recruited by exercise (e.g., the abdomen). The response to structured exercise and/or moderate-to-vigorous PA in the patient with DM taking insulin depends on a number of variables, including the adequacy of control by exogenous insulin. Accordingly, DM must be under adequate control before the patient begins an exercise program, regardless of whether the patient is type 1 diabetes mellitus (T1DM) or T2DM. A blood glucose concentration above 300 mg/dL or above 240 mg/dL with urinary ketone bodies is considered a relative contraindication to exercise participation. In patients taking insulin, consideration should be given to the ingestion of 20 to 30 g of additional carbohydrate before exercise when the preexercise blood glucose is below 100 mg/dL.

Exercise during the evening hours increases the risk of nocturnal hypoglycemia, which may occur up to 4 to 6 h after an exercise bout. To decrease the likelihood of this response during the night (or day), the patient with diabetes may need to reduce their insulin dose or increase carbohydrate intake before or after exercise. Finally, recognize the signs and symptoms of hypoglycemia. These include heart palpitations, confusion, weakness, and visual disturbances. If hypoglycemia is left untreated, it could lead to unconsciousness or convulsions. To reduce the likelihood of complications, patients with diabetes should always carry a form of fast-acting carbohydrate (e.g., juice, candy, glucose tables), exercise with a partner, and wear a diabetes identification tag.

Physical activity, fitness, and risk of cardiovascular events in DM. CVD represents an important long-term complication of DM and accounts for >75% of total mortality among patients with DM. In a pooled analysis from 19 prospective observational cohort studies, physical inactivity in the general population was associated with a 16% higher risk of stroke (hazard ratio [HR], 1.16; 95% confidence interval [CI], 1.05–1.27), a 24% higher risk of CHD (HR, 1.24; 95% CI, 1.13–1.36), and a 42% higher risk of incident DM (HR, 1.42; 95% CI, 1.25–1.61).[94] A pooled analysis of 10 population-based cohort studies showed an inverse association of PA with CVD or all-cause mortality in adults with DM.[95] Compared with inactive participants, those who reported some activity or met contemporary PA recommendations had a 26% and 35% lower all-cause mortality, respectively.[95] Similarly, a meta-analysis of 17 studies in patients with DM reported that a 1 MET-h/day incrementally higher PA was associated with reductions in all-cause mortality (9.5% [5.0%–13.8%]) and CVD risk (7.9% [4.3%–11.4%]).[96]

There are several physiologic mechanisms by which higher PA and CRF levels can lower the risk of acute cardiac events in patients with DM. First, higher levels of PA can reduce CV risk factors, including elevated blood pressure, insulin resistance, glucose intolerance, elevated triglyceride concentrations, low HDL-C, and obesity.[47] Another mechanism by which PA can be protective against CVD in DM is through favorable adaptations on cardiac structure and function. Accordingly, in a meta-analysis of six clinical trials (n = 441 patients), exercise training in individuals with DM in the preclinical stage, that is, without overt CHD or heart failure, significantly improved measures of cardiac function, including early diastolic mitral annular velocity, systolic function as measured by the global longitudinal strain, and CRF signified by increased peak $\dot{V}O_2$.[97]

LIFESTYLE MODIFICATION FOR THE MANAGEMENT OF DIABETES

The Look AHEAD trial, a large, randomized controlled trial, evaluated an intensive lifestyle intervention in overweight or obese adults with T2DM compared with a T2DM support and education control group.[18] Over a median follow-up of almost 10 years, the intensive lifestyle intervention group, which included dietary modification and increased PA (aimed at achieving and maintaining a weight loss of ≥7%), demonstrated significantly greater improvements in CRF, glycated hemoglobin, weight loss (intervention group vs. controls, 8.6% vs. 0.7% at 1 year; 6.0% vs. 3.5% at study end), and waist circumference. Other health benefits that were identified during the early years of the trial included improved biomarkers of glucose and lipid control, reduced sleep apnea, less depression, improved insulin sensitivity, decreased need for antihyperglycemic medications, improved quality of life, and lower health care costs. However, major CV events (i.e., death from CV causes, nonfatal myocardial infarction, nonfatal stroke, or hospitalization for angina) were similar in both groups, 403 patients in the intervention group and 418 in the control group, with no significant between-group difference (P = .51).[18] This may be partially explained by the provision of educational sessions and greater use of cardioprotective statins in the control group.[18] Although the treatment for T2DM commonly involves oral antihyperglycemic medication and dietary modification, these interventions do not augment CRF, which is crucial to increase exercise capacity, glycemic control, and survival among this escalating patient population.[36–39,98]

COUNSELING PATIENTS TO FAVORABLY MODIFY UNHEALTHY LIFESTYLE HABITS

Results from behavioral studies have shown that change is often not a linear, gradual movement over time. Instead, lifestyle change is progressive, regressive, spiraling, or static. Although most people believe that a single behavioral change is easier to make and sustain, multiple simultaneous changes are often easier because they quickly yield benefits.[99]

Assessing patients' readiness to change behaviors. Patients should be evaluated for their stage of readiness before being counseled to change a specific lifestyle behavior. The Transtheoretical Stages of Change Model can help identify patients who are positively interested in or, on the other hand, absolutely unwilling to change their health behavior.[100] This model includes six stages of intentional (or unintentional) behavior change that may sequentially occur: *precontemplation*: patient is not thinking about making lifestyle changes; *contemplation*: patient is "thinking" about making a desired change; *determination*: patient has taken some behavioral steps and intends to take action in the next 30 days; *action*: patient begins to consistently demonstrate the new behavior for <6 months; *maintenance*: patient has been in action for ≥6 months; and *relapse*: patient returns to former (unhealthy) lifestyle habits (Fig. 17.6).[100] Accordingly, while a precontemplator may need perception alteration, the contemplator may require a critical analysis of the pros and cons of changing the behavior.

Facilitating behavior change. The likelihood that patients will or will not embrace a new lifestyle behavior is determined by a myriad of socioeconomic, attitudinal, and cultural factors, including their expectations of the benefits, costs, and consequences of that behavior.[101] Identifying and then removing or attenuating the barriers to lifestyle modification are integral to achieving successful change. Lack of or a suboptimal social support system, social isolation, or financial difficulties are often cited as common barriers to achieving lasting lifestyle behavior changes. Practitioners should also anticipate patients declaring that they are too busy to make certain lifestyle changes (e.g., a structured exercise program). Strategizing with the patient to identify realistic options to overcome these barriers, real or perceived, is integral to changing unhealthy behaviors. Finally, failure to address underlying psychosocial factors such as depression, anger, denial, apathy,

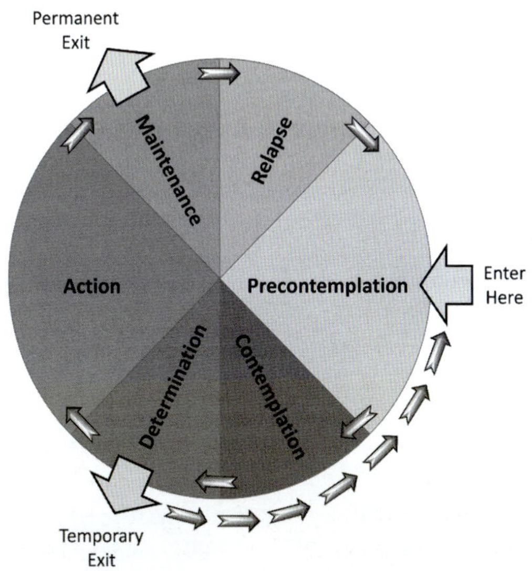

FIG. 17.6 Progressive stages of readiness for behavior change. Deviations from serial progression (i.e., either temporary or permanent exits) are most likely to occur during the determination and maintenance phases, respectively. Adapted from Prochaska JO, DiClemente C. Transtheoretical therapy, toward a more integrative model of change. *Psychother Theory Res Pract*. 1982;19:276–288.

chronic stress, personality factors, and potentially harmful character traits—factors commonly clustered in patients with CVD—can be obstacles to a healthy lifestyle as well as directly promote CHD.[102,103]

Emphasize to patients that the 10 most empowering two-letter words are, "If it is to be, it is up to me."[101] In other words, take responsibility. Patients need to understand that they have the single greatest influence on their destiny relative to health outcomes. It is not genetic predisposition, social circumstances, environmental exposures, or, for that matter, access to quality health care. It is the decisions they make on a day-to-day basis, predominantly their lifestyle behavioral choices.[8] Thus, for lifestyle and risk factor modification to work, they simply need to know where they are on the behavior continuum and where they need to go—that is, the foundation in setting goals.

The 5As approach has been reported to produce significant improvements in a variety of health behaviors, including smoking cessation, dietary practices, and PA (Fig. 17.7).[104–106] Fortunately, progress has been made in that more clinicians now perform the first 2As, that is, assess the risk behavior and advise behavior change. On the other hand, it is the less frequently performed As (agree, assist, arrange), which require more time to implement, and specific counseling skill sets to administer, that have the greatest impact on healthful behavior change. The core of effective counseling is a patient-centered approach, whereby clinicians work with patients, helping them to create an "action plan" to reach their self-stated goals, resulting from carefully crafted questions posed by the clinician.[107]

Motivational interviewing. Spring et al.[108] highlighted the important role of motivational interviewing as a form of talk therapy used by the clinician during patient encounters to encourage a behavioral transformation. To accomplish this, the practitioner must convey understanding, acceptance, and interest in the patient as an individual.[109] The first step is to open the door to change by using empathy to identify what causes unhealthy behaviors. The next step is getting the individual to understand and accept the need for change. This is best achieved using specific questions directed at the patient about why they need to change this behavior. Most importantly, the patient needs to be allowed (and encouraged) to speak. The next step is to help the patient become independent and self-motivating. Setting appropriate goals is the final step.

Overcoming inertia with downscaled goals. For many patients, setting initial goals for lifestyle modification (e.g., body weight reduction, increasing PA, healthy dietary practices) may be unrealistic and discouraging, especially if contemporary guidelines are literally embraced. Using conventional norms, the patient who is 173 cm tall and weighs 137 kg (BMI, 45.5 kg/m^2) might be counseled to reduce their body weight to a "normal" range (i.e., to 76 kg) since this approximates a BMI corresponding to 25 kg/m^2. Our approach would be to ask this patient about an initial goal weight they felt they could achieve. Regardless of their response, if it moved them in the right direction (i.e., <137 kg), we would strongly agree with and support their objective. Similarly, rather than counseling the habitually sedentary patient to exercise for 30 or even 60 min/day on most days of the week, as current guidelines suggest, we would recommend 10-min exercise bouts, three times per week, over the initial month of an exercise regimen. Considering dietary modification, we suggest initially replacing two unhealthy foods or snacks each day with fruits or vegetables (e.g., eating a salad instead of pizza for lunch or selecting an apple instead of potato chips). This approach gets patients moving in the right direction, many of whom may subsequently find themselves not only meeting but exceeding these goals.[101]

Although inertia is a major barrier to making permanent lifestyle changes, it is also one of the easiest obstacles to overcome. We simply need to get patients to *act*. The easier we make it for patients to act, no matter how trivial, the easier it will be to overcome inertia. Recognize that in many ways, lifestyle modification may be analogous to the law of inertia: a body at rest tends to remain at rest, whereas a body in motion tends to remain in motion. Indeed, there is an enduring axiom of success in the field of personal achievement that says, "The universe rewards action." This also represents a key tenet of lifestyle modification. Finally, it is important to emphasize that time is an ally to successful lifestyle modification. Ordinary effort, on a day-to-day basis, can ultimately yield extraordinary results.

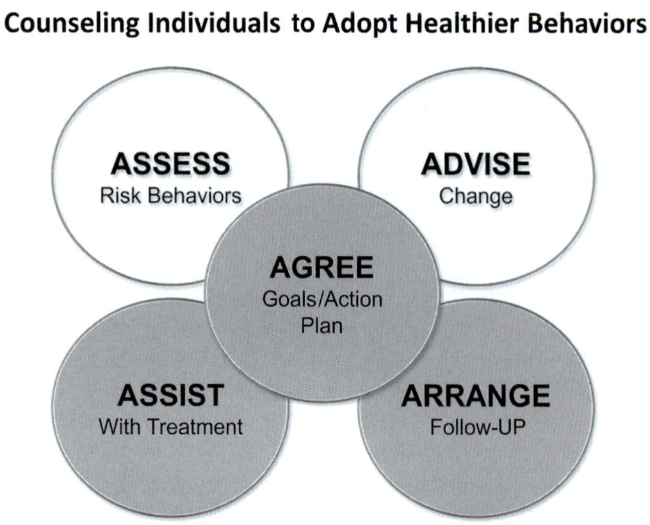

FIG. 17.7 The 5 As to facilitate effective health behavior change during a medical visit.

SUMMARY

Diabetes is associated with an increased risk of CVD morbidity and mortality. An estimated 463 million individuals are currently living with DM. In the United States, up to 95% of those with DM are classified as T2DM,[110] which is associated with pathological changes to the CV system including micro- and macrovascular abnormalities.[111] The increasing burden of T2DM is largely attributed to the growing prevalence of lifestyle-related cardiometabolic risk factors due to obesity and physical inactivity. In this chapter, we reviewed the beneficial impact of favorably modifying CHD risk factors in patients with T2DM, with specific reference to a reduced calorie, largely plant-based diet, weight loss, smoking cessation, regular PA, and improved CRF, with proven behavior modification approaches to achieve these outcomes.

Obesity is an independent risk factor for CVD, increasing the risk of CV events and mortality in patients with DM. Among overweight/obese individuals with T2DM, the health benefits of losing even 3% to 5% of body weight are well documented,[13,112] whereas greater weight losses (>10%) further increase the magnitude of CV risk reduction, and may even promote remission of the associated metabolic derangements.[14]

Cigarette smoking is another risk factor for CV and all-cause mortality in patients with DM.[113] There is also a high risk of stroke in patients with DM who smoke as compared with their counterparts who do not smoke.[114] Smoking is also associated with elevated total cholesterol and LDL-cholesterol levels, low-serum HDL-cholesterol levels, insulin resistance, and poor glycemic control.[115,116] In patients with T1DM, smokers are more likely to exhibit evidence of endothelial dysfunction compared with nonsmokers.[117] Accordingly, the ADA recommends including smoking cessation counseling and other forms of treatment as routine components of DM care.[16,21]

Multiple epidemiological cohort studies have demonstrated a protective association with higher levels of PA and CRF on CV outcomes in patients with T2DM. Furthermore, previous studies have shown that regular PA plays an important role in preventing or delaying many of macrovascular complications of T2DM.[118] A pooled analysis of 10 population-based cohort studies showed an inverse association of PA with CVD or all-cause mortality in patients with DM.[95] Similarly, CRF and mortality in patients with T2DM appear to be inversely related. In one study, males with DM referred for exercise testing with an exercise capacity <5 METs had a 2.5-fold risk of death as compared with their more fit counterparts (>8 MET capacity).[98] In another cohort of males with DM, low CRF was associated with an increased risk of mortality within normal weight, overweight, and obese categories.[37]

Collectively, these data suggest that aggressive lifestyle and risk factor modification in patients with T2DM improve CV outcomes. Although many patients and clinicians believe that a single behavior change is preferred at any given time, multiple simultaneous changes may be easier to adopt because they quickly yield perceptible benefits.[99] Using research-based counseling strategies, including readiness to change, motivational interviewing, the 5As approach, and overcoming inertia with downscaled goals can be helpful in achieving this objective.[101,106]

REFERENCES

1. Lloyd-Jones D, Adams RJ, Brown TM, et al. Heart disease and stroke statistics—2010 update: a report from the American Heart Association. *Circulation*. 2010;121(7):e46–e215.
2. Gregg EW, Cheng YJ, Cadwell BL, et al. Secular trends in cardiovascular disease risk factors according to body mass index in US adults. *JAMA*. 2005;293(15):1868–1874.
3. Mozaffarian D, Wilson PW, Kannel WB. Beyond established and novel risk factors: lifestyle risk factors for cardiovascular disease. *Circulation*. 2008;117(23):3031–3038.
4. Heidenreich PA, Trogdon JG, Khavjou OA, et al. Forecasting the future of cardiovascular disease in the United States: a policy statement from the American Heart Association. *Circulation*. 2011;123(8):933–944.
5. Weintraub WS, Daniels SR, Burke LE, et al. Value of primordial and primary prevention for cardiovascular disease: a policy statement from the American Heart Association. *Circulation*. 2011;124(8):967–990.
6. Asch DA, Muller RW, Volpp KG. Automated hovering in health care—watching over the 5000 hours. *N Engl J Med*. 2012;367(1):1–3.
7. Marvasti FF, Stafford RS. From sick care to health care—reengineering prevention into the U.S. system. *N Engl J Med*. 2012;367(10):889–891.
8. Schroeder SA. Shattuck lecture. We can do better—improving the health of the American people. *N Engl J Med*. 2007;357(12):1221–1228.
9. Chiuve SE, McCullough ML, Sacks FM, et al. Healthy lifestyle factors in the primary prevention of coronary heart disease among men: benefits among users and nonusers of lipid-lowering and antihypertensive medications. *Circulation*. 2006;114(2):160–167.
10. Wilson PW, D'Agostino RB, Sullivan L, et al. Overweight and obesity as determinants of cardiovascular risk: the Framingham experience. *Arch Intern Med*. 2002;162(16):1867–1872.
11. Goldstein DJ. Beneficial health effects of modest weight loss. *Int J Obes Relat Metab Disord*. 1992;16(6):397–415.
12. Klein S, Wadden T, Sugerman HJ. AGA technical review on obesity. *Gastroenterology*. 2002;123:882–932.
13. Jensen MD, Ryan DH, Apovian CM, et al. American College of Cardiology/American Heart Association Task Force on Practice Guidelines; Obesity Society. 2013 AHA/ACC/TOS guideline for the management of overweight and obesity in adults: a report of the American College of Cardiology/American Heart Association Task Force on Practice Guidelines and The Obesity Society. *Circulation*. 2014;129(25 Suppl 2):S102–38.
14. Dambha-Miller H, Day AJ, Strelitz J, Irving G, Griffin SJ. Behaviour change, weight loss and remission of type 2 diabetes: a community-based prospective cohort study. *Diabet Med*. 2020;37(4):681–688.
15. Sacks FM, Bray GA, Carey VJ, et al. Comparison of weight-loss diets with different compositions of fat, protein, and carbohydrates. *N Engl J Med*. 2009;360(9):859–873.
16. American Diabetes Association Professional Practice Committee. 5. Facilitating positive health behaviors and well-being to improve health outcomes: standards of care in diabetes–2023. *Diabetes Care*. 2022;46:S68–S96. https://doi.org/10.2337/dc23-S005.
17. Look AHEAD Research Group. Eight-year weight losses with an intensive lifestyle intervention: the Look AHEAD study. *Obesity (Silver Spring)*. 2014;22:5–13.
18. Wing RR, Bolin P, Brancati FL, et al. for the Look AHEAD Research Group Cardiovascular effects of intensive lifestyle intervention in type 2 diabetes. *N Engl J Med*. 2013;369:145–154.
19. Evert AB, Dennison M, Gardner CD, et al. Nutrition therapy for adults with diabetes or prediabetes: a consensus report. *Diabetes Care*. 2019;42(5):731–754.
20. Vitale M, Masulli M, Calabrese I, et al. on behalf of the TOSCA.IT Study Group Impact of a Mediterranean dietary pattern and its components on cardiovascular risk factors, glucose control, and body weight in people with type 2 diabetes: a real-life study. *Nutrients*. 2018;10(8):1067.
21. American Diabetes Association. 5. Lifestyle management: standards of medical care in diabetes—2019. *Diabetes Care*. 2019;42(Suppl. 1):S46–S60.
22. Duncan MS, Freiberg MS, Greevy Jr RA, et al. Association of smoking cessation with subsequent risk of cardiovascular disease. *JAMA 20*. 2019;322(7):642–650.
23. Barua RS, Rigotti NA, Benowitz NL, et al. 2018 ACC Expert consensus decision pathway on tobacco cessation treatment: a report of the American College of Cardiology Task Force on Clinical Expert Consensus Documents. *J Am Coll Cardiol*. 2018;72(25):3332–3365.
24. Kelley DE, Goodpaster BH:. Effects of physical activity on insulin action and glucose tolerance in obesity. *Med Sci Sports Exerc*. 1999;31(11 Suppl):S619–S623.
25. Loimaala A, Groundstroem K, Rinne M, et al. Effect of long-term endurance and strength training on metabolic control and arterial elasticity in patients with type 2 diabetes mellitus. *Am J Cardiol*. 2009;103(7):972–977.
26. Balducci S, Zanuso S, Nicolucci A, et al. Effect of an intensive exercise intervention strategy on modifiable cardiovascular risk factors in subjects with type 2 diabetes mellitus: a randomized controlled trial: the Italian Diabetes and Exercise Study (EDES). *Arch Intern Med*. 2010;170(20):1794–1803.
27. Balducci S, Zanuso S, Cardelli P, et al. Changes in physical fitness predict improvements in modifiable cardiovascular risk factors independently of body weight loss in subjects with type 2 diabetes participating in the Italian Diabetes and Exercise Study (IDES). *Diabetes Care*. 2012;35(6):1347–1354.
28. Umpierre D, Ribeiro PA, Kramer CK, et al. Physical activity advice only or structured exercise training and association with HbA1c levels in type 2 diabetes: a systematic review and meta-analysis. *JAMA*. 2011;305(17):1790–1799.
29. Chudyk A, Petrella RJ. Effects of exercise on cardiovascular risk factors in type 2 diabetes: a meta-analysis. *Diabetes Care*. 2011;34(5):1228–1237.
30. Carnethon MR, De Chavez PJ, Biggs ML, et al. Association of weight status with mortality in adults with incident diabetes. *JAMA*. 2012;308(6):581–590.
31. Florez H, Castillo-Florez S. Beyond the obesity paradox in diabetes: fitness, fatness, and mortality. *JAMA*. 2012;308(6):619–620.

32. Wei M, Kampert JB, Barlow CE, et al. Relationship between low cardiorespiratory fitness and mortality in normal-weight, overweight, and obese men. *JAMA*. 1999;282(16):1547–1553.
33. Fogelholm M. Physical activity, fitness and fatness: relations to mortality, morbidity and disease risk factors. A systematic review. *Obes Rev*. 2010; 11(3):202–221.
34. Kokkinos P, Myers J, Faselis C, et al. BMI-mortality paradox and fitness in African American and Caucasian men with type 2 diabetes. *Diabetes Care*. 2012;35(5):1021–1027.
35. Lee S, Kuk JL, Katzmarzyk PT, et al. Cardiorespiratory fitness attenuates metabolic risk independent of abdominal subcutaneous and visceral fat in men. *Diabetes Care*. 2005;28(4):895–901.
36. Wei M, Gibbons LW, Kampert JB, et al. Low cardiorespiratory fitness and physical inactivity as predictors of mortality in men with type 2 diabetes. *Ann Intern Med*. 2000;132(8):605–611.
37. Church TS, LaMonte MJ, Barlow CE, et al. Cardiorespiratory fitness and body mass index as predictors of cardiovascular disease mortality among men with diabetes. *Arch Intern Med*. 2005;165(18):2114–2120.
38. Sluik D, Buijsse B, Muckelbauer R, et al. Physical activity and mortality in individuals with diabetes mellitus: a prospective study and meta-analysis. *Arch Intern Med*. 2012;172(17):1285–1295.
39. Lyerly GW, Sui X, Lavie CJ, et al. The association between cardiorespiratory fitness and risk of all-cause mortality among women with impaired fasting glucose or undiagnosed diabetes mellitus. *Mayo Clin Proc*. 2009;84(9): 780–786.
40. Rejeski WJ, Ip EH, Bertoni AG, et al. Lifestyle change and mobility in obese adults with type 2 diabetes. *N Engl J Med*. 2012;366(13):1209–1217.
41. Hu FB, Sigal RJ, Rich-Edwards JW, et al. Walking compared with vigorous physical activity and risk of type 2 diabetes in women: a prospective study. *JAMA*. 1999;282(15):1433–1439.
42. Tuomilehto J, Lindstrom J, Eriksson JG, et al. Prevention of type 2 diabetes mellitus by changes in lifestyle among subjects with impaired glucose tolerance. *N Engl J Med*. 2001;344(18):1343–1350.
43. Knowler WC, Barrett-Connor E, Fowler SE, et al. Reduction in the incidence of type 2 diabetes with lifestyle intervention or metformin. *N Engl J Med*. 2002;346(6):393–403.
44. Gregg EW, Gerzoff RB, Caspersen CJ, et al. Relationship of walking to mortality among US adults with diabetes. *Arch Intern Med*. 2003;163(12): 1440–1447.
45. Hu FB, Stampfer MJ, Solomon C, et al. Physical activity and risk for cardiovascular events in diabetic women. *Ann Intern Med*. 2001;134(2):96–105.
46. Hu FB, Manson JE. Walking: the best medicine for diabetes? *Arch Intern Med*. 2003;163(12):1397–1398.
47. Kokkinos P, Narayan P, Meyers J, Franklin B. Cardiorespiratory fitness and the incidence of chronic disease. *J Clin Exerc Phys*. 2018;7(2):37–45.
48. Nocon M, Hiemann T, Müller-Riemenschneider F, et al. Association of physical activity with all-cause and cardiovascular mortality: a systematic review and meta-analysis. *Eur J Cardiovasc Prev Rehabil*. 2008;15(3): 239–246.
49. Li Y, Pan A, Wang DD, et al. Impact of healthy lifestyle factors on life expectancies in the US population. *Circulation*. 2018;138(4):345–355.
50. Quindry JC, Franklin BA. Exercise preconditioning as a cardioprotective phenotype. *Am J Cardiol*. 2021;148:8–15.
51. Thijssen DHJ, Redington A, George KP, et al. Association of exercise preconditioning with immediate cardioprotection: a review. *JAMA Cardiol*. 2018;3(2):169–176.
52. Shephard RJ, Balady GJ. Exercise as cardiovascular therapy. *Circulation*. 1999;99(7):963–972.
53. Blumenthal JA, Babyak MA, Moore KA, et al. Effects of exercise training on older patients with major depression. *Arch Intern Med*. 1999;159(19): 2349–2356.
54. Kokkinos P, Faselis C, Narayan P, et al. Cardiorespiratory fitness and incidence of type 2 diabetes in United States veterans on statin therapy. *Am J Med*. 2017;130(10):1192–1198.
55. Donnelly JE, Blair SN, Jakicic JM, et al. Appropriate physical activity intervention strategies for weight loss and prevention of weight regain for adults. *Med Sci Sports Exerc*. 2009;41(2):459–471.
56. Fletcher GF, Ades PA, Kligfield P, et al. Exercise standards for testing and training: a scientific statement from the American Heart Association. *Circulation*. 2013;128(8):873–934.
57. American College of Sports Medicine. *ACSM's Guidelines for Exercise Testing and Prescription*. 11th ed. Wolters Kluwer/Lippincott Williams & Wilkins; 2022:142–161.
58. Franklin BA, Thompson PD, Al-Zaiti SS, et al. Exercise-related acute cardiovascular events and potential deleterious adaptations following long-term exercise training: placing the risks into perspective: a scientific statement from the American Heart Association Physical Activity Committee of the Council of Lifestyle and Cardiometabolic Health; Council on Cardiovascular and Stroke Nursing; Council on Clinical Cardiology and Stroke Council. *Circulation*. 2020;141(13):e705–e736.
59. Williams MA, Haskell WL, Ades PA, et al. Resistance exercise in individuals with and without cardiovascular disease: 2007 update: a scientific statement from the American Heart Association Council on Clinical Cardiology and Council on Nutrition, Physical Activity, and Metabolism. *Circulation*. 2007;116(5):572–584.
60. FitzGerald SJ, Barlow CE, Kampert JB, et al. Muscular fitness and all-cause mortality: prospective observations. *J Phys Act Health*. 2004;1(1):7–18.
61. Franklin BA, Eijsvogels TMH, Pandey A, et al. Physical activity, cardiorespiratory fitness, and cardiovascular health: a clinical practice statement of the American Society for Preventive Cardiology Part II: physical activity, cardiorespiratory fitness, minimum and goal intensities for exercise training, prescriptive methods, and special patient populations. *Am J Prev Cardiol*. 2022;12:100425. https://doi.org/10.1016/j.ajpc.2022.100425. eCollection 2022 Dec.
62. Franklin BA, Brinks J, Berra K, et al. Using metabolic equivalents in clinical practice. *Am J Cardiol*. 2018;121(3):382–387.
63. Braith RW, Stewart KJ. Resistance exercise training: its role in the prevention of cardiovascular disease. *Circulation*. 2006;113(22):2642–2650.
64. McCartney N, McKelvie RS, Martin J, et al. Weight-training-induced attenuation of the circulatory response of older males to weight lifting. *J Appl Physiol*. 1993;74(3):1056–1060.
65. Grafe K, Bendick P, Burr M, et al. Effects of resistance training on vascular and hemodynamic responses in patients with coronary artery disease. *Res Q Exerc Sport*. 2018;89(4):457–464.
66. Brown EC, Franklin BA, Regensteiner JG, Stewart KJ. Effects of single bout resistance exercise on glucose levels, insulin action, and cardiovascular risk in type 2 diabetes: a narrative review. *J Diabetes Complications*. 2020;34(8): 107610.
67. Schoenfeld BJ, Grgic J, Krieger J. How many times per week should a muscle be trained to maximize muscle hypertrophy? A systematic review and meta-analysis of studies examining the effects of resistance training frequency. *J Sports Sci*. 2019;37(11):1286–1295.
68. Grgic J, Schoenfeld BJ, Latella C. Resistance training frequency and skeletal muscle hypertrophy: a review of available evidence. *J Sci Med Sport*. 2019;22(3):361–370.
69. U.S. Department of Health and Human Services. *Physical Activity and Health: A Report of the Surgeon General*. Department of Health and Human Services, Centers for Disease Control and Prevention, National Center for Chronic Disease and Health Promotion; 1996.
70. Dunn AL, Marcus BH, Kampert JB, et al. Comparison of lifestyle and structured interventions to increase physical activity and cardiorespiratory fitness: a randomized trial. *JAMA*. 1999;281(4):327–334.
71. Andersen RE, Wadden TA, Bartlett SJ, et al. Effects of lifestyle activity vs structured aerobic exercise in obese women: a randomized trial. *JAMA*. 1999;281(4):335–340.
72. Dunn AL, Andersen RE, Jakicic JM. Lifestyle physical activity interventions. History, short- and long-term effects, and recommendations. *Am J Prev Med*. 1998;15(4):398–412.
73. Pratt M. Benefits of lifestyle activity vs structured exercise. *JAMA*. 1999; 281(94):375–376.
74. Fan JX, Brown BB, Hanson H, et al. Moderate to vigorous physical activity and weight outcomes: does every minute count? *Am J Health Promot*. 2013;28(1):41–49.
75. Glazer NL, Lyass A, Esliger DW, et al. Sustained and shorter bouts of physical activity are related to cardiovascular health. *Med Sci Sports Exerc*. 2013; 45(1):109–115.
76. Levine JA. Nonexercise activity thermogenesis—liberating the life-force. *J Intern Med*. 2007;262(3):273–287.
77. Bey L, Hamilton MT. Suppression of skeletal muscle lipoprotein lipase activity during physical inactivity: a molecular reason to maintain daily low-intensity activity. *J Physiol*. 2003;551(Pt 2):673–682.
78. Levine JA, Lanningham-Foster LM, McCrady SK, et al. Interindividual variation in posture allocation: possible role in human obesity. *Science*. 2005;307(5709):584–586.
79. Bravata DM, Smith-Spangler C, Sundaram V, et al. Using pedometers to increase physical activity and improve health: a systematic review. *JAMA*. 2007;298(19):2296–2304.
80. Paluch AE, Gabriel KP, Fulton JE, et al. Steps per day and all-cause mortality in middle-aged adults in the Coronary Artery Risk Development in Young Adults Study. *JAMA Netw Open*. 2021;4(9):e2124516.
81. Leon AS, Norstrom J. Evidence of the role of physical activity and cardiorespiratory fitness in the prevention of coronary heart disease. *Quest*. 1995; 47(3):311–319.
82. Shahid SK, Schneider SH. Effects of exercise on insulin resistance syndrome. *Coron Artery Dis*. 2000;11(2):103–109.
83. Kraus WE, Houmard JA, Duscha BD, et al. Effects of the amount and intensity of exercise on plasma lipoproteins. *N Engl J Med*. 2002;347(19): 1483–1492.
84. Borg GA. Psychophysical bases of perceived exertion. *Med Sci Sports Exerc*. 1982;14(5):377–381.
85. Hordern MD, Dunstan DW, Prin JB, et al. Exercise prescription for patients with type 2 diabetes and pre-diabetes: a position statement from Exercise and Sport Science Australia. *J Sci Med Sport*. 2012;15(1):25–31.
86. Franklin BA, Arena R, Kaminsky LA, et al. Maximizing the cardioprotective benefits of exercise with age-, sex-, and fitness-adjusted target intensities for training. *Eur J Prev Cardiol*. 2022;29(1):e1–e3.
87. Haskell WL, Lee I-M, Pate RR, et al. Physical activity and public health: updated recommendation for adults from the American College of Sports Medicine and the American Heart Association. *Circulation*. 2007;116(9):1082–1093.
88. Garber CE, Blissmer B, Deschenes MR, et al. American College of Sports Medicine position stand. Quantity and quality of exercise for developing and maintaining cardiorespiratory, musculoskeletal, and neuromotor fitness in apparently healthy adults: guidance for prescribing exercise. *Med Sci Sports Exerc*. 2011;43(7):1334–1359.

89. Borghouts LB, Keizer HA. Exercise and insulin sensitivity: a review. *Int J Sports Med*. 2000;21(1):1–12.
90. Blair SN, Kohl 3rd HW, Paffenbarger Jr RS, et al. Physical fitness and all-cause mortality. A prospective study of healthy men and women. *JAMA*. 1989;262(17):2395–2401.
91. Martin BJ, Arena R, Haykowsky M, et al. Cardiovascular fitness and mortality after contemporary cardiac rehabilitation. *Mayo Clin Proc*. 2013;88(5): 455–463.
92. Barnard RJ, MacAlpin R, Kattus AA, et al. Ischemic response to sudden strenuous exercise in healthy men. *Circulation*. 1973;48(5):936–942.
93. Dimsdale JE, Hartley LH, Guiney T, et al. Postexercise peril. Plasma catecholamines and exercise. *JAMA*. 1984;251(5):630–632.
94. Kivimäki M, Singh-Manoux A, Pentti J, et al. Physical inactivity, cardiometabolic disease, and risk of dementia: an individual-participant meta-analysis. *BMJ*. 2019;365:l1495.
95. Sadarangani KP, Hamer M, Mindell JS, et al. Physical activity and risk of all-cause and cardiovascular disease mortality in diabetic adults from Great Britain: pooled analysis of 10 population-based cohorts. *Diabetes Care*. 2014;37(4):1016–1023.
96. Kodama S, Tanaka S, Heianza Y, et al. Association between physical activity and risk of all-cause mortality and cardiovascular disease in patients with diabetes: a meta-analysis. *Diabetes Care*. 2013;36(2):471–479.
97. Anand V, Garg S, Garg J, et al. Impact of exercise training on cardiac function among patients with type 2 diabetes: a systematic review and meta-analysis. *J Cardiopulm Rehabil Prev*. 2018;38(6):358–365.
98. Myers J, Prakash M, Froelicher V, et al. Exercise capacity and mortality among men referred for exercise testing. *N Engl J Med*. 2002;346(11): 793–801.
99. Hyman DJ, Pavlik VN, Taylor WC, et al. Simultaneous vs sequential counseling for multiple behavior change. *Arch Intern Med*. 2007;167(11):1152–1158.
100. Prochaska JO, DiClemente C. Transtheoretical therapy, toward a more integrative model of change. *Psychother Theory Res Pract*. 1982;19:276–288.
101. Franklin BA, Myers J, Kokkinos P. Importance of lifestyle modification on cardiovascular risk reduction: counseling strategies to maximize patient outcomes. *J Cardiopulm Rehabil Prev*. 2020;40(3):138–143.
102. Rozanski A, Blumenthal JA, Kaplan J. Impact of psychological factors on the pathogenesis of cardiovascular disease and implications for therapy. *Circulation*. 1999;99(16):2192–2217.
103. Williams RB, Barefoot JC, Schneiderman N. Psychosocial risk factors for cardiovascular disease: more than one culprit at work. *JAMA*. 2003;290(16): 2190–2192.
104. Chase EC, McMenamin SB, Halpin HA. Medicaid provider delivery of the 5A's for smoking cessation counseling. *Nicotine Tob Res*. 2007;9(11): 1095–1101.
105. Alexander SC, Cox ME, Boling Turer CL, et al. Do the five A's work when physicians counsel about weight loss?. *Fam Med*. 2011;43(3):179–184.
106. Lavie CJ, Franklin BA, Ferdinand KC. Improving behavioral counseling for primary cardiovascular disease prevention. *JAMA Cardiol*. 2022. https:// doi.org/10.1001/jamacardio.2022.2259. Published online.
107. Epstein RM, Franks P, Fiscella K, et al. Measuring patient-centered communications in patient-physician consultations: theoretical and practical issues. *Soc Sci Med*. 2005;61(7):1516–1528.
108. Spring B, Ockene JK, Gidding SS, et al. Better population health through behavior change in adults: a call to action. *Circulation*. 2013;128(19): 2169–2176.
109. Britt E, Hudson SM, Blampied NM. Motivational interviewing in health settings: a review. *Patient Edu Couns*. 2004;53(2):147–155.
110. Centers for Disease Control and Prevention. National diabetes statistics report. *National Center for Chronic Disease Prevention and Health Promotion*. 2017;2017
111. Fowler MJ. Microvascular and macrovascular complications of diabetes. *Clin Diabetes*. 2008;26:77–82.
112. Blackburn G. Effect of degree of weight loss on health benefits. *Obes Res*. 1995;3(Suppl 2):211s–216s.
113. Moy CS, LaPorte RE, Dorman JS, et al. Insulin-dependent diabetes mellitus mortality. The risk of cigarette smoking. *Circulation*. 1990;82(1):37–43.
114. Mulnier HE, Seaman HE, Raleigh VS, et al. Risk of stroke in people with type 2 diabetes in the UK: a study using the General Practice Research Database. *Diabetologia* 2006;49(12):2859–2865.
115. Facchini FS, Hollenbeck CB, Jeppesen J, Chen YD, Reaven GM. Insulin resistance and cigarette smoking. *Lancet*. 1992;339(8802):1128–1130.
116. Hofer SE, Rosenbauer J, Grulich-Henn J, et al. Smoking and metabolic control in adolescents with type 1 diabetes. *J Pediatr*. 2009;154(1):20–23.
117. Zoppini G, Targher G, Cacciatori V, Guerriero A, Muggeo M. Chronic cigarette smoking is associated with increased plasma circulating intercellular adhesion molecule 1 levels in young type 1 diabetic patients. *Diabetes Care*. 1999;22(11):1871–1874.
118. Stewart KJ. Exercise training and the cardiovascular consequences of type 2 diabetes and hypertension: plausible mechanisms for improving cardiovascular health. *JAMA*. 2002;288(13):1622–1631.

18 Effect of Blood Pressure Management on Coronary Heart Disease Risk in Patients With Type 2 Diabetes

CLARE ARNOTT AND ANUSHKA A. PATEL

The effects of blood pressure (BP) management on the risks of coronary heart disease (CHD) and other vascular outcomes among individuals with type 2 diabetes mellitus (T2DM) have been extensively investigated. This chapter reviews the epidemiologic associations between BP and CHD in diabetes and the efficacy of BP lowering on CHD outcomes, focusing on evidence about the direct and off-target effects of different classes of BP-lowering drugs, the results of relevant clinical trials evaluating different levels of intensity of BP lowering, and the potential role of new and emerging clinical interventions and pharmacotherapies. Finally, these will be placed within the context of the effects of BP lowering on other clinical outcomes, the role of absolute risk assessment for guiding BP management, and a global perspective of current levels of success in achieving adequate BP control in patients with T2DM.

EPIDEMIOLOGIC ASSOCIATIONS BETWEEN BLOOD PRESSURE AND CORONARY HEART DISEASE IN PEOPLE WITH TYPE 2 DIABETES MELLITUS

On average, systolic BP (SBP) and diastolic BP (DBP) are consistently higher among individuals with T2DM compared with those without T2DM, with some evidence to suggest a causal link between T2DM and increasing BP.[1–3] Nonoptimal BP is a well-established risk factor for people with and without diabetes. In general populations, there is log-linear association between both SBP and DBP and CHD, evident within any adult age group. This association appears continuous across the range of BP, down to at least SBP of 115 mm Hg and DBP of 75 mm Hg, such that for adults aged 40 to 89 years, a 20-mm Hg difference in SBP is associated with an approximate 45% difference in risk of CHD.[4] A systematic review and meta-analysis of 4.5 million individuals aged 18 to 45 years also supports a graded and progressive association between increasing BP increments and vascular events in young adults.[5]

Further, in 386,307 people with diabetes included in the Asia Pacific Cohort Studies Collaboration,[6] a similar continuous association was observed for both Asian and non-Asian populations. Among those with diabetes, a 10 mm Hg lower level of SBP was associated with an 18% lower level of CHD, which was not statistically different from the 23% lower level of CHD observed in people without diabetes (Fig. 18.1).

Further data relating to epidemiologic associations have been derived from observational analyses of clinical trial populations.[7,8] The United Kingdom Prospective Diabetes Study (UKPDS) demonstrated that a higher level of average SBP within a range from below 120 mm Hg to above 160 mm Hg was associated with a greater risk of myocardial infarction (MI) of approximately 12% per 10 mm Hg increment.[8] In the Action in Diabetes and Vascular Disease: Preterax and Diamicron MR Controlled Evaluation (ADVANCE) trial, a similar positive continuous association between SBP and CHD was observed down to 85 mm Hg.[9] Observational subgroup analyses of the International Verapamil SR Trandolapril Study (INVEST) suggested a possible J-curve relationship with a threshold on-treatment SBP level of 125 to 130 mm Hg in diabetic patients with established stable coronary artery disease with respect to all-cause mortality.[10] By and large, however, the epidemiologic data have formed a credible basis for the hypothesis that benefits of BP-lowering therapy might accrue to individuals with T2DM down to levels of SBP well below currently accepted thresholds for the diagnosis of hypertension.

Although these epidemiologic data provide a basis for expecting a reduction in CHD events from interventions that reduce BP in people with T2DM, the results from well-designed and appropriately powered randomized trials should inform recommendations for clinical and public health practice.

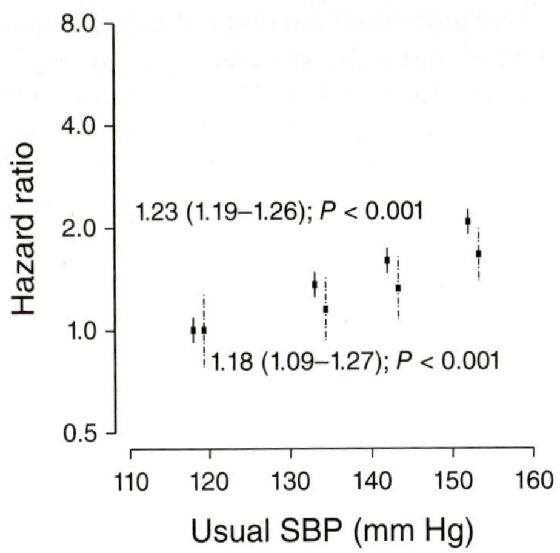

FIG. 18.1 Association between usual systolic blood pressure (*SBP*) and coronary heart disease (*CHD*) events by diabetes status in the Asia Pacific Cohort Studies Collaboration. For each association, the hazard ratio (95% confidence interval [CI]) for a 10 mm Hg higher level of SBP compared with SBP 120 mm Hg as reference and the *P* value for linear trend are indicated (upper value for those without diabetes; lower value for those with diabetes). Usual: baseline values corrected for regression dilution bias (using repeated measures). Reproduced with permission from Asia Pacific Cohort Studies Collaboration; Kengne AP, Patel A, Barzi F, et al. Systolic blood pressure, diabetes and the risk of cardiovascular diseases in the Asia-Pacific region. *J Hypertens.* 2007;25:1205–1213.

EFFICACY OF NONPHARMACOLOGICAL INTERVENTIONS ON BLOOD PRESSURE LEVELS AND CORONARY HEART DISEASE RISK IN PATIENTS WITH TYPE 2 DIABETES MELLITUS

Behavioral Modification

Initial attempts at BP reduction through nonpharmacological behavioral modification are emphasized in guidelines for the management of hypertension worldwide in individuals with or without diabetes.[11–17] These principally focus on increasing physical activity, reducing body weight and/or adiposity, and dietary modification, including sodium restriction and adequate potassium consumption. Although a number of studies have evaluated the effects of lifestyle interventions on diabetes incidence, the Look AHEAD (Action for Health in Diabetes) trial examined the sustained effects of an intensive lifestyle intervention compared to diabetes support and education in 5145 overweight or obese adults with T2DM.[18] The trial was prematurely discontinued on the basis of futility after a median of 9.6 years follow-up with respect to the primary composite cardiovascular disease outcome.[19] The intensive lifestyle intervention was associated with significant improvements for a number of vascular risk factors, including net reductions in BP that diminished over time with an average postrandomization difference in SBP of −1.9 mm Hg. The intervention evaluated and targeted both physical activity and diet, and separate effects of individual components of the lifestyle intervention on BP cannot be estimated (see also Chapters 5 and 12).

Although not restricted to people with diabetes, the Dietary Approaches to Stop Hypertension (DASH) trials provide some indication of the likely effects of certain diets on BP.[20,21] Allocation to the DASH diet (rich in fruits, vegetables, and low-fat dairy foods and with reduced saturated and total fat) in 459 adults over an 8-week intervention period was associated with significant reductions in SBP and DBP of 5.5 and 3.0 mm Hg, respectively, compared with a "typical" control diet.[20] In the subsequent DASH-sodium trial,[21] participants were randomly assigned different levels of sodium intake, within DASH or control diets. The effects of different levels of sodium intake in addition to the DASH diet were evaluated. Greatest benefits were observed with a low-sodium DASH diet, which compared with a control high-sodium diet, reduced SBP by 11.5 mm Hg in participants with hypertension and 7.1 mm Hg in those without a diagnosis of hypertension. With small numbers of participants, analysis in the subgroup with diabetes was not possible. Recent systematic reviews have concluded that reductions in dietary sodium were associated with significant reductions in BP, with a dose-response relationship and greater effects among older people, those with higher blood pressure and in non-White populations.[22,23] In a cluster randomized trial of salt substitute (75% sodium chloride and 25% potassium chloride) versus regular salt (100% sodium chloride) conducted among 20,995 participants with a history of stroke or who were aged 60 years and older with hypertension in rural China, salt substitute was associated with significant relative risk reductions over 4.7 years in stroke (14%), major cardiovascular events (13%), and death (12%).[23] Salt substitute was also associated with reduced rates of nonfatal acute coronary syndrome, without any excess in serious adverse events attributed to hyperkalemia. The mean reduction in systolic BP with salt substitute was 3.3 mm Hg. In prespecified subgroup analyses, there was no evidence of heterogeneity of intervention effect by baseline diabetes status.

RENAL SYMPATHETIC DENERVATION

Treatment of hypertension using endovascular catheter technology that allows selective sympathetic renal denervation (RDN) by transluminal radiofrequency or ultrasound ablation has been evaluated in clinical practice since the first in man trials in 2011.[24,25] The evaluation of efficacy and safety of this approach was initially limited to populations with "resistant" primary hypertension, with persistently high levels of BP despite comprehensive combination drug therapy, but has now also been evaluated in hypertensive populations in the absence of antihypertensive medications.[26] The Symplicity HTN-2 trial was the first randomized study reported, including 106 patients (approximately 30% with T2DM) with baseline SBP levels of 160 mm Hg or greater (≥150 mm Hg in the presence of diabetes), despite the use of at least three BP-lowering agents. The between-group difference in the primary outcome of office-measured BP level at 6 months was large and highly statistically significant (33/11 mm Hg, $P < 0.0001$).[27] No separate analyses were reported for the subgroup with T2DM. No serious safety concerns were identified in this small study; however, the absence of a sham procedure in the control arm raised concerns. In a subsequent systematic review and meta-analysis of randomized sham-controlled trials (9 trials, 1555 patients),[25] the proportion of T2DM patients in included studies ranged from 5% to 45%. Key findings were that RDN reduced 24-hour ambulatory blood pressure by 3.3 mm Hg compared to sham ($P < 0.001$) with a 5.25 mm Hg reduction in office systolic blood pressure and consistent benefits across both medicated and unmedicated patients. More recent data from one trial showing minimal or modest improvements in blood pressure with RDN relative to a sham procedure with short-term follow-up described more substantive effects with 36-month follow-up.[28] Even more recent small trials have suggested that second-generation RDN may have a differential effect on blood pressure, compared to sham, depending on concurrent use of antihypertensive therapy.[29]

It has been suggested that conditions associated with higher sympathetic activation or individuals at higher baseline CV risk may potentially derive a greater benefit from RDN. Data from the observational Global SYMPLICITY Registry[30] reported on the efficacy and safety of RDN in high-risk patients, including those with T2DM, over 3 years of follow-up. They reported a reduction in 24-hour systolic blood pressure in those with T2DM, which was numerically greater than was seen in those without T2DM at 3 years (−10.5 vs. −7.6 mm Hg), but the difference was not statistically significant ($P = 0.06$). While RDN was generally associated with acceptably low rates of adverse events, it was noted that those with T2DM experienced higher rates of subsequent MI (4.0% vs. 1.6%; $P = 0.002$) and end-stage renal disease (2.8% vs. 1.0%; $P = 0.005$).[30] These conclusions need confirmation in prospective randomized studies.

RDN is thus best described as a possibly effective and relatively safe intervention in resistant hypertension, requiring more reliable data on long-term efficacy and safety across specific patient populations, including in people with diabetes. Reflecting this, RDN has been included in the updated European Society of Hypertension guidelines as a Class II recommendation for the management of uncontrolled resistant hypertension (when estimated Glomerular Filtration Rate (eGFR) > 40 mL/min/1.73 m^2) that is "additive or alternative to increasing medications."[17]

EFFICACY AND SAFETY OF BLOOD PRESSURE–LOWERING DRUGS ON CORONARY HEART DISEASE IN PATIENTS WITH TYPE 2 DIABETES MELLITUS

Multiple guidelines for pharmacologic lowering of BP in patients with T2DM exist worldwide, with some major examples summarized in Table 18 1. Some of the evidence on which these recommendations are based is outlined here.

Overall Efficacy

Several meta-analyses have examined the relationship between pharmacological BP lowering and incident cardiovascular events. The most comprehensive overview of the effects of BP-lowering medications on vascular outcomes is provided by individual participant data (IPD) meta-analyses conducted in the Blood Pressure Lowering Treatment Trialists' Collaboration (BPLTTC).[31] The most recent analyses, published in 2022, included IPD from 51 studies and 358,533 individuals (29% with T2DM).[32] Over a median of 4.2 years follow-up, each 5 mm Hg reduction in systolic blood pressure resulted in a 6% relative reduction in major cardiovascular events in those with T2DM (HR, 0.94; 95% CI, 0.91–0.98) with a greater reduction observed in those without T2DM (HR, 0.89; 95% CI, 0.87–0.92; P for interaction 0.001). This heterogeneity was driven primarily by a smaller reduction in fatal and nonfatal coronary events in those with T2DM. Absolute risk reductions, however, were similar across those with and without T2DM due to the higher baseline risk of the T2DM cohort[32] (Fig. 18 2).

While most trials of BP lowering in diabetes focused on patients with hypertension, ADVANCE, the largest ever conducted placebo-controlled trial of BP lowering among individuals with T2DM (n = 11,140) addressed a question of routine BP lowering, regardless of initial BP level.[33,34] Participants with known cardiovascular or microvascular disease or with at least one major risk factor for cardiovascular disease and any initial level of BP were randomly assigned to a fixed combination of the ACE inhibitor perindopril and the thiazide-like diuretic indapamide (4/1.25 mg) or matching placebo. The mean BP of participants at study baseline was 145/81 mm Hg. Over the course of active treatment, BP was reduced by a mean of 5.6/2.2 mm Hg compared with a placebo. At the end of a mean 4.3 years follow-up, active treatment reduced the risk of the combined composite primary outcome of major microvascular and macrovascular (cardiovascular) events by 9% (95% CI, 0%–17%, P = 0.043). For prespecified secondary outcomes, there was an 18% (2%–32%; P = 0.027) reduction in cardiovascular mortality and a 14% (2%–24%; P = 0.020) reduction in CHD events (defined as death caused by CHD, nonfatal MI, silent MI, coronary revascularization, or hospital admission for unstable angina). The effects of the combination of perindopril and indapamide treatment were similar across a range of initial BP levels, pointing to an alternative strategy for the provision of BP therapy to patients with T2DM, not limited to those with arbitrarily defined "hypertension."

Comparative Efficacy of Blood Pressure-Lowering Drugs

There has been considerable debate about the potential existence of BP-independent beneficial effects of various classes of drugs used to lower BP in a broad group of high-risk patients, including those with diabetes and with respect to different vascular beds. Data from both large clinical trials and meta-analyses help to inform this debate and are summarized below.

Although not limited to patients with diabetes, the results of three large trials raised questions about potential differential effects of BP-lowering regimens in patients with T2DM. The Anglo-Scandinavian Cardiac Outcomes Trial (ASCOT) investigated 19,257 people with hypertension and additional risk factors for cardiovascular disease (27% with diabetes), and compared the effects of combinations of atenolol with a thiazide diuretic versus amlodipine with

TABLE 18.1 Summary of Select Major Guideline Recommendations for the Use of BP-Lowering Drugs in Patients With T2DM

GUIDELINE	PRINCIPLES FOR COMMENCING BP-LOWERING TREATMENT	RECOMMENDED CLASSES OF BP-LOWERING DRUG	RECOMMENDED TARGET BP LEVELS
Global: International Diabetes Federation Clinical Practice Recommendations for Managing Type 2 Diabetes in Primary Care, 2017 (https://idf.org/e-library/guidelines/128-idf-clinical-practice-recommendations-for-managing-type-2-diabetes-in-primary-care.html)	High blood pressure is recognized by all major guidelines as a major risk factor for CVD and CKD.	Patients with high blood pressure should start treatment with an ACE inhibitor or an ARB and then add a calcium channel blocker of a thiazide diuretic if targets are not achieved. An ACE inhibitor or an ARB should also be started when the patient has persistent microalbuminuria in the absence of high blood pressure.	Patients with T2D and hypertension should be treated to a DBP target of 80 mm Hg and an SBP target of 130–140 mm Hg. Consider the lower target when they are younger or when additional cardiovascular risk factors or microvascular disease are present.
Global: 2020 International Society of Hypertension Global Hypertension Practice Guidelines (https://www.ahajournals.org/doi/10.1161/HYPERTENSIONAHA.120.15026)	BP should be lowered if ≥140/90 mm Hg.	Treatment strategy should include an RAS inhibitor (and a CCB and/or thiazide-like diuretic).	BP should be treated to a target of <130/80 mm Hg (<140/80 in older patients).
United States: American Diabetes Association Standards of Medical Care in Diabetes, 2022 (https://doi.org/10.2337/dc22-S010)	People with BP between 140–150/90–99 mm Hg may begin with a single drug. For people with BP ≥160/100 mm Hg, initial pharmacologic treatment with two antihypertensive medications is recommended.	Alongside lifestyle modifications, in people with diabetes, ACE inhibitor or an ARB is recommended as first-line therapy. Multiple-drug therapy is generally required to achieve BP targets. However, combinations of ACE inhibitors and ARBs and combinations of ACE inhibitors or ARBs with direct renin inhibitors should not be used.	The goal of treatment is a BP target of <130/80 mm Hg if it can be safely attained.
United States: 2017 ACC/AHA/AAPA/ABC/ACPM/AGS/APhA/ASH/ASPC/NMA/PCNA Guideline for the Prevention, Detection, Evaluation, and Management of High Blood Pressure in Adults. (https://www.ahajournals.org/doi/10.1161/hyp.0000000000000065)	Antihypertensive drug treatment should be initiated at a BP ≥130/80 mm Hg.	All first-line classes of antihypertensive agents (i.e., diuretics, ACE inhibitors, ARBs, and CCBs) are useful and effective. ACE inhibitors or ARBs may be considered in the presence of albuminuria.	Treatment goal is <130/80 mm Hg.
Europe: European Society of Cardiology/European Society of Hypertension Guidelines for the Management of Arterial Hypertension, 2018 (https://doi.org/10.1093/eurheartj/ehy339)	Antihypertensive drug treatment is recommended for people with diabetes when office BP is ≥140/90 mm Hg.	Alongside lifestyle interventions, treatment should usually be initiated with a two-drug combination of an ACE inhibitor or ARB with a CCB or diuretic. For those requiring three drugs, a combination of an ACE inhibitor or ARB with a CCB and a diuretic is recommended.	Lowering SBP to a range of 120–129 mm Hg (16–65 age group) and 130–139 mm Hg (>65 age group) is recommended in patients with diabetes. The DBP target in patients with diabetes is recommended to be 70–79 mm Hg (all ages).
Europe: 2019 ESC Guidelines on diabetes, prediabetes, and cardiovascular diseases developed in collaboration with EASD. (https://academic.oup.com/eurheartj/article/41/2/255/5556890)	Antihypertensive drug treatment is recommended when office BP is >140/90 mm Hg.	An RAAS blocker (ACEI or ARB) is recommended, particularly in the presence of microalbuminuria, albuminuria, proteinuria, or LV hypertrophy. It is recommended that treatment is initiated with a combination of a RAAS blocker with a calcium channel blocker or thiazide/thiazide-like diuretic. The effects of GLP1-RAs and SGLT2 inhibitors on BP should be considered.	The BP goal is to target SBP to 130 mm Hg and <130 mm Hg if tolerated but not < 120 mm Hg. In older people (aged > 65 years), SBP goal is to a range of 130–139 mmHg.

ACE, Angiotensin-converting enzyme; *ARB*, angiotensin receptor blocker; *BB*, beta blockers; *CCB*, calcium channel blocker; *RAS*, renin angiotensin system.

perindopril on the primary outcome of fatal and nonfatal CHD events.[35] The point estimate of treatment effect favored the amlodipine-perindopril combination for the primary outcome, but this was not statistically significant. However, there were significant reductions in all secondary outcomes associated with the amlodipine-perindopril combination, ranging from a relative risk reduction of 11% to 24%, and including all-cause mortality (which led to early termination of the trial), all coronary events, and nonfatal MI and fatal CHD. However, the amlodipine-based regimen was associated with a significant 2.7/1.9 mm Hg lower BP over the duration of follow-up. There was no evidence of heterogeneity of the treatment effect by the presence or absence of diabetes, evaluated on the basis of total cardiovascular outcomes.

	Intervention		Comparator		Percentage of absolute risk reduction (95% CI)
	Events	Total	Events	Total	
Major cardiovascular events					
Diabetes	7441	47151	9335	53,981	−1·54 (−2·04 to −1·04)
No diabetes	11, 370	12,055,1	14,785	13,359,5	−1·61 (−1·86 to −1·36)
Overall	**18, 811**	**16,770,2**	**24,120**	**18,757,6**	**−1·63 (−1·86 to −1·40)**
$P_{interaction}$=1·00					
Stroke					
Diabetes	2238	47,183	2872	54,029	−0·58 (−0·86 to −0·30)
No diabetes	4229	12,069,5	5429	13,372,5	−0·56 (−0·71 to −0·40)
Overall	**6467**	**16,787,8**	**8301**	**18,775,4**	**−0·57 (−0·70 to −0·44)**
$P_{interaction}$=1·00					
Ischaemic heart disease					
Diabetes	3557	47, 159	4590	53, 997	−0·97 (−1·32 to −0·62)
No diabetes	5563	12, 062, 9	7383	13, 365, 5	−0·91 (−1·08 to −0·73)
Overall	**9120**	**16, 778, 8**	**11,973**	**18, 765, 2**	**−0·95 (−1·11 to −0·79)**
$P_{interaction}$=1·00					
Heart failure					
Diabetes	1666	43,685	2314	50, 886	−0·77 (−1·03 to −0·51)
No diabetes	1620	10, 473, 4	2308	11, 780, 9	−0·39 (−0·51 to −0·28)
Overall	**3286**	**14, 841, 9**	**4622**	**16, 869, 5**	**−0·52 (−0·63 to −0·41)**
$P_{interaction}$=0·018					
Cardiovascular death					
Diabetes	2084	43, 924	2466	51, 069	−0·09 (−0·37 to 0·19)
No diabetes	3109	11, 196, 3	4062	12, 500, 7	−0·48 (−0·62 to −0·34)
Overall	**5193**	**15, 588, 7**	**6532**	**17, 612, 9**	**−0·38 (−0·51 to −0·25)**
$P_{interaction}$=0·029					
All-cause death					
Diabetes	5379	48,357	6331	54, 627	−0·47 (−0·89 to −0·06)
No diabetes	8521	12, 070, 8	10, 427	13, 372, 3	−0·74 (−0·96 to −0·53)
Overall	**13, 900**	**16, 906, 5**	**16, 758**	**18, 835, 0**	**−0·68 (−0·87 to −0·49)**
$P_{interaction}$=0·5					

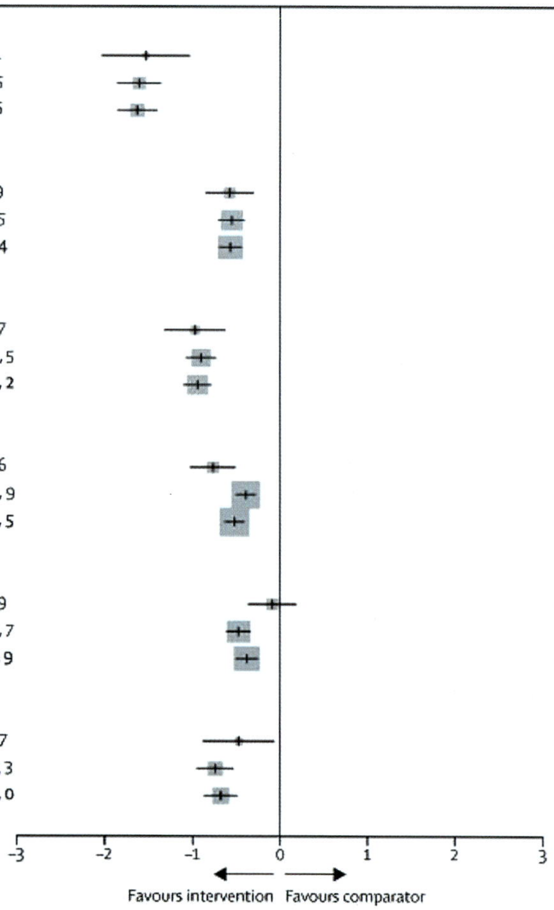

FIG. 18.2 Absolute treatment effects of blood pressure (*BP*)-lowering regimens on ischemic heart disease and other cardiovascular outcomes in people with and without diabetes. Absolute risk reduction was estimated using a Poisson regression model with identity link. The unit is the percentage of absolute risk difference (treatment vs. comparator) over follow-up time and reflects the mean of blood pressure reduction across all trials. $p_{interaction}$ was adjusted for multiple comparisons. Reproduced from Nazarzadeh M, Bidel Z, Canoy D, et al. Blood pressure-lowering treatment for prevention of major cardiovascular diseases in people with and without type 2 diabetes: an individual participant-level data meta-analysis. *Lancet Diabetes Endocrinol*. 2022;10:645–654.

The Ongoing Telmisartan Alone and in Combination with Ramipril Global Endpoint Trial (ONTARGET) included 25,620 patients (~40% with diabetes) at increased risk for cardiovascular disease.[36] Patients were randomized to ramipril alone, to telmisartan alone, or to both drugs. The mean BP level at study entry was 142/82 mm Hg. Over the course of follow-up, BP was 2.4/1.4 mm Hg lower in the combination therapy group compared with the ramipril-alone group. The incidence of the primary outcome (cardiovascular death, nonfatal MI, nonfatal stroke, or hospitalized heart failure) did not differ between the ramipril-alone group and each of the other randomized groups. As expected, participants allocated to telmisartan alone experienced less cough and angioedema than those who were randomized to ramipril. However, symptoms of hypotension occurred more frequently in the telmisartan group (2.7%) and in the combination group (4.8%) compared with the ramipril-alone group (1.7%). Renal dysfunction was observed most often in the combination group. There was no heterogeneity in treatment effects by diabetes status for the primary outcome. In summary, the results of ONTARGET confirmed comparable efficacy of the ACE inhibitor and the ARB, with evidence of no additional benefit and increased harm from combination therapy.

The Avoiding Cardiovascular Events through Combination Therapy to Patients Living with Systolic Hypertension (ACCOMPLISH) trial included 11,506 high-risk patients (~60% with diabetes) with hypertension.[37] Participants were randomly allocated to receive one of two combination drug regimens—the ACE inhibitor benazepril plus the calcium channel blocker amlodipine, or benazepril with the diuretic hydrochlorothiazide (HCT). The mean baseline BP level was 145/80 mm Hg. Over the duration of follow-up, a 0.9/1.1 mm Hg lower BP was observed in the benazepril-amlodipine group compared with the benazepril-HCT group. This study was stopped prematurely after a mean follow-up period of 3 years because of an observed statistically significant 20% reduction in the primary outcome (cardiovascular death, nonfatal MI, nonfatal stroke, hospitalization for angina, resuscitation after cardiac arrest, and coronary revascularization) in the benazepril-amlodipine group compared with the benazepril-HCT group. There was no evidence of heterogeneity based on the baseline diagnosis of diabetes. Although early concerns had been expressed about potential underestimation of the BP difference between treatment arms using on-trial measurements, subsequent results of 24-hour ambulatory BP monitoring in a subset of 573 participants did not show any significant differences.[38]

A 2015 systematic review restricted to trials of patients with diabetes identified few differences of the effects on clinical outcomes based on drug regimen, the key exceptions being for heart failure and stroke[39] (Fig. 18 3). In a more recent BPLTTC meta-analysis using IPD from 51 randomized trials, the magnitude of benefits on clinical outcomes produced by different regimens of BP-lowering therapy was assessed using a network meta-analysis by drug class and meta-regression stratified by T2DM status. In this overview, a smaller relative risk reduction in clinical events in those with T2DM, compared to those without T2DM, was consistently seen, irrespective of individual antihypertensive drug class, with no heterogeneity of treatment effect observed between drug classes.[32]

By and large, current hypertension and diabetes management guidelines worldwide acknowledge that achieving BP reduction is more pressing than decisions about which class of drug should be used, particularly given that two or more agents are frequently required in patients with diabetes.[11–17] In general, the use of a regimen that includes an ACE inhibitor or an ARB is recommended, particularly in the presence of albuminuria. Although thiazide or thiazide-like diuretics as well as beta-blockers have been associated with adverse effects on glucose homeostasis, the clinical relevance of this is doubtful and it does not preclude the use of these drugs in people with T2DM. Indeed, the indications for use of beta-blockers in patients with existing CHD or systolic heart failure (particularly vasodilating or cardioselective beta-blockers, such as carvedilol, nebivolol, or metoprolol succinate, which may also have more favorable metabolic effects than older beta-blockers)[40,41] and thiazide or thiazide-like diuretics in those with cerebrovascular disease are compelling.[42,43] For much of the world, affordability is also a key issue that must be considered in the choice of antihypertensive therapy.

More Versus Less Blood Pressure Lowering and Target Blood Pressure Levels

Most guidelines worldwide currently recommend more aggressive management of hypertension (mostly, a target of 130/80 mm Hg or lower) among people with diabetes compared with those without diabetes.[11–17]

The BPLTTC evaluation of the effects of more versus less BP lowering included 48 trials and 344,716 patients, of whom 28% had T2DM. For the primary outcome of major adverse CV events (MACE), the relative effects of

Medication Class vs. All Other Classes of Hypertensives	No. of Studies	Specified Medication, No.		Any Active Comparator, No.		SBP Reduction, Mean (95% CI), mm Hg[a]	Relative Risk (95% CI)
		Events	Participants	Events	Participants		
Mortality							
CCB[21, 22, 28, 40, 41, 66, 69, 70, 75-81]	11	1482	15,117	1910	17,665	0.5 (−2.0 to 1.1)	0.98 (0.92–1.05)
ACE[22, 28, 64, 65, 76-81]	6	615	4617	972	7154	1.7 (0.8 to 2.6)	1.02 (0.93–1.12)
Diuretics[22, 66, 69]	3	956	9649	634	7339	−1.5 (−2.4 to −0.7)	1.00 (0.91–1.10)
β-Blocker[21, 64, 65, 70, 72]	4	768	6770	753	6720	−0.7 (−1.8 to 0.5)	1.02 (0.92–1.13)
ARB[40, 41, 72]	2	150	1165	187	1176	2.5 (1.5 to 3.5)	0.81 (0.66–0.99)
Cardiovascular disease							
CCB[21, 22, 40, 41, 66, 69, 70, 75-81]	10	2035	14,814	2672	17,364	0.5 (−1.0 to 1.2)	0.98 (0.93–1.03)
ACE[22, 76-81]	4	862	3916	1406	6493	1.8 (1.0 to 2.6)	1.06 (0.99–1.15)
Diuretics[22, 66, 69]	3	1675	9649	1137	7339	−1.5 (−2.4 to −0.7)	0.98 (0.85–1.12)
β-Blocker[21, 70, 72]	3	792	6412	722	6320	−0.8 (−2.1 to 0.6)	1.24 (0.94–1.62)
ARB[40, 41, 72]	2	275	1165	300	1176	2.5 (1.5 to 3.5)	0.93 (0.80–1.08)
Coronary heart disease							
CCB[21, 22, 40, 41, 66, 69, 70, 75-81]	10	751	14,814	1002	17,364	0.5 (−1.0 to 1.2)	1.00 (0.91–1.09)
ACE[22, 64, 65, 76-81]	5	404	4316	668	6851	1.6 (0.6 to 2.6)	0.96 (0.85–1.08)
Diuretics[22, 66, 69]	3	635	9649	406	7339	−1.5 (−2.4 to −0.0)	1.02 (0.90–1.15)
β-Blocker[21, 64, 65, 70, 72]	4	308	6770	304	6720	−0.7 (−1.8 to 0.5)	1.03 (0.87–1.20)
ARB[40, 41, 72]	2	85	1165	77	1176	2.5 (1.5 to 3.5)	1.09 (0.80–1.48)
Stroke							
CCB[21, 22, 40, 41, 66, 69, 70, 75-81]	10	484	14,814	726	17,364	0.5 (−1.0 to 1.2)	0.86 (0.77–0.97)
ACE[22, 64, 65, 76-81]	5	257	4316	412	6851	1.6 (0.6 to 2.6)	1.03 (0.89–1.20)
Diuretics[22, 66, 69]	3	394	9649	270	7339	−1.5 (−2.4 to −0.7)	0.98 (0.84–1.14)
β-Blocker[21, 64, 65, 70, 72]	4	273	6770	220	6720	−0.7 (−1.8 to 0.5)	1.25 (1.05–1.50)
ARB[40, 41, 72]	2	79	1165	80	1176	2.5 (1.5 to 3.5)	0.98 (0.71–1.34)
Heart failure							
CCB[21, 22, 40, 41, 66, 69, 75-81]	9	612	11,645	643	14,133	0.7 (−1.0 to 1.4)	1.32 (1.18–1.47)
ACE[22, 64, 65, 76-81]	5	317	4316	454	6851	1.6 (0.6 to 2.6)	1.17 (1.02–1.35)
Diuretics[22, 66, 69]	3	448	9649	349	7339	−1.5 (−2.4 to −0.7)	0.83 (0.72–0.95)
β-Blocker[21, 64, 65, 72]	3	129	3539	110	3551	−1.3 (−2.8 to 0.2)	1.20 (0.92–1.56)
ARB[40, 41, 72]	2	92	1165	148	1176	2.5 (1.5 to 3.5)	0.61 (0.48–0.78)

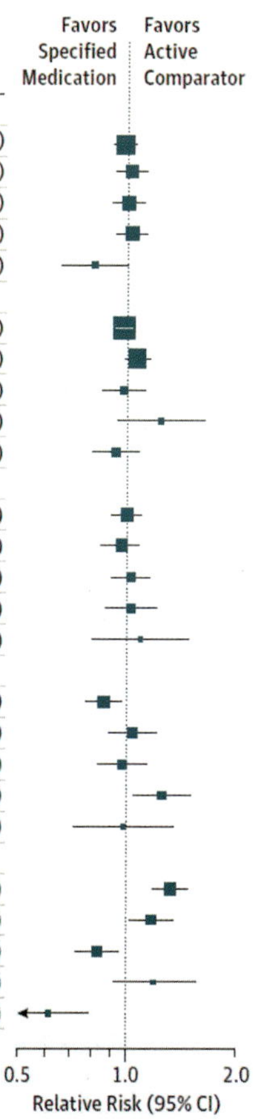

FIG. 18.3 Blood pressure-lowering drug class effects on CHD and other clinical outcomes from trials of participants with diabetes. [a]Systolic blood pressure (*SBP*) reduction is reported as a 95% CI for the mean reduction at the trial level, not a range of reduction among trials. The area of each square is proportional to the inverse variance of the estimate. Horizontal lines indicate 95% CIs of the estimate. *ACE*, Angiotensin-converting enzyme; *ARB*, angiotensin II receptor blocker; *CCB*, calcium channel blocker; *CHD*, coronary heart disease; *CI*, confidence interval. Reproduced from Emdin CA, Rahimi K, Neal B, et al. Blood pressure lowering in type 2 diabetes: a systematic review and meta-analysis. *JAMA*. 2015;313(6):603–615. https://doi.10.1001/jama.2014.18574.

BP lowering were shown on a meta-regression analysis to be proportional to the degree of SBP reduction achieved.[44] These analyses were not undertaken separately in those with T2DM; however, in meta-regression analyses performed in the most recent BPLTTC overview, similar correlations between the degree of BP lowering achieved and reductions in CV events were observed for individuals with and without diabetes (Fig. 18 4).[32]

The Action to Control Cardiovascular Risk in Diabetes (ACCORD) trial in people with T2DM and the Systolic Blood Pressure Intervention (SPRINT) trial,[45] in those without T2DM, are two pivotal trials addressing optimal blood pressure targets.

ACCORD was a factorial randomized trial of 10,251 individuals with T2DM from 77 centers in North America.[46–48] Participants with a hemoglobin A1c (HbA1c) of 7.5% or more and aged 40 years or older with cardiovascular disease or 55 years or older with anatomic evidence of significant atherosclerosis, albuminuria, left ventricular hypertrophy, or at least two additional risk factors for cardiovascular disease (dyslipidemia, hypertension, smoking, or obesity) were randomized to two glucose control targets (see also Chapter 13). A subset of 4733 participants (with SBP between 130 and 180 mm Hg on three or fewer antihypertensive medications and with no evidence of greater than 1.0 g of proteinuria per day or the equivalent) were also included in a randomized evaluation of a BP-lowering intervention targeting two different SBP levels (an SBP target of 120 mm Hg or less, compared with 140 mm Hg or less). The BP-lowering regimen was at the physician's discretion but included any class of drug therapy known to produce cardiovascular benefits (ACE inhibitors, ARBs, diuretics, calcium channel blockers, or beta-blockers). The primary outcome was a composite of major cardiovascular events defined as nonfatal MI, nonfatal stroke, and cardiovascular death. Secondary outcomes included all coronary events, all stroke events, and all-cause death, considered separately. The mean baseline BP in ACCORD was 139/76 mm Hg, and at study entry, 87% of participants were already taking some form of antihypertensive therapy. Over a mean follow-up of 4.7 years, intensive therapy achieved a mean SBP of 119 mm Hg compared with 134 mm Hg in the standard therapy group, resulting in a mean between-group difference of 14.2 mm Hg. However, intensive therapy did not result in a statistically significant reduction in major cardiovascular events (relative risk reduction [RRR] 12%; 95% CI, −6% to 27%; $P = 0.20$). When the components of the composite outcome were considered separately, intensive therapy did not reduce major coronary events (which included unstable angina) or cardiovascular death, but significantly reduced major strokes by 41% (95% CI, 11%–61%). There was no statistically significant effect of intensive BP therapy on all-cause mortality or heart failure. There was no evidence of heterogeneity in treatment effect in subgroups of participants defined by age, sex, baseline history of cardiovascular disease, and the use of BP-lowering therapy at study entry.

Many have interpreted the ACCORD trial as being "negative" with respect to the BP-lowering component, stimulating discussion that the current target of 130/80 mm Hg or lower promulgated by many guidelines may not be justified. However, notwithstanding the clear benefits of a more aggressive approach to BP lowering for stroke well below this threshold, the study was not sufficiently powered to detect substantial and clinically important beneficial effects on other cardiovascular events, including CHD (approximately one-quarter reduction, which would be broadly consistent with a 14 mm Hg difference in SBP based on epidemiologic data). Intensive BP lowering in ACCORD was associated with an increased number of serious adverse events attributed to BP-lowering drugs, compared with the standard therapy group; however, overall rates over an average period of almost 5 years of follow-up were low (3.3% vs. 1.3%). Particular concerns have been

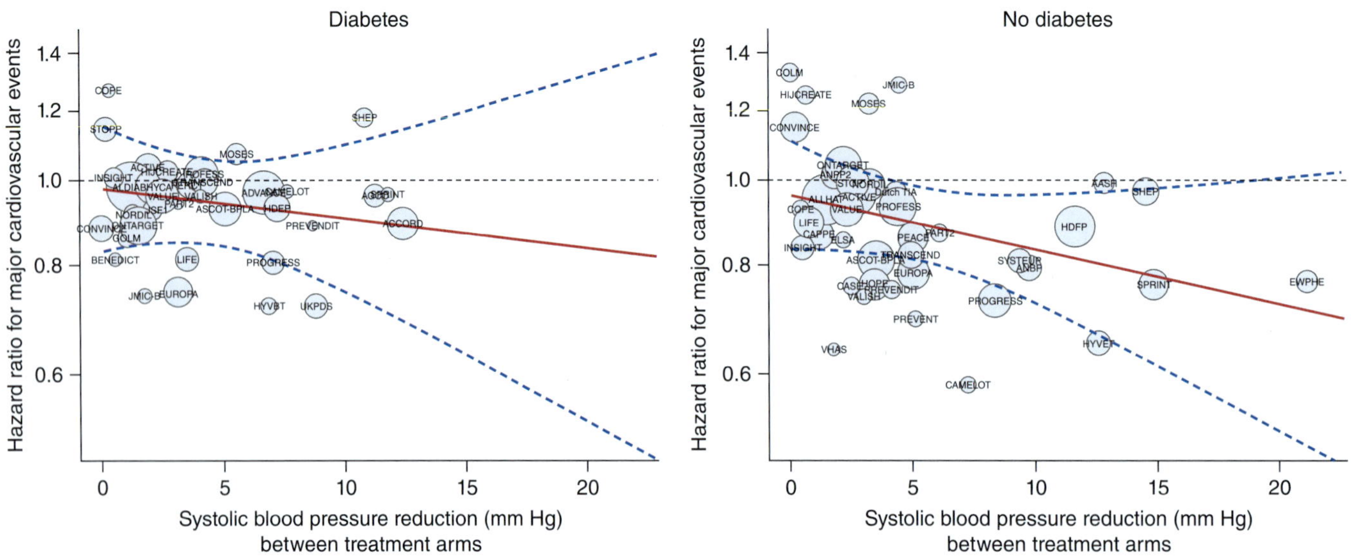

FIGURE 18.4 Meta-regression of intensity of blood pressure reduction and hazard ratio of major cardiovascular events by diabetes status at baseline. The hazard ratio for each trial is shown by the center of the bubbles, with the size of the bubble inversely related to the respective standard error. The solid red line is the fitted regression line; the dotted blue lines represent the 95 percent confidence intervals; the dashed gray line represents the hazard ratio = 1. Regression coefficients and 95 percent confidence intervals in people with and without diabetes at the baseline were −0.007 (−0.036 to 0.0205) and −0.014 (−0.035 to 0.006), respectively. Reproduced from Nazarzadeh M, Bidel Z, Canoy D, et al. Blood pressure-lowering treatment for prevention of major cardiovascular diseases in people with and without type 2 diabetes: an individual participant-level data meta-analysis. *Lancet Diabetes Endocrinol.* 2022;10:645–654.

raised about higher levels of serum creatinine and lower levels of estimated glomerular filtration rate postrandomization among intensive BP treatment participants. This did not translate to differences in end-stage renal disease (2.5% vs. 2.4%), and intensive BP-lowering therapy was associated with the development of numerically fewer cases of microalbuminuria and macroalbuminuria, the latter being significantly lower than the rates observed in the standard therapy group.

The SPRINT trial[45] also evaluated the cardioprotective value of intensive (<120 mm Hg systolic) versus standard blood pressure (<140 mm Hg systolic) control in 9361 individuals at elevated baseline cardiovascular risk; however, people with T2DM were excluded. Over 3.3 years, median follow-up SBP separation between groups was achieved (mean of 121.5 vs. 134.6 mm Hg), with intensive treatment resulting in a 25% lower rate of cardiovascular events (defined as MI, acute coronary syndromes, stroke, heart failure, and CV death) compared to the standard control (HR, 0.75; 95% CI, 0.64–0.89; $P < 0.001$). As was seen in the ACCORD trial, there was an increase in serious adverse events with intensive treatment, including hypotension, syncope, acute kidney injury/failure, and electrolyte abnormalities.

A post hoc analysis combining participants from the SPRINT trial with prediabetes and "SPRINT-eligible" participants from ACCORD with T2DM suggested a benefit for intensive systolic blood pressure control.[49] These analyses reported a 21% reduction (HR, 0.79; 95% CI, 0.65–0.96) in composite cardiovascular events (nonfatal MI, nonfatal stroke, CV death, revascularization, and heart failure) with intensive as compared to standard control. Again, an increase in adverse events was noted with intensive control (4.1% vs. 2.1%; $P = 0.003$).

In addition, a post hoc high-CV-risk subgroup analysis of the ACCORD trial and of the long-term observational follow-up "ACCORD Follow-on" (ACCORDION) was performed to determine the longer-term cardiovascular impacts of intensive BP control in those with T2DM. Over 9 years of follow-up, intensive BP control as compared to standard control, reduced MACE by 25% (HR, 0.75; 95% CI, 0.60–0.95), mainly driven by a reduction in nonfatal MI.[50]

Taken together, these data suggest a likely cardiovascular benefit for intensive systolic BP control in those with T2DM, which must be balanced against an increase in adverse events.

Legacy Effects of Blood Pressure Lowering

In 2008 the UKPDS study reported data from posttrial annual follow-up for an additional 6 years undertaken for all study participants, without attempts to maintain therapies based on the original randomization.[51,52] Long-term posttrial observational follow-up of the blood glucose-lowering arm demonstrated sustained, and in some cases newly emerged, reductions in clinical events associated with original randomization to intensive glucose control[52] (see also Chapter 13). These benefits were observed despite convergence of HbA1c values within a year of posttrial monitoring. Similarly, the BP difference achieved between randomized arms during the trial was no longer apparent within 2 years of the longer-term follow-up.[51] However, unlike the blood glucose intervention, the significant reductions in clinical events were lost during the additional observational period, without the emergence of any new benefits. Long-term observational data are also available for the ADVANCE trial. With posttrial follow-up of 5.9 years in the ADVANCE cohort, between-group BP differences were no longer evident, and the hazard ratios in favor of routine BP lowering for the outcomes of all-case and CV death were still significant but attenuated.[53]

Overall, notwithstanding post hoc subgroup analyses of ACCORDION,[48] a reasonable interpretation of these findings is that BP reduction needs to be maintained for the long-term benefits of such treatment to continue.

New Drugs

Over the last 2 years, potential new drug classes specifically developed for BP lowering have emerged from early-phase clinical trials. There have also been some important developments in pharmacological management of hypertension related to the use of fixed dose combination therapies and "off-target" BP-lowering effects of newer treatments initially developed for blood glucose lowering or other cardiometabolic disease indications.

FIXED-DOSE COMBINATION THERAPY

The use of fixed-dose combination (FDC) therapy (inclusion of two or more BP-lowering medications of different classes in a single pill) has increased rapidly over the past decade. Initially this focused on "substitution indications," whereby FDCs are used as a replacement of all individual components in the same doses taken separately, for reasons of improving convenience, reducing costs, and promoting adherence to therapy. However, evidence is increasingly emerging around the benefits of FDC therapy for the initial or early treatment of hypertension, compared to conventional approaches using monotherapy. Systematic reviews have shown greater BP lowering with initial dual combinations, even with each component at less-than-standard dose, compared with standard-dose monotherapy.[54] These benefits have been observed without evidence of an excess in withdrawal of drug therapy due to adverse effects. These findings have led to US and European guidelines recommending the consideration of FDCs as initial therapy for hypertension since 2017, and more definitive such recommendations by the World Health Organization guidelines in 2021.[11,14,55] No differential recommendations on the use of FDCs in people with T2DM is provided by any of these guidelines. Evidence has also emerged supporting the safety and efficacy of initial or early use of low-dose triple FDC therapy[56,57] and ultra-low-dose quadruple FDC therapy[58] compared to usual or standard care and monotherapy, respectively. In one of the trials evaluating triple FDC therapy, there was no evidence of heterogeneity by baseline diabetes status, while very few T2DM patients were included in the other triple therapy study or the study investigating quadruple FDC therapy. In a randomized trial comparing a novel low-dose formulation of telmisartan, amlodipine, and indapamide with each dual combination of component drugs, significant reductions in SBP were observed for each comparison, without an increase in treatment withdrawals with 3 months of follow-up.[59] While heterogeneity by diabetes status has not been systematically assessed, the additional BP-lowering effects of low-dose FDCs with three or four components compared to usual care, standard care, monotherapy, or dual therapy may be particularly relevant for achieving the lower BP goals often promulgated for people with T2DM.

NEW DRUG CLASSES

Two novel drug classes initially developed for hypoglycemic effects, sodium glucose cotransporter 2 (SGLT2) inhibitors and glucagon-like peptide 1 (GLP-1) receptor agonists, have entered the market over the last decade. In addition to blood glucose lowering, they have demonstrated important effects on blood pressure, body weight, and cardiovascular outcomes.[60–62]

The first SGLT2 inhibitor to be approved by the Food and Drug Administration in 2013 was canagliflozin, with several other drugs in the class now approved. In addition to reducing plasma glucose levels, these drugs reduce MI (fatal and nonfatal),[60] hospitalization for heart failure, MACE, adverse kidney events, and mortality in those with T2DM, as shown in several landmark cardiovascular and renal outcome trials.[63–66] Furthermore, SGLT2 inhibitors have demonstrated BP-lowering effects in those with T2DM. For example, a secondary analysis from the placebo-controlled CREDENCE trial (participants with T2DM and chronic kidney disease) identified a 3.5 mm Hg (95% CI, −4.27 to −2.72) reduction in systolic blood pressure with canagliflozin treatment, which was evident within 3 weeks and sustained throughout the trial. These BP-lowering effects were consistent, irrespective of baseline BP level and number of concomitant antihypertensive therapies (Fig 18 5).[67] This suggests that this drug class may be an important adjunct to traditional BP-lowering therapies in T2DM.

GLP-1 receptor agonists have been shown to reduce MACE as well as other important cardiovascular and mortality outcomes in those with T2DM. When looking specifically at CHD, a meta-analysis of eight cardiovascular outcome trials in T2DM demonstrated a 10% reduction in myocardial infarction (HR, 0.90; 95% CI, 0.83–0.98) with this drug class.[68] Further, these agents are associated with large reductions in body weight in both those with T2DM and those with obesity. For example, in the placebo-controlled STEP-2 trial, weekly semaglutide 2.4 mg in those with obesity and T2DM was associated with a 6.2% reduction in body weight after 68 weeks.[69] This drug class's BP-lowering effects are more modest, with chronic administration resulting in an average of 2.4 mm Hg reduction in SBP on meta-analysis.[70] Reflecting the clear and consistent reductions in atheroembolic events seen with GLP-1 receptor agonists, coupled with their effects on body weight, glucose control, and blood pressure, international guidelines and professional societies strongly recommend this drug class to reduced CV and CHD risk in high-risk individuals with T2DM.[68]

Subsequently, the dual GLP-1 and glucose-dependent insulinotropic polypeptide (GIP) receptor agonist tirzepatide has been developed for both glucose control and weight loss in those with obesity and T2DM. Studies have demonstrated impressive effects of tirzepatide on body weight and HbA1c with reductions in SBP also noted.[71] The impacts of this drug on CHD and broader CV outcomes are less well known with conflicting findings reported. A recent retrospective cohort analysis of almost 15,000 adults in the United States, however, suggests that tirzepatide as compared to the GLP-1 receptor agonist semaglutide was associated with a lower risk of the composite of MI and composite MACE.[72] Further prospective data are required, however, to better understand the effect of this drug on CHD outcomes in those with T2DM.

Finerenone is a novel, selective, nonsteroidal mineralocorticoid receptor agonist that has emerged as a new treatment option for those with T2DM and chronic kidney disease (CKD). The clinical benefits and safety of this drug were defined in the sister trials FIDELIO-DKD[73] (renal outcome trial) and FIGARO-DKD[74] (CV outcome trial) with a combined population of 13,026 patients with T2D and CKD, already taking an ACE or ARB, with no symptomatic heart failure with reduced ejection fraction. Key findings were that finerenone reduced CKD progression (kidney failure, sustained ≥40% decrease in eGFR from baseline, or renal death) by 23% (HR, 0.77; 95% CI, 0.67–0.88) and CV events (MACE or hospitalization for heart failure) by 14% (HR, 0.86; 95% CI, 0.78–0.95). A reduction in nonfatal MI was not identified (HR, 0.99; 95% CI, 0.76–1.31); however, it is important to note that the study was not powered to this secondary endpoint. This was coupled with an increase in hyperkalemia (18.3% finenerone vs. 9% placebo) but very few hyperkalemic events leading to hospitalization (1.4% vs. 0.3%) or permanent drug discontinuation and none leading to death. While there is an overall view that the clinical benefits of finerenone are largely mediated by downregulation of inflammatory and fibrotic pathways in the heart and kidneys, this drug does result in small reductions in systolic and diastolic blood pressure. In FIDELIO-DKD, the mean difference in the change in office SBP between finerenone and placebo groups over the course of the trial was −2.71 mm Hg (95% CI, −3.29 to −2.12). Mediation analysis suggests that approximately 14% of the primary kidney outcome and 13% of the secondary composite CV outcome could be explained by the observed changes in blood pressure.[75,76]

Aldosterone synthase inhibitors are relatively new agents for the management of treatment-resistant hypertension. The Phase 2 placebo-controlled trial of baxdrostat in 275 patients with treatment-resistant hypertension was recently reported, with the primary outcome of change in mean SBP over 12 weeks.[77] The patient population included 38% with T2DM. The trial was terminated early for efficacy, with baxdrostat associated with a dose-dependent reduction in the least-squares mean (±SE) SBP of −20.3 ± 2.1, −17.5 ± 2.0, and −12.1 ± 1.9 mm Hg at the 2-, 1-, and 0.5-mg doses, respectively. Additional analyses by T2DM status were not performed.[77] Similarly, early-phase trials of an RNA interference therapeutic agent targeting hepatic synthesis of angiotensinogen and zilebesiran have shown considerable promise for the treatment of uncontrolled hypertension but are yet to be assessed in populations with T2DM.[78]

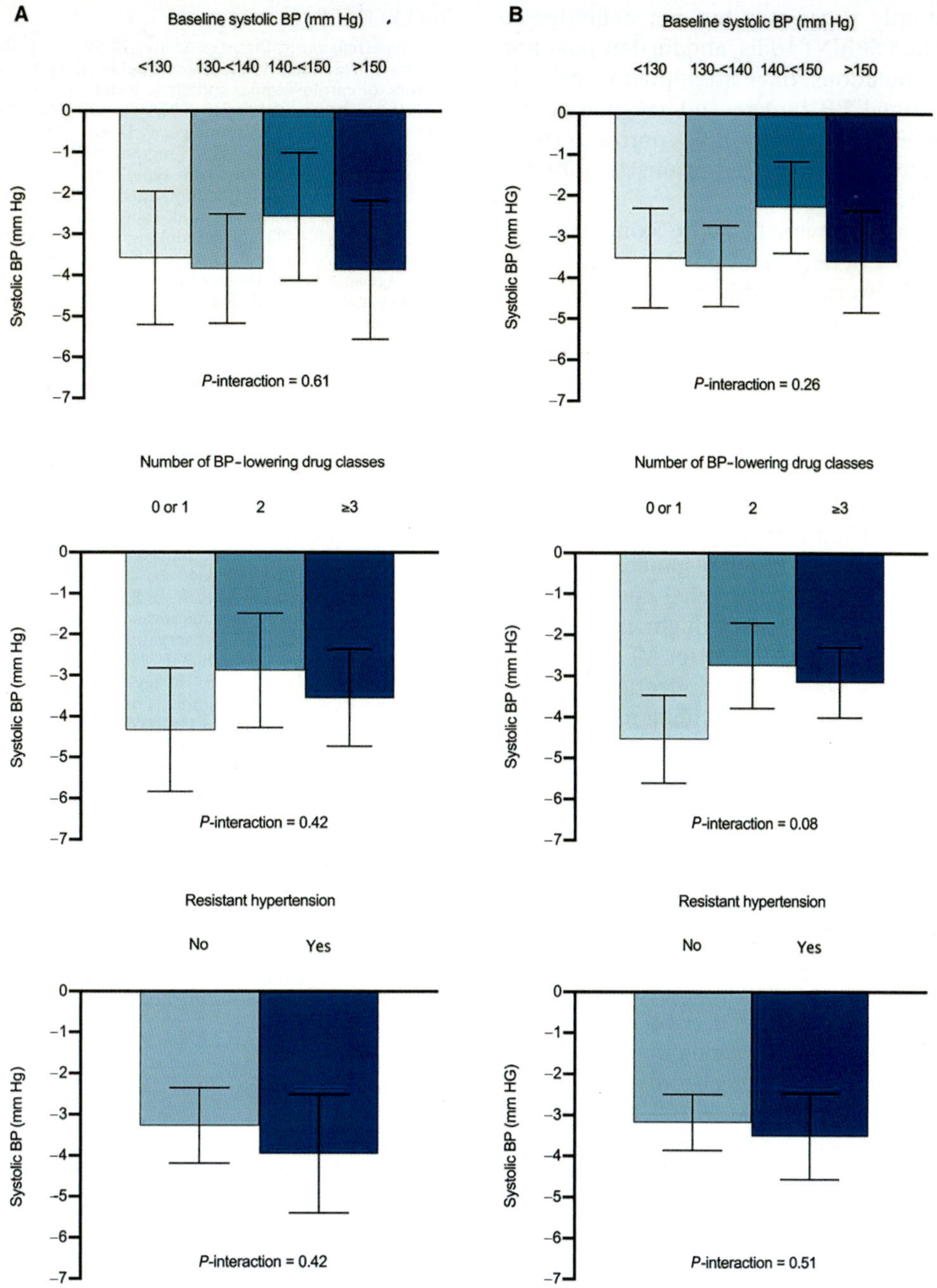

FIG. 18.5 Changes in systolic blood pressure (*SBP*) with canagliflozin versus placebo (A) from baseline to week 3 and (B) over the duration of the trial according to baseline SBP, number of classes of BP-lowering drug classes, and history of resistant hypertension. *BP*, Blood pressure. Reproduced from: Ye N, Jardine MJ, Oshima M, et al. Blood pressure effects of canagliflozin and clinical outcomes in type 2 diabetes and chronic kidney disease: insights from the CREDENCE trial. *Circulation*. 2021;143:1735–1749.

SUMMARY

Available evidence about the effect of BP management on CHD risk in patients with T2DM can be reasonably summarized in the following way.

Lifestyle interventions (targeting physical activity and dietary modification) in people with T2DM can favorably affect BP levels, and in the case of low-sodium/high-potassium salt substitute, clinical outcomes. However, effective implementation strategies to enact sustained positive changes are generally currently lacking.

Placebo-controlled trials provide clear evidence that BP lowering among individuals with diabetes and hypertension results in a reduction in CHD incidence. The findings of the largest of these trials suggest that routine provision of BP-lowering therapy to patients with T2DM, regardless of initial BP level, is an effective strategy for reducing CHD risk. Systematic reviews of BP-lowering trials suggest that relative risk reductions on CHD and other clinical outcomes may be less in people with diabetes compared to people without diabetes, although absolute risk reductions are similar. The variations in clinical effects of different BP-lowering classes of drugs in people with T2DM are likely to be modest, in the absence of other compelling indications for specific agents.

Specifically for the outcome of CHD, trial evidence of the benefits of more-intensive versus less-intensive BP lowering is consistently suggestive but not definitive to date. The ACCORD and SPRINT trials, and further post hoc analyses of these populations, have attempted to provide more clarity on optimal BP targets and taken together suggest a likely benefit for intensive SBP control in those with T2DM which should be balanced against a potential increase in adverse events.

These conclusions, however, must be considered in the context of a number of important points. First, recommendations about BP-lowering treatment should take into account the known or likely effects on all relevant health outcomes and not just CHD. For example, the evidence that more-intensive versus less-intensive BP lowering provides greater protection against stroke in patients with or without diabetes is unequivocal, including large beneficial effects in preventing stroke observed in the ACCORD trial. Similarly, calcium channel blocker or thiazide-based regimens may be more important for the prevention of stroke, whereas ACE inhibitor or ARB-based regimens are more protective against the microvascular renal complications of diabetes. The use of beta-blockers might be regarded as essential in certain patients with a prior MI and in individuals with heart failure with reduced ejection fraction. Thus consideration of a number of individual patient characteristics that may be relevant to a broad range of clinical outcomes is appropriate in making choices about the use of particular BP-lowering drug regimens in patients with T2DM.

Second, and related to this, is an understanding of the general paradigm of using an assessment of an individual's projected absolute risk of developing CHD (or stroke, or any CV disease) to help guide therapy. In the context of T2DM, this might be most relevant where uncertainty exists about the balance of potential risks and benefits in relation to the intensity of BP lowering in an individual patient. There are a number of clinical tools available to estimate CHD or CVD risk in people with T2DM, derived either from general populations or from specific populations with diabetes.[79] All have potential limitations and, given the heterogeneity of T2DM, contemporary models in more diverse populations are needed to better guide clinical practice.[80]

Finally, any ongoing uncertainty about the relative efficacy of therapeutic regimens or appropriate targets for BP reduction in people with T2DM closer to the "normotensive" range is dwarfed by the lack of knowledge about effective strategies to ensure that people with T2DM receive any BP-lowering therapy in the first place, let alone what might be considered ideal regimens or acceptable levels of BP control. The "practice gaps" are very large, particularly in the low- and middle-income countries that have the highest numbers of people with T2DM, but also in countries with richer economies.[81,82] From a global perspective, these issues will not be addressed by clinical trials establishing the efficacy of new drugs or new combinations of drugs. Rather, the development, implementation, and rigorous evaluation of interventions at the level of policy, systems, and services will be crucial to ensure maximal gains in human health from what we already know about the treatment of BP in people with T2DM.

REFERENCES

1. Hypertension in Diabetes Study (HDS): I. Prevalence of hypertension in newly presenting type 2 diabetic patients and the association with risk factors for cardiovascular and diabetic complications. *J Hypertens*. 1993;11(3): 309–317. https://doi.org/10.1097/00004872-199303000-00012.
2. Pechere-Bertschi A, Greminger P, Hess L, Philippe J, Ferrari P. Swiss Hypertension and Risk Factor Program (SHARP): cardiovascular risk factors management in patients with type 2 diabetes in Switzerland. *Blood Press*. 2005;14(6):337–344. https://doi.org/10.1080/08037050500340018.
3. Sun D, Zhou T, Heianza Y, et al. Type 2 diabetes and hypertension. *Circ Res*. 2019;124(6):930–937. https://doi.org/10.1161/CIRCRESAHA.118.314487.
4. Lewington S, Clarke R, Qizilbash N, Peto R, Collins R. Prospective Studies C. Age-specific relevance of usual blood pressure to vascular mortality: a meta-analysis of individual data for one million adults in 61 prospective studies. *Lancet*. 2002;360(9349):1903–1913. https://doi.org/10.1016/s0140-6736(02)11911-8.
5. Luo D, Cheng Y, Zhang H, et al. Association between high blood pressure and long term cardiovascular events in young adults: systematic review and meta-analysis. *BMJ*. 2020;370:m3222. https://doi.org/10.1136/bmj.m3222.
6. Asia Pacific Cohort Studies C, et al.Kengne AP, Patel A, et al. Systolic blood pressure, diabetes and the risk of cardiovascular diseases in the Asia-Pacific region. *J Hypertens*. 2007;25(6):1205–1213. https://doi.org/10.1097/HJH.0b013e3280dce59e.
7. Stamler J, Vaccaro O, Neaton JD, Wentworth D. Diabetes, other risk factors, and 12-yr cardiovascular mortality for men screened in the Multiple Risk Factor Intervention Trial. *Diabetes Care*. 1993;16(2):434–444. https://doi.org/10.2337/diacare.16.2.434.
8. Adler AI, Stratton IM, Neil HA, et al. Association of systolic blood pressure with macrovascular and microvascular complications of type 2 diabetes (UKPDS 36): prospective observational study. *BMJ*. 2000;321(7258):412–419. https://doi.org/10.1136/bmj.321.7258.412.
9. Kengne AP, Czernichow S, Huxley R, et al. Blood pressure variables and cardiovascular risk: new findings from ADVANCE. *Hypertension*. 2009;54(2): 399–404. https://doi.org/10.1161/HYPERTENSIONAHA.109.133041.
10. Cooper-DeHoff RM, Gong Y, Handberg EM, et al. Tight blood pressure control and cardiovascular outcomes among hypertensive patients with diabetes and coronary artery disease. *JAMA*. 2010;304(1):61–68. https://doi.org/10.1001/jama.2010.884.
11. Whelton PK, Carey RM, Aronow WS, et al. 2017 ACC/AHA/AAPA/ABC/ACPM/AGS/APhA/ASH/ASPC/NMA/PCNA Guideline for the Prevention, Detection, Evaluation, and Management of High Blood Pressure in Adults: A Report of the American College of Cardiology/American Heart Association Task Force on Clinical Practice Guidelines. *Hypertension*. 2018;71(6):e13–e115. https://doi.org/10.1161/HYP.0000000000000065.
12. Cosentino F, Grant PJ, Aboyans V, et al. 2019 ESC Guidelines on diabetes, pre-diabetes, and cardiovascular diseases developed in collaboration with the EASD. *Eur Heart J*. 2020;41(2):255–323. https://doi.org/10.1093/eurheartj/ehz486.
13. American Diabetes Association Professional Practice C 10. Cardiovascular disease and risk management: standards of medical care in diabetes-2022. *Diabetes Care*. 2022;45(Suppl 1):S144–S174. https://doi.org/10.2337/dc22-S010.
14. Williams B, Mancia G, Spiering W, et al. 2018 ESC/ESH Guidelines for the management of arterial hypertension. *Eur Heart J*. 2018;39(33):3021–3104. https://doi.org/10.1093/eurheartj/ehy339.
15. IDFGGfTDlu, 2005. Available from: https://wwwidforg/e-library/guidelines/79-global-guideline-for-type-2-diabetes.
16. Unger T, Borghi C, Charchar F, et al. 2020 International Society of Hypertension Global Hypertension Practice Guidelines. *Hypertension*. 2020;75(6):1334–1357. https://doi.org/10.1161/HYPERTENSIONAHA.120.15026.
17. Mancia G, Kreutz R, Brunstrom M, et al. 2023 ESH Guidelines for the management of arterial hypertension The Task Force for the management of arterial hypertension of the European Society of Hypertension: Endorsed by the International Society of Hypertension (ISH) and the European Renal Association (ERA). *J Hypertens*. 2023;41(12):1874–2071. https://doi.org/10.1097/HJH.0000000000003480.
18. Ryan DH, Espeland MA, Foster GD, et al. Look AHEAD (Action for Health in Diabetes): design and methods for a clinical trial of weight loss for the prevention of cardiovascular disease in type 2 diabetes. *Control Clin Trials*. 2003;24(5):610–628. https://doi.org/10.1016/s0197-2456(03)00064-3.
19. Look ARG, Wing RR, Bolin P, et al. Cardiovascular effects of intensive lifestyle intervention in type 2 diabetes. *N Engl J Med*. 2013;369(2):145–154. https://doi.org/10.1056/NEJMoa1212914.
20. Appel LJ, Moore TJ, Obarzanek E, et al. A clinical trial of the effects of dietary patterns on blood pressure. DASH Collaborative Research Group. *N Engl J Med*. 1997;336(16):1117–1124. https://doi.org/10.1056/NEJM199704173361601.
21. Sacks FM, Svetkey LP, Vollmer WM, et al. Effects on blood pressure of reduced dietary sodium and the Dietary Approaches to Stop Hypertension (DASH) diet. DASH-Sodium Collaborative Research Group. *N Engl J Med*. 2001;344(1):3–10. https://doi.org/10.1056/NEJM200101043440101.
22. Graudal NA, Hubeck-Graudal T, Jurgens G. Effects of low sodium diet versus high sodium diet on blood pressure, renin, aldosterone, catecholamines, cholesterol, and triglyceride. *Cochrane Database Syst Rev*. 2020;12:CD004022. https://doi.org/10.1002/14651858.CD004022.pub5.
23. Huang L, Trieu K, Yoshimura S, et al. Effect of dose and duration of reduction in dietary sodium on blood pressure levels: systematic review

and meta-analysis of randomised trials. *BMJ.* 2020;368:m315. https://doi.org/10.1136/bmj.m315.

24. Schlaich MP, Sobotka PA, Krum H, Lambert E, Esler MD. Renal sympathetic-nerve ablation for uncontrolled hypertension. *N Engl J Med.* 2009;361(9):932–934. https://doi.org/10.1056/NEJMc0904179.
25. Ogoyama Y, Tada K, Abe M, et al. Effects of renal denervation on blood pressures in patients with hypertension: a systematic review and meta-analysis of randomized sham-controlled trials. *Hypertens Res.* 2022;45(2):210–220. https://doi.org/10.1038/s41440-021-00761-8.
26. Townsend RR, Mahfoud F, Kandzari DE, et al. Catheter-based renal denervation in patients with uncontrolled hypertension in the absence of antihypertensive medications (SPYRAL HTN-OFF MED): a randomised, sham-controlled, proof-of-concept trial. *Lancet.* 2017;390(10108):2160–2170. https://doi.org/10.1016/S0140-6736(17)32281-X.
27. Symplicity HTNI, Esler MD, Krum H, et al. Renal sympathetic denervation in patients with treatment-resistant hypertension (The Symplicity HTN-2 Trial): a randomised controlled trial. *Lancet.* 2010;376(9756):1903–1909. https://doi.org/10.1016/S0140-6736(10)62039-9.
28. Bhatt, et al.Vaduganathan DL, Kandzari DE M, et al. Long-term outcomes after catheter-based renal artery denervation for resistant hypertension: final follow-up of the randomised SYMPLICITY HTN-3 Trial. *Lancet.* 2022;400(10361):1405–1416. https://doi.org/10.1016/S0140-6736(22)01787-1.
29. Kandzari DE, Townsend RR, Kario K, et al. Safety and efficacy of renal denervation in patients taking antihypertensive medications. *J Am Coll Cardiol.* 2023;82(19):1809–1823. https://doi.org/10.1016/j.jacc.2023.08.045.
30. Mahfoud F, Mancia G, Schmieder R, et al. Renal denervation in high-risk patients with hypertension. *J Am Coll Cardiol.* 2020;75(23):2879–2888. https://doi.org/10.1016/j.jacc.2020.04.036.
31. Turnbull F. Blood Pressure Lowering Treatment Trialists C Effects of different blood-pressure-lowering regimens on major cardiovascular events: results of prospectively-designed overviews of randomised trials. *Lancet.* 2003;362(9395):1527–1535. https://doi.org/10.1016/s0140-6736(03)14739-3.
32. Nazarzadeh M, Bidel Z, Canoy D, et al. Blood pressure-lowering treatment for prevention of major cardiovascular diseases in people with and without type 2 diabetes: an individual participant-level data meta-analysis. *Lancet Diabetes Endocrinol.* 2022;10(9):645–654. https://doi.org/10.1016/S2213-8587(22)00172-3.
33. Patel A, Group AC, MacMahon S, et al. Effects of a fixed combination of perindopril and indapamide on macrovascular and microvascular outcomes in patients with type 2 diabetes mellitus (the ADVANCE trial): a randomised controlled trial. *Lancet.* 2007;370(9590):829–840. https://doi.org/10.1016/S0140-6736(07)61303-8.
34. Zoungas S, de Galan BE, Ninomiya T, et al. Combined effects of routine blood pressure lowering and intensive glucose control on macrovascular and microvascular outcomes in patients with type 2 diabetes: new results from the ADVANCE trial. *Diabetes Care.* 2009;32(11):2068–2074. https://doi.org/10.2337/dc09-0959.
35. Dahlof B, Sever PS, Poulter NR, et al. Prevention of cardiovascular events with an antihypertensive regimen of amlodipine adding perindopril as required versus atenolol adding bendroflumethiazide as required, in the Anglo-Scandinavian Cardiac Outcomes Trial-Blood Pressure Lowering Arm (ASCOT-BPLA): a multicentre randomised controlled trial. *Lancet.* 2005;366(9489):895–906. https://doi.org/10.1016/S0140-6736(05)67185-1. Sep 10-16.
36. Yusuf S, Diener HC, Sacco RL, et al. Telmisartan to prevent recurrent stroke and cardiovascular events. *N Engl J Med.* 2008;359(12):1225–1237. https://doi.org/10.1056/NEJMoa0804593.
37. Jamerson K, Weber MA, Bakris GL, et al. Benazepril plus amlodipine or hydrochlorothiazide for hypertension in high-risk patients. *N Engl J Med.* 2008;359(23):2417–2428. https://doi.org/10.1056/NEJMoa0806182.
38. Jamerson KA, Devereux R, Bakris GL, et al. Efficacy and duration of benazepril plus amlodipine or hydrochlorothiazide on 24-hour ambulatory systolic blood pressure control. *Hypertension.* 2011;57(2):174–179. https://doi.org/10.1161/HYPERTENSIONAHA.110.159939.
39. Emdin CA, Rahimi K, Neal B, Callender T, Perkovic V, Patel A. Blood pressure lowering in type 2 diabetes: a systematic review and meta-analysis. *JAMA.* 2015;313(6):603–615. https://doi.org/10.1001/jama.2014.18574.
40. Bakris GL, Fonseca V, Katholi RE, et al. Metabolic effects of carvedilol vs metoprolol in patients with type 2 diabetes mellitus and hypertension: a randomized controlled trial. *JAMA.* 2004;292(18):2227–2236. https://doi.org/10.1001/jama.292.18.2227.
41. Brixius K, Middeke M, Lichtenthal A, Jahn E, Schwinger RH. Nitric oxide, erectile dysfunction and beta-blocker treatment (MR NOED study): benefit of nebivolol versus metoprolol in hypertensive men. *Clin Exp Pharmacol Physiol.* 2007;34(4):327–331. https://doi.org/10.1111/j.1440-1681.2007.04551.x.
42. Bell DS, Lukas MA, Holdbrook FK, Fowler MB. The effect of carvedilol on mortality risk in heart failure patients with diabetes: results of a meta-analysis. *Curr Med Res Opin.* 2006;22(2):287–296. https://doi.org/10.1185/030079906X80459.
43. Group PC. Randomised trial of a perindopril-based blood-pressure-lowering regimen among 6,105 individuals with previous stroke or transient ischaemic attack. *Lancet.* 2001;358(9287):1033–1041. https://doi.org/10.1016/S0140-6736(01)06178-5.
44. Blood Pressure Lowering Treatment Trialists C Pharmacological blood pressure lowering for primary and secondary prevention of cardiovascular disease across different levels of blood pressure: an individual participant-level data meta-analysis. *Lancet.* 2021;397(10285):1625–1636. https://doi.org/10.1016/S0140-6736(21)00590-0.
45. Group SR, Wright Jr. JT, Williamson JD, et al. A randomized trial of intensive versus standard blood-pressure control. *N Engl J Med.* 2015;373(22):2103–2116. https://doi.org/10.1056/NEJMoa1511939.
46. Group AS, Cushman WC, Evans GW, et al. Effects of intensive blood-pressure control in type 2 diabetes mellitus. *N Engl J Med.* 2010;362(17):1575–1585. https://doi.org/10.1056/NEJMoa1001286.
47. Gerstein HC, Miller ME, et al. Action to Control Cardiovascular Risk in Diabetes Study G Effects of intensive glucose lowering in type 2 diabetes. *N Engl J Med.* 2008;358(24):2545–2559. https://doi.org/10.1056/NEJMoa0802743.
48. Group AS, Ginsberg HN, Elam MB, et al. Effects of combination lipid therapy in type 2 diabetes mellitus. *N Engl J Med.* 2010;362(17):1563–1574. https://doi.org/10.1056/NEJMoa1001282.
49. Buckley LF, Dixon DL, Wohlford GFt, Wijesinghe DS, Baker WL, Van Tassell BW. Intensive versus standard blood pressure control in SPRINT-eligible participants of ACCORD-BP. *Diabetes Care.* 2017;40(12):1733–1738. https://doi.org/10.2337/dc17-1366.
50. Buckley LF, Dixon DL, Wohlford GFt, Wijesinghe DS, Baker WL, Van Tassell BW. Effect of intensive blood pressure control in patients with type 2 diabetes mellitus over 9 years of follow-up: a subgroup analysis of high-risk ACCORDION trial participants. *Diabetes Obes Metab.* 2018;20(6):1499–1502. https://doi.org/10.1111/dom.13248.
51. Holman RR, Paul SK, Bethel MA, Neil HA, Matthews DR. Long-term follow-up after tight control of blood pressure in type 2 diabetes. *N Engl J Med.* 2008;359(15):1565–1576. https://doi.org/10.1056/NEJMoa0806359.
52. Holman RR, Paul SK, Bethel MA, Matthews DR, Neil HA. 10-year follow-up of intensive glucose control in type 2 diabetes. *N Engl J Med.* 2008;359(15):1577–1589. https://doi.org/10.1056/NEJMoa0806470.
53. Zoungas S, Chalmers J, Neal B, et al. Follow-up of blood-pressure lowering and glucose control in type 2 diabetes. *N Engl J Med.* 2014;371(15):1392–1406. https://doi.org/10.1056/NEJMoa1407963.
54. Salam A, Kanukula R, Atkins E, et al. Efficacy and safety of dual combination therapy of blood pressure-lowering drugs as initial treatment for hypertension: a systematic review and meta-analysis of randomized controlled trials. *J Hypertens.* 2019;37(9):1768–1774. https://doi.org/10.1097/HJH.0000000000002096.
55. Organization WH. *Guideline for the pharmacological treatment of hypertension in adults: web annex A: summary of evidence.* World Health Organization; 2021.
56. Webster R, Salam A, de Silva HA, et al. Fixed Low-Dose Triple Combination Antihypertensive Medication vs Usual Care for Blood Pressure Control in Patients With Mild to Moderate Hypertension in Sri Lanka: A Randomized Clinical Trial. *JAMA.* 2018;320(6):566–579. https://doi.org/10.1001/jama.2018.10359.
57. Ojji DB, Salam A, Sani MU, et al. Low-dose triple-pill vs standard-care protocols for hypertension treatment in Nigeria: a randomized clinical trial. *JAMA.* 2024;332(13):1070–1079. https://doi.org/10.1001/jama.2024.18080.
58. Chow CK, Atkins ER, Hillis GS, et al. Initial treatment with a single pill containing quadruple combination of quarter doses of blood pressure medicines versus standard dose monotherapy in patients with hypertension (QUARTET): a phase 3, randomised, double-blind, active-controlled trial. *Lancet.* 2021;398(10305):1043–1052. https://doi.org/10.1016/S0140-6736(21)01922-X.
59. Rodgers A, Salam A, Schutte AE, et al. Efficacy and safety of a novel low-dose triple single-pill combination of telmisartan, amlodipine and indapamide, compared with dual combinations for treatment of hypertension: a randomised, double-blind, active-controlled, international clinical trial. *Lancet* (in press) 2024;404(10462):1536–1546. https://doi.org/10.1016/S0140-6736(24)01744-6.
60. Arnott C, Li Q, Kang A, et al. Sodium-glucose cotransporter 2 inhibition for the prevention of cardiovascular events in patients with type 2 diabetes mellitus: a systematic review and meta-analysis. *J Am Heart Assoc.* 2020;9(3):e014908. https://doi.org/10.1161/JAHA.119.014908.
61. Giugliano D, Scappaticcio L, Longo M, et al. GLP-1 receptor agonists and cardiorenal outcomes in type 2 diabetes: an updated meta-analysis of eight CVOTs. *Cardiovasc Diabetol.* 2021;20(1):189. https://doi.org/10.1186/s12933-021-01366-8.
62. Kristensen SL, Rorth R, Jhund PS, et al. Cardiovascular, mortality, and kidney outcomes with GLP-1 receptor agonists in patients with type 2 diabetes: a systematic review and meta-analysis of cardiovascular outcome trials. *Lancet Diabetes Endocrinol.* 2019 https://doi.org/10.1016/S2213-8587(19)30249-9.
63. Neal B, Perkovic V, Matthews DR. Canagliflozin and cardiovascular and renal events in type 2 diabetes. *N Engl J Med.* 2017;377(21):2099. https://doi.org/10.1056/NEJMc1712572.
64. Wiviott SD, Raz I, Bonaca MP, et al. Dapagliflozin and cardiovascular outcomes in type 2 diabetes. *N Engl J Med.* 2018 https://doi.org/10.1056/NEJMoa1812389.
65. Perkovic V, Jardine MJ, Neal B, et al. Canagliflozin and renal outcomes in type 2 diabetes and nephropathy. *N Engl J Med.* 2019 https://doi.org/10.1056/NEJMoa1811744.
66. Zinman B, Wanner C, Lachin JM, et al. Empagliflozin, cardiovascular outcomes, and mortality in type 2 diabetes. *N Engl J Med.* 2015;373(22):2117–2128. https://doi.org/10.1056/NEJMoa1504720.
67. Ye N, Jardine MJ, Oshima M, et al. Blood pressure effects of canagliflozin and clinical outcomes in type 2 diabetes and chronic kidney disease: insights from the CREDENCE trial. *Circulation.* 2021;143(18):1735–1749. https://doi.org/10.1161/CIRCULATIONAHA.120.048740.
68. Marx N, Husain M, Lehrke M, Verma S, Sattar N. GLP-1 receptor agonists for the reduction of atherosclerotic cardiovascular risk in patients with type 2 diabetes. *Circulation.* 2022;146(24):1882–1894. https://doi.org/10.1161/CIRCULATIONAHA.122.059595.

69. Davies M, Faerch L, Jeppesen OK, et al. Semaglutide 2.4 mg once a week in adults with overweight or obesity, and type 2 diabetes (STEP 2): a randomised, double-blind, double-dummy, placebo-controlled, phase 3 trial. *Lancet.* 2021;397(10278):971–984. https://doi.org/10.1016/S0140-6736(21)00213-0.
70. Abd El Aziz MS, Kahle M, Meier JJ, Nauck MA. A meta-analysis comparing clinical effects of short- or long-acting GLP-1 receptor agonists versus insulin treatment from head-to-head studies in type 2 diabetic patients. *Diabetes Obes Metab.* 2017;19(2):216–227. https://doi.org/10.1111/dom.12804.
71. Frias JP, Davies MJ, Rosenstock J, et al. Tirzepatide versus semaglutide once weekly in patients with type 2 diabetes. *N Engl J Med.* 2021;385(6):503–515. https://doi.org/10.1056/NEJMoa2107519.
72. Chuang MH, Chen JY, Wang HY, Jiang ZH, Wu VC. Clinical outcomes of tirzepatide or GLP-1 receptor agonists in individuals with type 2 diabetes. *JAMA Netw Open.* 2024;7(8):e2427258. https://doi.org/10.1001/jamanetworkopen.2024.27258.
73. Bakris GL, Agarwal R, Anker SD, et al. Effect of finerenone on chronic kidney disease outcomes in type 2 diabetes. *N Engl J Med.* 2020;383(23):2219–2229. https://doi.org/10.1056/NEJMoa2025845.
74. Pitt B, Filippatos G, Agarwal R, et al. Cardiovascular events with finerenone in kidney disease and type 2 diabetes. *N Engl J Med.* 2021;385(24):2252–2263. https://doi.org/10.1056/NEJMoa2110956.
75. Ruilope LM, Agarwal R, Anker SD, et al. Blood pressure and cardiorenal outcomes with finerenone in chronic kidney disease in type 2 diabetes. *Hypertension.* 2022;79(12):2685–2695. https://doi.org/10.1161/HYPERTENSIONAHA.122.19744.
76. Georgianos PI, Kourtidou C, Divani M, Liakopoulos V. BP-lowering effects of SGLT-2 inhibitors and finerenone: an indirect comparison in patients with chronic kidney disease and type 2 diabetes. *Expert Opin Pharmacother.* 2024;25(2):127–130. https://doi.org/10.1080/14656566.2024.2322527.
77. Freeman MW, Halvorsen YD, Marshall W, et al. Phase 2 trial of baxdrostat for treatment-resistant hypertension. *N Engl J Med.* 2023;388(5):395–405. https://doi.org/10.1056/NEJMoa2213169.
78. Bakris GL, Saxena M, Gupta A, et al. RNA interference with zilebesiran for mild to moderate hypertension: the KARDIA-1 randomized clinical trial. *JAMA.* Mar 5 2024;331(9):740–749. https://doi.org/10.1001/jama.2024.0728.
79. Dziopa K, Asselbergs FW, Gratton J, Chaturvedi N, Schmidt AF. Cardiovascular risk prediction in type 2 diabetes: a comparison of 22 risk scores in primary care settings. *Diabetologia.* 2022;65(4):644–656. https://doi.org/10.1007/s00125-021-05640-y.
80. Pylypchuk R, Wells S, Kerr A, et al. Cardiovascular risk prediction in type 2 diabetes before and after widespread screening: a derivation and validation study. *Lancet.* 2021;397(10291):2264–2274. https://doi.org/10.1016/S0140-6736(21)00572-9.
81. Khunti K, Ceriello A, Cos X, De Block C. Achievement of guideline targets for blood pressure, lipid, and glycaemic control in type 2 diabetes: a meta-analysis. *Diabetes Res Clin Pract.* 2018;137:137–148. https://doi.org/10.1016/j.diabres.2017.12.004.
82. Flood D, Seiglie JA, Dunn M, et al. The state of diabetes treatment coverage in 55 low-income and middle-income countries: a cross-sectional study of nationally representative, individual-level data in 680 102 adults. *Lancet Healthy Longev.* 2021;2(6):e340–e351. https://doi.org/10.1016/s2666-7568(21)00089-1.

19 Effect of Lipid Management on Coronary Heart Disease Risk in Persons With Type 2 Diabetes

JULIA BRANDTS AND KAUSIK K. RAY

INTRODUCTION

The fundamental principles of lipid management in the prevention of cardiovascular events are as follows: firstly, apolipoprotein B100 (apoB)-carrying lipoproteins are causal for atherosclerosis, and secondly, their effect is cumulative. The former means reducing any apoB100-carrying lipoproteins decreases the risk of atherosclerotic cardiovascular disease (ASCVD). The latter is quantified by a log-linear relationship between risk reduction and the absolute magnitude of lipid lowering. The latter is, in turn, determined by both the treatment intensity (potency) and the timing of treatment, equally influencing the achieved risk reduction. These principles are often abridged to "the lower, the better," but our current understanding of lifetime trajectories of risk has evolved, and the implications of the "cumulative exposure" hypothesis go far beyond this simple paradigm.

The relative risk of a CV event is decreased by a fifth for every 1 mmol/L (38.67 mg/dL) LDL-C reduction independent of the approach used and the population studied.[1] Apparent differences in relative benefits between cardiovascular outcome trials of statins, ezetimibe, and proprotein convertase subtilisin/kexin type 9 (PCSK9) inhibitors result from the difference in achieved absolute LDL-C reductions and duration of treatment. Differences in absolute benefit derive from differences in the baseline risk of the study population and the absolute reductions in LDL-C between trials. For instance, similar absolute LDL-C reductions translate into higher rates of avoided CV events and lower numbers needed to treat in individuals with high baseline risk compared with low-risk individuals. Therefore lipid management may effectively compensate for part of the excess risk evoked by the atherogenic metabolic alterations defining and accompanying type 2 diabetes mellitus (T2DM) if adequate absolute LDL-C reductions are achieved. Hence, the use of high-intensity treatment regimens (rather than high-intensity statins) is desirable to mitigate the risk of CV events and keep the vascular system healthy in these high-risk individuals.

As cardiovascular risk reduction is agnostic to how LDL-C is lowered, adjunct therapies like ezetimibe, bempedoic acid, and PCSK9-targeting medications may be added to the first-line statin treatment to achieve the desirable LDL-C reduction to offset (in part) the excess absolute risk. Although escalation of treatment intensity might be limited by tolerability, accessibility, or costs, an alternative approach is to consider starting lipid-lowering therapy earlier. This approach, based on genetic, observational, and trial data, posits that a small reduction in LDL-C over a long time horizon and started earlier in life where atherosclerosis is less advanced produces similar relative benefits as a larger absolute reduction maintained over a shorter time interval. Hence an early, modest reduction approach would be as effective as a late, more-intensive approach.

However, in clinical practice, the lifetime risk is difficult to predict, and the adverse impact of T2DM is often underestimated. Risk is heterogeneous in those with diabetes, so it is now considered, for instance, by European Society of Cardiology (ESC) guidelines at least a moderate to very-high-risk state rather than a very-high-risk state in the short term. That said, the lifetime risk is considerable as diabetes is often progressive in its pathophysiological sequelae. Moreover, diabetic metabolic alterations may cause the occurrence of mixed dyslipidaemia, in which the routinely used lipid parameter of atherogenic risk, LDL-C, becomes a less reliable surrogate for atherogenic apoB-carrying lipoproteins and risk of ASCVD events. Thus treatment initiation is often delayed and intensity not adequate, resulting in progression of atherosclerosis and its clinical manifestation, which in turn necessitates even greater intensification of treatment.

In the following, we will discuss the nature of diabetic dyslipidemia and its implications on recommended treatment goals and targets, followed by a summary of available therapies and a discussion of treatment strategies.

DIABETIC DYSLIPIDEMIA

The form of dyslipidemia that occurs in persons with T2DM is comparable to the changes that characterize the metabolic syndrome or can be present in persons with obesity and insulin resistance. Diabetic dyslipidemia or mixed dyslipidemia is characterized by increased triglycerides, decreased HDL cholesterol (HDL-C), a high non-HDL-C, and higher apoB, while LDL-C mass is normal or only slightly increased in the setting of a shift to small, dense LDL-C particles, and therefore for any level of LDL-C, there is a greater concentration of apoB particles.

Pathophysiology

The development of mixed dyslipidemia in insulin resistance results from different dysregulated mechanisms in adipose tissue, muscle, liver, and intestine (see also Chapters 2, 4, and 7). The starting point is often a long-term positive net energy balance of the body, leading to exhaustion of the physiological energy storage capacities, especially those of the white adipose tissue. According to the overflow hypothesis, this causes ectopic fat deposition and increased circulating free fatty acids (FFA).

Due to peripheral insulin resistance, lipolysis in adipose tissue is no longer sufficiently inhibited, which leads to a further increase in circulating FFAs.

The characteristic hypertriglyceridemia is an expression of increased triglyceride-rich lipoprotein (TRL) production[2] and decreased TRL degradation (Figure 19.1).[3] TRLs include chylomicrons, very-low-density lipoprotein (VLDL) particles, intermediate-density lipoprotein particles, and their remnants.[4]

FFAs, hepatic insulin resistance, and compensatory hyperinsulinemia inhibit apoB degradation[5] and promote de novo lipid synthesis through increased expression of Carbohydrate-Responsive Element-Binding Protein (ChREBP) and SREBP-1c. This induces the formation of TRL, predominantly the larger VLDL1 particles. Their TG content is particularly high.[6] The occurrence of elevated VLDL1 levels can even be considered a predictor for the development of T2DM.[6]

Enhanced activity of cholesteryl ester transfer protein (CETP) facilitates the enrichment of VLDL with cholesteryl esters from LDL and HDL particles in exchange for TG. Following hepatic lipase–mediated TG removal, secreted HDL and LDL particles are small and dense, the former becoming less atheroprotective and the latter more atherogenic.

Accelerated Atherogenesis Through Mixed Dyslipidemia

TRLs are atherogenic by penetrating the vessel wall, and thus, analogous to LDL, cholesterol can accumulate in the intima, promoting the formation of foam cells and, ultimately, atherosclerosis.[7] A major difference from LDL, which must be oxidized before it can enter the vessel wall, is that the remnants can be taken up without prior modification.[8] In addition, remnant particles are larger than LDL and transport 20 to 40 times as much cholesterol, possibly making them even more atherogenic than LDL.[9]

HDL cholesterol is not only reduced but also limited in its function of cholesterol efflux. This is partly explained by the reduced expression of ABCA1, a membranous transporter of reverse cholesterol transport,[10] and its glycosylation, which reduces its activity.[11]

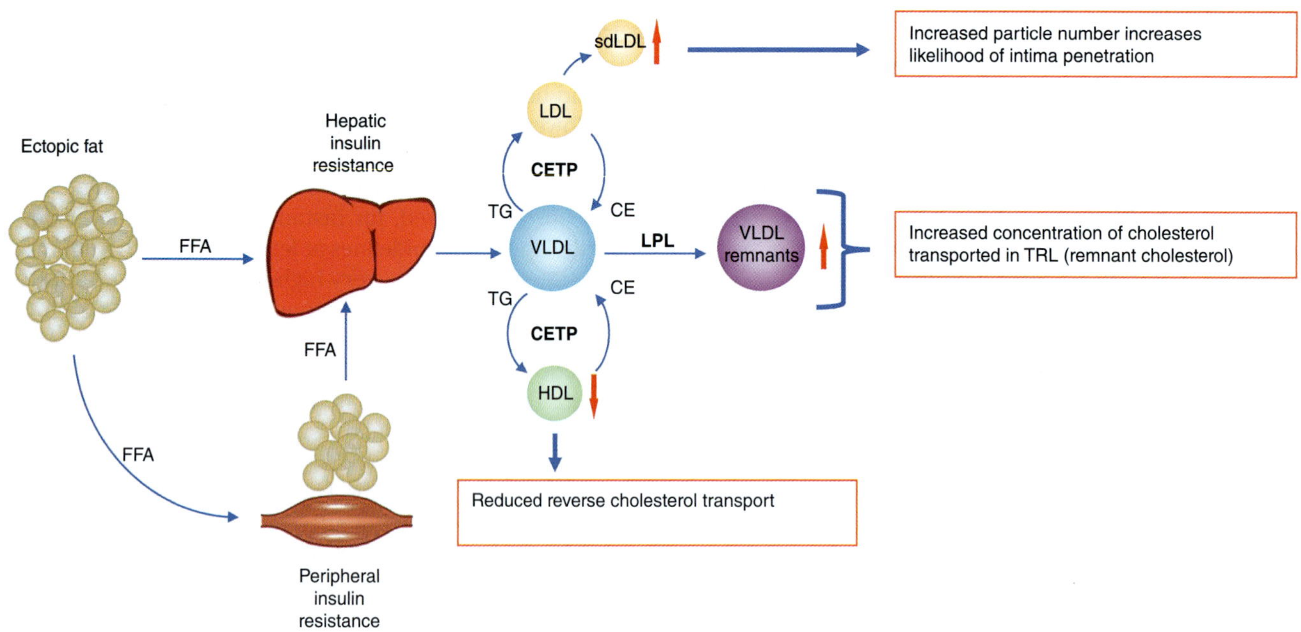

FIG. 19.1 Development of atherogenic dyslipidemia in insulin resistance. *CE*, Cholesteryl ester; *CETP*, cholesteryl ester transfer protein; *FFA*, free fatty acids; *HDL*, high-density lipoprotein; *LPL*, lipoprotein lipase; *sdLDL*, small dense low-density lipoprotein; *TG*, triglycerides; *TRL*, triglyceride-rich lipoprotein; *VLDL*, very low-density lipoprotein. Adjusted from Häring HU, Gallwitz B, Müller-Wieland D, et al. *Diabetologie in Klinik und Praxis*. Thieme Verlag; 2011; Gouni-Berthold I, Merkel M, Müller-Wieland D, Krone W. *Kapitel 28 Diabetische Dyslipidämie*.

Insulin resistance–induced changes include markedly reduced LDL particle catabolism. At least partly responsible for this is a reduced number of LDL B/E surface receptors in the cells.[12] In addition, increased glycosylation of LDL leads to a reduced affinity to its receptor. As a result, the individual LDL lipoprotein particles remain in the serum longer, increasing the likelihood of deposition in the vessel wall. The increased presence of sdLDL is associated with increased cardiovascular risk and atherosclerotic progression.[13] The particles are more likely to be glycosylated and oxidized and show an increased affinity for proteoglycans of the intima, leading to facilitated penetration of the arterial wall.[14] Glycosylated LDL particles are additionally preferentially taken up by macrophages, contributing to foam cell formation.

Atherogenic Lipid Burden and Lipid Treatment Targets in Type 2 Diabetes

The cholesterol in TRL is also called remnant cholesterol (RC) and is an independent cardiovascular risk factor that explains part of the residual risk seen in individuals with T2DM and mixed dyslipidemia. The RC subfraction increases with rising TG levels, while LDL-C remains roughly unaltered (Figure 19.2).[15] If not measured directly, RC is calculated as the difference of total cholesterol (TC) minus LDL-C and HDL-C (Figure 19.3) or in line with the Friedewald formula by TG(mg/dL)/5. The latter should not be applied if TG > 400 mg/dL. Therefore to omit analytical errors and account for all cholesterol transported in atherogenic, apoB-carrying lipoproteins, guidelines recommend using non-HDL-C, which can be simply calculated by subtracting HDL-C from TC, instead of LDL-C as the treatment target.

Different organizations have established LDL-C and non-HDL-C targets for persons with T2DM to manage cardiovascular risk effectively.

The 2022 ADA guidelines recommend primary prevention with statin therapy for persons with diabetes aged 40 and older.[16] For those under 40, statins are recommended if diabetes-specific risk enhancers are present, such as long duration of diabetes, albuminuria, reduced eGFR, retinopathy, neuropathy, or low ABI, with decisions made through shared decision-making.

The American Association of Clinical Endocrinology guidelines classify persons with T2DM into high, very high, or extreme ASCVD–risk categories.[17] Extreme-risk individuals should achieve LDL-C < 55 mg/dL, non-HDL-C < 80 mg/dL, and apoB < 70 mg/dL. Very-high-risk individuals, including those with diabetes or stage 3 or 4 CKD with one or more risk factors, should aim for LDL-C < 70 mg/dL, non-HDL-C < 100 mg/dL, and apoB < 80 mg/dL.

The 2019 ESC/EAS guidelines categorized individuals with diabetes into moderate, high, or very high risk based on age, diabetes duration, target organ damage, and ASCVD risk factors.[18] For very-high-risk individuals, an LDL-C goal of < 55 mg/dL and a secondary non-HDL-C goal < 85 mg/dL was recommended. The 2023 ESC CVD and diabetes guidelines also set an LDL-C goal of < 55 mg/dL for persons with ASCVD or severe target organ damage and for those with a 10-year CVD risk ≥20% using SCORE2-Diabetes.[19]

Asian Indian people with T2DM are considered to present unique dyslipidemia and ASCVD risk features.[20] Therefore the Lipid Association of India proposed updated risk stratification recommendations and LDL-C treatment goals as low as 30 mg/dL in those at especially high risk.[21] Risk stratification is based on major ASCVD risk factors like age, family history of premature ASCVD, smoking, hypertension, and low HDL-C but also nonconventional ASCVD risk factors such as coronary artery calcium score, CIMT, Lp(a), fasting glucose, waist circumference, and hsCRP. LDL-C is the primary target, with non-HDL-C as a coprimary target. Persons with diabetes are categorized into low, moderate, high, very high, and extreme risk, each with progressively aggressive LDL-C and non-HDL-C goals. For those without ASCVD and no target organ damage or ≤1 risk factor, an LDL-C goal of < 70 mg/dL is recommended. Persons without ASCVD but with target organ damage or ≥2 risk factors are categorized as very high risk with an LDL-C goal of < 50 mg/dL. People with ASCVD and zero to one other major ASCVD risk factor, without target organ damage, are classified as extreme-risk category A, while those with ≥2 major ASCVD risk factors or target organ damage fall under extreme-risk category B, with an LDL-C goal of < 30 mg/dL.

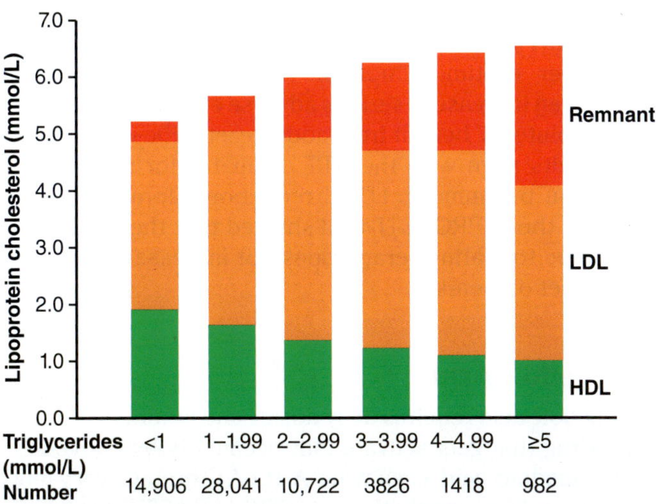

FIG. 19.2 Lipoprotein cholesterol as a function of increasing levels of nonfasting triglycerides. *HDL*, High-density lipoprotein; *LDL*, low-density lipoprotein. From Varbo A, Benn M, Tybjærg-Hansen A, et al. Remnant cholesterol as a causal risk factor for ischemic heart disease. *J Am Coll Cardiol*. 2013;61(4):427–436.

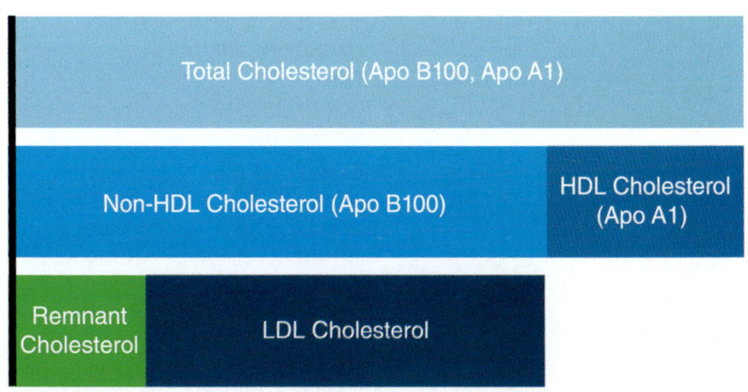

FIG. 19.3 Composition of the different cholesterol-carrying lipoprotein subgroups and their relationship to each other in a fasting blood sample. *Apo*, Apolipoprotein; *HDL*, high-density lipoprotein; *non-HDL*, non-high-density lipoprotein; *LDL*, low-density lipoprotein; *VLDL*, very-low-density lipoprotein.

LIPID-LOWERING AGENTS

Statins

Statins are the first-line pharmacological treatment in persons with T2DM to benefit from LDL-C lowering. Statins inhibit the HMG-Co reductase, a key enzyme in the cholesterol synthesis pathway. The decrease of intracytosolic cholesterol leads to compensatory LDL-R upregulation and consequently enhanced LDL-C and RC clearance. Several statins, differing in intensity and tolerability, are available (Table 19.1).

CTT meta-analysis, including almost 20,000 individuals with diabetes, showed a similar 21% reduction of major adverse cardiovascular events (cardiovascular death/MI/stroke; MACE) per mmol/L (38.67 mg/dL) LDL-C as in persons without diabetes.[23] However, the absolute risk reduction is significantly greater in persons with diabetes because of their higher baseline risk. In persons with diabetes, every mmol/L LDL-C reduction maintained over 5 years among 1000 persons would avoid 42 MACE, ranging from 36 in those without CHD to 57 in those with CHD. For comparison, among persons without diabetes and a previous MI, the same treatment would avoid 25 MACE and 48 in those with a previous MI.[1,24] The Treating to New Targets (TNT) trial compared moderate-intensity (atorvastatin 10 mg) versus high-intensity statin (atorvastatin 80 mg) treatment. In consideration of diabetic dyslipidemia, post hoc analysis explored the association of RC with CV event rates and modification through lipid lowering.[25] It demonstrated a greater CV benefit with larger RC reduction, independent of the achieved LDL-C reduction.

Despite being mostly well tolerated and considered safe, the use of statins is limited in some individuals because of real or perceived adverse effects, primarily muscle-related symptoms, ranging from myalgia with or without elevation of muscle enzymes (creatine kinase) to, rarely, rhabdomyolysis. A meta-analysis including 19 randomized placebo-controlled statin trials with a median follow-up of 4.3 years estimated a slight increase of 7% excess risk for muscle pain and weakness during the first year of statin treatment and no increase in the following years.[26] Moreover, the data suggest that only 1 in 15 reports of muscle symptoms would be causally attributable to statins. However, the inability to tolerate statins often necessitates either dose reduction or drug discontinuation, meaning that people achieve insufficient reductions in LDL-C and RC for their level of risk.

TABLE 19.1 Overview of Statins by Intensity and LDL-C Lowering Capacity

	HIGH INTENSITY	MODERATE INTENSITY	LOW INTENSITY
LDL-C[a] Lowering	≥50%	30%–49%	<30%
	Atorvastatin (40 mg) 80 mg Rosuvastatin 20 mg (40 mg)	Atorvastatin 10 mg (20 mg) Rosuvastatin (5 mg) 10 mg Simvastatin 20–40 mg	Simvastatin 10 mg
		Pravastatin 40 mg (80 mg) Lovastatin 40 mg (80 mg) Fluvastatin XL 80 mg Fluvastatin 40 mg twice daily Pitavastatin 1–4 mg	Pravastatin 10–20 mg Lovastatin 20 mg Fluvastatin 20–40 mg

[a]Reductions with the primary statin medications (atorvastatin, rosuvastatin, simvastatin) estimated using median reduction from the VOYAGER database; for other statin medications (fluvastatin, lovastatin, pitavastatin, pravastatin) identified according to FDA-approved product labeling in adults with hyperlipidemia, primary hypercholesterolemia, and mixed dyslipidemia.[22]

Furthermore, concerns regarding the use of statins and incident T2DM arose from meta-analyses, where statin therapy and its intensity were associated with a 9% to 12% increase in risk for new-onset T2DM.[27–29] However, compared with the gained CV event reduction through lipid lowering by statins, the overall benefit outweighs the harm. Therefore recommendations for the use of statins in those with sufficiently elevated cardiovascular risk remained unchanged.

Ezetimibe

Second-line treatment is the addition of ezetimibe, available as a generic. Ezetimibe, an inhibitor of intestinal cholesterol absorption, binds to the Niemann-Pick C1-like 1 (NPC1L1)-cholesterol complex and prevents its endocytosis by the enterocyte. This decreases intestinal cholesterol uptake by 54% and consequently circulating LDL-C levels by 18% to 20%.[30,31] Ezetimibe monotherapy is known to produce average LDL-C reductions of between 20% and 25%.

In the Improved Reduction of Outcomes: Vytorin Efficacy International Trial (IMPROVE-IT), lowering LDL-C through ezetimibe as an add-on to statins has been shown to reduce cardiovascular events by 6%, proportional to the absolute reduction in LDL-C of 17 mg/dL in those treated with the combination of ezetimibe with simvastatin compared with simvastatin alone.[32] On-treatment LDL-C levels were 55 mg/dL in the combination treatment group and 70 mg/dL in the simvastatin group. Among enrolled participants, 27% had concomitant diabetes, and subgroup analysis suggested a more pronounced cardiovascular benefit in these individuals with a 14% lower risk of MACE during the mean 4 years of follow-up.

Neither ezetimibe nor the further LDL-C reduction showed an increase in serious adverse events. Even though the absolute CV benefit from added ezetimibe was modest, the results align with the CTT estimates for relative risk reduction per mmol/L LDL-C reduction. Moreover, analysis from the IMPROVE-IT trial showed that the addition of ezetimibe to statin therapy does not increase the risk for new-onset diabetes.[23]

Bempedoic Acid

Bempedoic acid requires daily dosing and is administered as a prodrug that gets activated intracellularly by conversion to bempedoic acid coenzyme A (CoA) through very-long-chain acetyl-CoA synthetase-1 (ACSVL1).[33] ACSVL1 is mainly expressed in the liver and in smaller amounts in the kidney but not muscle. Therefore bempedoic acid can act with a high organ specificity. The active form, bempedoic acid-CoA thioester, acts similarly to statins in the cholesterol biosynthesis pathway. The target enzyme of empedoic acid is adenosine triphosphate-citrate lyase (ACL), which acts two steps upstream of the statin target HMG-CoA reductase. ACL converts citrate and CoA to oxaloacetate and acetyl-CoA, the substrate for fatty acid and cholesterol synthesis. Hence, inhibition of ACL by bempedoic acid decreases the cytosolic cholesterol concentration, which activates the sterol recognition element binding protein (SREBP) pathway leading to increased expression of LDL receptors (LDL-R).

Furthermore, bempedoic acid increases AMPK activity, presumably by an allosteric mechanism. AMPK activation leads to the downregulation of gluconeogenesis and acutely inhibits fatty acid and cholesterol synthesis.[34] Moreover, decreased AMPK activity is associated with insulin resistance. However, in vivo studies have shown that the primary pathway contributing to LDL-C and atherosclerosis reduction is ACL inhibition.[33]

Bempedoic acid 180 mg daily given orally reduces LDL-C by 18.1% in addition to statin background therapy[35] and by 24.5% in the absence of a statin background therapy.[36] Interestingly, a phase 2 study suggested a modestly greater treatment effect in persons with T2DM. In individuals with T2DM and elevated LDL-C after discontinuing all antihyperglycemic and lipid-lowering therapy for 6 weeks, 120 mg bempedoic acid monotherapy reduced LDL-C levels by 43% after 4 weeks of treatment, compared with 4% in the placebo group.[37] In contrast, pooled data from phase 3 trials showed no interaction of LDL-C reductions achieved with bempedoic acid with the baseline glycemic status.[38] Mean LDL-C and non-HDL-C reductions in persons with diabetes were 19.2% and 13.5% when bempedoic acid was added to a statin background therapy and 19.1% and 15.4%, respectively, in statin-intolerant individuals.

The CLEAR Outcomes trial evaluated the effect of bempedoic acid effect on cardiovascular events in 13,970 participants with established or high risk of CVD and a history of statin intolerance with a median follow-up duration of 40.6 months.[39] Bempedoic acid lowered LDL cholesterol levels by 21.1% compared to placebo and reduced the incidence of primary major adverse cardiovascular events by 11.7% versus 13.3% in the placebo group (hazard ratio, 0.87; 95% Confidence Interval, 0.79–0.96; $P = 0.004$). These results are consistent with the expected MACE reduction predicted per mmol/L LDL-C reduction by the Cholesterol Treatment Trialists' (CTT) meta-analysis.[23] However, bempedoic acid was associated with higher incidences of gout, cholelithiasis, and slight increases in serum creatinine, uric acid, and hepatic enzymes.[39]

So far, bempedoic acid has been shown to be safe and well tolerated.[35] A modest increase in uric acid and a more frequent occurrence of gout (1.2% vs. 0.3%) were found in the bempedoic acid treatment group compared with the placebo group. Even though bempedoic acid acts on the same pathway as statins, there was no observed increase in the occurrence of muscle-related symptoms or creatine kinase compared with the placebo, irrespective of whether participants had a history of statin intolerance or not. Bempedoic acid's good tolerability with respect to muscle symptoms may be attributed to the absence of the activating enzyme ACSVL1 in myocytes.

Further exploration of pooled phase 3 study safety data found no worsening or increased rates of new-onset T2DM for bempedoic acid compared with placebo.[38] Instead, rates of progression from prediabetes to T2DM were numerically lower in the bempedoic acid arm with 4.5% compared with the placebo arm with 5.9%. The plausibility of a protective effect of bempedoic acid might be supported through its AMPK-activating capability. Therefore, further exploration of bempedoic acid's effect in individuals with T2D and prediabetes may be worthwhile.

Proprotein Convertase Subtilisin/Kexin Type 9–Targeting Therapies

MONOCLONAL ANTIBODIES AGAINST PROPROTEIN CONVERTASE SUBTILISIN/KEXIN TYPE 9—ALIROCUMAB AND EVOLOCUMAB

Monoclonal antibodies (mAbs) bind to circulating PCSK9 and hinder it sterically from forming a complex with the LDL-R and LDL particles. Thereby the PCSK9-induced lysosomal degradation of the LDL-R is inhibited, and instead, LDL-Rs are recycled to cells' surfaces (Figure 19.4). Hence, PCSK9-targeting medications facilitate LDL-C clearance through increased longevity of the LDL-R.

mAbs against PCSK9 are applied subcutaneously (SC) by patients every 2 to 4 weeks. Alirocumab is available at doses of 75 and 150 mg every 2 weeks and reduces LDL-C by approximately 59.6% and 69.1%, respectively. Evolocumab is available at doses of 140 mg SC every 2 weeks or 420 mg monthly and lowers LDL-C by 63% to 75%.

Lowering LDL-C, using mAbs targeting PCSK9, has been shown to reduce cardiovascular events in two CV outcomes trials; the ODYSSEY OUTCOMES trial, assessing

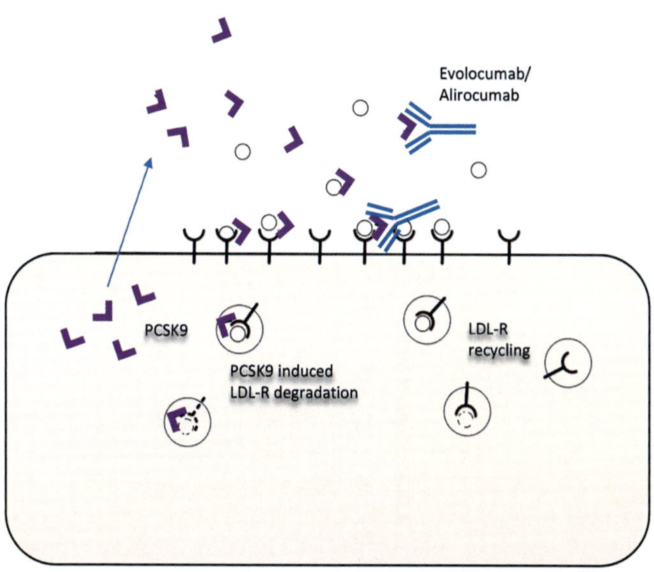

FIG. 19.4 Mechanism of action of monoclonal antibodies targeting PCSK9. Monoclonal antibodies (*mAbs*) bind to the circulating PCSK9 and hinder it sterically from forming a complex with the LDL-R and LDL particles. This inhibition prevents PCSK9-induced lysosomal degradation of the LDL-R, allowing LDL-Rs to be recycled to the cell surface. Consequently, PCSK9-targeting medications facilitate LDL-C clearance through increased longevity of the LDL-R, enhancing the removal of LDL cholesterol from the bloodstream. *LDL-C*, Low-density lipoprotein cholesterol; *LDL-R*, low-density lipoprotein receptor; *PCSK9*, proprotein convertase subtilisin/kexin type 9.

alirocumab, and the Further Cardiovascular Outcomes Research with PCSK9 (FOURIER) trial, assessing evolocumab.[40,41] These benefits were proportional to absolute reductions in LDL-C and duration of exposure.

In ODYSSEY OUTCOMES and FOURIER, 28.8% and 40% of participants had diabetes, respectively. In both studies, the achieved percentage LDL-C lowering and relative risk reductions were similar for persons with and without diabetes. However, the absolute risk reduction for MACE was about twofold higher with alirocumab in persons with diabetes compared with those without diabetes. Correspondingly, based on the results from FOURIER, 37 individuals with diabetes would need to be treated with evolocumab for 3 years, versus 62 of those without, to prevent a major cardiovascular event. The FOURIER-OLE extension study, involving 6635 participants, extended follow-up to a median of 5 years and up to 8.4 years of evolocumab exposure. At 12 weeks, the median LDL-C was 30 mg/dL, with 63.2% of persons achieving LDL-C < 40 mg/dL on evolocumab (Figure 19.5).[42] Long-term use of evolocumab showed no increase in adverse events compared to the placebo. Evolocumab-treated individuals had a 15% lower risk of major cardiovascular events and a 23% lower risk of cardiovascular death compared to those originally given a placebo.

An open-label study, ODYSSEY DM-DYSLIPIDEMIA, was dedicated to assessing alirocumab's effect specifically on diabetic dyslipidemia by comparing it to usual care in addition to maximally tolerated statins.[43] Usual care was defined as no additional lipid-lowering therapy, fenofibrate, ezetimibe, omega-3 fatty acid, or nicotinic acid. At week 24, individuals in the treatment arm showed greater reductions in non-HDL-, LDL-C, and apoB compared with usual care with 32.5%, 43.0%, and 32.2%, respectively, translating into non-HDL-C goal attainment of 67% in the alirocumab group versus only 18% in the usual care group. Interestingly, even though usual care included fibrate treatment, no difference in TG-level changes was observed between the two groups; in both treatment arms, TGs were reduced by about 10%. Evolocumab's effect, in addition to at least moderate statin background therapy among people with T2DM with and without mixed dyslipidemia compared with a placebo, was investigated in the BANTING[44] and BERSON[45] trials. Pooled analysis of both trials showed that a biweekly dosing of 140 mg evolocumab reduced non-HDL-C, LDL-C, and apoB by 63.9%, 72.4%, and 57.8%, respectively, in persons without mixed dyslipidemia and by 59.2%, 69.8%, and 57.8%, respectively, in those with high TG and low HDL-C compared with a placebo.[46] Both available monoclonal antibodies appeared to be safe and well tolerated. The most frequently occurring adverse events were related to the injection site, like rashes and discomfort. Alirocumab and evolocumab are human antibodies; neutralizing antibodies are extremely rare and were not associated with reductions in their LDL-C-lowering effect. Furthermore, no adverse or impairing effect was found for alirocumab and concomitant insulin treatment.[47] Moreover, the safety analysis of individual trials and pooled trial data showed no increase in new-onset diabetes and no significant reports of muscle-related adverse events.[48,49] The EBBINGHAUS trial has largely allayed initial concerns regarding the onset of neurocognitive disease through mAbs against PCSK9 based on patient self-reported changes in neurocognitive function in phase 3 studies.[50]

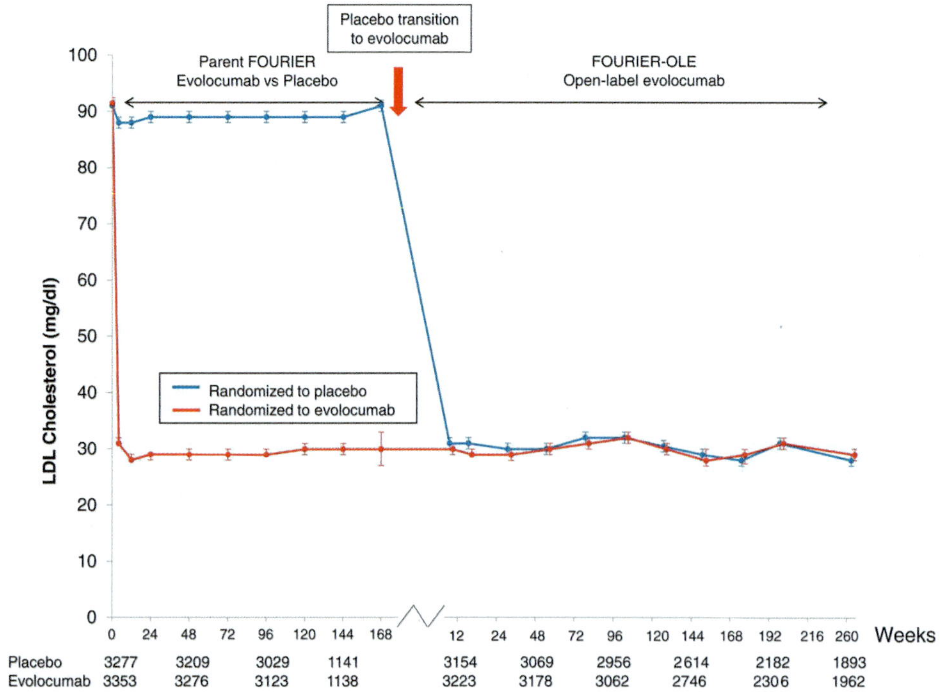

FIG. 19.5 LDL-C reductions under long-term treatment with evolocumab in the FOURIER-OLE extension study. Extended follow-up to a median of 5 years and up to 8.4 years of evolocumab exposure compared to placebo. *LDL-C*, Low-density lipoprotein cholesterol. From O'Donoghue ML, Giugliano RP, Wiviott SD, et al. Long-term evolocumab in patients with established atherosclerotic cardiovascular disease. *Circulation*. 2022;146(15):1109–1119.

mAbs against PCSK9 added to oral background therapy substantially augment the efficacy of combination treatment regimens to reduce apoB-carrying lipoproteins further; the high-risk population of individuals with T2DM may especially benefit from their use. However, because of higher treatment costs, their use is strictly regulated and only considered cost-effective in those with very-high-risk and/or established ASCVD, not reaching their LDL-C goals.

SYNTHETIC SMALL-INTERFERING RNA AGAINST PROPROTEIN CONVERTASE SUBTILISIN/KEXIN TYPE 9—INCLISIRAN

Inclisiran is a synthetic small-interfering RNA (siRNA) targeting PCSK9 administered subcutaneously. Inclisiran consists of a double-stranded RNA conjugated to triantennary N-acetylgalactosamine (GalNAc) carbohydrates. The GalNAc-terminus facilitates rapid and liver-specific uptake via asialoglycoprotein receptors.[51] Within 48 hours after administration, inclisiran is completely cleared from the systemic circulation[52] and taken up by the liver. siRNAs act through the natural cellular process of RNA interference. It is an intrinsic endogenous regulation mechanism for sequence-specific gene silencing and inhibition of protein synthesis. Therefore PCSK9 protein translation is inhibited through PCSK9 mRNA degradation by the inclisiran-induced RNA-induced silencing complex. Specific synthetic modifications to inclisiran's RNA increased the molecular stability of the complex, allowing long-acting target-specific silencing of PCSK9 gene expression. As approximately 80% of circulating PCSK9 in blood arises from the liver, inhibiting hepatic synthesis with a siRNA produces reductions in circulating LDL-C broadly comparable to mAbs, with the convenience of less frequent dosing. In contrast to mAbs directed against PCSK9, which work “downstream,” binding circulating PCSK9, thus preventing the binding of PCSK9 to the LDL-R, inclisiran reduces both intra- and extracellular PCSK9 levels.

Initial dosing 90 days apart followed by regular administration every 6 months is considered optimal to provide a sustained-average 50% LDL-C reduction. Non-HDL-C was reduced by 46%; apoB and VLDL-C were decreased by 41% and 16%, respectively, with two doses of 300 mg inclisiran; and TG levels were reduced by about 14%. For HDL-C, an increase of 9% was observed compared with a placebo.[53]

Fourteen percent of participants in ORION-1, randomized to the treatment arm, had diabetes mellitus at baseline (n = 76).[54] In subgroup analysis, no differences in inclisiran's LDL-C-lowering effect were observed when participants with and without diabetes were compared. Moreover, glycemia and inflammatory markers in persons with diabetes were similar between inclisiran and a placebo. As with LDL-C, inclisiran treatment significantly altered all lipoprotein levels.

In the two largest phase 3 trials, ORION-10 and -11, inclisiran reduced LDL-C by about 50% similarly among individuals with established ASCVD and high-risk primary prevention, irrespective of the intensity of the statin background therapy and whether it was combined with or without ezetimibe (Figure 19.6).[55] Additionally, adverse event rates were similar to the placebo group, including muscle symptoms and the risk of new-onset T2DM.

Through inclisiran's long-lasting effect (Figure 19.7), a lower intraindividual LDL-C variability is achieved compared with oral medications that require daily dosing and may be impaired in efficacy by suboptimal adherence. As LDL-C variability is associated with greater cardiovascular benefits,[56] inclisiran may achieve even greater reductions in cardiovascular events compared with treatments with a similar-percentage LDL-C-lowering effectiveness but higher inherent on-treatment LDL-C variability from therapies requiring more frequent dosing (e.g., high-intensity statins). Furthermore, the infrequent dosing regimen combined with administration through a healthcare professional may achieve almost optimal adherence and

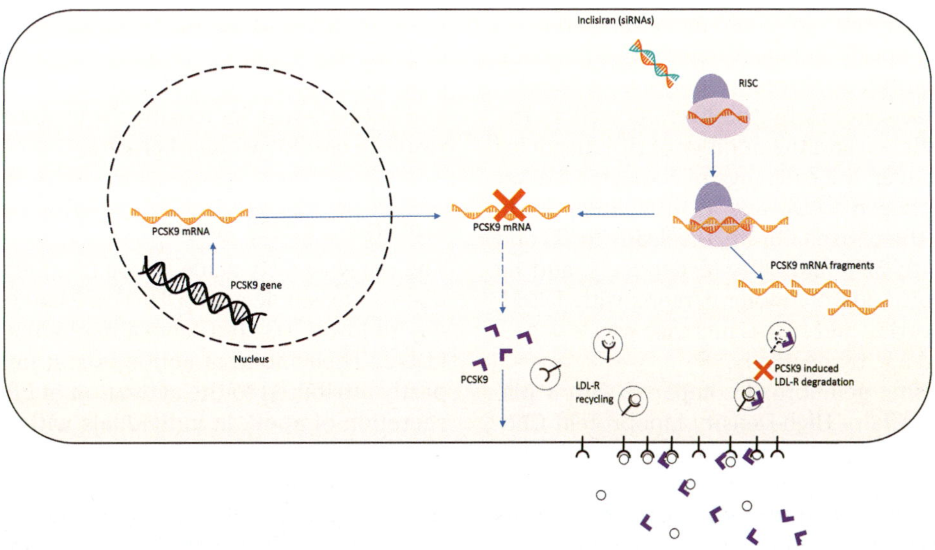

FIG. 19.6 Mechanism of action of siRNA inclisiran. Inclisiran utilizes small interfering RNA (*siRNA*) technology to target PCSK9 mRNA. By binding to PCSK9 mRNA, inclisiran induces its degradation through the RNA-induced silencing complex (*RISC*), preventing the translation of PCSK9 protein. This reduction in PCSK9 levels decreases the degradation of LDL receptors (*LDL-R*) in the liver. With more LDL-R available on the cell surface, there is an increased uptake and clearance of LDL cholesterol from the bloodstream, thereby lowering plasma LDL-C levels. *LDL-C*, Low-density lipoprotein cholesterol; *PCSK9*, proprotein convertase subtilisin/kexin type 9.

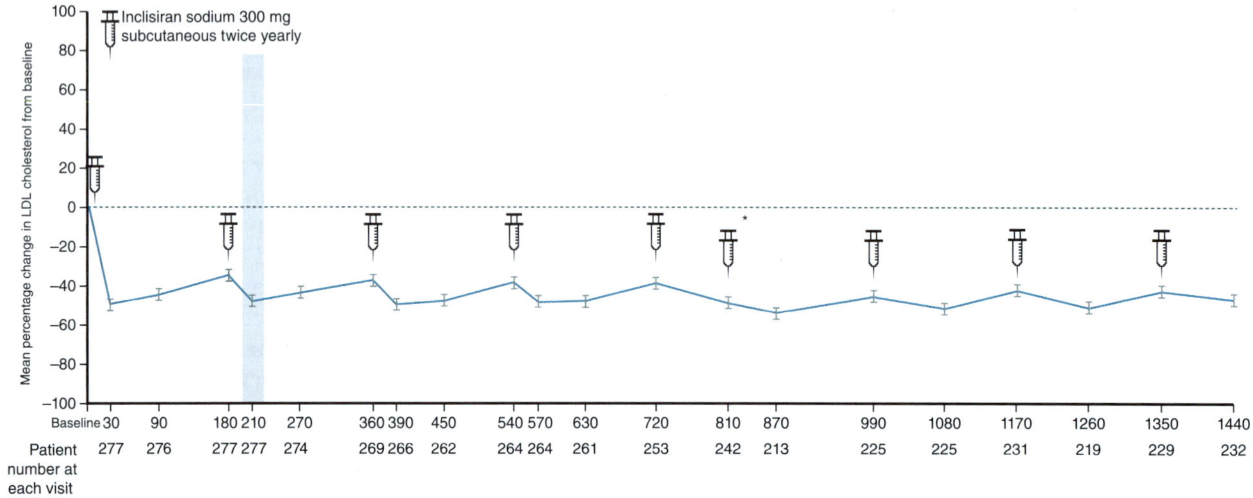

FIG. 19.7 Mean percentage change in LDL cholesterol from baseline with twice-yearly inclisira. Data from the ORION-3 extension study illustrates the long-term effects of twice-yearly subcutaneous inclisiran sodium (300 mg) on LDL cholesterol levels in patients with high cardiovascular risk and elevated LDL cholesterol. From Ray KK, Troquay RP, Visseren FL, et al. Long-term efficacy and safety of inclisiran in patients with high cardiovascular risk and elevated LDL cholesterol (ORION-3): results from the 4-year open-label extension of the ORION-1 trial. *Lancet Diabetes Endocrinol.* 2023;11(2):109–119.

maximize cardiovascular benefits.[57] However, the cardiovascular outcome trial, ORION 4 (NCT03705234), is still ongoing. Here, approximately 15,000 participants aged 55 years or older with preexisting ASCVD will be randomized to inclisiran or a placebo and followed for 5 years. The first results are expected in 2026–2027. Moreover, VICTORION-2 PREVENT is evaluating the benefits of inclisiran on MACE in participants with established ASCVD, age > 40 years, and LDL-C > 70 mg/dL (1.8 mmol/L), despite a high-intensity statin background therapy. Its estimated completion date is in 2027.

Fibrates

Fibrates have been used since the 1960s and were the primary agent for lipid management in the prestatin era. Fibrates are activating ligands to the peroxisome proliferator-activated receptor-α (PPAR-α). Its binding to PPAR-α induces the transcription of lipid-metabolism-related genes, like LPL and apoA1 but decreases the expression of apoC3. Consequently, lipoprotein lipolysis, FA uptake, and conversion to acetyl-CoA by the liver, as well as the removal of LDL particles, and the number of HDL particles are increased. Moreover, the exchange of cholesteryl ester and triglyceride between VLDL and HDL is reduced. In sum, depending on the chosen fibrate, this leads to TG and LDL-C lowering up to 50% and 20%, respectively, and an increase in HDL-C of < 20%.[58] Among persons with T2DM, the effect on TG lowering and HDL-C increase was less pronounced at 20% and 5%, respectively.[59,60]

Two trials assessing gemfibrozil compared with a placebo, The Veterans Affairs High-Density Lipoprotein Cholesterol Intervention Trial in men with CHD and low HDL-C and the Helsinki Heart Study in men without CHD and elevated non-HDL-C, demonstrated significant reductions in cardiovascular risk for gemfibrozil. Notably, this effect appeared to be independent of the reduction in TG concentration.[61] However, it is important to note that these trials were conducted prior to the prevalent use of statins. Two subsequent trials investigating fibric acids in persons with diabetes, the Fenofibrate Intervention and Event Lowering in Diabetes trial and the Action to Control Cardiovascular Risk in Diabetes study, found no effect on cardiovascular risk as a primary endpoint. Only among those with the highest baseline TG and simultaneously low HDL-C levels was a reduction in cardiovascular events observed.[59,60]

The latest study, PROMINENT, assessing the effect of pemafibrate on the risk of CV events in 10,497 persons with T2DM at high CV risk and mixed dyslipidemia, was stopped for futility after a planned interim analysis.[62] Pemafibrate reduced triglycerides by 26.2%, VLDL cholesterol by 25.8%, remnant cholesterol by 25.6%, and apoC3 by 27.6% but increased apoB by 4.8% compared to a placebo. The incidence of primary endpoint events was similar between the pemafibrate and placebo groups, with 572 and 560 events, respectively (HR, 1.03; 95% CI, 0.91–1.15). While the overall incidence of serious adverse events did not differ significantly, pemafibrate was associated with higher adverse renal events and venous thromboembolism but a lower incidence of nonalcoholic fatty liver disease. This suggests that reducing TG and VLDL-C, per se, through remodeling and lipolysis with increasing the clearance of TRLs, will not result in cardiovascular benefits.

Omega-3 Fatty Acids

The omega-3 fatty acids (eicosapentaenoic acid [EPA] and docosahexaenoic acid [DHA]) are used in doses of 2 to 4 g/day to lower TGs but have a minimal effect on HDL-C and LDL-C. Their mode of action is still unknown but may be partly attributed to the activation of PPARs and decreased secretion of apoB. In individuals with high TG levels, EPA reduced TGs by up to 45% in a dose-dependent manner.

Since results from a Japanese open-label randomized trial suggested that 1800 mg of pure icosapent ethyl, an EPA, reduces CV events by 19%,[63] three large CVO trials assessing omega-3 fatty acids followed with mixed results. The first was the A Study of Cardiovascular Events iN Diabetes trial, which enrolled individuals with diabetes but without atherosclerotic CV disease and randomized them to 1 g of omega-3 fatty acids or a placebo.[64] This trial failed to demonstrate cardiovascular benefits of omega-3 fatty acids. The dose used was arguably too low to achieve a significant clinical effect.

In the Reduction of Cardiovascular Events with EPA-Intervention Trial (REDUCE-IT), which included persons with CVD or diabetes (58%) and elevated TG above 1.7 mmol/L (150 mg/dL), 4 g of highly purified EPA reduced the risk of major cardiovascular events by 25%.[65] Interestingly, reductions in TG levels were modest at 17% with EPA, and hence the benefits were disproportionate to the reduction in TG. However, concerns regarding the magnitude of effect were raised by the fact that the chosen comparator, a mineral oil, increases inflammatory biomarkers associated with ASCVD and worsens the absorption of statins, causing an increase in LDL-C and raises hSCRP.[66] The sum of these effects in the mineral oil comparator group would bias the results in favor of EPA. However, even accounting for these effects, modeling the potential harm from the effects on inflammation and LDL-C rise would not be expected to totally abolish the cardiovascular benefits.[67] Furthermore, in a smaller open-labeled study from Japan, RESPECT EPA, 2 g of EPA provided reductions in cardiovascular events, supporting the findings of REDUCE-IT.[68] In addition, results from the EVAPORATE trial, including 47 (69.1%) persons with diabetes, suggested that icosapent ethyl slowed down coronary artery atherosclerosis progression and potentially induced plaque regression assessed through coronary computed tomographic angiography.[69]

Another randomized placebo-controlled trial, Outcomes Study to Assess STatin Residual Risk Reduction with EpaNova in HiGh CV Risk PatienTs with Hypertriglyceridemia (STRENGTH), investigated a mixture of n-3 fatty acids (EPA and DHA) compared with corn oil in 13,078 persons, of which 70% had diabetes.[70] In contrast to REDUCE-IT, this study did not find a beneficial effect on CVD risk reduction by omega-3 fatty acids in statin-treated secondary prevention and high-risk primary prevention persons with high TGs and low HDL-C. These mixed results may be partly explained by the differences in molecular structure and effects of EPA and DHA. While comparisons between trial results generate hypotheses rather than facts, potential reasons for the findings in STRENGTH could be that the beneficial effects of EPA are offset by potential harm from DHA or that the achieved serum EPA levels in STRENGTH might be insufficient. However, a secondary analysis of the STRENGTH trial suggested that there was no benefit or harm from higher EPA or DHA levels in STRENGTH;[71] in meta-regression, a dose-dependent risk reduction was found for EPA.[72] The same study showed that DHA was associated with nonfatal myocardial infarction at low but not at high doses. Interestingly, in bivariate meta-regression, including both EPA and DHA, EPA but not DHA conferred a reduced risk for nonfatal MI.

Moreover, in vitro studies suggest that the cardiovascular benefits of EPA may be due to its antiinflammatory effects and its influence on inflammatory signaling within the vessel wall. EPA has been shown to stabilize cell membranes, reduce oxidative stress, and inhibit proinflammatory pathways, which may contribute to its protective cardiovascular effects.[73]

Therefore current data suggest potential beneficial effects of purified EPA at high doses beyond reductions in lipid parameters, but not for omega-3 fatty acid mixtures.

TREATMENT STRATEGIES

Taken together, genetic studies and pharmacological therapies support the causal role of apoB-carrying lipoproteins in ASCVD and that lowering through different pathways provides near identical benefits. Therefore from a practical standpoint, treatments can be added as needed to achieve the desired level of non-HDL-C, considering cost, safety, availability, and patient preference.

Hence, many national and international guidelines recommend a stepwise approach (Figure 19.8), where statin treatment remains the first-line treatment because of its robustly proven clinical efficacy in reducing cardiovascular events and low cost. However, in persons with T2DM, given their high risk of ASCVD, starting with an oral combination of statin and ezetimibe may be reasonable in most cases. The effect of statin therapy can be approximated roughly in advance (Table 19.1) if pretreatment LDL-C and non-HDL-C levels are known. Thus it can be estimated at the beginning of therapy whether and which (Table 19.2) combination therapy would be necessary to achieve recommended treatment goals. Starting with a statin and adding ezetimibe later may cause unnecessary additional exposure to atherogenic lipoproteins. Even though ezetimibe's effect is modest compared with PCSK9-targeting medications, delaying its use may cause avoidable CV

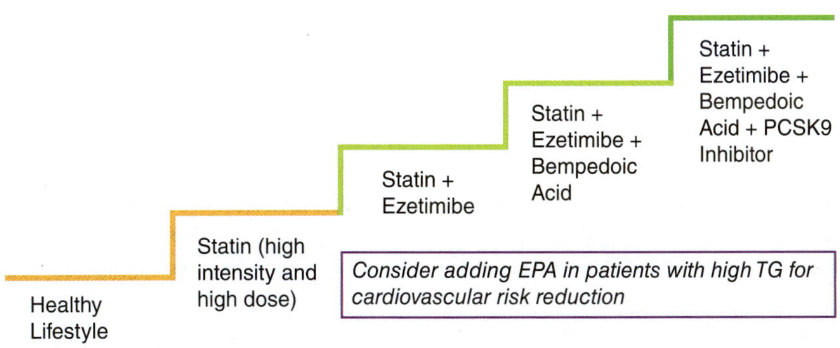

FIG. 19.8 Stepwise approach for lipid management. Each step builds upon the previous, incorporating statins, ezetimibe, bempedoic acid, and PCSK9 inhibitors, as necessary to reduce LDL-C, non-HDL-C, and apoB levels. For patients with high triglycerides (*TG*), adding EPA (eicosapentaenoic acid) could be considered.

TABLE 19.2 Average Placebo-Controlled Percentage Change in Lipid Parameters of Adjunct Lipid-Lowering Medications

TREATMENT	LDL-C CHANGE (%)	NON-HDL-C CHANGE (%)	TG CHANGE (%)
Ezetimibe	−21 to −27	−13	-8
Bempedoic acid	−18 to −21	−13 to 18	−0.4 to −4.9
Alirocumab	−61	−54	−15
Evolocumab	−59	−51	−16
Inclisiran	−52	−45	−10
Fibrates	≥−20	−14	−50
Icosapent ethyl	7	−13	−20
EPA + DHA	0.1	−5	−18

DHA, Docosahexaenoic acid; *EPA*, eicosapentaenoic acid; *LDL-C*, low-density lipoprotein cholesterol; *non-HDL-C*, non-high-density lipoprotein cholesterol; *TG*, triglycerides.

events, at least on a population level. Recent European real-world data demonstrated the widespread underutilization of combination therapy among individuals on lipid-lowering medication across all risk categories.[74] Overall, only 9% of persons received combination therapy with moderate- to high-intensity statins and ezetimibe, despite 76% not reaching their recommended LDL-C goal. Therefore clinicians should actively review their patients' needs for improving lipid management.

Adding bempedoic acid may be considered to further lower non-HDL-C, LDL-C, and cardiovascular events.

Among those at highest risk, PCSK9-directed therapy is already considered cost-effective, and with falling costs, it may also be regarded as a specific treatment for diabetic dyslipidemia. Currently, pharmacological adjunct treatment might be sought through EPA in persons with hypertriglyceridemia. Despite the controversy, a significant CV benefit probably remains, even if the effect magnitude might be smaller than reported in the cardiovascular outcomes trial.

Given the high absolute risk of ASCVD-related morbidity and mortality in persons with T2DM, prevention through lipid management is improving the quality and length of life, especially in these persons.

REFERENCES

1. Efficacy and safety of cholesterol-lowering treatment: prospective meta-analysis of data from 90056 participants in 14 randomised trials of statins. *Lancet.* 2005;366(9493):1267–1278. https://doi.org/10.1016/S0140-6736(05)67394-1.
2. Shojaee-Moradie F, Ma Y, Lou S, Hovorka R, Umpleby AM. Prandial hypertriglyceridemia in metabolic syndrome is due to an overproduction of both chylomicron and VLDL triacylglycerol. *Diabetes.* 2013;62(12):4063–4069.
3. Adiels M, Matikainen N, Westerbacka J, et al. Postprandial accumulation of chylomicrons and chylomicron remnants is determined by the clearance capacity. *Atherosclerosis.* 2012;222(1):222–228.
4. Stahel P, Xiao C, Hegele RA, Lewis GF. The atherogenic dyslipidemia complex and novel approaches to cardiovascular disease prevention in diabetes. *Can J Cardiol.* 2018;34(5):595–604.
5. Vergès B. Abnormal hepatic apolipoprotein B metabolism in type 2 diabetes. *Atherosclerosis.* 2010;211(2):353–360.
6. Adiels M, Borén J, Caslake MJ, et al. Overproduction of VLDL1 driven by hyperglycemia is a dominant feature of diabetic dyslipidemia. *Arterioscler Thromb Vasc Biol.* 2005;25(8):1697–1703.
7. Nordestgaard BG. Triglyceride-rich lipoproteins and atherosclerotic cardiovascular disease: new insights from epidemiology, genetics, and biology. *Circ Res.* 2016;118(4):547–563.
8. Nakajima K, Nakano T, Tanaka A. The oxidative modification hypothesis of atherosclerosis: the comparison of atherogenic effects on oxidized LDL and remnant lipoproteins in plasma. *Clin Chim Acta.* 2006;367(1-2):36–47.
9. Borén J, Williams KJ. The central role of arterial retention of cholesterol-rich apolipoprotein-B-containing lipoproteins in the pathogenesis of atherosclerosis: a triumph of simplicity. *Curr Opin Lipidol.* 2016;27(5):473–483.
10. Patel DC, Albrecht C, Pavitt D, et al. Type 2 diabetes is associated with reduced ATP-binding cassette transporter A1 gene expression, protein and function. *PLoS One.* 2011;6(7):e22142.
11. Passarelli M, Tang C, McDonald TO, O'Brien KD, Gerrity RG, Heinecke JW, Oram JF. Advanced glycation end product precursors impair ABCA1-dependent cholesterol removal from cells. *Diabetes.* 2005;54(7):2198–2205.
12. Duvillard L, Florentin E, Lizard G, et al. Cell surface expression of LDL receptor is decreased in type 2 diabetic patients and is normalized by insulin therapy. *Diabetes Care.* 2003;26(5):1540–1544.
13. Vakkilainen J, Steiner G, Ansquer J-C, et al. Relationships between low-density lipoprotein particle size, plasma lipoproteins, and progression of coronary artery disease: the Diabetes Atherosclerosis Intervention Study (DAIS). *Circulation.* 2003;107(13):1733–1737.
14. Tani M, Kawakami A, Mizuno Y, et al. Small dense LDL enhances THP-1 macrophage foam cell formation. *J Atherosclerosis Thrombosis.* 2011:1104200369-1104200369.
15. Varbo A, Benn M, Tybjærg-Hansen A, Jørgensen AB, Frikke-Schmidt R, Nordestgaard BG. Remnant cholesterol as a causal risk factor for ischemic heart disease. *J Am Coll Cardiology.* 2013;61(4):427–436. 2013/01/29/. https://doi.org/10.1016/j.jacc.2012.08.1026.
16. Committee ADAPP, Committee: ADAPP. 10. Cardiovascular disease and risk management: Standards of Medical Care in Diabetes—2022. *Diabetes Care.* 2022;45(Supplement_1):S144–S174.
17. Jellinger PS, Handelsman Y, Rosenblit PD, et al. American Association of Clinical Endocrinologists and American College of Endocrinology guidelines for management of dyslipidemia and prevention of cardiovascular disease. *Endocr Pract.* 2017;23:1–87.
18. Members TF, Societies ENC, Guidelines ECfP. 2019 ESC/EAS guidelines for the management of dyslipidaemias: lipid modification to reduce cardiovascular risk. *Atherosclerosis.* 2019;290:140–205.
19. Marx N, Federici M, Schütt K, et al. 2023 ESC Guidelines for the management of cardiovascular disease in patients with diabetes: Developed by the task force on the management of cardiovascular disease in patients with diabetes of the European Society of Cardiology (ESC). *Eur Heart J.* 2023;44(39):4043–4140.
20. Puri R, Mehta V, Duell PB, et al. Management of diabetic dyslipidemia in Indians: Expert consensus statement from the Lipid Association of India. *J Clin Lipidol.* 2023;17(2):e1–e14. 2023/03/01/. https://doi.org/10.1016/j.jacl.2022.11.002.
21. Puri R, Mehta V, Iyengar S, et al. Lipid association of India expert consensus statement on management of dyslipidemia in Indians 2020: Part III. *J Assoc Physicians India.* 2020;68(11 [Special]):8–9.
22. Grundy SM, Stone NJ, Bailey AL, et al. 2018 AHA/ACC/AACVPR/AAPA/ABC/ACPM/ADA/AGS/APhA/ASPC/NLA/PCNA Guideline on the Management of Blood Cholesterol: A Report of the American College of Cardiology/American Heart Association Task Force on Clinical Practice Guidelines. *J Am Coll Cardiology.* 2019;73(24):e285–e350. 2019/06/25/. https://doi.org/10.1016/j.jacc.2018.11.003.
23. Shah NP, McGuire DK, Cannon CP, et al. Impact of ezetimibe on new-onset diabetes: a substudy of IMPROVE-IT. *J Am Heart Assoc.* 2023;12(13):e029593.
24. Cholesterol Treatment Trialists C. Efficacy of cholesterol-lowering therapy in 18 686 people with diabetes in 14 randomised trials of statins: a meta-analysis. *Lancet.* 2008;371(9607):117–125. https://doi.org/10.1016/S0140-6736(08)60104-X.
25. Vallejo-Vaz AJ, Fayyad R, Boekholdt SM, et al. Triglyceride-rich lipoprotein cholesterol and risk of cardiovascular events among patients receiving statin therapy in the TNT trial. *Circulation.* 2018;138(8):770–781. https://doi.org/10.1161/CIRCULATIONAHA.117.032318.
26. Cholesterol Treatment Trialists' Collaboration, Effect of statin therapy on muscle symptoms: an individual participant data meta-analysis of large-scale, randomised, double-blind trials. *Lancet.* 2022;400(10355):832–845. doi:10.1016/S0140-6736(22)01545-8
27. Sattar N, Preiss D, Murray HM, et al. Statins and risk of incident diabetes: a collaborative meta-analysis of randomised statin trials. *Lancet.* 2010;375(9716):735–742. https://doi.org/10.1016/S0140-6736(09)61965-6.
28. Preiss D, Seshasai SRK, Welsh P, et al. Risk of incident diabetes with intensive-dose compared with moderate-dose statin therapy: a meta-analysis. *JAMA.* 2011;305(24):2556–2564. https://doi.org/10.1001/jama.2011.860.
29. Reith C, Preiss D, Blackwell L, et al. Effects of statin therapy on diagnoses of new-onset diabetes and worsening glycaemia in large-scale randomised blinded statin trials: an individual participant data meta-analysis. *Lancet Diabetes Endocrinol.* 2024;12(5):306–319.
30. Sudhop T, Lütjohann D, Kodal A, et al. Inhibition of intestinal cholesterol absorption by ezetimibe in humans. *Circulation.* 2002;106(15):1943–1948.
31. Bays HE, Moore PB, Drehobl MA, et al. Effectiveness and tolerability of ezetimibe in patients with primary hypercholesterolemia: pooled analysis of two phase II studies. *Clin Ther.* 2001;23(8):1209–1230.
32. Cannon CP, Blazing MA, Giugliano RP, et al. Ezetimibe added to statin therapy after acute coronary syndromes. *N Engl J Med.* 2015;372(25):2387–2397. https://doi.org/10.1056/NEJMoa1410489.
33. Pinkosky SL, Newton RS, Day EA, et al. Liver-specific ATP-citrate lyase inhibition by bempedoic acid decreases LDL-C and attenuates atherosclerosis. *Nat Commun.* 2016;7(1):1–13.
34. Herzig S, Shaw RJ. AMPK: guardian of metabolism and mitochondrial homeostasis. *Nat Rev Mol Cell Biol.* 2018;19(2):121–135.

35. Ray KK, Bays HE, Catapano AL, et al. Safety and efficacy of bempedoic acid to reduce LDL cholesterol. *N Engl J Med*. 2019;380(11):1022–1032.
36. Banach M, Duell PB, Gotto Jr AM, et al. Association of bempedoic acid administration with atherogenic lipid levels in phase 3 randomized clinical trials of patients with hypercholesterolemia. *JAMA Cardiol*. 2020;5(10):1124–1135. https://doi.org/10.1001/jamacardio.2020.2314.
37. Gutierrez MJ, Rosenberg NL, MacDougall DE, et al. Efficacy and safety of ETC-1002, a novel investigational low-density lipoprotein-cholesterol-lowering therapy for the treatment of patients with hypercholesterolemia and type 2 diabetes mellitus. *Arterioscler Thromb Vasc Biol*. 2014;34(3):676–683.
38. Leiter LA, Banach M, Catapano AL, et al. Bempedoic acid in patients with type 2 diabetes mellitus, prediabetes, and normoglycaemia: a post hoc analysis of efficacy and glycaemic control using pooled data from phase 3 clinical trials. *Diabetes Obes Metab*. 2022;24(5):868–880. https://doi.org/10.1111/dom.14645.
39. Nissen SE, Lincoff AM, Brennan D, et al. Bempedoic acid and cardiovascular outcomes in statin-intolerant patients. *N Engl J Med*. 2023;388(15):1353–1364. https://doi.org/10.1056/NEJMoa2215024.
40. Sabatine MS, Giugliano RP, Keech AC, et al. Evolocumab and clinical outcomes in patients with cardiovascular disease. *N Engl J Med*. 2017;376(18):1713–1722. https://doi.org/10.1056/NEJMoa1615664.
41. Schwartz GG, Steg PG, Szarek M, et al. Alirocumab and cardiovascular outcomes after acute coronary syndrome. *N Engl J Med*. 2018;379(22):2097–2107. https://doi.org/10.1056/NEJMoa1801174.
42. O'Donoghue ML, Giugliano RP, Wiviott SD, et al. Long-term evolocumab in patients with established atherosclerotic cardiovascular disease. *Circulation*. 2022;146(15):1109–1119. https://doi.org/10.1161/CIRCULATIONAHA.122.061620.
43. Ray KK, Leiter LA, Müller-Wieland D, et al. Alirocumab vs usual lipid-lowering care as add-on to statin therapy in individuals with type 2 diabetes and mixed dyslipidaemia: The ODYSSEY DM-DYSLIPIDEMIA randomized trial. *Diabetes Obes Metab*. 2018;20(6):1479–1489. https://doi.org/10.1111/dom.13257.
44. Rosenson RS, Daviglus ML, Handelsman Y, et al. Efficacy and safety of evolocumab in individuals with type 2 diabetes mellitus: primary results of the randomised controlled BANTING study. *Diabetologia*. 2019;62(6):948–958. https://doi.org/10.1007/s00125-019-4856-7.
45. Lorenzatti AJ, Eliaschewitz FG, Chen Y, et al. Randomised study of evolocumab in patients with type 2 diabetes and dyslipidaemia on background statin: Primary results of the BERSON clinical trial. *Diabetes Obes Metab*. 2019;21(6):1455–1463. https://doi.org/10.1111/dom.13680.
46. Lorenzatti AJ, Monsalvo ML, López JAG, Wang H, Rosenson RS. Effects of evolocumab in individuals with type 2 diabetes with and without atherogenic dyslipidemia: An analysis from BANTING and BERSON. *Cardiovasc Diabetol*. 2021;20(1):94. https://doi.org/10.1186/s12933-021-01287-6.
47. Leiter LA, Cariou B, Müller-Wieland D, et al. Efficacy and safety of alirocumab in insulin-treated individuals with type 1 or type 2 diabetes and high cardiovascular risk: The ODYSSEY DM-INSULIN randomized trial. *Diabetes Obes Metab*. 2017;19(12):1781–1792. https://doi.org/10.1111/dom.13114.
48. Sattar N, Toth PP, Blom DJ, et al. Effect of the proprotein convertase subtilisin/kexin type 9 inhibitor evolocumab on glycemia, body weight, and new-onset diabetes mellitus. *Am J Cardiol*. 2017;120(9):1521–1527.
49. Colhoun HM, Ginsberg HN, Robinson JG, et al. No effect of PCSK9 inhibitor alirocumab on the incidence of diabetes in a pooled analysis from 10 ODYSSEY Phase 3 studies. *Eur Heart J*. 2016;37(39):2981–2989. https://doi.org/10.1093/eurheartj/ehw292.
50. Giugliano RP, Mach F, Zavitz K, et al. Cognitive function in a randomized trial of evolocumab. *N Engl J Med*. 2017;377(7):633–643.
51. Nair JK, Willoughby JL, Chan A, et al. Multivalent N-acetylgalactosamine-conjugated siRNA localizes in hepatocytes and elicits robust RNAi-mediated gene silencing. *J Am Chem Soc*. 2014;136(49):16958–16961.
52. Wright RS, Collins MG, Stoekenbroek RM, et al. Effects of renal impairment on the pharmacokinetics, efficacy, and safety of inclisiran: an analysis of the ORION-7 and ORION-1 studies. *Elsevier*. 2020:77–89.
53. Ray KK, Stoekenbroek RM, Kallend D, et al. Effect of an siRNA therapeutic targeting PCSK9 on atherogenic lipoproteins: prespecified secondary end points in ORION 1. *Circulation*. 2018;138(13):1304–1316.
54. Leiter LA, Teoh H, Kallend D, et al. Inclisiran lowers LDL-C and PCSK9 irrespective of diabetes status: the ORION-1 randomized clinical trial. *Diabetes Care*. 2019;42(1):173–176.
55. Ray KK, Wright RS, Kallend D, et al. Two phase 3 trials of inclisiran in patients with elevated LDL cholesterol. *N Engl J Med*. 2020;382(16):1507–1519.
56. Bangalore S, Breazna A, DeMicco DA, Wun C-C, Messerli FH. Visit-to-visit low-density lipoprotein cholesterol variability and risk of cardiovascular outcomes: insights from the TNT trial. *J Am Coll Cardiology*. 2015;65(15):1539–1548. 2015/04/21/. https://doi.org/10.1016/j.jacc.2015.02.017.
57. Brandts J, Ray KK. Low density lipoprotein cholesterol–lowering strategies and population health: time to move to a cumulative exposure model. *Circulation*. 2020;141(11):873–876.
58. Chapman MJ, Redfern JS, McGovern ME, Giral P. Niacin and fibrates in atherogenic dyslipidemia: pharmacotherapy to reduce cardiovascular risk. *Pharmacol Ther*. 2010;126(3):314–345. https://doi.org/10.1016/j.pharmthera.2010.01.008.
59. The FIELD study investigators. Effects of long-term fenofibrate therapy on cardiovascular events in 9795 people with type 2 diabetes mellitus (the FIELD study): randomised controlled trial. *Lancet*. 2005;366(9500):1849–1861. https://doi.org/10.1016/S0140-6736(05)67667-2.
60. ACCORD Study Group. Effects of combination lipid therapy in type 2 diabetes mellitus. *N Engl J Med*. 2010;362(17):1563–1574. doi:10.1056/NEJMoa1001282
61. Frick MH, Elo O, Haapa K, et al. Helsinki Heart Study: primary-prevention trial with gemfibrozil in middle-aged men with dyslipidemia. *N Engl J Med*. 1987;317(20):1237–1245.
62. Pradhan AD, Glynn RJ, Fruchart J-C, et al. Triglyceride lowering with pemafibrate to reduce cardiovascular risk. *N Engl J Med*. 2022;387(21):1923–1934. https://doi.org/10.1056/NEJMoa2210645.
63. Yokoyama M, Origasa H, Matsuzaki M, et al. Effects of eicosapentaenoic acid on major coronary events in hypercholesterolaemic patients (JELIS): a randomised open-label, blinded endpoint analysis. *Lancet*. 2007;369(9567):1090–1098. https://doi.org/10.1016/S0140-6736(07)60527-3.
64. ASCEND Study Collaborative Group. Effects of n-3 fatty acid supplements in diabetes mellitus. *N Engl J Med*. 2018;379(16):1540–1550. doi:10.1056/NEJMoa1804989
65. Bhatt DL, Steg PG, Miller M, et al. Cardiovascular risk reduction with icosapent ethyl for hypertriglyceridemia. *N Engl J Med*. 2018;380(1):11–22. https://doi.org/10.1056/NEJMoa1812792.
66. Kastelein JJ, Stroes ES. FISHing for the miracle of eicosapentaenoic acid. *Mass Med Soc*. 2019:89–90.
67. Doi T, Langsted A, Nordestgaard BG. A possible explanation for the contrasting results of REDUCE-IT vs. STRENGTH: cohort study mimicking trial designs. *Eur Heart J*. 2021;42(47):4807–4817. https://doi.org/10.1093/eurheartj/ehab555.
68. Miyauchi K, Iwata H, Nishizaki Y, et al. Randomized trial for evaluation in secondary prevention efficacy of combination therapy–statin and eicosapentaenoic acid (RESPECT-EPA). *Circulation*. 2024;150(6):425–434. doi:10.1161/CIRCULATIONAHA.123.065520
69. Budoff MJ, Bhatt DL, Kinninger A, et al. Effect of icosapent ethyl on progression of coronary atherosclerosis in patients with elevated triglycerides on statin therapy: final results of the EVAPORATE trial. *Eur Heart J*. 2020;41(40):3925–3932. https://doi.org/10.1093/eurheartj/ehaa652.
70. Nicholls SJ, Lincoff AM, Garcia M, et al. Effect of high-dose omega-3 fatty acids vs corn oil on major adverse cardiovascular events in patients at high cardiovascular risk: the STRENGTH randomized clinical trial. *JAMA*. 2020;324(22):2268–2280. https://doi.org/10.1001/jama.2020.22258.
71. Nissen SE, Lincoff AM, Wolski K, et al. Association between achieved ω-3 fatty acid levels and major adverse cardiovascular outcomes in patients with high cardiovascular risk: a secondary analysis of the STRENGTH trial. *JAMA Cardiol*. 2021;6(8):910–917. https://doi.org/10.1001/jamacardio.2021.1157.
72. Sarajlic P, Artiach G, Larsson SC, Bäck M. Dose-dependent risk reduction for myocardial infarction with eicosapentaenoic acid: a meta-analysis and meta-regression including the STRENGTH trial. *Cardiovasc Drugs Ther*. 2021;35(5):1079–1081.
73. Mason RP, Libby P, Bhatt DL. Emerging mechanisms of cardiovascular protection for the omega-3 fatty acid eicosapentaenoic acid. *Arterioscler Thromb Vasc Biol*. 2020;40(5):1135–1147. https://doi.org/10.1161/ATVBAHA.119.313286.
74. Ray KK, Molemans B, Schoonen WM, et al. EU-wide cross-sectional observational study of lipid-modifying therapy use in secondary and primary care: the DA VINCI study. *Eur J Prevent Cardiol*. 2020;28(11):1279–1289. https://doi.org/10.1093/eurjpc/zwaa047.

20 Effect of Antithrombotic Therapy on Coronary Heart Disease Risk in People With Diabetes Mellitus

MICHELLE L. O'DONOGHUE AND DEEPAK L. BHATT

Platelets play a central role in the pathobiology of atherogenesis and atherothrombosis. Therefore therapies that are directed toward platelet inhibition are widely used in patients with established coronary heart disease (CHD) or in moderate- to high-risk individuals for primary prevention of cardiovascular (CV) events.[1] As our armamentarium of potent antiplatelet therapies continues to expand, there is growing interest in identifying the appropriate groups of patients who will derive the greatest benefit from more potent therapies. To that end, several studies over the past few decades have highlighted that individuals with diabetes mellitus (DM) exhibit abnormalities in platelet function that place them at increased risk of adverse outcomes, as compared with their nondiabetic counterparts (see also Chapter 10).[2] Although the mechanisms that contribute to platelet hyperreactivity in patients with diabetes continue to be elucidated, it appears that diabetic platelets are characterized by the dysregulation of several signaling pathways that occur both at the level of the platelet receptor and with subsequent downstream signaling.[3,4] In addition, glycosylation may impair endothelial function and promote oxidative stress, thereby further promoting platelet reactivity and procoagulant activity.[1] There is therefore a priori biologic plausibility to support the concept that patients with diabetes may derive enhanced benefit from particular therapies directed toward blocking the platelet. However, differences in platelet biology in patients with diabetes may also contribute to diminished antiplatelet drug responsiveness. This chapter reviews the use of established and novel oral antiplatelet therapies in patients with diabetes for use in primary or secondary prevention of CV events.

ACETYLSALICYLIC ACID

Acetylsalicylic acid (ASA) selectively acetylates the hydroxyl group of a serine residue leading to irreversible inhibition of the cyclooxygenase-1 (COX-1) enzyme.[5] In turn, inhibition of the COX-1 enzyme blocks downstream production of thromboxane A_2 (TXA_2; Fig. 20.1), thereby preventing thromboxane-mediated platelet aggregation and vasoconstriction. Because the platelet is enucleate, it is unable to resynthesize COX-1 and the effects of ASA persist throughout the lifetime of the platelet.[5]

Acetylsalicylic Acid in Persons Without Known Atherosclerotic Cardiovascular Disease

Although its role in persons with atherosclerotic cardiovascular disease (ASCVD) is well established, the net clinical benefit of ASA in those without known atherosclerosis continues to be debated. Several large trials of ASA have been conducted in the general population without known ASCVD, and investigators have subsequently evaluated the benefit of ASA within their diabetic subgroups.[6–8] Although limited by small numbers of patients with diabetes and by post hoc design, many trials were able to demonstrate a consistent benefit of ASA in the prevention of first CV events for both patients with and without diabetes.[6,7] These results were supported by the Early Treatment Diabetic Retinopathy Study (ETDRS), which included a mixed population of 3711 patients with DM with or without a history of CHD who were randomized to ASA 650 mg daily or placebo.[9] Although ASA did not reduce the primary endpoint of all-cause death (hazard ratio [HR] 0.91, 95% confidence interval [CI] 0.75–1.11), a favorable trend was observed toward a reduction in fatal or nonfatal myocardial infarction (MI) at 5 years that did not achieve statistical significance (HR, 0.83; 95% CI, 0.66–1.04).[9]

In contrast, a benefit for ASA could not be definitively demonstrated in patients with diabetes enrolled in the Primary Prevention Project (PPP), a randomized trial of low-dose ASA (100 mg daily) versus a placebo in 4495 patients with one or more CV risk factors.[8] Although underpowered to detect a significant benefit within the diabetic subgroup ($n = 1031$), the investigators were unable to demonstrate a

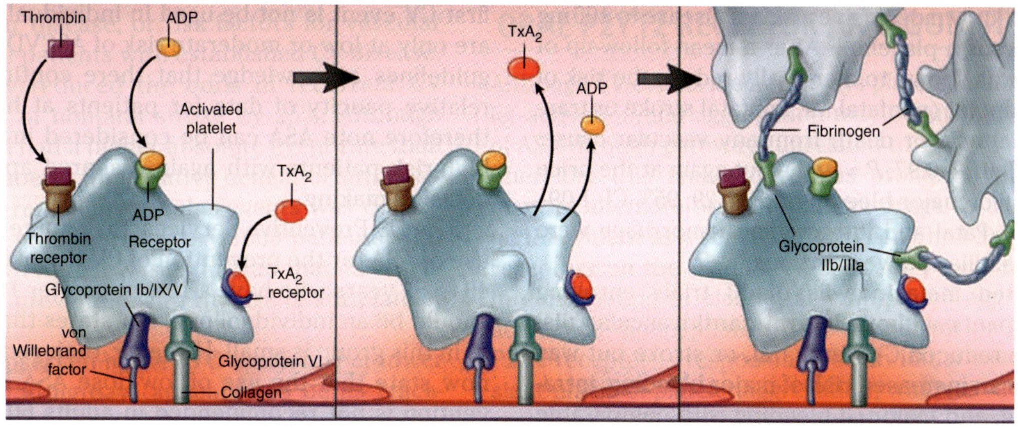

FIG. 20.1 The platelet has multiple ligands that contribute to pathways leading to platelet activation including thrombin, adenosine diphosphate (ADP), von Willebrand factor, and thromboxane A_2 (TXA_2). The activated platelet then releases prothrombotic factors, including ADP and TXA_2, thereby further amplifying platelet activation. A platelet latticework is formed when fibrinogen cross-links activated platelets via the glycoprotein IIb/IIIa receptor. The P2Y12 subtype of the ADP receptor is the site of action for established and novel compounds, including ticlopidine, clopidogrel, prasugrel, ticagrelor, and cangrelor. Modified from Bhatt DL. Intensifying platelet inhibition—navigating between Scylla and Charybdis, *N Engl J Med.* 2007;357:2078–2081.

significant reduction in CV death, MI, or stroke in patients with diabetes (HR, 0.90; 95% CI, 0.50–1.62) or in total CV events (HR, 0.89; 95% CI, 0.62–1.26). Moreover, an unfavorable trend was observed toward an increased risk of CV death (HR, 1.23; 95% CI, 0.69–2.19) in ASA-treated patients with diabetes. In contrast, a more consistent benefit was seen with ASA in patients without diabetes with regard to reduction in the risk of CV death, MI, or stroke (HR, 0.59; 95% CI, 0.37–0.94); total CV events (HR, 0.69; 95% CI, 0.53–0.90); and CV death (HR, 0.32; 95% CI, 0.14–0.72).[8]

Because subgroup analyses from randomized trials may yield spurious results, dedicated trials of ASA for primary prevention in patients with diabetes have since been completed. The Japanese Primary Prevention of Atherosclerosis with Aspirin for Diabetes (JPAD) study was the first prospectively designed trial to evaluate the use of low-dose ASA (81 or 100 mg daily) versus a placebo in 2539 type 2 patients with diabetes in Japan aged 30 to 85 years and without a known history of ASCVD.[10] After a median of 4.37 years, only 154 atherosclerotic events (including fatal or nonfatal ischemic heart disease, fatal or nonfatal stroke, and peripheral arterial disease [PAD]) occurred during follow-up and the trial was therefore unable to demonstrate clinical efficacy with ASA in patients with diabetes despite a directional trend (HR, 0.80; 95% CI, 0.58–1.10; P = 0.16).[10] In addition to being underpowered, other limitations of the trial included its open-label design, which introduced the possibility of bias. However, among the subgroup of patients older than 65 years, ASA reduced the risk of atherosclerotic events by 32% (P = 0.047). The incidence of hemorrhagic stroke or gastrointestinal (GI) bleeding was low and did not differ significantly between groups.[10]

Subsequently, the Prevention of Progression of Arterial Disease and Diabetes (POPADAD) trial evaluated the efficacy of low-dose ASA (100 mg daily) versus a placebo in 1276 adults in Scotland older than 40 years with type 1 or type 2 diabetes and an ankle brachial pressure index below 0.99 in the absence of symptomatic CV disease.[11] Although the trial was relatively small, the incidence of CV events (death from congestive heart failure [CHF] or stroke, nonfatal MI or stroke, or amputation because of critical limb ischemia) was almost identical between treatment arms during a median of 6.7 years of follow-up (116 vs. 117 events; HR, 0.98, 95% CI, 0.76–1.26). ASA did not reduce the risk of death from CHD or stroke (HR, 1.23; 95% CI, 0.79–1.93). GI bleeding was infrequent, and its incidence did not differ between groups.[11]

The Japanese Primary Prevention Project (JPPP)[12] was an open-label trial that randomized 14,464 patients in Japan aged 60 to 85 years with hypertension, dyslipidemia, or diabetes mellitus to enteric-coated ASA (100 mg/d) or none. The trial was stopped for futility after a median follow-up of ~5 years. The primary outcome of CV death, MI, or stroke was neutral (HR, 0.94; 95% CI, 0.77–1.15; P = 0.54), despite a significant reduction in MI (HR, 0.53; 95% CI, 0.31–0.91; P = 0.02) and TIA (HR, 0.57; 95% CI, 0.32–0.99; P = 0.04). There was an observed increase in extracranial hemorrhage requiring transfusion or hospitalization (HR, 1.85; 95% CI, 1.22–2.81; P = 0.004).

Although not a dedicated trial for individuals with diabetes mellitus, the use of ASA in older persons without known ASCVD was more broadly challenged by the results of the ASPREE (Aspirin in Reducing Events in the Elderly) trial. The trial randomized 19,114 participants from Australia or the United States aged ≥70 years old (≥65 years old for Hispanic and African American patients within the United States) without life-limiting chronic illness, dementia, physical disability, or documented cardiovascular or cerebrovascular disease (11% with diabetes mellitus) to ASA 100 mg daily or placebo.[13] After a median follow-up of 4.7 years, the trial was stopped early for futility. The primary endpoint of disability-free survival (survival free from dementia or persistent physical disability) was not reduced with ASA (HR, 1.01; 95% CI, 0.92–1.11; P = 0.79), nor was the risk of CV events.[14] ASA increased the risk of major bleeding (HR, 1.38; 95% CI, 1.18–1.62; P < 0.001). A higher risk of all-cause mortality was observed with ASA, mainly due to cancer-related mortality, although no longer significant after statistical correction for multiple comparisons.

In contrast, the ASCEND (A Study of Cardiovascular Events in Diabetes) trial randomized 15,480 patients with

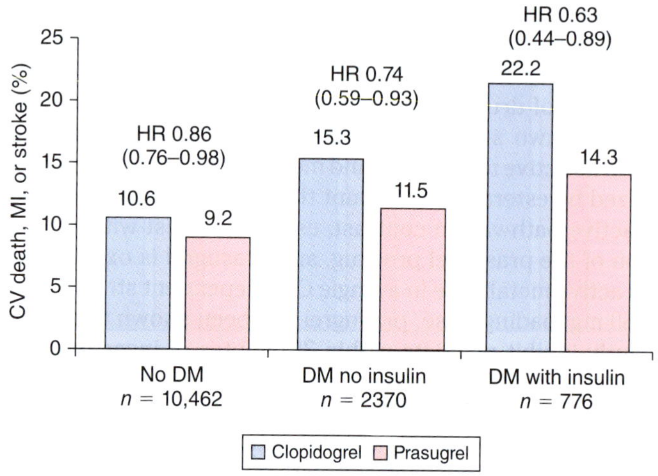

FIG. 20.5 Clinical events and relative benefit (hazard ratio [HR], 95% confidence interval [CI]) of prasugrel versus clopidogrel for patients without diabetes mellitus (DM), patients with diabetes not treated with insulin, and insulin-treated patients with diabetes in the TRITON-TIMI 38 trial. The relative benefit of prasugrel versus clopidogrel appeared to be enhanced in patients with diabetes, and further benefit was observed in those patients requiring insulin therapy.[52] *CV*, Cardiovascular; *MI*, myocardial infarction. Modified from Wiviott SD, Braunwald E, Angiolillo DJ, et al. Greater clinical benefit of more intensive oral antiplatelet therapy with prasugrel in patients with diabetes mellitus in the trial to assess improvement in therapeutic outcomes by optimizing platelet inhibition with prasugrel—Thrombolysis in Myocardial Infarction 38. *Circulation*. 2008;118:1626–1636.

this high-risk patient group (2.6% vs. 2.5%; HR, 1.06; 95% CI, 0.66–1.69). Because of the higher event rate and greater benefit of prasugrel in insulin-treated patients, the absolute risk reduction in CV events with prasugrel was 8%, indicating that only 13 insulin-treated patients with diabetes would need to be treated to prevent one ischemic event, contrasted with a number-needed-to-treat of 26 for DM patients not on insulin. The observations from the diabetic subgroup of the TRITON-TIMI 38 trial therefore support the hypothesis that the achieved degree of platelet reactivity is an important predictor of outcome. Because individuals with DM have higher baseline platelet reactivity and diminished pharmacodynamic response to clopidogrel, it is plausible that patients with diabetes derive enhanced benefit from this more potent antiplatelet therapy that is able to attain lower levels of on-treatment platelet reactivity.

The Prasugrel in Comparison to Clopidogrel for Inhibition of Platelet Activation and Aggregation—Thrombolysis in Myocardial Infarction 44 (PRINCIPLE-TIMI 44) trial was a two-phase study of 201 patients undergoing PCI that compared the pharmacodynamic response to prasugrel (60-mg loading dose, 10 mg daily) with higher-dose clopidogrel (600-mg loading dose, 150 mg daily).[47] Prasugrel achieved greater IPA as compared with higher-dose clopidogrel in both the loading dose and maintenance dose phases. The rate of patients who were hyporesponsive to clopidogrel (IPA $\leq$20% in response to 20 μM ADP) was higher in patients with diabetes than in those without diabetes at all timepoints. In contrast, no hyporesponders were observed for patients on prasugrel at 6 hours, regardless of diabetes status.[47] Consistent findings were observed in the OPTIMUS-3 trial, which exclusively enrolled patients with DM.[53] In OPTIMUS-3, individuals with DM and coronary artery disease (CAD) were randomized to prasugrel (60-mg loading dose, 10 mg daily) or clopidogrel (600-mg loading dose, 150 mg daily) over two 1-week treatment periods separated by a 2-week washout. Prasugrel achieved greater platelet inhibition than high-dose clopidogrel at 4 hours after a loading dose. This difference was maintained throughout the loading dose and maintenance phase (from 1 hour through 7 days; $P < 0.001$). Prasugrel reduced the number of patients with diabetes with an inadequate response to thienopyridine therapy as compared with high-dose clopidogrel.[53]

After the publication of the TRITON-TIMI 38 trial findings, the Targeted Platelet Inhibition to Clarify the Optimal Strategy to Medically Manage Acute Coronary Syndromes (TRILOGY ACS) trial compared the long-term efficacy of prasugrel (10 mg daily) versus clopidogrel (75 mg daily) in 7243 patients with ACS who were managed medically without coronary revascularization (see also Chapter 21).[54] A lower dose of prasugrel (5 mg daily) was used in patients who weighed less than 60 kg or were older than 75 years. The primary analysis was restricted to patients younger than 75 years. In this patient group, prasugrel did not significantly reduce the risk of CV death, MI, or stroke as compared with clopidogrel (HR, 0.91; 95% CI, 0.79–1.05). The findings were consistent in the subset of 2811 patients with DM (HR, 0.90; 95% CI, 0.73–1.09; *P* interaction = 0.71). The prespecified analysis of first or recurrent ischemic events (all components of the primary endpoint) suggested a lower risk for prasugrel among patients under the age of 75 years (HR, 0.85; 95% CI, 0.72–1.00; $P = 0.04$). Rates of severe and intracranial bleeding were similar in the two groups in all age groups.[54] Therefore the findings of the TRILOGY ACS trial do not support the use of prasugrel in patients who are managed without coronary revascularization.

The 2025 AHA/ACC Guidelines for the Management of Patients with ACS offers a class I recommendation for the use of clopidogrel, prasugrel, or ticagrelor (see later) on a background of ASA in patients with ACS who are undergoing PCI, with consideration to be given to preferential use of prasugrel or ticagrelor as a class I recommendation.[55] There is no distinction in the recommendations with regard to drug of choice based on DM status (see also Chapter 21).[56] If prasugrel is used, it should be given promptly and no later than 1 hour after PCI once the coronary anatomy is defined and the decision is made to proceed with PCI (see also Chapters 17 and 22). There is no apparent benefit and possible risk of harm if prasugrel is administered prior to coronary catheterization in patients with non-ST-elevation acute coronary syndromes.[57] Based on the findings from TRITON-TIMI 38, prasugrel should not be administered to patients with a history of stroke or transient ischemic attack (TIA). In patients over the age of 75 years, the use of prasugrel is generally not recommended but may be considered in high-risk patients such as those with DM. A lower dose of 5 mg daily can be considered in patients over the age of 75 or who weigh less than 60 kg. It is generally recommended that prasugrel be continued for at least 12 months in ACS patients who undergo PCI. Earlier discontinuation of ASA or a P2Y12 receptor inhibitor or "de-escalation" of prasugrel or ticagrelor to clopidogrel can be considered in patients in whom the anticipated morbidity from bleeding exceeds its benefits.

Ticagrelor

Ticagrelor is the first reversibly binding oral P2Y12 receptor antagonist.[58] It is a nonthienopyridine and does not require metabolism to form its active metabolite. It has been shown to bind the P2Y12 receptor with a noncompetitive binding mechanism toward ADP. Similar to prasugrel, ticagrelor demonstrates rapid onset of action and decreased interpatient variability as compared with clopidogrel. Because of an elimination half-life of 7 hours and its reversible binding characteristics, it is administered twice daily. However, its antiplatelet effects have been shown to extend to approximately 120 hours.[58] Although it is more potent than clopidogrel, its ability to inhibit platelet aggregation is roughly equivalent to that of clopidogrel at 24 hours after drug discontinuation because of its faster offset kinetics. Ticagrelor may therefore be less likely than clopidogrel to increase the risk of bleeding in patients who require surgery 48 to 120 hours after the last dose.[58]

The Study of Platelet Inhibition and Patient Outcomes (PLATO) trial evaluated the safety and efficacy of ticagrelor in 18,624 patients across the spectrum of ACS (see also Chapter 21).[59] Patients were randomized to clopidogrel (300- to 600-mg loading dose, 75 mg daily) or ticagrelor (180-mg loading dose, 90 mg daily). At 12 months, ticagrelor reduced the risk of vascular death, MI, or stroke by 16% (HR, 0.84; 95% CI, 0.77–0.92), as compared with clopidogrel. In addition, ticagrelor reduced the risk of death from vascular causes (4.0% vs. 5.1%; $P = 0.001$) and all-cause mortality (4.5% vs. 5.9% with clopidogrel; $P < 0.001$), but increased the risk of non-CABG-related Thrombolysis in Myocardial Infarction (TIMI) major bleeding by 25% ($P = 0.03$). Of the P2Y12 inhibitors that have been evaluated to date, ticagrelor is the only drug to have demonstrated a mortality benefit across the spectrum of ACS. However, ticagrelor did not increase the risk of fatal bleeding ($P = 0.66$) or CABG-related major bleeding ($P = 0.32$).

The relative benefit of ticagrelor appeared to be comparable in patients with and without diabetes in PLATO, although the absolute benefits were greater in insulin-treated patients with diabetes.[60] Ticagrelor reduced the risk of vascular death, MI, or stroke by 12% in patients with diabetes (HR, 0.88; 95% CI, 0.76–1.03) versus 17% in patients without diabetes (HR, 0.83; 95% CI, 0.74–0.92; *P* interaction = 0.49; Fig. 20.6). Similarly, in patients with diabetes, ticagrelor reduced the risk of all-cause mortality (HR, 0.82; 95% CI, 0.66–1.01) and stent thrombosis (HR, 0.65; 95% CI, 0.36–1.17) to an extent that was consistent with the overall cohort. Ticagrelor tended to increase non–CABG-related PLATO major bleeding in both patients with and without diabetes (HR, 1.13; 95% CI, 0.86–1.49; HR, 1.22; 95% CI, 1.01–1.46, respectively; *P* interaction = 0.69). There was no heterogeneity in the efficacy or safety of ticagrelor with regard to patients who were or were not treated with insulin.[60]

If patients with diabetes indeed derive enhanced benefit from more potent antiplatelet therapy after ACS, it is unclear why these findings were not observed in the PLATO trial. In patients who are hyporesponsive to clopidogrel, switching to ticagrelor has been shown to inhibit platelet aggregation to the same extent as it does when clopidogrel-responsive patients are treated with ticagrelor.[62] In this same study, almost all patients treated with ticagrelor (25% of whom had diabetes) achieved platelet reactivity levels below the threshold that has been shown to be associated with an increased risk of ischemic events, regardless of their clopidogrel response status.[62]

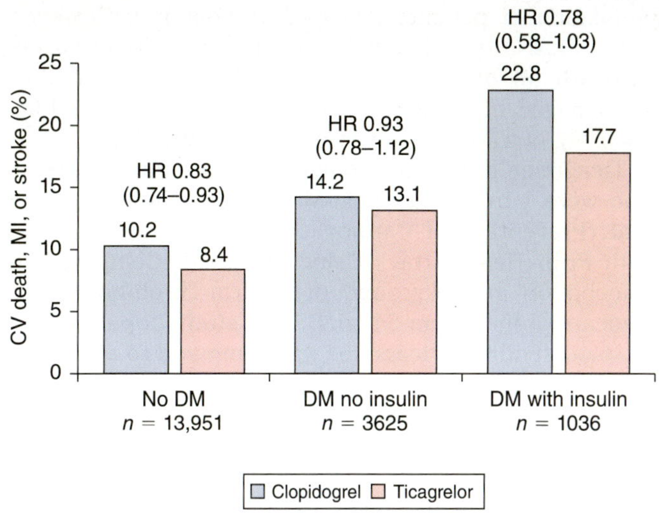

FIG. 20.6 Clinical events and comparative efficacy (hazard ratio [HR], 95% confidence interval [CI]) of ticagrelor versus clopidogrel for patients without diabetes mellitus (DM), patients with diabetes not treated with insulin, and patients with diabetes treated with insulin in the PLATO trial. The absolute benefit of ticagrelor appeared largest in patients with diabetes treated with insulin, although the relative benefits were similar in all three groups.[61] *CV*, Cardiovascular; *MI*, myocardial infarction. Modified from James S, Angiolillo DJ, Cornel JH, et al. Ticagrelor vs. clopidogrel in patients with acute coronary syndromes and diabetes: a substudy from the PLATelet inhibition and patient Outcomes (PLATO) trial. *Eur Heart J.* 2010;31:3006–3016.

There are relatively limited head-to-head data to compare the pharmacodynamic or clinical efficacy of prasugrel with that of ticagrelor. In a study of 44 patients with ACS (23% of whom had DM) and high on-treatment platelet reactivity on clopidogrel, patients were randomized in a double-blind crossover design to either ticagrelor 90 mg twice daily or prasugrel 10 mg daily without a loading dose for 15 days before crossing over to the alternate therapy.[63] At the end of the two treatment periods, ticagrelor achieved a greater degree of platelet inhibition than prasugrel ($P < 0.001$). Both drugs were effective at reducing platelet reactivity below the predefined threshold for poor response.[63] In the open-label ISAR-REACT (Intracoronary Stenting and Antithrombotic Regimen: Rapid Early Action for Coronary Treatment)-5 trial, 4018 persons with ACS and a planned invasive approach were randomized to prasugrel or ticagrelor. Although the investigator had hypothesized that ticagrelor would yield superior results, those treated with ticagrelor were at excess risk of MACE (death, MI, or stroke) when compared to ticagrelor (HR, 1.36; 95% CI, 1.09–1.70; $P = 0.006$). Despite the lower risk of MACE for patients treated with prasugrel, the risk of major bleeding with ticagrelor versus prasugrel was grossly similar (HR, 1.12; 95% CI, 0.83–1.51; $P = 0.46$).[64] Based on these findings, the European Society of Cardiology guidelines now state that prasugrel can be considered preferentially over ticagrelor in patients with NSTE-ACS,[52] though this remains a controversial recommendation.

Unlike with prasugrel, the benefit of ticagrelor has not been directly assessed in a dedicated trial of an ACS population of patients managed without PCI. However, in the PLATO trial, ticagrelor reduced the risk of vascular death, MI, or stroke in patients who were intended to be managed noninvasively (HR, 0.85; 95% CI, 0.73–1.00; $P = 0.04$), of whom 29% eventually underwent PCI.[65]

Ticagrelor has been studied in more stable patients who were 1 to 3 years post-MI in the PEGASUS-TIMI 54 trial (Prevention of Cardiovascular Events in Patients With Prior Heart Attack Using Ticagrelor Compared to Placebo on a Background of Aspirin-Thrombolysis in Myocardial Infarction 54 trial). In a study population of 21,162 individuals, ticagrelor was compared to a placebo at the standard dose of 90 mg twice daily and a reduced dose of 60 mg twice daily. Both doses of ticagrelor significantly reduced the risk of MACE (HR, 0.85; 95% CI, 0.75–0.96; $P = 0.008$; HR, 0.84; 95% CI, 0.74–0.95; $P = 0.004$, respectively), but increased the risk of major bleeding. The relative excess in bleeding was lower with 60 mg twice daily, thereby supporting the concept that ticagrelor can be reduced to a lower dose 12 months after ACS without diminishing its efficacy.[66] In those with DM (n = 6806), ticagrelor reduced cardiovascular death by 22% and CHD death by 34%. Although the overall efficacy and safety of ticagrelor were similar for those with or without DM, the number needed to treat to prevent a MACE event was smaller for those with DM than those without over 3 years (67 vs. 91), owing to a higher event rate[67] in those with DM.

Ticagrelor has also been studied in 19,220 persons with DM and stable coronary disease in the THEMIS (Effect of Ticagrelor on Health Outcomes in Diabetes Mellitus Patients Intervention Study) trial who were at high risk for cardiovascular events, but who had not had prior MI or stroke. Over a median follow-up time of 39.9 months, ticagrelor reduced the risk of CV death, MI, or stroke by 10% (HR, 0.90; 95% CI, 0.81–0.99; $P = 0.04$). The risk of TIMI major bleeding (HR, 2.32; 95% CI, 1.82–2.94; $P < 0.001$) and intracranial hemorrhage (HR, 1.71; 95% CI, 1.18–2.48; $P = 0.005$) was increased when compared to a placebo.[68] When the types of MIs were examined, ticagrelor reduced spontaneous MI (type 1) and MI related to stent thrombosis (type 4b), in addition to the risk of STEMI.[61] In those patients who had undergone PCI (n = 11,154), ticagrelor demonstrated greater net clinical benefit (HR, 0.85; 95% CI, 0.75–0.95; $P = 0.005$)[69] and that net benefit was consistent across diabetes-related factors, including DM duration, HbA1c, and background use of antihyperglycemic therapies.[70]

OTHER ORAL ANTIPLATELET MEDICATIONS

Cilostazol

Cilostazol is a phosphodiesterase III inhibitor that raises cyclic adenosine monophosphate (cAMP) levels in platelets and vascular smooth muscle cells, leading to inhibition of platelet activation and arteriolar vasodilation.[71] When cilostazol was added to a background of dual antiplatelet therapy, nonrandomized studies demonstrated that this agent appeared to reduce the risk of stent thrombosis[72,73] and ischemic events,[73,74] without a significant increase in bleeding. Thus far, randomized trials of triple antiplatelet therapy in patients after PCI have yielded conflicting results, although most trials have been underpowered for clinical outcomes (see also Chapter 17).[75] In the Efficacy of Cilostazol on Ischemic Complications after Drug-Eluting Stent Implantation (CILON-T) trial, the addition of cilostazol failed to reduce the risk of cardiac death, nonfatal MI, ischemic stroke, or target lesion revascularization in patients after DES implantation (8.5% vs. 9.2%; $P = 0.74$), despite achieving a reduction in platelet reactivity.[75] In contrast, in a second trial of patients after ACS undergoing PCI, cilostazol reduced the risk of cardiac death, nonfatal MI, stroke, or target vessel revascularization (10.3% vs. 15.1%; $P = 0.011$) when added to ASA and clopidogrel.[76] In the latter study, the benefit of cilostazol appeared to be enhanced in patients with high-risk clinical or angiographic features, including DM (n = 263; 9.9% vs. 18.9%; HR, 0.47; 95% CI, 0.23–0.96).[76]

These findings are supported by pharmacodynamic data that have shown that cilostazol enhances inhibition of P2Y12 signaling in patients with diabetes.[77] Cilostazol, combined with standard-dose clopidogrel, reduces platelet reactivity to a greater extent than clopidogrel 150 mg daily in patients with type 2 DM.[78] The greater pharmacodynamic effect of cilostazol in patients with diabetes was observed, regardless of whether or not patients carried genetic polymorphisms that have been shown to influence response to clopidogrel.[78] These findings may, in part, explain the ability of cilostazol to reduce the risk of ischemic events in high-risk patients. To that end, the antiplatelet effects of cilostazol appear to be enhanced in patients with diabetes[79] and patients with high on-treatment platelet reactivity.[80,81]

In addition to its antiplatelet effects, cilostazol is hypothesized to exert pleiotropic effects, including inhibition of neointimal hyperplasia. Supporting this concept, a systematic review that combined data from 23 randomized trials of cilostazol suggested that it may reduce the risk of in-stent restenosis (RR, 0.60; 95% CI, 0.49–0.73) and need for repeat revascularization (RR, 0.69; 95% CI, 0.55–0.86) without a significant increase in bleeding (RR, 0.71; 95% CI, 0.43–1.16) in patients after PCI.[82] In a dedicated trial of patients with diabetes receiving a DES, the addition of cilostazol to ASA and clopidogrel reduced angiographic restenosis and extent of late luminal loss, thereby leading to a lower rate of target lesion revascularization at 9 months as compared with dual antiplatelet therapy alone.[83] Although the study was underpowered for clinical events, the incidence of MACE tended to be lower in the triple than in the dual antiplatelet therapy group (3.0% vs. 7.0%; $P = 0.066$).[83] However, the use of cilostazol is limited by a high frequency of side effects, including headache, GI disturbance, and palpitations. Larger, more definitive studies of cilostazol are therefore needed before it can be routinely used as an adjunct to dual antiplatelet therapy after coronary stenting. A planned large trial of cilostazol was terminated early due to slow enrollment, but again suggested a lower risk of target-vessel revascularization.[84] The European Medicines Agency issued a warning in 2018 to restrict the use of cilostazol on the basis of bleeding concerns.[85]

Dipyridamole

Dipyridamole exhibits a number of properties that contribute to platelet inhibition and vasodilation. Dipyridamole inhibits thromboxane synthase, leading to reduced TXA_2 production and thereby reduced platelet activation.[86] It inhibits adenosine deaminase and cellular reuptake of adenosine into platelets, erythrocytes, and endothelial cells causing extracellular adenosine levels to rise.[86] Dipyridamole is also a phosphodiesterase inhibitor leading to higher cAMP and cyclic guanosine monophosphate (cGMP) levels within platelets and endothelial cells and thereby blocking response to ADP via the P2Y12 receptor and enhancing nitric oxide signaling.[86,87]

Although there are limited data to support the use of dipyridamole in patients with CHD, its use has been extensively studied in patients with cerebrovascular disease in combination with ASA. In the European Stroke Prevention Study (ESPS), the combination of ASA (330 mg) and dipyridamole (75 mg) three times daily reduced the risk of all-cause mortality or stroke by 33.5%, compared with a placebo in patients with a recent stroke or TIA.[88] Moreover, the benefit appeared to be further enhanced in patients with diabetes versus those without diabetes (48% vs. 32%, respectively).[89] Furthermore, it appears that the effects of dipyridamole and ASA are additive.[90] In patients with recent stroke or TIA, the combination of dipyridamole (400 mg daily) and ASA (50 mg daily) reduced the risk of stroke by 37% compared with a placebo, whereas dipyridamole alone reduced the risk of stroke by 16% and ASA alone by 18%.[90] In the open-label European/Australasian Stroke Prevention in Reversible Ischaemia Trial (ESPRIT), the combination of ASA plus dipyridamole (200 mg twice daily) reduced the risk of CV death, MI, stroke, or major bleeding by 20% (HR, 0.80; 95% CI, 0.66–0.98), as compared with ASA alone (30–325 mg daily) in patients with a history of an acute cerebrovascular event.[91] An increased frequency of headache contributed to a higher rate of discontinuation in the dipyridamole group.[91] Currently, there is no role for dipyridamole for the purpose of reduction of coronary risk.

PROTEASE-ACTIVATED RECEPTOR-1 ANTAGONISTS

Vorapaxar

Thrombin stimulates platelet activation via protease-activated receptor-1 (PAR-1), the major thrombin receptor on the platelet cell surface. Although extensive research has been directed toward the ADP-dependent P2Y12 receptor, thrombin is the most potent platelet agonist.[92] Because ASA and clopidogrel do not interfere with PAR-1–dependent platelet activation, patients on standard dual antiplatelet therapy remain at risk of recurrent CV events via alternate pathways of platelet activation.

Vorapaxar is a competitive and selective antagonist of PAR-1 that acts by binding at or near the tethered ligand binding site.[92] Because PAR-1 receptor antagonists selectively interfere with thrombin-mediated platelet activation without disrupting the coagulation cascade or ADP-dependent platelet activation, it was hypothesized that PAR-1 receptor antagonists might reduce the risk of ischemic events without significantly increasing the risk of bleeding. This hypothesis was supported by phase II studies that suggested trends toward efficacy with increasing doses of vorapaxar and without a significant increase in major bleeding.[93]

Vorapaxar was subsequently evaluated in two large-scale clinical trials of patients with stable atherosclerotic disease or ACS, the Trial to Assess the Effects of SCH 530348 in Preventing Heart Attack and Stroke in Patients with Atherosclerosis (TRA2°P-TIMI 50) and the Trial to Assess the Effects of SCH 530348 in Preventing Heart Attack and Stroke in Patients with Acute Coronary Syndrome (TRA-CER), respectively. In January 2011, the joint Data and Safety Monitoring Board for the two trials reported an excess in intracranial hemorrhage in patients with a history of stroke. As a consequence, the study drug was discontinued in the TRA2°P-TIMI 50 trial for patients with a history of stroke, but the trial continued to completion in patients with a history of MI or PAD. The TRA-CER trial was stopped prematurely after reaching its prespecified number of primary endpoints.

In the 26,449 patients with stable atherosclerotic disease enrolled in the TRA2°P-TIMI 50 trial, vorapaxar (2.5 mg daily) significantly reduced the risk of CV death, MI, or stroke by 13% and the risk of CV death, MI, stroke, or urgent coronary revascularization by 12% (HR, 0.88; 95% CI, 0.82–0.95) as compared with a placebo during a median follow-up of 2.5 years.[94] Although vorapaxar reduced the risk of recurrent CV events, vorapaxar increased the risk of moderate or severe bleeding by 66% (HR, 1.66; 95% CI, 1.43–1.93), including a significant increase in the risk of intracranial hemorrhage. The rate of fatal bleeding was not significantly increased in the vorapaxar group. The efficacy and safety of vorapaxar were consistent in patients with or without DM (*P* interaction = 0.61 for CV death, MI, or stroke; *P* interaction = 0.79 for Global Utilization of Streptokinase and Tissue Plasminogen Activator for Occluded Coronary Arteries [GUSTO] moderate or severe bleeding). No heterogeneity was observed on the basis of background thienopyridine use. In patients with peripheral artery disease, vorapaxar reduced acute limb ischemia and peripheral revascularization.[95]

The balance between efficacy and safety appeared to be most favorable for vorapaxar in patients with a history of MI more than 1 month before randomization in the TRA°2P-TIMI 50 trial.[96] Of the 17,779 patients within this prespecified subgroup, vorapaxar significantly reduced the risk of CV death, MI, or stroke by 20% (HR, 0.80; 95% CI, 0.72–0.89), including a 21% reduction in the risk of MI (HR, 0.79; 95% CI, 0.70–0.89) and a 34% reduction in the risk of ischemic stroke (HR, 0.66; 95% CI, 0.48–0.89). Moderate or severe bleeding remained more common in patients treated with vorapaxar as compared with patients on placebo (HR, 1.61; 95% CI, 1.31–1.97). Within this subgroup of patients, intracranial hemorrhage was infrequent and not statistically increased for patients on vorapaxar (0.6% vs. 0.4%; *P* = 0.076).[96]

Despite an observed trend toward efficacy, vorapaxar was not superior to a placebo for the management of patients with ACS in the TRA-CER trial.[97] Vorapaxar (40-mg loading dose, 2.5 mg daily) did not significantly reduce the risk of the primary endpoint of CV death, MI, recurrent ischemia with hospitalization, or urgent coronary revascularization (HR, 0.92; 95% CI, 0.85–1.017) in patients after ACS. Vorapaxar did reduce the key secondary endpoint of CV death, MI, or stroke by 11% compared with placebo (HR, 0.89; 95% CI, 0.81–0.98), including a 12% reduction in MI (HR, 0.88; 95% CI, 0.79–0.98). Consistent with the findings from the TRA°2P-TIMI 50 trial, vorapaxar increased the risk of GUSTO moderate or severe bleeding (HR, 1.35; 95% CI, 1.16–1.58) and intracranial hemorrhage (HR, 3.39; 95% CI, 1.78–6.45) in patients after ACS.

FUTURE DIRECTIONS

As the prevalence of DM continues to grow, there will be an urgent need to develop therapies that may help to attenuate CV risk in this high-risk population. In addition to the antiplatelet drugs reviewed in this chapter, several novel antiplatelet drugs remain in development. These include therapies that target the PAR-1 and PAR-4 receptors, as well as GPVI antagonists and C-type Lectin-like Receptors (CLEC-2). Inhibitors of the von Willebrand factor and GPIbα are an additional area of investigation. An extended-release ASA formulation is now available in some countries that allows for more prolonged absorption and more prolonged platelet exposure to the drug.[98] As more potent or alternate antiplatelet therapies undergo clinical evaluation, continued emphasis will need to be placed on achieving the optimal balance between efficacy and safety.

REFERENCES

1. Ferreiro JL, Angiolillo DJ. Diabetes and antiplatelet therapy in acute coronary syndrome. *Circulation*. 2011;123:798–813.
2. Bhatt DL. What makes platelets angry: diabetes, fibrinogen, obesity, and impaired response to antiplatelet therapy? *J Am Coll Cardiol*. 2008;52:1060–1061.
3. Vinik AI, Erbas T, Park TS, Davi G. Platelet dysfunction in type 2 diabetes. *Diabetes Care*. 2001;24:1476–1485.
4. Ferroni P, Basili S, Falco A, et al. Platelet activation in type 2 diabetes mellitus. *J Thromb Haemost*. 2004;2:1282–1291.
5. Patrono C, Garcia Rodriguez LA, Landolfi R, Baigent C. Low-dose aspirin for the prevention of atherothrombosis. *N Engl J Med*. 2005;353:2373–2383.
6. Steering Committee of the Physicians' Health Study Research Group. Final report on the aspirin component of the ongoing Physicians' Health Study. *N Engl J Med*. 1989;321:129–135.
7. Hansson L, Zanchetti A, Carruthers SG, et al. Effects of intensive blood-pressure lowering and low-dose aspirin in patients with hypertension: principal results of the Hypertension Optimal Treatment (HOT) randomised trial. HOT Study Group. *Lancet*. 1998;351:1755–1762.
8. de Gaetano G. Low-dose aspirin and vitamin E in people at cardiovascular risk: a randomised trial in general practice. Collaborative Group of the Primary Prevention Project. *Lancet*. 2001;357:89–95.
9. Aspirin effects on mortality and morbidity in patients with diabetes mellitus. Early Treatment Diabetic Retinopathy Study report 14. ETDRS Investigators. *JAMA*. 1992;268:1292–1300.
10. Ogawa H, Nakayama M, Morimoto T, et al. Low-dose aspirin for primary prevention of atherosclerotic events in patients with type 2 diabetes: a randomized controlled trial. *JAMA*. 2008;300:2134–2141.
11. Belch J, MacCuish A, Campbell I, et al. The prevention of progression of arterial disease and diabetes (POPADAD) trial: factorial randomised placebo controlled trial of aspirin and antioxidants in patients with diabetes and asymptomatic peripheral arterial disease. *BMJ*. 2008;337:a1840.
12. Yasuo Ikeda, Kazuyuki Shimada, Tamio Teramoto, et al. Low-dose aspirin for primary prevention of cardiovascular events in Japanese patients 60 years or older with atherosclerotic risk factors: a randomized clinical trial. *JAMA*. 2014;312(23):2510–2520. https://doi.org/10.1001/jama.2014.15690. PMID: 25401325.
13. McNeil JJ, Woods RL, Nelson MR, et al. ASPREE Investigator Group. Effect of aspirin on disability-free survival in the healthy elderly. *N Engl J Med*. 2018;379:1499–1508. https://doi.org/10.1056/NEJMoa1800722.
14. McNeil JJ, Wolfe R, Woods RL, et al. ASPREE Investigator Group Effect of aspirin on cardiovascular events and bleeding in the healthy elderly. *N Engl J Med*. 2018;379:1509–1518. https://doi.org/10.1056/NEJMoa1805819.
15. Bowman L, Mafham M, Wallendszus K, et al. Effects of aspirin for primary prevention in persons with diabetes mellitus. *N Engl J Med*. 2018;379:1529–1539. https://doi.org/10.1056/NEJMoa180498.
16. Zheng Sean L, Roddick Alistair J. Association of aspirin use for primary prevention with cardiovascular events and bleeding events: a systematic review and meta-analysis. *JAMA*. 2019;321(3):277–287. https://doi.org/10.1001/jama.2018.20578. PMID: 30667501 PMCID: PMC6439678.
17. American Diabetes Association 9. Cardiovascular disease and risk management: standards of medical care in diabetes-2018. *Diabetes Care*. 2018;41(suppl 1):S86–S104. https://doi.org/10.2337/dc18-S009. (January).
18. Arnett DK, Blumenthal RS, Albert MA. ACC/AHA Guideline on the primary prevention of cardiovascular disease: a report of the American College of Cardiology/American Heart Association Task Force on Clinical Practice Guidelines. *Circulation*. 2019;140:e596–e646. https://doi.org/10.1161/CIR.0000000000000678.
19. US Preventive Services Task Force; Davidson KW, Barry MJ, Mangione CM, et al. Aspirin use to prevent cardiovascular disease: US Preventive Services Task Force recommendation statement. *JAMA*. 2022;327(16):1577–1584. https://doi.org/10.1001/jama.2022.4983.
20. Visseren et al. 2021 ESC Guidelines on cardiovascular disease prevention in clinical practice. *Eur Heart J*. 2021;42(34):3227–3337. https://doi.org/10.1093/eurheartj/ehab484
21. American Diabetes Association 10. Cardiovascular disease and risk management: standards of medical care in diabetes 2019. *Diabetes Care*. 2019;42:S103–S123. https://doi.org/10.2337/dc19-S010.
22. Cosentin F, Grant PJ, Aboyans V, et al. 2019 ESC Guidelines on diabetes, prediabetes, and cardiovascular diseases developed in collaboration with the EASD. *Eur Heart J*. 2020;41:255–323.
23. Randomised trial of intravenous streptokinase oral aspirin, both, or neither among 17,187 cases of suspected acute myocardial infarction: ISIS-2. ISIS-2 (Second International Study of Infarct Survival) Collaborative Group. *Lancet*. 1988;2:349–360.
24. Antithrombotic Trialists' Collaboration. Collaborative meta-analysis of randomised trials of antiplatelet therapy for prevention of death, myocardial infarction, and stroke in high risk patients. *BMJ*. 2002;324:71–86.
25. Steinhubl SR, Bhatt DL, Brennan DM, et al. Aspirin to prevent cardiovascular disease: the association of aspirin dose and clopidogrel with thrombosis and bleeding. *Ann Intern Med*. 2009;150:379–386.
26. Mehta SR, Bassand JP, Chrolavicius S, et al. CURRENT-OASIS 7 Investigators. Dose comparisons of clopidogrel and aspirin in acute coronary syndromes. *N Engl J Med*. 2010;363:930–942.
27. Jones WSchuyler, Mulder Hillary, Wruck Lisa M, et al. ADAPTABLE Team. Comparative effectiveness of aspirin dosing in cardiovascular disease. *N Engl J Med*. 2021 May 27;384(21):1981–1990. https://doi.org/10.1056/NEJMoa2102137. Epub 2021 May 15. PMID: 33999548 PMCID: PMC9908069.
28. Gachet C. ADP receptors of platelets and their inhibition. *Thromb Haemost*. 2001;86:222–232.
29. CAPRIE Steering Committee. A randomised, blinded, trial of clopidogrel versus aspirin in patients at risk of ischaemic events (CAPRIE). *Lancet*. 1996;348:1329–1339.
30. Bhatt DL, Marso SP, Hirsch AT, et al. Amplified benefit of clopidogrel versus aspirin in patients with diabetes mellitus. *Am J Cardiol*. 2002;90:625–628.
31. Colwell JA. Aspirin therapy in diabetes. *Diabetes Care*. 2004;27(Suppl 1):S72–S73.
32. Bon-Kwon Koo, Jeehoon Kang, Kyung Woo Park, et al. HOST-EXAM investigators. Aspirin versus clopidogrel for chronic maintenance monotherapy after percutaneous coronary intervention (HOST-EXAM): an investigator-initiated, prospective, randomised, open-label, multicentre trial. *Lancet*. 2021 Jun 26;397(10293):2487–2496. https://doi.org/10.1016/S0140-6736(21)01063-1. Epub 2021 May 16. PMID: 34010616.
33. Yusuf S, Zhao F, Mehta SR, et al. Effects of clopidogrel in addition to aspirin in patients with acute coronary syndromes without ST-segment elevation. *N Engl J Med*. 2001;345:494–502.
34. Angiolillo DJ, Shoemaker SB, Desai B, et al. Randomized comparison of a high clopidogrel maintenance dose in patients with diabetes mellitus and coronary artery disease: results of the Optimizing Antiplatelet Therapy in Diabetes Mellitus (OPTIMUS) study. *Circulation*. 2007;115:708–716.
35. Angiolillo DJ, Bernardo E, Ramírez C, et al. Insulin therapy is associated with platelet dysfunction in patients with type 2 diabetes mellitus on dual oral antiplatelet treatment. *J Am Coll Cardiol*. 2006;48:298–304.
36. Bhatt DL, Fox KA, Hacke W, et al. Clopidogrel and aspirin versus aspirin alone for the prevention of atherothrombotic events. *N Engl J Med*. 2006;354:1706–1717.
37. Bhatt DL, Flather MD, Hacke W, et al. Patients with prior myocardial infarction, stroke, or symptomatic peripheral arterial disease in the CHARISMA trial. *J Am Coll Cardiol*. 2007;49:1982–1988.
38. Shuldiner AR, O'Connell JR, Bliden KP, et al. Association of cytochrome P450 2C19 genotype with the antiplatelet effect and clinical efficacy of clopidogrel therapy. *JAMA*. 2009;302:849–857.
39. O'Donoghue M, Wiviott SD. Clopidogrel response variability and future therapies: clopidogrel: does one size fit all? *Circulation*. 2006;114:e600–e606.

40. Angiolillo DJ, Bernardo E, Sabate M, et al. Impact of platelet reactivity on cardiovascular outcomes in patients with type 2 diabetes mellitus and coronary artery disease. *J Am Coll Cardiol*. 2007;50:1541–1547.
41. Gurbel PA, Bliden KP, Hiatt BL, O'Connor CM. Clopidogrel for coronary stenting: response variability, drug resistance, and the effect of pretreatment platelet reactivity. *Circulation*. 2003;107:2908–2913.
42. Mega JL, Simon T, Collet JP, et al. Reduced-function CYP2C19 genotype and risk of adverse clinical outcomes among patients treated with clopidogrel predominantly for PCI: a meta-analysis. *JAMA*. 2010;304:1821–1830.
43. Michno A, Bielarczyk H, Pawelczyk T, et al. Alterations of adenine nucleotide metabolism and function of blood platelets in patients with diabetes. *Diabetes*. 2007;56:462–467.
44. Ferreira IA, Mocking AI, Feijge MA, et al. Platelet inhibition by insulin is absent in type 2 diabetes mellitus. *Arterioscler Thromb Vasc Biol*. 2006;26: 417–422.
45. Li Y, Woo V, Bose R. Platelet hyperactivity and abnormal $Ca(2^{+})$ homeostasis in diabetes mellitus. *Am J Physiol Heart Circ Physiol*. 2001;280:H1480–H1489.
46. Guthikonda S, Alviar CL, Vaduganathan M, et al. Role of reticulated platelets and platelet size heterogeneity on platelet activity after dual antiplatelet therapy with aspirin and clopidogrel in patients with stable coronary artery disease. *J Am Coll Cardiol*. 2008;52:743–749.
47. Wiviott SD, Trenk D, Frelinger AL, et al. Prasugrel compared with high loading- and maintenance-dose clopidogrel in patients with planned percutaneous coronary intervention: the Prasugrel in Comparison to Clopidogrel for Inhibition of Platelet Activation and Aggregation-Thrombolysis in Myocardial Infarction 44 trial. *Circulation*. 2007;116:2923–2932.
48. Jakubowski JA, Winters KJ, Naganuma H, Wallentin L. Prasugrel: a novel thienopyridine antiplatelet agent. A review of preclinical and clinical studies and the mechanistic basis for its distinct antiplatelet profile. *Cardiovasc Drug Rev*. 2007;25:357–374.
49. Wiviott SD, Braunwald E, McCabe CH, et al. Prasugrel versus clopidogrel in patients with acute coronary syndromes. *N Engl J Med*. 2007;357:2001–2015.
50. Bhatt DL. Intensifying platelet inhibition—navigating between Scylla and Charybdis. *N Engl J Med*. 2007;357:2078–2081.
51. Wiviott SD, Braunwald E, Angiolillo DJ, et al. Greater clinical benefit of more intensive oral antiplatelet therapy with prasugrel in patients with diabetes mellitus in the trial to assess improvement in therapeutic outcomes by optimizing platelet inhibition with prasugrel-Thrombolysis in Myocardial Infarction 38. *Circulation*. 2008;118:1626–1636.
52. Collet JP, Thiele H, Barbato E, et al. 2020 ESC Guidelines for the management of acute coronary syndromes in patients presenting without persistent ST-segment elevation. *Eur Heart J*. 2021;42(14):1289–1367. https://doi.org/10.1093/eurheartj/ehaa575.
53. Angiolillo DJ, Badimon JJ, Saucedo JF, et al. A pharmacodynamic comparison of prasugrel vs. high-dose clopidogrel in patients with type 2 diabetes mellitus and coronary artery disease: results of the Optimizing anti-Platelet Therapy In diabetes MellitUS (OPTIMUS)-3 Trial. *Eur Heart J*. 2011;32: 838–846.
54. Roe MT, Armstrong PW, Fox KA, et al. Prasugrel versus clopidogrel for acute coronary syndromes without revascularization. *N Engl J Med*. 2012.
55. Rao SV, O'Donoghue ML, Ruel M, Rab T, et al. 2025 ACC/AHA/ACEP/NAEMSP/SCAI guideline for the management of patients with acute coronary syndromes: A report of the American College of Cardiology/American Heart Association Joint Committee on Clinical Practice Guidelines. *Circulation*. 2025;151(13):e771–e862. https://doi.org/10.1161/CIR.0000000000001309.
56. Jneid H, Anderson JL, Wright RS, et al. 2012 Writing Committee Members 2012 ACCF/AHA focused update of the guideline for the management of patients with unstable angina/non-ST-elevation myocardial infarction (updating the 2007 guideline and replacing the 2011 focused update): a report of the American College of Cardiology Foundation/American Heart Association Task Force on practice guidelines. *Circulation*. 2012;126:875–910.
57. Gilles M, Leonardo B, Dariusz D, et al. ACCOAST Investigators. Pretreatment with prasugrel in non-ST-segment elevation acute coronary syndromes. *N Engl J Med*. 2013;369:999–1010. https://doi.org/10.1056/NEJMoa1308075. Epub 2013 Sep 1. PMID: 23991622.
58. Gurbel PA, Bliden KP, Butler K, et al. Randomized double-blind assessment of the ONSET and OFFSET of the antiplatelet effects of ticagrelor versus clopidogrel in patients with stable coronary artery disease: the ONSET/OFFSET study. *Circulation*. 2009;120:2577–2585.
59. Wallentin L, Becker RC, Budaj A, et al. Ticagrelor versus clopidogrel in patients with acute coronary syndromes. *N Engl J Med*. 2009;361:1045–1057.
60. James S, Angiolillo DJ, Cornel JH, et al. Ticagrelor vs. clopidogrel in patients with acute coronary syndromes and diabetes: a substudy from the PLATelet inhibition and patient Outcomes (PLATO) trial. *Eur Heart J*. 2010;31:3006–3016.
61. Abtan Jeremie, Bhatt Deepak L, Held Claes, et al. Incidence of myocardial infarction types in patients treated with ticagrelor in the THEMIS trial. *Circ Cardiovasc Interv*. 2021;14(12):e011035. https://doi.org/10.1161/CIRCINTERVENTIONS.120.011035. Epub 2021 Nov 24. PMID: 34814698.
62. Gurbel PA, Bliden KP, Butler K, et al. Response to ticagrelor in clopidogrel nonresponders and responders and effect of switching therapies: the RESPOND study. *Circulation*. 2010;121:1188–1199.
63. Alexopoulos D, Galati A, Xanthopoulou I, et al. Ticagrelor versus prasugrel in acute coronary syndrome patients with high on-clopidogrel platelet reactivity following percutaneous coronary intervention: a pharmacodynamic study. *J Am Coll Cardiol*. 2012;60:193–199.
64. Stefanie Schüpke, Franz-Josef Neumann, Maurizio Menichelli, et al. ISAR-REACT 5 Trial Investigators. Ticagrelor or prasugrel in patients with acute coronary syndromes. *N Engl J Med*. 2019;381(16):1524–1534. https://doi.org/10.1056/NEJMoa1908973. Epub 2019 Sep 1. PMID: 31475799.
65. James SK, Roe MT, Cannon CP, et al. Ticagrelor versus clopidogrel in patients with acute coronary syndromes intended for non-invasive management: substudy from prospective randomised PLATelet inhibition and patient Outcomes (PLATO) trial. *BMJ*. 2011;342:d3527.
66. Bonaca Marc P, Bhatt Deepak L, Cohen Marc, et al. Long-term use of ticagrelor in patients with prior myocardial infarction. *N Engl J Med*. 2015;372(19):1791–1800. https://doi.org/10.1056/NEJMoa1500857. Epub 2015 Mar 14. PMID: 25773268.
67. Bhatt Deepak L, Bonaca Marc P, Bansilal Sameer, et al. Reduction in ischemic events with ticagrelor in diabetic patients with prior myocardial infarction in PEGASUS-TIMI 54. *J Am Coll Cardiol*. 2016;67(23):2732–2740. https://doi.org/10.1016/j.jacc.2016.03.529. Epub 2016 Apr 1. PMID: 27046160.
68. Steg PGabriel, Bhatt Deepak L, Simon Tabassome, et al. THEMIS Steering Committee and Investigators. Ticagrelor in patients with stable coronary disease and diabetes. *N Engl J Med*. 2019;381(14):1309–1320. https://doi.org/10.1056/NEJMoa1908077. Epub 2019 Sep 1. PMID: 31475798.
69. Bhatt DL, Steg PG, Mehta SR, et al. Ticagrelor in patients with diabetes and stable coronary artery disease with a history of previous percutaneous coronary intervention (THEMIS-PCI): a phase 3, placebo-controlled, randomised trial. *Lancet*. 2019;394(10204):1169–1180. https://doi.org/10.1016/S0140-6736(19)31887-2.
70. Leiter Lawrence A, Bhatt Deepak L, McGuire Darren K, et al. THEMIS Steering Committee and Investigators. Diabetes-related factors and the effects of ticagrelor plus aspirin in the THEMIS and THEMIS-PCI trials. *J Am Coll Cardiol*. 2021 May 18;77(19):2366–2377. https://doi.org/10.1016/j.jacc.2021.03.298. PMID: 33985681.
71. Schrör K. The pharmacology of cilostazol. *Diab Obes Metab*. 2002;4(Suppl 2): S14–S19.
72. Lee SW, Park SW, Hong MK, et al. Triple versus dual antiplatelet therapy after coronary stenting: impact on stent thrombosis. *J Am Coll Cardiol*. 2005; 46:1833–1837.
73. Lee SW, Park SW, Yun SC, et al. Triple antiplatelet therapy reduces ischemic events after drug-eluting stent implantation: Drug-Eluting stenting followed by Cilostazol treatment REduces Adverse Serious cardiac Events (DECREASE registry). *Am Heart J*. 2010;159:284–291.e1.
74. Chen KY, Rha SW, Li YJ, et al. Triple versus dual antiplatelet therapy in patients with acute ST-segment elevation myocardial infarction undergoing primary percutaneous coronary intervention. *Circulation*. 2009;119:3207–3214.
75. Suh JW, Lee SP, Park KW, et al. Multicenter randomized trial evaluating the efficacy of cilostazol on ischemic vascular complications after drug-eluting stent implantation for coronary heart disease: results of the CILON-T (influence of CILostazol-based triple antiplatelet therapy ON ischemic complication after drug-eluting stenT implantation) trial. *J Am Coll Cardiol*. 2011; 57:280–289.
76. Han Y, Li Y, Wang S, et al. Cilostazol in addition to aspirin and clopidogrel improves long-term outcomes after percutaneous coronary intervention in patients with acute coronary syndromes: a randomized, controlled study. *Am Heart J*. 2009;157:733–739.
77. Angiolillo DJ, Capranzano P, Goto S, et al. A randomized study assessing the impact of cilostazol on platelet function profiles in patients with diabetes mellitus and coronary artery disease on dual antiplatelet therapy: results of the OPTIMUS-2 study. *Eur Heart J*. 2008;29:2202–2211.
78. Jeong YH, Tantry US, Park Y, et al. Pharmacodynamic effect of cilostazol plus standard clopidogrel versus double-dose clopidogrel in patients with type 2 diabetes undergoing percutaneous coronary intervention. *Diabetes Care*. 2012.
79. Angiolillo DJ, Capranzano P, Ferreiro JL, et al. Impact of adjunctive cilostazol therapy on platelet function profiles in patients with and without diabetes mellitus on aspirin and clopidogrel therapy. *Thromb Haemost*. 2011;106: 253–262.
80. Capranzano P, Ferreiro JL, Ueno M, et al. Pharmacodynamic effects of adjunctive cilostazol therapy in patients with coronary artery disease on dual antiplatelet therapy: impact of high on-treatment platelet reactivity and diabetes mellitus status. *Catheter Cardiovasc Interv*. 2012.
81. Jeong YH, Lee SW, Choi BR, et al. Randomized comparison of adjunctive cilostazol versus high maintenance dose clopidogrel in patients with high post-treatment platelet reactivity: results of the ACCEL-RESISTANCE (Adjunctive Cilostazol Versus High Maintenance Dose Clopidogrel in Patients With Clopidogrel Resistance) randomized study. *J Am Coll Cardiol*. 2009;53:1101–1109.
82. Biondi-Zoccai GG, Lotrionte M, Anselmino M, et al. Systematic review and meta-analysis of randomized clinical trials appraising the impact of cilostazol after percutaneous coronary intervention. *Am Heart J*. 2008;155:1081–1089.
83. Lee SW, Park SW, Kim YH, et al. Drug-eluting stenting followed by cilostazol treatment reduces late restenosis in patients with diabetes mellitus the DECLARE-DIABETES Trial (A Randomized Comparison of Triple Antiplatelet Therapy with Dual Antiplatelet Therapy After Drug-Eluting Stent Implantation in Diabetic Patients). *J Am Coll Cardiol*. 2008;51:1181–1187.
84. Lee CH, Lee JY, Park GM, et al. Comparison of 1-year outcomes of triple (aspirin + clopidogrel + cilostazol) versus dual antiplatelet therapy (aspirin + clopidogrel + placebo) after implantation of second-generation drug-eluting stents into one or more coronary arteries: from the DECREASE-PCI trial. *Am J Cardiol*. 2018;121(4):423–429. https://doi.org/10.1016/j.amjcard.2017.11.005.

85. European Medicines Agency. European Medicines Agency recommends restricting use of cilostazol-containing medicines. London: European Medicines Agency. Available at: http://www.ema.europa.eu/docs/en_GB/document_library/Referrals_document/Cilostazol_31/WC500140675.pdf.
86. Kim HH, Liao JK. Translational therapeutics of dipyridamole. *Arterioscler Thromb Vasc Biol*. 2008;28:s39–s42.
87. Aktas B, Utz A, Hoenig-Liedl P, et al. Dipyridamole enhances NO/cGMP-mediated vasodilator-stimulated phosphoprotein phosphorylation and signaling in human platelets: in vitro and in vivo/ex vivo studies. *Stroke*. 2003; 34:764–769.
88. ESPS Group. European stroke prevention study. *Stroke*. 1990;21:1122–1130.
89. Sivenius J, Laakso M, Riekkinen Sr. P, et al. European stroke prevention study: effectiveness of antiplatelet therapy in diabetic patients in secondary prevention of stroke. *Stroke*. 1992;23:851–854.
90. Diener HC, Cunha L, Forbes C, et al. European stroke prevention study. 2. Dipyridamole and acetylsalicylic acid in the secondary prevention of stroke. *J Neurol Sci*. 1996;143:1–13.
91. Halkes PH, van Gijn J, Kappelle LJ, et al. Aspirin plus dipyridamole versus aspirin alone after cerebral ischaemia of arterial origin (ESPRIT): randomised controlled trial. *Lancet*. 2006;367:1665–1673.
92. O'Donoghue ML, Bhatt DL, Wiviott SD, et al. Safety and tolerability of atopaxar in the treatment of patients with acute coronary syndromes: the lessons from antagonizing the cellular effects of Thrombin-Acute Coronary Syndromes Trial. *Circulation*. 2011;123:1843–1853.
93. Becker RC, Moliterno DJ, Jennings LK, et al. Safety and tolerability of SCH 530348 in patients undergoing non-urgent percutaneous coronary intervention: a randomised, double-blind, placebo-controlled phase II study. *Lancet*. 2009;373:919–928.
94. Morrow DA, Braunwald E, Bonaca MP, et al. Vorapaxar in the secondary prevention of atherothrombotic events. *N Engl J Med*. 2012;366:1404–1413.
95. Bonaca Marc P, Scirica Benjamin M, Creager Mark A, et al. Vorapaxar in patients with peripheral artery disease: results from TRA2°P-TIMI 50. *Circulation*. 2013;127(14):1522–1529. https://doi.org/10.1161/CIRCULATIONAHA.112.000679. Epub 2013 Mar 15. PMID: 23501976.
96. Scirica BM, Bonaca MP, Braunwald E, et al. Vorapaxar for secondary prevention of thrombotic events for patients with previous myocardial infarction: a prespecified subgroup analysis of the TRA 2 P-TIMI 50 trial. *Lancet*. 2012.
97. Tricoci P, Huang Z, Held C, et al. Thrombin-receptor antagonist vorapaxar in acute coronary syndromes. *N Engl J Med*. 2012;366:20–33.
98. https://www.accessdata.fda.gov/drugsatfda_docs/label/2015/200671s000lbl.pdf.

21 Role of Percutaneous Coronary Intervention in Patients With Diabetes

BARIS GENCER, JUAN F. IGLESIAS, AND MARCO ROFFI

Diabetes mellitus (DM) is a major risk factor for atherosclerosis,[1] thereby affecting multiple vascular territories and increasing the risk of major adverse cardiovascular events.[2,3] At the cardiac level, it is associated with a risk of coronary artery disease (CAD) equivalent to 15 years of aging.[4]

The aims of coronary revascularization in stable CAD are symptom relief and, in a selected subgroup of patients, improvement of the prognosis.[5] The fundamental role of optimal medical treatment—independent of the revascularization modality—is especially true for the patient population with diabetes.[6] In the current context of a worldwide increasing prevalence of diabetes, within the percutaneous revascularization arena particular attention is needed in the development of new strategies in the field of adjuvant pharmacologic therapies and drug-eluting stents (DESs).[7] As summarized in Tables 21.1 and 21.2, major achievements were made in the development of percutaneous coronary intervention (PCI) and stent technology. Despite all the advances in the field, patients with diabetes undergoing revascularization—both surgical and through PCI—continue to have worse outcomes compared with nondiabetic individuals, likely due to the diffuse nature of the coronary involvement and the associated comorbidities.[8,9]

For patients with diabetes, assessment of several clinical parameters, such as coronary anatomy, complexity of lesions, clinical presentation, left ventricular function, comorbidities, and patient preference, may help to determine the best revascularization option (Fig. 21.1).[10] The myocardial revascularization guidelines of the European Society of Cardiology recommend revascularization in all stable patients with diabetes and extensive CAD (Class I, level of evidence A).[5,11] The use of an invasive strategy in patients with acute coronary syndromes (ACSs) is recommended in patients with diabetes similarly as in patients without diabetes.[12,13] The management of patients with ACS is covered more thoroughly in another chapter.

SPECIFIC CHARACTERISTICS OF DIABETES-ASSOCIATED ATHEROTHROMBOSIS

Patients with diabetes constitute a subgroup of patients at increased risk of unfavorable outcomes after PCI because of more severe and extensive CAD, as well as a higher rate of restenosis.[8,14,15]

In addition, patients with diabetes are characterized by prothrombotic and proinflammatory states induced by a variety of metabolic disturbances that may lead, among other complications, to increased plaque vulnerability, platelet reactivity, and thrombotic complications after PCI.[10]

Hyperglycemia, insulin resistance, and oxidative stress are the major abnormalities that contribute to the dysfunction of extracellular and intracellular molecular pathways of endothelial cells, platelets, and blood coagulant factors.[16,17] In the bare-metal stent (BMS) era, the most evident adverse effect of diabetes after PCI was the increased risk of restenosis which was strongly attenuated by the development of DESs.[18] Although diabetes remained a risk factor for increased risk of restenosis with DESs, the increased risk of stent thrombosis (ST) with first-generation DESs became a greater concern in the context of diabetes.[19] Accordingly, diabetes has been identified as an independent predictor of ST in a variety of studies addressing the use of first-generation DESs (Fig. 21.2).[10]

CONSERVATIVE STRATEGY VERSUS REVASCULARIZATION

A few studies have compared a conservative strategy versus revascularization in patients with CAD. The only trial focusing specifically on patients with diabetes was the Bypass Angioplasty Revascularization Investigation 2 Diabetes (BARI 2D) trial, which enrolled 2368 individuals with

TABLE 21.1 Summary of Percutaneous Coronary Intervention History

YEAR	IMPORTANT STEPS IN PERCUTANEOUS CORONARY INTERVENTION
1977	First percutaneous coronary angioplasty
1986	First BMS implantation
1993	Superiority of BMS vs. balloon documented
1996	Adoption of dual antiplatelet therapy after BMS to prevent ST
2002	Superiority of DES vs. BMS in terms of restenosis documented
2002	Approval of SES in Europe
2003	Approval of SES by the FDA
2003	Superiority of PES vs. BMS documented
2004	Approval of PES by the FDA
2005	Superiority of SES vs. PES documented in patients with diabetes in terms of restenosis
2007	Superiority of SES vs. BMS documented in patients with diabetes in terms of clinical outcomes
2008	Approval of ZES by the FDA
2008	Approval of EES by the FDA
2011	Noninferiority of EES vs. SES documented in patients with diabetes
2012	Superiority of BES with biodegradable polymer vs. BMS documented in patients with STEMI
2012	IPD suggesting improvement of safety and efficacy with biodegradable polymer DES vs. durable polymer SES

BES, Biolimus-eluting stent; *BMS*, bare-metal stent; *DES*, drug-eluting stent; *EES*, everolimus-eluting stent; *FDA*, US Food and Drug Administration; *IPD*, individual participant data; *PCI*, percutaneous coronary intervention; *PES*, paclitaxel-eluting stent; *SES*, sirolimus-eluting stent; *STEMI*, ST-segment elevation myocardial infarction; *ST*, stent thrombosis; *ZES*, zotarolimus-eluting stent.

TABLE 21.2 Types of Coronary Stents

	COMPANY	SUBSTANCE	BIODEGRADABLE POLYMER
Newer-Generation Drug-Eluting Stents			
PROMUS	Boston Scientific	Everolimus	
XIENCE	Abbot Vascular	Everolimus	
RESOLUTE	Medtronic	Zotarolimus	
EkuNIR (BioNIR)	Medinaol Ltd	Ridaforolimus	
BIOMATRIX	Biosensors	Biolimus	X
ORSIRO	Biotronik	Sirolimus	X
NOBORI	Terumo	Biolimus	X
SYNERGY	Boston Scientific	Everolimus	X
ULTIMASTER	Terumo	Sirolimus	X
Polymer-free			
BIOFREEDOM	Biosensors	Biolimus	
Bioabsorbable Scaffolding			
ABSORB	Abbot Vascular	Everolimus	X (bioabsorbable)

type 2 diabetes and stable CAD confirmed by angiography (stenosis ≥50% with a positive stress test or ≥70% with classic symptoms).[20] Patients with unstable symptoms, left main coronary disease, creatinine level of more than 2.0 mg/dL (177 μmol/L), a glycated hemoglobin level of more than 13.0%, class III or IV heart failure, or PCI or coronary artery bypass grafting (CABG) within the previous 12 months were excluded. Patients were randomized to treatment with optimal medical therapy plus revascularization versus optimal medical therapy alone, while the modality of revascularization (PCI or CABG) was left at the discretion of the treating physicians but selected before randomization. The revascularization group included patients treated with PCI ($n = 765$) and with CABG ($n = 347$). This trial showed that intensive medical therapy alone was not significantly different from immediate revascularization plus intensive medical therapy in terms of major averse cardiovascular events (MACEs) (death, myocardial infarction [MI], and stroke) after 5 years of follow-up (77.2% for the revascularization group vs. 75.9% for the medical group, $P = .70$). The corresponding survival rates were 88.3% and 87.8%, respectively.[20]

A secondary analysis showed that patients selected to undergo CABG—that is, those with more advanced disease—derived a benefit from revascularization in terms of MACEs (22.5% CABG vs. 30.4% medical therapy, $P = .01$). In those chosen to undergo PCI, medical treatment seemed to be an appropriate first-line strategy, particularly in those with less severe CAD. In the overall cohort, 23% of patients initially allocated to medical therapy underwent revascularization within the 5 years.[20] The revascularization strategy reduced the occurrence of symptoms and subsequent revascularization at 3 years—lower rates of worsening angina (8% vs. 13%, $P < .001$), new angina (37% vs. 51%, $P = .001$), and coronary revascularization (18% vs. 33%, $P < .001$), and higher rate of angina-free status (66% vs. 58%, $P = .003$). While medical treatment seems an appropriate first-line strategy in patients with diabetes with CAD, particularly in those with less severe disease, the results of BARI 2D may be difficult to reproduce in clinical practice. Accordingly, patients enrolled in the study were highly adherent to medical treatment and the majority achieved all secondary prevention therapeutic goals. Finally, a secondary analysis of BARI 2D showed that, independent of the revascularization type, complete revascularization was associated with lower MACE rates.[21]

The International Study of Comparative Health Effectiveness with Medical and Invasive Approaches (ISCHEMIA) trial randomized chronic coronary disease patients with evidence of ischemia but no left main disease to an invasive (medical therapy plus angiography and revascularization if feasible) or a conservative approach (medical therapy alone with revascularization if medical therapy failed). Among the 5900 participants, 2553 (43%) had a diabetes defined by history, hemoglobin $A1_c$ ≥6.5%, or use of glucose-lowering medication and 30% were treated with insulin. The risk for the primary endpoint of all-cause death or MI with a median follow-up

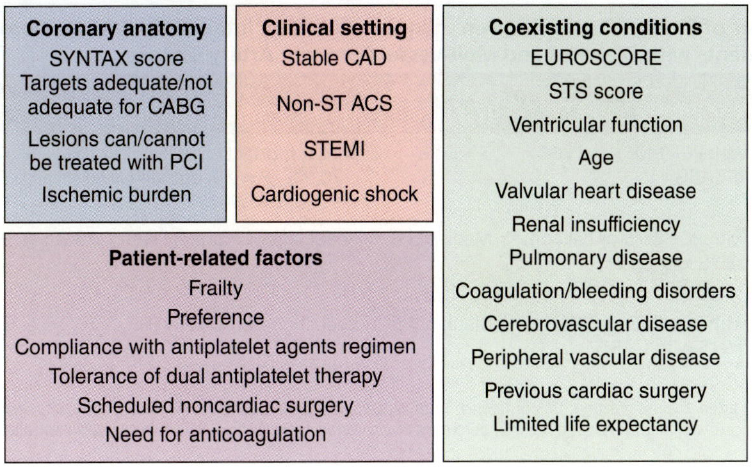

FIG. 21.1 Parameters guiding the choice of revascularization strategy in patients with diabetes. *CABG*, Coronary artery bypass grafting; *ACS*, acute coronary syndrome; *CAD*, coronary artery disease; *PCI*, percutaneous coronary intervention; *STEMI*, ST-segment elevation myocardial infarction; *STS*, Society of Thoracic Surgeons; *SYNTAX*, Synergy Between Percutaneous Coronary Intervention with Taxus and Cardiac Surgery trial. (Modified from Roffi M, Angiolillo DJ, Kappetein AP. Current concepts on coronary revascularization in patients with diabetes. *Eur Heart J*. 2011;32:2748–2757.)

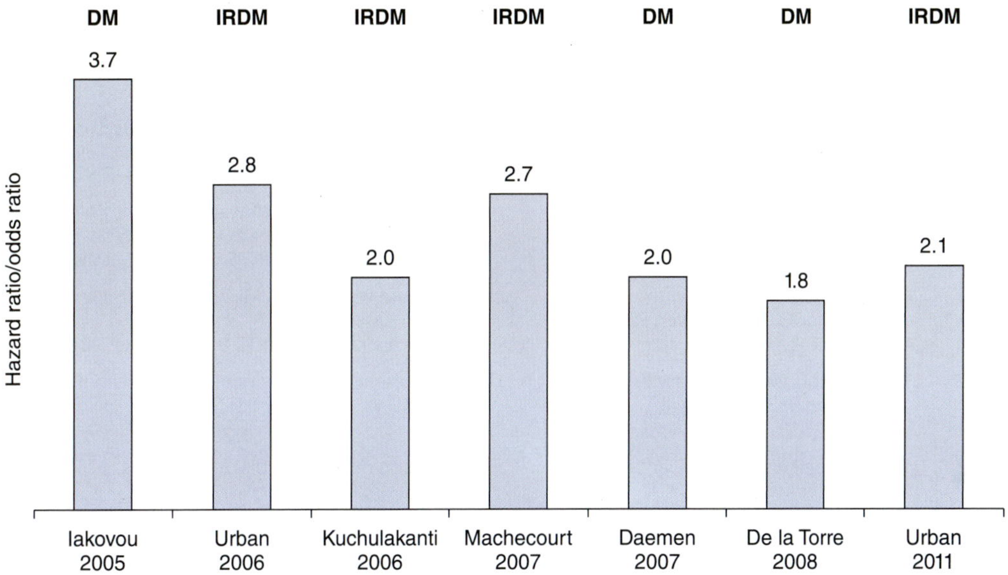

FIG. 21.2 Studies have demonstrated the incremental independent risk associated with diabetes mellitus (*DM*) and insulin-requiring diabetes mellitus (*IRDM*) for stent thrombosis among patients treated with percutaneous coronary intervention using drug-eluting stents. The results are reported with the hazard ratio or odds ratio of multivariable analyses. (Modified from Roffi M, Angiolillo DJ, Kappetein AP. Current concepts on coronary revascularization in patients with diabetes. *Eur Heart J*. 2011;32:2748–2757.)

of 3.2 years was significantly higher in patients with diabetes (hazard ratio [HR], 1.49; 95% confidence interval [CI], 1.31–1.70; $P < .001$) compared with nondiabetic individuals.[22] No benefit of an invasive versus conservative strategy was observed in patients with diabetes (HR, 1.00; 95% CI, 0.87–1.17) or without diabetes (HR, 1.01; 95% CI, 0.86–1.17).[22]

In conclusion, in low-risk patients with diabetes (e.g., moderate CAD on coronary angiogram, stable symptoms, normal left ventricular and renal function) with excellent compliance with medical therapy, an initially conservative strategy is a valuable option. However, the results of the randomized clinical trial (RCT) cannot be extrapolated to higher-risk patients, to those with ACS, or to patients with unknown coronary anatomy. Independent of the revascularization strategy, optimal medical management remains the cornerstone of treatment.

Percutaneous Coronary Intervention Versus Bypass Surgery

The optimal revascularization modality in patients with multivessel CAD has been a source of debate for decades in patients with diabetes, and this debate is expected to continue with the new era of DESs and antithrombotic and antiplatelet therapies.[23] In this section, we consider studies that have addressed the issue of revascularization in patients with diabetes with multivessel CAD (PCI vs. CABG). Tables 21.3 and 21.4 summarize the results from RCTs, meta-analyses, and registries.

The SYNTAX RCT compared PCI (paclitaxel-eluting stent [PES]) versus CABG in a study population of 1800 patients with left main and/or multivessel CAD. The results were statistically not different in terms of the primary composite endpoint at 1 year (death, stroke, MI) between both

TABLE 21.3 Pooled Analysis of Studies Comparing Percutaneous Coronary Intervention Versus Coronary Artery Bypass Graft Surgery in Population of Patients with Diabetes and Multivessel Coronary Artery Disease

STUDY DESIGN	YEAR	DIABETIC POPULATION	FOLLOW-UP (YEARS)	EFFECT OF TREATMENT ON OUTCOMES
IPD from 4 RCTs[24]	2008	275 with PCI (BMS) and 268 with CABG	5	Similar mortality (7.9% vs. 12.4%, *P* = .09) and MACEs (21.4% vs. 20.9%, *P* = .9), but increased revascularization with PCI (29.7% vs. 9.2%, *P* < .001)
IPD from 10 RCTs[25]	2009	618 with PCI (BMS or balloon) and 615 with CABG	Median 5.9	Reduction of mortality with CABG (HR, 0.70; 95% CI, 0.56–0.87)
IPD from 3 registries[26]	2012	846 with PCI (DES or BMS) and 915 with CABG	Median 5.5	Reduction of mortality (HR, 0.70; 95% CI, 0.55–0.88) and MACEs (HR, 0.71; 95% CI, 0.57–0.89), but increased revascularization with PCI (HR, 4.55; 95% CI, 3.27–6.32)

BMS, Bare-metal stent; *CABG*, coronary artery bypass grafting; *CI*, confidence interval; *DES*, drug-eluting stent; *HR*, hazard ratio; *IPD*, individual participant data; *MACE*, major averse cardiovascular event (death, myocardial infarction, or stroke); *PCI*, percutaneous coronary intervention; RCT, randomized controlled trial.

TABLE 21.4 Recent Randomized Controlled Trials Comparing Percutaneous Coronary Intervention Versus Coronary Artery Bypass Graft Surgery in Population of Patients with Diabetes and Multivessel Coronary Artery Disease

STUDIES	YEAR	DIABETIC POPULATION	FOLLOW-UP (YEARS)	EFFECT OF TREATMENT ON OUTCOMES
SYNTAX[27]	2009	452 patients (221 treated with CABG and 231 treated with PES)	1	All-cause death, CVA, MI: 10.3% CABG vs. 10.1% PES (*P* = .96) Revascularization rate: 6.4% CABG vs. 20.3% PCI (*P* < .001)
CARDIA[28]	2010	510 patients (254 treated with CABG and 256 treated with PCI including both BMS and DES)	1	Composite rate of death, MI, CVA: 10.5% CABG vs. 13.0% PCI (HR, 1.25; 95% CI, 0.75–2.09; *P* = .39) Rates of death, MI, CVA, or repeat revascularization: 11.3% CABG vs. 19.3% PCI (HR, 1.77; 95% CI, 1.11–2.82)
ARTS I and II[29]	2011	367 patients (159 SES, 96 CABG, 112 BMS)	5	Rate of MACE and CVA was significantly higher with BMS (BMS 53.6% vs. CABG 23.4% vs. SES 40.5%, *P* < .01), but not mortality (BMS 13.6% vs. CABG 8.6% vs. SES 9.0%, *P* > .05)
SYNTAX[30]	2011	452 patients (221 treated with CABG and 231 treated with PES)	3	All-cause death, CVA, MI, and TVR: 22.9% CABG vs. 37.0% PES (*P* = .002) Revascularization rate: 12.9% CABG vs. 28.0% for PES (*P* < .001)
FREEDOM[31]	2012	1900 patients (947 treated with CABG and 953 treated with DES)	5	Death from any cause, nonfatal MI, or nonfatal CVA: 18.7% for CABG vs. 26.6% for PCI (*P* = .005)
VA CARDS[32]	2013	198 (97 treated with CABG and 101 treated with DES)	2	All-cause mortality: 5.0% for CABG vs. 21.0% for PCI (HR, 0.30; 95% CI, 0.11–0.80) Nonfatal MI: 15.0% for CABG vs. 6.2% for PCI (HR, 3.32; 95% CI, 1.07–10.30)

BMS, Bare-metal stent; *CABG*, coronary artery bypass grafting; *CI*, confidence interval; *CVA*, cerebrovascular accident; *DES*, drug-eluting stent; *HR*, hazard ratio; *MI*, myocardial infarction; *PCI*, percutaneous coronary intervention; *PES*, paclitaxel-eluting stent; *SES*, sirolimus-eluting stent; TVR, target-vessel revascularization.

revascularization methods in patients without diabetes (6.8% CABG vs. 6.8% PES, *P* = .97) and patients with diabetes (10.3% CABG vs. 10.1% PES, *P* = .96).[27] However, in subgroup analyses, mortality was higher after PES in patients with diabetes and highly complex lesions (13.5% PCI vs. 4.1% CABG, *P* = .04), and PES resulted in higher target-vessel revascularization (TVR) in patients with diabetes (20.3% vs. 6.4% CABG, *P* > .001). The SYNTAX follow-up at 3 years showed that patients with diabetes treated initially with PCI-PES experienced a higher risk of MACEs (37.0% PES vs. 22.9% CABG, *P* = .002) or repeat revascularization (28.0% PES vs. 12.9% CABG, *P* < .001) compared with the CABG-treated group.[30] After exclusion of the clinically less impactful TVR component endpoint, the composite endpoint of death, stroke, and MI was not statistically different between the groups (16.3% for PCI vs. 14.0% for CABG, *P* = .53). The authors concluded that PCI might be preferred for patients with less complex left main and/or three-vessel lesions (SYNTAX scores ≤22), but CABG should be the option of choice for patients with more complex left main CAD or three-vessel anatomic disease, especially for patients with diabetes.[33] The 5-year follow-up from the overall population has been published, and results confirmed that CABG should be the choice for patients with complex lesions (intermediate and high SYNTAX scores) and that PCI is an acceptable treatment for less complex lesions (low SYNTAX scores).[34]

The FREEDOM RCT compared PCI (DES) with CABG in 1900 patients with diabetes with multivessel CAD and showed an increased risk of the primary outcome of MACEs in the PCI group compared with the CABG group after 5 years of follow-up (26.6% vs. 18.7%, *P* = .005).[31] CABG was superior to PCI in terms of a reduced overall death rate (16.3% vs. 10.9%, *P* = .049) and MI (13.9% vs. 6.0%, *P* < .001) but inferior to PCI in terms of a higher rate of stroke at 5 years (2.4% in the PCI group and 5.2% in the CABG group, *P* = .03). However, debate persists because the PCI option yielded comparable results to CABG during

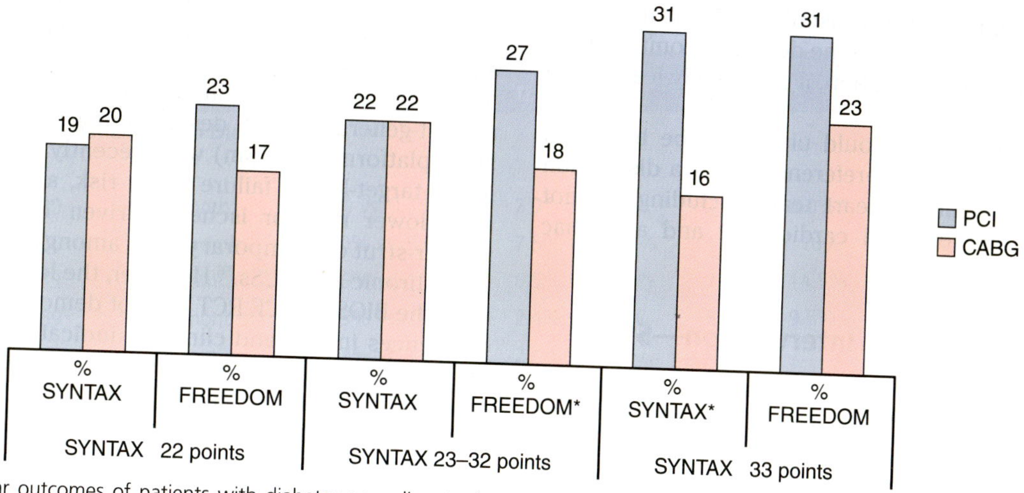

FIG. 21.3 Five-year outcomes of patients with diabetes according to the anatomic lesion complexity (SYNTAX score) and revascularization treatment (PCI vs. CABG). Binary event rates of the composite endpoint of death, stroke, and myocardial infarction in the SYNTAX[53] and FREEDOM trials. *CABG*, Coronary artery bypass grafting; *PCI*, percutaneous coronary intervention. *$P < .05$.

the first 2 years of follow-up, with event curves thereafter diverging ultimately to reveal an absolute 5-year survival benefit of 5.4% for CABG (95% CI, 1.5–9.2). Fig. 21.3 summarizes the findings of the 5-year follow-up of the SYNTAX and FREEDOM trials in patients with diabetes according to the baseline anatomic complexity. Both studies reported a benefit of treatment with CABG in patients with complex disease (SYNTAX score ≥33 points) in terms of composite endpoint reduction (death, stroke, MI). In patients with less complex disease (SYNTAX score <22 points), PCI and CABG results did not differ significantly, suggesting that PCI is an acceptable alternative. In patients with intermediate disease (SYNTAX score 23–32 points), the FREEDOM trial reported a benefit of CABG not confirmed in the SYNTAX trial, suggesting that a consensus for the optimum treatment should be discussed by the "heart team," including both cardiac surgeons and interventional cardiologists.

In the Evaluation of XIENCE versus Coronary Artery Bypass Surgery for Effectiveness of Left Main Revascularization (EXCEL Trial), the 3-year composite primary endpoint (composite of all-cause death, stroke, or MI) was significantly higher in patients with compared to those without diabetes (20.0% vs. 12.9%; $P < .001$). The rate of the 3-year primary endpoint was similar after treatment with PCI and CABG in patients with diabetes (20.7% vs. 19.3%; HR, 1.03; 95% CI, 0.71–1.50; $P = .87$) and without diabetes (12.9% vs. 12.9%; HR, 0.98; 95% CI, 0.73–1.32; $P = .89$).[35]

In current practice, patients with diabetes and multivessel CAD deemed to be at a standard surgical risk based on comorbidities and coronary anatomy should be informed about the potential survival benefit with CABG as well as the lower need for repeat revascularization and MI.[31,36] This shared-decision discussion at this stage is aimed at offering patients the most appropriate and evidence-based treatment recommendations with all the transparency of the available current evidence. Overall, the revascularization strategy should be based on and guided by anatomic and clinical characteristics, as well as an interventional SYNTAX score (http://syntaxscore.com) and surgical EUROSCORE (www.euroscore.org) reflecting the complexity and its influence on anticipated results from each revascularization modality and its risks. Recently, the SYNTAX II score has been developed and estimates the 4-year mortality for each treatment (PCI vs. CABG). The score contains eight variables: anatomic SYNTAX score, age, creatinine clearance, left ventricular ejection fraction, presence of unprotected left main CAD, peripheral artery disease, female sex, and chronic obstructive pulmonary disease.[37] Although the impact of newer-generation DESs needs to be fully evaluated, the threshold for CABG should be definitively lower in patients with diabetes than in their nondiabetic counterparts.

In the 2019 European Society of Cardiology (ESC) myocardial revascularization guidelines, PCI was the preferred approach for patients with diabetes with multivessel disease and low complex CAD defined as a SYNTAX score equal or less than 22 points, including patients with left main disease (class I).[5] In a recent meta-analysis of 4394 patients (also without diabetes) with left main CAD at low or intermediate CAD complexity (median SYNTAX score 25 points), the 5-year all-cause death was similar between PCI and CABG.[36] Whereas PCI is a valuable option in a patient with one- or two-vessel CAD, including left main disease, CABG remained the favored approach of revascularization in diabetes patients with three-vessel CAD at low complexity.[11]

In the 2021 US revascularization guidelines, CABG with an arterial graft on the left anterior descending artery is recommended in preference to PCI to reduce mortality and repeat revascularizations in patients with diabetes and multivessel CAD (Class of Recommendation I, Level of Evidence A). In patients amenable to PCI who have an indication for revascularization and are poor candidates for surgery, PCI can be useful to reduce long-term ischemic outcomes (Class of Recommendations 2a, Level of Evidence B). In patients with diabetes who have left main stenosis and low- or intermediate-complexity CAD in the rest of the coronary anatomy, PCI may be an alternative to CABG to reduce major adverse cardiovascular events (Class of Recommendations 2b, Level of Evidence B).

In patients with intermediate or high complex CAD defined as SYNTAX score more than 22 points, the

An exploratory superiority analysis suggests that PF-AES might even be superior to ZES with regard to the TLF at 1 year,[63] but these hypothesis-generating findings need to be confirmed by the powered superiority analysis planned at the 2-year follow-up. Importantly, SUGAR is the first adequately powered RCT to compare newer-generation DES in diabetes patients, and the first to demonstrate significant reductions in event rates after DES implantation in patients with diabetes. Similarly, the 3040-patient DIAB8 RCT is currently investigating the superior efficacy of PF-AES compared to second-generation DP-EES with respect to the primary endpoint of TLR at 1 year among all-comer patients with diabetes undergoing PCI. Finally, the ABILITY Diabetes Global (*NCT04236609*) RCT is currently assessing the clinical performance of an innovative hybrid DES concept that combines a newer-generation thin-strut BP-DES with a sirolimus-coated balloon compared with a contemporary polymer-based EES with respect to the primary endpoint of clinically indicated TLR at 1 year, according to a non-inferiority and sequentially superiority hypothesis among 3000 all-comer patients with diabetes undergoing PCI. The long-term outcome results from these ongoing large-scale RCTs are eagerly awaited to provide novel insights into the potential clinical benefits of these recent DES designs compared to contemporary newer-generation DES for PCI in diabetic individuals.

ADJUNCTIVE PHARMACOLOGIC TREATMENT

Antiplatelet Therapy Acute Coronary Syndrome

In the post-MI setting, in the PEGASUS-TIMI 54, a prolonged duration of $P2Y_{12}$ inhibition with ticagrelor was shown to be effective to reduce ischemic events for a median treatment duration of 33 months both in patients with diabetes (10.1% vs. 11.6%; HR, 0.85; 95% CI, 0.71–1.03) and without diabetes (6.8% vs. 7.8%; HR, 0.85; 95% CI 0.73–0.99).[64] The Optimizing Antiplatelet Therapy in Diabetes Mellitus (OPTIMUS) trial was a prospective, randomized, double-blind, crossover study designed to perform serial measures of platelet inhibition in patients with diabetes treated with (1) prasugrel (60-mg loading dose and 10-mg maintenance dose) compared with (2) clopidogrel (600-mg loading dose and 150-mg maintenance dose). Prasugrel was associated with a greater degree of platelet inhibition (89.3% vs. 27.7%, $P < .0001$), both with loading and maintenance periods, compared with clopidogrel.[65]

The benefit of prasugrel was confirmed in the Trial to Assess Improvement in Therapeutic Outcomes by Optimizing Platelet Inhibition with Prasugrel—Thrombolysis in Myocardial Infarction (TRITON-TIMI 38) in patients with ACS, with a significant reduction in clinically relevant MACEs compared with the use of clopidogrel.[66] Ticagrelor was assessed in the Study of Platelet Inhibition and Patient Outcomes (PLATO) in patients with ACS in comparison with clopidogrel. Despite the larger population of patients with diabetes enrolled in PLATO compared with TRITON-TIMI 38, the benefit observed in patients with diabetes with ticagrelor did not reach statistical significance.[67]

Stable Patients

In patients with diabetes ($N = 749$) and CAD (stable or unstable), a longer duration of clopidogrel therapy (>9 months) after BMS or DES implantation was associated with a lower incidence of death or MI compared with patients who discontinued taking the drug within 6 months and within 6 to 9 months.[68] In a large cohort after DES implantation, the continuation of clopidogrel (for at least 24 months) was associated with a reduction in risk for death and death or MI compared with patients who discontinued clopidogrel at 6 or 12 months. Dual-antiplatelet therapies are recommended as adjuncts to PCI in stable CAD with a loading dose administration of aspirin (150–300 mg) and clopidogrel (600 mg) in the periprocedural management. The routine use of pretreatment with $P2Y_{12}$ inhibitors is not recommended in patients in whom coronary anatomy is unknown.[13] In stable patients with CAD, the continuation daily dose should be 75 to 150 mg acetylsalicylic acid (ASA) and 75 mg clopidogrel for a usual duration of 6 months, in contrast to 12 months for patients after an ACS.[69,70] A recent meta-analysis of 16 RCTs comprising 16,376 diabetic adults did not show major differences in MACE and net adverse clinical event between comparisons of dual antiplatelet therapy duration, except for lower bleeding risk with 3 months than with 12 months, suggesting that individualization of therapy is also a good approach in patients with diabetes. Since patients with diabetes more frequently have a suboptimal platelet response to clopidogrel compared with patients without diabetes, more potent $P2Y_{12}$ inhibitors (prasugrel and ticagrelor) may be of particular benefit in patients with diabetes.

The 2021 American College of Cardiology (ACC)/American Heart Association (AHA) guidelines for coronary artery revascularization had a similar approach, proposing 12 months in duration of treatment after ACS and 6 months after a stable disease revascularized with a DES and the possibility of extending or discontinuing according to the risk of bleeding. Here also, recommendations for antiplatelet therapy are both applicable for patients with and without diabetes.[70]

Whereas newer $P2Y_{12}$ inhibitors (prasugrel and ticagrelor) are superior to clopidogrel in patients with diabetes and ACS, comparative data in the setting of stable or elective PCI are now available. In the Effect of Ticagrelor on Health Outcomes in Diabetes Patients Intervention Study (THEMIS), 19,220 patients with stable coronary heart disease and diabetes were randomized to ticagrelor plus aspirin versus aspirin alone. After a median follow-up of 39 months, the risk of the primary endpoint of the composite of CV death, MI, or stroke was lower in the ticagrelor group compared with aspirin (7.7% vs. 8.5%; HR, 0.90; 95% CI, 0.81–0.99; $P = .04$), while the risk of thrombolysis in myocardial infarction (TIMI) major bleeding was higher (2.2% vs. 1.0%; HR, 2.32; 95% CI, 1.82–2.94; $P < .001$).[71] In the THEMIS-PCI trial, 11.154 patients (58% of THEMIS) had a history of PCI. The primary endpoint was significantly reduced with ticagrelor compared with a placebo (7.3% vs. 8.6%; HR, 0.85; 95% CI, 0.74–0.97; $P = .013$).[72] This trial was a landmark study providing the evidence of a longer use of antithrombotic regimen after PCI in the diabetic population in terms of ischemic event reduction. However, the increased bleeding risk should be weighted against the potential benefit in terms of ischemic events reduction using a metric integrating the number needed to treat (NNT) to the number needed to harm (NNH). In THEMIS, the NNT was 125 compared to an NNH of 63 over a duration of 39 months. Thus an unfavorable benefit-risk profile (almost 2.0) might be associated with the use of ticagrelor in this setting.

Recommendations

The 2023 guidelines on the management of ACSs recommend a standard duration of 12 months of antiplatelet therapy with the possibility of deescalation or prolongation depending on the benefit/risk ratio. The recommendations are valid both for diabetic and nondiabetic populations.[69]

On top of antithrombotic therapies, the effect of lipid-lowering therapy after PCI and on the risk of revascularization is an increasing area of investigations. In the Further Cardiovascular Outcomes Research with PCSK9 Inhibition in Subjects with Elevated Risk (FOURIER) trial, an intensive lipid-lowering therapy with evolocumab on top of statin decreased the risk of complex revascularization in the diabetic subpopulation ($N = 10{,}081$) with established atherosclerotic cardiovascular disease. Over a median follow-up of 3 years, the risk of complex revascularization, defined as complex PCI (multivessel PCI with at least three stents and three lesions, bifurcation, or a total stent length of 60 mm at least) or CABG, was significantly lowered with evolocumab compared to standard care (2.6% vs. 4.0%; HR, 0.64; 0.50–0.82) compared to a strategy with statin alone.[73]

FUTURE STRATEGIES TO IMPROVE PERCUTANEOUS CORONARY INTERVENTION RESULTS

In terms of medical devices, the initial encouraging data from bioabsorbable scaffolds suggest that this strategy may further improve PCI-related outcomes, such as ST and target-vessel MI. However, no compromise in terms of efficacy (i.e., restenosis and TVR) will be acceptable, particularly in patients with diabetes. Therefore large-scale RCTs against newer, conventional DESs are needed before this technology may be broadly applied.

With respect to revascularization strategy, the mechanisms of the survival benefit of CABG versus PCI in patients with diabetes with advanced CAD still need to be fully understood.[74] In the future, this may allow selection of the best revascularization strategy for the individual patient. Aggressive secondary prevention based on strict control of associated cardiovascular risk factors remains the cornerstone of the treatment of patients with diabetes with CAD, independent of the revascularization strategy.

SUMMARY

Patients with diabetes constitute a subgroup of patients at increased risk of unfavorable outcomes following PCI because of more severe and extensive CAD, as well as higher rates of restenosis and ST. Improvements in technology and design in coronary stenting have resulted in improved clinical results, and PCI has become the major therapeutic option for coronary revascularization in patients with diabetes. DESs have dramatically changed the approach to CAD treatment, especially in patients with multivessel disease, reducing stent restenosis and the need for surgical procedures. In low-risk patients with diabetes with excellent compliance with medical therapy, an initial conservative strategy is a valuable option. In patients with diabetes and multivessel CAD, PCI might be preferred for patients with less-complex lesions, but CABG should be the option of choice for most patients with complex multivessel coronary disease.

REFERENCES

1. Wild S, Roglic G, Green A, Sicree R, King H. Global prevalence of diabetes: estimates for the year 2000 and projections for 2030. *Diabetes Care*. 2004;27:1047–1053. https://doi.org/10.2337/diacare.27.5.1047.
2. Krempf M, Parhofer KG, Steg PG, et al. Reach Registry I. Cardiovascular event rates in diabetic and nondiabetic individuals with and without established atherothrombosis (from the REduction of Atherothrombosis for Continued Health [REACH] Registry). *Am J Cardiol*. 2010;105:667–671. https://doi.org/10.1016/j.amjcard.2009.10.048.
3. Donahoe SM, Stewart GC, McCabe CH, et al. Diabetes and mortality following acute coronary syndromes. *JAMA*. 2007;298:765–775. https://doi.org/10.1001/jama.298.7.765.
4. Booth GL, Kapral MK, Fung K, Tu JV. Relation between age and cardiovascular disease in men and women with diabetes compared with non-diabetic people: a population-based retrospective cohort study. *Lancet*. 2006;368:29–36. https://doi.org/10.1016/S0140-6736(06)68967-8.
5. Cosentino F, Grant PJ, Aboyans V, et al. 2019 ESC Guidelines on diabetes, pre-diabetes, and cardiovascular diseases developed in collaboration with the EASD. *Eur Heart J*. 2020;41:255–323. https://doi.org/10.1093/eurheartj/ehz486.
6. Preis SR, Hwang SJ, Coady S, et al. Trends in all-cause and cardiovascular disease mortality among women and men with and without diabetes mellitus in the Framingham Heart Study, 1950 to 2005. *Circulation*. 2009;119:1728–1735. https://doi.org/10.1161/CIRCULATIONAHA.108.829176.
7. Garg P, Normand SL, Silbaugh TS, et al. Drug-eluting or bare-metal stenting in patients with diabetes mellitus: results from the Massachusetts Data Analysis Center Registry. *Circulation*. 2008;118:2277–2285. https://doi.org/10.1161/CIRCULATIONAHA.108.820159. 2277p following 2285.
8. Frobert O, Lagerqvist B, Carlsson J, Lindback J, Stenestrand U, James SK. Differences in restenosis rate with different drug-eluting stents in patients with and without diabetes mellitus: a report from the SCAAR (Swedish Angiography and Angioplasty Registry). *J Am Coll Cardiol*. 2009;53:1660–1667. https://doi.org/10.1016/j.jacc.2009.01.054.
9. Syed AI, Ben-Dor I, Li Y, et al. Outcomes in diabetic versus nondiabetic patients who present with acute myocardial infarction and are treated with drug-eluting stents. *Am J Cardiol*. 2010;105:819–825. https://doi.org/10.1016/j.amjcard.2009.11.010.
10. Roffi M, Angiolillo DJ, Kappetein AP. Current concepts on coronary revascularization in diabetic patients. *Eur Heart J*. 2011;32:2748–2757. https://doi.org/10.1093/eurheartj/ehr305.
11. Neumann FJ, Sousa-Uva M, Ahlsson A, et al. 2018 ESC/EACTS Guidelines on myocardial revascularization. *Eur Heart J*. 2019;40:87–165. https://doi.org/10.1093/eurheartj/ehy394.
12. O'Donoghue ML, Vaidya A, Afsal R, et al. An invasive or conservative strategy in patients with diabetes mellitus and non-ST-segment elevation acute coronary syndromes: a collaborative meta-analysis of randomized trials. *J Am Coll Cardiol*. 2012;60:106–111. https://doi.org/10.1016/j.jacc.2012.02.059.
13. Collet JP, Thiele H, Barbato E, et al. 2020 ESC Guidelines for the management of acute coronary syndromes in patients presenting without persistent ST-segment elevation. *Eur Heart J*. 2021;42:1289–1367. https://doi.org/10.1093/eurheartj/ehaa575.
14. Iijima R, Ndrepepa G, Mehilli J, et al. Impact of diabetes mellitus on long-term outcomes in the drug-eluting stent era. *Am Heart J*. 2007;154:688–693. https://doi.org/10.1016/j.ahj.2007.06.005.
15. Mathew V, Holmes DR. Outcomes in diabetics undergoing revascularization: the long and the short of it. *J Am Coll Cardiol*. 2002;40:424–427. https://doi.org/10.1016/s0735-1097(02)02025-9.
16. Creager MA, Luscher TF, Cosentino F, Beckman JA. Diabetes and vascular disease: pathophysiology, clinical consequences, and medical therapy: Part I. *Circulation*. 2003;108:1527–1532. https://doi.org/10.1161/01.CIR.0000091257.27563.32.
17. Luscher TF, Creager MA, Beckman JA, Cosentino F. Diabetes and vascular disease: pathophysiology, clinical consequences, and medical therapy: Part II. *Circulation*. 2003;108:1655–1661. https://doi.org/10.1161/01.CIR.0000089189.70578.E2.

18. Bangalore S, Kumar S, Fusaro M, et al. Outcomes with various drug eluting or bare metal stents in patients with diabetes mellitus: mixed treatment comparison analysis of 22,844 patient years of follow-up from randomised trials. *BMJ.* 2012;345:e5170. https://doi.org/10.1136/bmj.e5170.
19. Holmes Jr. DR, Kereiakes DJ, Garg S, et al. Stent thrombosis. *J Am Coll Cardiol.* 2010;56:1357–1365. https://doi.org/10.1016/j.jacc.2010.07.016.
20. Group BDS, Frye RL, August P, et al. A randomized trial of therapies for type 2 diabetes and coronary artery disease. *N Engl J Med.* 2009;360:2503–2515. https://doi.org/10.1056/NEJMoa0805796.
21. Schwartz L, Bertolet M, Feit F, et al. Impact of completeness of revascularization on long-term cardiovascular outcomes in patients with type 2 diabetes mellitus: results from the Bypass Angioplasty Revascularization Investigation 2 Diabetes (BARI 2D). *Circ Cardiovasc Interv.* 2012;5:166–173. https://doi.org/10.1161/CIRCINTERVENTIONS.111.963512.
22. Newman JD, Anthopolos R, Mancini GBJ, et al. Outcomes of participants with diabetes in the ISCHEMIA trials. *Circulation.* 2021;144:1380–1395. https://doi.org/10.1161/CIRCULATIONAHA.121.054439.
23. Flaherty JD, Davidson CJ. Diabetes and coronary revascularization. *JAMA.* 2005;293:1501–1508. https://doi.org/10.1001/jama.293.12.1501.
24. Daemen J, Boersma E, Flather M, et al. Long-term safety and efficacy of percutaneous coronary intervention with stenting and coronary artery bypass surgery for multivessel coronary artery disease: a meta-analysis with 5-year patient-level data from the ARTS, ERACI-II, MASS-II, and SoS trials. *Circulation.* 2008;118:1146–1154. https://doi.org/10.1161/CIRCULATIONAHA.107.752147.
25. Hlatky MA, Boothroyd DB, Bravata DM, et al. Coronary artery bypass surgery compared with percutaneous coronary interventions for multivessel disease: a collaborative analysis of individual patient data from ten randomised trials. *Lancet.* 2009;373:1190–1197. https://doi.org/10.1016/S0140-6736(09)60552-3.
26. Park DW, Kim YH, Song HG, et al. Long-term outcome of stents versus bypass surgery in diabetic and nondiabetic patients with multivessel or left main coronary artery disease: a pooled analysis of 5775 individual patient data. *Circ Cardiovasc Interv.* 2012;5:467–475. https://doi.org/10.1161/CIRCINTERVENTIONS.112.969915.
27. Banning AP, Westaby S, Morice MC, et al. Diabetic and nondiabetic patients with left main and/or 3-vessel coronary artery disease: comparison of outcomes with cardiac surgery and paclitaxel-eluting stents. *J Am Coll Cardiol.* 2010;55:1067–1075. https://doi.org/10.1016/j.jacc.2009.09.057.
28. Kapur A, Hall RJ, Malik IS, et al. Randomized comparison of percutaneous coronary intervention with coronary artery bypass grafting in diabetic patients. 1-Year results of the CARDia (Coronary Artery Revascularization in Diabetes) trial. *J Am Coll Cardiol.* 2010;55:432–440. https://doi.org/10.1016/j.jacc.2009.10.014.
29. Onuma Y, Wykrzykowska JJ, Garg S, Vranckx P, Serruys PW, Arts I. Investigators II. 5-Year follow-up of coronary revascularization in diabetic patients with multivessel coronary artery disease: insights from ARTS (arterial revascularization therapy study)-II and ARTS-I trials. *JACC Cardiovasc Interv.* 2011;4:317–323. https://doi.org/10.1016/j.jcin.2010.12.004.
30. Mack MJ, Banning AP, Serruys PW, et al. Bypass versus drug-eluting stents at three years in SYNTAX patients with diabetes mellitus or metabolic syndrome. *Ann Thorac Surg.* 2011;92:2140–2146. https://doi.org/10.1016/j.athoracsur.2011.06.028.
31. Farkouh ME, Domanski M, Fuster V. Revascularization strategies in patients with diabetes. *N Engl J Med.* 2013;368:1455–1456. https://doi.org/10.1056/NEJMc1301244.
32. Kamalesh M, Sharp TG, Tang XC, et al. Percutaneous coronary intervention versus coronary bypass surgery in United States veterans with diabetes. *J Am Coll Cardiol.* 2013;61:808–816. https://doi.org/10.1016/j.jacc.2012.11.044.
33. Ellis SG. Coronary revascularization for patients with diabetes: updated data favor coronary artery bypass grafting. *J Am Coll Cardiol.* 2013;61:817–819. https://doi.org/10.1016/j.jacc.2012.12.003.
34. Mohr FW, Morice MC, Kappetein AP, et al. Coronary artery bypass graft surgery versus percutaneous coronary intervention in patients with three-vessel disease and left main coronary disease: 5-year follow-up of the randomised, clinical SYNTAX trial. *Lancet.* 2013;381:629–638. https://doi.org/10.1016/S0140-6736(13)60141-5.
35. Milojevic M, Serruys PW, Sabik 3rd JF, et al. Bypass surgery or stenting for left main coronary artery disease in patients with diabetes. *J Am Coll Cardiol.* 2019;73:1616–1628. https://doi.org/10.1016/j.jacc.2019.01.037.
36. Sabatine MS, Bergmark BA, Murphy SA, et al. Percutaneous coronary intervention with drug-eluting stents versus coronary artery bypass grafting in left main coronary artery disease: an individual patient data meta-analysis. *Lancet.* 2021;398:2247–2257. https://doi.org/10.1016/S0140-6736(21)02334-5.
37. Farooq V, van Klaveren D, Steyerberg EW, et al. Anatomical and clinical characteristics to guide decision making between coronary artery bypass surgery and percutaneous coronary intervention for individual patients: development and validation of SYNTAX score II. *Lancet.* 2013;381:639–650. https://doi.org/10.1016/S0140-6736(13)60108-7.
38. Koskinas KC, Siontis GC, Piccolo R, et al. Impact of diabetic status on outcomes after revascularization with drug-eluting stents in relation to coronary artery disease complexity: patient-level pooled analysis of 6081 patients. *Circ Cardiovasc Interv.* 2016;9:e003255. https://doi.org/10.1161/CIRCINTERVENTIONS.115.003255.
39. Lee SW, Park SW, Kim YH, et al. A randomized comparison of sirolimus- versus paclitaxel-eluting stent implantation in patients with diabetes mellitus. *J Am Coll Cardiol.* 2008;52:727–733. https://doi.org/10.1016/j.jacc.2008.04.056.
40. Lee SW, Park SW, Kim YH, et al. A randomized comparison of sirolimus-versus paclitaxel-eluting stent implantation in patients with diabetes mellitus: 4-year clinical outcomes of DES-DIABETES (drug-eluting stent in patients with DIABETES mellitus) trial. *JACC Cardiovasc Interv.* 2011;4:310–316. https://doi.org/10.1016/j.jcin.2010.12.006.
41. Maeng M, Jensen LO, Galloe AM, et al. Comparison of the sirolimus-eluting versus paclitaxel-eluting coronary stent in patients with diabetes mellitus: the diabetes and drug-eluting stent (DiabeDES) randomized angiography trial. *Am J Cardiol.* 2009;103:345–349. https://doi.org/10.1016/j.amjcard.2008.09.084.
42. Hong SJ, Kim MH, Cha KS, et al. Comparison of three-year clinical outcomes between sirolimus-versus paclitaxel-eluting stents in diabetic patients: prospective randomized multicenter trial. *Catheter Cardiovasc Interv.* 2010;76:924–933. https://doi.org/10.1002/ccd.22369.
43. Kim MH, Hong SJ, Cha KS, et al. Effect of paclitaxel-eluting versus sirolimus-eluting stents on coronary restenosis in Korean diabetic patients. *J Interv Cardiol.* 2008;21:225–231. https://doi.org/10.1111/j.1540-8183.2008.00353.x.
44. Briguori C, Airoldi F, Visconti G, et al. Novel approaches for preventing or limiting events in diabetic patients (Naples-diabetes) trial: a randomized comparison of 3 drug-eluting stents in diabetic patients. *Circ Cardiovasc Interv.* 2011;4:121–129. https://doi.org/10.1161/CIRCINTERVENTIONS.110.959924.
45. Billinger M, Beutler J, Taghetchian KR, et al. Two-year clinical outcome after implantation of sirolimus-eluting and paclitaxel-eluting stents in diabetic patients. *Eur Heart J.* 2008;29:718–725. https://doi.org/10.1093/eurheartj/ehn021.
46. Kirtane AJ, Patel R, O'Shaughnessy C, et al. Clinical and angiographic outcomes in diabetics from the ENDEAVOR IV trial: randomized comparison of zotarolimus- and paclitaxel-eluting stents in patients with coronary artery disease. *JACC Cardiovasc Interv.* 2009;2:967–976. https://doi.org/10.1016/j.jcin.2009.08.008.
47. Maeng M, Jensen LO, Tilsted HH, et al. Outcome of sirolimus-eluting versus zotarolimus-eluting coronary stent implantation in patients with and without diabetes mellitus (a SORT OUT III Substudy). *Am J Cardiol.* 2011;108:1232–1237. https://doi.org/10.1016/j.amjcard.2011.06.037.
48. Kim WJ, Lee SW, Park SW, et al. Randomized comparison of everolimus-eluting stent versus sirolimus-eluting stent implantation for de novo coronary artery disease in patients with diabetes mellitus (ESSENCE-DIABETES): results from the ESSENCE-DIABETES trial. *Circulation.* 2011;124:886–892. https://doi.org/10.1161/CIRCULATIONAHA.110.015453.
49. Mahmud E, Bromberg-Marin G, Palakodeti V, Ang L, Creanga D, Demaria AN. Clinical efficacy of drug-eluting stents in diabetic patients: a meta-analysis. *J Am Coll Cardiol.* 2008;51:2385–2395. https://doi.org/10.1016/j.jacc.2008.03.028.
50. Stettler C, Allemann S, Egger M, Windecker S, Meier B, Diem P. Efficacy of drug eluting stents in patients with and without diabetes mellitus: indirect comparison of controlled trials. *Heart.* 2006;92:650–657. https://doi.org/10.1136/hrt.2005.070698.
51. Kufner S, de Waha A, Tomai F, et al. A meta-analysis of specifically designed randomized trials of sirolimus-eluting versus paclitaxel-eluting stents in diabetic patients with coronary artery disease. *Am Heart J.* 2011;162:740–747. https://doi.org/10.1016/j.ahj.2011.07.003.
52. Stettler C, Allemann S, Wandel S, et al. Drug eluting and bare metal stents in people with and without diabetes: collaborative network meta-analysis. *BMJ.* 2008;337:a1331. https://doi.org/10.1136/bmj.a1331.
53. Stone GW, Kedhi E, Kereiakes DJ, et al. Differential clinical responses to everolimus-eluting and paclitaxel-eluting coronary stents in patients with and without diabetes mellitus. *Circulation.* 2011;124:893–900. https://doi.org/10.1161/CIRCULATIONAHA.111.031070.
54. Bavishi C, Baber U, Panwar S, et al. Efficacy and safety of everolimus and zotarolimus-eluting stents versus first-generation drug-eluting stents in patients with diabetes: a meta-analysis of randomized trials. *Int J Cardiol.* 2017;230:310–318. https://doi.org/10.1016/j.ijcard.2016.12.116.
55. Park KW, Lee JM, Kang SH, et al. Everolimus-eluting Xience v/Promus versus zotarolimus-eluting resolute stents in patients with diabetes mellitus. *JACC Cardiovasc Interv.* 2014;7:471–481. https://doi.org/10.1016/j.jcin.2013.12.201.
56. Iglesias JF, Degrauwe S, Cimci M, et al. Differential effects of newer-generation ultrathin-strut versus thicker-strut drug-eluting stents in chronic and acute coronary syndromes. *JACC Cardiovasc Interv.* 2021;14:2461–2473. https://doi.org/10.1016/j.jcin.2021.09.028.
57. Iglesias JF, Heg D, Roffi M, et al. Five-year outcomes in patients with diabetes mellitus treated with biodegradable polymer sirolimus-eluting stents versus durable polymer everolimus-eluting stents. *J Am Heart Assoc.* 2019;8:e013607. https://doi.org/10.1161/JAHA.119.013607.
58. Ploumen EH, Buiten RA, Kok MM, et al. Treating diabetic all-comers with contemporary drug-eluting stents: prespecified comparisons from the BIO-RESORT and the BIONYX randomized trials. *Int J Cardiol.* 2021;325:37–44. https://doi.org/10.1016/j.ijcard.2020.10.051.
59. Joner M, Finn AV, Farb A, et al. Pathology of drug-eluting stents in humans: delayed healing and late thrombotic risk. *J Am Coll Cardiol.* 2006;48:193–202. https://doi.org/10.1016/j.jacc.2006.03.042.
60. Iqbal J, Serruys PW, Silber S, et al. Comparison of zotarolimus- and everolimus-eluting coronary stents: final 5-year report of the RESOLUTE all-comers trial. *Circ Cardiovasc Interv.* 2015;8:e002230. https://doi.org/10.1161/CIRCINTERVENTIONS.114.002230.
61. Bavishi C, Chugh Y, Kimura T, et al. Biodegradable polymer drug-eluting stent vs. contemporary durable polymer drug-eluting stents in patients with

diabetes: a meta-analysis of randomized controlled trials. *Eur Heart J Qual Care Clin Outcomes*. 2020;6:81–88. https://doi.org/10.1093/ehjqcco/qcz031.

62. Koch T, Lenz T, Joner M, et al. Ten-year clinical outcomes of polymer-free versus durable polymer new-generation drug-eluting stent in patients with coronary artery disease with and without diabetes mellitus: results of the Intracoronary Stenting and Angiographic Results: Test Efficacy of Sirolimus- and Probucol- and Zotarolimus-Eluting Stents (ISAR-TEST 5) trial. *Clin Res Cardiol*. 2021;110:1586–1598. https://doi.org/10.1007/s00392-021-01854-7.
63. Romaguera R, Salinas P, Gomez-Lara J, et al. Amphilimus- vs. zotarolimus-eluting stents in patients with diabetes mellitus and coronary artery disease: the SUGAR trial. *Eur Heart J*. 2022;43:1320–1330. https://doi.org/10.1093/eurheartj/ehab790.
64. Bhatt DL, Bonaca MP, Bansilal S, et al. Reduction in ischemic events with ticagrelor in diabetic patients with prior myocardial infarction in PEGASUS-TIMI 54. *J Am Coll Cardiol*. 2016;67:2732–2740. https://doi.org/10.1016/j.jacc.2016.03.529.
65. Angiolillo DJ, Badimon JJ, Saucedo JF, et al. A pharmacodynamic comparison of prasugrel vs. high-dose clopidogrel in patients with type 2 diabetes mellitus and coronary artery disease: results of the Optimizing anti-Platelet Therapy In diabetes MellitUS (OPTIMUS)-3 Trial. *Eur Heart J*. 2011;32:838–846. https://doi.org/10.1093/eurheartj/ehq494.
66. Wiviott SD, Braunwald E, Angiolillo DJ, et al. Greater clinical benefit of more intensive oral antiplatelet therapy with prasugrel in patients with diabetes mellitus in the trial to assess improvement in therapeutic outcomes by optimizing platelet inhibition with prasugrel-Thrombolysis in Myocardial Infarction 38. *Circulation*. 2008;118:1626–1636. https://doi.org/10.1161/CIRCULATIONAHA.108.791061.
67. James S, Angiolillo DJ, Cornel JH, et al. Ticagrelor vs. clopidogrel in patients with acute coronary syndromes and diabetes: a substudy from the PLATelet inhibition and patient Outcomes (PLATO) trial. *Eur Heart J*. 2010;31:3006–3016. https://doi.org/10.1093/eurheartj/ehq325.
68. Brar SS, Kim J, Brar SK, et al. Long-term outcomes by clopidogrel duration and stent type in a diabetic population with de novo coronary artery lesions. *J Am Coll Cardiol*. 2008;51:2220–2227. https://doi.org/10.1016/j.jacc.2008.01.063.
69. Byrne RA, Rossello X, Coughlan JJ, et al. 2023 ESC guidelines for the management of acute coronary syndromes. *Eur Heart J*. 2023;44:3720–3826. https://doi.org/10.1093/eurheartj/ehad191.
70. Lawton JS, Tamis-Holland JE, Bangalore S, et al. 2021 ACC/AHA/SCAI guideline for coronary artery revascularization: a report of the American College of Cardiology/American Heart Association Joint Committee on Clinical Practice Guidelines. *Circulation*. 2022;145:e18–e114. https://doi.org/10.1161/CIR.0000000000001038.
71. Steg PG, Bhatt DL, Simon T, et al. Ticagrelor in patients with stable coronary disease and diabetes. *N Engl J Med*. 2019;381:1309–1320. https://doi.org/10.1056/NEJMoa1908077.
72. Bhatt DL, Steg PG, Mehta SR, et al. Ticagrelor in patients with diabetes and stable coronary artery disease with a history of previous percutaneous coronary intervention (THEMIS-PCI): a phase 3, placebo-controlled, randomised trial. *Lancet*. 2019;394:1169–1180. https://doi.org/10.1016/S0140-6736(19)31887-2.
73. Oyama K, Furtado RHM, Fagundes Jr. A, et al. Effect of evolocumab on complex coronary disease requiring revascularization. *J Am Coll Cardiol*. 2021;77:259–267. https://doi.org/10.1016/j.jacc.2020.11.011.
74. Kappetein AP, Head SJ, Morice MC, et al. Treatment of complex coronary artery disease in patients with diabetes: 5-year results comparing outcomes of bypass surgery and percutaneous coronary intervention in the SYNTAX trial. *Eur J Cardiothorac Surg*. 2013;43:1006–1013. https://doi.org/10.1093/ejcts/ezt017.

PART V **OTHER CARDIOVASCULAR CONSIDERATIONS FOR PATIENTS WITH TYPE 2 DIABETES**

22 Peripheral Artery Disease in Persons With Type 2 Diabetes

AARON W. ADAY AND JOSHUA A. BECKMAN

Peripheral artery disease (PAD) is defined as partial or complete obstruction of one or more lower extremity arteries that significantly reduces ankle perfusion pressure and is usually caused by atherosclerosis. Classic symptoms of PAD include leg pain with ambulation, termed *intermittent claudication*, resulting, in part, from an inadequate blood supply relative to demand in the lower extremities. In severe cases, termed *chronic limb-threatening ischemia (CLTI)*, symptoms occur at rest, and tissue ischemia may lead to ulceration or gangrene. Patients with PAD may also have atypical limb symptoms or functional limitations without reported limb symptoms. Regardless, PAD is associated with a significant risk of functional decline, limb revascularization, amputation, and death. Patients with diabetes are among those most likely to develop PAD and also among those most likely to develop complications resulting from both disease processes.

This chapter provides a framework for the diagnosis and management of patients with PAD, focusing on the overlap and special characteristics of patients with concomitant diabetes.

EPIDEMIOLOGY AND PROGNOSIS OF PERIPHERAL ARTERY DISEASE AND DIABETES—OVERLAPPING EPIDEMICS

The reported prevalence of PAD varies as a function of the population tested, the diagnostic method used, and whether symptoms are included to derive estimates. The ankle-brachial index (ABI) is the most commonly used noninvasive measurement in epidemiologic studies and is described in more detail later. The ABI is the ratio of the higher ankle pressure in a given limb to the higher of either brachial systolic blood pressure. Global data suggest that the overall prevalence of PAD, defined as an ABI ≤0.9, is 5.56%; the prevalence is greatest in high-income countries (7.37%). Modeling estimates suggest up to 30% of Black individuals and 20% of White or Hispanic individuals will develop PAD over their lifetime.[1,2] The prevalence of PAD also increases with age[3] (Fig. 22.1). Only a small proportion of those with ABI-defined PAD have claudication, with estimates ranging from approximately 10% to 30%.[4–6] The prevalence of PAD increases with age[6,7] (Fig. 22.2). There is less information about the true incidence of CLTI. However, data from 2003 to 2008 suggest the prevalence of CLTI is 1.3% among individuals older than age 40.[8]

Major risk factors for PAD overlap with, but are not identical to, those for coronary artery disease (CAD) and cerebrovascular disease. It is important to note that diabetes, smoking, older age, elevated triglyceride-rich lipoprotein concentrations, and elevated systolic blood pressure are particularly potent risk factors for PAD.[2] Meta-analysis data suggest active smoking is associated with a 2.8-fold increased risk of PAD, and this was greater than the other risk factors studied.[1] In the Atherosclerosis Risk in Communities (ARIC) study, the relative risk (RR) for PAD for those with a ≥25 pack-year history of smoking compared to[9] those who have never smoked was ~4 compared to 1.5 to 2 for CAD and stroke.[9] Mendelian randomization analyses have also shown that smoking is more[10] potently linked to developing PAD than CAD or stroke.[10]

Similar to smoking, diabetes increases the risk of PAD nearly twofold in contemporary meta-analyses.[11] Even in those without diabetes, insulin resistance has also been linked to the development of PAD.[12] The duration and severity of diabetes correlate with the incidence and extent of PAD. Among 48,607 males in the prospective

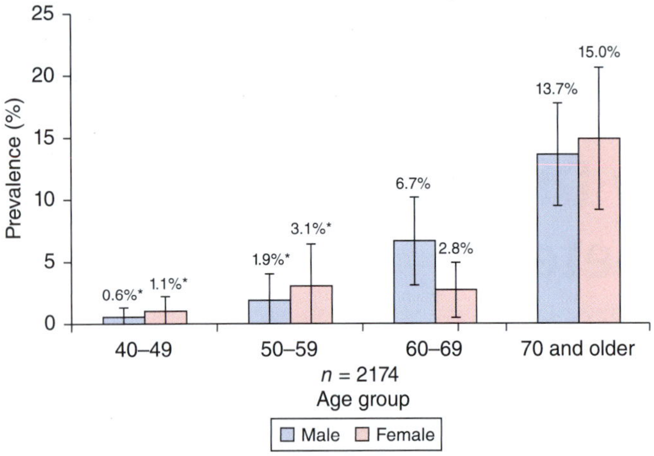

FIG. 22.1 Peripheral artery disease (PAD) prevalence and age from the National Health and Nutrition Examination Survey (NHANES).[4] (Modified from Selvin E, Erlinger TP. Prevalence of and risk factors for peripheral arterial disease in the United States: results from the National Health and Nutrition Examination Survey, 1999–2000. *Circulation*. 2004;110:738–743.)

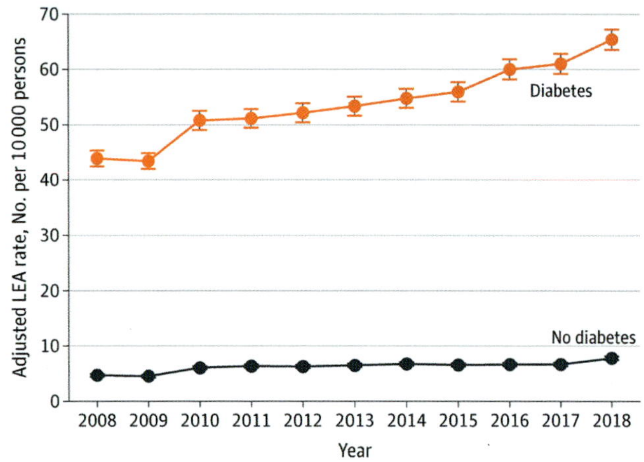

FIG. 22.3 Incidence rate for lower extremity amputation adjusted for age, sex, and race among diabetic and nondiabetic patients. (Modified from Cai M, Xie Y, Bowe B, et al. Temporal trends in incidence rates of lower extremity amputation and associated risk factors among patients using veterans health administration services from 2008 to 2018. *JAMA Netw Open*. 2021;4(1):e2033953.)

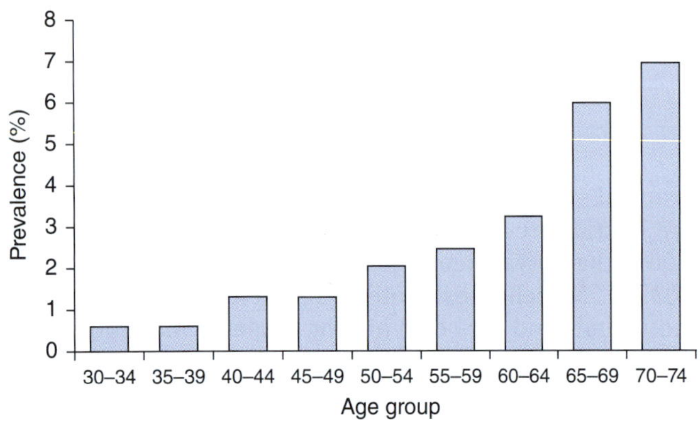

FIG. 22.2 The prevalence of claudication with age. From TransAtlantic Inter-Society Consensus Document on Management of Peripheral Arterial Disease II (TASC II).[6] (From Norgren L, Hiatt WR, Dormandy JA, et al. Inter-society consensus for the management of peripheral arterial disease [TASC II]. *Eur J Vasc Endovasc Surg*. 2007;33(Suppl 1):S1–S75.)

Health Professionals Follow-up Study, 1 to 5 years of a diabetes diagnosis was associated with a hazard ratio (HR) for PAD of 1.39 (95% CI, 0.82–2.36); this increased to 4.53 (95% CI, 2.39–8.58) with >25 years of diabetes.[13] The degree of diabetic glycemic control is also an independent risk factor for PAD; with every 1% increase in glycosylated hemoglobin (HbA1c), the risk of PAD increases by 28%.[14]

Patients with diabetes and PAD have a sixfold increased risk of CLTI compared to nondiabetic patients,[15] and up to 76% of patients with CLTI have diabetes.[16,17] Individuals with diabetes are approximately 15 times more likely to have an amputation than those without diabetes,[18] and the rate of lower extremity amputations is increasing, particular among those with diabetes.[19] From 2009 to 2015, the age-adjusted rate among those with diabetes increased from 3.1 per 1000 adults to 4.6 per 1000 adults (Fig. 22.3).[20] Patients with diabetes often have extensive and severe PAD and a greater propensity for arterial calcification.[21,22] Involvement of the femoral and popliteal arteries often resembles that of nondiabetics, but distal disease affecting the tibial and peroneal arteries occurs more frequently in diabetics.[23]

CLINICAL PRESENTATION, DIAGNOSIS, AND NATURAL HISTORY OF PERIPHERAL ARTERY DISEASE IN DIABETES

The hallmark features of clinical PAD include intermittent claudication and rest pain. The location of the symptoms often relates to the site of the most proximal stenosis. In general, buttock, hip, or thigh claudication typically occurs in patients with aortic or iliac stenosis. Calf claudication characterizes femoral or popliteal involvement. Ankle or foot claudication occurs in patients with tibial or peroneal disease. Claudication symptoms should be brought on by exertion and should resolve within minutes after cessation of effort. Leg pain that occurs at rest, such as nocturnal cramping in the calf or thigh, should not be confused with claudication.

Symptoms may occur at rest in patients with CLTI. Typically, patients complain of paresthesias or pain in the foot or toes of the affected limb. This discomfort worsens with limb elevation and often improves when the limb is lowered, as would be expected because of the increased perfusion pressure to the distal limb by the effect of gravity. The pain can be particularly severe at sites of skin breakdown, and often the skin is exquisitely sensitive to light touch. These symptoms may be absent, however, in diabetic patients with significant peripheral neuropathy, who may have important limb ischemia but experience few symptoms.

A complete cardiovascular physical examination is necessary to detect all the findings of PAD in patients with diabetes. Pulse abnormalities and bruits increase the likelihood of PAD.[24] The legs of patients with chronic aortoiliac disease may demonstrate muscular atrophy. Hair loss, thick or brittle toenails, and smooth and shiny skin on the legs can also indicate PAD. Patients with severe limb ischemia often have cool skin and may have petechiae, cyanosis or pallor, dependent rubor, skin fissures, ulceration, or gangrene. Ulcers that result from PAD often have a pale base with irregular borders and usually involve the tips

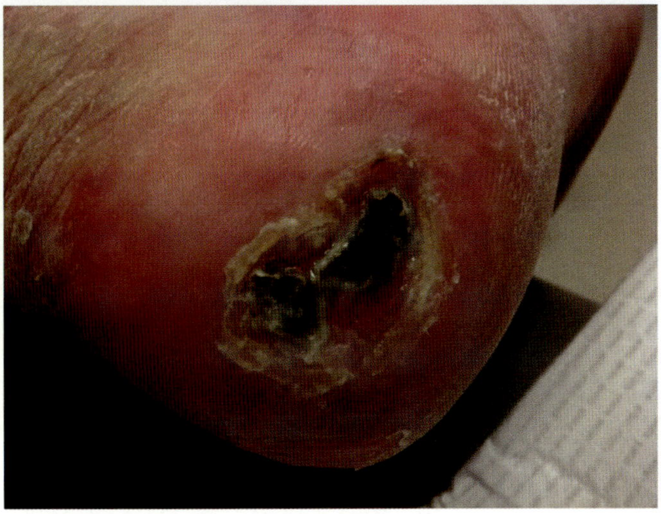

FIG. 22.4 A typical nonhealing arterial ulcer.

TABLE 22.1 Clinical Classification Schemes for Peripheral Artery Disease

FONTAINE CLASSIFICATION		RUTHERFORD CLASSIFICATION		
STAGE	CLINICAL DESCRIPTION	GRADE	CATEGORY	CLINICAL DESCRIPTION
I	Asymptomatic	0	0	Asymptomatic
IIa	Mild claudication	I	1	Mild claudication
IIb	Moderate-to-severe claudication	I, I	2, 3	Moderate claudication, severe claudication
III	Rest pain	II	4	Rest pain
IV	Ulceration or gangrene	III, IV	5, 6	Minor tissue loss, ulceration or gangrene

Data from White CJ, Gray WA. Endovascular therapies for peripheral arterial disease: an evidence-based review. *Circulation.* 2007;116:2203–2215.

of the toes, the heel of the foot, or other sites that bear chronic pressure (Fig. 22.4).

The clinical stage of symptomatic PAD can be classified according to the Fontaine or Rutherford scoring systems.[25,26] Fontaine stage I represents those who have PAD but are asymptomatic. Stages IIa and IIb include patients with mild and moderate-to-severe intermittent claudication. Patients with ischemic rest pain are classified as stage III, and those with ulceration or gangrene are stage IV. In the Rutherford classification, asymptomatic patients are classified as category 0. Patients with mild claudication are category 1. Patients with moderate claudication are category 2 and patients with severe claudication are category 3. Patients with rest pain are category 4. Patients with minor tissue loss, ulceration, or gangrene are categories 5 and 6 (Table 22.1).

The main reasons to diagnose PAD in diabetic individuals are to initiate therapies that decrease the risk of atherothrombotic events, to improve the overall quality of life, and to decrease disability. A diagnosis of PAD indicates the presence of systemic atherosclerosis that confers additional cardiovascular risk to the patient with diabetes, which gives further impetus to aggressively manage vascular risk factors in this high-risk group.[27] Although the physical examination provides important information, additional noninvasive testing is necessary to formally diagnose PAD. The ABI is a reproducible and reasonably accurate measurement for the detection of PAD. The American Heart Association has published a consensus scientific statement regarding use of the ABI and suggested standard definitions and interpretation.[28] The ABI is normally between 1.00 and 1.40.[28,29] In PAD, atherosclerotic lesions in the leg arteries cause a decrease in the ankle systolic blood pressure, and the ABI is reduced to below 1.00. PAD is defined as an ABI of 0.90 or lower, with values from 0.91 to 1.00 classified as borderline.[28,30] Lower ABI values indicate more severe PAD. Patients with symptoms of leg claudication often have ABIs from 0.5 to 0.8, and patients with CLTI usually have an ABI below 0.5. The ABI has been shown to correlate inversely with walking distance and walking speed. For example, less than 40% of patients with an ABI below 0.4 can complete a 6-minute walking test.[31] One limitation of the ABI in patients with diabetes, however, is that leg blood pressure recordings cannot be reliably interpreted in patients with calcified vessels because these vessels are not reliably compressed during inflation of the blood pressure cuff. Because diabetic patients are more likely than nondiabetics to have arterial calcifications, ABI measurements in certain individuals can be difficult to interpret, and other noninvasive tests, such as a toe-brachial index, should be used to make the diagnosis.[29] The diagnostic measurement of the ABI for the detection of lower-extremity PAD varies according to the population studied, the cutoff threshold, and the reference gold standard test (i.e., invasive angiography or duplex ultrasound). The sensitivity and specificity of the ABI range from 0.17 to 1.0 and from 0.8 to 1.0, respectively.[28] Overall, lower sensitivities are reported in diabetic patients.[32–34]

The American Diabetes Association (ADA) consensus statement recommends that an ABI be performed in all diabetic individuals with symptoms of claudication or abnormal pedal pulses on exam.[35] For the general, nondiabetic population, screening ABI testing is currently not recommended by the United States Preventive Services Task Force.[36] In general, PAD is underdiagnosed in the primary care setting.[5] A large-scale PAD screening study demonstrated that only one-third of patients with documented PAD had classical claudication symptoms.[37] These data suggest that classic symptoms are inadequate in determining a person's health status with regard to PAD. Particularly in diabetic patients with peripheral neuropathy, ABI screening of asymptomatic individuals represents an important tool in diagnosing PAD and allowing for an appropriately tailored strategy for therapeutic decisions.

Patients with PAD remain undertreated even after diagnosis. Among 250,103 patients with PAD in the MarketScan database, 40.0% were not receiving lipid-lowering therapy at baseline.[38] Patients with PAD are less likely to receive a statin than those with CAD or cerebrovascular disease.[39] In the Best endovascular versus best surgical therapy in patients with CLTI (BESTCLI) clinical trial of patients with PAD and CLTI, only 25% were receiving optimal medical therapy defined as a controlled blood pressure, no active smoking, and use of both lipid-lowering and antiplatelet therapy.[40]

In a patient with confirmed PAD for whom further investigation is required, usually at a time when revascularization is considered, there are other modalities available for investigating the extent and nature of the PAD. Segmental pressures and pulse volume recordings are both noninvasive hemodynamic studies that aid in the localization of arterial occlusive disease.[29] Other noninvasive imaging techniques, including magnetic resonance angiography and computed tomographic angiography, or duplex ultrasonography can provide more precise anatomic information for revascularization planning purposes. Conventional, contrast-based angiography is also useful, particularly when other modalities are inconclusive.

Overall, patients with PAD have an increased risk of adverse cardiovascular events, as well as impaired quality of life, and an increased risk of limb loss. In addition, patients with PAD and concomitant diabetes are at risk for higher cardiovascular and cerebrovascular event rates than comparable nondiabetics.[41] The combination of PAD and diabetes causes most nontraumatic lower-extremity amputations in the United States.[42] In the Exenatide Study of Cardiovascular Event Lowering trial, patients with diabetes and PAD had a 5.5-fold greater risk of amputation than those with diabetes alone.[41] Up to 30% of patients with diabetes and CLTI require amputation, and this trend is worsening.[43]

Diabetes is also commonly associated with microvascular disease. Each of the major manifestations of microvascular disease is associated with higher rates of amputation. In the Wisconsin Epidemiologic Study of Diabetic Retinopathy, proliferative retinopathy increased the risk of amputation 5-fold in young persons and 20-fold in older patients. An increasing risk of amputation has been directly associated with worsening proteinuria as well. Neuropathy increases the risk of amputation, like other manifestations of microvascular disease, but also heightens the risk of foot injury as a result of impaired sensation, muscle wasting with a swan neck deformity from motor neuropathy, and decreased sweating with skin dryness and cracking from autonomic neuropathy. The presence of microvascular disease potentiates the risk of amputation beyond PAD alone from 14-fold to 24-fold compared with healthy persons (Fig. 22.5).[44] The presence of microvascular disease independently increases the risk of amputation and the onset of PAD magnifies that risk markedly.

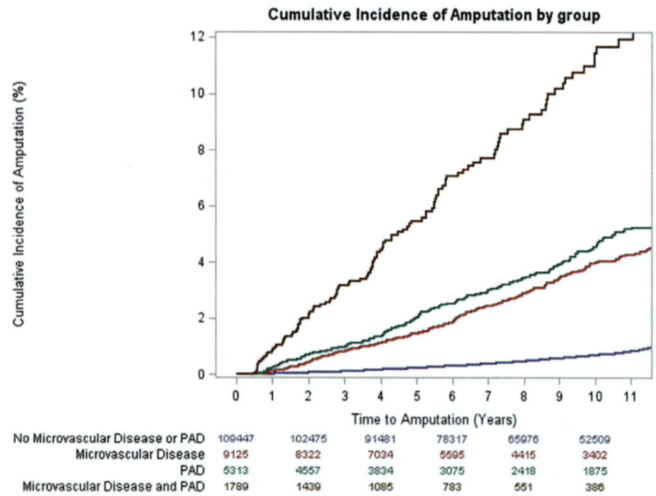

FIG. 22.5 Cumulative incidence of amputation among US veterans based on the presence of microvascular disease and/or peripheral artery disease PAD. (Modified from Beckman JA, Duncan MS, Damrauer SM, et al. Microvascular disease, peripheral artery disease, and amputation. *Circulation*. 2019;140(6):449–458.)

RISK FACTOR IDENTIFICATION, LIFESTYLE MODIFICATION, AND PHARMACOTHERAPY

Once diabetic individuals with PAD have been identified, the aim of medical management is to aggressively modify cardiovascular risk factors for the prevention of adverse cardiovascular events and to relieve symptoms related to PAD to improve functional status and quality of life. These two goals should be addressed simultaneously in every patient.

Lowering Cardiovascular Morbidity and Mortality

The risk factors for PAD largely overlap those of other forms of atherosclerotic vascular disease, and PAD is similarly associated with an increased risk of coronary, cerebrovascular, and renovascular disease. As a result, PAD is considered a coronary heart disease equivalent, elevating it to the highest category of cardiovascular risk.[45] The 2024 American Heart Association/American College of Cardiology (ACC/AHA) practice guidelines on the management of PAD recommend smoking cessation, lipid-lowering therapy with statins, and the treatment of diabetes and hypertension.[29] Data from a Dutch prospective cohort study of 2420 patients with PAD (ABI 0.90 or lower) support these conclusions and demonstrate that a comprehensive approach to risk factor modification can have additive benefits.[46] In this study, after adjustment for risk factors and propensity scores, statins (HR, 0.46; 95% CI, 0.36–0.58), beta-blockers (HR, 0.68; 95% CI, 0.58–0.80), aspirin (HR, 0.72; 95% CI, 0.61–0.84), and angiotensin-converting enzyme (ACE) inhibitors (HR, 0.80; 95% CI, 0.69–0.94) were significantly associated with a reduced risk of long-term mortality. The benefits of these therapies appear additive, and these data support the universal nature of atherosclerotic vascular disease, whether in the form of PAD or elsewhere.

DYSLIPIDEMIA

Several cholesterol-lowering trials in patients with dyslipidemia and CAD and/or PAD have evaluated the effects of lipid lowering on PAD. Among 155,647 patients with incident PAD in the Veterans Affairs health care system, high-intensity statin use was associated with a 33% reduction in amputation and a 26% reduction in mortality compared to a control group on antiplatelet therapy alone.[47] This benefit extended to low- and moderate-intensity statins, although to a lesser degree. Among 3642 patients with PAD in the Further Cardiovascular Outcomes Research with PCSK9 Inhibition in Subjects with Elevated

Risk (FOURIER) trial, which randomized patients to the PCSK9 inhibitor evolocumab or placebo, treatment with evolocumab led to a 27% reduction in a composite of cardiovascular death, myocardial infarction (MI), or stroke.[48]

Independent of cholesterol-lowering effects, statin use improves pain-free walking distance and walking speed in patients with PAD and claudication.[49] Two studies randomized patients with claudication to simvastatin 40 mg daily or a placebo. Aronow and colleagues reported an improvement in pain-free walking distance of a 24% increase at 6 months and of a 42% increase at 1 year after initiation of treatment, although total walking distance and ABI did not improve.[50] In contrast, Mondillo and colleagues reported increases in ABI, total walking distance, and pain-free survival in patients randomized to simvastatin (Fig. 22.6).[51] Mohler and colleagues randomized 354 patients with claudication to atorvastatin 10 mg or 80 mg or a placebo.[52] Patients receiving atorvastatin had an increased pain-free walking distance, but not total walking distance or ABI. Patients with PAD who take statins have been shown to have less annual decline in lower-extremity performance than those who do not.[53] Overall, the aggregate data suggest that statin use may increase the walking distance until the onset of pain, but statin use does not clearly affect total walking time or change lower-extremity blood flow as measured by ABI.

There is also a role for fibrate therapy in the treatment of PAD. The Fenofibrate Intervention and Event Lowering in Diabetes study randomized 9795 patients aged 50 to 75 years with type 2 diabetes to either fenofibrate 200 mg/day or a placebo for 5 years' duration. The risks of first amputation (45 vs. 70 events; HR, 0.64; 95% CI, 0.44–0.94; $P = 0.02$) and minor amputation events without known large-vessel disease (18 vs. 34 events; HR, 0.53; 95% CI, 0.30–0.94; $P = 0.027$) were lower for patients assigned to fenofibrate than for patients assigned to a placebo, with no difference between groups in risk of major amputations.[54]

Current AHA/ACC guidelines advocate a goal LDL-C reduction of ≥50% for all patients with PAD using high-intensity statins or maximally tolerated statin therapy.[29] For the highest-risk individuals, including those with both PAD and diabetes, guidelines recommend using nonstatin agents to target an LDL-C below 70 mg/dL. The European Society of Cardiology guidelines recommend an LDL-C reduction of ≥50% or an LDL target of <1.4 mmol/L (<55 mg/dL) for patients with diabetes and PAD.[55]

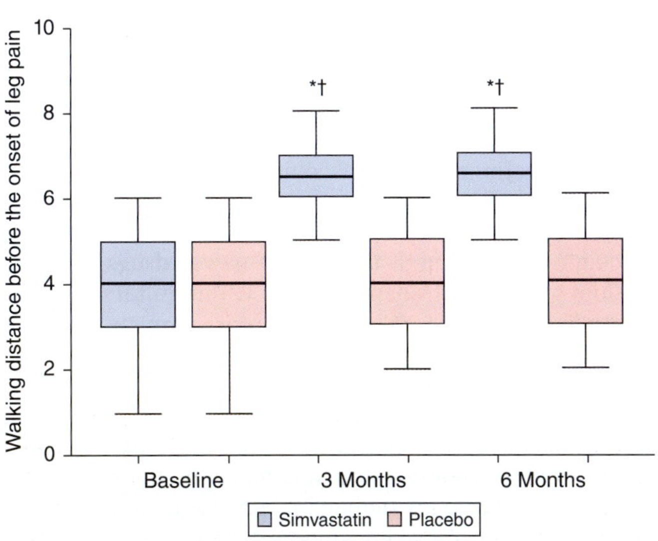

FIG. 22.6 Simvastatin can improve walking distance in patients with PAD.[46] (Modified from Mondillo S, Ballo P, Barbati R, et al. Effects of simvastatin on walking performance and symptoms of intermittent claudication in hypercholesterolemic patients with peripheral vascular disease. *Am J Med.* 2003;114:359–364.)

SMOKING CESSATION

Several nonrandomized studies have shown that patients who successfully quit smoking have decreased rates of PAD progression, CLTI, amputation, MI, and stroke, and have an increased survival.[56] Unfortunately, the spontaneous cessation rates without intervention range from 2% to 5% in the United States, despite nearly 75% of smokers expressing a desire to stop. Given the importance of smoking cessation, it is important for health care providers to consistently convey to patients that discontinuation of tobacco products is extremely important to overall survival, well-being, and limb preservation.[57,58] Behavioral interventions can improve cessation rates, but only modestly. Only 5% of patients who receive physician advice, follow-up correspondence, phone calls, and supplementary visits will quit smoking.[59] Randomized trial evidence, however, has demonstrated that a 10-week intervention that results in just a 21.7% smoking cessation rate at 5 years significantly improves survival in patients with chronic lung disease compared with those treated with usual care.[60] Thus efforts at cessation should be made.

Hennrikus and colleagues have specifically demonstrated that individuals with PAD respond to intensive counseling and education in a randomized trial of 124 patients. These researchers compared an intensive tobacco cessation counseling program with a minimal educational program over 6 months. Study participants assigned to the intensive intervention group were significantly more likely to be abstinent from tobacco at 6-month follow-up: 21.3% versus 6.8% in the minimal intervention group ($P = 0.023$).[61]

Smoking cessation can be aided in many ways, including the use of pharmacotherapy, such as short-term nicotine replacement products including gums, long-acting nicotine replacement patches, bupropion, or varenicline. Pharmacologic interventions are more effective than medical advice alone. In controlled studies, the rates of stopping smoking with the use of pharmacologic treatment interventions have varied from 17% to 48% at 6 months and from 11% to 34% at 1 year.[62]

Bupropion is a norepinephrine and dopamine reuptake inhibitor that diminishes the desire for smoking via a poorly understood mechanism. It is associated with cessation rates of 27% to 35% at 6 months and 23% to 30% at 1 year.[63] Varenicline, a partial agonist selective for the alpha$_4$, beta$_2$ nicotinic acetylcholine receptor, is the most effective pharmacologic smoking cessation agent. In a study of 1025 smokers where participants were randomized to a placebo, sustained-release bupropion, or varenicline, abstinence rates from weeks 9 to 52 were significantly elevated in the two drug arms compared with placebo. Cessation rates were 8.4%, 16.1%, and 21.9%, respectively, for individuals taking placebo, bupropion, and varenicline.[64]

In a second large, randomized trial, investigators found similar abstinence rates in individuals treated with placebo, bupropion, or varenicline.[65]

The current Expert Consensus Decision Pathway from the American College of Cardiology recommends either varenicline or combination nicotine replacement therapy (patch plus lozenge, gum, inhaler, or spray) as a first-line therapy.[66] Although earlier studies raised concern for neuropsychiatric side effects with varenicline, a subsequent randomized, placebo-controlled clinical trial designed to investigate this issue found no increased risk of such side effects with varenicline compared to nicotine replacement therapy or placebo.[67]

Despite multiple options for the approach to tobacco cessation in individuals with PAD, there appears to be continued risk in individuals who successfully abstain. Data from the Women's Health Study demonstrate that although smoking cessation substantially reduces risk for PAD events in females, there remains an increased occurrence of PAD events in former smokers compared with individuals who never smoked.[68] In ARIC, individuals were at a heightened risk for PAD 30 years after smoking cessation compared to those who had never smoked, whereas the risk for CAD persisted to 20 years after cessation.[9]

HYPERTENSION

In a large number of clinical trials involving thousands of patients, antihypertensive drug therapy has been associated with a 35% to 40% mean reduction in the rate of stroke, a 20% to 25% reduction in MI, more than a 50% reduction in heart failure, and a significant reduction in the development of chronic kidney disease.[69] Although the treatment of hypertension has been studied in many contexts, there are limited data available to determine whether the treatment of hypertension prevents the development of claudication or alters the course of PAD itself.

The Treatment of Mild Hypertension Study showed that drug treatment in addition to nutritional interventions was superior to nutritional interventions alone in preventing the development of intermittent claudication and PAD over an average follow-up of 4.4 years.[70] Reports on the effect of blood pressure lowering on the ability to walk in patients with intermittent claudication are mixed.[71–73] However, these small studies have demonstrated that the ACE inhibitor captopril maintains and may increase walking distance in patients with claudication. Alpha-adrenergic blockers, beta-blockers, and calcium channel blockers may adversely affect walking distance, particularly if there is a substantial decrease in systolic blood pressure. In a 6-month crossover trial of 20 hypertensive patients with PAD randomized to atenolol, labetalol, pindolol, captopril, or a placebo, only individuals treated with captopril maintained a walking distance.[73] This appears to be a class effect, as enalapril and ramipril also seem to improve lower-extremity blood flow in patients with claudication.[74] Among 33,357 patients in the Antihypertensive and Lipid-Lowering Treatment to Prevent Heart Attack Trial (ALLHAT), a target systolic blood pressure <120 mm Hg was associated with a 26% increased risk of limb events compared to a target blood pressure of 120 to 129 mm Hg.[75] Thus while antihypertensive therapy is important in patients with PAD, aggressive blood pressure lowering may come at the cost of worsened limb perfusion.

In patients with both PAD and diabetes, the Appropriate Blood Pressure Control in Diabetes (ABCD) study supports intensive management of hypertension.[76] The ABCD study randomized 480 normotensive patients (baseline diastolic blood pressure of 80–89 mm Hg) with type 2 diabetes to either an intensive blood pressure regimen with enalapril or nisoldipine or a placebo. Individuals were followed for 5 years. Fifty-three of the patients had PAD as defined by an ABI below 0.90. In patients with PAD, there were 3 cardiovascular events (13.6%) in the intensive treatment group compared with 12 events (38.7%) in patients taking a placebo ($P = 0.046$). After an adjustment for multiple cardiovascular risk factors, an inverse relationship between ABI and cardiovascular events was observed with a placebo ($P = 0.009$), but not with intensive treatment ($P = 0.91$). Thus with intensive blood pressure control, the risk of an event was not increased, even at the lowest ABI values, and was the same as in patients without PAD. The conclusion from the trial was that intensive blood pressure lowering to a mean of 128/75 mm Hg resulted in a marked reduction in cardiovascular events.

Current guidelines recommend antihypertensive therapy be administered to hypertensive patients with PAD to achieve a blood pressure less than 130/80 mm Hg to reduce the risk of MI, stroke, heart failure, and cardiovascular death.[77]

DIABETES MELLITUS

To date, no prospective trials have been performed to assess whether improved glycemic control decreases the cardiovascular risk associated with PAD, the walking distance of patients with claudication, or the frequency of amputation among those with PAD. In a retrospective review of the Diabetes Control and Complications Trial of patients with type 1 diabetes mellitus, there was a 22% risk reduction in the development of PAD in the group that received intensive insulin therapy.[78] Epidemiologic studies also support the benefit of tight glycemic control. The prospective Belfast Diet Study of type 2 diabetic patients demonstrated an increasing risk for MI of 1.04 per mmol increase in fasting plasma glucose.[79] In the UK Prospective Diabetes Study of 2693 patients followed for nearly 8 years, patients in the highest tertile of HbA1c had a 1.5-fold greater risk for MI compared with those in the lowest tertile.[80] Although no prospective trial has demonstrated the noncoronary vascular benefits of improved glycemic control, meta-analyses of newer drugs, such as sodium glucose cotransport-2 (SGLT2) inhibitors and glucagon-like peptide-1 (GLP-1) receptor agonists, suggest their cardiovascular benefits may be even greater in the setting of tight glycemic control.[81]

Further reductions in goal HbA1c levels have been tested in several recent trials.[82–85] Although intensive glycemic control reduced the incidence of microvascular events, there were no significant reductions in macrovascular outcomes between standard and intensive glycemic control. The Action to Control Cardiovascular Risk in Diabetes trial, for example, randomized 10,251 patients with a history of a cardiovascular event or significant cardiovascular risk to intensive glycemic control (target HbA1c below 6.0%) or standard glycemic control (target HbA1c 7.0%–7.9%). Within 12 months of randomization, the intensive glycemic group reached a median HbA1c of 6.4% (from a baseline median of 8.1%) compared with a median HbA1c of 7.5% in the standard glycemic group. However, the glycemic control arm was stopped because of an increased mortality rate in the intensive glycemic control group.[82] At this time, the optimal HbA1c goal for individuals with PAD has not been clearly defined for all patients.

SGLT2 inhibitors are a mainstay of diabetes treatment due to their broad cardiovascular benefits.[86] However, an early concern from large, placebo-controlled randomized trials of SGLT2 inhibitors was an increased risk of lower limb amputation. In the Canagliflozin Cardiovascular Assessment Study (CANVAS), therapy with canagliflozin led to a nearly twofold increased risk of amputation compared to a placebo,[87] and there was speculation that this may be due to a class effect.[88,89] However, a meta-analysis examining more than 41,000 participants in randomized, placebo-controlled trials of SGLT2 inhibitors found no increased risk of amputation with other drugs in this class (RR, 1.06; 95% CI, 0.93–1.21), suggesting this risk is unique to canagliflozin.[90]

GLP-1 receptor agonists have similarly revolutionized the medical therapy of diabetes, in part due to a reduction in cardiovascular risk demonstrated in multiple placebo-controlled trials of drugs in this class.[91] The impact of these medications on lower limb outcomes remains unclear. In a Danish cohort study of 309,116 patients with diabetes, treatment with GLP-1 receptor agonists was associated with a reduced amputation risk (HR, 0.50; 95% CI, 0.54–0.74). This reduction was largely seen in those treated with liraglutide.[92] In a small, open-label clinical trial of patients with diabetes and PAD, liraglutide increased pedal transcutaneous oxygen pressure, a measure of peripheral perfusion.[93] Randomized, placebo-controlled trials of GLP-1 receptor antagonists in patients with PAD and diabetes that include limb-specific outcomes are ongoing.

Current recommendations from the ADA support a target HbA1c of <7%, regardless of PAD status.[94] Despite a paucity of clinical trial evidence, meticulous foot care is also recommended for patients with diabetes and PAD to reduce the risk of skin ulceration, necrosis, and subsequent amputation. This includes the use of appropriate footwear to avoid pressure injury, daily inspection and cleansing by the patient, and the use of moisturizing cream to prevent dryness and fissuring. Frequent foot inspection by patients and health care providers is thought to enable early identification of foot lesions and ulcerations and facilitate prompt referral for treatment.[95]

OBESITY AND WEIGHT REDUCTION

The reported association between obesity and PAD is inconsistent. Obesity, as determined by a body mass index (BMI) over 30 kg/m^2, was not a risk factor for PAD or intermittent claudication in the Edinburgh Artery Study, Whitehall study, or Lipid Research Clinics study.[96–98] In contrast, among 3,250,350 individuals who underwent commercial ABI screening, body mass index (BMI) > 40 kg/m^2 was associated with a greater prevalence of an abnormal ABI < 0.90 among men (odds ratio [OR] = 2.98) and females (OR 1.37) compared to those with a BMI of 25 to 29.9 kg/m^2.[99] Despite the mixed evidence for a direct relationship between obesity and PAD, obesity may heighten the risk for PAD by increasing the prevalence of other previously established risk factors. For example, in a study of 8688 males followed for 5 years, being overweight was the most significant predictor of who was going to develop type 2 diabetes mellitus.[98] McDermott and colleagues have shown that over 4 years of follow-up, patients with intermittent claudication and a BMI over 30 kg/m^2 had significantly more functional decline.[100] Thus it stands to reason that any decrease in weight will decrease the work required for walking and will improve exercise capacity. Therefore maintenance of a normal weight is recommended for patients with PAD.

ANTIPLATELET THERAPY

There is substantial evidence that the cardiovascular morbidity and mortality related to PAD in patients with diabetes is related to platelet activity and inflammation. Platelet activity can be modified by the use of antiplatelet agents. The data supporting the use of antiplatelet agents for the prevention of cardiovascular events in patients with PAD in general is mixed, as is described here.

A meta-analysis of approximately 150 prospective controlled trials of antiplatelet therapy (mostly aspirin) has been reported as part of the Antithrombotic Trialists' Collaborative. This analysis combined data from more than 135,000 individuals with evidence of cardiovascular disease, including PAD. Investigators demonstrated a 22% reduction in the odds ratio in the composite primary endpoint of MI, stroke, and vascular death in patients taking antiplatelet therapy compared with controls. When the subset of approximately 9000 patients with claudication was analyzed, the protective effect of antiplatelet therapy was similar.[101] A more recent meta-analysis of 18 prospective trials totaling 5269 patients with PAD found that aspirin therapy compared with placebo was not associated with significant reductions in all-cause or cardiovascular mortality, MI, or major bleeding.[102]

The Aspirin for Asymptomatic Atherosclerosis trial enrolled asymptomatic patients with ABI of 0.95 or lower (instead of the standard cutoff value of 0.90 used in the multisociety guidelines) to 100 mg of aspirin daily or placebo. After a mean 8.2-year follow-up there were no differences in the composite number of vascular events, defined as MI, stroke, or coronary revascularization, between groups treated with aspirin or placebo.[103]

Specifically with regard to diabetic patients and PAD, the Prevention of Progression of Arterial Disease and Diabetes (POPADAD) trial enrolled diabetic patients with asymptomatic PAD. This study did not find a beneficial effect of aspirin compared with placebo on a primary endpoint of death from coronary disease, nonfatal MI, nonfatal stroke, or amputation.[104]

Clopidogrel has also been studied in patients with PAD. The Clopidogrel Versus Aspirin in Patients at Risk of Ischaemic Events (CAPRIE) trial compared aspirin versus clopidogrel in patients with recent stroke, recent MI, or established PAD.[105] Patients treated with clopidogrel had an 8.7% relative risk reduction (5.3% vs. 5.8%, $P = 0.043$) in the primary endpoint of stroke, MI, or vascular death compared with those treated with aspirin. In the subset analysis of patients with PAD who were enrolled in the trial, there was a 23.8% relative risk reduction in favor of clopidogrel. The Clopidogrel for High Atherothrombotic Risk and Ischemic Stabilization, Management, and Avoidance (CHARISMA) trial compared the efficacy of dual antiplatelet therapy with clopidogrel plus aspirin versus aspirin alone in patients with established CAD, cerebrovascular disease, or PAD, as well as in patients with multiple atherosclerotic risk factors.[106] Overall, dual antiplatelet therapy produced no significant benefit compared with aspirin alone on the primary endpoint of MI, stroke, or cardiovascular death. Among the 3096 patients with PAD who enrolled, clopidogrel plus aspirin did reduce the rates of MI and hospitalization for ischemic events compared with aspirin alone.[107] In the Examining Use of Ticagrelor in Peripheral Artery Disease (EUCLID) trial, patients with symptomatic PAD were randomized to either clopidogrel 75 mg daily or ticagrelor, a newer platelet $P2Y_{12}$ receptor inhibitor, 90 mg twice daily. Treatment with ticagrelor reduced neither the risk of cardiovascular nor limb events compared to clopidogrel.[108]

Oral anticoagulation with warfarin has also been studied in patients with PAD. The Warfarin Antiplatelet Vascular Evaluation study evaluated antiplatelet therapy in addition to warfarin compared with antiplatelet therapy alone in patients with PAD.[109] There was no significant improvement with warfarin therapy; however, patients treated with warfarin and antiplatelet agent together had more life-threatening bleeding than those treated with warfarin alone.

More recently, low-dose antithrombotic therapy with the clotting factor Xa inhibitor rivaroxaban has demonstrated marked efficacy in patients with PAD. In the Cardiovascular Outcomes for People Using Anticoagulation Strategies (COMPASS) trial, 27,395 participants with stable atherosclerotic disease, including 5551 with lower extremity PAD, were randomized to rivaroxaban 5 mg twice daily, aspirin 100 mg daily, or rivaroxaban 2.5 mg twice daily plus aspirin 100 mg daily.[110] The trial was stopped early due to a 24% reduction in the composite of cardiovascular death, stroke, or MI in the rivaroxaban plus aspirin versus aspirin alone arm. Among participants with a history of diabetes, low-dose rivaroxaban plus aspirin led to threefold reduction in the risk of all-cause mortality compared to aspirin alone.[111] This drug regimen also led to a 46% reduction in lower extremity amputation.[112] In the Vascular Outcomes Study of ASA (acetylsalicylic acid) Along with Rivaroxaban in Endovascular or Surgical Limb Revascularization for PAD (VOYAGER PAD) trial, participants with PAD who were undergoing either surgical or percutaneous lower extremity arterial revascularization were randomized to rivaroxaban 2.5 mg twice daily plus aspirin versus aspirin alone.[113] As in COMPASS, the addition of low-dose rivaroxaban led to a 15% reduction in the primary outcome of acute limb ischemia, major amputation for vascular causes, MI, ischemic stroke, or cardiovascular death.

Current guidelines recommend that patients with PAD be treated with a single antiplatelet drug, such as aspirin or clopidogrel (recommended as a class I recommendation for symptomatic patients and a class IIa recommendation for asymptomatic patients) to reduce the risk of MI, stroke, or vascular death. A combination of low-dose aspirin and low-dose rivaroxaban is recommended to reduce risk of MI, stroke, vascular death, and adverse limb outcomes.[29] In the absence of another indication, full-dose anticoagulation is not recommended to reduce cardiovascular events.

RENIN ANGIOTENSIN SYSTEM ANTAGONISM IN PERIPHERAL ARTERY DISEASE

Although the achievement of target blood pressure levels outweighs the use of a specific class of antihypertensive agents, renin-angiotensin system antagonists should be considered an initial drug class of choice, and professional guidelines recommend their use in patients with PAD to reduce the risk of cardiovascular events.

Both ACE inhibitors and angiotensin II receptor blockers (ARBs) have favorable effects on the cardiovascular system beyond their ability to lower blood pressure. Based on the Heart Outcomes Prevention Evaluation (HOPE) study, patients with diabetes or evidence of vascular disease plus one other cardiovascular risk factor who received ramipril had a 22% relative risk reduction of the combined endpoint of stroke, MI, and death compared with patients who received placebo, despite a baseline blood pressure considered at goal for most patients. These outcomes were seen, despite a modest overall blood pressure reduction of 3/2 mm Hg.[114] Overall, 17.8% of patients in the placebo group reached the primary study endpoint of MI, stroke, or cardiovascular death. The rate was 22% for the 4051 patients with PAD compared with 14.3% for the 5246 patients without PAD.

In the European Trial on Reduction of Cardiac Events with Perindopril in Patients with Stable Coronary Artery Disease, 12,218 patients with stable CAD were randomly assigned to perindopril or placebo. After a mean follow-up of 4.2 years, cardiovascular events were significantly decreased in patients treated with perindopril. All predefined subgroups, including the 883 patients who had documented PAD, benefited from perindopril.[115] These data concurred with the findings of the HOPE trial. Thus based on two studies of patients with normal blood pressure at rest and only modest changes in blood pressure with therapy, ACE inhibitors decrease cardiovascular morbidity and mortality more than expected with the observed blood pressure lowering.

Similar to ACE inhibitors, ARBs have documented cardiovascular benefits beyond their antihypertensive properties. In particular, ARBs have been shown to improve endothelial function through decreased vascular inflammation.[116] Patients with high cardiovascular risk, including those with PAD, are likely to benefit from ARBs. ARBs, such as losartan and candesartan, have shown morbidity and mortality benefits either alone or in combination with ACE inhibitors, as demonstrated in the Losartan Intervention for Endpoint Reduction in Hypertension (LIFE) and the Candesartan in Heart Failure: Assessment of Reduction in Mortality and Morbidity (CHARM) studies.[117,118] In the LIFE study, losartan was compared with atenolol in hypertensive patients with electrocardiographic evidence of left ventricular hypertrophy. Overall, losartan significantly lowered the incidence of cardiovascular events, particularly stroke, despite similar decreases in blood pressure. Thus similar to ACE inhibitors, ARBs should be thought of as having cardiovascular benefits beyond blood pressure reduction. It is interesting to note that in Swedish National Registry data, patients treated with candesartan were less likely to develop PAD compared with patients treated with losartan despite similar blood pressure lowering.[119] However, a small, randomized, controlled study of telmisartan did not show a benefit in a 6-minute walk beyond a placebo.[120]

BETA-ADRENERGIC BLOCKERS IN PERIPHERAL ARTERY DISEASE

The commonly held belief that beta-blocking agents worsen claudication and shorten the amount of exercise required to bring on discomfort in the legs has been well challenged. In a carefully performed meta-analysis of 11 randomized, controlled trials, Radack and Deck demonstrated that beta-adrenergic blocker therapy does not worsen claudication symptoms in people with PAD.[121] Only 1 of 11 studies in this meta-analysis showed that pain-free and maximal treadmill walking distances were decreased by atenolol, labetalol, or pindolol, but not captopril. However, beta-blockers should not be considered as first-line agents in the treatment of hypertension and PAD, given the beneficial effects of ACE inhibitors and ARBs already discussed. If there are clear indications for beta-blocker use, such as congestive heart failure, post-MI status, angina pectoris, or arrhythmias, then beta-blockers can and should be used.[122]

Therapy for the Treatment of Claudication

In addition to modifying risk factors to improve overall cardiovascular morbidity and mortality, there are noninvasive strategies available to treat the mobility limitations caused by PAD.

PENTOXIFYLLINE

Pentoxifylline is a rheologic modifier approved by the FDA for symptomatic relief of claudication. It is thought to act by improving red blood cell and leukocyte flexibility, inhibiting neutrophil activation and adhesion, decreasing fibrinogen concentrations, and reducing blood viscosity, permitting improved muscular perfusion. Studies investigating the efficacy of pentoxifylline have yielded conflicting results. A meta-analysis found that pentoxifylline improved the walking distance by 29 meters compared with a placebo.[123] The improvement was approximately 50% in the placebo group, whereas pentoxifylline added an additional 30%. The benefit was substantially less, however, than that achieved with a supervised exercise program.[124]

The beneficial response to pentoxifylline is small in most patients, and the overall data are insufficient to support its widespread use in patients with claudication.[125] Professional guidelines recommend against its use in patients with PAD.[29]

CILOSTAZOL

Cilostazol is a phosphodiesterase-3 inhibitor that suppresses platelet aggregation and is a direct arterial dilator.[126] The efficacy of cilostazol has been demonstrated in several studies[127–129] and in a meta-analysis[130] of eight randomized, placebo-controlled trials that included 2702 patients with stable moderate-to-severe claudication. In the meta-analysis, treatment with 100 mg twice daily for 12 to 24 weeks increased maximal and pain-free walking distances by 50% and 67%, respectively. Because cilostazol is a phosphodiesterase inhibitor similar to milrinone, it is contraindicated in patients with symptomatic congestive heart failure or patients with a left ventricular ejection fraction less than 40%.

Cilostazol is more effective than pentoxifylline when compared directly. Superiority was illustrated in a trial of 698 patients randomized to cilostazol, pentoxifylline, or placebo for 24 weeks. The increase in mean walking distance over baseline with pentoxifylline and placebo was the same (30% and 34%, respectively), but the increase with cilostazol was significantly greater (54%).[131] The most common adverse effects with cilostazol are headache, palpitations, and diarrhea. The optimal dose of cilostazol is 100 mg twice daily, and the medication should be given on an empty stomach. Because of the inhibitory effects of cilostazol on drug metabolism, the dose should be halved in patients taking medications that inhibit the cytochrome P-450 isoenzymes CYP3A4 and CYP2C19 (e.g., erythromycin, diltiazem, omeprazole).[132]

OTHER PHARMACOLOGIC AGENTS

Multiple other agents have been used in the treatment of claudication. Naftidrofuryl, a 5-hydroxytryptamine serotonin receptor inhibitor, has been available in Europe for a number of years. The mechanism of action of this drug is not clear, but it is thought to promote glucose uptake and increase adenosine triphosphate levels. A meta-analysis of four trials showed an increase in the time to initial pain development with treadmill walking over a 3- to 6-month period.[133]

Buflomedil is an alpha-adrenolytic agent available in Europe, but not the United States, that has been used in the treatment of claudication. The Limbs International Medicinal Buflomedil trial evaluated the efficacy and safety of buflomedil in 2078 patients with claudication and an ABI of 0.3 to 0.8, in a randomized, placebo-controlled trial. At a median follow-up of 2.8 years, the rate of a composite endpoint of cardiovascular death, nonfatal MI, nonfatal stroke, symptomatic deterioration in PAD, or leg amputation was significantly lower in the patients who received buflomedil (9.1% vs. 12.4%). The benefit was largely driven by a reduction in symptoms of PAD.[134]

Ginkgo biloba has also been studied in the treatment of claudication with some modest success. Ginkgo is thought to act via an antioxidant mechanism that inhibits vascular injury. It is also thought to have some antithrombotic effects. The effect of ginkgo has been reviewed in a meta-analysis that showed that patients receiving ginkgo extract increased pain-free walking by approximately 34 meters, a significant increase compared with a placebo.[135]

Many other agents have been tried in the treatment of symptomatic claudication. These include estrogen replacement therapy, chelation therapy with intravenous ethylenediaminetetraacetic acid, and vitamin E supplementation. None have been shown to have a significant benefit, and none are recommended by current therapy guidelines.

EXERCISE

Many prospective trials have demonstrated that supervised exercise is an effective method of treating patients with claudication.[136] The magnitude of the effect from a supervised exercise program exceeds that achieved with any of the pharmacologic agents available. A meta-analysis of 21 studies,[137] which included both randomized and nonrandomized trials, showed that pain-free walking time improved by an average of 180% and maximal walking time by 120% in patients with claudication who underwent supervised exercise training (Table 22.2). Furthermore, a meta-analysis from the Cochrane Collaboration that included only randomized, controlled trials showed that exercise improved maximal walking ability by an average of 150% (range 74%–230%).[138] In the Claudication: Exercise Versus Endoluminal Revascularization (CLEVER) study, investigators randomized 111 patients with aortoiliac disease to medical therapy, medical therapy plus supervised exercise, or medical therapy plus endovascular revascularization.[139] Patients in the medical therapy plus supervised exercise therapy group were able to increase their peak walking time by 5.8 ± 4.9 minutes compared with 1.2 ± 2.6 minutes for those in the medical therapy alone group. It is interesting to note that the increase in peak walking time was intermediate in the revascularization group, but quality of life as measured by the Peripheral Artery Questionnaire improved most in the revascularization group. Subsequent clinical trials have similarly shown an improvement in walking capacity and quality of life with exercise therapy.[140–142]

There are several mechanisms by which exercise training may improve claudication, although the available data are not sufficient to render firm conclusions regarding their relative importance. These mechanisms include improved endothelial function via increases in nitric oxide synthase and prostacyclin; reduction of local inflammation; increased exercise pain tolerance; induction of vascular angiogenesis; improved muscle metabolism by favorable effects on muscle carnitine metabolism; and reductions in blood viscosity and red cell aggregation.[143]

Although less well studied, exercise may also improve survival in PAD. This idea was addressed in a prospective, observational study of 225 males with PAD in whom physical activity was measured with a vertical accelerometer. Patients were followed for a mean duration of 57 months, over which time 33% of patients died. Individuals in the highest quartile of accelerometer-measured activity had a significantly lower mortality than those in the lowest quartile (HR, 0.29; 95% CI, 0.10–0.83).[144]

The current PAD guidelines state that a program of supervised exercise training is recommended as an initial treatment modality for patients with claudication (class I,

TABLE 22.2 Effect of Supervised Exercise From a Meta-Analysis of 21 Studies

COMPONENTS OF EXERCISE PROGRAMS	NO. OF STUDIES	CHANGE IN THE DISTANCE TO ONSET OF PAIN, m	*P*	CHANGE IN THE DISTANCE TO MAXIMAL PAIN, m	*P*
Exercise Duration					
≤30 min/session	8	143.1 ± 162.8	0.039	143.6 ± 418.9	0.007
>30 min/session	6	314.2 ± 172.4		652.6 ± 363.9	
Exercise Frequency					
<3 sessions/week	7	177.8 ± 129.6	0.048	249.0 ± 349.5	0.045
≥3 sessions/week	11	270.7 ± 221.4		541.5 ± 253.2	
Length of Program					
<26 week	10	131.9 ± 158.6	0.008	275.1 ± 228.3	0.009
≥26 week	11	345.6 ± 161.7		518.5 ± 409.2	
Claudication Pain Endpoint Used During Training Sessions					
Onset of pain	15	104.7 ± 91.2	0.007	195.5 ± 78.3	0.005
Near-maximal pain	6	350.2 ± 246.2		606.8 ± 426.6	
Mode of Exercise					
Walking	6	294.3 ± 289.7	0.042	511.9 ± 483.2	0.023
Combination of exercises	15	152.1 ± 158.4		286.9 ± 127.4	
Level of Supervision					
Supervised	11	238.3 ± 120.5	0.476	448.6 ± 291.7	0.518
Combination of home and supervised	8	208.4 ± 198.4		339.8 ± 471.9	

Values for each component are adjusted means ± standard deviations (SDs) of the change in the distances to onset and to maximal claudication pain after the other five exercise program components were controlled for.
Data from Gardner AW, Poehlman ET: Exercise rehabilitation programs for the treatment of claudication pain: a meta-analysis. *JAMA*. 1995;274:975–980.

level of evidence A).[29] Supervised exercise training should be performed for a minimum of 30 to 60 minutes, in sessions performed at least three times per week for a minimum of 12 weeks.[145]

Exercise programs have several important limitations. Patients must be motivated, which is often difficult when they experience claudication-related pain whenever they walk. Although the best results occur when patients enroll in a supervised program as with cardiac rehabilitation, structured home-based programs are important options for patients who are unable to attend a formal community-based program or for those who completed a 12-week community program.[145]

REVASCULARIZATION

Many patients do not experience optimal improvement in symptoms related to PAD from medical therapy or risk factor modification alone. Two general revascularization strategies exist: endovascular interventions and open surgical techniques. As in the coronary circulation, the success of revascularization in the lower extremities depends on many variables including lesion location, lesion length, and the nature of the distal runoff. Diabetes alters the distribution of lower-extremity atherosclerosis so that these patients tend to have severe arterial occlusive disease below the knee in the runoff vessels. As the distal runoff declines, the results of endovascular interventions worsen and the need for surgery increases.

Endovascular Management

In general, endovascular revascularization is more appropriate in patients with relatively focal disease in arteries above the knee.[146] However, short-term success rates for opening long totally occluded vessels and below-the-knee arteries are improving.[147] Thus far, the best results have been seen in aortoiliac vessels, in which 1-year patency rates of 80% to 90% have been demonstrated.[148–150] Femoral interventions have 1-year patency rates that vary widely, from approximately 30% to 80%, with diabetes adversely affecting the long-term rates of success.[151–155] However, in diabetic patients with reasonable runoff, patency rates are similar to those in nondiabetics.[156] Newer technologies, such as angioplasty with drug-coated balloons, may also improve long-term patency.[157]

Surgical Management

In diabetes, open surgical revascularization tends to have greater durability than endovascular procedures. Bypass to the tibial or pedal vessels with autogenous vein is the most predictable method of improving blood flow to the

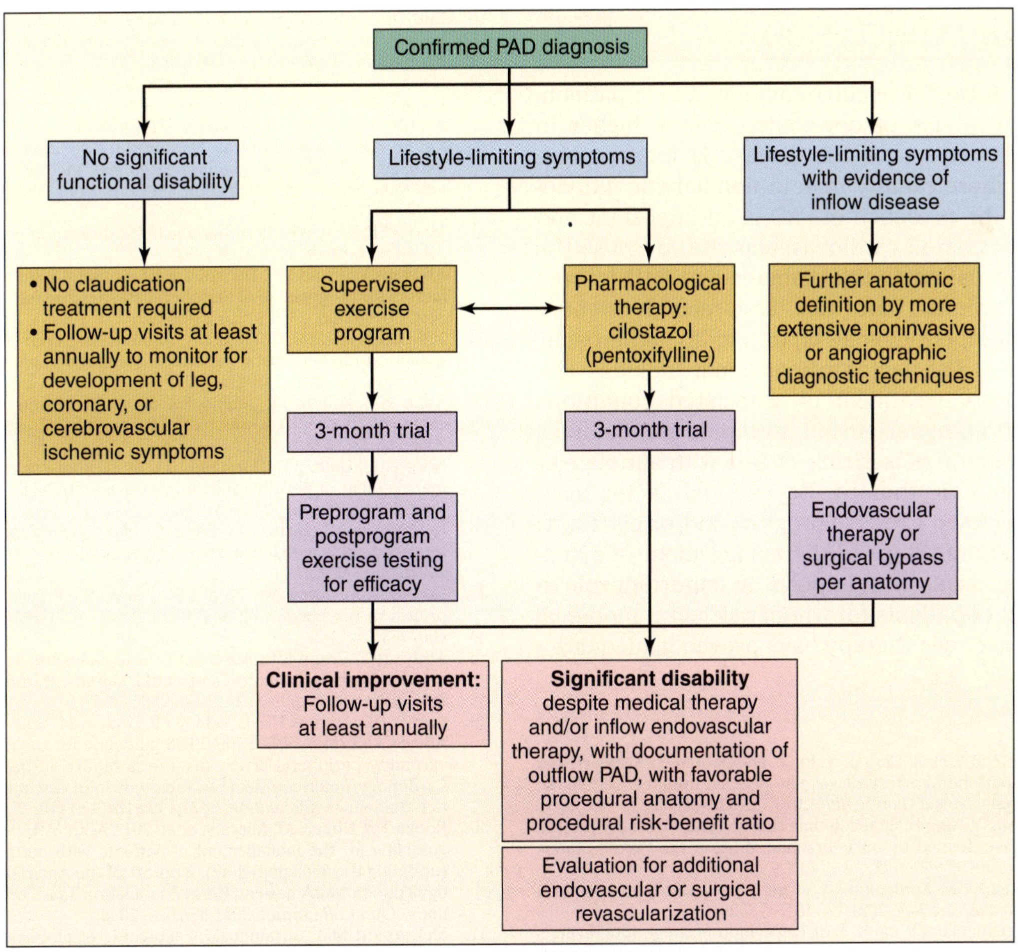

FIG. 22.7 Treatment algorithm for peripheral artery disease (PAD). (Modified from Gornik HL, Aronow HD, Goodney PP, Arya S, Brewster LP, Byrd L, et al. 2024 ACC/AHA/AACVPR/APMA/ABC/SCAI/SVM/SVN/SVS/SIR/VESS guideline for the management of lower extremity peripheral artery disease: a report of the American College of Cardiology/American Heart Association Joint Committee on Clinical Practice Guidelines. *Circulation*, 2024;149(24):e1313–e410.).

threatened limb. Surgical bypass with greater saphenous vein is the procedure of choice for patients with diabetes and tibial disease; however, this comes at the price of increased periprocedural cardiovascular morbidity and mortality.[150] The specific operation must take into account the anatomic location of the arterial lesions and the presence of comorbid conditions. The surgical procedure is planned after identification of the arterial obstruction by imaging, ensuring that there is sufficient arterial inflow to and outflow from the graft to maintain patency.

Revascularization is the definitive therapy for the management of patients with CLTI, with the aim of healing ischemic ulcers and preventing limb loss. Although most limbs can be revascularized, the lack of target vessel, the unavailability of autogenous vein, or irreversible gangrene means that some cannot. In these patients, amputation is often a better option than prolonged, but failing, medical therapy.

APPROACH TO THE TREATMENT OF DIABETIC PATIENTS WITH PERIPHERAL ARTERY DISEASE

Overall, the approach to treatment of the diabetic patient with PAD is similar to that of other patients with PAD. A schematic of the overall approach is presented in Fig. 22.7.

SUMMARY AND CONCLUSION

PAD is a common cardiovascular complication in patients with diabetes. The risk of developing PAD is higher in patients with diabetes, and the disease is more severe and progresses more rapidly than in nondiabetic individuals. Moreover, the presence of PAD is an important and potent marker of overall cardiovascular risk. Because the greater threat to patients with diabetes and PAD is from cardiovascular events (and not limb-related events), the primary therapeutic goal is to modify atherosclerotic risk factors. Risk factor management includes lifestyle modifications, treatment of associated conditions (tobacco cessation, hypertension, dyslipidemia, diabetes itself), and prevention of ischemic events with antiplatelet and/or antithrombotic therapy. Beyond risk factor management, a supervised exercise program and/or cilostazol are the preferred first steps in the management of symptomatic PAD. Revascularization plays an important role in the management of patients for whom risk factor modification and pharmacologic therapy have proven inadequate.

REFERENCES

1. Song P, Rudan D, Zhu Y, et al. Global, regional, and national prevalence and risk factors for peripheral artery disease in 2015: an updated systematic review and analysis. *Lancet Glob Health*. 2019;7:e1020–e1030.
2. Matsushita K, Sang Y, Ning H, et al. Lifetime risk of lower-extremity peripheral artery disease defined by ankle-brachial index in the United States. *J Am Heart Assoc*. 2019;8:e012177.
3. Aday AW, Matsushita K. Epidemiology of peripheral artery disease and polyvascular disease. *Circ Res*. 2021;128:1818–1832.
4. McDermott MM, Greenland P, Liu K, et al. Leg symptoms in peripheral arterial disease: associated clinical characteristics and functional impairment. *JAMA*. 2001;286:1599–1606.
5. Hirsch AT, Criqui MH, Treat-Jacobson D, et al. Peripheral arterial disease detection, awareness, and treatment in primary care. *JAMA*. 2001;286:1317–1324.
6. Eraso LH, Fukaya E, Mohler 3rd ER, Xie D, Sha D, Berger JS. Peripheral arterial disease, prevalence and cumulative risk factor profile analysis. *Eur J Prev Cardiol*. 2014;21:704–711.
7. Norgren L, Hiatt WR, Dormandy JA, et al. Inter-society consensus for the management of peripheral arterial disease (TASC II). *J Vasc Surg*. 2007;45(Suppl S):S5–67.
8. Nehler MR, Duval S, Diao L, et al. Epidemiology of peripheral arterial disease and critical limb ischemia in an insured national population. *J Vasc Surg*. 2014;60:686–695. e682.
9. Ding N, Sang Y, Chen J, et al. Cigarette smoking, smoking cessation, and long-term risk of 3 major atherosclerotic diseases. *J Am Coll Cardiol*. 2019;74:498–507.
10. Levin MG, Klarin D, Assimes TL, et al. Genetics of smoking and risk of atherosclerotic cardiovascular diseases: a mendelian randomization study. *JAMA Netw Open*. 2021;4:e2034461.
11. Fowkes FG, Rudan D, Rudan I, et al. Comparison of global estimates of prevalence and risk factors for peripheral artery disease in 2000 and 2010: a systematic review and analysis. *Lancet*. 2013;382:1329–1340.
12. Pande RL, Perlstein TS, Beckman JA, Creager MA. Association of insulin resistance and inflammation with peripheral arterial disease: the National Health and Nutrition Examination Survey, 1999 to 2004. *Circulation*. 2008;118:33–41.
13. Al-Delaimy WK, Merchant AT, Rimm EB, Willett WC, Stampfer MJ, Hu FB. Effect of type 2 diabetes and its duration on the risk of peripheral arterial disease among men. *Am J Med*. 2004;116:236–240.
14. Selvin E, Marinopoulos S, Berkenblit G, et al. Meta-analysis: glycosylated hemoglobin and cardiovascular disease in diabetes mellitus. *Ann Intern Med*. 2004;141:421–431.
15. Howard DP, Banerjee A, Fairhead JF, et al. Population-based study of incidence, risk factors, outcome, and prognosis of ischemic peripheral arterial events: implications for prevention. *Circulation*. 2015;132:1805–1815.
16. Kornitzer M, Dramaix M, Sobolski J, Degre S, De Backer G. Ankle/arm pressure index in asymptomatic middle-aged males: an independent predictor of ten-year coronary heart disease mortality. *Angiology*. 1995;46:211–219.
17. Dick F, Diehm N, Galimanis A, Husmann M, Schmidli J, Baumgartner I. Surgical or endovascular revascularization in patients with critical limb ischemia: influence of diabetes mellitus on clinical outcome. *J Vasc Surg*. 2007;45:751–761.
18. Bild DE, Selby JV, Sinnock P, Browner WS, Braveman P, Showstack JA. Lower-extremity amputation in people with diabetes. Epidemiology and prevention. *Diabetes Care*. 1989;12:24–31.
19. Geiss LS, Li Y, Hora I, Albright A, Rolka D, Gregg EW. Resurgence of diabetes-related nontraumatic lower-extremity amputation in the young and middle-aged adult U.S. Population. *Diabetes Care*. 2019;42:50–54.
20. Cai M, Xie Y, Bowe B, et al. Temporal trends in incidence rates of lower extremity amputation and associated risk factors among patients using veterans health administration services from 2008 to 2018. *JAMA Netw Open*. 2021;4:e2033953.
21. Marso SP, Hiatt WR. Peripheral arterial disease in patients with diabetes. *J Am Coll Cardiol*. 2006;47:921–929.
22. Aboyans V, Criqui MH, Denenberg JO, Knoke JD, Ridker PM, Fronek A. Risk factors for progression of peripheral arterial disease in large and small vessels. *Circulation*. 2006;113:2623–2629.
23. Jude EB, Oyibo SO, Chalmers N, Boulton AJ. Peripheral arterial disease in diabetic and nondiabetic patients: a comparison of severity and outcome. *Diabetes Care*. 2001;24:1433–1437.
24. Khan NA, Rahim SA, Anand SS, Simel DL, Panju A. Does the clinical examination predict lower extremity peripheral arterial disease? *JAMA*. 2006;295:536–546.
25. Norgren L, Hiatt WR, Dormandy JA, et al. Inter-society consensus for the management of peripheral arterial disease (TASC II). *Eur J Vasc Endovasc Surg*. 2007;33(Suppl 1):S1–75.
26. Rutherford RB, Baker JD, Ernst C, et al. Recommended standards for reports dealing with lower extremity ischemia: revised version. *J Vasc Surg*. 1997;26:517–538.
27. Gutierrez JA, Aday AW, Patel MR, Jones WS. Polyvascular disease: reappraisal of the current clinical landscape. *Circ Cardiovasc Interv*. 2019;12:e007385.
28. Aboyans V, Criqui MH, Abraham P, et al. Measurement and interpretation of the ankle-brachial index: a scientific statement from the American Heart Association. *Circulation*. 2012;126:2890–2909.
29. Gornik HL, Aronow HD, Goodney PP, et al. 2024 ACC/AHA/AACVPR/APMA/ABC/SCAI/SVM/SVN/SVS/SIR/VESS guideline for the management of lower extremity peripheral artery disease: a report of the American College of Cardiology/American Heart Association Joint Committee on Clinical Practice Guidelines. *Circulation*. 2024;149:e1313–e1410.
30. Rooke TW, Hirsch AT, Misra S, et al. 2011 ACCF/AHA focused update of the guideline for the management of patients with peripheral artery disease (updating the 2005 guideline): a report of the American College of Cardiology Foundation/American Heart Association Task Force on Practice Guidelines. *J Am Coll Cardiol*. 2011;58:2020–2045.
31. McDermott MM, Guralnik JM, Ferrucci L, et al. Physical activity, walking exercise, and calf skeletal muscle characteristics in patients with peripheral arterial disease. *J Vasc Surg*. 2007;46:87–93.

32. Premalatha G, Ravikumar R, Sanjay R, Deepa R, Mohan V. Comparison of colour duplex ultrasound and ankle-brachial pressure index measurements in peripheral vascular disease in type 2 diabetic patients with foot infections. *J Assoc Physicians India*. 2002;50:1240–1244.
33. Alnaeb ME, Crabtree VP, Boutin A, Mikhailidis DP, Seifalian AM, Hamilton G. Prospective assessment of lower-extremity peripheral arterial disease in diabetic patients using a novel automated optical device. *Angiology*. 2007;58:579–585.
34. Clairotte C, Retout S, Potier L, Roussel R, Escoubet B. Automated ankle-brachial pressure index measurement by clinical staff for peripheral arterial disease diagnosis in nondiabetic and diabetic patients. *Diabetes Care*. 2009; 32:1231–1236.
35. American Diabetes Association Professional Practice C. 12. Retinopathy, neuropathy, and foot care: standards of care in diabetes-2024. *Diabetes Care*. 2024;47:S231–S243.
36. Beckman JA. The U.S. Preventive Services Task Force: objectivity as authority. *Am Coll Cardiol*. 2019;73:1719–1722.
37. Criqui MH, Fronek A, Klauber MR, Barrett-Connor E, Gabriel S. The sensitivity, specificity, and predictive value of traditional clinical evaluation of peripheral arterial disease: results from noninvasive testing in a defined population. *Circulation*. 1985;71:516–522.
38. Hess CN, Cannon CP, Beckman JA, et al. Effectiveness of blood lipid management in patients with peripheral artery disease. *J Am Coll Cardiol*. 2021; 77:3016–3027.
39. Colantonio LD, Hubbard D, Monda KL, et al. Atherosclerotic risk and statin use among patients with peripheral artery disease. *J Am Coll Cardiol*. 2020;76:251–264.
40. Menard MT, Jaff MR, Farber A, et al. Baseline modern medical management in the BEST-CLI trial. *J Vasc Surg*. 2023;78:711–718. e715.
41. Badjatiya A, Merrill P, Buse JB, et al. Clinical outcomes in patients with type 2 diabetes mellitus and peripheral artery disease: results from the EXSCEL trial. *Circ Cardiovasc Interv*. 2019;12:e008018.
42. Centers for Disease Control and Prevention. Diabetes-related amputations of lower extremities in the Medicare population—Minnesota, 1993–1995. *MMWR Morb Mortal Wkly Rep*. 1998;47:649–652.
43. Humphries MD, Brunson A, Li CS, Melnikow J, Romano PS. Amputation trends for patients with lower extremity ulcers due to diabetes and peripheral artery disease using statewide data. *J Vasc Surg*. 2016;64:1747–1755. e1743.
44. Beckman JA, Duncan MS, Damrauer SM, et al. Microvascular disease, peripheral artery disease, and amputation. *Circulation*. 2019;140:449–458.
45. Grundy SM, Stone NJ, Bailey AL, et al. 2018 AHA/ACC/AACVPR/AAPA/ABC/ACPM/ADA/AGS/APhA/ASPC/NLA/PCNA guideline on the management of blood cholesterol: a report of the American College of Cardiology/American Heart Association Task Force on Clinical Practice Guidelines. *Circulation*. 2019;139:e1082–e1143.
46. Feringa HHH, van Waning VH, Bax JJ, et al. Cardioprotective medication is associated with improved survival in patients with peripheral arterial disease. *J Am Coll Cardiol*. 2006;47:1182–1187.
47. Arya S, Khakharia A, Binney ZO, et al. Association of statin dose with amputation and survival in patients with peripheral artery disease. *Circulation*. 2018;137:1435–1446.
48. Bonaca MP, Nault P, Giugliano RP, et al. Low-density lipoprotein cholesterol lowering with evolocumab and outcomes in patients with peripheral artery disease: insights from the FOURIER Trial (Further Cardiovascular Outcomes Research With PCSK9 Inhibition in Subjects With Elevated Risk). *Circulation*. 2018;137:338–350.
49. McDermott MM, Guralnik JM, Greenland P, et al. Statin use and leg functioning in patients with and without lower-extremity peripheral arterial disease. *Circulation*. 2003;107:757–761.
50. Aronow WS, Nayak D, Woodworth S, Ahn C. Effect of simvastatin versus placebo on treadmill exercise time until the onset of intermittent claudication in older patients with peripheral arterial disease at six months and at one year after treatment. *Am J Cardiol*. 2003;92:711–712.
51. Mondillo S, Ballo P, Barbati R, et al. Effects of simvastatin on walking performance and symptoms of intermittent claudication in hypercholesterolemic patients with peripheral vascular disease. *Am J Med*. 2003;114:359–364.
52. Mohler 3rd ER, Hiatt WR, Creager MA. Cholesterol reduction with atorvastatin improves walking distance in patients with peripheral arterial disease. *Circulation*. 2003;108:1481–1486.
53. Giri J, McDermott MM, Greenland P, et al. Statin use and functional decline in patients with and without peripheral arterial disease. *J Am Coll Cardiol*. 2006;47:998–1004.
54. Rajamani K, Colman PG, Li LP, et al. Effect of fenofibrate on amputation events in people with type 2 diabetes mellitus (FIELD study): a prespecified analysis of a randomised controlled trial. *Lancet*. 2009;373:1780–1788.
55. Cosentino F, Grant PJ, Aboyans V, et al. 2019 ESC Guidelines on diabetes, pre-diabetes, and cardiovascular diseases developed in collaboration with the EASD. *Eur Heart J*. 2020;41:255–323.
56. Quick CR, Cotton LT. The measured effect of stopping smoking on intermittent claudication. *Br J Surg*. 1982;69(Suppl):S24–26.
57. Hobbs SD, Bradbury AW. Smoking cessation strategies in patients with peripheral arterial disease: an evidence-based approach. *Eur J Vasc Endovasc Surg*. 2003;26:341–347.
58. Hobbs SD, Wilmink AB, Adam DJ, Bradbury AW. Assessment of smoking status in patients with peripheral arterial disease. *J Vasc Surg*. 2005;41: 451–456.
59. Law M, Tang JL. An analysis of the effectiveness of interventions intended to help people stop smoking. *Arch Intern Med*. 1995;155:1933–1941.
60. Anthonisen NR, Skeans MA, Wise RA, Manfreda J, Kanner RE, Connett JE. The effects of a smoking cessation intervention on 14.5-year mortality: a randomized clinical trial. *Ann Intern Med*. 2005;142:233–239.
61. Hennrikus D, Joseph AM, Lando HA, et al. Effectiveness of a smoking cessation program for peripheral artery disease patients: a randomized controlled trial. *J Am Coll Cardiol*. 2010;56:2105–2112.
62. Okuyemi KS, Ahluwalia JS, Harris KJ. Pharmacotherapy of smoking cessation. *Arch Fam Med*. 2000;9:270–281.
63. Dalsgareth OJ, Hansen NC, Soes-Petersen U, et al. A multicenter, randomized, double-blind, placebo-controlled, 6-month trial of bupropion hydrochloride sustained-release tablets as an aid to smoking cessation in hospital employees. *Nicotine Tob Res*. 2004;6:55–61.
64. Gonzales D, Rennard SI, Nides M, et al. Varenicline, an alpha4beta2 nicotinic acetylcholine receptor partial agonist, vs sustained-release bupropion and placebo for smoking cessation: a randomized controlled trial. *JAMA*. 2006;296:47–55.
65. Jorenby DE, Leischow SJ, Nides MA, et al. A controlled trial of sustained-release bupropion, a nicotine patch, or both for smoking cessation [see comments]. *N Engl J Med*. 1999;340:685–691.
66. Barua RS, Rigotti NA, Benowitz NL, et al. 2018 ACC expert consensus decision pathway on tobacco cessation treatment: a report of the American College of Cardiology Task Force on Clinical Expert Consensus Documents. *J Am Coll Cardiol*. 2018;72:3332–3365.
67. Anthenelli RM, Benowitz NL, West R, et al. Neuropsychiatric safety and efficacy of varenicline, bupropion, and nicotine patch in smokers with and without psychiatric disorders (EAGLES): a double-blind, randomised, placebo-controlled clinical trial. *Lancet*. 2016;387:2507–2520.
68. Conen D, Everett BM, Kurth T, et al. Smoking, smoking cessation, and risk for symptomatic peripheral artery disease in women: a cohort study. *Ann Intern Med*. 2011;154:719–726.
69. James PA, Oparil S, Carter BL, et al. 2014 evidence-based guideline for the management of high blood pressure in adults: report from the panel members appointed to the Eighth Joint National Committee (JNC 8). *JAMA*. 2014;311:507–520.
70. The Treatment of Mild Hypertension Research Group. The treatment of mild hypertension study. A randomized, placebo-controlled trial of a nutritional-hygienic regimen along with various drug monotherapies. *Arch Intern Med*. 1991;151:1413–1423.
71. Novo S, Abrignani MG, Pavone G, et al. Effects of captopril and ticlopidine, alone or in combination, in hypertensive patients with intermittent claudication. *Int Angiol*. 1996;15:169–174.
72. Solomon SA, Ramsay LE, Yeo WW, Parnell L, Morris-Jones W. Beta blockade and intermittent claudication: placebo controlled trial of atenolol and nifedipine and their combination. *BMJ*. 1991;303:1100–1104.
73. Roberts DH, Tsao Y, McLoughlin GA, Breckenridge A. Placebo-controlled comparison of captopril, atenolol, labetalol, and pindolol in hypertension complicated by intermittent claudication. *Lancet*. 1987;2:650–653.
74. Sonecha TN, Nicolaides AN, Kyprianou P, et al. The effect of enalapril on leg muscle blood flow in patients with claudication. *Int Angiol*. 1990;9: 22–24.
75. Itoga NK, Tawfik DS, Lee CK, Maruyama S, Leeper NJ, Chang TI. Association of blood pressure measurements with peripheral arterial disease events: a reanalysis of the ALLHAT data. *Circulation*. 2018
76. Mehler PS, Coll JR, Estacio R, Esler A, Schrier RW, Hiatt WR. Intensive blood pressure control reduces the risk of cardiovascular events in patients with peripheral arterial disease and type 2 diabetes. *Circulation*. 2003;107: 753–756.
77. Whelton PK, Carey RM, Aronow WS, et al. 2017 ACC/AHA/AAPA/ABC/ACPM/AGS/APhA/ASH/ASPC/NMA/PCNA guideline for the prevention, detection, evaluation, and management of high blood pressure in adults: a report of the American College of Cardiology/American Heart Association Task Force on Clinical Practice Guidelines. *Circulation*. 2018;138:e484–e594.
78. Anonymous. Effect of intensive diabetes management on macrovascular events and risk factors in the Diabetes Control and Complications Trial. *Am J Cardiol*. 1995;75:894–903.
79. Hadden DR, Patterson CC, Atkinson AB, et al. Macrovascular disease and hyperglycaemia: 10-year survival analysis in Type 2 diabetes mellitus: the Belfast Diet Study. *Diabet Med*. 1997;14:663–672.
80. Diabetes C, Complications Trial Research G, Nathan DM, et al. The effect of intensive treatment of diabetes on the development and progression of long-term complications in insulin-dependent diabetes mellitus. *N Engl J Med*. 1993;329:977–986.
81. Giugliano D, Maiorino MI, Bellastella G, Chiodini P, Esposito K. Glycemic control, preexisting cardiovascular disease, and risk of major cardiovascular events in patients with type 2 diabetes mellitus: systematic review with meta-analysis of cardiovascular outcome trials and intensive glucose control trials. *J Am Heart Assoc*. 2019;8:e012356.
82. Gerstein HC, Miller ME, Byington RP, et al. Effects of intensive glucose lowering in type 2 diabetes. *N Engl J Med*. 2008;358:2545–2559.
83. Gerstein HC, Miller ME, et al. Action to Control Cardiovascular Risk in Diabetes Study Effects of intensive glucose lowering in type 2 diabetes. *N Engl J Med*. 2008;358:2545–2559.
84. Patel A, MacMahon S, Chalmers J, et al. Intensive blood glucose control and vascular outcomes in patients with type 2 diabetes. *N Engl J Med*. 2008; 358:2560–2572.

85. Duckworth W, Abraira C, Moritz T, et al. Glucose control and vascular complications in veterans with type 2 diabetes. *N Engl J Med*. 2009;360:129–139.
86. Cowie MR, Fisher M. SGLT2 inhibitors: mechanisms of cardiovascular benefit beyond glycaemic control. *Nat Rev Cardiol*. 2020;17:761–772.
87. Neal B, Perkovic V, Mahaffey KW, et al. Canagliflozin and cardiovascular and renal events in type 2 diabetes. *Engl J Med*. 2017;377:644–657.
88. Ueda P, Svanstrom H, Melbye M, et al. Sodium glucose cotransporter 2 inhibitors and risk of serious adverse events: nationwide register based cohort study. *BMJ*. 2018;363:k4365.
89. Khouri C, Cracowski JL, Roustit M. SGLT-2 inhibitors and the risk of lower-limb amputation: is this a class effect? *Diabetes Obes Metab*. 2018;20:1531–1534.
90. Nuffield Department of Population Health Renal Studies Group, Consortium SiM-AC-RT. Impact of diabetes on the effects of sodium glucose co-transporter-2 inhibitors on kidney outcomes: collaborative meta-analysis of large placebo-controlled trials. *Lancet*. 2022;400:1788–1801.
91. Marx N, Husain M, Lehrke M, Verma S, Sattar N. GLP-1 receptor agonists for the reduction of atherosclerotic cardiovascular risk in patients with type 2 diabetes. *Circulation*. 2022;146:1882–1894.
92. Schafer Z, Mathisen A, Thomsen TR, Rossing P, Kirketerp-Moller K. Glucagon-like peptide-1 treatment reduces the risk of diabetes-type 2 related amputations: a cohort study in Denmark. *Diabetes Res Clin Pract*. 2023;202:110799.
93. Caruso P, Maiorino MI, Longo M, et al. Liraglutide for lower limb perfusion in people with type 2 diabetes and peripheral artery disease: the STARDUST randomized clinical trial. *JAMA Netw Open*. 2024;7:e241545.
94. American Diabetes Association Professional Practice C 6. Glycemic goals and hypoglycemia: standards of care in diabetes-2024. *Diabetes Care*. 2024;47:S111–S125.
95. Draznin B, Aroda VR, et al. American Diabetes Association Professional Practice C 12. Retinopathy, neuropathy, and foot care: standards of medical care in diabetes-2022. *Diabetes Care*. 2022;45:S185–S194.
96. Housley E, Leng GC, Donnan PT, Fowkes FG. Physical activity and risk of peripheral arterial disease in the general population: Edinburgh Artery Study. *J Epidemiol Community Health*. 1993;47:475–480.
97. Smith GD, Shipley MJ, Rose G. Intermittent claudication, heart disease risk factors, and mortality. The Whitehall Study. *Circulation*. 1990;82:1925–1931.
98. Medalie JH, Papier CM, Goldbourt U, Herman JB. Major factors in the development of diabetes mellitus in 10,000 men. *Arch Intern Med*. 1975;135:811–817.
99. Heffron SP, Dwivedi A, Rockman CB, et al. Body mass index and peripheral artery disease. *Atherosclerosis*. 2020;292:31–36.
100. McDermott MM, Criqui MH, Ferrucci L, et al. Obesity, weight change, and functional decline in peripheral arterial disease. *J Vasc Surg*. 2006;43:1198–1204.
101. Antithrombotic Trialists' Collaboration Collaborative meta-analysis of randomised trials of antiplatelet therapy for prevention of death, myocardial infarction, and stroke in high risk patients. *BMJ*. 2002;324:71–86.
102. Berger JS, Krantz MJ, Kittelson JM, Hiatt WR. Aspirin for the prevention of cardiovascular events in patients with peripheral artery disease: a meta-analysis of randomized trials. *JAMA*. 2009;301:1909–1919.
103. Fowkes FG, Price JF, Stewart MC, et al. Aspirin for prevention of cardiovascular events in a general population screened for a low ankle brachial index: a randomized controlled trial. *JAMA*. 2010;303:841–848.
104. Belch J, MacCuish A, Campbell I, et al. The prevention of progression of arterial disease and diabetes (POPADAD) trial: factorial randomised placebo controlled trial of aspirin and antioxidants in patients with diabetes and asymptomatic peripheral arterial disease. *BMJ*. 2008;337:a1840.
105. Committee CS. A randomised, blinded, trial of clopidogrel versus aspirin in patients at risk of ischaemic events (CAPRIE). CAPRIE Steering Committee. *Lancet*. 1996;348:1329–1339.
106. Bhatt DL, Fox KA, Hacke W, et al. Clopidogrel and aspirin versus aspirin alone for the prevention of atherothrombotic events. *N Engl J Med*. 2006;354:1706–1717.
107. Cacoub PP, Bhatt DL, Steg PG, Topol EJ, Creager MA. CHARISMA Investigators Patients with peripheral arterial disease in the CHARISMA trial. *Eur Heart J*. 2009;30:192–201.
108. Hiatt WR, Fowkes FG, Heizer G, et al. Ticagrelor versus clopidogrel in symptomatic peripheral artery disease. *N Engl J Med*. 2017;376:32–40.
109. Anand S, Yusuf S, et al. Warfarin Antiplatelet Vascular Evaluation Trial Investigators Oral anticoagulant and antiplatelet therapy and peripheral arterial disease. *N Engl J Med*. 2007;357:217–227.
110. Eikelboom JW, Connolly SJ, Bosch J, et al. Rivaroxaban with or without aspirin in stable cardiovascular disease. *N Engl J Med*. 2017;377:1319–1330.
111. Bhatt DL, Eikelboom JW, Connolly SJ, et al. Role of combination antiplatelet and anticoagulation therapy in diabetes mellitus and cardiovascular disease: insights from the COMPASS trial. *Circulation*. 2020;141:1841–1854.
112. Anand SS, Bosch J, Eikelboom JW, et al. Rivaroxaban with or without aspirin in patients with stable peripheral or carotid artery disease: an international, randomised, double-blind, placebo-controlled trial. *Lancet*. 2018;391:219–229.
113. Bonaca MP, Bauersachs RM, Anand SS, et al. Rivaroxaban in peripheral artery disease after revascularization. *N Engl J Med*. 2020;382:1994–2004.
114. Yusuf S, Sleight P, Pogue J, Bosch J, Davies R, Dagenais G. Effects of an angiotensin-converting-enzyme inhibitor, ramipril, on cardiovascular events in high-risk patients. The Heart Outcomes Prevention Evaluation Study Investigators. *N Engl J Med*. 2000;342:145–153.
115. Fox KM. Efficacy of perindopril in reduction of cardiovascular events among patients with stable coronary artery disease: randomised, double-blind, placebo-controlled, multicentre trial (the EUROPA study). *Lancet*. 2003;362:782–788.
116. Navalkar S, Parthasarathy S, Santanam N, Khan BV. Irbesartan, an angiotensin type 1 receptor inhibitor, regulates markers of inflammation in patients with premature atherosclerosis. *J Am Coll Cardiol*. 2001;37:440–444.
117. Dahlof B, Devereux RB, Kjeldsen SE, et al. Cardiovascular morbidity and mortality in the Losartan Intervention For Endpoint reduction in hypertension study (LIFE): a randomised trial against atenolol. *Lancet*. 2002;359:995–1003.
118. Pfeffer MA, Swedberg K, Granger CB, et al. Effects of candesartan on mortality and morbidity in patients with chronic heart failure: the CHARM-Overall programme. *Lancet*. 2003;362:759–766.
119. Kjeldsen SE, Stalhammar J, Hasvold P, Bodegard J, Olsson U, Russell D. Effects of losartan vs candesartan in reducing cardiovascular events in the primary treatment of hypertension. *J Hum Hypertens*. 2010;24:263–273.
120. McDermott MM, Bazzano L, Peterson CA, et al. Effect of telmisartan on walking performance in patients with lower extremity peripheral artery disease: the TELEX randomized clinical trial. *JAMA*. 2022;328:1315–1325.
121. Radack K, Deck C. Beta-adrenergic blocker therapy does not worsen intermittent claudication in subjects with peripheral arterial disease. A meta-analysis of randomized controlled trials. *Arch Intern Med*. 1991;151:1769–1776.
122. Olin JW. Hypertension and peripheral arterial disease. *Vasc Med*. 2005;10:241–246.
123. Hood SC, Moher D, Barber GG. Management of intermittent claudication with pentoxifylline: meta- analysis of randomized controlled trials. *CMAJ*. 1996;155:1053–1059.
124. Hiatt WR, Regensteiner JG, Hargarten ME, Wolfel EE, Brass EP. Benefit of exercise conditioning for patients with peripheral arterial disease. *Circulation*. 1990;81:602–609.
125. Broderick C, Forster R, Abdel-Hadi M, Salhiyyah K. Pentoxifylline for intermittent claudication. *Cochrane Database Syst Rev*. 2020;10:CD005262.
126. Reilly MP, Mohler 3rd. ER. Cilostazol: treatment of intermittent claudication. *Ann Pharmacother*. 2001;35:48–56.
127. Dawson DL, Cutler BS, Meissner MH, Strandness Jr. DE. Cilostazol has beneficial effects in treatment of intermittent claudication: results from a multicenter, randomized, prospective, double-blind trial. *Circulation*. 1998;98:678–686.
128. Money SR, Herd JA, Isaacsohn JL, et al. Effect of cilostazol on walking distances in patients with intermittent claudication caused by peripheral vascular disease. *J Vasc Surg*. 1998;27:267–274. discussion 274-265.
129. Beebe HG, Dawson DL, Cutler BS, et al. A new pharmacological treatment for intermittent claudication: results of a randomized, multicenter trial. *Arch Intern Med*. 1999;159:2041–2050.
130. Thompson PD, Zimet R, Forbes WP, Zhang P. Meta-analysis of results from eight randomized, placebo-controlled trials on the effect of cilostazol on patients with intermittent claudication. *Am J Cardiol*. 2002;90:1314–1319.
131. Dawson DL, Cutler BS, Hiatt WR, et al. A comparison of cilostazol and pentoxifylline for treating intermittent claudication. *Am J Med*. 2000;109:523–530.
132. Dobesh PP, Stacy ZA, Persson EL. Pharmacologic therapy for intermittent claudication. *Pharmacotherapy*. 2009;29:526–553.
133. Girolami B, Bernardi E, Prins MH, et al. Treatment of intermittent claudication with physical training, smoking cessation, pentoxifylline, or nafronyl: a meta-analysis. *Arch Intern Med*. 1999;159:337–345.
134. Limbs International Medicinal Buflomedil Study G, Leizorovicz A, Becker F. Oral buflomedil in the prevention of cardiovascular events in patients with peripheral arterial obstructive disease: a randomized, placebo-controlled, 4-year study. *Circulation*. 2008;117:816–822.
135. Pittler MH, Ernst E. Ginkgo biloba extract for the treatment of intermittent claudication: a meta-analysis of randomized trials. *Am J Med*. 2000;108:276–281.
136. Regensteiner JG, Gardner A, Hiatt WR. Exercise testing and exercise rehabilitation for patients with peripheral arterial disease: status in 1997. *Vasc Med*. 1997;2:147–155.
137. Gardner AW, Poehlman ET. Exercise rehabilitation programs for the treatment of claudication pain: a meta-analysis. *JAMA*. 1995;274:975–980.
138. Lane R, Harwood A, Watson L, Leng GC. Exercise for intermittent claudication. *Cochrane Database Syst Rev*. 2017;12:CD000990.
139. Murphy TP, Cutlip DE, Regensteiner JG, et al. Supervised exercise versus primary stenting for claudication resulting from aortoiliac peripheral artery disease: six-month outcomes from the claudication: exercise versus endoluminal revascularization (CLEVER) study. *Circulation*. 2012;125:130–139.
140. McDermott MM, Ferrucci L, Tian L, et al. Effect of granulocyte-macrophage colony-stimulating factor with or without supervised exercise on walking performance in patients with peripheral artery disease: the PROPEL randomized clinical trial. *JAMA*. 2017;318:2089–2098.
141. McDermott MM, Ades P, Guralnik JM, et al. Treadmill exercise and resistance training in patients with peripheral arterial disease with and without intermittent claudication: a randomized controlled trial. *JAMA*. 2009;301:165–174.
142. McDermott MM, Spring B, Tian L, et al. Effect of low-intensity vs high-intensity home-based walking exercise on walk distance in patients with peripheral artery disease: the LITE randomized clinical trial. *JAMA*. 2021;325:1266–1276.

143. Hamburg NM, Balady GJ. Exercise rehabilitation in peripheral artery disease: functional impact and mechanisms of benefits. *Circulation*. 2011;123:87–97.
144. Garg PK, Tian L, Criqui MH, et al. Physical activity during daily life and mortality in patients with peripheral arterial disease. *Circulation*. 2006;114: 242–248.
145. Treat-Jacobson D, McDermott MM, Beckman JA, et al. Implementation of supervised exercise therapy for patients with symptomatic peripheral artery disease: a science advisory from the American Heart Association. *Circulation*. 2019;140:e700–e710.
146. White CJ, Gray WA. Endovascular therapies for peripheral arterial disease: an evidence-based review. *Circulation*. 2007;116:2203–2215.
147. Mahmud E, Cavendish JJ, Salami A. Current treatment of peripheral arterial disease: role of percutaneous interventional therapies. *J Am Coll Cardiol*. 2007;50:473–490.
148. Sullivan TM, Childs MB, Bacharach JM, Gray BH, Piedmonte MR. Percutaneous transluminal angioplasty and primary stenting of the iliac arteries in 288 patients. *J Vasc Surg*. 1997;25:829–838. discussion 838-829.
149. Dormandy JA, Rutherford RB. Management of peripheral arterial disease (PAD). TASC Working Group. TransAtlantic Inter-Society Concensus (TASC). *J Vasc Surg*. 2000;31:S1–S296.
150. Norgren L, Hiatt WR, Dormandy JA, Nehler MR, Harris KA, Fowkes FG. Inter-society consensus for the management of peripheral arterial disease (TASC II). *J Vasc Surg*. 2007;45(Suppl S):S5–67.
151. Capek P, McLean GK, Berkowitz HD. Femoropopliteal angioplasty. Factors influencing long-term success. *Circulation*. 1991;83:I70–80.
152. Zeller T. Current state of endovascular treatment of femoro-popliteal artery disease. *Vasc Med*. 2007;12:223–234.
153. Holmvang L, Kelbaek H, Kaltoft A, et al. Long-term outcome after drug-eluting versus bare-metal stent implantation in patients with ST-segment elevation myocardial infarction: 5 years follow-up from the randomized DEDICATION trial (Drug Elution and Distal Protection in Acute Myocardial Infarction). *JACC Cardiovasc Interv*. 2013;6:548–553.
154. Miura T, Miyashita Y, Soga Y, et al. Drug-eluting versus bare-metal stent implantation with or without cilostazol in the treatment of the superficial femoral artery. *Circ Cardiovasc Interven*. 2018;11:e006564.
155. Fahrni G, Farah A, Engstrom T, et al. Long-term results after drug-eluting versus bare-metal stent implantation in saphenous vein grafts: randomized controlled trial. *J Am Heart Assoc*. 2020;9:e017434.
156. Stokes KR, Strunk HM, Campbell DR, Gibbons GW, Wheeler HG, Clouse ME. Five-year results of iliac and femoropopliteal angioplasty in diabetic patients. *Radiology*. 1990;174:977–982.
157. Tepe G, Laird J, Schneider P, et al. Drug-coated balloon versus standard percutaneous transluminal angioplasty for the treatment of superficial femoral and popliteal peripheral artery disease: 12-month results from the IN.PACT SFA Randomized Trial. *Circulation*. 2015;131:495–502.

23 Cerebrovascular Disease in Persons With Diabetes

FRANK JOACHIM ERBGUTH

Stroke—in particular the ischemic subtype—is one of the major vascular manifestations of diabetes, together with coronary heart disease (CHD), peripheral arterial occlusive disease, and diabetic retinopathy. The relationship between hyperglycemia and stroke is bidirectional: on the one hand, patients with diabetes exhibit more than a twofold risk of ischemic stroke compared with patients without diabetes (see the next discussion on epidemiology of stroke in diabetes), even after statistical correction for other diabetes-associated vascular risk factors. On the other hand, acute stroke can generate both acute and persistent disturbances of glucose metabolism with poststroke hyperglycemia (PSH) (see the discussion on PSH below), which is associated with an approximate twofold risk of an unfavorable outcome. Treatment of hyperglycemia in patients with diabetes combined with multiple vascular risk factor management can substantially decrease the rate of stroke in primary as well as in secondary prevention. However, diabetes-associated end-organ damage to the brain is not only restricted to neuronal damage by strokes but also involves chronic and insidious damage of the brain, resulting in cognitive decline and dementia. Dementia in patients with diabetes not only results from vascular-mediated neuronal damage manifesting as vascular dementia (VD) but also is caused by an enhancement of neurodegenerative changes in the brain manifesting as Alzheimer disease (AD). In addition, between diabetes and dementia, bidirectional relations are likely as follows: on the one hand, people with diabetes have double the risk of developing dementia by mechanisms that are not yet fully understood; and on the other hand, the cognitive and behavioral manifestations of dementia such as lack of physical exercise and interference with therapeutic compliance may lead to disturbances of glucose metabolism, resulting in lability of glucose control, including an increased frequency of episodes of severe hypoglycemia.

EPIDEMIOLOGY OF STROKE IN DIABETES

Epidemiology of Stroke: General Observations and Time Trends

Stroke is the second most frequent cause of death worldwide and the second leading cause of long-term disability in industrialized countries. The incidence of stroke is considerable across the United States and European countries, with the subtypes of ischemic stroke and transient ischemic attack (TIA) being the most common events (80%–85%). Stroke incidence in European epidemiologic studies ranges from 114 cases/100,000 persons per year in France for first-ever stroke to 350 cases/100,000 persons per year in Germany for all stroke subtypes. Stroke prevalence estimates range from 1.5% in Italy to 3% in the United Kingdom and United States.[1]

The epidemiologic Oxford Vascular Study[2] analyzed the frequency of three types of vascular events (acute coronary, cerebrovascular, and peripheral) in a population of 91,106 inhabitants in Oxfordshire, United Kingdom, from 2002 to 2005. Cerebrovascular events (618 strokes and 300 TIAs), with a proportion of 45%, were more frequent than coronary vascular events, which affected 42% of the

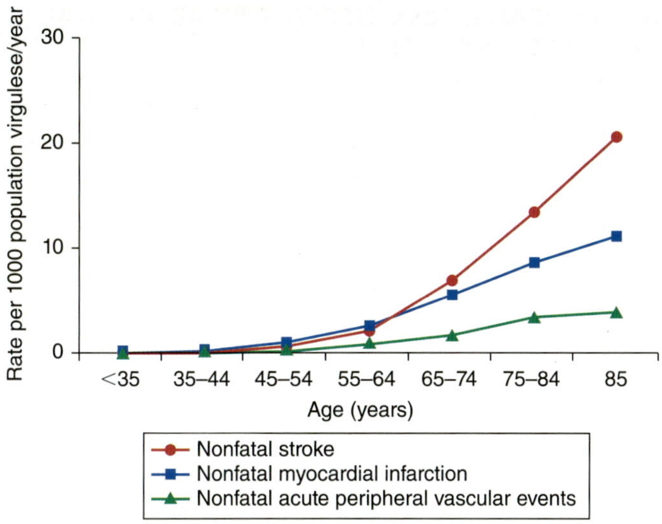

FIG. 23.1 Age-specific event rates for nonfatal stroke *(red line)*, nonfatal myocardial infarction *(blue line)*, and nonfatal acute peripheral vascular events *(green line)*. (From Rothwell PM, Coull AJ, Silver LE, et al. Population-based study of event-rate, incidence, case fatality, and mortality for all acute vascular events in all arterial territories [Oxford Vascular Study]. *Lancet.* 2005;366:1773–1783.)

cohort and peripheral vascular events, with an incidence of 9%. The relative incidence of cerebrovascular events compared with coronary events was 1.19 (95% confidence interval [CI] 1.06–1.33) overall and 1.40 (1.23–1.59) for nonfatal events. Event and incidence rates rose steeply with age in all arterial territories (Fig. 23.1). Similar data were shown by French investigators.[3]

The stroke incidence is higher in males than in females of the same age, based on age-adjusted data. The Global Burden of Disease (GBD) Study 2019 found that the age-standardized rate of stroke incidence globally decreased by 17.0% between 1990 and 2019 and was most pronounced in high-income countries, with a 33% decrease.[4] The positive changes in stroke incidence are the result of a marked increase in primary care prescription of primary and secondary vascular preventive medications such as lipid-lowering, antihypertensive, and antithrombotic drugs and of some positive changes in lifestyle. Despite these positive developments, problems remain with patients' lack of adherence to prevention strategies and with underuse of oral anticoagulation in patients with atrial fibrillation (AF) at high risk of stroke.

Stroke mortality rates have been decreasing consistently over time, with recent reports indicating a 56% reduction in stroke mortality between 1990 and 2019 in high-income countries.[4] Such increased survival of stroke patients may be linked to advances in preclinical and hospital treatment in acute stroke (e.g., intravenous thrombolysis [IVT] and mechanical thrombectomy [MT]) and in neurorehabilitation.

Diabetes and Other Risk Factors for Stroke

The risk of stroke associated with diabetes has been assessed predominantly in people with type 2 diabetes because stroke is more common in that population than in the age group typical of persons with type 1 diabetes.

TABLE 23.1 Duration of Diabetes and Ischemic Stroke Risk

DIABETES DURATION (YEARS)	ADJUSTED HAZARD RATIO (HR)	95% CONFIDENCE INTERVAL (CI)
0–5	1.7	1.1–2.7
5–10	1.8	1.1–3.0
> 10	3.2	2.4–4.5

Data from Banerjee C, Moon YP, Paik MC, et al. Duration of diabetes and risk of ischemic stroke: the Northern Manhattan Study. *Stroke.* 2012;43:1212–1217.

Epidemiologic studies identified a twofold to fourfold increase in stroke risk for persons with diabetes, regardless of concomitant risk factors.[5] In females, the risk is about 30% higher than in males.[6] During the longest observation period of 30 years in the Framingham Heart Study, a 2.5- to 3.6-fold increased risk of stroke in patients with diabetes was found.[6] The risk of stroke in people with diabetes is as high as that of people without diabetes who have already had a stroke.[7]

Stroke risk in diabetes increases with diabetes duration: The duration of diabetes was independently associated with ischemic stroke risk according to data from the Northern Manhattan Study, adjusting for other risk factors. The observed risk increase associated with diabetes overall was 3% each year and tripled with diabetes duration of 10 years or longer (Table 23.1).[8]

Assuming a population-wide prevalence of diabetes of 10%, these epidemiologic findings indicate a diabetes-attributable risk of stroke of approximately 12%. Hence, one in eight cases of stroke may be attributable to diabetes. Taking into account overall stroke mortality in general and its observed increased risk in diabetes, cerebrovascular disease causes approximately 20% of deaths of patients with diabetes.[5]

COMPARISON OF VASCULAR RISK FACTORS BETWEEN STROKE AND CORONARY HEART DISEASE

The case-control study INTERSTROKE[9]—analogous to the INTERHEART study[10]—examined the worldwide burden of stroke and the quantitative impact of known risk factors in different countries, in particular in developing countries. Of all fatal strokes worldwide, 85% occur in countries with low to middle income, and the number of strokes worldwide is massively driven by the increase in stroke incidence in developing and newly industrialized countries. Comparing 3000 stroke patients (78% ischemic stroke, 22% hemorrhagic stroke) and 3000 controls, the study extracted the 10 risk factors listed in decreasing order in Table 23.2 (odds ratios [ORs] and percentage of the population attributable risk [PAR]). For comparison, the corresponding numbers from the INTERHEART study are given in a third column.

Collectively the listed 10 risk factors account for 90% of all strokes, and the first 5 risk factors—namely, arterial hypertension, smoking, abdominal adiposity, diet habits, and little physical exercise—explain 80% of all strokes. Hypertension was the most important individual epidemiologic risk factor, which tripled the stroke risk, and therefore has a higher relative importance for the risk of

TABLE 23.2 Impact of Ten Vascular Risk Factors on Stroke and Myocardial Infarction: Odds Ratios and Percentage of the Population Attributable Risk (PAR)

RISK FACTOR/BEHAVIOR	ODDS RATIO	PAR (%) FOR STROKE	PAR (%) FOR MYOCARDIAL INFARCTION
1. Arterial hypertension	2.64	34.6	17.9
2. Waist-to-hip ratio	1.65	26.5	20.1
3. Regular physical activity	0.69	28.5	12.2
4. Smoking	2.09	18.9	35,7
5. Diet risk score	1.35	18.8	13.7
6. Diabetes	1.36	5.0	9.9
7. Alcohol intake	1.51	3.8	6.7
8. Psychosocial factors (stress, depression)	1.3	9.8	32.5
9. Cardiac causes	2.38	6.7	—
10. Ratio of apolipoproteins B to A1	1.89	24.9	49.2

stroke than for the risk of CHD. Diabetes mellitus (DM) as the sixth strongest risk factor by PAR% was placed in the middle field, being surrounded by diabetes-related risk factors such as adiposity, lack of physical exercise, and diet habits. The 2016 data from the INTERSTROKE study[11] showed a similar impact of diabetes for the risk of stroke, and in the GBD study, high fasting plasma glucose levels ranked third among population attributable fraction of disability-adjusted life years.[4]

From the mentioned epidemiologic data, an individual stroke risk calculation can be deduced. Kothari et al.[12] developed a mathematical model from the United Kingdom Prospective Diabetes Study (UKPDS) data to calculate an individual's risk of stroke within the following 5 years. In this model, for example, a 67-year-old smoker with arterial hypertension, hypercholesterolemia, and diabetes duration of 12 years has a 10.5% risk of stroke within the next 5 years.

It is not surprising that diabetes not only doubles the risk for a first-ever stroke but in the same manner doubles the risk for a recurrent stroke after a first event.[13]

DIABETES AS A STROKE RISK FACTOR IN YOUNGER PATIENTS

Type 1 and type 2 diabetes play an important role as stroke risk factors, particularly in younger, and middle-aged patients, because in these age groups other competing stroke risk factors are less prevalent and henceforth contribute less attributable risk than at older ages. Therefore in persons aged 18 to 44 years, diabetes raised the relative stroke risk to more than sixfold, depending on sex and race or ethnicity.[14] In general, in patients younger than 60 years, the relative risk (RR) of stroke in those with diabetes versus without diabetes is approximately double that of individuals older than 70 years. According to calculations from several studies, diabetes leads to an advanced cerebrovascular aging of approximately 10 to 15 years.

MULTIPLICATIVE RISK INCREASE BY ADDITIONAL VASCULAR RISK FACTORS

Patients with diabetes almost always have additional vascular risk factors such as arterial hypertension, dyslipidemia, obesity, lack of physical exercise, and nonvalvular AF. These comorbidities not only add to the risk of stroke from diabetes but multiplicatively affect the risk of stroke. Some studies, for example, found that the combination of diabetes and hypertension was associated with a 5-fold to 10-fold increased risk of stroke, suggesting a more than additive effect on stroke risk.[15]

Stroke Risk in Prediabetes- and Diabetes-Associated Metabolic Risk Configurations (Insulin Resistance, Impaired Glucose Tolerance, Glycated Hemoglobin, Metabolic Syndrome, Adiposity)

Not only in diabetes per se but also in prediabetic states, the risk for cerebrovascular disease is increased, although in general more modestly than with fully established diabetes. Prediabetes is defined as the condition in which glycemic variables are higher than normal but lower than the established diabetes thresholds. Prediabetes is a high-risk state for diabetes development: 5% to 10% of people with prediabetes will convert to diabetes each year.

A meta-analysis of 129 studies involving 10,069,955 individuals prediabetes[16] showed a significant higher risk ratio for stroke of 1.14 compared with normoglycemic controls. Impaired glucose tolerance carried a higher risk stroke than impaired fasting glucose.

When impaired glucose tolerance was measured by oral glucose tolerance test (OGTT) as in the Japanese Hisayama study,[17] 2-hour values of the OGTT of 11.1 mmol/L were associated with a more-than-doubled risk for stroke (in males, hazard ratio [HR] 2.71; in females, HR 2.19).

Glycated hemoglobin (HbA1c) concentrations are also associated with the risk of stroke even below diabetes thresholds. In an analysis of adults without diabetes participating in the community-based Atherosclerosis Risk in Communities (ARIC) study,[18] HbA1c concentrations—adjusted for potential confounders and for other vascular risk factors—of greater than 6% were associated with two to three times increased risk of stroke. The adjusted HRs for ischemic stroke according to baseline HbA1c are displayed in Fig. 23.2.

METABOLIC RISK CONFIGURATIONS (INSULIN RESISTANCE, METABOLIC SYNDROME, ADIPOSITY)

Insulin resistance (IR), a state in which cells fail to respond to the normal actions of insulin, has also been found to be associated with an increased risk of stroke. The RR for the highest quartile versus the lowest quartile of IR calculations (e.g., GUTT-Index, $ISI_{0,120}$-Index) ranged between 1.5 and 2.0, adjusted for demographics and prevalent cardiovascular disease[19]

The US National Health and Nutrition Examination Survey (NHANES) revealed the homeostatic model assessment of IR (HOMA-IR; equation: Fasting glucose [mmol/L] × Fasting insulin [mU/L]/22.5) as a measure for IR[20] to be

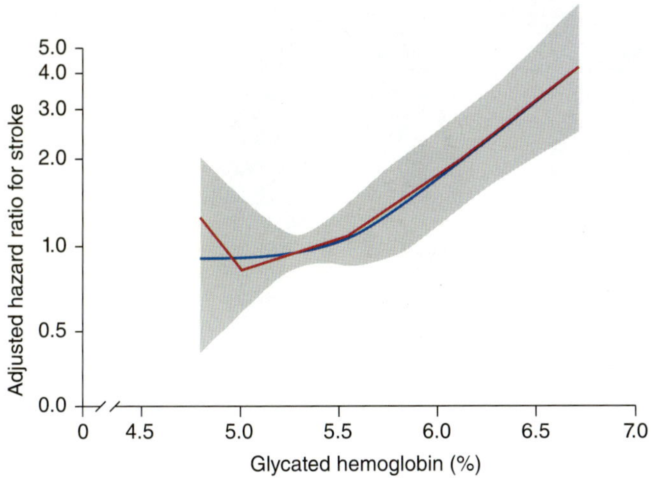

FIG. 23.2 Adjusted hazard ratios for ischemic stroke according to baseline glycated hemoglobin. *Blue line*: Restricted-cubic-spline model with 4 knost; *red line*: 3-Knot linear spline model (knots at 5.0%, 5.5%, and 6.0%). (Modified with permission from Selvin E, Steffes MW, Zhu H, et al. Glycated hemoglobin, diabetes, and cardiovascular risk in nondiabetic adults. *N Engl J Med.* 2010;362:800–811.)

independently and significantly associated with stroke risk with an OR of 1.06 (95% CI, 1.01–1.12) for each HOMA-IR unit, after adjustment for age, history of myocardial infarction (MI), the presence of hypertension or claudication, activity level, and HbA1c.[21] It seems clear that IR is a risk factor for stroke, but it remains controversial whether insulin concentrations themselves or markers of glucose tolerance convey the highest risk.

The impact of the metabolic syndrome (MetS), a clustering of disturbed glucose and insulin metabolism, obesity, and abdominal fat distribution, dyslipidemia, and hypertension on stroke risk remains controversial. While some studies showed increases in stroke with risk ratios up to 2.5,[22,23] other studies failed to demonstrate significant associations.[13,24]

All together, the available data support the consideration of MetS as an independent risk factor for stroke, depending on the metabolic and vascular risk configuration of the affected person on the whole and depending on the definition of MetS. The fact that the incremental stroke risk associated with MetS appears greater than the sum of its components suggests potential biologic interaction among MetS components, generating a risk that is more than additive. According to the type of study and the definition of MetS, its relation to increased risk of stroke is most commonly statistically significant.

The methodologic problems of such association studies with MetS are also obvious, if one notes the variability of the proportion of patients with diabetes included, which ranged from 0% to 100%.

Obesity in most studies is associated with an increased risk of stroke by 50% to 100%, whether measured by body mass index (BMI), waist-to-hip ratio, waist-to-height ratio, or waist circumference.[25,26] In the INTERSTROKE study,[9] persons with a waist-to-hip ratio in the highest tertile had a 65% increased risk of stroke (OR, 1.65; 99% CI, 1.36–1.99) compared with those in the lowest tertile.

However, all measures of adiposity and obesity such as BMI, waist-to-hip ratio, and waist circumference do not consistently improve the prediction of stroke risk when added to the most robustly associated stroke risk factors such as arterial hypertension and diabetes. This can be shown by the 2021 HUNT-Study, where obesity and overweight even over an extended period of time were not independent ischemic stroke risk factors, and the risk depended more on the metabolic consequences of obesity.[27] Despite these often discordant observations, excess adiposity remains a major modifiable determinant of these causal risk factors for stroke.

PATHOPHYSIOLOGY AND SUBTYPES OF ISCHEMIC STROKE IN DIABETES

Stroke in diabetes is the clinical culmination of atherosclerotic changes in the extracranial and intracranial large and small arteries associated with hyperglycemia. The proatherogenic effects in diabetes on cerebral blood vessels are not different from effects on coronary arteries and encompass advanced glycation end products, oxidative stress, endothelial dysfunction, inflammation, and hypercoagulability. In addition, the increased rate of CHD among patients with diabetes causes cardiomyopathy and AF, both of which predispose to cardioembolic stroke. AF is responsible for at least 20% to 30% of ischemic strokes.[28] AF is relatively common in patients with diabetes, with an increased prevalence of 30% to 40% compared to individuals without diabetes.[29] The severity of cardioembolic strokes and the resulting disability are greater than with noncardioembolic stroke, and hospital mortality is doubled.

Diabetes is one of the risk items counting as one point in the nine-point CHA_2DS_2-VASc score, which is used to calculate an individual's stroke risk in AF and to inform clinical decision-making with regard to antithrombotic therapies.

Because of its impact on cerebrovascular and cardiac systems, diabetes incrementally increases the risk for all three subtypes of ischemic stroke: lacunar, large artery occlusive, and thromboembolic. The distribution of these stroke subtypes among patients with diabetes is similar to that in the general population; however, those with diabetes have a greater burden of small-vessel, or lacunar, infarcts, which sometimes are clinically silent.[30] In addition, the proportion of ischemic strokes with infratentorial localization is relatively increased in patients with diabetes (Fig. 23.3).

PRIMARY AND SECONDARY PREVENTION OF STROKE IN DIABETES

Glucose Control

Since it is not possible for ethical reasons to prospectively compare an antiglycemic treatment with an untreated control group, the only way to assess the therapeutic effect is to prospectively compare a group of conventionally treated patients with diabetes with a group of intensively treated patients. In the 1441 patients with type 1 diabetes (aged 13–40 years) enrolled in the Diabetes Control and Complications Trial (DCCT) and Epidemiology of Diabetes Interventions and Complications (EDIC) study,[31] intensive

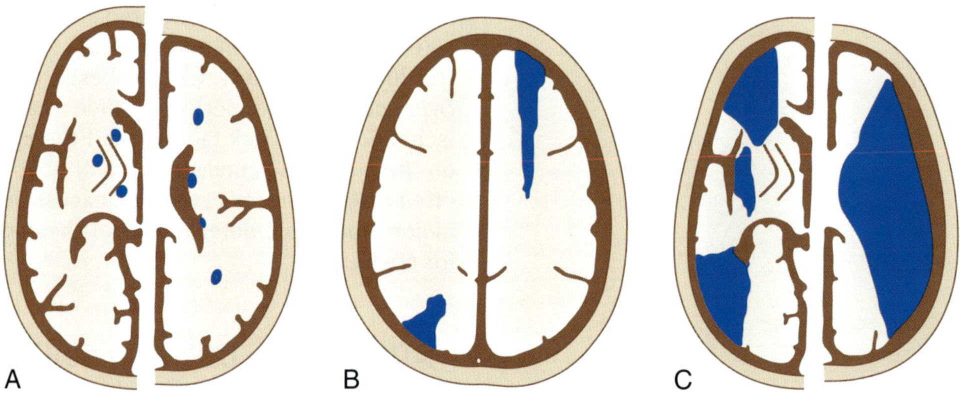

FIG. 23.3 Diabetes increases the risk for all subtypes of ischemic stroke: (A) lacunar; (B) hemodynamic by large artery occlusion; and (C) cardioembolic.

glucose management for 6.5 years reduced the risk of cardiovascular composite events (nonfatal MI, stroke, or cardiovascular deaths) significantly by 57% over a mean follow-up period of 17 years, compared with individuals under conventional treatment. However, the absolute numbers of stroke were low, with only one event in the intensive treatment group and five in the conventional treatment group. The target preprandial blood glucose in the intensively treated group was 70 to 120 mg/dL (<180 mg/dL postprandial); the mean HbA1c values were approximately 2% lower than in the conventional treatment group (7.4% vs. 9.1%).

In patients with type 2 diabetes in the UKPDS study,[32] intensive treatment with sulfonylureas or insulin did not significantly reduce cardiovascular outcomes compared with conventional diet therapy. However, in the substudy within the UKPDS in which obese patients received metformin as a first-line treatment, the generally small risk of stroke was reduced significantly by 42% compared with the group receiving conventional treatment (3.3 vs. 6.2 events per 1000 patient-years).[33]

Three more recent large long-term trials (Action in Diabetes and Vascular Disease: Preterax and Diamicron MR Controlled Evaluation [ADVANCE]; Action to Control Cardiovascular Risk in Diabetes [ACCORD]; Veterans Affairs Diabetes Trial [VADT]) also compared the effects of intensive versus standard treatment in individuals with long-standing type 2 diabetes and a high risk of cardiovascular and cerebrovascular events.[34–36] In the ADVANCE, VADT, and the ACCORD studies, no difference in cardiovascular outcomes—including stroke—could be found between the two glucose-lowering strategies.

No beneficial effects of tight glucose management over a mean period of 5 years could be found in a meta-analysis of 34,533 patients with type 2 diabetes (HR, 0.96; 95% CI, 0.83–1.1).[37] A similar result was communicated in a Cochrane review summarizing the findings from 34,912 patients with type 2 diabetes from 28 randomized trials.[38] The duration of intervention varied from 3 days to 12.5 years. Targeting intensive glycemic control did not reduce the risk ratio (RR) of nonfatal stroke significantly (95% CI, 0.84–1.19).

Taken together, to date, insufficient data are available to prove that intensive and tight glycemic control per se improves occurrence of stroke—in particular in type 2 diabetes. Treatment of patients with a high risk of stroke must balance the risk of recurrent hypoglycemia against the potential advantages of lower targets of HbA1c.

Management of Diabetes-Associated Vascular Risk Factors

In the UKPDS, the variables that predicted the 188 incident strokes in DM included duration of diabetes, age, sex, smoking, systolic blood pressure (SBP), dyslipidemia, and the presence of AF. Modifiable risk factors for stroke accompanying diabetes have been targeted for stroke prevention in several randomized controlled trials.

HYPERTENSION

Hypertension has long been recognized as the major modifiable risk factor for stroke. Lowering of blood pressure in patients with type 2 diabetes had a significant effect on the risk of stroke. The most pronounced risk reduction was seen in the UKPDS, where better blood pressure control among patients with type 2 diabetes was associated with a 44% reduction in stroke incidence for each 10-mm Hg reduction in mean SBP.[39] Other studies showed lower positive effects of more intensive blood pressure control.[40] The stroke-preventing effect of blood pressure lowering was mainly detected in those trials, in which the initial SBP was higher and the target was 130 to 135 mm Hg.

In the ACCORD-BP trial, a total of 4733 participants with type 2 diabetes were randomly assigned to intensive blood pressure treatment targeting a systolic pressure of less than 120 mm Hg or standard therapy targeting a systolic pressure of less than 140 mm Hg.[41] After 1 year, a mean SBP of 119.3 mm Hg was achieved in the intensive therapy group and 133.5 mm Hg in the standard therapy group. The annual risk rates of stroke after a mean follow-up of 4.7 years were 0.32% and 0.53% in the two groups, respectively (HR, 0.59; 95% CI, 0.39–0.89). However, the intensive blood pressure management did not reduce the rate of the composite outcome of fatal and nonfatal major cardiovascular events and led to an increase in adverse events such as syncope and hyperkalemia.

A summary meta-analysis concluded that among patients with type 2 diabetes, SBP lowering among those with baseline values of 140 mm Hg and greater led to a

TABLE 23.3 Various Interventions for Stroke Reduction in Diabetes

INTERVENTION (REFERENCE)	NUMBER OF STUDIES	RR/HR (95% CI)
Blood pressure lowering in diabetes (meta-analysis per 10-mm Hg lower SBP)[42]	19	RR 0.73 (0.64–0.83)
Statins in diabetes (meta-analysis per mmol/L reduction in LDL-C)[43]	14	RR 0.79 (0.67–0.93) (99% CI)
Evolocumab plus statin vs. placebo plus statin (FOURIER trial—diabetes subgroup)[19]	1	HR 0.72 (0.56–0.93)
Aspirin vs. placebo in secondary prevention (meta-analysis)[44]	16	RR 0.81 (0.71–0.92)
Rivaroxaban 2.5 mg BID plus aspirin vs. placebo plus aspirin (COMPASS trial—diabetes subgroup)[17]	1	HR 0.63 (0.43–0.90)
GLP-1RA vs. placebo (meta-analysis)[13]	8	HR 0.83 (0.76–0.92)

RR, Relative risk; *HR*, Hazard ratio; *CI*, confidence interval; *GLP-1RA*, glucagon-like peptide 1 receptor agonist; *LDL-C*, low-density lipoprotein cholesterol.

27% lower stroke rate (RR, 0.73; 95% CI, 0.64–0.83) with an absolute rate of 4.06% (95% CI, 2.53–5.40)[42] (Table 23.3). Most guidelines for stroke prevention recommend a blood pressure less than 130/80 mm Hg. Reaching these target levels is probably more important than the choice of antihypertensive drug. However, for stroke prevention, beta-blockers seem to be inferior to other antihypertensives, and in contrast, calcium channel blockers have been shown to be superior. As a potential explanation for such observed differences in efficacy in stroke prevention by drug classes, different effects on within-individual blood pressure variability across the classes have been proposed, which seems to be an independent risk predictor for stroke.[43,44]

LIPIDS

For primary prevention of stroke in patients with diabetes, many studies showed a significant reduction in ischemic stroke rates between 20% and 50%, depending on the composition of the study population[45] (Table 23.3).

For secondary stroke prevention, the 2006 SPARCL trial found that atorvastatin 80 mg daily versus placebo reduced the stroke risk in patients with a recent stroke or TIA and no known CHD by 16% with a 5-year absolute reduction in stroke risk of 2.2%.[46] In the secondary analysis of the study for the subgroup of individuals with type 2 diabetes and MetS, no treatment-by-subgroup interactions were found, indicating a similar stroke preventive effect for the subgroup of patients with diabetes. The 2020 "Treat Stroke to Target Investigators" study[48] demonstrated that after an ischemic stroke or TIA with evidence of atherosclerosis, patients who had a target low-density lipoprotein (LDL) cholesterol level of less than 70 mg/dL had a significant 22% lower risk of subsequent cardiovascular events (ischemic stroke, MI, coronary or carotid revascularization, or death from cardiovascular causes) than those who had a target range of 90 to 110 mg/dL. In the subgroup of patients with diabetes (23%), the preventive effect of the statin therapy was even more pronounced, with a risk reduction of 40%. The 2860 patients had been followed for a median of 3.5 years. Because the study was stopped early before reaching the intended number of cases, there was no significant effect for the single secondary endpoint "stroke." Given the much-discussed adverse long-term effects of statin treatment on the development of diabetes or an increased risk of intracerebral hemorrhage, it is meaningful that no increased incidences of diabetes or intracerebral hemorrhage were shown in this study.

The PCSK9 inhibitor Evolocumab added to statin treatment in a risk population with atherosclerotic cardiovascular disease showed a significant 28% stroke reduction compared with statins alone in the diabetes subgroup.[49]

Platelet Inhibition

In meta-analyses on the use of aspirin for primary prevention in persons with diabetes, no consistent significant benefits could be recorded with respect to the reduction of serious vascular events, including stroke.

In a randomized trial with 15,480 participants with diabetes and no evident cardiovascular disease,[50] serious vascular events occurred in a significantly lower percentage of participants in the aspirin group than in the placebo group (8.5% vs. 9.6%; RR, 0.88; 95% CI, 0.79–0.97; $P = .01$). In contrast, major bleeding events—mostly of gastrointestinal location—occurred more often in the aspirin group (4.1% vs. 3.2%; RR, 1.29; 95% CI, 1.09–1.52; $P = .003$). Because the absolute benefits were largely counterbalanced by the bleeding hazard, no general recommendation for aspirin in primary prevention of vascular events including stroke can be given.

For secondary prevention of stroke, no major studies specifically for individuals with diabetes have been performed. But there are no hints that the general recommendation of platelet inhibition after stroke in patients with diabetes is different from other patients. A meta-analysis of 16 studies by the Antithrombotic Trialists' Collaboration, for example, showed a significant 19% risk reduction of stroke recurrence equally pronounced in subjects with and without diabetes.[51]

Although there is no clear proof for a substantial effect of platelet inhibition on the risk of stroke in primary prevention, antiplatelet agents—mostly aspirin—should be considered for all those patients with diabetes who are identified to be at increased risk of future cerebrovascular complications.

MULTIFACTOR RISK FACTOR MANAGEMENT

Various studies showed a significant reduction of vascular events, including stroke by multifactorial and intense risk factor management, compared with usual care. Absolute risk reductions for stroke in the 2019 published ADDITION-Leicester study were 6.3% and 8.8% within 10 and 20 years, respectively.[47]

The most pronounced substantial benefit of multifactorial management was found in the Steno-2 landmark trial,[52] in which the 7.8-year multifactorial approach encompassed

TABLE 23.4 Numbers of Events After 13.3 Years with Intensive Versus Conventional Multifactorial Cardiovascular Risk-Modifying Therapy Among 160 High-Risk Patients with Diabetes

	INTENSIVE THERAPY (NUMBER OF EVENTS)	CONVENTIONAL THERAPY (NUMBER OF EVENTS)
Death from any cause	24	40
Myocardial infarction	9	35
Stroke	6	30
All cardiovascular events	51	158

the use of statins, angiotensin-converting enzyme (ACE) inhibitors, angiotensin II receptor blockers, platelet inhibition, glucose control, and lifestyle modification. At the end of the 13.3 years of follow-up, among 160 high-risk individuals with long-standing type 2 diabetes and microalbuminuria who participated in the study, a reduction in cardiovascular events by 59% (HR, 0.41; 95% CI, 0.25–0.67] was found. The number of all types of stroke was reduced by 80% (6 vs. 30 events) (Table 23.4). The beneficial effect of the aggressive multirisk factor approach in the primary study could also be demonstrated for the observation period extended to 21 years, during which an HR for stroke occurrence was 0.31, and micro- and macrovascular complications were significantly reduced.[53]

These findings underscore that multifactorial risk factor management may be key for a substantial reduction of stroke in diabetes.

EFFECTS OF DIFFERENT ANTIHYPERGLYCEMIC MEDICATIONS ON THE RISK OF STROKE

In response to the development of the two new classes of antihyperglycemic agents, namely glucagon-like peptide 1 receptor agonists (GLP-1RAs), and sodium glucose cotransporter 2 (SGLT2) inhibitors, various guidelines recommend the addition of these substances when prevention of further vascular events is the priority and therefore should then be added to metformin independently of baseline HbA1c. Although the two classes of agents show similar reductions in the combined vascular endpoint (major averse cardiovascular event [MACE]), they differ in their effects on individual endpoints, such as stroke. Whereas no effect on the secondary endpoint of stroke was found with all SGLT2 inhibitors, GLP-1RAs consistently showed such a beneficial effect. A meta-analysis of eight studies with GLP-1RAs revealed statistically significant reductions in the combined outcome of fatal/nonfatal stroke versus placebo (HR, 0.83; 95% CI, 0.76–0.92) as well as decreases in MACE, cardiovascular death, fatal/nonfatal MI, and hospitalization for heart failure[54] (Table 23.3). Therefore GLP-RAs added to metformin should be considered for individuals with type 2 DM (T2DM) who have experienced a prior stroke/TIA or are at high risk for stroke.

Oral Anticoagulation in Atrial Fibrillation in Patients With Diabetes

Twenty to thirty percent of ischemic strokes are caused by cardiac embolism, most commonly from the left atrium and its appendage in nonvalvular AF. Diabetes, together with previous stroke, hypertension, advancing age, congestive heart failure, female sex, and atherosclerosis, is one of the major risk factors for stroke in individuals with AF (see the discussion of pathophysiology and subtypes of ischemic stroke in diabetes) and counts for one point in the nine-point CHA_2DS_2-VASc score, which is used for the calculation of an individual's stroke risk in AF.

Primary stroke prevention with adjusted-dose warfarin, a vitamin K antagonist (VKA), with a target international normalized ratio (INR) of 2.0 to 3.0, reduces the RR of first-ever stroke in individuals with AF with a moderate vascular risk profile by approximately two-thirds compared with a placebo (annual stroke risk 1.8% vs. 4.6%), with a slight increase in the annual rates of intracranial hemorrhage (0.4% vs. 0.2%) or major extracranial bleeding (approximately 2% vs. 1%). For secondary stroke prevention, warfarin with a target INR of 2.0 to 3.0 also reduces the risk of recurrent stroke significantly by approximately two-thirds compared with placebo (annual stroke risk 3.9% vs. 12.3%) and is associated with an annual increase in major bleeding (2.8% vs. 0.7%; HR, 3.20, 95% CI, 0.91–11.3).[55] Aspirin is not an adequate strategy to replace warfarin or direct oral anticoagulants (DOACs) because it does not significantly reduce the risk of stroke. Particularly in older patients, aspirin is often prescribed with the assumption that it will cause fewer bleeding complications than warfarin. However, not only is aspirin not efficacious in stroke prevention in AF, but it also causes a similar rate of intracranialbleeding compared with warfarin. The Birmingham Atrial Fibrillation Treatment of the Aged (BAFTA) trial compared warfarin and aspirin in patients aged 75 years or older with a 14% prevalence of diabetes and demonstrated a twofold increased stroke rate with aspirin versus warfarin without a significant difference in major intracranial or extracranial hemorrhage (1.9% vs. 2.0%).[56]

Despite its great efficacy in stroke prevention, oral anticoagulation with VKAs such as warfarin is sometimes poorly managed; register data show that only approximately 50% to 70% of suitable patients receive no or inadequate anticoagulant treatment.

Four DOACs have been proven to be successful competitors with warfarin. The direct thrombin inhibitor dabigatran etexilate and the factor Xa inhibitors rivaroxaban, apixaban, and edoxaban were shown in large prospective trials to be at least as efficacious and safe as warfarin.[57] These four DOACs have all shown noninferiority in prevention of ischemic stroke compared with VKAs, with better safety, consistently limiting the number of intracranial hemorrhages by about 50%.

The impact of diabetes on stroke preventive therapy with DOACs where evaluated in a meta-analysis, which showed that in patients with DM the relative and absolute risk reduction of the composite outcome of stroke and systemic embolism, CVD death, and intracranial bleeding compared with warfarin were even more pronounced than in patients without diabetes.[58]

In general, oral anticoagulants are not used for prevention of strokes caused by arteriosclerosis. The only possible exception is a combination of low-dose rivaroxaban (2.5 mg twice daily) and aspirin (100 mg once daily), which showed superiority over rivaroxaban (5 mg twice daily) or aspirin alone in the COMPASS trial in risk patients with clinical atherosclerosis.[59] In a stroke outcome-focused subgroup analysis, there was a significant better stroke prevention by the combination rivaroxaban plus aspirin in patients with DM compared with patients without DM with an RR of 0.63 (95% CI, 0.43–0.90)[60] (Table 23.3).

Carotid Artery Interventions in Diabetes: Carotid Endarterectomy and Carotid Artery Stenting

Carotid artery stenosis is one of the macrovascular complications of diabetes. The presence of an atherosclerotic stenotic lesion in the extracranial internal carotid artery or carotid bulb has been associated with an increased risk of stroke. Randomized trials have shown that carotid endarterectomy (CEA) in appropriately selected patients with carotid stenosis modestly reduces stroke risk compared with patients treated by medical management alone.

However, the risk of stroke in patients undergoing intensive contemporary medical treatment has fallen significantly since the mid-1980s. Recent estimates suggest that the stroke risk in patients undergoing contemporary best medical treatment is overlapping that of patients who have undergone surgery in historical randomized trials such that the advantages of CEA demonstrated in older trials in such patients are the subject of controversies.[61,62]

In patients with symptomatic carotid artery stenoses, CEA was of some benefit for participants with 50% to 69% symptomatic stenosis (moderate-quality evidence) and highly beneficial for those with 70% to 99% stenosis (moderate-quality evidence).[63] Therefore the 2021 guidelines from the American Heart Association/American Stroke Association (AHA/ASA) recommend CEA after nondisabling ischemic stroke within the past 6 months and ipsilateral severe (70%–99%) carotid artery stenosis, provided that perioperative morbidity and mortality risk is lower than 6%. Patients with asymptomatic carotid artery stenosis should receive lifestyle interventions and intensive treatment of all vascular risk factors. Prophylactic CEA performed with less than 3% morbidity and mortality is regarded as useful in highly selected patients with asymptomatic carotid stenosis of minimum 60%.

Carotid artery stenting (CAS) as an alternative to CEA has shown higher rates of periprocedural strokes, which were largely driven by more minor strokes following CAS than CEA. Rates of death, major stroke, ipsilateral stroke, and MI were comparable between CEA and CAS.

CAS as an alternative to CEA is reasonable in patients in whom anatomic or medical conditions are present that increase the risk for surgery (such as radiation-induced stenosis or restenosis after CEA). CAS may be considered particularly in patients with significant cardiovascular comorbidities predisposing to cardiovascular complications with CEA.[64]

Both intervention methods, CEA and CAS, had not been studied in randomized trials exclusively in patients with diabetes. In CEA, both periprocedural and long-term risks are higher in patients with diabetes than without; for example, pooled data[65] from the European Carotid Surgery Trial (ECST)[66] and North American Symptomatic Carotid Endarterectomy Trial (NASCET)[67] found a significant 1.45 periprocedural risk of complications for patients with versus without diabetes (9.7% vs. 7.0%; RR, 1.45; 95% CI, 1.05–2.02). For CAS in patients with diabetes, a meta-analysis showed a nonsignificantly increased risk of perioperative and long-term complications compared with patients without diabetes.[68] However, the benefit of both carotid interventions for stroke reduction remains despite the potentially higher risk in patients with diabetes, as a higher rate of vascular events is also seen in the control arms without diabetes. Thus, in part, even a higher absolute risk reduction of strokes could be observed.

Mechanical Revascularization of Severe Intracranial Arterial Stenosis

Patients with a recent cerebrovascular event and severe stenosis (70%–99%) of major intracranial arteries are at a high annual risk of approximately 23% for recurrent stroke in the territory of the stenotic artery, despite treatment with aspirin and standard management of vascular risk factors. As a promising prevention strategy, percutaneous transluminal angioplasty and stenting (PTAS) was studied in the Stenting and Aggressive Medical Management for Preventing Recurrent Stroke in Intracranial Stenosis (SAMMPRIS) trial with early and long-term results.[69,70] The enrollment of the study was halted after 451 randomized patients because of the high risk of stroke or death within 30 days of enrollment in the PTAS arm (self-expanding wingspan stent) relative to the medical arm. Of the participants, 46% had type 2 diabetes. The 30-day rate of stroke or death was 14.7% in the PTAS group (nonfatal stroke, 12.5%; fatal stroke, 2.2%), almost threefold higher than in the medically managed group with 5.8% (nonfatal stroke, 5.3%; nonstroke-related death, 0.4%). Beyond 30 days, stroke in the same brain territory occurred in 13 patients in each group. An analysis of patient and procedural factors that may have been associated with periprocedural cerebrovascular events in the trial found that diabetes was one of the major factors that were significantly associated with ischemic events, with an OR of 4.5 (95% CI, 1.3–16.1) associated with diabetes. The early benefit of aggressive medical management over stenting with the wingspan stent for high-risk patients with intracranial stenosis persisted over the extended follow-up period of 32.4 months.[70] Based on this study, in severe intracranial stenosis, the following aggressive medical management is recommended: dual platelet inhibition with aspirin at a dose of 325 mg/day together with clopidogrel at a dose of 75 mg/day for the first 90 days after the incident event; management of the primary risk factors such as elevated SBP and elevated LDL cholesterol levels; and management of secondary risk factors (diabetes, elevated nonhigh-density lipoprotein cholesterol levels, smoking, excess weight, and insufficient exercise) with the help of a lifestyle modification program. The corresponding targets of intervention were SBP of less than 140 mm Hg (<130 mm Hg in patients with diabetes) and an LDL cholesterol level of less than 70 mg/dL. Thus stenting in intracranial stenosis cannot be recommended at this time.

HYPOGLYCEMIA AND STROKE

The brain is directly and rapidly affected by a critical decrease in blood glucose because its metabolism relies exclusively on glucose supply. In this context, repeated episodes of severe hypoglycemia are thought to contribute to the development of cognitive decline and dementia, because of their cumulative neurotoxic effect (see the later discussion of diabetes as a vascular risk factor for cognitive impairment and dementia).

However, hypoglycemia may also cause adverse cerebrovascular events. Acute hypoglycemia provokes profound physiologic changes affecting the cardiovascular system and several hematologic parameters, as a consequence of sympathoadrenal activation and counterregulatory hormonal secretion. Many of these responses have an important role in protecting the brain from neuroglycopenia, through altering regional blood flow and promoting metabolic changes that will restore blood glucose to normal. Some of these effects are potentially pathophysiologic, and in people with diabetes who have not yet developed endothelial dysfunction, they may have an adverse impact on a vasculature that is already damaged. The acute hemodynamic and hematologic changes may increase the risk of localized tissue ischemia, and major vascular events can certainly be precipitated by acute hypoglycemia. These include myocardial and cerebral ischemia and occasionally infarction. The possible mechanisms underlying these hypoglycemia-induced cerebrovascular effects include hemorrheologic changes, white cell activation, vasoconstriction, and the release of inflammatory mediators and cytokines. Therefore it is suggested that acute and repeated hypoglycemia could aggravate cerebrovascular complications associated with diabetes by enhancing atherosclerotic vascular and proembolic changes.[71]

DIABETES AND ACUTE STROKE—POSTSTROKE HYPERGLYCEMIA

Epidemiology and Definition of Poststroke Hyperglycemia

If one analyzes the patient characteristics in acute stroke studies, approximately one-fifth of all stroke patients have diabetes. The prevalence of DM ranges between 10% and 30%, depending on the cohort studied.

PSH occurs not only in the acute stroke phase in patients with preexisting DM but also in patients without a prior diagnosis of diabetes.[72] PSH can occur in all subtypes of strokes. The frequency found in various studies depends on the following:

1. The definition of the threshold of hyperglycemia (fasting glucose from 6.0 to 7.8 mmol/L)
2. The definition of the duration of the acute poststroke period (12–96 hours)
3. The frequency of blood glucose testing (single test on admission vs. repeated single tests vs. continuous glucose monitoring)
4. The nutritional status of patients (no nutrition vs. parenteral nutrition vs. intravenous nutrition)

With a glucose limit value of 7.0 mmol/L, the frequency of PSH is approximately 40% to 50%,[73,74] at least twice as high as the diabetes prevalence in stroke patients. PSH may have a dynamic progression with various patterns with respect to latency and duration of PSH, namely, "initial" or "delayed" PSH peaks as well as "two peaks" and permanent hyperglycemia.[75,76] The PSH pattern distribution varied significantly between patients with and without diabetes; whereas patients with diabetes more frequently had permanent hyperglycemia, patients without diabetes more frequently had initial PSH peaks (Table 23.5.[76] Only 15% of patients with diabetes but 70% of those without diabetes showed a permanent normoglycemic state within 24 hours poststroke.

This possible variability of PSH over time explains that frequencies and patterns of PSH in various studies depend on the respective times of glucose measures. This makes it difficult to interpret and compare different studies.

Causes of Poststroke Hyperglycemia

If one takes the previously described prevalence rates, half of patients with PSH have a preexisting disturbance of glucose metabolism such as diabetes or prediabetes. In nonpreexisting diabetes, a postulated cause of PSH is a neurometabolic "stress hyperglycemia" with the activation of the hypothalamus-pituitary-adrenal (HPA) axis with the release of cortisol and adrenaline and subsequent glycolysis and gluconeogenesis.[77] The neuroanatomic correlates of central autonomic dysregulation in PSH were studied with magnetic resonance imaging (MRI) in 229 affected patients without diabetes with stroke. A clear and significant correlation between the occurrence of PSH and the location of the infarct in the right insular and operculum region could be detected. Both brain structures are involved in the regulation of the sympathetic nervous system.[77]

Neurotoxicity in Poststroke Hyperglycemia

The findings with regard to neuronal damage mechanisms of PSH mainly result from experimental studies performed on animals and a few patient examinations with functional cerebral imaging. These have shown that there is not one single damage mechanism but rather a complex interaction of various "neurotoxic" effects. Table 23.6 summarizes the potential direct and indirect mechanisms

TABLE 23.5 Distribution of Patients With and Without Diabetes in the Four Progression Patterns of Poststroke Hyperglycemia

	DIABETES (*N* = 161) *N* (%)	NO DIABETES (*N* = 587) *N* (%)
Initial hyperglycemia	21 (13%)	79 (13%)
Hyperglycemia after 24 hours	16 (10%)	54 (9%)
Persistent hyperglycemia	100 (62%)	46 (8%)
Persistent normoglycemia	24 (15%)	408 (70%)

Data from Yong M, Kaste M. Dynamic of hyperglycemia as a predictor of stroke outcome in the ECASS-II trial. *Stroke.* 2008;39:2749–2755.

of neuronal damage by hyperglycemia during the acute phase of ischemic stroke.[78–80]

Poststroke Hyperglycemia as a Global Negative-Outcome Predictor

In animal models, the extent of hyperglycemia in acute cerebral ischemia determined the size of cerebral lesions

TABLE 23.6 Hyperglycemic Damage Mechanisms in Acute Ischemic Stroke

Parenchyma toxicity (anaerobic/glucose metabolism)	Acidosis Lactate accumulation Increase of the NMDA receptor–dependent cellular calcium flux Inflammation Increased formation of free radicals Increased expression of matrix metalloproteinase 9 (MMP-9)
Vascular damage and perfusion defect	Endothelial dysfunction Reduced vessel reactivity Inflammation Prothrombotic state—for example, activation of plasminogen activator inhibitor 1 (PAI-1) Reduced NO production
Impairment of the blood-brain barrier	Edema formation Increased rate of hemorrhage
Noncerebral effects	Immune system Shift in fluid balance Disruption in peripheral perfusion
Consequences of the insulin deficit	Increased formation of free fatty acids with prothrombotic effect and reduction in vessel reactivity

MMP-9, Matrix metalloproteinase 9; *NMDA*, *N*-methyl-D-aspartate; *PAI-1*, plasminogen activator inhibitor 1.

and mortality. In patient studies, the negative prognostic impact of PSH was identified after adjustment for other variables such as age, severity, and extent of stroke with a factor between 1.5 and 2 for all negative outcome endpoints.[81] It is interesting to note that the negative effect of PSH in clinical studies was lower in patients with diabetes compared with those without diabetes (OR 1.3 vs. 3).[81–83]

In general, the negative implications of PSH have not been studied specifically with regard to the various types of strokes. However, there are some indications that PSH does not necessarily have an unfavorable effect in small lacunar infarctions or even could be favorable in terms of prognosis. The analysis of the patient population participating in the studies with the neuroprotectant lubeluzole (LUB-INT-9 and LUB-INT-5])[84] showed that glucose levels in excess of 8 mmol/L within 6 hours after the stroke event coincided with larger infarctions with an expected lower functional outcome (OR, 0.60; 95% CI, 0.41–0.88), whereas in lacunar ischemia the chance for a good functional outcome was almost three times better (OR, 2.70; 95% CI, 1.01–7.13). However, this positive correlation turned negative with higher glucose levels (>12 mmol/L) (Fig. 23.4).

Influence of Diabetes on Acute Stroke Treatments

The two standard therapies for vascular recanalization in ischemic strokes are IVT with alteplase and MT. IVT has demonstrated efficacy beyond the generally recommended time window of 4.5 hours after stroke onset, up

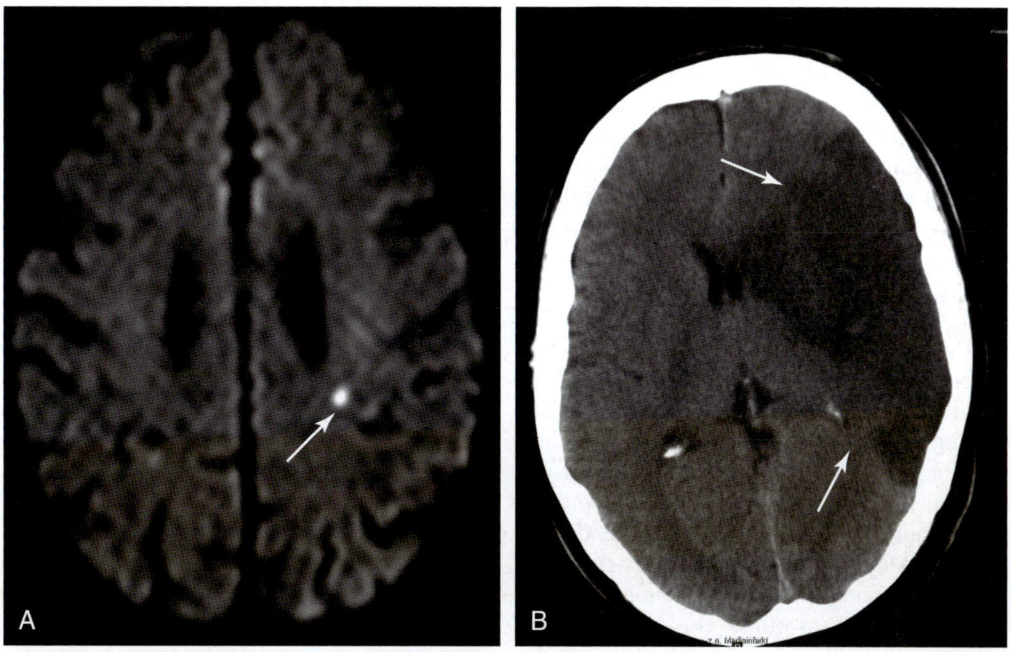

FIG. 23.4 (A) In small lacunar infarctions (white dot in the diffusion-weighted magnetic resonance imaging scan; *white arrow*), poststroke hyperglycemia has a less negative effect on functional outcome than in large territorial infarctions; (B) large, dark gray infarction demarcation between the two *white arrows* in the computed tomography scan.

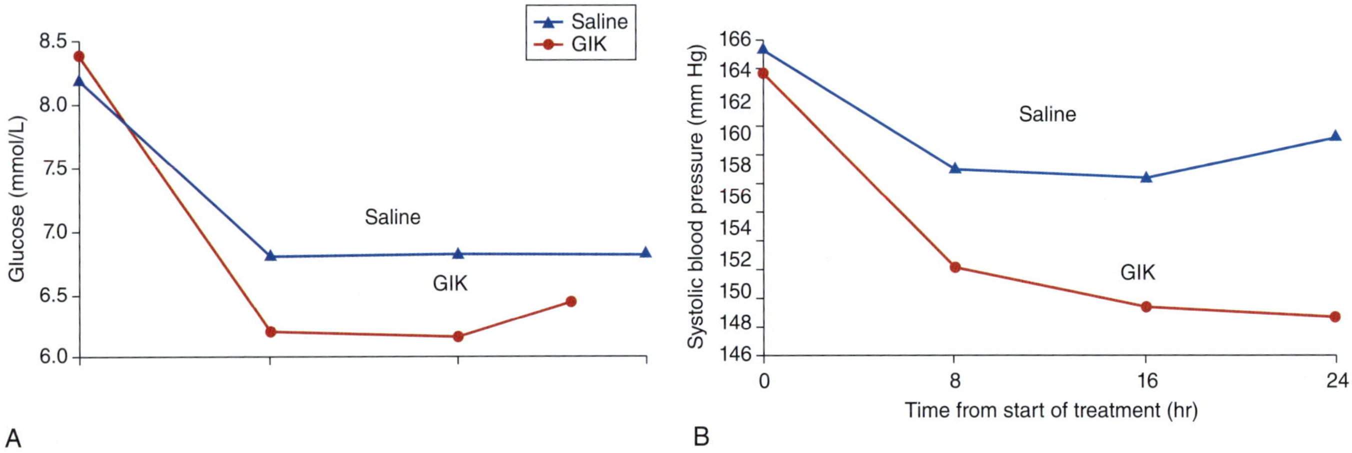

FIG. 23.5 Mean glucose levels (A) and systolic blood pressure values (B) initially and 8, 16, and 24 hours later in both study arms of the GIST-UK study. *GIK*, Glucose-insulin-potassium infusion. (From Gray CS, Hildreth AJ, Sandercock PA, et al. Glucose-potassium-insulin infusions in the management of post-stroke hyperglycaemia: the UK Glucose Insulin in Stroke Trial (GIST-UK). *Lancet Neurol.* 2007;6:397–406.)

to 9 hours using mismatch imaging showing (MRI or computed tomography) salvageable brain tissue for patient selection.[85] Although there are some hints that patients with diabetes or PSH have poorer recanalization rates and higher intracerebral hemorrhage complications, the superiority over conservative therapy still remains.[86,87]

MT in large-vessel occlusion, meanwhile widely used after good results from randomized trials in 2015, improves the rate of good functional outcome in usually severely affected patients by a factor of two to three.[88] The proportion of patients with diabetes in the different studies was about 15%. Similar to IVT, diabetes is a risk predictor for worse outcome also with MT, but it does not affect the relative rates of improvement for good functional outcome compared with no intervention.[89]

As early recurrence prophylaxis for mild ischemic strokes (with a National Institutes of Health Stroke Scale [NIHSS] score with 3 or less) and high-risk TIAs (with an ABCD2 score of 4 or more), dual antiplatelet therapy with ASA and clopidogrel for 21 days is now recommended based on study evidence.[90] With longer administration, the increasing risk of cerebral hemorrhage neutralizes the positive effect. In the ABCD2 risk score with a maximum of seven points, existing diabetes contributes one risk point in addition to the other characteristics of TIA (age, clinical features, duration of symptoms, blood pressure).

Glucose-Lowering Treatment of Poststroke Hyperglycemia

There is no consensus regarding the best type of glycemic control, the best method for achieving it, and the necessary monitoring in the setting of acute stroke. The mentioned fluctuating course of PSH includes the risk of induced hypoglycemia when strict control by intravenous insulin infusions is attempted. The type of insulin delivery has differed in reported studies; for example, whereas intravenous glucose-insulin-potassium infusions were administered in the intervention study the UK Glucose Insulin in Stroke Trial (GIST-UK) (Fig. 23.5),[91] other studies used staggered perfusion rates of insulin in NaCl 0.9% strictly applied according to the measured glucose levels, or they used 5% glucose or insulin in individual intravenous bolus dosages.

Two systematic reviews are available, which are used as the basis for various international guideline recommendations. Both evaluations consistently report a lack of benefit from intensified therapy with intravenous insulin for tight glycemic control, with an increased rate of complications in terms of hypoglycemia. The Cochrane review included 11 RCTs involving 1583 adult patients with blood glucose levels > 110 mg/dL (6.1 mmol/L) within 24 hours of stroke.[92] Blood glucose–lowering treatment was not associated with a reduction in death or dependence or permanent neurologic deficit. However, the rate of symptomatic hypoglycemia was higher in the intervention group with a significant OR of 14.6. The other review included nine studies with $N = 1491$ participants on the control of elevated blood glucose levels with intravenous insulin.[93] There was no significant difference in mortality or functional outcome between patients treated with intravenous insulin and controls. Rates of hypoglycemia (OR 8.19) and symptomatic hypoglycemia (OR 6.15) were significantly higher in patients treated with intravenous insulin (8.19 and 6.15, respectively).

The GLycemia in Acute Stroke (GLIAS) study results[83] allow speculation that there is a U-shaped curve of correlation between the prognosis and the blood glucose level. Accordingly, both hypoglycemic and near-hypoglycemic values would be just as negatively predictive as significantly hyperglycemic values, and the best prognosis would be within the moderately hyperglycemic and normoglycemic ranges. If the hypothesis for such a correlation were to be tested prospectively, it remains plausible that lowering glucose levels from the moderately hyperglycemic to the hypoglycemic range would have a negative effect, whereas interventions to lower hyperglycemia to less-severe hyperglycemia or to normoglycemia could have a favorable effect on clinical outcomes. It is probable that the effectiveness of glycemic control is decisively dependent on the quality of glucose monitoring and the avoidance of hypoglycemia.

The 2019 AHA/ASA guidelines recommend the treatment of hyperglycemia to achieve blood glucose levels in a range of 140 to 180 mg/dL and to closely monitor to prevent hypoglycemia in patients in the acute phase of stroke. It is also recommended to treat hypoglycemia (<60 mg/dL) with slow intravenous administration of 25 mL of 50% dextrose solution.[94]

DIABETES AS A RISK FACTOR FOR COGNITIVE IMPAIRMENT AND DEMENTIA

Because type 2 diabetes doubles the risk of stroke, and stroke alone causes cognitive impairment by strategic cognition-relevant brain lesions in approximately 20% of patients, one might expect a statistical and clinical association between diabetes and cognitive impairment. However, the brains of patients with diabetes, in addition to having the obvious cerebrovascular pathology, may also be affected by the neurodegenerative Alzheimer pathology, leading to dementia. Although the influence of diabetes on cognitive function has been suggested since the 1930s and a large number of studies have been conducted in this area since then, no consensus has emerged regarding the role of diabetes in the development of dementia or whether optimal blood glucose control yields a protective effect. In general, the association between type 2 diabetes and dementia seems to be stronger for VD than for AD.

Epidemiology on the link between diabetes and different types of dementia type 2 diabetes disproportionally affects older adults in whom dementia is also a common condition. Large population-based studies examining people at an older age (>70 years) demonstrate that patients with type 2 diabetes are overrepresented among individuals with dementia. Dementia is one of the most devastating diseases of late life; approximately 5 million new cases of dementia are estimated to occur worldwide every year. In the general population, mild cognitive impairment and dementia are most prevalent in people older than 60 years of age: mild cognitive impairment affects about 6%, and dementia affects about 5%, and the prevalence rises substantially with increasing age. An increase of prevalence of about 200% to 300% by 2050 in developed countries is expected, but a much larger increase (~500%) is expected in the more heavily populated, newly urbanized, and developing regions of the world. Up to 20% of persons older than 60 years with T2DM develop dementia. The incidence rate of dementia in people with T2DM ranges from 83 per 10,000 person-years in those aged between 60 and 64 years to as high as 1000 per 10,000 person-years in those older than 85 years of age. DM is a prevalent comorbidity in people with dementia, with a prevalence of up to 40%, depending on the type of cohort studied.[95,96] Alzheimer dementia (AD) is the most common form of dementia, accounting for approximately 80% of all cases, followed by VD. In most patients with dementia, multiple causes are most likely to be involved, with marked interindividual variations. In people with dementia, a mixture of pathologies often exists, including AD with its accumulation of brain amyloid and tau proteins with consequent neuronal loss on the one hand and vascular brain injury on the other hand. Notably, many molecular and pathological consequences of diabetes overlap with those that might lead to dementia. So-called mixed dementia describes a combination of clinical and radiologic features of AD and VD. The proportion of these major types of dementia depends on criteria used for the differentiation, which vary widely. Diabetes has been linked not only to the full picture of dementia but also to more subtle forms of cognitive impairment below the threshold of dementia, defined by neuropsychological testing. People with mild cognitive impairment are at increased risk of developing dementia, although the

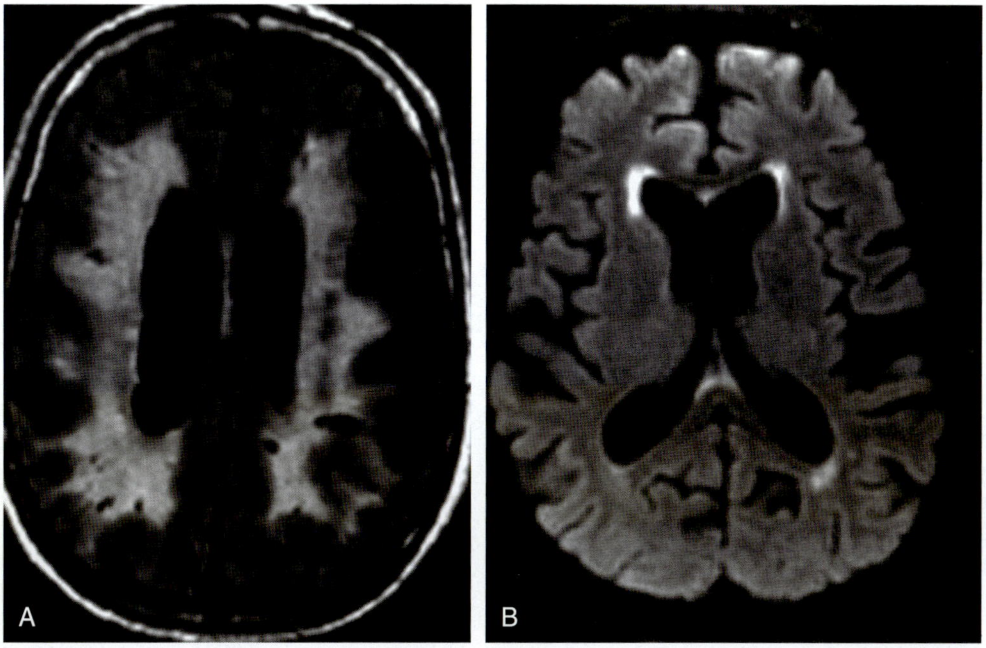

FIG. 23.6 Magnetic resonance imaging scans of patients with diabetes-related types of dementia. (A) A patient with vascular dementia with extensive white matter lesion and lacunar infarctions *(black holes)*. (B) A patient with only small white matter lesions but pronounced brain atrophy.

conversion rates reported range from 1% to 25% or more per year.[95] The determination of cognitive deficits and the diagnosis of the type of dementia are also not always easy. Thus the boundaries among cognitive deficit, early dementia, and more severe stages of dementia are sometimes difficult to discern.

DM is associated with cognitive dysfunction and has been related to accelerated cognitive decline in older adults, development of mild cognitive impairment, and increased risk of dementia, including both AD and VD (Fig. 23.6). The association between DM and risk of mild cognitive impairment and dementia is robust, and diabetes also seems to increase the risk of progression from such impairment to dementia. However, bidirectional relationships also exist between diabetes and dementia: decreased cognitive function leads to a less favorable and thus diabetogenic lifestyle and to poorer diabetes self-care.

Mild cognitive decline in patients with diabetes without dementia showed worse cognitive performance in patients across age groups between 50 and 80 years with type 2 diabetes compared with age-, sex-, and education-matched controls. The affected cognitive functions were verbal memory, information processing speed, perception, visuoconstruction, language attention, and executive performance. Cross-sectional population-based cohort studies and case-control studies indicate a 1.5-fold increased risk for development of mild cognitive impairment in patients with type 2 diabetes.[97–99] Meta-analyses of the association between type 2 diabetes and dementia report a significantly elevated risk ratio between 1.15 and 1.9.[100,101] This wide range results from the different durations of diabetic disease in the different studies. The duration of type 2 diabetes is crucial for the risk of dementia development; thus the following HRs of dementia associated with diabetes versus control subjects were found during the 32-year Whitehall II prospective cohort study: at 0 to 5 years of diabetes duration, HR 1.11; at 6 to 10 years, HR 1.49; and at > 10 years, HR 2.12.[102]

Higher glucose levels have a negative effect on cognition, regardless of whether or not diabetes is present. In the Adult Changes in Though study,[103] during a median follow-up of 6.8 years, even in participants without diabetes, higher average glucose levels within the preceding 5 years were related to an increased risk of dementia (115 mg/dL/6.4 mmol/L) as compared with 100 mg/dL (5.5 mmol/L) with a significant adjusted HR for dementia of 1.18. Among participants with diabetes, higher average glucose levels (190 mg/dL/10.5 mmol/L) were also related to an increased risk of dementia as compared to lower levels (160 mg/dL/8.9 mmol/L) with an HR of 1.40.[103] Overall, type 2 diabetes is associated with a 2-fold to 4-fold increased risk of VD and a 1.5- to 2-fold increased risk of AD. However, in studies, differentiation between the dementia subtypes of VD and AD is difficult, especially when it is based only on a clinical diagnosis. Moreover, many patients may be affected by both vascular and neurodegenerative pathology. On the basis of these numbers, 6% to 8% of all cases of late-life dementia would be attributable to type 2 diabetes.

As with the relationship between prediabetic metabolic abnormalities and stroke, cognitive decrements have also been found in prediabetic stages and its vascular risk escorts such as hyperinsulinemia, impaired glucose tolerance, and MetS. They are all associated with an approximately 1.5- to 2-fold increased risk of development of cognitive impairment or dementia.[104]

Similarly, as with the relationship between diabetes and stroke, additional vascular risk factors and predispositions that are associated with type 2 diabetes (e.g., hypertension, dyslipoproteinemia, depression, stroke, genetics, demographic and lifestyle characteristics) may modulate or mediate cognitive functioning. One longitudinal study, for example, found that cognitive functioning in patients with type 2 diabetes was related to long-term exposure to hypertension, even in prediabetic stages.[105]

Genetic predisposition might contribute to the association among type 2 diabetes, cognitive decrements, and dementia. The most widely examined risk factor is the apolipoprotein E (apo E) ε4 allele, an important risk factor for CVD and late-onset AD in the general population. Some studies have shown interaction effects between type 2 diabetes and the apo E ε4 allele, further aggravating the diabetes-associated risk of cognitive decline and dementia,[106] whereas others could not confirm such an interaction.[107] Another genetic relationship between type 2 diabetes and AD may be mediated by the insulin-degrading enzyme, which in the brain degrades both insulin and amyloid beta, the main component of amyloid plaques and pathologic hallmark of AD. Variations in the insulin-degrading enzyme gene were associated with an increased risk of type 2 diabetes and AD.[108] It is interesting to note that these associations were only observed in individuals who do not carry the apo E ε4 allele.

Brain Imaging and Autopsy Studies

Brain imaging studies have been used to analyze vascular lesions including infarcts, white matter hyperintensities (WMHs) and microbleeds, and cerebral atrophy as possible structural correlates of impaired cognition in type 2 diabetes. According to the increased risk of stroke in DM, it is not surprising that population-based studies found a 1.5- to 2-fold higher prevalence and incidence of associated lacunar infarcts. There is also an increased occurrence of lacunes and a modest increase in the volume of WMHs and microbleeds in patients with T2DM.[109]

However, WML, for example, can develop not only as a result of an underlying vascular brain pathology but also as a consequence of nonvascular processes such as inflammation. Modest degrees of global and focal cerebral atrophy in patients with diabetes have been reported from cross-sectional studies. Findings of atrophy in specific brain regions such as the frontal or medial temporal lobe, including the hippocampus and amygdala—a typical pattern in AD—suggest a possible association between type 2 diabetes and neurodegenerative brain changes and dementia.[110]

The extent of brain atrophy in DM is approximately equivalent to 3 to 5 years of advanced brain aging in individuals without diabetes. Another emerging marker of brain injury in T2DM is the imaging technique of diffusion tensor imaging (DTI), which allows to explore microstructural integrity of the white matter and related changes in brain networks. DTI studies show widespread changes in white matter microstructure and connectivity in relation to T2DM, which are clearly related to cognitive dysfunction.[110] In line with the findings from imaging studies, autopsy studies in patients with diabetes have revealed an approximately 2.5-fold increased risk for cortical and subcortical cerebral infarctions. Diabetes was also associated with changes in the cerebral microvasculature, including amyloid angiopathy and capillary basement thickening.

In contrast, large autopsy studies could not demonstrate a significantly higher prevalence of the Alzheimer core pathology of neuritic amyloid plaques and tau tangles.[111] Studies on in vivo biomarkers of AD pathology using cerebrospinal fluid analyses or brain Amyloid-PET (positron emission tomography) are completely in line with these observations. Yet, despite these findings, DM is associated with a higher expression of MRI and PET biomarkers of neurodegeneration per se, suggesting that DM accelerates neurodegeneration via nonclassical AD mechanisms.

Vascular and Degenerative Mechanisms in Diabetes-Related Dementia

Mechanisms through which type 2 diabetes may adversely affect cognitive function include vascular disturbances, glucose toxicity, hypoglycemic episodes, and disturbances of cerebral insulin signaling and amyloid metabolism. As one potential noncerebrovascular mechanism in the relationship between diabetes and dementia, peripheral hyperinsulinemia with impaired cerebral insulin signaling leading to a type of "cerebral IR" affecting amyloid-beta clearance in the brain has been suggested.[112,113]

A summary of the discussed relationships between diabetes and dementia is shown in Fig. 23.7.

Prevention and Treatment of Diabetes-Related Dementia

In addition to the widely used symptomatic medications against AD, such as cholinesterase inhibitors and *N*-methyl-D-aspartate (NMDA) receptor antagonists, monoclonal antibodies selective for amyloid β aggregates (aducanumab, donanemab, and lecanemab) showed moderate, significant positive effects in prospective controlled trials and became the first causally acting drugs targeting the pathophysiology of AD approved by the US Food and Drug Administration (FDA) between 2021 and 2024 (aducanumab is no longer on sale). [114,115]

There is no evidence that approved symptomatic or causally acting medical treatments used in the treatment of AD, such as cholinesterase inhibitors, NMDA receptor antagonists, or monoclonal antibodies, have different effects on patients with diabetes versus without diabetes. However, the beneficial effects of these antidementive medications are limited.

The low potential of diabetes management on the overall risk of developing dementia was shown in a publication of the Lancet Commission on dementia prevention, intervention, and care.[116] Here, 12 potentially modifiable risk factors for dementia were identified with a potential cumulative 40% risk reduction. The 12 factors were hypertension, diabetes, excessive alcohol consumption, head injury, air pollution, less education, hearing impairment, smoking, obesity, depression, physical inactivity, and infrequent social contact. Only 1% of the potential 40% risk reduction was attributed to diabetes control.

Although good glycemic control reduces the risk of diabetes-associated complications in general, it remains unclear whether it has beneficial effects on cognitive function. The results of the ACCORD MIND substudy reported similar cognitive performance with intensive versus treatment strategies, with greater mortality rate in the

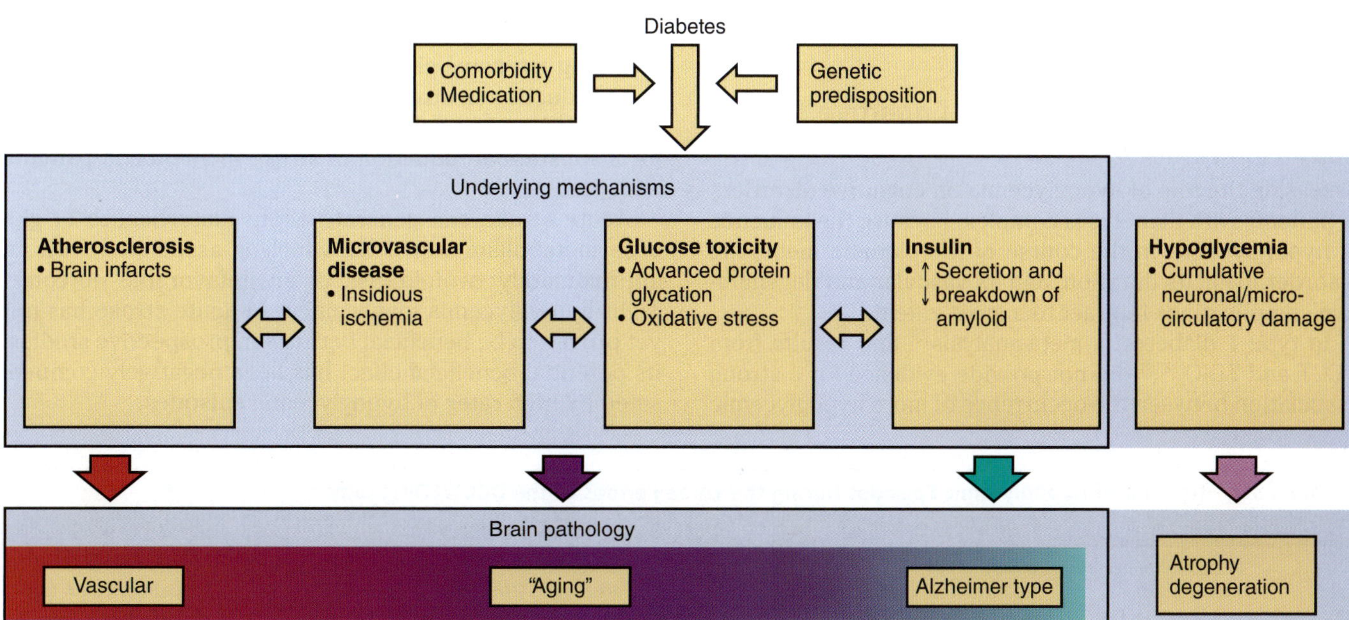

FIG. 23.7 Proposed pathophysiologic interaction between diabetes and advanced brain aging or dementia including vascular mechanisms, glucose-mediated neuronal toxicity, interference with Alzheimer-typical cerebral amyloid deposition, and cerebral damage by episodes of hypoglycemia. (Modified from Biessels GJ, Staekenborg S, Brunner E, et al. Risk of dementia in diabetes mellitus: a systematic review. *Lancet Neurol.* 2006;5:64–74.)

intensively treated group, possibly because of an increased risk of severe hypoglycemia.[117] Also in the 47 months of observational extension study (ACCORDION MIND), no differences between the two groups could be observed.[118] These negative results have been supported by other randomized trials. To date, there is no evidence that different diabetes medications have a specific beneficial effect on cognitive function in DM. The results from five pooled population-based cohort studies showed no association between the use of metformin, sulfonylurea, or insulin in people with type 2 DM and cognitive function, dementia prevalence, or brain imaging.[119] Similarly, there is no evidence of specific antidementia efficacy for newer antidiabetic drugs, such as GLP-1RAs, DPP4-inhibitors, or SGLT-2 inhibitors. In the randomized prospective TOMMORROW trial, pioglitazone did not delay the onset of mild cognitive impairment in nondiabetic persons.[120] There is only one prospective randomized study showing a positive effect of an antidiabetic drug on neurodegeneration: in patients with Parkinson disease, the GLP-1RA exenatide delayed progression of motor symptoms over 1 year.[121]

Hopes for a beneficial antidementive effect of intranasal insulin, supported by results of smaller studies, were disappointed by a negative randomized placebo-controlled study in this regard.[122]

Ultimately, similar to stroke prevention, dementia prevention in diabetic persons depends not only on diabetes management but mainly on multifactorial management of all dementia risk factors, as it was presented by the Lancet Commission.[116] Two studies confirm this approach and may serve as examples: The Finnish Finger Study with 1260 participants (13% with DM)[123] showed that multifactorial lifestyle interventions for only 2 years were associated with a lower dementia rate in the studied elderly high-risk population. In an observational study of 301 individuals during a mean follow-up of 2.3 years, multiple vascular risk factor intervention (hypertension, dyslipidemia, hyperglycemia, tobacco smoking) was found to slow cognitive decline in patients with preexisting AD.[124]

The Role of Hypoglycemia on Cognitive Impairment and Dementia

Assessing the role of hypoglycemia on cognitive disorders in patients with diabetes is complex, because the influence of hyperglycemia in the course of the diabetic metabolic disorder itself, its duration, and its vascular and degenerative complications interact to a great extent.

In type 1 diabetes, a meta-analysis[125] and results from DCCT and EDIC[126,127] did not provide evidence for a strong association between the occurrence of more hypoglycemic episodes in the intensive treatment group (Table 23.7) and impaired cognition in young adult patients.

In type 2 diabetes, two longitudinal studies show, exemplarily, that the positive association between hypoglycemic episodes and cognitive deficits probably is bidirectional in nature. Data from the large diabetes registry of the Kaiser-Permanente Northern California Diabetes Registry showed a dose-response relationship between the number of severe hypoglycemic episodes and the risk of development of dementia up to 17 years after the events.[128]

In contrast, the Fremantle diabetes study[129] found no evidence that severe hypoglycemia contributes to cognitive decline in older patients with type 2 diabetes but suggested a reverse direction of causality: People with dementia were at increased risk of further severe hypoglycemic episodes over the subsequent 5 years of follow-up. Thus a bidirectional relationship between diabetes-associated hypoglycemia episodes and cognitive disturbances is likely. Differential vulnerability of the brain to hypoglycemia in young and older patient populations may be another reason for the observed discrepancy between type 1 and type 2 diabetes.

SUMMARY

Patients with diabetes have a twofold to fourfold risk of ischemic stroke compared with patients without diabetes. This increased risk encompasses all four subtypes: ischemic, lacunar, large artery occlusive, and thromboembolic strokes. Comorbid vascular risk factors in patients with diabetes not only add to the stroke risk from diabetes but multiplicatively affect this risk. The risk for cerebrovascular disease is already increased in prediabetic states.

Interventional studies that focused exclusively on glucose control in patients with diabetes could not demonstrate a significant reduction in stroke rates. However, approaches using multifactorial risk factor management—including intensive glucose control—have shown a significant reduction in stroke rates. These findings underscore that multifactorial risk factor management may be the key for a substantial reduction of stroke incidence in patients with diabetes.

Acute stroke can generate acute disturbances of glucose metabolism with PSH, which is associated with an approximately twofold risk of an unfavorable outcome. Tight hyperglycemia management in acute stroke has not yet proven to be beneficial because in prospective studies, its potential beneficial effect has been negatively compensated by high rates of hypoglycemic episodes.

TABLE 23.7 Number of Hypoglycemic Episodes During the Three Periods of the DCCT/EDIC Study

EPISODES	DCCT (6.5 YEARS)		EDIC FOLLOW-UP (12 YEARS)		18 YEARS FOLLOW-UP	
	Intensive treatment ($N = 588$)	Conventional treatment ($N = 556$)	Intensive treatment ($N = 588$)	Conventional treatment ($N = 556$)	Intensive treatment ($N = 588$)	Conventional treatment ($N = 556$)
0	364	445	465	424	326	365
1–5	190	104	119	127	212	175
> 5	34	7	4	4	50	16

In addition to increasing the risk of stroke, diabetes similarly leads to chronic and insidious damage of the brain, resulting in cognitive decline and dementia. Dementia in patients with diabetes results not only from cerebrovascular-mediated neuronal damage but also from neurodegenerative processes manifesting as AD.

There are hints regarding a bidirectional relationship between diabetes and dementia. On the one hand, people with diabetes have double the risk of developing dementia; on the other hand, cognitive and behavioral manifestations of dementia lead to disturbances in glucose control and metabolism.

REFERENCES

1. Zhang Y, Chapman AM, Plested M, et al. The incidence, prevalence, and mortality of stroke in France, Germany, Italy, Spain, the UK, and the US: a literature review. *Stroke Res Treat.* 2012:ID 436125, doi:10.1155/2012/436125. Epub
2. Rothwell PM, Coull AJ, Silver LE, et al. Population-based study of event-rate, incidence, case fatality, and mortality for all acute vascular events in all arterial territories (Oxford Vascular Study). *Lancet.* 2005;366:1773–1783.
3. Gentil A, Bejot Y, Lorgis L, et al. Comparative epidemiology of stroke and acute myocardial infarction: the Dijon Vascular project (Diva). *J Neurol Neurosurg Psychiatry.* 2009;80:1006–1011.
4. GBD 2019 Stroke Collaborators. Global, regional, and national burden of stroke and its risk factors, 1990-2019: a systematic analysis for the Global Burden of Disease Study 2019. *Lancet Neurol.* 2021;20:795–820.
5. Luitse MJ, Biessels GJ, Rutten GE, et al. Diabetes, hyperglycaemia, and acute ischaemic stroke. *Lancet Neurol.* 2012;11:261–271.
6. Kannel WB, McGee DL. Diabetes and cardiovascular disease. The Framingham study. *JAMA.* 1979;241:2035–2038.
7. Hu G, Jousilahti P, Sarti C, et al. The effect of diabetes and stroke at baseline and during follow-up on stroke mortality. *Diabetologia.* 2006;49:2309–2316.
8. Banerjee C, Moon YP, Paik MC, et al. Duration of diabetes and risk of ischemic stroke: the Northern Manhattan Study. *Stroke.* 2012;43:1212–1217.
9. O'Donnell MJ, Xavier D, Liu L, et al. Risk factors for ischaemic and intracerebral haemorrhagic stroke in 22 countries (the INTERSTROKE study): a case-control study. *Lancet.* 2010;376:112–123.
10. Yusuf S, Hawken S, Ounpuu S, et al. Effect of potentially modifiable risk factors associated with myocardial infarction in 52 countries (the INTERHEART study): case-control study. *Lancet.* 2004;364:937–952.
11. O'Donnell MJ, Chin SL, Rangarajan S, et al. Global and regional effects of potentially modifiable risk factors associated with acute stroke in 32 countries (INTERSTROKE): a case-control study. *Lancet.* 2016;388:761–775.
12. Kothari V, Stevens RJ, Adler AI, et al. UKPDS 60: risk of stroke in type 2 diabetes estimated by the UK Prospective Diabetes Study risk engine. *Stroke.* 2002;33:1776–1781.
13. Callahan A, Amarenco P, Goldstein LB, et al. Risk of stroke and cardiovascular events after ischemic stroke or transient ischemic attack in patients with type 2 diabetes or metabolic syndrome: secondary analysis of the Stroke Prevention by Aggressive Reduction in Cholesterol Levels (SPARCL) trial. *Arch Neurol.* 2011;68:1245–1251.
14. Rohr J, Kittner S, Feeser B, et al. Traditional risk factors and ischemic stroke in young adults: the Baltimore-Washington Cooperative Young Stroke Study. *Arch Neurol.* 1996;53:603–607.
15. Hu G, Sart C, Jousilahti P, et al. The impact of history of hypertension and type 2 diabetes at baseline on the incidence of stroke and stroke mortality. *Stroke.* 2005;21:18–25.
16. Cai X, Zhang Y, Li M, et al. Association between prediabetes and risk of all cause mortality and cardiovascular disease: updated meta-analysis. *BMJ.* 2020;370:m2297. https://doi.org/10.1136/bmj.m2297.
17. Doi Y, Ninomiya T, Hata J, et al. Impact of glucose tolerance status on development of ischemic stroke and coronary heart disease in a general Japanese population: the Hisayama study. *Stroke.* 2010;41:203–209.
18. Selvin E, Steffes MW, Zhu H, et al. Glycated hemoglobin, diabetes, and cardiovascular risk in nondiabetic adults. *N Engl J Med.* 2010;362:800–811.
19. Thacker EL, Psaty BM, McKnight B, et al. Fasting and post-glucose load measures of insulin resistance and risk of ischemic stroke in older adults. *Stroke.* 2011;42:3347–3351.
20. Rudenski AS, Matthews DR, Levy JC, et al. Understanding insulin resistance: both glucose resistance and insulin resistance are required to model human diabetes. *Metabolism.* 1991;40:908–917.
21. Bravata DM, Wells CK, Kernan WN, et al. Association between impaired insulin sensitivity and stroke. *Neuroepidemiology.* 2005;25:69–74.
22. Wang J, Ruotsalainen S, Moilanen L, et al. The metabolic syndrome predicts incident stroke: a 14-year follow-up study in elderly people in Finland. *Stroke.* 2008;39:1078–1083.
23. Boden-Albala B, Sacco RL, Lee HS, et al. Metabolic syndrome and ischemic stroke risk: Northern Manhattan Study. *Stroke.* 2008;39:30–35.
24. Protopsaltis I, et al. Metabolic syndrome and its components as predictors of ischemic stroke in type 2 patients with diabetes. *Stroke.* 2008;39:1036–1038.
25. Hankey GJ. Nutrition and the risk of stroke. *Lancet Neurol.* 2012;11:66–81.
26. Guo Y, Yue XJ, Li HH, et al. Overweight and obesity in young adulthood and the risk of stroke: a meta-analysis. *J Stroke Cerebrovasc Dis.* 2016;25:2995–3004.
27. Horn JW, Feng T, Mørkedal B, et al. Obesity and risk for first ischemic stroke depends on metabolic syndrome: the HUNT study. *Stroke.* 2021;52:3555–3561.
28. Migdady I, Russman A, Buletko AB. Atrial fibrillation and ischemic stroke: a clinical review. *Semin Neurol.* 2021;41:348–364.
29. Wang A, Green JB, Halperin JL, et al. Atrial fibrillation and diabetes mellitus: JACC review topic of the week. *J Am Coll Cardiol.* 2019;74:1107–1115.
30. Cui R, Iso H, Yamagishi K, et al. Diabetes mellitus and risk of stroke and its subtypes among Japanese: the Japan public health center study. *Stroke.* 2011;42:2611–2614.
31. Nathan DM, Cleary PA, Backlund JY, et al. Diabetes control and complications trial/epidemiology of diabetes interventions and complications (DCCT/EDIC) Study Research Group: intensive diabetes treatment and cardiovascular disease in patients with type 1 diabetes. *N Engl J Med.* 2005;353:2643–2653.
32. UKPDS-Study Group. Intensive blood-glucose control with sulphonylureas or insulin compared with conventional treatment and risk of complications in patients with type 2 diabetes (UKPDS 33). UK Prospective Diabetes Study (UKPDS) Group. *Lancet.* 1998;352:837–853.
33. UK Prospective Diabetes Study (UKPDS) Group. Effect of intensive blood-glucose control with metformin on complications in overweight patients with type 2 diabetes (UKPDS 34). *Lancet.* 1998;352:854–865.
34. Action to Control Cardiovascular Risk in Diabetes Study Group. Effects of intensive glucose lowering in type 2 diabetes. *N Engl J Med.* 2008;358:2545–2559.
35. ADVANCE Collaborative Group. Intensive blood glucose control and vascular outcomes in patients with type 2 diabetes. *N Engl J Med.* 2008;358:2560–2572.
36. Duckworth W, Abraira C, Moritz T, et al. VADT Investigators: glucose control and vascular complications in veterans with type 2 diabetes. *N Engl J Med.* 2009;360:129–139.
37. Boussageon R, Bejan-Angoulvant T, Saadatian-Elahi M, et al. Effect of intensive glucose lowering treatment on all cause mortality, cardiovascular death, and microvascular events in type 2 diabetes: meta-analysis of randomised controlled trials. *BMJ.* 2011;343:d4169.
38. Hemmingsen B, Lund SS, Gluud C, et al. Targeting intensive glycaemic control versus targeting conventional glycaemic control for type 2 diabetes mellitus. *Cochrane Database Syst Rev* Nov 11, (11): doi: 10.1002/14651858
39. UKPDS. Tight blood pressure control and risk of macrovascular and microvascular complications in type 2 diabetes: UKPDS 38. *UK Prospective Diabetes Study Group, BMJ.* 1998;317:703–713.
40. Bangalore S, Kumar S, Lobach I, et al. Blood pressure targets in subjects with type 2 diabetes mellitus/impaired fasting glucose: observations from traditional and Bayesian random-effects meta-analyses of randomized trials. *Circulation.* 2011;123:2799–2810.
41. ACCORD Study Group. Effects of intensive blood-pressure control in type 2 diabetes mellitus. *N Engl J Med.* 2010;362:1575–1585.
42. Emdin CA, Rahimi K, Neal B, et al. Blood pressure lowering in type 2 diabetes: a systematic review and meta-analysis. *JAMA.* 2015;313:603–615.
43. Rothwell PM, Howard SC, Dolan E, et al. Effects of beta blockers and calcium-channel blockers on within-individual variability in blood pressure and risk of stroke. *Lancet Neurol.* 2010;9:469–480.
44. Heshmatollah A, Ma Y, Fani L, et al. Visit-to-visit blood pressure variability and the risk of stroke in the Netherlands: a population-based cohort study. *PLoS Med.* 2022;19:e1003942. https://doi.org/10.1371/journal.pmed.1003942.
45. Kearney PM, Blackwell L, Collins R, et al. Cholesterol Treatment Trialists' (CTT) collaborators: efficacy of cholesterol-lowering therapy in 18,686 people with diabetes in 14 randomised trials of statins: a meta-analysis. *Lancet.* 2008;371:117–125.
46. Amarenco P, Bogousslavsky J, Callahan 3rd A, et al. Stroke Prevention by Aggressive Reduction in Cholesterol Levels (SPARCL) investigators: high-dose atorvastatin after stroke or transient ischemic attack. *N Engl J Med.* 2006;355:549–559.
47. Webb D, Dales J, Zaccardi F, et al. Intensive versus standard multifactorial cardiovascular risk factor control in screen-detected type 2 diabetes: 5-year and longer-term modelled outcomes of the ADDITION-Leicester study. *Diabetes Metab Res Rev.* 2019;35:e3111. https://doi.org/10.1002/dmrr.3111.
48. Amarenco P, Kim JS, Labreuche J, et al. A comparison of two LDL cholesterol targets after ischemic stroke. *N Engl J Med.* 2020;382:9–19.
49. Giugliano RP, Pedersen TR, Saver JL, et al. Stroke prevention with the PCSK9 (Proprotein Convertase Subtilisin-Kexin Type 9) inhibitor evolocumab added to statin in high-risk patients with stable atherosclerosis. *Stroke.* 2020;51:1546–1554.
50. ASCEND Study Collaborative Group, et al.Bowman L, Mafham M, Wallendszus K, et al. Effects of aspirin for primary prevention in persons with diabetes mellitus. *N Engl J Med.* 2018;379:1529–1539.
51. Antithrombotic Trialists Collaboration, et al.Baigent C, Blackwell L, Collins R, et al. Aspirin in the primary and secondary prevention of vascular

disease: collaborative meta-analysis of individual participant data from randomised trials. *Lancet*. 2009;373:1849–1860.
52. Gæde P, Lund-Andersen H, Parving H-H, et al. Effect of a multifactorial intervention on mortality in type 2 diabetes. *N Engl J Med*. 2008;358:580–591.
53. Gæde P, Oellgaard J, Kruuse C, et al. Beneficial impact of intensified multifactorial intervention on risk of stroke: outcome of 21 years of follow-up in the randomised Steno-2 Study. *Diabetologia*. 2019;62:1575–1580.
54. Sattar N, Lee MMY, Kristensen SL, et al. Cardiovascular, mortality, and kidney outcomes with GLP-1 receptor agonists in patients with type 2 diabetes: a systematic review and meta-analysis of randomised trials. *Lancet Diabetes Endocrinol*. 2021;9:653–662.
55. Alberts MJ, Eikelboom JW, Hankey GJ. Antithrombotic therapy for stroke prevention in non-valvular atrial fibrillation. *Lancet Neurol*. 2012;11:1066–1081.
56. Mant J, Hobbs FDR, Fletcher K, et al. Warfarin versus aspirin for stroke prevention in an elderly community population with atrial fibrillation (the Birmingham Atrial Fibrillation Treatment of the Aged Study, BAFTA): a randomised controlled trial. *Lancet*. 2007;370:493–503.
57. Ruff CT, Giugliano RP, Braunwald E, et al. Comparison of the efficacy and safety of new oral anticoagulants with warfarin in patients with atrial fibrillation: a meta-analysis of randomised trials. *Lancet*. 2014;383:955–962.
58. Abdool M, Kunutsor SK, Khunti K, et al. Does the presence of diabetes mellitus confer an increased risk of stroke in patients with atrial fibrillation on direct oral anticoagulants? A systematic review and meta-analysis. *Diabetes Metab Syndr*. 2020;14:1725–1733.
59. Eikelboom JW, Connolly SJ, Bosch J, et al. Rivaroxaban with or without aspirin in stable cardiovascular disease. *N Engl J Med*. 2017;377:1319–1330.
60. Sharma M, Hart RG, Connolly SJ, et al. Stroke outcomes in the COMPASS trial. *Circulation*. 2019;139:1134–1145.
61. Marquardt L, Geraghty OC, Mehta Z, et al. Low risk of ipsilateral stroke in patients with asymptomatic carotid stenosis on best medical treatment: a prospective, population-based study. *Stroke*. 2010;41:e11–e17.
62. Howard DPJ, Gaziano L, Rothwell PM. Oxford Vascular Study. Risk of stroke in relation to degree of asymptomatic carotid stenosis: a population-based cohort study, systematic review, and meta-analysis. *Lancet Neurol*. 2021;20:193–202.
63. Rerkasem A, Orrapin S, Howard DP, et al. Carotid endarterectomy for symptomatic carotid stenosis. *Cochrane Database Syst Rev 9*. 2020(9). https://doi.org/10.1002/14651858.CD001081.pub4.
64. Kleindorfer DO, Towfighi A, Chaturvedi S, et al. 2021 Guideline for the prevention of stroke in patients with stroke and transient ischemic attack: a guideline from the American Heart Association/American Stroke Association. *Stroke*. 2021;52:e364–e467.
65. Rothwell PM, Eliasziw M, Gutnikov SA, et al. Endarterectomy for symptomatic carotid stenosis in relation to clinical subgroups and timing of surgery. *Lancet*. 2004;363:915–924.
66. ECST Collaborative Group. Randomised trial of endarterectomy for recently symptomatic carotid stenosis: final results of the MRC European Carotid Surgery Trial (ECST). *Lancet*. 1998;351:1379–1387.
67. North American Symptomatic Carotid Endarterectomy Trial Collaborators. Beneficial effect of carotid endarterectomy in symptomatic patients with high-grade carotid stenosis. *N Engl J Med*. 1991;325:445–453.
68. Chu SS, Hu J, Tang LW, et al. The impact of diabetes mellitus on carotid artery stenting: a meta-analysis. *Neurosurg Rev*. 2021;44:3039–3046.
69. Chimowitz MI, Lynn MJ, Derdeyn CP, et al. Stenting versus aggressive medical therapy for intracranial arterial stenosis. *N Engl J Med*. 2011;365:993–1003.
70. Derdeyn CP, Chimowitz MI, Lynn MJ, et al. Stenting and Aggressive Medical Management for Preventing Recurrent Stroke in Intracranial Stenosis Trial Investigators. Aggressive medical treatment with or without stenting in high-risk patients with intracranial artery stenosis (SAMMPRIS): the final results of a randomised trial. *Lancet*. 2014;383:333–341.
71. Wright RJ, Frier BM. Vascular disease and diabetes: is hypoglycaemia an aggravating factor? *Diabetes Metab Res Rev*. 2008;24:353–363.
72. Ferrari F, Moretti A, Villa RF. Hyperglycemia in acute ischemic stroke: physiopathological and therapeutic complexity. *Neural Regen Res*. 2022;17:292–299.
73. Allport L, Baird T, Butcher K, et al. Frequency and temporal profile of post stroke hyperglycaemia using continuous glucose monitoring. *Diabetes Care*. 2006;29:1839–1844.
74. Scott JF, Robinson GM, French JM, et al. Prevalence of admission hyperglycaemia across clinical subtypes of acute stroke. *Lancet*. 1999;353:376–377.
75. Wong AA, Schluter PJ, Henderson RD, et al. Natural history of blood glucose within the first 48 hours after ischemic stroke. *Neurology*. 2008;70:1036–1041.
76. Yong M, Kaste M. Dynamic of hyperglycemia as a predictor of stroke outcome in the ECASS-II trial. *Stroke*. 2008;39:2749–2755.
77. Winder K, Seifert F, Ohnemus T, et al. Neuroanatomic correlates of post-stroke hyperglycemia. *Ann Neurol*. 2015;77:262–268.
78. Garg R, Chaudhuri A, Munschauer F, et al. Hyperglycaemia, insulin and acute ischaemic stroke. *Stroke*. 2006;37:267–273.
79. Gilmore RM, Stead LG. The role of hyperglycemia in acute ischemic stroke. *Neurocrit Care*. 2006;5:153–158.
80. Quinn TJ, Lees KR. Hyperglycaemia in acute stroke–to treat or not to treat. *Cerebrovasc Dis*. 2009;27(Suppl 1):148–155.
81. Stead LG, Gilmore RM, Bellolio MF, et al. Hyperglycemia as an independent predictor of worse outcome in non-diabetic patients presenting with acute ischemic stroke. *Neurocrit Care*. 2009;10:181–186.
82. Capes SE, Hunt D, Malmberg K, et al. Stress hyperglycemia and prognosis of stroke in nondiabetic and diabetic patients: a systematic overview. *Stroke*. 2001;32:2426–2432.
83. Fuentes B, Castillo J, San JosØ B, et al. The prognostic value of capillary glucose levels in acute stroke. The GLycemia in Acute Stroke (GLIAS) study. *Stroke*. 2009;40:562–568.
84. Uyttenboogaart M, Koch MW, Stewart RE, et al. Moderate hyperglycaemia is associated with favourable outcome in acute lacunar stroke. *Brain*. 2007;130:1626–1630.
85. Thomalla G, Simonsen CZ, Boutitie F, et al. WAKE-UP Investigators. MRI-guided thrombolysis for stroke with unknown time of onset. *N Engl J Med*. 2018;379:611–622.
86. Ribo M, Molina C, Montaner J, et al. Acute hyperglycaemia state is associated with lower tPA-induced recanalization rates in stroke patients. *Stroke*. 2005;36:1705–1709.
87. Ahmed N, Davalos A, Eriksson N, et al. for the SITS Investigators Association of admission blood glucose and outcome in patients treated with intravenous thrombolysis: results from the Safe Implementation of Treatments in Stroke International Stroke Thrombolysis Register (SITS-ISTR). *Arch Neurol*. 2010;67:1123–1130.
88. Roaldsen MB, Jusufovic M, Berge E, et al. Endovascular thrombectomy and intra-arterial interventions for acute ischaemic stroke. *Cochrane Database Syst Rev*. 2021;6 https://doi.org/10.1002/14651858.CD007574.pub3.
89. Perez-Vega C, Domingo RA, Tripathi S, et al. Influence of glucose levels on clinical outcome after mechanical thrombectomy for large-vessel occlusion: a systematic review and meta-analysis. *J Neurointerv Surg*. 2022;14 https://doi.org/10.1136/neurintsurg-2021-017771. Epub 2021 Aug 6. PMID: 34362794.
90. Prasad K, Siemieniuk R, Hao Q, et al. Dual antiplatelet therapy with aspirin and clopidogrel for acute high risk transient ischaemic attack and minor ischaemic stroke: a clinical practice guideline. *BMJ*. 2018;363:k5130.
91. Gray CS, Hildreth AJ, Sandercock PA, et al. Glucose-potassium-insulin infusions in the management of post-stroke hyperglycaemia: the UK Glucose Insulin in Stroke Trial (GIST-UK). *Lancet Neurol*. 2007;6:397–406.
92. Bellolio MF, Gilmore RM, Ganti L. Insulin for glycaemic control in acute ischaemic stroke. *Cochrane Database Syst Rev*. 2014:CD005346.
93. Ntaios G, Papavasileiou V, Bargiota A, et al. Intravenous insulin treatment in acute stroke: a systematic review and meta-analysis of randomized controlled trials. *Int J Stroke*. 2014;9:489–493.
94. Powers WJ, Rabinstein AA, Ackerson T, et al. Guidelines for the early management of patients with acute ischemic stroke: 2019 update to the 2018 guidelines for the early management of acute ischemic stroke: a guideline for healthcare professionals from the American Heart Association/American Stroke Association. *Stroke*. 2019;50:e344–e418.
95. Velayudhan LV, Poppe M, Archer N, et al. Risk of developing dementia in people with diabetes and mild cognitive impairment. *Br J Psychiatry*. 2010;196:36–40.
96. Srikanth V, Sinclair AJ, Hill-Briggs F, et al. Type 2 diabetes and cognitive dysfunction-towards effective management of both comorbidities. *Lancet Diabetes Endocrinol*. 2020;8:535–545.
97. Reijmer YD, van den Berg E, Ruis C, et al. Cognitive dysfunction in patients with type 2 diabetes. *Diabetes Metab Res Rev*. 2010;26:507–519.
98. Cerhan JR, Folsom AR, Mortimer JA, et al. Correlates of cognitive function in middle-aged adults. *Gerontology*. 1998;44:95–105.
99. Elias PK, Elias MF, D'Agostino RB, et al. NIDDM and blood pressure as risk factors for poor cognitive performance. The Framingham Study. *Diabetes Care*. 1997;20:1388–1395.
100. Xue M, Xu W, Ou YN, et al. Diabetes mellitus and risks of cognitive impairment and dementia: A systematic review and meta-analysis of 144 prospective studies. *Ageing Res Rev*. 2019;55:100944. https://doi.org/10.1016/j.arr.2019.100944.
101. Biessels GJ, Staekenborg S, Brunner E, et al. Risk of dementia in diabetes mellitus: a systematic review. *Lancet Neurol*. 2006;5:64–74.
102. Barbiellini Amidei C, Fayosse A, Dumurgier J, et al. Association between age at diabetes onset and subsequent risk of dementia. *JAMA*. 2021;325:1640–1649.
103. Crane PK, Walker R, Hubbard RA, et al. Glucose levels and risk of dementia. *N Engl J Med*. 2013;369:540–548.
104. Yaffe K, Blackwell T, Kanaya AM, et al. Diabetes, impaired fasting glucose, and development of cognitive impairment in older women. *Neurology*. 2004;63:658–663.
105. van den Berg E, Dekker JM, Nijpels G, et al. Blood pressure levels in pre-diabetic stages are associated with worse cognitive functioning in patients with type 2 diabetes. *Diabetes Metab Res Rev*. 2009;25:657–664.
106. Luchsinger JA, Reitz C, Patel B, et al. Relation of diabetes to mild cognitive impairment. *Arch Neurol*. 2007;64:570–575.
107. Kanaya AM, Barrett-Connor E, Gildengorin G, et al. Change in cognitive function by glucose tolerance status in older adults: a 4-year prospective study of the Rancho Bernardo study cohort. *Arch Intern Med*. 2004;164:1327–1333.
108. Edland SD. Insulin-degrading enzyme, apolipoprotein E, and Alzheimer's disease. *J Mol Neurosci*. 2004;23:213–217.
109. van Harten B, de Leeuw FE, Weinstein HC, et al. Brain imaging in patients with diabetes: a systematic review. *Diabetes Care*. 2006;29:2539–2548.
110. Biessels GJ, Despa F. Cognitive decline and dementia in diabetes mellitus: mechanisms and clinical implications. *Nat Rev Endocrinol*. 2018;14:591–604.

111. Dos Santos Matioli MNP, Suemoto CK, Rodriguez RD, et al. Diabetes is not associated with Alzheimer's disease neuropathology. *J Alzheimers Dis*. 2017; 60:1035–1043.
112. Messier C, Gagnon M. Cognitive decline associated with dementia and type 2 diabetes: the interplay of risk factors. *Diabetologia*. 2009;52:2471–2474.
113. Craft S. Insulin resistance and Alzheimer's disease pathogenesis: potential mechanisms and implications for treatment. *Curr Alzheimer Res*. 2007;4 147–152.
114. Sims JR, Zimmer JA, Evans CD, et al. TRAILBLAZER-ALZ 2 Investigators: Donanemab in early symptomatic Alzheimer disease: the TRAILBLAZER-ALZ 2 randomized clinical trial. *JAMA*. 2023;330:512–527.
115. van Dyck CH, Swanson CJ, Aisen P, et al. Lecanemab in early Alzheimer's disease. *N Engl J Med*. 2023;388:9–21.
116. Livingston G, Huntley J, Sommerlad A, et al. Dementia prevention, intervention, and care: 2020 report of the Lancet Commission. *Lancet 896*. 2020(10248):413–446.
117. Launer LJ, Miller ME, Williamson JD, et al. Effects of intensive glucose lowering on brain structure and function in people with type 2 diabetes (ACCORD MIND): a randomised open-label substudy. *Lancet Neurol*. 2011;10:969–977.
118. Murray AM, Hsu FC, Williamson JD, et al. ACCORDION MIND: results of the observational extension of the ACCORD MIND randomised trial. *Diabetologia*. 2017;60:69–80.
119. Weinstein G, Davis-Plourde KL, Conner S, et al. Association of metformin, sulfonylurea and insulin use with brain structure and function and risk of dementia and Alzheimer's disease: pooled analysis from 5 cohorts. *PLoS ONE*. 2019;14:e0212293.
120. Burns DK, Alexander RC, Welsh-Bohmer KA, et al. Safety and efficacy of pioglitazone for the delay of cognitive impairment in people at risk of Alzheimer's disease (TOMMORROW): a prognostic biomarker study and a phase 3, randomised, double-blind, placebo-controlled trial. *Lancet Neurol*. 2021;20: 537–547.
121. Athauda D, Maclagan K, Skene SS, et al. Exenatide once weekly versus placebo in Parkinson's disease: a randomised, double-blind, placebo-controlled trial. *Lancet*. 2017;390:1664–1675. 120.
122. Craft S, Raman R, Chow TW, et al. Safety, efficacy, and feasibility of intranasal insulin for the treatment of mild cognitive impairment and alzheimer disease dementia: a randomized clinical trial. *JAMA Neurol*. 2020;77:1099–1109.
123. Ngandu T, Lehtisalo J, Solomon A, et al. A 2 year multidomain intervention of diet, exercise, cognitive training, and vascular risk monitoring versus control to prevent cognitive decline in at-risk elderly people (FINGER): a randomised controlled trial. *Lancet*. 2015;385:2255–2263.
124. Deschaintre Y, Richard F, Leys D, et al. Treatment of vascular risk factors is associated with slower decline in Alzheimer disease. *Neurology*. 2009;73:674–680.
125. Brands AMA, Biessels GJ, De Haan EHF, et al. The effects of type 1 diabetes on cognitive performance: a meta-analysis. *Diabetes Care*. 2005;28: 726–735.
126. Austin EJ, Deary IJ. Effects of repeated hypoglycemia on cognitive function: a psychometrically validated reanalysis of the Diabetes Control and Complications Trial data. *Diabetes Care*. 1999;22:1273–1277.
127. The Diabetes Control and Complications Trial Research Group. Long-term effect of diabetes and its treatment on cognitive function. *N Engl J Med*. 2007;356:1842–1852.
128. Whitmer RA, Karter AJ, Yaffe K, et al. Hypoglycemic episodes and risk of dementia in older patients with type 2 diabetes mellitus. *JAMA*. 2009;301:1565–1572.
129. Bruce DG, Davis WA, Casey GP, et al. Severe hypoglycaemia and cognitive impairment in older patients with diabetes: the Fremantle Diabetes Study. *Diabetologia*. 2009;52:1808–1815.

24 Atrial Fibrillation in Persons With Type 2 Diabetes

LAURENT FAUCHIER AND PIERRE HENRI DUCLUZEAU

Disclosures. LF: consultant or speaker fees of small amounts for AstraZeneca, Bayer, BMS/Pfizer, Boehringer Ingelheim, Medtronic, Novartis, Novo, and Zoll outside of this work.

KEY POINTS

- Opportunistic screening for AF by assessing the pulse and heart rate or by ECG recording is appropriate in persons ≥65 years of age and this needs to be carefully applied in persons with diabetes in view of their risk.
- Systematic screening with ECG should be considered to detect AF in persons ≥75 years of age or those at a high risk of stroke, and this deserves specific consideration in persons with diabetes in view of their risk.
- Oral anticoagulation is indicated for stroke prevention in AF persons with DM and with at least one additional (CHA_2DS_2-VASc) risk factor for stroke.
- Oral anticoagulation should be considered for stroke prevention in persons with DM and AF and no other risk factors for stroke (according to CHA_2DS_2-VASc), particularly in the case of inadequate chronic glycemic control.
- For stroke prevention in persons with AF with DM, DOACs should be preferred over vitamin K antagonists, with the exception of persons with mechanical valve prostheses or mild-to-moderate mitral stenosis.
- The HAS-BLED score helps identify modifiable and nonmodifiable risk factors for bleeding in persons with DM and AF and identify persons in need of closer follow-up.

INTRODUCTION

Atrial fibrillation (AF) and type 2 diabetes mellitus (DM) have emerged as global epidemics worldwide with significant effects on morbidity and mortality. The risk for thromboembolism is higher when AF and DM coexist. In the last decade, there have been significant improvements for stroke prevention in persons with AF with direct oral anticoagulants (DOACs), earlier detection of AF in at-risk populations, and for treating DM with noninsulin antihyperglycemic medications.

DIABETES AS A RISK FACTOR FOR ATRIAL FIBRILLATION

Prevalence and Incidence of Atrial Fibrillation in Persons With Type 2 Diabetes Mellitus

AF is common in persons with DM. The prevalence of AF is around twofold higher in persons with DM compared with persons without DM. AF incidence may be even higher in persons with microvascular complications (kidney disease, retinopathy). In a meta-analysis by Huxley et al., including prospective studies and case-control studies comprising data from 1.7 million persons, 109,000 of them had incident AF, and DM was associated with about 40% higher risk of AF. However, after adjusting for possible confounding factors, the effect appeared to be more limited with a risk only 24% higher.[1] The proportion of AF attributable to DM in the population was estimated to be only 2.5%. Persons with both T2DM and high blood pressure may have a threefold higher risk of associated AF compared with persons without DM or hypertension, but this association was no longer significant after adjusting for presence of insulin resistance, which therefore appeared to be a major determinant for the development of AF.[2] Insulin resistance is also a mechanism by which hypertension and obesity might be associated with an increased risk of AF. DM and glucose intolerance are also associated with an increased risk of left ventricular hypertrophy (LVH), which could be one of the factors promoting AF.[3] Long-term inflammation is also a suspected link between DM and AF: inflammation may be found in the two conditions, it can partly predict the development of DM and of AF, and antiinflammatory treatments have shown to be efficient on a few indirect parameters for some persons with DM and/or with AF (Fig. 24.1).[3]

In a subsequent analysis carried out in 35,000 healthcare professionals and followed for 16 years, females with T2DM had a doubled risk of developing AF during follow-up, but the attributable risk of DM was quite lower (15%) after adjusting for possible confounding factors from the baseline characteristics.[4]

In a study about the risk for AF in T2DM, 421,855 persons with T2DM from the Swedish National Diabetes Register and 2,131,223 controls from the Swedish Population Registry were studied and followed for 13 years.[5] In the fully adjusted risk regression model, the risk of incident AF was 28% greater with T2DM versus controls (HR, 1.28; 95% CI, 1.26–1.30; $p < 0.0001$). The risk of AF in persons with T2DM increased with poor glycemic control and kidney complications.[5]

Although males usually have higher absolute rates for incident AF, the relative rates of incident AF associated with T2DM are higher in females than in males, and the excess risk in females is mainly seen in middle-aged persons.[6]

This suggests that persons with T2DM have a higher risk of prevalent AF (around 15%) and then of incident AF (around 0.8%/year), which seems in part related to some other associated risk factors commonly seen in these persons. Persons with type 1 are also at a higher risk of AF (HR 1.32 in females vs. males), suggesting that DM per se would also be an independent risk factor for AF.[6] By contrast, when assessing for AF after a stroke, since DM may be more closely associated with noncardioembolic ischemic stroke, the evaluation may not find as much AF.[7]

T2DM has been associated with atrial electrical and structural remodeling that may underlie increased vulnerability for AF.[3] In persons with T2DM, calcium handling may be altered and may further result in AF mediation. Furthermore, atrial fibroblasts from persons with T2DM have a more profibrotic phenotype compared with fibroblasts of persons without DM, evident from increased expression of collagen type 1, which adds to structural remodeling of the atrium.

Therapy for Diabetes Mellitus and Risk of Atrial Fibrillation

The risk of new-onset AF is sometimes associated with diabetes duration and glycemic control (Fig. 24.2)[8,9] and may be affected by specific antihyperglycemic therapies. The impact of antihyperglycemic therapy on the risk for AF has been discussed in recent years (Table 24.1).[3,9,10] While some glucose-lowering therapies decrease the incidence of heart failure (HF) and chronic kidney disease (CKD) in persons with DM, in many cardiovascular outcome studies, AF was not a prespecified outcome. It has been reported that metformin and pioglitazone may be associated with a lower risk for AF.[11] In the DECLARE TIMI-58 trial, dapagliflozin reduced the risk of AF events by 19% (HR, 0.81; 95% CI, 0.68–0.95; $p = 0.009$). The risk reduction for AF events was consistent regardless of a history of previous AF or cardiovascular disease at baseline.[12] In a meta-analysis of 34 randomized studies, SGLT2i were also associated with 19% lower risk of incident AF in persons with DM or HF.[13] Glucagon-like peptide-1 receptor agonists (GLP1-RAs) have been investigated in various populations with an increased cardiovascular risk, but only a few studies reported effects on new onset of AF, with no significant differences when using GLP1-RA.[3,9]

Screening for Atrial Fibrillation in Diabetes

Considering the high prevalence of AF in T2DM and the estimated incidence of nearly 1%/year, more efficient screening of persons with T2DM for AF might be associated with improved therapeutic management. For symptomatic

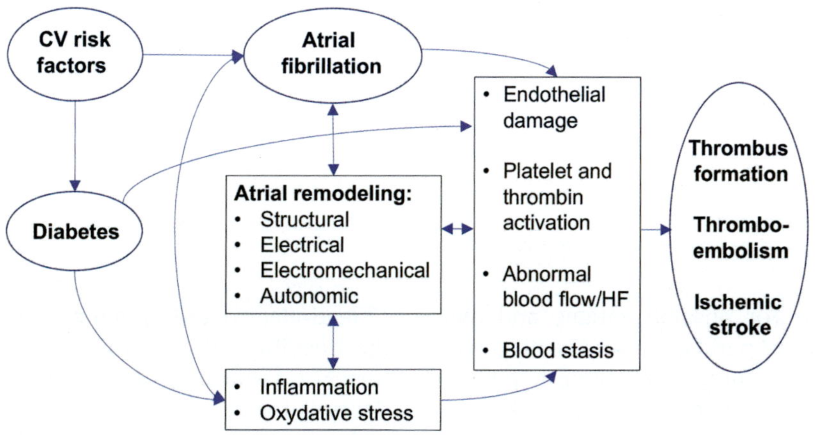

FIG. 24.1 Pathophysiology of possible links between diabetes, atrial fibrillation, heart failure, and thromboembolic events. *CV*, cardiovascular; *HF*, heart failure.

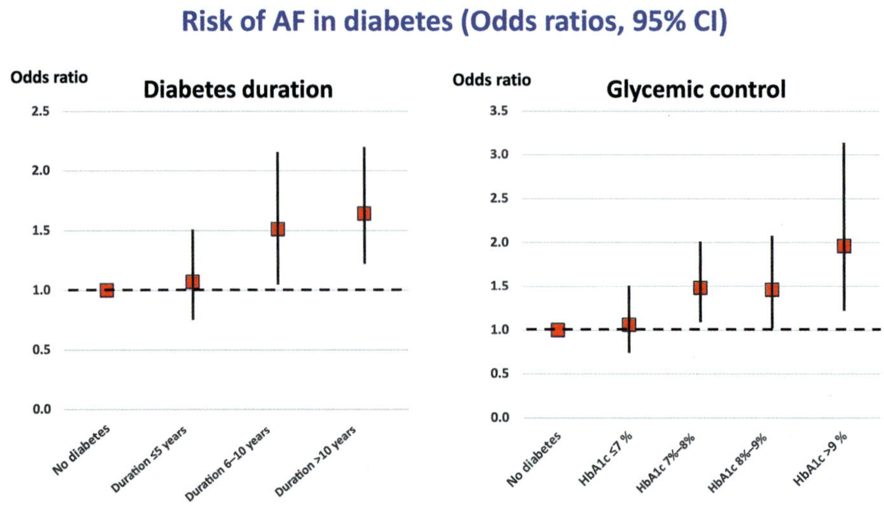

FIG. 24.2 Effect of duration of diabetes and glycemic control on risk of atrial fibrillation (*AF*). *CI*, Confidence interval. Adapted from Dublin S, Glazer NL, Smith NL, et al. Diabetes mellitus, glycemic control, and risk of atrial fibrillation. *J Gen Intern Med*. 2010;25:853–858.

TABLE 24.1 Selected Studies Over Time About Glucose-Lowering Drugs Use and Incident Atrial Fibrillation

FIRST AUTHOR, YEAR	STUDY DESIGN	PATIENTS, *N*	MEDICATION	FINDINGS
Chao et al., 2012	Cohort	12,065	Thiazolidinedione	Lower risk of new-onset AF with thiazolidinediones use vs. nonuse (HR, 0.69; 95% CI, 0.49–0.91; $p = 0.03$)
Chang et al., 2014	Cohort	645,710	Metformin	Lower risk of new-onset AF with metformin use (HR, 0.81; 95% CI, 0.76–0.86; $p < 0.0001$)
Chen et al., 2017	Case-control	9790	Antihyperglycemic agents	Higher risk of AF in insulin users (vs. nonusers; OR, 1.58; 95% CI 1.37–1.82). Lower risk of AF in dipeptidyl peptidase-4 inhibitors users (vs. nonusers; OR, 0.65; 95% CI, 0.45–0.93)
Zhang et al., 2017	Meta-analysis	130,854	Thiazolidinedione	Lower risk of AF with thiazolidinedione compared to controls in observational studies (OR, 0.73; 95% CI 0.62–0.87; $p = 0.0003$)
Chang et al., 2017	Cohort	90,880	DPP4i	DPP4i use associated with a lower risk of new-onset AF compared with nonuse (HR, 0.65; $p < 0.0001$)
Monami et al., 2017	Meta-analysis	33,271	GLP1-RA	No association with AF incidence (OR, 0.87; 95% CI 0.71–1.05; $p = 0.15$)
Liou et al., 2018	Case-control	14,410	Antihyperglycemic agents	Higher risk of developing AF in insulin users vs. nonusers (OR, 1.19; 95% CI, 1.06–1.35). Lower risk of AF in biguanides users (OR, 0.81; 95% CI, 0.71–0.95) and thiazolidinediones users (OR, 0.72; 95% CI, 0.63–0.83) vs. nonusers
Usman et al., 2018	Meta-analysis	34,987	SGLT2i	Lower risk of AF with SGLT2i use (OR, 0.61; 95% CI, 0.31–1.19; $p = 0.15$)
Zelniker et al., 2020	RCT	17,160	SGLT2i	Lower risk of AF with SGLT2i use (HR, 0.81; 95% CI 0.68–0.95; $p = 0.009$)
Fernandes et al., 2021	Meta-analysis	63,166	SGLT2i	Lower risk of incident atrial arrhythmias with SGLT2i use (OR, 0.81; 95% CI, 0.69–0.95; $p = 0.008$)
Lee et al., 2022	Cohort	43,426	SGLT2i vs. DPP4i	Lower risk of incident AF with SGLT2i compared to DPP4i use (HR, 0.68; 95% CI, 0.56–0.83; $p = 0.0001$)
Engström et al., 2023	Cohort	136,956	SGLT2i vs. GLP1-RA	Lower risk of AF with SGLT2i compared to GLP1-RA use (adjusted HR, 0.89; 95% CI, 0.81–0.96)
Fawzy et al., 2023	Cohort	262,376	SGLT2i	Lower risk of incident AF with SGLT2i use vs. nonuse (HR, 0.81; 95% CI, 0.76–0.84)

AF, Atrial fibrillation; *CI*, confidence interval; *DPP-4*, dipeptidyl peptidase-4; *GLP-1RA*, glucagon-like peptide-1 receptor antagonist; *HR*, hazard ratio; *OR*, odds ratio; *RCT*, randomized control trial; *SGLT2i*, sodium-glucose cotransporter-2 inhibitors.

persons with palpitations (or possibly fatigue and dyspnea) related to persistent or permanent AF, the diagnosis is likely to be made during an outpatient visit or in the hospital if the patient presents emergently. However, AF may also be asymptomatic in 30% to 50% of cases, as mentioned above. It can be found in different ways: on a conventional 12-lead electrocardiogram at a routine consultation or in the hospital, on a 24-hour (sometimes 72-hour) ambulatory ECG recording, or in a patient with a pacemaker or a defibrillator by analyzing the diagnostic functions (serving as long-term ambulatory ECG) during a check in-office or during remote monitoring or by wearable technology that assess heart rate and rhythm. Subcutaneously implantable loop recorders with long-term information over 24 to 36 months have the technical capacity to diagnose AF independent of symptoms, but their use is only approved in most countries for the evaluation of persons with unexplained syncope or for those with ischemic stroke and no documented AF. AF detection with an implantable loop recorder in persons with DM may have a similar clinical impact regarding the need for oral anticoagulation. Also, AF may currently be detected by consumer devices and wearables detecting an irregular pulse (e.g., photoplethysmography). In these cases, there is a need for a definite diagnosis of AF by a direct recording of an ECG tracing (e.g., using the recent version of smartwatches).[14]

Potential advantages and disadvantages of detecting undiagnosed AF through screening have been identified.[14] Specific recommendations on strategies and tools for routine screening of AF in persons with DM who are asymptomatic might be included in future guidelines, since data are consistent on two points:

1. When T2DM is associated with other risk factors (more particularly when the CHA_2DS_2-VASc score is high), the risk of developing AF increases during follow-up and may reach nearly 20% per year in some very-high-risk subgroups.[15]
2. At the same time, the annual thromboembolic risk increases exponentially in these persons in the case of AF and can reach 8% to 10% per year.[16]

It would seem logical on a population scale to systematically screen for AF in persons without AF with a CHA_2DS_2-VASc score of 2 or higher to identify subclinical AF that would inform therapy to reduce the risk of stroke, which is the major complication in this setting.[17] This approach has not been validated in a specific randomized study dedicated to persons with T2DM. The ESC guidelines for the management of AF currently recommend opportunistic screening for any patient over 65 years and systematic screening for persons at high risk of developing AF.[14,18] Thus both opportunistic and systematic screenings for AF in persons with diabetes are appropriate, and this may include using a prolonged noninvasive ECG-based approach and should be considered in individuals aged ≥65 years with diabetes to ensure earlier detection of AF.[18–21]

The association between AF and DM appears to be well established at the population level.[6] DM associated with AF result in a worse prognosis, and several reports from health authorities indicate that efforts must be made for the prevention of AF, although there is not a strong level of evidence that this strategy will result in a significant benefit regarding morbidity (particularly ischemic stroke) or mortality.

DIABETES AS A RISK FACTOR FOR WORSE PROGNOSIS IN PERSONS WITH ATRIAL FIBRILLATION

DM and AF frequently coexist, and when this occurs, there is a substantially higher risk of all-cause death, cardiovascular death, stroke, CKD, and HF.[22,23] The risk of death may be 25% to 60% higher in persons with AF with DM (vs. AF and no DM). Risk factors frequently associated with DM, such as hypertension and obesity, may also worsen prognosis. The association of DM and kidney impairment is associated with a higher risk of cardiovascular events and mortality than each condition alone, emphasizing the role of cardiovascular prevention in persons with T2DM when AF is also present. AF is associated with higher risks and cardiovascular events in persons with T2DM, strongly suggesting that AF further increases the already elevated cardiovascular risk in these persons. AF identifies persons with DM likely to obtain greater absolute benefits from efficient blood pressure-lowering treatment.[3] AF in persons with T2DM should be considered as a marker of adverse outcome, suggesting prompt and aggressive management of all risk factors.

The detection of AF in persons with DM has major clinical consequences because the risk of stroke is markedly higher in these persons. In the absence of other comorbidities, the annual risk of stroke can be estimated at 2.2% per year in isolated DM.[24] It is also higher in persons with diabetes due to the common association with other risk factors for stroke, including the existence of hypertension, an age over 65 or 75, associated vascular disease, or HF. All of them are identified in the items of the CHA_2DS_2-VASc score. Although there may be some disparities in the literature, several analyses reported that the presence of DM was an independent predictor for ischemic stroke in persons with AF.[25] However, the incremental risk for stroke in older persons associated with DM is attenuated, most likely due to a contributing risk of comorbidities.[26] Overall, DM is probably not the most potent independent risk factor for stroke in AF compared with the other items in the CHA_2DS_2-VASc score widely used to guide anticoagulation therapy, but it is included in this risk stratification tool, giving a point as well as for most other items.[27]

Beyond the higher risk of mortality and cardiovascular events, DM in persons with AF is likely to modify symptoms, particularly breathlessness, which is linked to the higher prevalence of obesity and higher risk of HF. However, one part of the adverse influence of DM in persons with AF might be sometimes related to a masking of AF-related palpitations, which can cause a delay in the initiation of treatment and consequently poorer outcomes in persons with T2DM. Compared with persons with AF with no DM, those with DM less often reported palpitations (29% vs. 34%) or syncope (3% vs. 5%), but they reported significantly more frequent dyspnea on exertion (30% vs. 27%) or at rest (11% vs. 10%), exercise intolerance (12% vs. 9%), and fatigue (28% vs. 26%). Although these differences were statistically significant, they may not be apparent from a clinical point of view. Persons with AF with DM had worse functional status with higher European Heart Rhythm Association scores (although the percent of persons with no symptoms was similar) and also had marginally lower quality-of-life scores than those with no DM.[23] DM has also been identified as an independent predictor of AF recurrence after AF ablation. While AF ablation usually reduces palpitations and improves NYHA functional class in persons without DM, persons with DM may report less improvement of NYHA class, despite a reduction of palpitations (Table 24.2).

TABLE 24.2 Studies on Diabetes and Outcomes After Catheter Ablation of Atrial Fibrillation (AF)

FIRST AUTHOR, YEAR	STUDY DESIGN	PATIENTS, *N* (DM)	FINDINGS
Tang et al., 2006	Cohort	263 (31)	No difference in AF recurrence between DM and non-DM patients after the procedure (mean follow-up of 13 months, 32.3% vs. 22.4%; $p = 0.24$)
Chao et al., 2010	Cohort	228 (65)	Abnormal glucose metabolism associated with increased postablation AF recurrence (mean follow-up of 19 months, 18.5% vs. 8.0%; HR, 3.25; 95% CI, 1.21–8.72; $p = 0.02$)
Wokhlu et al., 2010	Cohort	774 (47)	Diabetes independent predictor of AF recurrence (median follow-up of 3.0 years; HR, 1.9; 95% CI, 1.3–2.9; $p = 0.002$)
Lin et al., 2014	Meta-analysis	12,924 (N/A)	No difference in postablation AF recurrence between DM and non-DM patients (OR, 1.11; 95% CI, 0.97–1.26)
Anselmino et al., 2015	Meta-analysis	1464 (1464)	Higher HbA1c, older age, higher BMI, related to higher risk of AF recurrence ($p < 0.001$)
Bogossian et al., 2016	Cohort	8175 (944)	No increased periprocedural risk and no increased arrhythmia recurrence after ablation of atrial flutter or AF. Reduced palpitations with ablation in both DM and no DM. Improved NYHA class only in patients with no DM
Donnellan et al., 2019	Cohort	298 (298)	Higher HbA1c at the time of ablation associated with higher postablation AF recurrence rates (69% if HbA1c > 9% vs. 32% if HbA1c < 7%; $P < 0.0001$)
Creta et al., 2020	Cohort	2504 (234)	DM associated with higher rate of atrial arrhythmia relapse (32% vs. 25%; $p = 0.03$), particularly for patients with persistent AF
Zhao et al., 2023	Cohort	525 (525)	Lower risk of AF recurrence after AF ablation with SGLT2i use among patients with DM (HR, 0.63; 95% CI, 0.44–0.90; $p = 0.007$)
Abu-Qaoud et al., 2023	Cohort	4450 (4450)	Lower risk of arrhythmia recurrence after AF ablation with SGLT2i use among patients with DM (HR, 0.85; 95% CI, 0.77–0.95; $p = 0.003$)

AF, Atrial fibrillation; *CI,* confidence interval; *DM,* diabetes mellitus; *HR,* hazard ratio; *OR,* odds ratio; *SGLT2i,* sodium-glucose cotransporter-2 inhibitors.

CARDIOVASCULAR COMPLICATIONS AND RISK OF STROKE IN ATRIAL FIBRILLATION WITH DIABETES

The Risk of Cardiovascular Complications When Diabetes and Atrial Fibrillation Coexist

Type 2 DM is linked to lifestyle and is therefore usually associated with additional cardiovascular risk factors for stroke such as obesity, hypertension, and dyslipidemia, creating a complex interaction of adverse effects with an increased risk of cerebrovascular events.[28] In epidemiological studies performed in different populations, the relative risk of stroke in DM ranged between 1.4 and 5.8,[29] being 2.5 for males and 3.6 for females in the 20-year follow-up of the cohort of the historical Framingham study, aged 30 to 62 years at study entry.[30]

The patterns of strokes associated with T2DM may be different from those of cardioembolic strokes related to AF, since most of the ischemic strokes in persons with T2DM correspond to lacunar infarcts, related to microvascular disease and the coexistence of hypertension.[31] Moreover, the strokes associated with DM are associated with a higher risk of mortality, as well as more stroke recurrences and stroke-related dementia as compared with non-diabetic patients.[29]

Considering the interactions between AF and DM (around 15% of persons with DM presenting with AF according to data from a meta-analysis on T2DM and around 30% of persons with AF affected by DM), it may be challenging to assess the effects of T2DM control and antihyperglycemic medications on the risk of stroke in persons with AF.[3] There is controversy on whether better glycemic control results affect stroke rates in persons with DM. A longer duration of DM has been associated with an increased risk of embolic stroke but was not associated with a higher risk of bleeding during anticoagulant treatment.[32] In an analysis of a group of persons enrolled in the ATRIA (Anticoagulation and Risk Factors in AF) study, focusing on periods where persons were not anticoagulated,[33] a longer duration of DM was associated with an increased rate of ischemic stroke. The analyses regarding the relationship between the magnitude of increased HbA1c and the risk of ischemic stroke in persons with AF with DM resulted in conflicting results.[3]

Beyond the level of glycemic control, analyses from the PREFER in AF (European Prevention of Thromboembolic Events–European Registry in AF) study showed that the risk of stroke was higher in individuals with DM treated with insulin compared with those not treated with insulin and to persons with no DM.[34] Whether this association reflects a causal effect or a clustering of risk factors and long DM duration in persons treated with insulin compared with other glucose-lowering agents is not clear. Apart from insulin, the effects of other medications for glycemic control on stroke risk are still objects of investigation, with a lower risk of stroke when using metformin and thiazolidinediones.[3]

Beyond stroke, DM is associated with worse outcomes in persons with AF enrolled in contemporary registries.[23] In interpreting these associations, the higher prevalence of persistent and permanent AF, as well as the higher prevalence of HF, CKD, and coronary artery disease (CAD) among persons with DM, has to be considered. The worst profile of persons with T2DM and AF was also reported in the EORP-AF (EURObservational Research Program Atrial Fibrillation) General Registry, where persons with DM had a higher prevalence of most comorbidities and a higher risk of all-cause, cardiovascular, and noncardiovascular mortality.[35] The reciprocal relationship was also found in persons with DM, in whom AF was associated with worse outcomes. In the ADVANCE study, persons with diabetes with AF had increased risks of major coronary events, stroke, HF, cardiovascular death, and all-cause mortality compared with persons with T2 DM without AF.[36]

Diabetic retinopathy is a typical microvascular complication of DM, and in the Loire Valley AF project,[37] crude rates of stroke/thromboembolism increased in a stepwise fashion when persons with AF and no DM were compared with persons with AF with DM with no retinopathy and persons with AF with DM and retinopathy.[37] However, the presence of retinopathy associated with DM was not an independent predictor for stroke or severe bleeding in multivariable analyses.

Diabetes Subtypes, Diabetes Severity, and the Risk of Cardiovascular Events in Atrial Fibrillation

DM is a heterogeneous chronic metabolic disease that is characterized by hyperglycemia that may be caused by several different mechanisms, such as low insulin production and/or decreased insulin sensitivity. Compared with T1DM (10%–15% of cases) usually seen in younger persons and characterized by a lack of insulin production that is associated with autoimmunity, T2DM (80%–85% of cases) has an older age of onset and is characterized by abnormally high circulating insulin-to-glucose ratio and high levels of Homeostatic Model Assessment of Insulin Resistance (HOAM-IR) that are closely associated with central obesity-related insulin resistance. Furthermore, additional rare forms of DM exist, which often have a genetic background, such as maturity-onset DM of the young (MODY) and neonatal DM.[3]

When applying the CHA_2DS_2-VASc score to assess the risk for a stroke in AF, the "D" (diabetes) is defined as fasting blood glucose ≥7 mmol/L (or ≥126 mg/dL) or treatment with oral antihyperglycemic medications and/or insulin.[14] In addition to the different DM types, DM may have heterogeneous and different degrees of target organ damage for eyes, nerves, and kidneys, which may also affect the risk for cardiovascular complications. The risk for stroke in persons with DM and AF increases with longer DM duration, as well as with more DM comorbidities such as nephropathy and retinopathy.[37]

The characterization of DM types may actually be more complex. In 8980 adults with newly diagnosed DM, Ahlqvist et al. identified five patient clusters based on six preselected parameters: age at diagnosis, body mass index (BMI), absence or presence of glutamate decarboxylase antibodies identifying autoimmune DM, HbA1c levels for assessment of glycemic control, Homeostatic Model Assessment 2 (HOMA2)-B to assess β-cell function on the basis of C-peptide and glucose concentration, and HOMA2-IR to assess insulin sensitivity. The severe, insulin-resistant diabetes (SIRD) cluster had the highest risk of coronary events (HR, 1.76; 95% CI, 1.36–2.27) and stroke (HR, 1.72; 95% CI, 1.20–2.48) compared with the mild age-related diabetes (MARD) cluster,[38] but the relevance in the context of AF for the risk of stroke is unknown.

ANTICOAGULATION IN PERSONS WITH DIABETES AND ATRIAL FIBRILLATION

Treatment with an oral anticoagulant of persons with AF at high risk of stroke leads to a substantial reduction in stroke and systemic embolism (SE). The original data concerned vitamin K antagonists (VKAs). It is today fully established that the efficacy of anticoagulant therapy is far superior than antiplatelet therapy for stroke prevention in AF. Oral anticoagulation is the main part in the "A" pillar of the "ABC" AF management ("A," Anticoagulation/Avoid stroke).[14]

Persons with AF can be stratified according to their risk for stroke and systemic embolism. The preferred cardioembolic risk stratification tool is the CHA_2DS_2-VASc score, specifically for excluding from anticoagulation those persons at very low risk of stroke.[14] The CHA_2DS_2-VA score (excluding sex category for simplicity) is proposed in the most recent European guidelines to decide the initiation of long-term anticoagulation.[18] These scoring systems include DM as a risk factor for stroke because the likelihood of developing a thromboembolic event is substantially increased in persons with diabetes with AF. The use of VKAs in persons with DM is effective in reducing strokes and systemic embolism, but anticoagulation control may be more difficult to obtain than in persons without diabetes, and adverse bleeding events may be more frequent in persons with T2DM.[3]

Randomized Trials With Direct Oral Anticoagulants Compared With Warfarin

The development of DOACs included evaluation in several randomized controlled trials (RCTs). In four of these, the DOAC was compared with dose-adjusted warfarin. In each of the trials comparing a DOAC with warfarin, the results have been reported for the trial as a whole and in the subgroup of persons with DM. There are however significant differences in patient characteristics between the trials (Table 24.3). The proportion of persons with DM in these trials totaled between 23% and 40%. Persons with DM in these trials were generally younger and had a higher BMI than persons without DM. Comorbidities such as coronary disease and peripheral arterial disease were more common in persons with DM, and the rates of stroke, systemic embolism, mortality, and major bleeding were higher.

Several meta-analyses of these major trials reported that DOACs reduce the risk of stroke for persons with DM to a similar extent as for persons with no DM (p-int = 0.73).[39,40] There was no significant modification of effect of DM on the relative reduction of major bleeding with DOACs versus warfarin (p-int = 0.12). Cardiovascular mortality and

TABLE 24.3 Hazard Ratios With Direct Oral Anticoagulants (*DOACs*) Compared With Warfarin in Persons With Atrial Fibrillation According to the Presence of Diabetes or Not in Four Randomized Controlled Trials

TRIAL		RE-LY	ROCKET-AF	ARISTOTLE	ENGAGE AF – TIMI 48	COMBINED
DOAC		Dabigatran 150 mg	Rivaroxaban 20 mg	Apixaban 5 mg	Edoxaban 60/30 mg	
Mean CHADS2 score		2.1	3.5	2.1	2.8	2.6
N (No diabetes)		13,892	8569	3654	8991	35,106
N (Diabetes)		4221	5695	4547	5080	19,543
Stroke/SE	No diabetes	0.67 (0.51–0.86)	0.92 (0.75–1.13)	0.81 (0.65–1.00)	0.83 (0.70–1.02)	0.82 (0.74–0.91)
	Diabetes	0.61 (0.41–0.91)	0.82 (0.63–1.08)	0.75 (0.53–1.05)	0.93 (0.71–1.23)	0.80 (0.69–0.93)
Major bleeds	No diabetes	0.86 (0.73–1.02)	1.12 (0.93-1.35)	0.60 (0.51–0.72)	0.81 (0.69–0.96)	0.83 (0.55–1.24)
	Diabetes	1.12 (0.87–1.44)	1.00 (0.81–1.24)	0.96 (0.74–1.25)[a]	0.79 (0.65–0.96)	0.95 (0.75–1.20)
ICH	No diabetes	0.36 (0.23–0.57)	0.72 (0.46–1.12)	0.40 (0.28–0.58)	0.50 (0.35–0.73)	0.47 (0.39–0.58)
	Diabetes	0.58 (0.29–1.16)	0.62 (0.36–1.05)	0.49 (0.25–0.95)	0.40 (0.23–0.69)	0.51 (0.38–0.69)
CV mortality	No diabetes	0.84 (0.69–1.03)	1.08 (0.89–1.30)	0.89 (0.74–1.06)	0.83 (0.71–0.96)	0.90 (0.82–0.98)
	Diabetes	0.86 (0.65–1.13)	0.80 (0.64–0.99)	0.89 (0.66–1.20)	0.93 (0.77–1.13)	0.87 (0.77–0.98)

CV, Cardiovascular; *ICH*, intracranial hemorrhage; *SE*, systemic embolism.
[a]*p* value for interaction < 0.01 (all other values of *p* for interaction are nonstatistically significant

intracranial hemorrhage were significantly and to a similar extent reduced by DOACs in both the presence and absence of DM.

Of note, in the ARISTOTLE trial, the primary efficacy endpoint (reduction of stroke/SE) was similarly reduced with apixaban in persons with DM and those with no DM. By contrast, there was a statistical interaction for safety endpoint (major bleeding) with apixaban; there was a trend toward a more pronounced reduction of bleeding in persons with no DM.

In these four DOAC trials, Patti and colleagues observed that vascular death rates were reduced in persons with diabetes with DOAC treatment compared with warfarin (4.97% vs. 5.99%, respectively; RR, 0.83; 95% CI, 0.72–0.96; $p = 0.01$), but not in those without DM, maybe because the absolute death rate reduction was higher in persons with DM than in those with no DM (1.02% vs. 0.27%).[41]

Dabigatran was the only DOAC that significantly reduced stroke/SE in both persons with and without DM, and edoxaban was the only DOAC to significantly reduce major bleeding in both groups of persons with and without DM. It was also noted that although persons with DM treated with insulin had higher rates of bleeding and stroke, both rivaroxaban and edoxaban were effective in reducing these outcome events in persons with DM treated with or without insulin, while data for dabigatran and apixaban regarding this issue were lacking.

Regarding the more specific setting of postacute coronary syndrome/revascularization, the RE-DUAL trial included 2725 persons with AF of whom 993 had DM. Dabigatran plus clopidogrel or ticagrelor, compared with conventional triple therapy, was equally effective at reducing bleeding and had comparable efficacy endpoints in persons with DM compared with those with no DM after angioplasty.[42] However, this trial was not designed to specifically demonstrate differences in persons with DM and was underpowered for this purpose.

Large Observational and "Real-Life" Analyses With DOACs Compared With VKAs

The characteristics of persons in the randomized trials may contrast with the data from real-world studies. Several reports have appeared based on large registries. Any comparison from registry data needs adjustments to balance confounding factors between groups, and residual confounders may still be present after complex adjustments. Nevertheless, information from these so-called "real-world" settings are valuable to assess risks and outcomes in nonclinical trial situations and to confirm or question differences between treatments or interventions previously studied in more formal trial environments.

Registry data have largely confirmed the results from RCTs. In EORP-AF, 21% of persons with AF had DM. Persons with DM were significantly older than those without DM, had more CKD and cardiovascular comorbidities, and were more often prescribed oral anticoagulants. Persons with DM had a higher rate of all-cause mortality, cardiovascular mortality, and noncardiovascular mortality.[43] The analyses of the FANTASIIA Spanish cohort reported that time in therapeutic range in persons treated with VKA was lower in persons with DM compared with persons without DM. Persons with DM had the same age as non-diabetic patients; a much higher CHA_2DS_2-VASc score; and a higher risk for major bleeding, myocardial infarction, cardiovascular mortality, and total mortality but no differences in stroke rates.[44]

In contrast, 30% of persons in ORBIT had DM, and they were younger; had a higher BMI; and were more likely to have hypertension, kidney disease, HF, coronary artery disease, and stroke.[23]

The largest observational study of anticoagulation in persons with DM (n = 154,324) compared warfarin with three DOACs. A lower risk of stroke was seen with apixaban (HR, 0.67; 95% CI, 0.57–0.77) and rivaroxaban (HR, 0.79; 95% CI, 0.71–0.89), whereas dabigatran was associated with a similar risk of stroke (HR, 0.84; 95% CI, 0.67–1.07), and both apixaban (HR, 0.60; 95% CI, 0.56–0.65) and dabigatran (HR, 0.78; 95% CI, 0.69–0.88) were associated with a lower risk of major bleeding, but rivaroxaban (HR, 1.02; 95% CI, 0.94–1.10) was associated with a similar risk of bleeding events by comparison to warfarin.[45] Since there were potential residual confounders in such an observational analysis, only statistical associations (and not causal relationships) could be concluded.

Baker et al. studied 10,700 persons with DM taking rivaroxaban compared with a matched group of 13,946 warfarin users. In addition to validating the previous findings of lower risk of MACE associated with DOAC use, they found that major adverse limb events were lower with rivaroxaban than with warfarin. Rivaroxaban was associated with a 25% lower risk of MACE and a 63% lower risk of major limb adverse events, with an 80% lower risk of limb amputation.[46]

Chan et al. analyzed persons from the Taiwan National Health Insurance Database. In this study of persons with DM, 5812 taking warfarin were compared using propensity weighting, with 20,967 persons taking a DOAC. The risk of major adverse limb events was 28% lower in persons treated with a DOAC. The beneficial effect on limb events seemed to apply to all four DOACs.[47]

Interestingly, it has been conjectured that DOAC treatment might suppress atrial fibrosis and collagen deposition induced by hypercoagulability and that AF may not recur or progress as quickly in persons treated with DOACs instead of VKAs. Conversely a recent registry study in persons with recent-onset AF reported that the development of diabetes was 20% less frequent in the group treated with DOAC than in those treated with VKAs. This difference was seen with rivaroxaban, apixaban, and dabigatran and was most obvious in persons older than 65 years and in those with good adherence to treatment.[48] A causal relationship between treatment with a VKA and more development of diabetes was not demonstrated, but such an effect might be related to an increase in vitamin K-dependent osteocalcin known to stimulate insulin and adiponectin.

Clinical Implications

All the randomized and observational data suggest that when comparing dose-adjusted warfarin to DOAC therapy, there is a similar relative risk reduction for all major efficacy outcomes, including all-cause mortality, cardiovascular mortality, life-threatening bleeding, and intracranial hemorrhage in populations without diabetes and in persons with DM, irrespective of their baseline stroke risk or the presence of other cardiovascular risk factors than diabetes.[40,49] Since DM is part of most risk-scoring schemes used to decide which persons with AF should be anticoagulated, most persons with diabetes do receive anticoagulation. One may encourage anticoagulating every person with DM and AF, especially when DM has been present for a long time or is associated with an insufficiently controlled glycemic status. Because of the higher risk for these adverse events in persons with DM, a similar relative risk reduction generally results in a greater absolute risk reduction in this population. As with persons with no diabetes, major bleeding and major gastrointestinal bleeding associated with different DOACs compared with warfarin seem to change similarly in persons with diabetes.

Obesity is an important risk factor for cardiovascular complications, but in the four DOAC trials, obesity was shown to protect against stroke/systemic embolism.[50] This effect was not demonstrated in observational studies, and others suggest that obesity may increase the risk of thromboembolism and bleeding.[3]

Since (a) CKD is a frequent comorbidity in persons with AF and DM and (b) treatment with a VKA leads to further progression of kidney impairment, stroke prevention with DOAC therapy seems preferable to the use of VKAs (see section 5). There have been some reports suggesting differences between DOACs, but there is no head-to-head comparison between the different DOACs, and when pooling data from controlled trials and observational studies, there is no sufficient evidence to distinguish between DOACs regarding their appropriateness for the management of persons with AF and DM.[3]

HEART FAILURE IN PERSONS WITH ATRIAL FIBRILLATION AND DIABETES

The role of HF for stroke risk in AF is important in persons with DM who are at increased risk for both stroke and HF.[14,22] The prevalence of DM in persons with HF is around 30% to 40% and similar in HF with preserved ejection fraction (HFpEF) and HF with reduced ejection fraction (HFpEF). Persons with DM are at a higher risk of developing HFrEF or HFpEF, and the risk increases with age. Conversely, HF itself is a risk factor for the development of DM, most likely related to insulin resistance and/or decreased physical activity.[22] The presence of HF results in a higher risk of HF hospitalization, cardiovascular death, and all-cause death in persons with DM, with the strongest predictive value of DM seen in persons with HFrEF.[22] At the time of new-onset AF, persons with DM are at increased risk for developing acute HF due to the loss of atrial kick and impaired LV filling. AF and acute HF frequently coexist and can exacerbate each other. In acute HF, the risk is amplified by the presence of DM, and DM significantly increases short-term risk, including in-hospital death, all-cause death within 1 year, and the risk for HF rehospitalization.[3]

In addition to the direct detrimental effect of insulin resistance and hyperglycemia on LV dysfunction, major risk factors promoting the development of HF in DM are CAD, CKD, and hypertension.[22] LV diastolic dysfunction is frequent in DM and already observed in persons with pre-DM, as it shows a strong correlation with insulin resistance and hyperglycemia.[22] HFpEF represents the most frequent form of HF in DM (about 75%), and its prevalence is higher with old age and women and in persons with both hypertension and DM.[51] Guideline-directed medical treatment and device therapies for HF are equally effective in persons with and without DM, as shown in RCTs in which on average about 30% to 40% of persons had DM.[22]

Beta-blockers play an important role for rate and symptom control in persons with AF.[14] They are a main part in the "B" pillar of the "ABC" AF management ("B," better symptom control with rate or rhythm control therapies)[14] and fully relevant for rate control in persons with AF with DM. Interestingly, while their treatment benefits strongly support their general use in persons with HFrEF and DM in sinus rhythm, their benefits in persons with AF have been debated.[14,22]

Nondihydropyridine calcium channel blocker (verapamil or diltiazem) can be used as an alternative to beta-blockers for rate control in persons with AF and for treatment of hypertension in persons with or without HFpEF, but their use is contraindicated in persons with HFrEF, and they may lead to higher drug levels of DOACs and thus an increased bleeding risk.[14,51] Among persons with permanent AF and symptoms of HF, low-dose digoxin may also be used, considering that this may result in a similar quality of life at 6 months than with bisoprolol.[52]

For several decades, the available evidence from clinical studies indicated that glycemic control in DM with glucose-lowering therapies had only moderate beneficial effects on macrovascular endpoints and on the risk for HF-related outcomes. However, the completion of several cardiovascular outcome trials with SGLT2 inhibitors and GLP1-RAs in recent years resulted in major changes.[22] Particularly, the SGLT2 inhibitors have been shown to significantly lower the risk for hospitalization for HF in persons with T2DM at high cardiovascular risk.[53] The risk reductions for HF hospital admission were consistent and in the range of 27% to 39% in these trials. However, the prevalence of persons with AF in these studies was relatively low or originally not reported. Nevertheless, a dedicated post hoc study compared persons with AF at baseline (n = 389) and persons without AF (n = 6631) in the EMPA-REG OUTCOME trial.[54] It indicated that empagliflozin compared with a placebo reduced cardiovascular death or hospitalization for HF in both group of persons with DM and AF (HR, 0.58; 95% CI, 0.36–0.92) and those with DM without AF (HR, 0.67; 95% CI, 0.55–0.82; p-int = 0.56).[54] Interestingly, the absolute number of events that were prevented was higher in persons with AF, resulting in larger absolute treatment effects of empagliflozin.

A subgroup analysis investigating the impact of AF (about 38% of the study population) is available in DAPA-HF.[55] It showed in persons with AF at baseline a somewhat weaker protective effect (HR, 0.82; 95% CI, 0.63–1.06) compared with persons without AF (HR, 0.72; 95% CI, 61–0.84) on the primary composite outcome of worsening HF or cardiovascular death.[55] These analyses included both HFrEF persons with and without DM as enrolled in DAPA-HF. A study investigating the effect of the combined SGLT2 and SGLT1 inhibitor sotagliflozin in persons with DM and a history of recent worsening of HF confirmed the protective effect of this treatment approach, and the subgroup analyses showed a similar risk reduction for the primary composite outcome of death from cardiovascular causes and hospitalizations or urgent visits for HF in persons with or without AF/atrial flutter.[56]

Importantly, SGLT2 inhibitors may also reduce the risk of cardiovascular death or hospitalization for HF in persons with HF and a preserved ejection fraction, regardless of the presence or absence of AF or DM.[57]

CHRONIC KIDNEY DISEASE IN PERSONS WITH ATRIAL FIBRILLATION AND DIABETES

In addition to being a risk factor for the development of AF and for a complicated stroke in the presence of AF, DM is associated with an increased risk for the development of kidney disease. In persons with AF and CKD treated with anticoagulants, there is an increased risk of bleeding, but there are also concerns about the risk of anticoagulation-related nephropathy. The latter is a recently recognized form of acute kidney injury in which overanticoagulation causes profuse glomerular hemorrhage, which manifests on kidney biopsy as numerous kidney tubules filled with red cells and red cell casts.

Although anticoagulation-related nephropathy may develop in response to any anticoagulant, including VKAs and DOACs, it has been particularly associated with overdosing of warfarin with INR levels > 3. Older persons with DM and diabetic kidney disease are particularly prone to develop anticoagulation-related nephropathy that may trigger episodes of acute kidney injury more frequently in persons with AF. These acute kidney injury episodes can in turn accelerate the progression of CKD and are associated with an increased mortality rate.[3]

In persons with significantly impaired kidney function (CrCl < 30 mL/min), a reduced dose of rivaroxaban, apixaban, or edoxaban is recommended in persons with a CrCl between 15 and 30 mL/min, but persons with a CrCl < 25 to 30 mL/min were not included in the randomized trials. The FDA approved a low 75-mg bid dose of dabigatran for persons with a CrCl < 30 mL/min, available in the United States, but it has not been tested in a prospective trial, and it is not approved for use within Europe. The use of VKA has been proposed when the time in therapeutic range (TTR) is above 70%, but harm may exceed benefit with an increased risk for bleeding, anticoagulation-nephropathy, and vascular calcification. Until ongoing studies clarify the optimal anticoagulation strategy in severe kidney disease, this has to be based on individual assessment of risk and benefits.

In persons with AF and particularly in persons with diabetic kidney disease, the use of VKAs may aggravate vascular calcification, including calcification in the vascular bed of the kidney, and thereby contribute to worsening kidney function in these persons. In contrast, DOACs, such as the factor Xa inhibitor rivaroxaban, due to their different mode of action, do not only lack this negative effect but may even provide beneficial protective effects against vascular injury and kidney function decline by decreasing vascular inflammation, remodeling, and vascular calcifications. Several observational studies and one randomized trial (RE-LY) suggested that kidney function may be progressively impaired when VKA therapy, as opposed to DOAC treatment, is prescribed.[58,59] Studies of persons with AF treated with VKAs versus DOACs found more progression of kidney disease (development of CKD stage 5, i.e., estimated glomerular filtration rate [eGFR] < 15 mL/min/1.73 m^2 or a need for kidney replacement therapy) with VKAs than DOACs.[59] Persons with AF with DM in addition to CKD may thus be protected from progressive kidney impairment by avoiding VKAs and favoring DOAC therapy.

Due to the high risk for CKD, screening for CKD is mandated in the regular follow-up of all persons with DM, with at least an annual assessment of kidney function (eGFR) and control of blood pressure. In diabetes with a fast decline in kidney function, even more frequent measurements may be needed. Declining kidney function increases the risk for bleeding, and the dose of DOACs should be adjusted according to the level of kidney clearance. In the trials comparing DOACs with VKAs, kidney function was evaluated as creatinine clearance estimated from creatinine, sex, age, and weight using the Cockcroft and Gault formula.

FUTURE DIRECTIONS

- Regarding recent developments for glucose-lowering therapies, the presence of AF at the baseline or during follow-up is mostly not systematically reported and information on whether strokes are AF-related is mostly lacking. Whether a reduction in the incidence of AF accompanies a proportional reduction of the risk of stroke in persons with DM is less well explored.
- The beneficial effects of SGLT2 inhibitors in HFrEF persons have been clearly documented in persons with diabetes. However, their impact on outcome in these persons with both diabetes and AF at the baseline is less clear. Thus more dedicated analyses on the effects of SGTL2 inhibitors in persons with AF and their potential differential impact in persons with HF and concomitant AF and diabetes are needed.
- The relation between the severity of DM, the level of glycemic control, and AF-related outcomes is not well documented.
- DM is associated with an increased risk of deterioration of kidney function. Persons with significantly impaired kidney function were largely excluded from the DOAC or recent glucose-lowering therapies trials. More data on the possible benefits of newer medications in persons with AF, DM, and CKD would be useful.
- In persons with AF and acute coronary syndrome, current treatment is based on anticoagulants plus antiplatelets (single or dual) for up to 1 year after the acute event. The general recommendation after 12 months is to omit antiplatelet medications and prescribe only oral anticoagulants. In view of the complexity of the coronary pattern in ischemic heart disease, more data are needed to assess if persons with AF, CAD, and DM could benefit from the combination of oral anticoagulants and antiplatelet therapy for a longer period.
- The potential beneficial effect of DOACs on the development of AF (or AF recurrences/progression) and diabetes has been hypothesized and is supported by data from both basic science and observational clinical studies, but a formal assessment in RCTs is needed. A specific study for persons with DM would be relevant.

REFERENCES

1. Huxley RR, Filion KB, Konety S, Alonso A. Meta-analysis of cohort and case-control studies of type 2 diabetes mellitus and risk of atrial fibrillation. *Am J Cardiol*. 2011;108:56–62.
2. Ostgren CJ, Merlo J, Råstam L, Lindblad U. Atrial fibrillation and its association with type 2 diabetes and hypertension in a Swedish community. *Diabetes Obes Metab*. 2004;6:367–374.
3. Fauchier L, Boriani G, de Groot JR, Kreutz R, Rossing P, Camm AJ. Medical therapies for prevention of cardiovascular and renal events in patients with atrial fibrillation and diabetes mellitus. *EP Europace*. 2021;23:1873–1891.
4. Schoen T, Pradhan AD, Albert CM, Conen D. Type 2 diabetes mellitus and risk of incident atrial fibrillation in women. *J Am Coll Cardiol*. 2012;60: 1421–1428.
5. Seyed Ahmadi S, Svensson AM, Pivodic A, Rosengren A, Lind M. Risk of atrial fibrillation in persons with type 2 diabetes and the excess risk in relation to glycaemic control and renal function: a Swedish cohort study. *Cardiovasc Diabetol*. 2020;19:9.
6. Bisson A, Bodin A, Fauchier G, et al. Sex, age, type of diabetes and incidence of atrial fibrillation in patients with diabetes mellitus: a nationwide analysis. *Cardiovasc Diabetol*. 2021;20:24.
7. Bisson A, Clementy N, Bodin A, et al. Relationship of preexisting cardiovascular comorbidities to newly diagnosed atrial fibrillation after ischemic stroke. *Stroke*. 2017;48:2878–2880.
8. Dublin S, Glazer NL, Smith NL, et al. Diabetes mellitus, glycemic control, and risk of atrial fibrillation. *J Gen Intern Med*. 2010;25:853–858.
9. Wang A, Green JB, Halperin JL, Piccini JP. Atrial fibrillation and diabetes mellitus: JACC review topic of the week. *J Am Coll Cardiol*. 2019;74:1107–1115.
10. Fauchier G, Bisson A, Bodin A, et al. Glucose-lowering drug use and new-onset atrial fibrillation in patients with diabetes mellitus. *Diabetologia*. 2021;64:2602–2605.
11. Liou YS, Yang FY, Chen HY, Jong GP. Antihyperglycemic drugs use and new-onset atrial fibrillation: a population-based nested case control study. *PLoS One*. 2018;13:e0197245.
12. Zelniker TA, Bonaca MP, Furtado RHM, et al. Effect of dapagliflozin on atrial fibrillation in patients with type 2 diabetes mellitus: insights from the DECLARE-TIMI 58 trial. *Circulation*. 2020;141:1227–1234.
13. Fernandes GC, Fernandes A, Cardoso R, et al. Association of SGLT2 inhibitors with arrhythmias and sudden cardiac death in patients with type 2 diabetes or heart failure: a meta-analysis of 34 randomized controlled trials. *Heart Rhythm*. 2021
14. Hindricks G, Potpara T, Dagres N, et al. 2020 ESC guidelines for the diagnosis and management of atrial fibrillation developed in collaboration with the European Association for Cardio-Thoracic Surgery (EACTS). *Eur Heart J*. 2021;42:373–498.
15. Fauchier L, Clementy N, Pelade C, Collignon C, Nicolle E, Lip GYH. Patients with ischemic stroke and incident atrial fibrillation: a nationwide cohort study. *Stroke*. 2015;46:2432–2437.
16. Lip GYH, Nieuwlaat R, Pisters R, Lane DA, Crijns HJGM. Refining clinical risk stratification for predicting stroke and thromboembolism in atrial fibrillation using a novel risk factor-based approach: the euro heart survey on atrial fibrillation. *Chest*. 2010;137:263–272.
17. Svennberg E, Friberg L, Frykman V, Al-Khalili F, Engdahl J, Rosenqvist M. Clinical outcomes in systematic screening for atrial fibrillation (STROKESTOP): a multicentre, parallel group, unmasked, randomised controlled trial. *Lancet (London, England)*. 2021;398:1498–1506.
18. Van Gelder IC, Rienstra M, Bunting KV, et al. 2024 ESC Guidelines for the management of atrial fibrillation developed in collaboration with the European Association for Cardio-Thoracic Surgery (EACTS). *Eur Heart J*. 2024;45: 3314–3414.
19. Elbadawi A, Sedhom R, Gad M, et al. Screening for atrial fibrillation in the elderly: A network meta-analysis of randomized trials. *Eur J Intern Med*. 2022; 105:38–45.
20. McIntyre WF, Diederichsen SZ, Freedman B, Schnabel RB, Svennberg E, Healey JS. Screening for atrial fibrillation to prevent stroke: a meta-analysis. *Eur Heart J Open*. 2022:2 oeac044.
21. Lyth J, Svennberg E, Bernfort L, et al. Cost-effectiveness of population screening for atrial fibrillation: the STROKESTOP study. *Eur Heart J*. 2023;44: 196–204.
22. Cosentino F, Grant PJ, Aboyans V, et al. 2019 ESC Guidelines on diabetes, pre-diabetes, and cardiovascular diseases developed in collaboration with the EASD. *Eur Heart J*. 2020;41:255–323.
23. Echouffo-Tcheugui JB, Shrader P, Thomas L, et al. Care patterns and outcomes in atrial fibrillation patients with and without diabetes: ORBIT-AF registry. *J Am Coll Cardiol*. 2017;70:1325–1335.
24. Olesen JB, Lip GYH, Hansen ML, et al. Validation of risk stratification schemes for predicting stroke and thromboembolism in patients with atrial fibrillation: nationwide cohort study. *BMJ*. 2011;342:d124–d124.
25. Hughes M, Lip GY. Stroke and thromboembolism in atrial fibrillation: a systematic review of stroke risk factors, risk stratification schema and cost effectiveness data. *Thromb Haemost*. 2008;99:295–304.
26. Aronow WS, Ahn C, Kronzon I, Gutstein H. Risk factors for new thromboembolic stroke in patients > or = 62 years of age with chronic atrial fibrillation. *Am J Cardiol*. 1998;82:119–121.
27. Fauchier L, Bodin A, Bisson A. Editorial commentary: The CHA2DS2VASc score and its black and white items. *Trends Cardiovasc Med*. 2019;29: 392–393.

28. Dutton GR, Lewis CE. The look AHEAD trial: implications for lifestyle intervention in type 2 diabetes mellitus. *Prog Cardiovasc Dis*. 2015;58:69–75.
29. Tun NN, Arunagirinathan G, Munshi SK, Pappachan JM. Diabetes mellitus and stroke: a clinical update. *World J Diabetes*. 2017;8:235–248.
30. Kannel WB, McGee DL. Diabetes and cardiovascular disease. The Framingham study. *JAMA*. 1979;241:2035–2038.
31. Vaidya V, Gangan N, Sheehan J. Impact of cardiovascular complications among patients with Type 2 diabetes mellitus: a systematic review. *Expert Rev Pharmacoecon Outcomes Res*. 2015;15:487–497.
32. Overvad TF, Skjøth F, Lip GY, et al. Duration of diabetes mellitus and risk of thromboembolism and bleeding in atrial fibrillation: nationwide cohort study. *Stroke*. 2015;46:2168–2174.
33. Ashburner JM, Go AS, Chang Y, et al. Effect of diabetes and glycemic control on ischemic stroke risk in AF patients: ATRIA study. *J Am Coll Cardiol*. 2016;67:239–247.
34. Patti G, Lucerna M, Cavallari I, et al. Insulin-requiring versus noninsulin-requiring diabetes and thromboembolic risk in patients with atrial fibrillation: PREFER in AF. *J Am Coll Cardiol*. 2017;69:409–419.
35. Fumagalli S, Said SA, Laroche C, et al. Management and prognosis of atrial fibrillation in diabetic patients: an EORP-AF General Pilot Registry report. *Eur Heart J Cardiovasc Pharmacother*. 2018;4:172–179.
36. Du X, Ninomiya T, de Galan B, et al. Risks of cardiovascular events and effects of routine blood pressure lowering among patients with type 2 diabetes and atrial fibrillation: results of the ADVANCE study. *Eur Heart J*. 2009;30:1128–1135.
37. Lip GYH, Clementy N, Pierre B, Boyer M, Fauchier L. The impact of associated diabetic retinopathy on stroke and severe bleeding risk in diabetic patients with atrial fibrillation. *Chest*. 2015;147:1103–1110.
38. Ahlqvist E, Storm P, Karajamaki A, et al. Novel subgroups of adult-onset diabetes and their association with outcomes: a data-driven cluster analysis of six variables. *Lancet Diabetes Endocrinol*. 2018;6:361–369.
39. Ruff CT, Giugliano RP, Braunwald E, et al. Comparison of the efficacy and safety of new oral anticoagulants with warfarin in patients with atrial fibrillation: a meta-analysis of randomised trials. *Lancet*. 2014;383:955–962.
40. Plitt A, Zelniker TA, Park JG, et al. Patients with diabetes mellitus and atrial fibrillation treated with NOACs: Meta-analysis of 8 outcomes in 58, 634 patients across 4 randomized controlled trials. *Eur Heart J Cardiovasc Pharmacother*. 2020
41. Patti G, Di Gioia G, Cavallari I, Nenna A. Safety and efficacy of nonvitamin K antagonist oral anticoagulants versus warfarin in diabetic patients with atrial fibrillation: A study-level meta-analysis of phase III randomized trials. *Diabetes Metab Res Rev*. 2017:33.
42. Maeng M, Steg PG, Bhatt DL, et al. Dabigatran dual therapy versus warfarin triple therapy post-PCI in patients with atrial fibrillation and diabetes. *JACC Cardiovasc Interv*. 2019;12:2346–2355.
43. Ding WY, Kotalczyk A, Boriani G, et al. Impact of diabetes on the management and outcomes in atrial fibrillation: an analysis from the ESC-EHRA EORP-AF Long-Term General Registry. *Eur J Intern Med*. 2022. https://doi.org/10.1016/j.ejim.2022.04.026. Online ahead of print.
44. García-Fernández A, Esteve-Pastor MA, Roldán-Rabadán I, et al. Relationship of adverse events to quality of anticoagulation control in atrial fibrillation patients with diabetes: real-world data from the FANTASIIA Registry. *Ann Med*. 2020;52:300–309.
45. Lip GYH, Keshishian AV, Kang AL, et al. Effectiveness and safety of oral anticoagulants in patients with nonvalvular atrial fibrillation and diabetes mellitus. *Mayo Clin Proc*. 2020;95:929–943.
46. Baker WL, Beyer-Westendorf J, Bunz TJ, et al. Effectiveness and safety of rivaroxaban and warfarin for prevention of major adverse cardiovascular or limb events in patients with non-valvular atrial fibrillation and type 2 diabetes. *Diabetes Obes Metab*. 2019;21:2107–2114.
47. Chan YH, Lee HF, Li PR, et al. Effectiveness, safety, and major adverse limb events in atrial fibrillation patients with concomitant diabetes mellitus treated with non-vitamin K antagonist oral anticoagulants. *Cardiovasc Diabetol*. 2020;19:63.
48. Huang HK, Liu PP, Lin SM, et al. Risk of developing diabetes in patients with atrial fibrillation taking non-vitamin K antagonist oral anticoagulants or warfarin: a nationwide cohort study. *Diabetes Obes Metab*. 2021;23:499–507.
49. Plitt A, McGuire DK, Giugliano RP. Atrial fibrillation, type 2 diabetes, and non-vitamin K antagonist oral anticoagulants: a review. *JAMA Cardiol*. 2017;2:442–448.
50. Proietti M, Guiducci E, Cheli P, Lip GY. Is there an obesity paradox for outcomes in atrial fibrillation? A systematic review and meta-analysis of non-vitamin K antagonist oral anticoagulant trials. *Stroke*. 2017;48:857–866.
51. McDonagh TA, Metra M, Adamo M, et al. 2021 ESC Guidelines for the diagnosis and treatment of acute and chronic heart failure. *Eur Heart J*. 2021;42:3599–3726.
52. Kotecha D, Bunting KV, Gill SK, et al. Effect of digoxin vs bisoprolol for heart rate control in atrial fibrillation on patient-reported quality of life. *JAMA*. 2020;324:2497.
53. McGuire DK, Shih WJ, Cosentino F, et al. Association of SGLT2 inhibitors with cardiovascular and kidney outcomes in patients with type 2 diabetes: a meta-analysis. *JAMA Cardiol*. 2021;6:148–158.
54. Böhm M, Slawik J, Brueckmann M, et al. Efficacy of empagliflozin on heart failure and renal outcomes in patients with atrial fibrillation: data from the EMPA-REG OUTCOME trial. *Eur J Heart Fail*. 2020;22:126–135.
55. McMurray JJV, Solomon SD, Inzucchi SE, et al. Dapagliflozin in patients with heart failure and reduced ejection fraction. *N Engl J Med*. 2019;381:1995–2008.
56. Bhatt DL, Szarek M, Steg PG, et al. Sotagliflozin in patients with diabetes and recent worsening heart failure. *N Engl J Med*. 2020.
57. Anker SD, Butler J, Filippatos G, et al. Empagliflozin in heart failure with a preserved ejection fraction. *N Engl J Med*. 2021;385:1451–1461.
58. Yao X, Tangri N, Gersh BJ, et al. Renal outcomes in anticoagulated patients with atrial fibrillation. *J Am Coll Cardiol*. 2017;70:2621–2632.
59. Hernandez AV, Bradley G, Khan M, et al. Rivaroxaban vs. warfarin and renal outcomes in non-valvular atrial fibrillation patients with diabetes. *Eur Heart J Qual Care Clin Outcomes*. 2020;6:301–307.

25 Chronic Kidney Disease: Implications for Cardiovascular Risk and Management in Patients With Type 2 Diabetes

WILLIAM GUY HERRINGTON AND RICHARD HAYNES

KEY POINTS

- Patients with diabetes mellitus (DM) need to be regularly (e.g., annually) screened for chronic kidney disease (CKD) or have their CKD staged using assessments of glomerular filtration rate (GFR) and albuminuria.
- CKD increases the risk of coronary artery disease, but is also particularly associated with structural heart disease, heart failure, arrhythmias, and sudden cardiac death. Most patients with CKD are more likely to die from cardiovascular disease (CVD) before progressing to the need for kidney replacement therapy.
- DM increases the risk of CVD mortality at any given level of GFR or albuminuria, and CKD appears to be a cause of CVD (directly or indirectly) independent of DM status.
- Additional complications of CKD commonly include effects on blood pressure, a characteristic atherogenic dyslipidemia, dysregulated salt-water balance and calcium-phosphate homeostasis, and renal anemia. These perturbations account for some of the links between CKD and CVD.
- Meta-analyses of trials of intensive glycemic control have suggested this strategy modestly reduces the risk of coronary artery disease and importantly reduces the risk of developing or worsening of diabetic nephropathy, but there may be no effect on the risk of heart failure, and effects on the risk of kidney failure are uncertain.
- In CKD, intensive statin-based regimens are safe and should be used to maximize the benefits. A meta-analysis has shown statin-based regimens safely reduce atherosclerotic CVD risk in CKD. Intensive regimens are recommended as in moderate-to-severe CKD (e.g., eGFR $< 45\,\text{mL/min}/1.73\ \text{m}^2$) a trend to smaller risk reductions per unit reduction in low-density lipoprotein cholesterol emerges when trial data are compared to patients without CKD. It is noteworthy that there is uncertainty about benefits in patients on dialysis among whom nonatherosclerotic CVD, including heart failure and sudden cardiac death, are common.
- A meta-analysis has shown intensive blood pressure regimens reduce the risk of CVD and albuminuria, but whether this translates into a reduced risk of kidney failure has not been demonstrated.
- Large placebo-controlled trials have shown renin-angiotensin-aldosterone system inhibitors, sodium-glucose cotransporter-2 inhibitors, and the nonsteroidal mineralocorticoid receptor antagonist finerenone may all reduce the risk of both kidney failure and CVD in patients with type 2 DM and proteinuric CKD. Most recently, the glucagon-like peptide-1 receptor agonist semaglutide has been shown to not only improve glycaemic control but also reduce cardiovascular risk and slow the rate of decline of kidney function in patients with type 2 DM and proteinuric CKD. These interventions should be started early and used in combination to prevent end-organ damage.
- In patients with DM and CKD, low-dose aspirin is indicated in patients with prior atherothrombotic CVD. In patients with type 2 DM and CKD but without CVD, the balance of CVD benefits versus major bleeding risk is finely balanced.
- Patients with DM and CKD are at high risk of stroke of all types. Intensive blood pressure control reduces the stroke risk, and statin-based therapy reduces the ischemic stroke risk. However, the optimum approach to thromboprophylaxis in atrial fibrillation in severe CKD is uncertain as the bleeding risk is high, warfarin may accelerate vascular calcification, and newer anticoagulants have been understudied in patients with severe CKD.
- Partial correction of dysregulated calcium-phosphate homeostasis with 1-alpha hydroxylated vitamin D and phosphate binders is a common clinical practice in nephrology but has not been shown to reduce CVD risk (and may even increase it).

- Partial correction of anemia caused by CKD with intravenous iron and erythropoiesis-stimulating agents is also common in nephrology practice as it reduces the need for blood transfusion and improves the quality of life. However, randomized trials have not confirmed that such practices prevent the development of structural heart disease, and aiming for a "normalized" hemoglobin increases the risk of stroke. Treating anemia in CKD therefore aims for partial correction and requires careful monitoring.

Chronic kidney disease (CKD) is defined as abnormalities of kidney structure or function, present for at least 3 months, with implications for health.[1,2] It has a major impact on global morbidity and mortality due to its associations both with the risk of kidney failure and cardiovascular disease (CVD). For most patients with CKD, the risk of dying from CVD exceeds that of progression to the need for kidney replacement therapy in their lifetime, and so the management of both of these risks is a cornerstone of general nephrology practice.

Diabetic kidney disease is a leading cause of CKD globally,[3] and is particularly common in regions where the prevalence of obesity is high. Diabetes mellitus (DM) and CKD both independently increase the risk of CVD, and their coexistence is associated with high risk, which can be extreme in severe CKD (i.e., eGFR < 30 mL/min/1.72 m^2).[4,5] Population data show that even mild-to-moderate CKD is associated with the risk of coronary artery disease risk, which is equivalent to someone with established atherosclerotic CVD,[6] but structural heart disease and heart failure,[7] central and peripheral artery disease,[8] arrhythmias, and sudden cardiac death are particular features of CVD in CKD.[9] This chapter provides details of internationally agreed-upon definitions and staging for CKD; introduces its epidemiology, pathology, and associated complications; and provides an evidence-based approach to the management of risk of both CVD and kidney failure for patients with both DM and CKD.

CHRONIC KIDNEY DISEASE NOMENCLATURE AND STAGING

The kidney disease improving global outcomes (KDIGO) organization has coordinated the development of clinical practice guidelines in nephrology, including comprehensive "CKD evaluation and management" and specific "diabetes management in CKD" guidelines[10] (www.kdigo.org). KDIGO "controversies conferences" also facilitate resolution of key nephrology-related issues,[7–9] and have tackled its complex nomenclature[11] (Table 25.1). The use of the term "kidney" rather than "renal" is encouraged, with

TABLE 25.1 Summary of Kidney Disease-Related Nomenclature[10,11]

CONCEPT OR TERM	RELATED TERMS	DEFINITION/MEANING
Glomerular filtration rate (*GFR*)	Estimated GFR (*eGFR*) Measured GFR	A specific measure of glomerular kidney function, which is a key component of CKD staging. eGFR is normalized to body surface area and estimated from blood creatinine (eGFR$_{Cr}$), cystatin C (eGFR$_{cys}$), or both (eGFR$_{cr\text{-}cys}$) using estimating formulas assuming a steady state. GFR is directly measured using time-consuming clearance methods or exogenous filtration markers in selected circumstances when precise knowledge of GFR is important (e.g., living kidney donor assessment).
Albuminuria	Urinary albumin-to-creatinine ratio (*uACR*) Albumin excretion rate Historical terms: Normoalbuminuria Microalbuminuria Macroalbuminuria	Urine dipsticks can provide semiquantitative assessments of the amount of albumin in the urine and are useful for screening and predicting risk. More specific quantification of any urinary albumin can be performed by spot or timed urine collections. A ratio of urinary albumin-to-creatinine concentrations helps account for urine concentration in a spot sample and is practical for clinical practice. A uACR < 30 mg/g (about <3 mg/mmol) is considered normoalbuminuria (A1); 30–300 mg/g (about 3–30 mg/mmol) is equivalent to an albumin excretion rate of 30–300 mg per day and historically referred to as microalbuminuria (A2); while a uACR ≥300 mg/g (about ≥30 mg/mmol) is equivalent to ≥300 mg per day and considered macroalbuminuria (A3). (Note: To formally convert a uACR from mg/g to mg/mmol, divide by 8.84.)
Proteinuria	Urinary protein-to-creatinine ratio (*uPCR*) Protein excretion rate	Proteinuria includes urinary excreted albumin and nonalbumin proteins and may be used clinically, particularly when quantifying high urinary concentrations of albumin. Formulas for converting uPCR to estimates of uACR exist.[12]
Chronic kidney disease (*CKD*)	Historical terms: Chronic renal failure or chronic renal insufficiency	CKD is defined as eGFR <60 mL/min/1.73 m^2 or markers of kidney damage present for at least 3 months (with implications for health). CKD is staged using GFR, albuminuria, and diagnosis.
Kidney failure	Historical terms: End-stage kidney disease End-stage renal disease	Kidney failure refers to patients with eGFR < 15 mL/min/1.73 m^2 or treated with dialysis for at least 3 months, or kidney transplantation (i.e., CKD stage G5). The suffix D denotes dialysis status, and the suffix T denotes transplant status.
Kidney replacement therapy		Treatment with a long-term dialysis modality (i.e., stage G5D) or kidney transplantation (i.e., stages G1-5T).
Acute kidney injury (*AKI*)	Historical term: Acute renal failure	AKI is defined clinically as oliguria for >6 hours, a rise in serum creatinine by >0.3 mg/dL in 2 days or by >50% in 1 week (Note: To convert serum creatinine from mg/dL to μmol/L, multiply by 88.4.)
Diabetes and kidney disease	Historical terms: Diabetic kidney disease (*DKD*) Diabetic nephropathy	The term "diabetic nephropathy" has been used to refer to patients with overt proteinuria (i.e., a uACR of ≥300 mg/g) attributed to traditional diabetic pathophysiology and/or histology. The term "diabetic kidney disease" recognizes the wider spectrum of renal pathological changes that DM and associated risk factors can cause. The term "diabetes and kidney disease" is suggested by KDIGO.

the term "kidney disease" encompassing both acute and chronic (i.e., present for >3 months) conditions.

The original 2012 KDIGO framework for staging CKD is based principally on both categories of glomerular filtration rate (GFR) and level of albuminuria. Although GFR can be directly measured, it is more practical to estimate GFR using equations based on serum creatinine.[13] An estimated GFR (eGFR) of at least 60 mL/min/1.73 m^2 may be considered "normal" in older adults and, in the absence of albuminuria or other evidence of kidney disease with implication for health, does not constitute CKD.[1,2]

Note that estimating formulas perform best below a GFR of about 60 mL/min/1.73 m^2, so directly measuring GFR (referred to as mGFR) is generally reserved for scenarios where knowledge of a precise GFR is important (e.g., planning live kidney donation or certain chemotherapy drug dosing).

A persistent decrease in eGFR below 60 mL/min/1.73 m^2 (i.e., stages G3–5) is sufficient to confirm CKD. Below this level of eGFR, the risk of kidney failure[4] and CVD[6,14] both progressively increases. An eGFR persistently less than 15 mL/min/1.73 m^2 is referred to as "kidney failure" (in preference to the term "end-stage kidney disease").[11] This is the eGFR threshold below which maintenance (i.e., long-term) kidney replacement therapy may become clinically necessary.

Historical eGFR formulas developed by the CKD-Epidemiology (CKD-EPI) collaboration took account of race because previous studies indicated a higher average serum creatinine level for the same measured GFR in Black individuals.[13] Race is not always available when laboratories report eGFR, and older formulas were more likely to be biased in Black individuals who suffer a disproportionate burden of kidney failure. The 2021 CKD-EPI eGFR formulas have been developed without race, share the bias more equitably between races, and were recommended for immediate implementation in the United States due to their potential to improve clinical decision-making for Black Americans.[13]

Albuminuria is an early marker of CKD. A spot urine sample measuring albumin-to-creatinine ratio is a simple method to detect albuminuria and also estimates an approximate 24-hour albumin excretion rate. It is clinically more practical than timed (e.g., 8-hour or 24-hour) urine collections. The ratio estimate relies on an assumption that urinary creatinine excretion is generally constant, enabling daily variation in urinary tonicity to be accounted for.[2] In patients with DM, a spot albumin-to-creatinine ratio is therefore an optimum method to regularly screen for, and quantify, albuminuria (e.g., annually).[2,15]

Albuminuria predicts both risk of kidney failure and CVD independently of eGFR.[4,16] CKD staging therefore incorporates both GFR (G1–5) and albuminuria (A1–3) into CKD risk categories. The KDIGO heat map depicts risk using green, yellow, orange, and red to represent low, moderately high, high, and very high risk (Fig. 25.1). Low-risk CKD is estimated to have a 0.04/1000 patient-years risk of kidney failure in general population data, and in the absence of important abnormalities in kidney structure, stages G1A1 and G2A1 represent normal kidneys (i.e., no CKD). Relative to the low-risk category, moderately high-, high-, and very high-risk categories (i.e., yellow, orange, and red), represent increased relative risk of kidney failure by about ~5 times, ~20 times, and ~150 times, respectively.

The CKD heat maps are also mirrored with respect to how decreased GFR and increased albuminuria independently predict a wide range of cardiovascular diseases, including myocardial infarction, stroke, heart failure, atrial fibrillation, and peripheral arterial disease.[17] The 2024 KDIGO Clinical Practice Guideline for the Evaluation and Management of CKD provides for full details of how their CKD heat maps can be used clinically.[1]

An individual's absolute risk of kidney failure is estimated using validated Kidney Failure Risk Equations which, as a minimum, include age, sex, eGFR, and uACR.[18] Any of the eGFR formulas used in these risk prediction equations provide excellent discrimination of risk.[19] KFRE equations could help personalize CKD monitoring and treatment, but the KDIGO risk categories/heat map provides a general guide: low-risk CKD is suggested to have annual assessments, moderately high-risk, high-risk, and very high-risk recommend at least one, two, and three to four annual assessments, respectively.

	Albuminuria stage (mg/mmol)		
eGFR stage (ML/min/1.73m^2)	A1 <30 mg/g	A2 30–300 mg/g	A3 >300 mg/g
G1 (≥90)			
G2 (60–89)			
G3a (45–59)			
G3b (30–44)			
G4 (15–29)			
G5 (<15)			

FIG. 25.1 KDIGO CKD staging by GFR and uACR categories with color heat map. *eGFR*, estimated glomerular filtration rate. When used to predict kidney failure risk, green represents low risk and represents no CKD in the absence of known structural or histological evidence of kidney disease with implications for health, yellow is moderately increased risk, orange is high risk, and red is very high risk. Adapted from Kidney Disease: Improving Global Outcomes CKD Working Group. KDIGO 2024 clinical practice guideline for the evaluation and management of chronic kidney disease. *Kidney Int. 2024;105(4S):S117–S314.*.

Once kidney failure develops, nephrology services generally set up intensive multidisciplinary low clearance clinic systems to provide predialysis counseling and make the necessary preparations for an organized start of kidney replacement therapy or supportive care (aiming to avoid "crash-landing" onto dialysis). Historical trends in eGFR decline predicting a need to start kidney replacement therapy, and referrals for preparations are suggested about 1 year in advance.

PREVALENCE OF CHRONIC KIDNEY DISEASE

Globally, the crude prevalence of CKD in adults is about 9% to 12%,[20] slightly higher in women and in low- and middle-income countries.[21] In the United States, CKD prevalence appeared to plateau between 2004 and 2012 after years of increase,[21,22] and has remained stable (although the recent change to 2021 CKD-EPI eGFR formulas could have an important implication for these prevalence estimates).[23] Survey data from 2015 to 2018 show that the prevalence of an eGFR below 60 mL/min/1.73 m^2 or albuminuria (i.e., uACR > 30 mg/g) is evident in 14.4% of US adults based on a single measurement from the National Health and Nutrition Examination Survey. This 14.4% prevalence estimate included ~6.3% of adults with CKD stages G3–5 and 0.12% with kidney failure (i.e., stage G5). The prevalence of DM among surveyed participants with CKD was 33%, increasing to 47% among those with CKD stages G4–5. The prevalence of DM among individuals without CKD was 10%.[23]

DIAGNOSIS OF DIABETIC KIDNEY DISEASE

CKD prevalence data do not distinguish between CKD caused by DM versus another cause, and in patients with DM and CKD, the etiological diagnosis of CKD is often presumed. This is because a kidney biopsy is rarely performed in patients with DM and CKD to avoid the risk of procedural bleeding and because a tissue diagnosis is unlikely to alter the management.[24] The 2020 KDIGO Clinical Practice Guideline for Diabetes Management in CKD recognized this diagnostic limitation and avoided diabetic nephropathy and diabetic kidney disease as terms, instead referring even more nonspecifically to "patients with diabetes and CKD."

Historically, the term "diabetic nephropathy" has been used to refer to patients with overt proteinuria (i.e., ≥300 mg per day) attributed to traditional DM pathophysiology (i.e., glomerular hyperfiltration) and/or histology (i.e., classical glomerular features). Glomerular features of diabetic nephropathy range from mild glomerular capillary basement membrane thickening through mesangial expansion to classical nodular sclerosis. The term "diabetic kidney disease" recognizes the wider spectrum of renal pathological changes that DM and associated risk factors can cause. International pathological classifications include these vascular and interstitial features: vascular changes can include large-vessel arteriosclerosis and/or arteriolar hyalinosis. Interstitial changes may include interstitial fibrosis and tubular atrophy (known as IFTA) and/or interstitial inflammation.[24]

A clinical diagnosis of diabetic kidney disease is presumed when there has been DM present for a sufficient duration (usually at least 5 years in patients with type 1 DM) and/or there is evidence of other microvascular involvement (e.g., retinopathy, neuropathy). Features suggestive of another cause of CKD may prompt a kidney biopsy if a tissue diagnosis is likely to change the management. Reasons to consider a tissue diagnosis may include a sudden decrease in GFR; a sudden substantial increase in albuminuria with the development of nephrotic syndrome (i.e., >3.5 g proteinuria per day with hypoalbuminemia); nephritic syndrome (i.e., microscopic hematuria with hypertension, edema, and progressively decreasing GFR); or clinical features of a systemic disease which can involve the kidney and which has specific immunological or other management which generally requires histology for confirmation and/or disease staging (e.g., lupus or vasculitis).[24] The specific primary kidney diagnosis is, however, unlikely to modify approaches to CVD risk management.

ASSOCIATIONS BETWEEN CHRONIC KIDNEY DISEASE AND RISK OF DIFFERENT TYPES OF CARDIOVASCULAR DISEASE

Below an eGFR of about 60 mL/min/1.73 m^2, CVD mortality risk increases progressively with a decreasing eGFR. This has been suggested as part of the justification for the staging eGFR threshold for stage G3 and the use of "disease" in the term "CKD" (although some nephrologists disagree with the use of the term "disease" given how common an eGFR of below 60 mL/min/1.73 m^2 is at older age).[16]

Patients with DM have a higher risk of kidney failure for a given level of eGFR or albuminuria, but the shape of associations between eGFR and CVD mortality risk is the same in patients with and without DM,[4] emphasizing the importance of CKD as a predictor or, in fact, a cause of CVD.

The CVD mortality risk in CKD results from a range of different atherosclerotic and nonatherosclerotic CVD pathologies, with sudden cardiac death a particular feature in severe CKD.[25–27] The presence of CKD appears to accelerate the presentation and progression of CVD, and CVD may accelerate CKD progression. The relationships between CKD and different types of CVD are introduced below.

Coronary and Central Artery Disease in Chronic Kidney Disease

Coronary artery disease is common in CKD, partly as a result of a characteristic dyslipidemia which is similar to that observed in patients with DM.[6] In addition to lipid deposition, calcification of atherosclerotic plaque and the vascular intima is also a feature of severe CKD,[28] with arterial disease also accompanied by accelerated vascular media calcification. Vascular calcification is attributed to disordered calcium-phosphate metabolism, referred to as CKD-mineral bone disorder (CKD-MBD).[29,30] Management

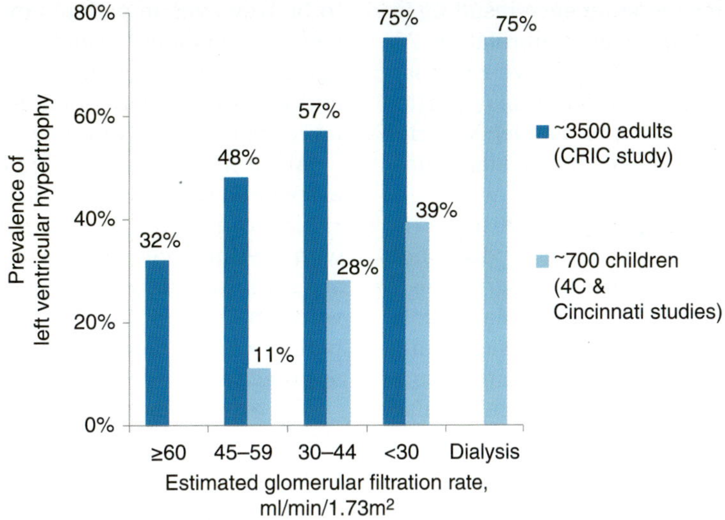

FIG. 25.2 Prevalence of left ventricular hypertrophy in adults and children with CKD. Data from Park M, Hsu CY, Li Y, et al. Associations between kidney function and subclinical cardiac abnormalities in CKD. *J Am Soc Nephrol*. 2012;23(10):1725–34. https://doi:10.1681/ASN.2012020145; Schaefer F, Doyon A, Azukaitis K, et al. Cardiovascular Phenotypes in Children with CKD: The 4C Study. *Clin J Am Soc Nephrol*. 2017;12(1):19–28. https://doi:10.2215/CJN.01090216 and Mitsnefes MM, Daniels SR, Schwartz SM, Meyer RA, Khoury P, Strife CF. Severe left ventricular hypertrophy in pediatric dialysis: prevalence and predictors. *Pediatr Nephrol*. 2000;14(10-11):898–902.

of the renal dyslipidemia and CKD-MBD are discussed in more detail later in this chapter.

A meta-analysis of observational studies shows that each 30% reduction in eGFR is associated with about a 30% increase in risk of atherosclerotic CVDs.[5] At a population level, the risk of myocardial infarction among patients with CKD and an eGFR of 45 mL/min/1.73 m^2 or more is similar to that of patients with established coronary artery disease or with DM, and exceeds that risk when eGFR declines to below 45 mL/min/1.73 m^2.[6] Furthermore, the risk of death after a myocardial infarction is increased three- to fourfold in patients with CKD compared to people free of both DM and CKD, and is increased fivefold in patients with both DM and CKD.[6]

In CKD, the initial clinical manifestation of coronary artery disease is also more likely to be a myocardial infarction than exertional angina.[31] Like in DM, myocardial infarction is more likely to present atypically, with less than half of patients with CKD reporting chest pain. Dyspnea and non-ST elevation electrocardiographic changes are common presentations.

In CKD, abdominal aortic aneurysm (AAA) risk is increased by about 30% compared to the general population (although this may be a bidirectional relationship with AAA and associated vascular disease causing CKD, as well as CKD and its associated-metabolic disturbances potentially causing AAAs). Experts suggest the indications for elective and emergent AAA repair are the same in people with and without CKD, although the risk of procedural complications is expected to be higher in CKD.[8]

Two moderately large trials found no important additional benefits of revascularization for renovascular disease above optimal medical therapy[8] (perhaps because proximal arterial disease represents a marker of more general ischemic nephropathy). Rare scenarios when revascularization may be considered have been proposed,[8] but well-meaning attempts to dilate renal artery stenoses may result in important complications, including permanent worsening of kidney function from distal cholesterol emboli. The revascularization of renal arteries should generally only be considered by experts or in a research setting.

Heart Failure in Chronic Kidney Disease

Heart failure in CKD may result from a combination of chronic pressure overload, including hypertension and increased arterial stiffness, progressive volume overload (from dysregulated sodium and water homeostasis), direct alterations in myocardial structure and function, as well as the potential for CKD to cause coronary artery disease, atrial fibrillation, and valvular disease.[7,32]

A recent cohort of patients with CKD and DM found a clinical history of heart failure to be apparent in about 14%,[33] but evidence of subclinical structural heart disease is much more common. Left ventricular hypertrophy emerges in early CKD stages and also affects children with CKD (Fig. 25.2).[34] After adjustment for confounders, CKD stages G4–5 in adults are associated with double the odds of left ventricular hypertrophy compared to individuals with an eGFR of at least 60 mL/min/1.73 m^2.[25] About one-half of adults with CKD stages G3–4 have structural abnormalities,[25] increasing to about three-quarters by the time kidney replacement therapy becomes indicated.[35,36] In children with CKD, about two-fifths with an eGFR below 30 mL/min/1.73 m^2 have evidence of left ventricular hypertrophy.[34] Cardiomyocyte death and myocardial fibrosis are also apparent in CKD, predisposing to both systolic and diastolic cardiac dysfunction.[32,37]

Valvular Disease in Chronic Kidney Disease

The risk of valvular calcification is approximately doubled in patients with CKD, with about one-quarter of patients exhibiting evidence of mitral or aortic calcification (compared to about 11% of patients with DM).[38] Progression of calcification is also often rapid in patients with CKD, with any subsequent development of symptomatic aortic stenosis with left ventricular pressure overload contributing to heart failure risk,[39] and any mitral valve annular calcification potentially causing incompetence resulting in volume overload and increased risk of atrial fibrillation. As many as one in five patients with CKD may have a history of atrial fibrillation.[9] In CKD, atrial fibrillation may particularly contribute to heart failure symptoms if left ventricular hypertrophy has resulted in left ventricular filling becoming more reliant on atrial contraction.

Optimal management of valvular heart disease in CKD remains uncertain. Statin-based therapy does not appear to influence valvular heart disease progression,[40] or indeed risk of heart failure.[41] Although valvular calcification is associated with arterial calcification, suggesting CKD-MBD is a common pathogenic mechanism,[42] suppressing parathyroid hormone levels with cinacalcet also does not appear to modify risk of CVD.[43] Furthermore, surgical interventions for aortic and mitral valve disease are associated with substantially higher risk of complications and mortality in CKD.[38] Strategies for managing atrial fibrillation in CKD are considered below.

Sudden Cardiac Death

As GFR declines below about 45 mL/min/1.73 m^2, nonatherosclerotic events begin to account for a relatively larger proportion of total CVD events than atherosclerotic CVD.[31] Arrhythmias associated with both nonatherosclerotic and atherosclerotic disease contribute to the high risk of sudden death in CKD. The hemodialysis population is an extreme phenotype of CKD, where sudden cardiac death accounts for a third of deaths.[9] Bradyarrythmias and asystole may be common, as well as ventricular tachyarrythmias. Rapid changes in volume and electrolytes which accompany hemodialysis may contribute to the excess risk of death after longer interdialytic intervals (e.g., before the first dialysis session of the week).[44] As already introduced, multiple predisposing factors for an arrythmogenic heart exist in predialysis CKD, including left ventricular hypertrophy and myocardial fibrosis, fluid overload, and myocardial ischemia with vascular calcification.[9] Decreased eGFR is a predictor of intracardiac conduction defects and also arrhythmias after a myocardial infarction.[45] Although more data are needed to assess long-term risk-benefits, recent expert opinion suggests patients with CKD should be considered for implantable cardioverter defibrillators for secondary prevention, and for primary prevention in patients with a left ventricular ejection fraction of ≤35%.[9]

Stroke and Atrial Fibrillation in Chronic Kidney Disease

CKD is also associated with increased risk of all forms of stroke, with incident stroke risk compared to the general population increased by three- to sevenfold through CKD stages G3–5. CKD is also associated with increased stroke severity, worse stroke outcomes, and vascular cognitive impairment.[46]

The evidence base for stroke treatment and prevention in CKD is limited, particularly in severe CKD where risk is highest. Intravenous thrombolysis administered within the first 4.5 hours after onset of an ischemic stroke results in better functional outcomes. A meta-analysis shows this to be true even in patients over the age of 80 years, when CKD is common.[47] Guidelines suggesting thrombolysis use in eligible patients with CKD without restriction are endorsed by expert opinion, despite some potential for increased risk of symptomatic intracerebral hemorrhage.[46]

Atrial fibrillation is common in CKD, and CKD is also associated with increased risk of thromboembolism.[9] Algorithms for rate versus rhythm control have been proposed, with rhythm control only suggested in CKD for those who are symptomatic with short duration of atrial fibrillation, with small left atrial size and/or reversible causes, with patient choice dictating medical versus catheter ablation approaches.[9]

There is major scope to improve thromboembolic stroke risk prediction in CKD,[46] but based on the currently available scores, most patients with DM and CKD will have a CHA_2DS_2-VASc score of ≥2 and be considered for prophylactic anticoagulation. Down to an eGFR of about 25 mL/min/1.73 m^2, direct oral anticoagulants (DOACs; e.g., apixaban) have been shown to be noninferior to warfarin with respect to ischemic stroke prevention, and may reduce the risk of intracranial hemorrhage compared to warfarin.[46] With appropriate dose reduction, some DOACs have regulatory approval to be used in CKD stage 5 (including those on dialysis).[9] DOACs also have the benefits of reduced need for monitoring and avoiding the potential for warfarin to accelerate vascular calcification through inhibition of phosphate scavenging by the vitamin K-dependent enzyme matrix gamma-carboxyglutamate Gla protein.[46]

Intensive blood pressure lowering and LDL-cholesterol lowering are expected to reduce ischemic stroke risk in CKD (see next section). Primary prevention of ischemic stroke with low-dose aspirin in patients with DM and CKD has not been demonstrated to be of net benefit (see section on antiplatelet therapy below).

GENERAL MANAGEMENT STRATEGIES TO LOWER THE RISK OF KIDNEY FAILURE OR CVD IN PATIENTS WITH DM AND CKD

The management of CVD risk in patients with CKD and DM considers both traditional[48,49] and CKD-specific risk factors which result from the associated-metabolic disturbances (summarized in Fig. 25.3).[61] In this section, we describe the evidence base for lifestyle modification, management of dyslipidemia, and intensive glycemic and blood pressure control.

Lifestyle Recommendations in Chronic Kidney Disease

A raised body mass index is independently associated with risk of CKD,[62,63] and a randomized trial of behavioral interventions to promote weight loss in patients with type 2 DM appeared to reduce the risk of developing very high-risk CKD over the long term.[64] In addition, it has been recommended that all patients with DM and CKD receive standard advice on smoking, nutrition, and exercise.[10]

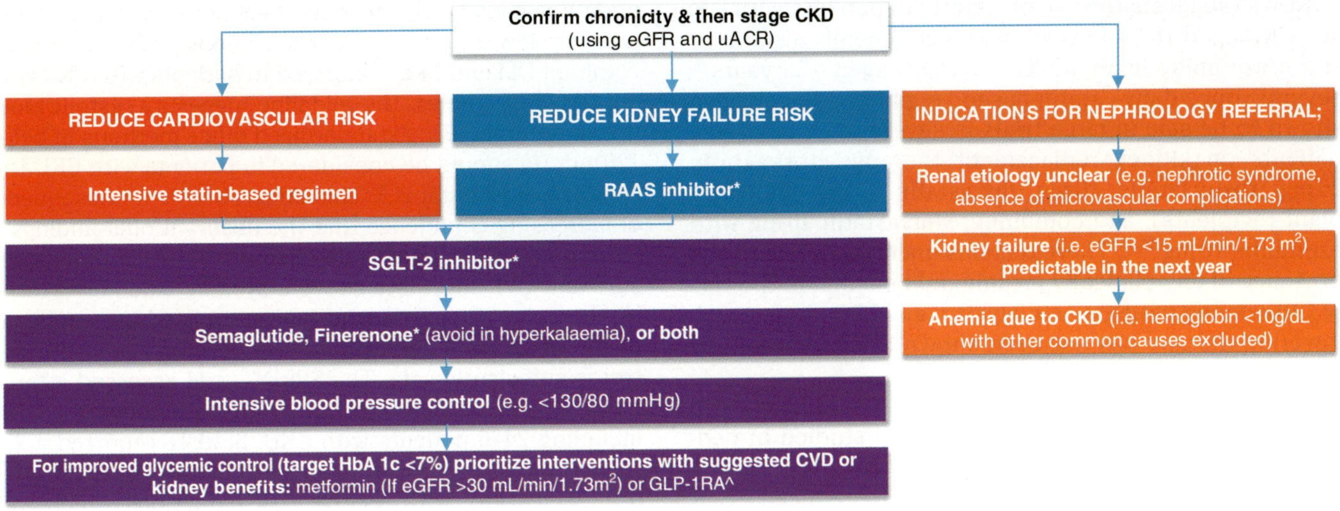

FIG. 25.3 Treatment algorithm for managing cardiovascular disease (*CVD*) and kidney failure risk in patients with type 2 diabetes mellitus (*DM*) and chronic kidney disease (*CKD*). *Sodium-glucose cotransporter-2 (*SGLT-2*) inhibitors,[50,51] renin-angiotensin-aldosterone system (*RAAS*) inhibitors[52,53] the nonsteroidal mineralocorticoid receptor antagonist finerenone[54] have been shown to be particularly effective at reducing risk of kidney failure when albuminuria is present (e.g., urine albumin-to-creatinine ratio ≥30 mg/g). Glucagon-like peptide-1 receptor agonist (*GLP-1RA*)[55] with semaglutide has been shown to reduce CVD risk and slow progression of kidney function loss in proteinuric diabetic kidney disease.[56] ^Metformin is suggested to have cardioprotective properties.[57] Antidiabetic medications with neutral or no proven benefit on risk of CVD or kidney failure in CKD include dipeptidyl peptidase-4 (*DPP-4*) inhibitors,[58] insulin, and sulfonylureas. Note that RAAS inhibitors may also reduce the risk of CVD in patients with type 2 DM and CKD, but definitive evidence from trials is limited to a possible reduction in the risk on hospitalization for heart failure from a single trial.[53] Intensive blood pressure–lowering regimens reduce the risk of CVD, but definitive evidence from a trial that it also reduces the risk of kidney failure is also unavailable.[59,60] Emdin CA, Rahimi K, Neal B, Callender T, Perkovic V, Patel A. Blood pressure lowering in type 2 diabetes: a systematic review and meta-analysis. *JAMA*. 2015;313(6):603–15. https://doi:10.1001/jama.2014.18574 and Ettehad D, Emdin CA, Kiran A, et al. Blood pressure lowering for prevention of cardiovascular disease and death: a systematic review and meta-analysis. *Lancet*. 2016;387(10022):957–967. https://doi:10.1016/S0140-6736(15)01225-8.

Management of Hyperglycemia in Chronic Kidney Disease

Hyperglycemia is strongly associated with the risk of mortality from CVD and kidney failure,[65–67] as are higher levels of glycosylated hemoglobin (HbA1c).[68] A meta-analysis of four large-scale trials of intensive versus standard glycemic control which includes 27,049 patients with type 2 DM by the Collaborators on Trials of Lowering Glucose (CONTROL) group has shown that the ~0.9% achieved average difference in HbA1c (lowered from 7.7% to 6.8%) over about 5 years reduced the risk of any major cardiovascular event of about 9% (hazard ratio [HR], 0.91; 95% confidence interval [CI], 0.84–0.99). This included a 15% relative risk reduction for myocardial infarction (HR, 0.85; 95% CI, 0.76–0.94), but no clear effects on risk of heart failure or stroke.[69] Five years of intensive glycemic control also reduced the risk of kidney events, particularly the risk of developing or worsening of "diabetic nephropathy" based on measures of albuminuria.[57,70,71] Definitive evidence that this translates into the reduced risk of kidney failure is unavailable, but personalized HbA1c glycemic targets between <6.5% (48 mmol/mol) and <8.0% (64 mmol/mol) are suggested for patients with CKD and DM, with a target <7.0% (53 mmol/mol) still recommended particularly to reduce microvascular complications, wherever possible.[57,70] How these targets might be safely achieved pharmacologically while maximizing CVD benefits is introduced later in this chapter.

In CKD, HbA1c monitoring may be less reliable at eGFRs below 30 mL/min/1.73 m^2 because of shortened red cell life span, and suggestions have been made to increase the use of self-monitoring or continuous glucose monitoring if trying to safely achieve tight glycemic control in such patients.[10]

Management of Dyslipidemia in Chronic Kidney Disease

The dyslipidemia in CKD is characterized by high circulating triglycerides with increased numbers of very-low-density lipoprotein and intermediate-density lipoprotein particles, plus low levels of high-density lipoprotein cholesterol. Low-density lipoprotein (LDL) cholesterol may not be particularly elevated, but an increased proportion of small oxidized LDL particles and increased apolipoprotein B are observed.[72]

Meta-analyses by the Cholesterol Treatment Trialists' Collaboration of large-scale trials of statin-based therapy including 183,419 participants have shown that the relative risk of major vascular events (i.e., coronary death, nonfatal myocardial infarction, ischemic stroke, and coronary revascularization) is reduced by 21% per 1.0 mmol/L (39 mg/dL) lower LDL-cholesterol in patients with or without DM (relative risk [RR], 0.79; 95% CI, 0.77–0.81).[73,74] In moderate-to-severe CKD a trend toward smaller relative reductions per unit reduction in LDL-cholesterol on major vascular events emerges, but clear benefits remain in patients not on dialysis. The high baseline vascular risk at lower eGFR means that these smaller proportion reductions translate into important absolute risk reductions. The diminution in relative risk reduction as GFR declines and the high risk of atherosclerotic CVD in CKD despite relatively normal levels of LDL-cholesterol implies that intensive LDL-cholesterol-lowering regimens are required to maximize the LDL-cholesterol reduction and confer maximum benefits. The dyslipidemia management strategy in patients with CKD and DM should be to achieve the largest possible absolute reduction in LDL-cholesterol safely.[74,75]

KDIGO suggests the use of a statin in patients with DM and CKD aged 18 to 49 years and recommends a statin or statin/ezetimibe in all adults with CKD aged ≥50 years.[76] Several once-daily statin-based regimens have been shown to be safe in large trials in severe CKD, including patients on kidney replacement therapy: atorvastatin 20 mg, rosuvastatin 10 mg, fluvastatin 40 mg (in transplant recipients), and combining simvastatin 20 mg with ezetimibe 10 mg.[77–81] There remains uncertainty about the presence of any clinically meaningful benefits on the risk of CVD among patients on dialysis,[74] and LDL-cholesterol-lowering therapy has not been shown to prevent kidney failure.[79,82]

The effects of proprotein convertase subtilisin/kexin type 9 (PCSK9) inhibitors have not been studied in dedicated trials of moderate-to-severe CKD, but 10,081 patients with DM and 4443 patients with reduced eGFR (i.e., CKD stage G3+, median eGFR 51 mL/min/173 m^2) were randomized into the 27,563 participant FOURIER placebo-controlled trial of evolocumab. A CKD subgroup analysis of FOURIER showed that evolocumab safely reduced LDL-C by 58% (below 40 mg/dL), and the overall 15% relative risk reduction on atherosclerotic CVD events (RR, 0.85; 0.79–0.92) was similar in participants with and without evidence of a decreased eGFR.[82]

Blood Pressure Lowering in Chronic Kidney Disease

Systemic hypertension usually accompanies decreased eGFR due to a range of mechanisms. These include shared causes, such as obesity, and CKD-associated changes in vascular biology, such as increased arterial stiffness and activation of the renin-angiotensin-aldosterone system with dysregulated salt and water homeostasis.

Increased systemic blood pressure is causally linked to the risk of CVD. Meta-analyses by the Blood Pressure Lowering Treatment Trialists' Collaboration of 152,290 participants from large trials have shown that lowering blood pressure reduces the risk of major cardiovascular events (i.e., death from CVD, nonfatal myocardial infarction, stroke, or heart failure) by about 17% per 5 mm Hg lower systolic blood pressure (RR, 0.89; 0.93–0.95). These relative benefits appeared to be irrespective of the choice of antihypertensive drug and are apparent in the 30,295 included participants with an eGFR < 60 mL/min/1.73 m^2.[49]

In other meta-analyses restricted to 100,354 trial participants with type 2 DM, the CVD benefits of intensive blood pressure lowering have been demonstrated, with particularly large reductions in the risk of stroke.[59] Relative risk reductions per 10 mm Hg lower systolic blood pressure on the risk of CVD were greater in those with a starting systolic value of at least 140 mm Hg, but reductions in the risk of stroke were evident with further reductions in systolic blood pressure among those with a baseline level of below 140 mm Hg.[59]

The randomized trial data in patients with DM and CKD suggest that a systolic blood pressure target of below 130 mm Hg is clinically appropriate. The 2021 KDIGO Management of Blood Pressure in the CKD Clinical Practice Guideline update acknowledged that the benefits of intensive blood pressure lowering are less certain among patients with concomitant DM and CKD compared to patients with CKD without DM. Nevertheless the guideline suggests a systolic blood pressure target using standardized office methods of below 120 mm Hg should be considered in patients with CKD irrespective of DM status.[83] This suggestion is a consequence of increasing confidence that the observational findings of clear positive log-linear relationships between blood pressure and CVD mortality above a systolic value of ~115 mm Hg represent causal associations (supported by genetic epidemiology),[84] and achieving intensive blood pressure control is sufficiently safe. The SPRINT trial assessed a target of <120 versus <140 mm Hg in 9361 patients without DM, including 2446 patients with CKD. SPRINT reported a 25% reduction in the risk of major cardiovascular events (HR, 0.75; 0.64–0.89), with relative risk reductions which were similar in participants with and without CKD.[85]

Higher blood pressure is observationally associated with risk of CKD progression[86] and kidney failure.[87,88] Accelerated phase hypertension causes histological glomerular arteriolar changes which can manifest as acute kidney injury and/or CKD. At such high levels of systemic blood pressure, protection from the kidney's blood flow autoregulation systems begins to be lost.

In DM, the presence of hyperglycemia dysregulates homeostatic tubuloglomerular feedback, blunting kidney blood flow autoregulation and increasing the kidney's susceptibility to moderate elevations in systemic blood pressure. The combination of DM and early hypertension may be sufficient to induce glomerular hyperfiltration and albuminuria. These changes are considered a precursor for the histological changes of diabetic kidney disease and later eGFR decline. Randomized trial data demonstrating that lowering systolic blood pressure below 140 mm Hg in patients with DM reduces albuminuria are consistent with this concept.[59] Whether such reductions in albuminuria translate into long-term prevention of kidney failure has not been confirmed.[59,60]

Prioritizing the use of blood pressure-lowering agents that favorably modify intraglomerular hemodynamics is recommended in patients with DM and CKD.[83] Inhibitors of sodium-glucose cotransporter-2 (SGLT-2) reduce intraglomerular pressure through restoring tubuloglomerular feedback and reducing glomerular afferent arteriolar tone.[89] Inhibitors of the renin-angiotensin-aldosterone system (RAAS) pathway act on the glomerular efferent arterioles, reducing tone and consequently also reducing intraglomerular pressure (Fig. 25.4).

SPECIFIC PHARMACOLOGICAL AGENTS SHOWN TO LOWER THE RISK OF KIDNEY FAILURE AND/OR CVD IN PATIENTS WITH CKD AND DM

Large placebo-controlled trials that specifically recruited patients with type 2 DM and CKD have confirmed important kidney benefits of RAAS inhibitors (i.e., angiotensin-converting enzyme inhibitors or angiotensin-II receptor

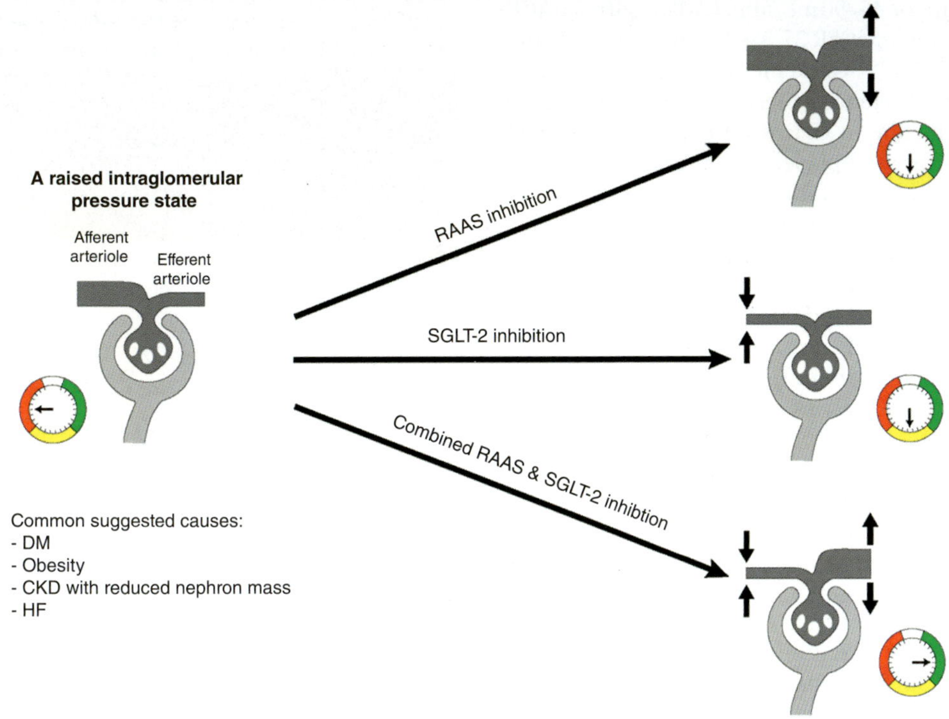

FIG. 25.4 Hemodynamic effects of RAAS inhibitors and SGLT-2 inhibitors on glomerular arterioles and intraglomerular pressure. *CKD*, Chronic kidney disease; *DM*, diabetes mellitus; *HF*, heart failure; *RAAS*, renin-angiotensin-aldosterone system; *SGLT-2*, sodium-glucose co-transporter-2. From Herrington et al. The potential for improving cardio-renal outcomes by sodium-glucose co-transporter-2 inhibition in people with chronic kidney disease: a rationale for the EMPA-KIDNEY study. *Clin Kidney J.* 2018;11(6):749–761.

blockers), SGLT-2 inhibitors, and the nonsteroidal mineralocorticoid receptor antagonist, finerenone. Semaglutide also slows the rate of kidney function loss in diabetic kidney disease.[56] These interventions could be started early to prevent the development and or progression of end-organ damage in those identified to be at risk (see Fig. 25.2).

Inhibitors of the Renin-Angiotensin-Aldosterone System in Chronic Kidney Disease

Three key randomized trials of inhibitors of the RAAS system with an angiotensin-converting enzyme inhibitor or angiotensin-receptor-2 blocker reduce the risk of kidney failure in patients with DM and overt nephropathy.[52,53,90] Two moderately sized trials have demonstrated that angiotensin-receptor-2 blockers slow the progression from microalbuminuria to overt nephropathy in patients with DM with less degrees of albuminuria.[91,92] RAAS inhibitors are therefore recommended for use in patients with DM as soon as the first clinical indication of CKD is evident and it is considered reasonable to treat patients with CKD with high blood pressure with a RAAS inhibitor in the absence of albuminuria.[83] Combining an angiotensin-converting enzyme inhibitor with an angiotensin-receptor-2 blocker, or with a direct renin-inhibitor, however, is not currently recommended. Large trials have identified an increased risk of hyperkalemia and acute kidney injury without demonstrable additional benefits of this "dual-blockade" approach on the risk of kidney failure or CVD.[93,94]

Neprilysin is an enzyme which cleaves peptides, including natriuretic peptides, and is particularly expressed in the kidney. Its inhibition results in both natriuresis and vasodilation, which lowers systemic blood pressure. As neprilysin inhibitors have the potential to activate the RAAS,[95] they are combined with an ARB. The combined angiotensin receptor-nephrilysin inhibitor sacubitril-valsartan reduces the risk of death from CVD or hospitalization for heart failure in patients with heart failure with reduced ejection fraction.[96] ARNis may be commonly used in heart failure clinics and are safe to use in CKD (down to at least 20 mL/min/1.73 m^2), but CKD is not an indication for ARNI prescription: in a phase 2 trial in CKD, sacubitril-valsartan safely reduced blood pressure and cardiac biomarkers, but there was no clear evidence that it offered nephroprotection above that provided by irbesartan alone.[97]

Sodium-Glucose Cotransporter-2 Inhibitors in Chronic Kidney Disease

Combining an SGLT-2 inhibitor with an RAAS inhibitor clearly reduces the risk of kidney failure and hospitalization for heart failure patients with type 2 DM and CKD.[50,51] The CREDENCE, DAPA-CKD, and EMPA-KIDNEY placebo-controlled trials were all stopped early for efficacy while testing cardiorenal primary outcomes with canagliflozin, dapagliflozin, and empagliflozin, respectively. CREDENCE recruited patients with diabetic kidney disease with an eGFR of 30 to 90 mL/min/1.73 m^2 and a uACR of 300 to 5000 mg/g (mean eGFR 56 $\pm$ 18 mL/min/1.73 m^2; median uACR 927 mg/g), while DAPA-CKD recruited patients with CKD and an eGFR of 25 to 75 mL/min/1.73 m^2 and a uACR of 200 to 5000 mg/g (mean eGFR 43 $\pm$ 18 mL/min/1.73 m^2; median uACR 949 mg/g),[50,51] and EMPA-KIDNEY provided evidence at low levels of eGFR and uACR (eligibility

20–45 mL/min/1.73 m² or 45–90 mL/min/1.73 m² with a uACR of at least 200 mg/g; mean eGFR 37.3 ± 14.5 mL/min/1.73 m²; median uACR 329 mg/g).[98,99] Once meta-analyzed according to a composite kidney disease progression outcome based on at least a 50% decline in GFR from baseline, the need for maintenance kidney replacement therapy or death from kidney failure, SGLT-2 inhibitors have been shown to reduce such renal risk by 37% (HR, 0.63; 0.58–0.69).[100] This reduction in relative risk was consistent irrespective of diabetes status and across the different types of kidney disease studied.[101] EMPA-KIDNEY demonstrated renal benefits across the full range of GFR included, even at the lowest levels.[98,99] This indicates that SGLT-2i should be prescribed widely in CKD to modify the risk of kidney failure and can be continued until the need to start kidney replacement therapy despite low eGFR substantially attenuating their HbA1c-lowering effect.[102] Although the EMPA-KIDNEY trial was too short to demonstrate key benefits on its primary outcome directly in those with low uACR, the exploration of the annual rate of progression of kidney function suggests renoprotection is evident even in the absence of albuminuria. We recommend the initiation of an SGLT-2 inhibitor in patients with type 2 DM following the first clinical evidence of CKD.[98] There are also clear benefits of SGLT-2i on the risk of hospitalization for heart failure (Table 25.2)[103] and CVD death.[100] The effect on CVD death appears to reduce from reductions in the risk of heart failure death and sudden cardiac death, with less clear effect on myocardial infarction (once data from large trials are combined) and no effect on stroke.[104]

SGLT-2 inhibitors also appear to reduce the risk of acute kidney injury,[100,103] and so any acute decline in eGFR on commencing an SGLT-2 inhibitor should not routinely prompt their cessation (and we suggest checking kidney function shortly after commencing an SGLT-2 inhibitor is not routinely needed).

From a safety perspective, SGLT-2 inhibitors approximately double the risk of ketoacidosis in patients with diabetes, but as the absolute risk is low in patients with type 2 DM, there is a clear net benefit of SGLT-2 inhibitors.[103] By virtue of their high absolute risk of cardiovascular death, heart failure complications, kidney disease progression, and acute kidney injury, the net absolute benefits may be particularly large in patients with type 2 DM and CKD, particularly if they have albuminuria (see Table 25.2).

In patients with type 1 DM and CKD, baseline ketoacidosis risk is high and so a doubling of an already high risk is a safety concern. There is an absence of large trials with sufficient follow-up time to assess whether any absolute benefits of SGLT-2 inhibitors on kidney failure and CVD outcomes are outweighed by the high absolute risk of ketoacidosis with SGLT-2 inhibitors.[103,105] There is a pathophysiological rationale and supportive GFR slope data from EMPA-KIDNEY to propose that renal benefits of SGLT2 inhibitors would be retained in diabetic kidney disease in type 1 DM,[99] but safety concerns means use of SGLT-2 inhibitors in type 1 DM is limited to specialists in selected patients, and requires availability of a ketone meter to facilitate rapid detection of ketosis.

TABLE 25.2 Estimates of Net Effects per 1000 Patient-Years of an SGLT-2 Inhibitor, by Types of Patient Recruited into Trials

	ESTIMATED ABSOLUTE EFFECTS PER 1000 PATIENT-YEARS OF AN SGLT-2 INHIBITOR (STANDARD ERROR)	
OUTCOMES	TYPE 2 DM AND HIGH CVD RISK TRIALS	PROTEINURIC CKD TRIALS (MAINLY TYPE 2 DM)
Benefits		
Kidney disease progression	−3 (0.3)	−18 (1)
Heart failure hospitalization	−3 (0.2)	−6 (0.4)
Cardiovascular death	−2 (0.4)	−3 (0.6)
Acute kidney injury	−1 (0.2)	−5 (0.7)
Harms		
Ketoacidosis	0.3 (0.1)	0.3 (0.1)
Amputation	0.7 (0.3)	1 (0.7)

Patient group-specific absolute effects estimated by applying the overall relative risk to the average event rate in the placebo arms.
Adapted from Staplin N, Roddick AJ, Emberson J, et al. Net effects of sodium-glucose co-transporter-2 inhibition in different patient groups: a meta-analysis of large placebo-controlled randomized trials. *EClinicalMedicine*. 2021;41:101163. doi:10.1016/j.eclinm.2021.101163

Nonsteroidal Mineralocorticoid Receptor Antagonists in Chronic Kidney Disease

Steroidal mineralocorticoid receptor antagonists reduce blood pressure and albuminuria in patients with CKD but have not been definitively shown to slow kidney disease progression.[106] Instead, placebo-controlled FIDELIO-DKD and FIGARO-DKD trials specifically tested a nonsteroidal mineralocorticoid receptor antagonist and demonstrated that finerenone reduced the risk of kidney failure and CVD in patients with CKD and type 2 DM already on maximal RAAS inhibition.[54,107,108] FIDELIO-DKD demonstrated reductions in the risk of a categorical kidney outcome, a composite combining kidney failure and a sustained decline in an eGFR of ≥40%, in patients with an eGFR 25 to 60 mL/min/1.73 m² and a uACR of 30 to 5000 mg/g, or an eGFR 60 to 75 mL/min/1.73 m² with a uACR of 300 to 5000 mg/g.[107] FIGARO-DKD demonstrated reductions in the risk of CVD, and particularly heart failure events, using a primary composite outcome of CVD death, nonfatal myocardial infarction, nonfatal stroke, or hospitalization for heart failure, in patients with eGFR 25 to 60 mL/min/1.73 m² and a uACR of 30 to 5000 mg/g, or an eGFR over 60 mL/min/1.73 m² with a uACR of 300 to 5000 mg/g.[108] Pooling data from the two trials found the kidney failure risk was reduced by 16% (HR, 0.84; 0.71–0.99) and hospitalization for heart failure by 22% (HR, 0.78; 0.66–0.92; Fig. 25.5).[54] Finerenone has not been studied in sufficient numbers of participants to confirm whether this translates into a reduced risk of death from CVD.

Information on the efficacy of combining mineralocorticoid receptor antagonists with SGLT-2 inhibitors in CKD are limited as only ~4% of FIDELIO-DKD, ~8% of FIGARO-DKD, ~5% of DAPA-CKD, and no CREDENCE participants were prescribed such a combination.[50,107,108,109] Subgroup analyses from the SGLT-2 inhibitor trials in

Outcome	Finerenone (n = 6519)		Placebo (n = 6507)		Hazard ratio (95% CI)		P-value[a]
	Number of patients with event (%)	Number of patients with event per 100 patient-years	Number of patients with event (%)	Number of patients with event per 100 patient-years			
Composite cardiovascular outcome[b]	825 (12.7)	4.34	939 (14.4)	5.01		0.86 (0.78–0.95)	0.0018
Death from cardiovascular causes	322 (4.9)	1.61	364 (5.6)	1.84		0.88 (0.76–1.02)	0.092
Non fatal myocardial infarction	173 (2.7)	0.88	189 (2.9)	0.97		0.91 (0.74–1.12)	0.36
Non fatal stroke	198 (3.0)	1.01	198 (3.0)	1.02		0.99 (0.82–1.21)	0.95
Hospitalization for heart failure	256 (3.9)	1.31	325 (5.0)	1.68		0.78 (0.66–0.92)	0.0030
eGFR ≥57% composite kidney outcome[c]	360 (5.5)	1.96	465 (7.1)	2.55		0.77 (0.67–0.88)	0.0002
Kidney failure	254 (3.9)	1.38	297 (4.6)	1.62		0.84 (0.71–0.99)	0.039
End-stage kidney disease[d]	151 (2.3)	0.76	188 (2.9)	0.96		0.80 (0.64–0.99)	0.040[e]
Sustained decrease in eGFR to <15 mL/min/1.73 m^2	195 (3.0)	1.06	237 (3.6)	1.29		0.81 (0.67–0.98)	0.026[e]
Sustained ≥57% decrease in eGFR from baseline	257 (3.9)	1.40	361 (5.5)	4.03		0.70 (0.60–0.83)	<0.0001
Renal death	2 (<0.1)	0.01	4 (<0.1)	0.02		0.53 (0.10–2.91)	0.46[e]
eGFR ≥40% composite kidney outcome[f]	854 (13.1)	4.81	995 (15.3)	5.64		0.85 (0.77–0.93)	0.0004
Sustained ≥40% decrease in eGFR from baseline	817 (12.5)	4.60	962 (14.8)	5.45		0.84 (0.76–0.92)	0.0002
Death from any cause	552 (8.5)	2.76	614 (9.4)	3.10		0.89 (0.79–>1.00[g])	0.051[e]
Hospitalization for any cause	2836 (43.5)	19.04	2926 (45.0)	19.91		0.96 (0.91–1.01)	0.087[e]

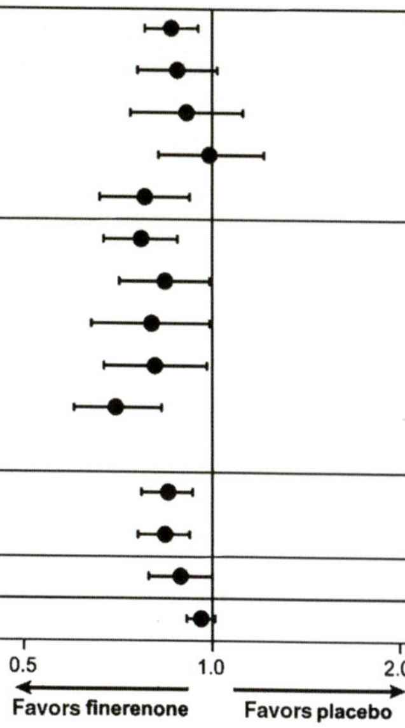

FIG. 25.5 Pooled analyses FIDELIO-DKD and FIGARO-DKD. *eGFR*, estimated glomerular filtration rate. Reproduced from Agarwal et al. *Eur Heart J*. 2022; 43(6):474–484.

heart failure, where mineralocorticoid receptor antagonist coprescription was more common, found that mineralocorticoid receptor antagonist use did not modify key analyses' findings.[110–112]

FIDELIO-DKD and FIGARO-DKD excluded patients with a potassium of >4.8 mmol/L, as mineralocorticoid receptor antagonists cause hyperkalemia.[107,108] Unlike dual RAAS blockade with an ACEi plus ARB, adding finerenone to a RAAS inhibitor did not increase the risk of serious acute kidney injury. The finerenone trials in proteinuric CKD attributed to type 2 DM implemented careful algorithmic potassium monitoring and found that whether based on laboratory data or investigator reports, the risk for hyperkalemia was approximately double compared to a placebo. Permanent withdrawal of finerenone versus a placebo for hyperkalemia was 1.7% versus 0.6%, but serious hyperkalemia was relatively rare, with a <1% excess risk for hospitalization for serious hyperkalemia over 3 years of follow-up. Risk factors for hyperkalemia were higher baseline potassium and lower eGFR. Concomitant diuretics or an SGLT-2 inhibitor were both associated with a lower risk for hyperkalemia. This observation is consistent with findings from trials of SGLT-2 inhibitors in heart failure populations where combining RAAS inhibitors and SGLT-2 inhibitors does not appear to cause hyperkalemia,[50,51,94,112,113,115] and SGLT-2 inhibitors may reduce the risk of severe hyperkalemia among MRA users.[112,113] Large trials combining an aldosterone synthase inhibitors and SGLT-2 inhibitors are planned.[116]

In summary, large trial evidence supports the addition of finerenone to treatment with a RAAS inhibitor in patients with type 2 DM and proteinuria (i.e., urine albumin-to-creatinine ratio of at least 30 mg/g) provided the additional blood monitoring and the risk of serious hyperkalemia are acceptable.[107,108] The trials of finerenone did not recruit patients with type 1 DM, but extrapolating the efficacy findings, the intervention may be useful in patients with type 1 DM at the risk of kidney disease progression, among whom the use of an SGLT-2 inhibitor may be considered unsafe.

CHOICE OF ANTIDIABETIC AGENTS IN PATIENTS WITH DIABETES MELLITUS AND CHRONIC KIDNEY DISEASE

GLUCAGON-LIKE PEPTIDE-1 RECEPTOR AGONIST (GLP-1 RA) IN CHRONIC KIDNEY DISEASE

SGLT-2 inhibitors should be prioritized for use in patients with type 2 DM and CKD. Their blood glucose-lowering effects are, however, substantially attenuated once eGFR falls below about 45 mL/min/1.73 m^2 (despite beneficial effects on CVD and kidney failure risk are clearly preserved at low eGFR).[102] We recommend prioritizing the use of GLP-1RA in diabetic kidney disease. Key evidence is provided by the FLOW trial which randomized 3533 participants with CKD at the risk of progression (mean body mass index is 32 kg/m^2) to subcutaneous semaglutide versus a matching placebo and was stopped early for efficacy. The prespecified composite primary outcome was kidney failure, a sustained decline of ≥50% in eGFR from the baseline, or death from kidney or cardiovascular causes. Over 3.4 years, the allocation to semaglutide resulted in a 24% (HR, 0.76; 0.88–0.66) reduction in the risk of the primary composite outcome. Semaglutide also reduced the risk of major cardiovascular events by 18% (HR, 0.82; 0.68–0.98), including cardiovascular death by 29% (HR, 0.71; 0.56–0.89).[56] There were notable reductions in weight by an average of 4.1 kg and improvements in glycated hemoglobin by −0.81%.[56] GLP-1RAs do cause nausea and other gastrointestinal disturbances,[117] yet with the semaglutide dose studied in FLOW (1.0 mg/week initiated with an 8-week dose escalation), the medication was reasonably tolerated.[56] Before FLOW, GLP1-RAs were already known to safely improve glycemic control and weight and reduce CVD risk in patients with type 2 diabetes and early CKD.[55] The GLP-1RA dulaglutide has been tested in CKD stages G3–4 in patients with type 2 DM. It was shown to be as effective at lowering HbA1c as insulin glargine and to have lower rates of symptomatic hypoglycemia, reduced weight, and a slowed rate of eGFR decline compared to insulin glargine.[118] These trials provide evidence to justify that GLP-1RAs are prioritized ahead of insulin in patients with type 2 DM and CKD (see Fig. 25.3), and semaglutide should be used for its effect on cardiorenal risk.

METFORMIN IN CHRONIC KIDNEY DISEASE

The evidence that metformin may favorably modify CVD risk comes from subgroup analyses and long-term follow-up of the United Kingdom Prospective Diabetes Study in a population of patients with newly diagnosed diabetes without CVD.[57,119,120] Extrapolating these data, an argument for prioritizing the use of metformin ahead of other sulfonylureas and insulin has been made. However, below an eGFR of 30 mL/min/1.73 m^2, metformin should generally be stopped to avoid the risk of lactic acidosis due to its accumulation.[120,121] Above an eGFR of 30 mL/min/1.73 m^2, metformin with an appropriate dose adjustment can still be used to manage hyperglycemia in CKD without the risk of hypoglycemia. If used at eGFRs between 30 and 45 mL/min/1.73 m^2, a maximum daily dose of about 500 to 1000 mg per day is suggested based on pharmacokinetic considerations (and 500 mg per day for selected patients with an eGFR < 30 mL/min/1.73 m^2).[122]

OTHER ANTIDIABETIC THERAPIES IN CHRONIC KIDNEY DISEASE

The dipeptidyl peptidase-4 (DPP-4) inhibitor linagliptin has been extensively studied in CKD and can be safely used even in severe CKD to lower blood glucose. Large-scale placebo-controlled trials show, however, that they do not meaningfully reduce the risk of CVD or kidney failure.[58] Sulfonylurea treatment (e.g., gliclazide) is a potentially cheaper alternative to DPP-4 inhibitors to improve glycemic control in CKD, with an appropriate dose reduction to avoid hypoglycemia. Sulfonylurea therapy has not been shown to favorably modify CVD risk or slow kidney disease progression. Direct comparisons of the sulfonylurea glimepiride versus an SGLT-2 inhibitor in a trial using eGFR slopes have shown the importance of prioritizing the use of an SGLT-2 inhibitor.[123]

THE USE OF ANTIPLATELET THERAPY IN CHRONIC KIDNEY DISEASE

In patients without CKD, low-dose aspirin 75 to ... is indicated for secondary prevention of athero... CVD in patients with DM and CKD who have ... CVD.[124] In patients with DM without evidence of prior atherosclerotic CVD, the absolute benefits of low-dose aspirin on CVD risk appear counterbalanced by the absolute risk of bleeding. The placebo-controlled ASCEND trial reported aspirin use in 15,480 patients with DM and no prior CVD reduced risk of serious vascular events (defined as myocardial infarction, stroke, or CVD death) by 12% (RR, 0.88; 0.79–0.97) and increased major bleeding by 29% (RR, 1.29; 1.09–1.52).[125] CKD is associated with both increased atherosclerotic CVD[6] and bleeding risk,[126] and the balance of risk and benefits of low-dose aspirin in patients with CKD without CVD may be similarly finely counterbalanced. A recent Cochrane collaboration meta-analysis of 40,597 patients with CKD from antiplatelet versus placebo trials, and 11,805 patients with CKD from antiplatelet agent comparison trials showed the relative effects of aspirin on risk of myocardial infarction (RR, 0.88; 0.79–0.99) and major bleeding (RR, 1.35; 1.10–1.65) are consistent with the results of ASCEND.[127]

In the large placebo-controlled ASPREE trial which recruited 19,114 presumed healthy individuals who were at least 70 years of age, there was no effect of allocation to aspirin 100 mg daily on a change in eGFR over time.[128] Some patients with CKD may still wish to accept the risk of major bleeding offered by aspirin to modestly reduce the risk of a first serious vascular event, and some may have a kidney diagnosis which supports considering the use of aspirin (e.g., presumed or proven renovascular disease). However, based on the current level of evidence, low-dose aspirin should not be routinely offered to patients with type 2 DM and CKD until the results of the dedicated ATTACK trial in CKD are known.[129]

MANAGEMENT OF THE METABOLIC CONSEQUENCES OF CHRONIC KIDNEY DISEASE AND THE IMPACT ON CARDIOVASCULAR DISEASE

Management of CKD-MBD

Serum phosphate may increase in severe CKD (e.g., eGFR < 30 mL/min/1.73 m^2) and has been associated with an increased risk of CVD.[61] Phosphate lowering, controlling parathyroid hormone,[43] and maintaining normal calcium levels is common practice in nephrology despite a lack of definitive evidence that it modifies the risk of CVD.[30] Some evidence suggests the dose of calcium-based phosphate binders should be restricted.[130,131] Kidney specialist advice can be sought for management of a persistently raised serum phosphate (>1.5 mmol/L) despite dietary advice.

Anemia in Chronic Kidney Disease

In CKD in patients with type 2 DM, correction of renal anemia with parenteral erythropoiesis-stimulating agents (ESA) improves quality of life, but has not been shown to reduce risk of CVD, and it does increase the risk of stroke.[132] Kidney specialist advice can be sought for management of renal anemia (e.g., hemoglobin < 10 g/dL) to improve symptoms, but ESAs are unlikely to meaningfully reduce the risk of clinical manifestations of CVD or left ventricular mass index.[133] Oral hypoxia-inducible factor prolyl hydroxylase inhibitors (HIF-PHIs), which slow the degradation of hypoxia inducible factor thereby increasing the production of erythropoietin, offer a potential oral method to correct renal anemia. HIF-PHIs may also facilitate iron absorption, mobilization, and recycling. However, uncertainty about long-term safety with their use exists.[134]

Intravenous iron preparation is widely used in nephrological practice to reduce the required dose of ESAs. There is large-scale randomized evidence from patients on dialysis that such an approach is safe, at least in the short to medium term, and may reduce the risk of cardiac events (myocardial infarction or heart failure).[135] This is consistent with data from trials of patients with heart failure and iron deficiency, in which parenteral iron use reduced the risk of heart failure rehospitalization.[136]

Antiinflammatory Agents in Chronic Kidney Disease

Inflammation is commonly identified in CKD, and a trial of canukinumab, an inhibitor of the interleukin-1 beta pathway, and with low-dose colchicine show that these antiinflammatory agents reduce CVD risk after myocardial infarction.[137,138] Whether inhibition of the interleukin-6 pathway reduces the risk of CVD in DM and CKD is being tested by a large-scale trial.[139,140]

OTHER CONSIDERATIONS FOR THE MANAGEMENT OF CARDIOVASCULAR DISEASE IN CHRONIC KIDNEY DISEASE

Coronary Artery Interventions

Invasive versus medical management strategies for moderate or severe coronary artery disease in CKD has been tested in the ISCHEMIA-CKD trial. Of the 777 participants, 444 had a history of DM.[141] The trial was conducted in parallel with the much larger ISCHEMIA trial, which found no evidence that an initial invasive strategy did not reduced the risk of ischemic CVD events or death over a median of 3.2 years (although findings were somewhat sensitive to different definitions of myocardial infarction).[142] When results from both ISCHEMIA and ISCHEMIA-CKD are considered together, ISCHEMIA-CKD also suggests that an initial conservative approach using intensive medical therapies to manage stable coronary artery disease is appropriate for patients with an eGFR < 30 mL/min/1.73 m^2.[141] ISCHEMIA found antianginal benefits of an initial invasive strategy, which ISCHEMIA-CKD did not replicate, but such benefits should not be ruled out due to ISCHEMIA-CKD's lower statistical power.[141,142] Further follow-up to an average of 5 years revealed the high rates of all-cause and cardiovascular mortality in this population (nearly 40% and 30%, respectively), with similar rates between the two initial management strategies. It should be noted that patients with acute or unstable coronary artery disease or with unacceptable levels of angina were excluded from both trials, meaning optimal management of such conditions in patients with CKD requires cardiological consultation and may still include an intensive strategy.

SUMMARY

In summary, CKD is particularly associated with the risk of heart failure, arrhythmias, and sudden cardiac death, as well as atherosclerotic CVDs, and most patients with CKD die from CVD before progressing to the need for kidney replacement therapy. Meta-analyses in patients with type 2 DM have shown that intensively controlling blood pressure and blood glucose safely reduces the risk of CVD (modestly) and albuminuria in patients with type 2 DM, and it is presumed that such strategies translate into a reduced risk of kidney failure (despite a lack of definitive trial evidence). Key treatments that placebo-controlled trials have shown to be effective at reducing the risk of CVD and/or kidney failure in patients with type 2 DM and CKD target systemic blood pressure and intraglomerular hypertension and include RAAS inhibitors, SGLT-2 inhibitors, GLP-1RA semaglutide, and the nonsteroidal mineralocorticoid receptor antagonist finerenone. Appropriately prescribing such interventions in combination and in those at risk reduces the risk of either the development or the progression of kidney end-organ damage and heart failure risk. Intensive statin-based regimens safely reduce atherosclerotic CVD risk in CKD.

REFERENCES

1. Kidney Disease: Improving Global Outcomes CKD Working Group. KDIGO 2024 clinical practice guideline for the evaluation and management of chronic kidney disease. *Kidney Int.* 2024;105(4S):S117–S314. https://doi.org/10.1016/j.kint.2023.10.018.
2. Kidney Disease: Improving Global Outcomes CKD Working Group. KDIGO 2012 clinical practice guideline for the evaluation and management of chronic kidney disease. *Kidney Int Suppl.* 2013;3(1–150):1–150.
3. Global Burden of Disease-CKD Collaboration. Global, regional, and national burden of chronic kidney disease, 1990-2017: a systematic analysis for the Global Burden of Disease Study 2017. *Lancet.* 2020;395(10225):709–733. https://doi.org/10.1016/S0140-6736(20)30045-3.
4. Fox CS, Matsushita K, Woodward M, et al. Associations of kidney disease measures with mortality and end-stage renal disease in individuals with and without diabetes: a meta-analysis. *Lancet.* 2012;380(9854):1662–1673. https://doi.org/10.1016/s0140-6736(12)61350-6.
5. Mafham M, Emberson J, Landray MJ, Wen CP, Baigent C. Estimated glomerular filtration rate and the risk of major vascular events and all-cause mortality: a meta-analysis. *PLoS One.* 2011;6(10):e25920. https://doi.org/10.1371/journal.pone.0025920.
6. Tonelli M, Muntner P, Lloyd A, et al. Risk of coronary events in people with chronic kidney disease compared with those with diabetes: a population-level cohort study. *Lancet.* 2012;380(9844):807–814. https://doi.org/10.1016/S0140-6736(12)60572-8. S0140-6736(12)60572-8 [pii].
7. House AA, Wanner C, Sarnak MJ, et al. Heart failure in chronic kidney disease: conclusions from a Kidney Disease: Improving Global Outcomes (KDIGO) Controversies Conference. *Kidney Int.* 2019;95(6):1304–1317. https://doi.org/10.1016/j.kint.2019.02.022.
8. Johansen KL, Garimella PS, Hicks CW, et al. Central and peripheral arterial diseases in chronic kidney disease: conclusions from a Kidney Disease: Improving Global Outcomes (KDIGO) Controversies Conference. *Kidney Int.* 2021;100(1):35–48. https://doi.org/10.1016/j.kint.2021.04.029.
9. Turakhia MP, Blankestijn PJ, Carrero JJ, et al. Chronic kidney disease and arrhythmias: conclusions from a Kidney Disease: Improving Global Outcomes (KDIGO) Controversies Conference. *Eur Heart J.* 2018;39(24):2314–2325. https://doi.org/10.1093/eurheartj/ehy060.
10. Kidney Disease: Improving Global Outcomes Diabetes Work Group KDIGO 2020 clinical practice guideline for diabetes management in chronic kidney disease. *Kidney Int.* 2020;98(4S):S1–S115. https://doi.org/10.1016/j.kint.2020.06.019.
11. Levey AS, Eckardt KU, Dorman NM, et al. Nomenclature for kidney function and disease: report of a Kidney Disease: Improving Global Outcomes

(KDIGO) Consensus Conference. *Kidney Int.* 2020;97(6):1117–1129. https://doi.org/10.1016/j.kint.2020.02.010.

12. Sumida K, Nadkarni GN, Grams ME, et al. Conversion of urine protein-creatinine ratio or urine dipstick protein to urine albumin-creatinine ratio for use in chronic kidney disease screening and prognosis: an individual participant-based meta-analysis. *Ann Intern Med.* 2020;173(6):426–435. https://doi.org/10.7326/M20-0529.
13. Inker LA, Eneanya ND, Coresh J, et al. New creatinine- and cystatin C-based equations to estimate GFR without race. *N Engl J Med.* 2021;385(19):1737–1749. https://doi.org/10.1056/NEJMoa2102953.
14. Go AS, Chertow GM, Fan D, McCulloch CE, Hsu C-y. Chronic kidney disease and the risks of death, cardiovascular events, and hospitalization. *N Engl J Med.* 2004;351(13):1296–1305.
15. Park JI, Baek H, Kim BR, Jung HH. Comparison of urine dipstick and albumin:creatinine ratio for chronic kidney disease screening: a population-based study. *PLoS One.* 2017;12(2):e0171106. https://doi.org/10.1371/journal.pone.0171106.
16. Matsushita K, van der Velde M, Astor BC, et al. Association of estimated glomerular filtration rate and albuminuria with all-cause and cardiovascular mortality in general population cohorts: a collaborative meta-analysis. *Lancet.* 2010;375(9731):2073–2081. https://doi.org/10.1016/S0140-6736(10)60674-5. 10.1016/S0140-6736(10)60674-5 [pii].
17. CKD-Prognosis Consortium. Estimated glomerular filtration rate, albuminuria, and adverse outcomes: an individual-participant data meta-analysis. *JAMA.* 2023;330(13):1266–1277. https://doi.org/10.1001/jama.2023.17002.
18. Tangri N, Grams ME, Levey AS, et al. Multinational assessment of accuracy of equations for predicting risk of kidney failure: a meta-analysis. *JAMA.* 2016;315(2):164–174. https://doi.org/10.1001/jama.2015.18202.
19. Bundy JD, Mills KT, Anderson AH, et al. Prediction of end-stage kidney disease using estimated glomerular filtration rate with and without race: a prospective cohort study. *Ann Intern Med.* 2022. https://doi.org/10.7326/M21-2928.
20. Hill NR, Fatoba ST, Oke JL, et al. Global prevalence of chronic kidney disease - a systematic review and meta-analysis. *PLoS One.* 2016;11(7):e0158765. https://doi.org/10.1371/journal.pone.0158765.
21. Coresh J. Update on the burden of CKD. *J Am Soc Nephrol.* 2017;28(4):1020–1022. https://doi.org/10.1681/ASN.2016121374.
22. Murphy D, McCulloch CE, Lin F, et al. Trends in prevalence of chronic kidney disease in the United States. *Ann Intern Med.* 2016;165(7):473–481. https://doi.org/10.7326/M16-0273.
23. United States Renal Data System. CKD in the general population. In *2021 USRDS Annual Data Report.* Available from: https://adr.usrds.org/2021/chronic-kidney-disease/1-ckd-in-the-general-population.
24. Alicic RZ, Rooney MT, Tuttle KR. Diabetic kidney disease: challenges, progress, and possibilities. *Clin J Am Soc Nephrol.* 2017;12(12):2032–2045. https://doi.org/10.2215/CJN.11491116.
25. Park M, Hsu CY, Li Y, et al. Associations between kidney function and subclinical cardiac abnormalities in CKD. *J Am Soc Nephrol.* 2012;23(10):1725–1734. https://doi.org/10.1681/ASN.2012020145.
26. Foley RN, Parfrey PS, Kent GM, Harnett JD, Murray DC, Barre PE. Long-term evolution of cardiomyopathy in dialysis patients. *Kidney Int.* 1998;54(5):1720–1725. https://doi.org/10.1046/j.1523-1755.1998.00154.x.
27. Suzuki T, Agarwal SK, Deo R, et al. Kidney function and sudden cardiac death in the community: the Atherosclerosis Risk in Communities (ARIC) Study. *Am Heart J.* 2016;180:46–53. https://doi.org/10.1016/j.ahj.2016.07.004.
28. Kono K, Fujii H, Nakai K, et al. Composition and plaque patterns of coronary culprit lesions and clinical characteristics of patients with chronic kidney disease. *Kidney Int.* 2012;82(3):344–351. https://doi.org/10.1038/ki.2012.118. ki2012118 [pii].
29. London GM, Guérin AP, Marchais SJ, Métivier F, Pannier B, Adda H. Arterial media calcification in end-stage renal disease: impact on all-cause and cardiovascular mortality. *Nephrol Dial Transplant.* 2003;18(9):1731–1740.
30. KDIGO. 2017 Clinical practice guideline update for the diagnosis, evaluation, prevention, and treatment of chronic kidney disease-mineral and bone disorder (CKD-MBD). *Kidney Int Suppl.* 2017;7(1):1–59. https://doi.org/10.1016/j.kisu.2017.04.001. *(*2011*).*
31. Sarnak MJ, Amann K, Bangalore S, et al. Chronic kidney disease and coronary artery disease: JACC state-of-the-art review. *J Am Coll Cardiol.* 2019;74(14):1823–1838. https://doi.org/10.1016/j.jacc.2019.08.1017.
32. Jankowski J, Floege J, Fliser D, Bohm M, Marx N. Cardiovascular disease in chronic kidney disease: pathophysiological insights and therapeutic options. *Circulation.* 2021;143(11):1157–1172. https://doi.org/10.1161/CIRCULATIONAHA.120.050686.
33. EMPA-KIDNEY Collaborative Group. Design, recruitment, and baseline characteristics of the EMPA-KIDNEY trial. *Nephrol Dial Transplant.* 2022. https://doi.org/10.1093/ndt/gfac040.
34. Schaefer F, Doyon A, Azukaitis K, et al. Cardiovascular phenotypes in children with CKD: the 4C study. *Clin J Am Soc Nephrol.* 2017;12(1):19–28. https://doi.org/10.2215/CJN.01090216.
35. Mitsnefes MM, Daniels SR, Schwartz SM, Meyer RA, Khoury P, Strife CF. Severe left ventricular hypertrophy in pediatric dialysis: prevalence and predictors. *Pediatr Nephrol.* 2000;14(10-11):898–902.
36. Foley RN, Parfrey PS, Harnett JD, et al. Clinical and echocardiographic disease in patients starting end-stage renal disease therapy. *Kidney Int.* 1995;47(1):186–192.
37. Alhaj E, Alhaj N, Rahman I, Niazi TO, Berkowitz R, Klapholz M. Uremic cardiomyopathy: an underdiagnosed disease. *Congest Heart Fail.* 2013;19(4):E40–E45. https://doi.org/10.1111/chf.12030.
38. Marwick TH, Amann K, Bangalore S, et al. Chronic kidney disease and valvular heart disease: conclusions from a Kidney Disease: Improving Global Outcomes (KDIGO) Controversies Conference. *Kidney Int.* 2019;96(4):836–849. https://doi.org/10.1016/j.kint.2019.06.025.
39. Rattazzi M, Bertacco E, Del Vecchio A, Puato M, Faggin E, Pauletto P. Aortic valve calcification in chronic kidney disease. *Nephrol Dial Transplant.* 2013;28(12):2968–2976. https://doi.org/10.1093/ndt/gft310.
40. Rossebø AB, Pedersen TR, Boman K, et al. Intensive lipid lowering with simvastatin and ezetimibe in aortic stenosis. *N Engl J Med.* 2008;359(13):1343–1356. https://doi.org/10.1056/NEJMoa0804602. NEJMoa0804602 [pii].
41. Kjekshus J, Apetrei E, Barrios V, et al. Rosuvastatin in older patients with systolic heart failure. *N Engl J Med.* 2007;357(22):2248–2261. https://doi.org/10.1056/NEJMoa0706201. NEJMoa0706201 [pii].
42. Leskinen Y, Paana T, Saha H, et al. Valvular calcification and its relationship to atherosclerosis in chronic kidney disease. *JHeart Valve Dis.* 2009;18(4):429–438.
43. Chertow GM, Block GA, Correa-Rotter R, et al. Effect of cinacalcet on cardiovascular disease in patients undergoing dialysis. *N Engl J Med.* 2012;367(26):2482–2494. https://doi.org/10.1056/NEJMoa1205624.
44. Foley RN, Gilbertson DT, Murray T, Collins AJ. Long interdialytic interval and mortality among patients receiving hemodialysis. *N Engl J Med.* 2011;365(12):1099–1107. https://doi.org/10.1056/NEJMoa1103313.
45. Beattie JN, Soman SS, Sandberg KR, et al. Determinants of mortality after myocardial infarction in patients with advanced renal dysfunction. *Am J Kidney Dis.* 2001;37(6):1191–1200.
46. Kelly DM, Ademi Z, Doehner W, et al. Chronic kidney disease and cerebrovascular disease: consensus and guidance from a KDIGO controversies conference. *Stroke.* 2021;52(7):e328–e346. https://doi.org/10.1161/STROKEAHA.120.029680.
47. Emberson J, Lees KR, Lyden P, et al. Effect of treatment delay, age, and stroke severity on the effects of intravenous thrombolysis with alteplase for acute ischaemic stroke: a meta-analysis of individual patient data from randomised trials. *Lancet.* 2014;384(9958):1929–1935. https://doi.org/10.1016/S0140-6736(14)60584-5.
48. Schiffrin EL, Lipman ML, Mann JF. Chronic kidney disease: effects on the cardiovascular system. *Circulation.* 2007;116(1):85–97. https://doi.org/10.1161/CIRCULATIONAHA.106.678342.
49. Ninomiya T, Perkovic V, Turnbull F, et al. Blood pressure lowering and major cardiovascular events in people with and without chronic kidney disease: meta-analysis of randomised controlled trials. *BMJ.* 2013;347:f5680. https://doi.org/10.1136/bmj.f5680.
50. Perkovic V, Jardine MJ, Neal B, et al. Canagliflozin and renal outcomes in type 2 diabetes and nephropathy. *N Engl J Med.* 2019;380(24):2295–2306. https://doi.org/10.1056/NEJMoa1811744.
51. Heerspink HJL, Stefansson BV, Correa-Rotter R, et al. Dapagliflozin in patients with chronic kidney disease. *N Engl J Med.* 2020;383(15):1436–1446. https://doi.org/10.1056/NEJMoa2024816.
52. Lewis EJ, Hunsicker LG, Clarke WR, et al. Renoprotective effect of the angiotensin-receptor antagonist irbesartan in patients with nephropathy due to type 2 diabetes. *N Engl J Med.* 2001;345(12):851–860. https://doi.org/10.1056/NEJMoa011303.
53. Brenner BM, Cooper ME, de Zeeuw D, et al. Effects of losartan on renal and cardiovascular outcomes in patients with type 2 diabetes and nephropathy. *N Engl J Med.* 2001;345(12):861–869. https://doi.org/10.1056/NEJMoa011161.
54. Agarwal R, Filippatos G, Pitt B, et al. Cardiovascular and kidney outcomes with finerenone in patients with type 2 diabetes and chronic kidney disease: the FIDELITY pooled analysis. *Eur Heart J.* 2022;43(6):474–484. https://doi.org/10.1093/eurheartj/ehab777.
55. Sattar N, Lee MMY, Kristensen SL, et al. Cardiovascular, mortality, and kidney outcomes with GLP-1 receptor agonists in patients with type 2 diabetes: a systematic review and meta-analysis of randomised trials. *Lancet Diabetes Endocrinol.* 2021;9(10):653–662. https://doi.org/10.1016/S2213-8587(21)00203-5.
56. Perkovic V, Tuttle KR, Rossing P, et al. Effects of semaglutide on chronic kidney disease in patients with type 2 diabetes. *N Engl J Med.* 2024. https://doi.org/10.1056/NEJMoa2403347.
57. Holman RR, Paul SK, Bethel MA, Matthews DR, Neil HA. 10-year follow-up of intensive glucose control in type 2 diabetes. *N Engl J Med.* 2008;359(15):1577–1589. https://doi.org/10.1056/NEJMoa0806470. NEJMoa0806470 [pii].
58. Rosenstock J, Perkovic V, Johansen OE, et al. Effect of linagliptin vs placebo on major cardiovascular events in adults with type 2 diabetes and high cardiovascular and renal risk: the CARMELINA randomized clinical trial. *JAMA.* 2019;321(1):69–79. https://doi.org/10.1001/jama.2018.18269.
59. Emdin CA, Rahimi K, Neal B, Callender T, Perkovic V, Patel A. Blood pressure lowering in type 2 diabetes: a systematic review and meta-analysis. *JAMA.* 2015;313(6):603–615. https://doi.org/10.1001/jama.2014.18574.
60. Ettehad D, Emdin CA, Kiran A, et al. Blood pressure lowering for prevention of cardiovascular disease and death: a systematic review and meta-analysis. *Lancet.* 2016;387(10022):957–967. https://doi.org/10.1016/S0140-6736(15)01225-8.
61. Palmer SC, Hayen A, Macaskill P, et al. Serum levels of phosphorus, parathyroid hormone, and calcium and risks of death and cardiovascular

disease in individuals with chronic kidney disease: a systematic review and meta-analysis. *JAMA*. 2011;305(11):1119–1127. https://doi.org/10.1001/jama.2011.308.

62. Zhu P, Herrington WG, Haynes R, et al. Conventional and genetic evidence on the association between adiposity and CKD. *J Am Soc Nephrol*. 2021;32(1):127–137. https://doi.org/10.1681/ASN.2020050679.
63. Herrington WG, Smith M, Bankhead C, et al. Body-mass index and risk of advanced chronic kidney disease: prospective analyses from a primary care cohort of 1.4 million adults in England. *PLoS One*. 2017;12(3):e0173515. https://doi.org/10.1371/journal.pone.0173515.
64. Look AHEAD Research Group. Effect of a long-term behavioural weight loss intervention on nephropathy in overweight or obese adults with type 2 diabetes: a secondary analysis of the Look AHEAD randomised clinical trial. *Lancet Diabetes Endocrinol*. 2014;2(10):801–809. https://doi.org/10.1016/S2213-8587(14)70156-1.
65. Sarwar N, Gao P, Seshasai SR, et al. Diabetes mellitus, fasting blood glucose concentration, and risk of vascular disease: a collaborative meta-analysis of 102 prospective studies. *Lancet*. 2010;375(9733):2215–2222. https://doi.org/10.1016/S0140-6736(10)60484-9. S0140-6736(10)60484-9 [pii].
66. Seshasai SR, Kaptoge S, Thompson A, et al. Diabetes mellitus, fasting glucose, and risk of cause-specific death. *N Engl J Med*. 2011;364(9):829–841. https://doi.org/10.1056/NEJMoa1008862.
67. Herrington WG, Alegre-Diaz J, Wade R, et al. Effect of diabetes duration and glycaemic control on 14-year cause-specific mortality in Mexican adults: a blood-based prospective cohort study. *Lancet Diabetes Endocrinol*. 2018;6(6):455–463. https://doi.org/10.1016/S2213-8587(18)30050-0.
68. Selvin E, Steffes MW, Zhu H, et al. Glycated hemoglobin, diabetes, and cardiovascular risk in nondiabetic adults. *N Engl J Med*. 2010;362(9):800–811. https://doi.org/10.1056/NEJMoa0908359.
69. Turnbull FM, Abraira C, Anderson RJ, et al. Intensive glucose control and macrovascular outcomes in type 2 diabetes. *Diabetologia*. 2009;52(11):2288–2298. https://doi.org/10.1007/s00125-009-1470-0.
70. Zoungas S, Arima H, Gerstein HC, et al. Effects of intensive glucose control on microvascular outcomes in patients with type 2 diabetes: a meta-analysis of individual participant data from randomised controlled trials. *Lancet Diabetes Endocrinol*. 2017;5(6):431–437. https://doi.org/10.1016/S2213-8587(17)30104-3.
71. Wong MG, Perkovic V, Chalmers J, et al. Long-term benefits of intensive glucose control for preventing end-stage kidney disease: ADVANCE-ON. *Diabetes Care*. 2016;39(5):694–700. https://doi.org/10.2337/dc15-2322.
72. Aguilar-Ramirez D, Alegre-Diaz J, Herrington WG, et al. Association of kidney function with NMR-quantified lipids, lipoproteins, and metabolic measures in Mexican adults. *J Clin Endocrinol Metab*. 2021;106(10):2828–2839. https://doi.org/10.1210/clinem/dgab497.
73. Kearney PM, Blackwell L, Collins R, et al. Efficacy of cholesterol-lowering therapy in 18,686 people with diabetes in 14 randomised trials of statins: a meta-analysis. *Lancet*. 2008;371(9607):117–125. https://doi.org/10.1016/S0140-6736(08)60104-X. S0140-6736(08)60104-X [pii].
74. Cholesterol Treatment Trialists Collaboration. Impact of renal function on the effects of LDL cholesterol lowering with statin-based regimens: a meta-analysis of individual participant data from 28 randomised trials. *Lancet Diabetes Endocrinol*. 2016;4(10):829–839. https://doi.org/10.1016/S2213-8587(16)30156-5.
75. Mach F, Baigent C, Catapano AL, et al. 2019 ESC/EAS Guidelines for the management of dyslipidaemias: lipid modification to reduce cardiovascular risk. *Eur Heart J*. 2020;41(1):111–188. https://doi.org/10.1093/eurheartj/ehz455.
76. KDIGO Clinical practice guideline for lipid management in chronic kidney disease. *Kidney Int Suppl*. 2013;3:263–264.
77. Fellström BC, Jardine AG, Schmieder RE, et al. Rosuvastatin and cardiovascular events in patients undergoing hemodialysis. *N Engl J Med*. 2009;360(14):1395–1407. https://doi.org/10.1056/NEJMoa0810177. NEJMoa0810177 [pii].
78. Wanner C, Krane V, März W, et al. Randomized controlled trial on the efficacy and safety of atorvastatin in patients with type 2 diabetes on hemodialysis (4D study): demographic and baseline characteristics. *Kidney Blood Press Res*. 2004;27(4):259–266. https://doi.org/10.1159/000080241. 80241 [pii].
79. Baigent C, Landray MJ, Reith C, et al. The effects of lowering LDL cholesterol with simvastatin plus ezetimibe in patients with chronic kidney disease (Study of Heart and Renal Protection): a randomised placebo-controlled trial. *Lancet*. 2011;377(9784):2181–2192. https://doi.org/10.1016/S0140-6736(11)60739-3. [pii].
80. Reith C, Staplin N, Herrington WG, et al. Effect on non-vascular outcomes of lowering LDL cholesterol in patients with chronic kidney disease: results from the Study of Heart and Renal Protection. *BMC Nephrol*. 2017;18(1):147. https://doi.org/10.1186/s12882-017-0545-2.
81. Holdaas H, Fellström B, Jardine AG, et al. Effect of fluvastatin on cardiac outcomes in renal transplant recipients: a multicentre, randomised, placebo-controlled trial. *Lancet*. 2003;361(9374):2024–2031. https://doi.org/10.1016/S0140-6736(03)13638-0. S0140-6736(03)13638-0 [pii].
82. Charytan DM, Sabatine MS, Pedersen TR, et al. Efficacy and safety of evolocumab in chronic kidney disease in the FOURIER trial. *J Am Coll Cardiol*. 2019;73(23):2961–2970. https://doi.org/10.1016/j.jacc.2019.03.513.
83. Kidney Disease: Improving Global Outcomes Blood Pressure Work Group: KDIGO 2021 clinical practice guideline for the management of blood pressure in chronic kidney disease. *Kidney Int*. 2021;99(3S):S1–S87. https://doi.org/10.1016/j.kint.2020.11.003.
84. Lewington S, Clarke R, Qizilbash N, Peto R, Collins R. P.S. Collaboration Age-specific relevance of usual blood pressure to vascular mortality: a meta-analysis of individual data for one million adults in 61 prospective studies. *Lancet*. 2002;360(9349):1903–1913. https://doi.org/10.1016/s0140-6736(02)11911-8. [pii].
85. SPRINT Research Group A randomized trial of intensive versus standard blood-pressure control. *N Engl J Med*. 2015. https://doi.org/10.1056/NEJMoa1511939.
86. Hunsicker LG, Adler S, Caggiula A, et al. Predictors of the progression of renal disease in the Modification of Diet in Renal Disease Study. *Kidney Int*. 1997;51(6):1908–1919.
87. Palit S, Chonchol M, Cheung AK, Kaufman J, Smits G, Kendrick J. Association of BP with death, cardiovascular events, and progression to chronic dialysis in patients with advanced kidney disease. *Clin J Am Soc Nephrol*. 2015;10(6):934–940. https://doi.org/10.2215/cjn.08620814.
88. Tozawa M, Iseki K, Iseki C, Kinjo K, Ikemiya Y, Takishita S. Blood pressure predicts risk of developing end-stage renal disease in men and women. *Hypertension*. 2003;41(6):1341–1345. https://doi.org/10.1161/01.hyp.0000069699.92349.8c.
89. Herrington WG, Preiss D, Haynes R, et al. The potential for improving cardio-renal outcomes by sodium-glucose co-transporter-2 inhibition in people with chronic kidney disease: a rationale for the EMPA-KIDNEY study. *Clin Kidney J*. 2018;11(6):749–761. https://doi.org/10.1093/ckj/sfy090.
90. Lewis EJ, Hunsicker LG, Bain RP, Rohde RD. The effect of angiotensin-converting-enzyme inhibition on diabetic nephropathy. The Collaborative Study Group. *N Engl J Med*. 1993;329(20):1456–1462. https://doi.org/10.1056/nejm199311113292004.
91. Parving HH, Lehnert H, Bröchner-Mortensen J, et al. The effect of irbesartan on the development of diabetic nephropathy in patients with type 2 diabetes. *N Engl J Med*. 2001;345(12):870–878. https://doi.org/10.1056/NEJMoa011489.
92. Makino H, Haneda M, Babazono T, et al. Prevention of transition from incipient to overt nephropathy with telmisartan in patients with type 2 diabetes. *Diabetes Care*. 2007;30(6):1577–1578. https://doi.org/10.2337/dc06-1998.
93. Parving HH, Brenner BM, McMurray JJ, et al. Cardiorenal end points in a trial of aliskiren for type 2 diabetes. *N Engl J Med*. 2012;367(23):2204–2213. https://doi.org/10.1056/NEJMoa1208799.
94. Fried LF, Emanuele N, Zhang JH, et al. Combined angiotensin inhibition for the treatment of diabetic nephropathy. *N Engl J Med*. 2013;369(20):1892–1903. https://doi.org/10.1056/NEJMoa1303154.
95. Judge P, Haynes R, Landray MJ, Baigent C. Neprilysin inhibition in chronic kidney disease. *Nephrol Dial Transplant*. 2015;30(5):738–743. https://doi.org/10.1093/ndt/gfu269.
96. McMurray JJ, Packer M, Desai AS, et al. Angiotensin-neprilysin inhibition versus enalapril in heart failure. *N Engl J Med*. 2014;71(11):993–1004. https://doi.org/10.1056/NEJMoa1409077.
97. UK HARP-III Collaborative Group. Effects of sacubitril/valsartan versus irbesartan in patients with chronic kidney disease. *Circulation*. 2018; 138(15):1505–1514. https://doi.org/10.1161/CIRCULATIONAHA.118.034818.
98. EMPA-KIDNEY Collaborative Group. Effects of empagliflozin on progression of chronic kidney disease: a prespecified secondary analysis from the empa-kidney trial. *Lancet Diabetes Endocrinol*. 2024;12(1):39–50. https://doi.org/10.1016/S2213-8587(23)00321-2.
99. EMPA-KIDNEY Collaborative Group, et al. Empagliflozin in patients with chronic kidney disease. *N Engl J Med*. 2023;388(2):117–127. https://doi.org/10.1056/NEJMoa2204233.
100. Nuffield Department of Population Health Renal Studies Group and SMART-Consortium. Impact of diabetes on the effects of sodium glucose co-transporter-2 inhibitors on kidney outcomes: collaborative meta-analysis of large placebo-controlled trials. *Lancet*. 2022;400(10365):1788–1801. https://doi.org/10.1016/S0140-6736(22)02074-8.
101. EMPA-KIDNEY Collaborative Group. Impact of primary kidney disease on the effects of empagliflozin in patients with chronic kidney disease: secondary analyses of the EMPA-KIDNEY trial. *Lancet Diabetes Endocrinol*. 2024;12(1):51–60. https://doi.org/10.1016/S2213-8587(23)00322-4.
102. Cherney DZI, Cooper ME, Tikkanen I, et al. Pooled analysis of Phase III trials indicate contrasting influences of renal function on blood pressure, body weight, and HbA1c reductions with empagliflozin. *Kidney Int*. 2018;93(1):231–244. https://doi.org/10.1016/j.kint.2017.06.017.
103. Staplin N, Roddick AJ, Emberson J, et al. Net effects of sodium-glucose co-transporter-2 inhibition in different patient groups: a meta-analysis of large placebo-controlled randomized trials. *EClinicalMedicine*. 2021;41:101163. https://doi.org/10.1016/j.eclinm.2021.101163.
104. Patel SM, Kang YM, Im K, et al. Sodium-glucose cotransporter-2 inhibitors and major adverse cardiovascular outcomes: a SMART-C collaborative meta–analysis. *Circulation*. 2024;149(23):1789–1801. https://doi.org/10.1161/CIRCULATIONAHA.124.069568.
105. Garg SK, Henry RR, Banks P, et al. Effects of sotagliflozin added to insulin in patients with type 1 diabetes. *N Engl J Med*. 2017;377(24):2337–2348. https://doi.org/10.1056/NEJMoa1708337.
106. Currie G, Taylor AH, Fujita T, et al. Effect of mineralocorticoid receptor antagonists on proteinuria and progression of chronic kidney disease: a systematic review and meta-analysis. *BMC Nephrol*. 2016;17(1):127. https://doi.org/10.1186/s12882-016-0337-0.

107. Bakris GL, Agarwal R, Anker SD, et al. Effect of finerenone on chronic kidney disease outcomes in type 2 diabetes. *N Engl J Med*. 2020;383(23):2219–2229. https://doi.org/10.1056/NEJMoa2025845.
108. Pitt B, Filippatos G, Agarwal R, et al. Cardiovascular events with finerenone in kidney disease and type 2 diabetes. *N Engl J Med*. 2021. https://doi.org/10.1056/NEJMoa2110956.
109. Wheeler DC, Stefansson BV, Batiushin M, et al. The dapagliflozin and prevention of adverse outcomes in chronic kidney disease (DAPA-CKD) trial: baseline characteristics. *Nephrol Dial Transplant*. 2020;35(10):1700–1711. https://doi.org/10.1093/ndt/gfaa234.
110. Bhatt DL, Szarek M, Pitt B, et al. Sotagliflozin in patients with diabetes and chronic kidney disease. *N Engl J Med*. 2021;384(2):129–139. https://doi.org/10.1056/NEJMoa2030186.
111. Docherty KF, Jhund PS, Inzucchi SE, et al. Effects of dapagliflozin in DAPA-HF according to background heart failure therapy. *Eur Heart J*. 2020;41(25):2379–2392. https://doi.org/10.1093/eurheartj/ehaa183.
112. Ferreira JP, Zannad F, Pocock SJ, et al. Interplay of mineralocorticoid receptor antagonists and empagliflozin in heart failure: EMPEROR-reduced. *J Am Coll Cardiol*. 2021;77(11):1397–1407. https://doi.org/10.1016/j.jacc.2021.01.044.
113. Shen L, Kristensen SL, Bengtsson O, et al. Dapagliflozin in HFrEF patients treated with mineralocorticoid receptor antagonists. An analysis of DAPA-HF. *JACC Heart Fail*. 2021;9(4):254–264. https://doi.org/10.1016/j.jchf.2020.11.009.
114. Bhatt DL, Szarek M, Steg PG, et al. Sotagliflozin in patients with diabetes and recent worsening heart failure. *N Engl J Med*. 2021;384(2):117–128. https://doi.org/10.1056/NEJMoa2030183.
115. Weir MR, Slee A, Sun T, et al. Effects of canagliflozin on serum potassium in the CANagliflozin cardioVascular Assessment Study (CANVAS) Program. *Clin Kidney J*. 2020;14(5):1396–1402. https://doi.org/10.1093/ckj/sfaa133.
116. Judge PK, Tuttle KR, Staplin N, et al. The potential for improving cardio-renal outcomes in chronic kidney disease with the aldosterone synthase inhibitor vicadrostat (BI 690517): a rationale for the EASi-KIDNEY trial. *Nephrol Dial Transplant*. 2024 Nov 12:gfae263. doi:10.1093/ndt/gfae263. Online ahead of print. DOI:10.1093/ndt/gfae263.
117. Lincoff AM, Brown-Frandsen K, Colhoun HM, et al. Semaglutide and cardiovascular outcomes in obesity without diabetes. *N Engl J Med*. 2023;389(24):2221–2232. https://doi.org/10.1056/NEJMoa2307563.
118. Tuttle KR, Lakshmanan MC, Rayner B, et al. Dulaglutide versus insulin glargine in patients with type 2 diabetes and moderate-to-severe chronic kidney disease (AWARD-7): a multicentre, open-label, randomised trial. *Lancet Diabetes Endocrinol*. 2018;6(8):605–617. https://doi.org/10.1016/S2213-8587(18)30104-9.
119. UK Prospective Diabetes Study (UKPDS) Group. Effect of intensive blood-glucose control with metformin on complications in overweight patients with type 2 diabetes (UKPDS 34). *Lancet*. 1998;352(9131):854–865. doi:S0140673698070378 [pii]
120. Graham GG, Punt J, Arora M, et al. Clinical pharmacokinetics of metformin. *Clin Pharmacokinet*. 2011;50(2):81–98. https://doi.org/10.2165/11534750-000000000-00000.
121. Duong JK, Kumar SS, Kirkpatrick CM, et al. Population pharmacokinetics of metformin in healthy subjects and patients with type 2 diabetes mellitus: simulation of doses according to renal function. *Clin Pharmacokinet*. 2013. https://doi.org/10.1007/s40262-013-0046-9.
122. Duong JK, Roberts DM, Furlong TJ, et al. Metformin therapy in patients with chronic kidney disease. *Diabetes Obes Metab*. 2012;14(10):963–965. https://doi.org/10.1111/j.1463-1326.2012.01617.x.
123. Heerspink HJ, Desai M, Jardine M, Balis D, Meininger G, Perkovic V. Canagliflozin slows progression of renal function decline independently of glycemic effects. *J Am Soc Nephrol*. 2017;28(1):368–375. https://doi.org/10.1681/ASN.2016030278.
124. Anti-thrombotic Trialists' Collaboration. Collaborative meta-analysis of randomised trials of antiplatelet therapy for prevention of death, myocardial infarction, and stroke in high risk patients. *BMJ*. 2002;324(7329):71–86.
125. ASCEND Study Collaborative Group. Effects of aspirin for primary prevention in persons with diabetes mellitus. *N Engl J Med*. 2018;379(16):1529–1539. https://doi.org/10.1056/NEJMoa1804988.
126. Molnar AO, Bota SE, Garg AX, et al. The risk of major hemorrhage with CKD. *J Am Soc Nephrol*. 2016;27(9):2825–2832. https://doi.org/10.1681/ASN.2015050535.
127. Natale P, Palmer SC, Saglimbene VM, Ruospo M, Razavian M, Craig JC, Jardine MJ, Webster AC, Strippoli GFM. Antiplatelet agents for chronic kidney disease. *Cochrane Database Syst Rev*. 2022;2(2):CD008834. https://doi.org/10.1002/14651858.CD008834.pub4. Art. No.
128. Polkinghorne KR, Wetmore JB, Phuong Thao LT, et al. Effect of aspirin on CKD progression in older adults: secondary analysis from the ASPREE randomized clinical trial. *Am J Kidney Dis*. 2022. https://doi.org/10.1053/j.ajkd.2022.02.019.
129. Aspirin to Target Arterial Events in Chronic Kidney Disease (ATTACK). https://clinicaltrials.gov/ct2/show/NCT03796156.
130. Jamal SA, Vandermeer B, Raggi P, et al. Effect of calcium-based versus non-calcium-based phosphate binders on mortality in patients with chronic kidney disease: an updated systematic review and meta-analysis. *Lancet*. 2013;382(9900):1268–1277. https://doi.org/10.1016/s0140-6736(13)60897-1.
131. Navaneethan SD, Palmer SC, Craig JC, Elder GJ, Strippoli GF. Benefits and harms of phosphate binders in CKD: a systematic review of randomized controlled trials. *Am J Kidney Dis*. 2009;54(4):619–637. https://doi.org/10.1053/j.ajkd.2009.06.004.
132. Pfeffer MA, Burdmann EA, Chen CY, et al. A trial of darbepoetin alfa in type 2 diabetes and chronic kidney disease. *N Engl J Med*. 2009;361(21):2019–2032. https://doi.org/10.1056/NEJMoa0907845. NEJMoa0907845 [pii].
133. Drüeke TB, Locatelli F, Clyne N, et al. Normalization of hemoglobin level in patients with chronic kidney disease and anemia. *N Engl J Med*. 2006;355(20):2071–2084. https://doi.org/10.1056/NEJMoa062276. 355/20/2071 [pii].
134. Tonelli M, Thadhani R. Anaemia in chronic kidney disease: what do new generation agents offer? *Lancet*. 2022;399(10326):702–703. https://doi.org/10.1016/S0140-6736(22)00120-9.
135. Macdougall IC, White C, Anker SD, et al. Intravenous iron in patients undergoing maintenance hemodialysis. *N Engl J Med*. 2019;380(5):447–458. https://doi.org/10.1056/NEJMoa1810742.
136. Ponikowski P, Kirwan BA, Anker SD, et al. Ferric carboxymaltose for iron deficiency at discharge after acute heart failure: a multicentre, double-blind, randomised, controlled trial. *Lancet*. 2020;396(10266):1895–1904. https://doi.org/10.1016/S0140-6736(20)32339-4.
137. Ridker PM, Everett BM, Thuren T, et al. Antiinflammatory therapy with canakinumab for atherosclerotic disease. *N Engl J Med*. 2017;377(12):1119–1131. https://doi.org/10.1056/NEJMoa1707914.
138. Tardif JC, Kouz S, Waters DD, et al. Efficacy and safety of low-dose colchicine after myocardial infarction. *N Engl J Med*. 2019;381(26):2497–2505. https://doi.org/10.1056/NEJMoa1912388.
139. Ridker PM, Devalaraja M, Baeres FMM, et al. IL-6 inhibition with ziltivekimab in patients at high atherosclerotic risk (RESCUE): a double-blind, randomised, placebo-controlled, phase 2 trial. *Lancet*. 2021;397(10289):2060–2069. https://doi.org/10.1016/S0140-6736(21)00520-1.
140. ZEUS. A Research Study to Look at How Ziltivekimab Works Compared to Placebo in People With Cardiovascular Disease, Chronic Kidney Disease and Inflammation (ZEUS). https://clinicaltrials.gov/ct2/show/NCT05021835.
141. Bangalore S, Maron DJ, O'Brien SM, et al. Management of coronary disease in patients with advanced kidney disease. *N Engl J Med*. 2020;382(17):1608–1618. https://doi.org/10.1056/NEJMoa1915925.
142. Maron DJ, Hochman JS, Reynolds HR, et al. Initial invasive or conservative strategy for stable coronary disease. *N Engl J Med*. 2020;382(15):1395–1407. https://doi.org/10.1056/NEJMoa1915922.
143. A Research Study to See How Semaglutide Works Compared to Placebo in People With Type 2 Diabetes and Chronic Kidney Disease (FLOW). https://clinicaltrials.gov/ct2/show/NCT03819153.
144. Wheeler DC, Stefansson BV, Jongs N, et al. Effects of dapagliflozin on major adverse kidney and cardiovascular events in patients with diabetic and non-diabetic chronic kidney disease: a prespecified analysis from the DAPA-CKD trial. *Lancet Diabetes Endocrinol*. 2021;9(1):22–31. https://doi.org/10.1016/S2213-8587(20)30369-7.
145. Neuen BL, Ohkuma T, Neal B, et al. Relative and absolute risk reductions in cardiovascular and kidney outcomes with canagliflozin across KDIGO risk categories: findings from the CANVAS program. *Am J Kidney Dis*. 2021;77(1):23–34.e1. https://doi.org/10.1053/j.ajkd.2020.06.018.

26 Disparities in Type 2 Diabetes Risk, Cardiovascular Consequences, and Care: Females, Racial/Ethnic Minorities, and the Elderly

LEONARD E. EGEDE, REBEKAH J. WALKER, AND JONI S. WILLIAMS

DIABETES AND CARDIOVASCULAR COMPLICATIONS

Diabetes is a worldwide epidemic, with 537 million adults living with it, and predictions show this will grow to 783 million by 2045.[1] In the United States (US), 14.7% of the adult population lives with diabetes, with an additional 38.0% of US adults living with prediabetes.[2] Diabetes affects all age, sex, and ethnic and racial groups but increases with age, with 29.2% of adults aged 65 or older living with diabetes (Fig. 26.1).[2] Trends over time show that diabetes disproportionately affects minority populations (Fig. 26.2), with the prevalence of diagnosed diabetes highest in American Indians and Alaska Natives (16.0%), followed by non-Hispanic Black/African Americans (12.5%), and Native Hawaiian or Other Pacific Islander adults (11.7%).[2,3] Prevalence estimates are slightly higher in males, with 12.6% of US males and 10.2% of US females diagnosed with diabetes (Fig. 26.3); however, females are more likely to have undiagnosed diabetes, which confers additional risk due to a lack of management of the disease.[2,3] In addition, when comparing prevalence stratified by both sex and race/ethnicity, diabetes is higher in American Indian/Alaskan Native and non-Hispanic Black/African American females compared to males (Fig. 26.4). Disparities extend beyond prevalence with differences by race/ethnicity in diabetes deaths (Fig. 26.5) and prevalence of comorbidities.[2]

Cardiovascular disease (CVD) is a group of heart and blood vessel diseases including coronary heart disease, cerebrovascular disease, peripheral artery disease (PAD), congenital heart disease, coronary artery disease, and heart failure.[4] Individuals with diabetes are two to four times more likely to develop CVD compared with the general population, making diabetes a major independent risk factor for CVD.[5–8] CVD is also widely documented as a leading cause of mortality in adults with diabetes, with the risk of death from cardiovascular causes two to six times higher than adults without diabetes.[5,8,9] Diabetes increases the risk of heart failure 40% and the risk of hemorrhagic stroke 50% and leads to a twofold increased risk for ischemic stroke.[5] Those with diabetes also have a two- to fourfold increased risk of PAD.[5] Studies over the past 5 years documented declines in the overall rates of myocardial infarction (MI), stroke, and heart failure, but stable or increasing CVD rates in those with diabetes.[10] As a result, more recent studies highlight that while improvements in care attenuate the risk between diabetes and CVD mortality, elevated risk remains.[7,8]

The American Diabetes Association publishes standards for diabetes screening and therapeutic care annually to provide targets for clinical care.[11] To prevent complications, such as CVD, it is recommended that most adults with diabetes target an HbA_{1c} of 7% or lower, blood pressure of 140/90 mm Hg or lower, and LDL cholesterol under 130 mg/dL and do not smoke.[3,11] Additionally, lifestyle change, weight reduction, and cardioprotective therapeutics are used as important tools to lower risk for CVD in individuals with diabetes.[4] In a pooled analysis of adults aged 28 to 86 with diabetes and no known CVD from the Atherosclerosis Risk in Communities, Multi-Ethnic Study of Atherosclerosis, and Jackson Heart Study, Wong and colleagues found that 41.1%, 26.5%, and 7.2% of the sample met targets for one, two, or all three diabetes targets (HbA_{1c}, blood pressure, LDL),[12] respectively. In a second study, based on a US

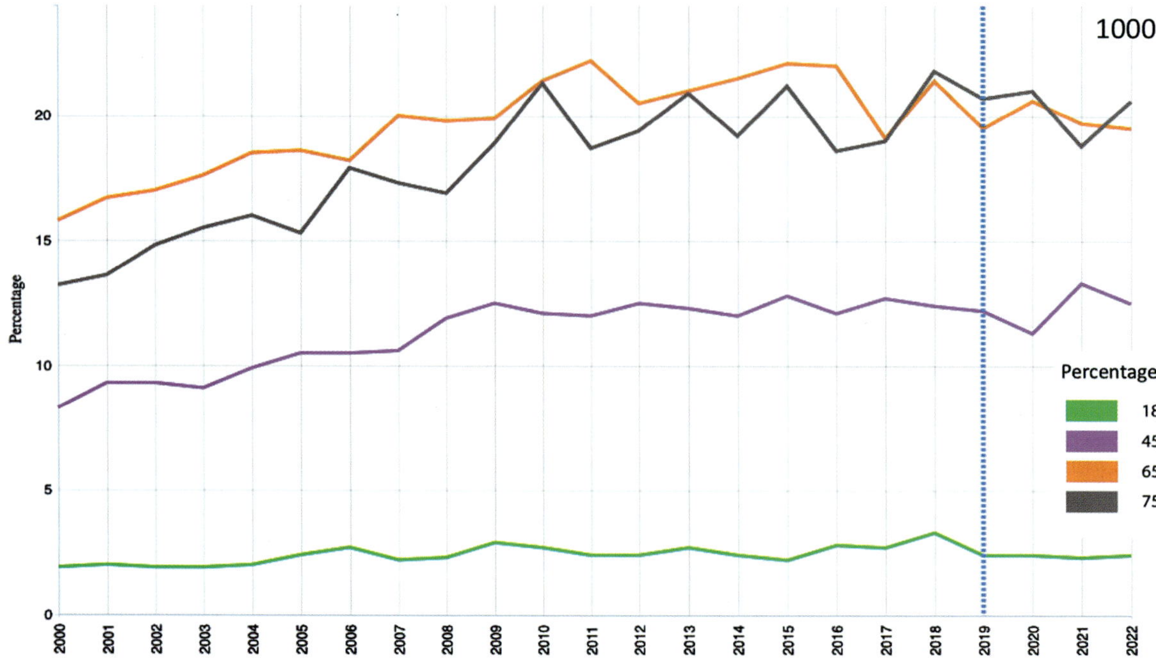

FIG. 26.1 Percentage of adults with self-reported physician-diagnosed diabetes, by age, United States, 2000–2022. Centers for Disease Control and Prevention (CDC). *National Diabetes Surveillance System Diabetes Atlas*. Vertical dotted line indicates major change to survey methods. Available from: https://gis.cdc.gov/grasp/diabetes/diabetesatlas-surveillance.html

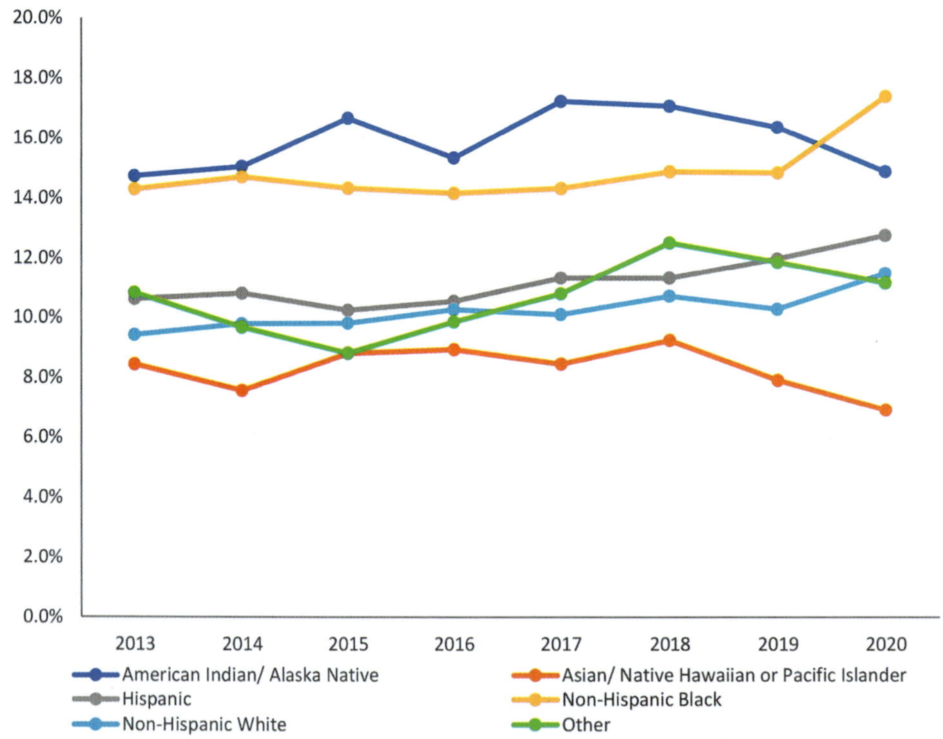

FIG. 26.2 Percentage of adults with self-reported physician-diagnosed diabetes, by race/ethnicity, United States, 2013–2020. Centers for Disease Control and Prevention (CDC). *National Diabetes Surveillance System Diabetes Atlas*. Available from: https://gis.cdc.gov/grasp/diabetes/diabetesatlas-surveillance.html

Diabetes Collaborative Registry, 21.6% of adults with diabetes were at target for all four measures (HbA_{1c}, blood pressure, LDL, and smoking).[13] Individuals with one, two, or all three (HbA_{1c}, blood pressure, and LDL) at target levels had incrementally lower adjusted risks of CVD events.[12] In addition, blood pressure control appears to be more difficult to achieve for adults with diabetes compared with those without.[14] A study investigating the relationship between systolic blood pressure (SBP) and CVD mortality noted a narrower beneficial range for aggressive SBP reduction in those with diabetes.[15] Therefore while treatment to target CVD risk factors has improved over the past decade, most adults with diabetes do not have concurrent risk factor control, increasing their risk for complications or mortality.[4,12]

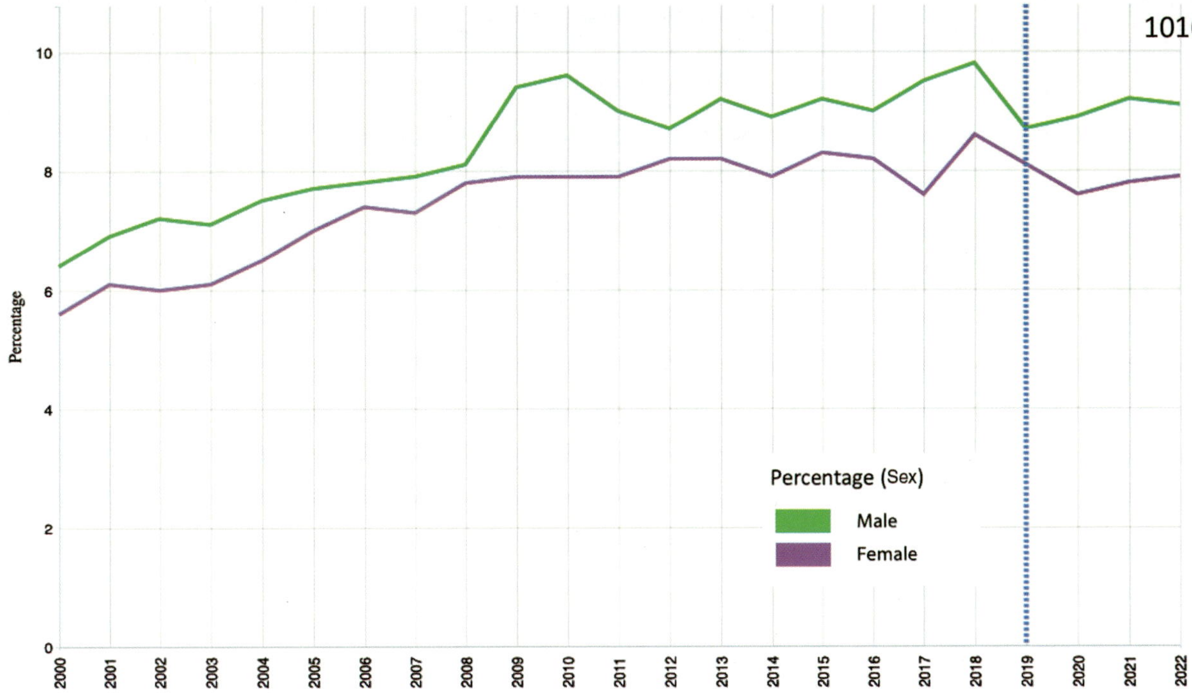

FIG. 26.3 Percentage of adults with self-reported physician-diagnosed diabetes, by sex, United States, 2013–2022. Centers for Disease Control and Prevention (CDC). *National Diabetes Surveillance System Diabetes Atlas*. Vertical dotted line indicates major change to survey methods. Available from: https://gis.cdc.gov/grasp/diabetes/diabetesatlas-surveillance.html

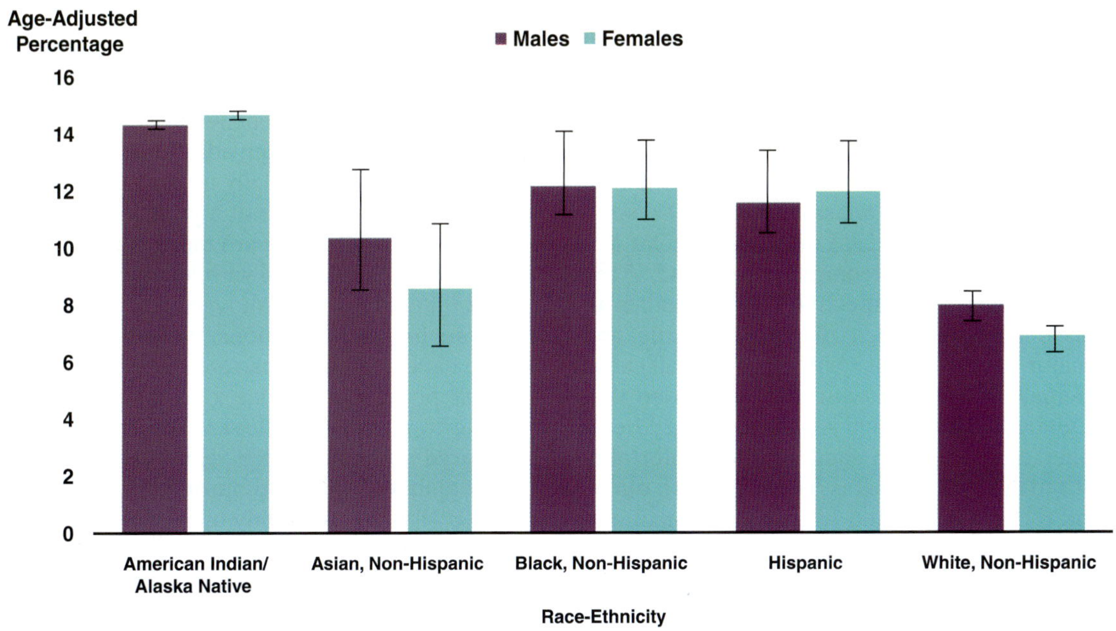

FIG. 26.4 Age-adjusted estimated prevalence of diagnosed diabetes by race/ethnicity group and sex for adults aged 18 or older, United States, 2019–2021 (purple, *men*; blue, *women*). Center for Disease Control and Prevention (CDC). *Diabetes Statistics Report; 2019-2021 National Health Interview Survey*. 2021. Indian Service National Data Warehouse (for American Indian/Alaskan Native group only). Available from: https://www.cdc.gov/diabetes/php/data-research/appendix.html#cdc_report_pub_study_section_3-table-3

Successful management of diabetes requires regular engagement with the healthcare system, patient knowledge and self-management skills, and regular completion of self-management behaviors such as maintaining a healthy diet and regular physical activity.[11] Several studies have highlighted improved screening and treatment, leading to declining trends of CVD events and mortality.[16] Unfortunately, this improvement has not been seen consistently across age, sex, or race/ethnicity, and therefore disparities in risk and complications continue.[16]

DISPARITIES IN CARDIOVASCULAR CONSEQUENCES

Females

Diabetes has been recognized as a strong risk factor for cardiovascular complications, more so among females than males.[17–22] Compared with only a twofold increase in males, diabetes increases the risk of cardiovascular disease by nearly fourfold in females.[2] Evidence points to less

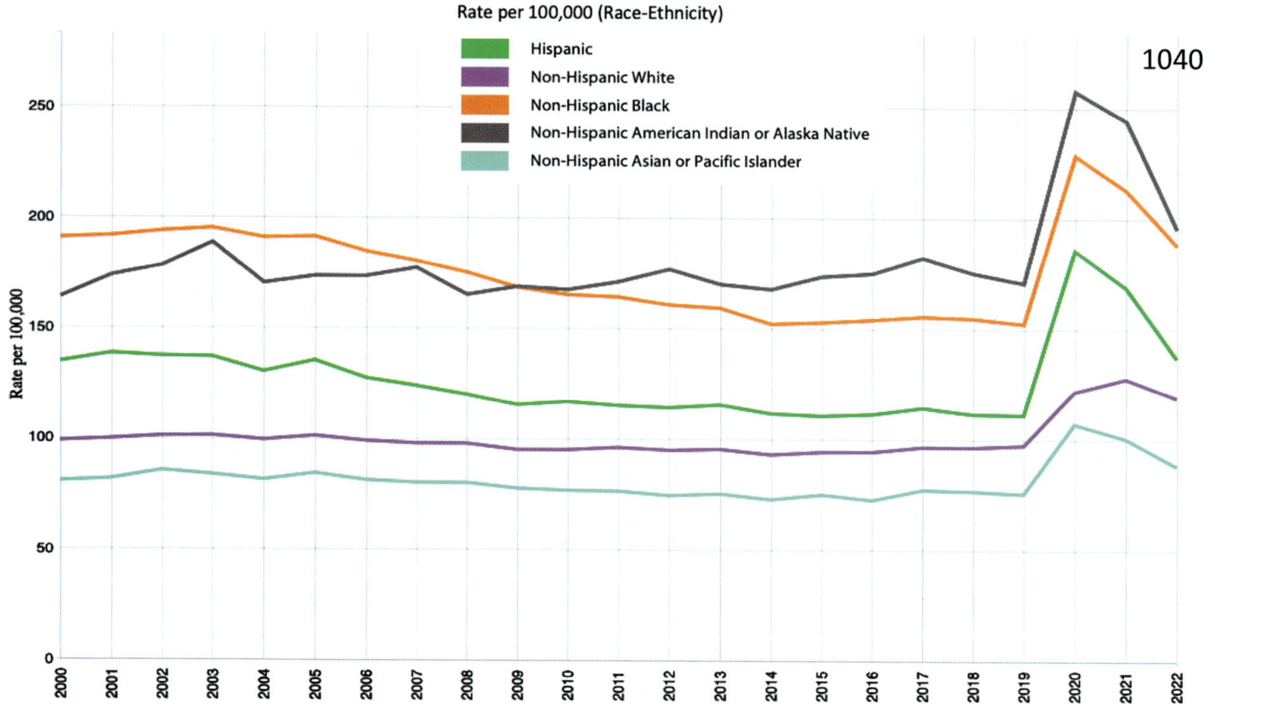

FIG. 26.5 Number of diabetes deaths per 100,000 population, by race/ethnicity, United States, 2000–2022. Centers for Disease Control and Prevention (CDC). *National Diabetes Surveillance System Diabetes Atlas*. Available from: https://gis.cdc.gov/grasp/diabetes/diabetesatlas-surveillance.html

favorable cardiovascular risk profiles and more adverse CVD risk factors and a faster development of these complications after initial diagnosis of type 2 diabetes in females compared with males.[21,23,24] In addition, females are reported to have poorer outcomes after experiencing a cardiovascular event such as a MI, suggesting that disparities in the diagnosis and treatment of cardiovascular disease may lead to worsened outcomes for females.[2,17,20,25,26] A recent meta-analysis of prospective cohort studies to assess the association between diabetes mellitus and the risk for major cardiovascular outcomes and all-cause mortality in females compared with men concluded that females with diabetes have a high risk for coronary heart disease, stroke, cardiac death, and all-cause mortality compared with males with diabetes.[27] Females with diabetes were found to have a 58% and 13% greater risk of coronary heart disease and all-cause mortality, respectively, compared with males with diabetes.[27] Despite extensive research in this area, the evidence explaining the etiologies and mechanisms underlying this disparity remain unclear. It has been postulated that females experience a greater increase in cardiovascular risk as they transition from a state of normoglycemia to one of hyperglycemia in diabetes due to sex differences in body anthropometrics, body hormones, fat storage, and body fat distribution.[17,20,25] CVD also often presents later in life for females, and unfortunately, this occurs during a time when they are more likely to be diagnosed with multiple comorbid conditions that include type 2 diabetes.[28] Cardiovascular conditions that include coronary artery disease, peripheral vascular disease, and strokes occur in higher rates among females with diabetes compared with females without diabetes.[21,22,29] Evidence shows that the longitudinal burden and cumulative exposure of cardiovascular disease risk factors from childhood to adulthood may contribute to the greater burden of CVD among females in adulthood who develop type 2 diabetes[30]; however, additional research in this area is needed. This is especially important given females with diabetes develop strokes at a younger age compared with males with diabetes and are more likely to have coronary artery disease compared with females without diabetes.[22]

Sex differences in cardiovascular consequences of diabetes such as complications, ischemic heart disease, and stroke have been demonstrated in the literature.[18,25] In the general population, being a female is cardioprotective, lending to a lower cardiovascular risk profile in females compared with males.[18,19,31] However, in the presence of type 2 diabetes, this cardioprotection for females is attenuated.[18,19,31] A growing body of evidence has demonstrated that females with diabetes have a higher relative risk of cardiovascular disease (i.e., incident and fatal coronary heart diseases, stroke, etc.) compared with males with diabetes and also compared with men and females without diabetes.[18,19,25,32–39] Differences in prescribing practices and the use of medications for cardiovascular disease management and treatment, the clustering of cardiovascular risk factors, and the disproportionate burden of other novel and emergent risk markers have been identified as causes for a higher relative risk of cardiovascular disease in females with diabetes.[18,21] In addition, some studies have shown that the relative risk of ischemic heart disease due to diabetes can be nearly 50% higher among females with diabetes compared with males with diabetes, and the relative risk of stroke has been reported as 27% higher for females with diabetes than males with diabetes.[25,33,35,36] While one systematic review reports limited evidence on the effects of diabetes on microvascular complications, one meta-analysis reports a 19% higher relative risk of vascular dementia among females with diabetes compared with males with diabetes.[25,40] The reasons for these disparities in vascular complications between males and females remain unclear; however, evidence suggests the uptake and provision of healthcare is a plausible explanation and that aggressive risk factor management is needed for females with diabetes.[22,25,32] Finally, some evidence points to females being less likely to be assessed for cardiovascular risk factors such as smoking[41,42]; therefore additional screening for diabetes-related complications in both men and females with diabetes is warranted. de Jong and colleagues suggest the higher relative risk of cardiovascular consequences conferred to females cannot be attributed solely to disparities in risk factor assessment and screening, since other factors including treatment and adherence centered around the uptake and provision of healthcare should also be considered.[25] Therefore there is an urgent need for developing risk assessment strategies and therapeutic interventions that are sex and gender specific to prevent further cardiovascular consequences.[42]

Obesity has been identified as the most prominent risk factor for type 2 diabetes.[18] Compared with males with diabetes, significantly more females with type 2 diabetes have obesity, which often manifests as a higher body mass index and an increased central adiposity.[18] Compared with males, females gain more weight to develop insulin resistance, which is associated with a greater reduction in protection from cardiovascular risk, increased endothelial dysfunction, more low-grade inflammation, and elevated factors resulting in hypercoagulability.[18] Sex differences have also been observed in the relative risk of CVD related to measures of obesity such as waist circumference and waist-to-hip ratio between adults with and without diabetes; however, females with diabetes have the worst outcomes in these areas even in comparison to males.[18]

Finally, females diagnosed with gestational diabetes comprise a unique population group that may be at increased risk for cardiovascular complications. A Canadian systematic review of more than 5,390,000 females who experienced approximately 101,000 cardiovascular events showed an increased risk for CVD (RR, 1.98; 95% CI, 1.57–2.50) for up to 10 years postpartum among females with gestational diabetes, who subsequently developed type 2 diabetes.[43] Similar to the short-term diabetes exposure of gestational diabetes, hypertensive disorders of pregnancy and polycystic ovarian syndrome are both associated with a higher increase for type 2 diabetes and CVD risk factors due to females reportedly having higher rates of overweight/obesity, including central adiposity and dyslipidemia.[31,43]

Racial/Ethnic Minorities

Racial/ethnic disparities are consistently reported in the age of diagnosis with diabetes, HbA_{1c} levels, body composition, and smoking, all which have been noted to influence development of CVD in adults with diabetes.[44,45] For example, African Americans were more likely to be diagnosed with diabetes in younger age groups (18–39 and 40–49 years, compared with < 50), suggesting that early-onset type 2 diabetes may play a role in differences in risk of CVD events in African Americans.[44] Among those with diabetes, MI rates were similar across most racial/ethnic groups, except Asians who had a lower rate of MI.[10] In addition, all racial ethnic groups saw declines in overall rate of MI over time.[10] Stroke rates, however, differed by racial/ethnic group, with non-Hispanic Blacks with diabetes having the highest rate of stroke and seeing no decline over time.[10] In comparison, stroke rates fell in non-Hispanic Whites, Asian, and Hispanic adults with diabetes.[10] Heart failure rates also declined across all racial/ethnic groups except Asians; however, the rate of heart failure remained twice as high for non-Hispanic Black adults with diabetes.[10] Finally, non-Hispanic Blacks are at higher risk of end-stage renal disease (ESRD) compared with non-Hispanic Whites, despite similar access to care and control for demographic differences, clinical conditions, medications, and quality-of-care measures.[46] Some differences in systolic blood pressure existed during follow-up in this group; however, these differences did not explain disparities in ESRD, suggesting work is needed to identify how to decrease disparity gaps noted in cardiovascular consequences of diabetes.[46]

A large body of recent research has focused on understanding disparities in cardiovascular outcomes for Asian adults with type 2 diabetes. Studies in the United Kingdom highlight the importance of considering different ethnicities within the larger Asian population, with South Asian ethnicities noted for a higher risk of CVD compared with Whites and other Asian ethnicities.[44,47,48] While diabetes was associated with a 5% increase in fatal and nonfatal CVD events in White Europeans, it was associated with a 28% increased risk in adults of South Asian ethnicity.[16] This increased risk was primarily driven by increased risk of MI.[16] Malay and Asian Indians with diabetes had a higher CVD risk compared with Chinese adults with diabetes in a study conducted in Singapore.[49] Significant differences were also noted in risk profiles including a higher HbA_{1c} and increased risk of cardiovascular events at a younger age for South Asian adults compared with White Europeans in the United Kingdom.[50] In a study conducted in Ontario, Canada, Chinese adults with diabetes developed fewer cardiovascular complications than Whites; however, the risk for South Asian adults with diabetes was similar to Whites.[47] Differences also existed for complications and mortality, with South Asians showing a lower risk for mortality despite a similar risk for cardiovascular complications.[47] A different pattern existed for a stroke, with Chinese adults showing a similar risk as white patients and South Asians with diabetes having a lower risk than Whites with diabetes.[47] Interethnic differences within Asian populations are likely to exist based on differences in risk profiles (Buljubasic 2020).[51] When using ethnic-specific BMI cutoffs, South Asian adults were more likely to have excess visceral fat associated with increased metabolic risk.[50] Using a matched cohort of Dutch White and Chinese adults with diabetes, Bulijubasic found lower levels of cholesterol (LDL and total cholesterol), cardiac Troponin T, and C-reactive protein in Chinese adults 1-year postacute coronary syndrome diagnosis (Buljubasic 2020). However, in a study conducted in Kuala Lumpur, Malaysia, Chinese ethnicity was associated with a higher risk of asymptomatic left ventricular diastolic dysfunction among adults with diabetes and no known heart disease, compared with other Southeast Asian ethnicities.[51] Differences also exist for macro- and microvascular complications of diabetes by Asian ethnicity, with higher risk for South Asians compared with whites.[52] South Asians with diabetes had a higher prevalence of ischemic heart disease and nephropathy, despite having lower lipid levels.[52] In addition, Pacific Islanders showed a higher prevalence of retinopathy and reduced renal function compared with whites.[52] In a study conducted in Scotland, adults of Pakistani ethnicity developed diabetes earlier, had a higher HbA_{1c}, and had a higher risk of developing CVD (ischemic heart or cerebrovascular disease) compared with whites, while Chinese had a lower risk.[44] The same incidence of CVD in Pakistanis occurred 10 years earlier than for whites or Chinese.[44] More work is needed to understand if the differences are the result of access to healthcare, medication use patterns, medication adherence, management of cardiovascular risk factors over time, or other health behaviors.[44]

To tailor interventions, some researchers have sought to test the utility of phenomapping groups with a higher risk.[53,54] In one study using baseline data from[55] the Action to control cardiovascular risk in diabetes (ACCORD) and Look Action for health in diabetes (AHEAD) trial cohorts, variables were clustered into those with the highest burden of comorbidities and complications, those with intermediate burden and complications, and those with the fewest comorbidities and complications.[53] Those in the group with the fewest comorbidities and complications responded most favorably to a reduction in risk through the interventions.[53] Racial/ethnic differences in unique subgroups have been observed, which may result in a differential risk of CVD over time.[54] In a separate study using data from the National Health and Nutrition Examination Survey, the authors identified four primary phenotypes: diabetes related to aging, severe obesity, severe hyperglycemia, and young adulthood onset.[54] Across all racial/ethnic groups, over half of individuals fit into a subgroup related to aging.[54] One-third of Hispanic individuals were best fit into the severe hyperglycemia subgroup, whereas non-Hispanic Whites and non-Hispanic Blacks fit more often into the severe obesity subgroup.[54] The subgroup related to young adulthood-onset diabetes had worse profiles for complications and worse lipid profiles, compared with the older age-related subgroup, but had similar prevalence across racial/ethnic groups.[54] Further research is needed to understand how diabetes phenotypes can be used to optimize treatment strategies and minimize cardiovascular complications.

Obesity and body composition are a common area of focus to explain racial/ethnic differences in CVD risk. In a longitudinal study conducted in the United Kingdom of adults with diabetes and no CVD at baseline, whites with normal weight developed CVD a half year earlier compared with obese whites, but the risk was similar for normal weight and obese African Caribbean or South Asian adults with diabetes.[56] Further, obese African Caribbean adults were more likely to develop CVD compared with overweight African Caribbean adults by 1.2 years, but there were no differences between obese and overweight whites.[56] An important confounder in this study was smoking, another CVD risk factor, which was more prevalent in the normal weight groups.[56] Many studies highlight the importance of considering metabolic markers beyond BMI in determining risk.[57] For example, abdominal obesity, a known risk factor for CVD independent of BMI differs by race/ethnicity.[57] In one study of US adults, non-Hispanic Black females and Mexican American females had the highest prevalence of abdominal obesity compared with other race/ethnicities.[57] In a second study conducted in the United Kingdom, South Asians were noted to have a higher risk of CVD events at a similar BMI and higher levels of abdominal fat at the same BMI compared with white individuals.[16] As accumulation of visceral fat is associated with higher CVD risk, this may explain some of the disparities in CVD outcomes for South Asian adults with diabetes.[16] Recent research also suggests that metabolically healthy obese individuals may be at a decreased risk of developing CVD, while metabolically unhealthy normal weight individuals may have increased risk for CVD and total mortality.[58] Non-Hispanic Blacks have a higher prevalence of having metabolically healthy obesity compared with non-Hispanic Whites.[57] As a result, metabolic abnormalities and obesity may need to be considered on a continuum, with metabolically healthy individuals at the lower-risk end and likely to progress to an unhealthy phenotype over time.[58]

Elderly

Though the risk for diabetes increases with age, there is far less research investigating age-related disparities compared with disparities by sex or race/ethnicity. In a study conducted across a large, integrated primary care system in Spain, the prevalence of cardiovascular complications increased with age, while the relative importance of traditional risk factors such as hypertension or dyslipidemia stayed the same or decreased with advancing age.[59] In addition, the only significant differences in CVD mortality were age over 80, higher Charlson score, presence of cognitive impairment, and no statin treatment.[59] Based on these results, treatment for older adults with diabetes should be adapted to consider not only lowering of cardiovascular risk but also remaining life expectancy, functional and cognitive impairments, and availability of caregiver support.[59] Finally, among older adult populations, females tend to demonstrate more adverse cardiovascular risk factor profiles compared with males, which suggests investigation of interactions between age and other sociodemographic factors may be of interest for future work.[60]

DISPARITIES IN CARE

Access to healthcare is defined by the Institute of Medicine as having "the timely use of personal health services to achieve the best health outcomes."[61] It requires entry into the healthcare system, receipt of needed services at healthcare sites, and the development of a relationship of mutual communication and trust with providers who meet the needs of individual patients. Equal access to care does not necessarily translate into equity in clinical outcomes. True equity is achieved when there is equity in access, utilization, and outcomes.[62]

Sex Disparities in Access to Care and Management

Sex differences in risk factor control have been well studied and documented; however, the results remain inconclusive in terms of hemoglobin A1c (HbA_{1c}), SBP, diastolic blood pressure (DBP), and low-density lipoprotein cholesterol (LDL-C) control by sex.[63,64] For differences in hypertension (SBP and DBP) and dyslipidemia, mainly LDL-C, differences between males and females may be due to declines in estrogen levels and signaling after menopause.[18] In addition, it has been shown that females are less likely to be prescribed medications such as aspirin, statins, and angiotensin-converting enzyme inhibitors in comparison to males and more likely to be prescribed diuretics.[25] Other evidence suggests that biological differences and differences in treatment adherence between females and males could contribute to sex differences in diabetes-conferred cardiovascular complications.[17,25] The duration of diabetes has been studied in some populations as a plausible cause for sex differences in cardiovascular consequences; however, it has not been shown to account for the observed differences between females and males and has not been as useful in understanding higher cardiovascular risk profiles among females with diabetes.[65] Despite these theories, additional research is needed to understand the sex differences in CVD risk factors and the underlying mechanisms.

When considering biological differences and differences in treatment adherence between females and males, dyslipidemia is a cardiovascular risk factor worth exploring more. Dyslipidemia in type 2 diabetes often manifests as a cluster of abnormalities that include elevated triglycerides, decreased high-density lipoprotein cholesterol, and increased LDL-C.[18] Typically occurring after 60 years of age, females with diabetes experience these abnormalities more frequently than their male counterparts.[18] In addition, females with type 2 diabetes have higher LDL-C levels that are more likely to be poorly controlled[17,18]; however, they are less likely to receive statin therapy or any other lipid-lowering medications compared with males with diabetes.[18] Some evidence suggests that these disparities may be partially attributed to females with diabetes conferring higher LDL-C levels compared with males with diabetes or that factors such as side effects that are less tolerable by females or the associated costs of statin medications could lead to suboptimal adherence among females compared with males.[18,29]

Females with type 2 diabetes have been underrepresented in clinical trials focused on understanding the effect of therapies such as statins and newer diabetes medications on the development of cardiovascular disease, where adherence tends to be poorer among females.[18,66–68] To address this gap, initiatives dedicated to increasing the participation by females with type 2 diabetes in clinical trials should be explored and implemented.[18] In addition, research should focus on understanding the differential impact of medication therapies and interventions by sex on cardiovascular disease development in diabetes.[18] Additional evidence is warranted to understand the biological and physiological mechanisms associated with differences, and work investigating the impact of more aggressive management of cardiovascular risk factors in females or sex-specific therapeutic guidelines would help inform clinical care.[18,22,31,42]

Racial/Ethnic Disparities in Access to Care and Management

Significant differences exist by race/ethnicity in cardiovascular risk factor control in adults with diabetes.[14,69–73] Based on a study comparing national US data from 1988 to 1994 and 1999 to 2008, control of CVD risk factors in adults with diabetes improved over time; however, racial/ethnic disparities increased over the same period.[70] African Americans and Mexican Americans with diabetes were over 50% more likely to have poor glycemic control compared with non-Hispanic White adults.[70] There were no significant differences in blood pressure or total cholesterol between the racial/ethnic groups, and Mexican Americans with diabetes were less likely to smoke compared with non-Hispanic Whites.[70] Similarly, in a study of low-income adults with diabetes in the United States, African Americans were less likely to meet individual or combined treatment goals.[72] In a cohort of US veterans with diabetes, it was also found that non-Hispanic Blacks had a 2-fold-higher odds and Hispanics 1.5-fold higher odds of having at least one risk factor out of control compared with non-Hispanic Whites.[69] When considering having multiple risk factors, non-Hispanic blacks were 1.4, 3.6, and 7.7 times more likely to have one, two, or three risk factors out of control.[69] Hispanics similarly were 1.2, 2.3, and 4.1 times more likely to have one, two, or three risk factors out of control compared with non-Hispanic Whites.[69] In the US Diabetes Collaborative Registry, only 14.7% of African Americans met HbA_{1c}, blood pressure, LDL, and smoking targets, compared with 22.5% of non-Hispanic Whites.[13] These differences were not explained by access to care, as in an insured sample, racial/ethnic differences were more apparent in HbA_{1c}.[71] Asian Indians, Filipinos, Hispanic, and African American adults all showed worse control of HbA_{1c} compared with non-Hispanic Whites.[71] While many studies group individuals of Hispanic/Latino descent into one group, an analysis of data from the ACCORD trial noted differences among Hispanic groups in glucose control.[74] In this sample, all Hispanic groups were less likely to achieve glucose control compared with non-Hispanic Whites.[74]

Racial disparities are also consistently noted in Indigenous populations, with Native American, First Nations, and Australian Aboriginal adults with diabetes experiencing higher rates of cardiovascular disease and poorer risk factor control compared with their non-Indigenous counterparts.[6,75,76] Using data from the California Health Interview Survey, Harjo et al. found that Native Americans with diabetes had a higher prevalence of high cholesterol, compared with non-Hispanic Whites, similar prevalence of hypertension, and a higher likelihood of being a current smoker.[77] Using linked administrative datasets from 1996 to 2015, Chu et al. found declines in incidence of cardiac events among First Nations people with diabetes over time. However, these rates remained higher than other racial groups.[75] Declines in incidence were hypothesized to result from increases in coronary artery revascularization procedures and prescriptions for cardioprotective medications within First Nations people over the same period.[75] In a study of Australian Aboriginal and Anglo-Celt adults with diabetes, both groups showed improvement in HbA_{1c} over time; however, the gap between groups persisted with 70.6% of Aboriginal adults compared with 37.7% of Anglo-Celt adults having an HbA_{1c} over 7%.[76] In addition, fewer Aboriginal patients received antihypertensive treatment or lipid-modifying treatment and were more likely to have retinopathy, microalbuminuria, and PAD compared with Anglo-Celt patients.[76] The higher rates of retinopathy and microalbuminuria are likely a result of worse glycemic control in this group, but the younger age of diabetes diagnosis in Aboriginal adults could also play a role.[76] Additionally, Aboriginal adults had significantly higher smoking rates, which may be a driver of disparities in macrovascular complications such as PAD.[76] As PAD is independently associated with risk of cardiac mortality, this may explain the higher rate of death in Aboriginal adults with diabetes.[76] Access to healthcare is an important consideration for indigenous populations as they are often located in more remote locations with fewer healthcare services. In a study of First Nations people in Ontario, Chu et al. found that while rates of admissions to the hospital for MI and heart failure decreased, the disparity between First Nations people and other adults remained.[75] They noted that current approaches to services are insufficient to close the disparity gap, and poor postdischarge management resulting from poor primary care access may contribute to the ongoing gap.[75] First Nations people face structural barriers such as limited access to facilities, higher levels of food insecurity, and more frequent negative interactions with healthcare providers, which must be addressed to make a meaningful change in outcomes.[75]

Age-Related Disparities in Access to Care and Management

Though potential overtreatment in adults aged 65 and older has received significant attention, studies continue to indicate HbA_{1c} between 6% and 6.9% results in optimal outcomes regardless of age.[7] Individuals aged 65 and older have a higher incidence of all-cause and CVD mortality compared with younger age groups.[7] Additionally, adjusted risk differences associated with increasing HbA_{1c} were larger in older individuals compared with younger, with each 1% increment of HbA_{1c} above 7% associated with higher short- and long-term all-cause and CVD mortality, regardless of age.[7] It will be important for future research to investigate the risks and benefits of more aggressive treatment in older adults, including a collection of the impacts of different treatment regimens on quality of life for older adults and caregivers.

Identification/Screening and Prevention in High-Risk Groups: Prediabetes

Based on the difficulty in preventing comorbidities once diabetes is clinically manifest, the focus is shifting to identifying individuals at high risk for diabetes. While a large body of evidence exists regarding the relationship between diabetes and CVD risk, less work has been conducted in individuals with prediabetes. The Centers for Disease Control and Prevention (CDC) estimates that over one-third of US adults have prediabetes, based on their fasting glucose or HbA_{1c} levels.[2] Of this number, only 19% have been told by a health professional they have prediabetes and therefore may be unaware of their increased risk of developing type 2 diabetes.[2] A higher proportion of males have prediabetes, compared with females (41.9% in males compared with 34.3% in females), and females are estimated to be more often aware of the diagnosis (20.9% in females compared with 17.4% in males).[2] It is worth noting that research has been conducted to assess cardiovascular risk profiles in females with prediabetes compared with males with prediabetes.[78] Similar data have been observed as for diabetes with females with prediabetes having worse cardiovascular risk profiles; however, more extensive research in this area is warranted.[78] As with diabetes, the prevalence of prediabetes increases with age; however, disparities by race/ethnicity are less pronounced than in diabetes.[3]

Due to the similar pathophysiology, the leading cause of morbidity and mortality in both diabetes and prediabetes is CVD.[79] Lifestyle modification is a critical aspect of cardiovascular risk reduction in adults with prediabetes, including physical activity and nutrition.[4] In a pilot study investigating the use of the Diabetes Prevention Program to lower Atherosclerotic cardiovascular disease (ASCVD) risk in adults with prediabetes, Kucera et al. found preliminary evidence for a decrease in cardiovascular risks using the nonpharmacological strategy.[80] In addition, psychosocial factors may influence prediabetes outcomes similar to diabetes. Elevated depressive symptoms were associated with a higher risk of all-cause and CVD mortality, with the strongest magnitude of effect in individuals with prediabetes, compared with those with diabetes.[81] This aligns with recommendations from the American Diabetes Association to provide depression screening for those at high risk of developing diabetes.[11] More work is needed in this area to understand how best to identify and engage individuals with prediabetes to reduce their risk of both diabetes and CVD complications.

Emerging Evidence on Role of Structural Racism, Structural Inequalities, and Social Determinants of Health on Cardiovascular Disease Risk, Cardiovascular Consequences, and Disparities in Care

A growing body of work highlights the importance of considering the role of structural racism, structural inequalities, and social determinants of health when developing strategies to reduce CVD risk in individuals with diabetes.[73,75,82–84] Social determinants of health are defined as the conditions in which people are born, grow, live, work, and age, which shape their health.[85] These include factors like socioeconomic status, neighborhood and physical environment, social support networks, and access to healthcare.[85] Social determinants also encompass more upstream factors that occur antecedent to social risks, including structural racism and structural inequalities.[86] Racism is increasingly recognized as an upstream social determinant of CVD health that must be addressed.[4,83] However, while a broad literature base highlights the influence of social determinants of health on outcomes in adults with diabetes, work is needed to understand the mechanisms of this relationship, interventions to improve the outcomes and minimize complications, and policies to target structural inequalities.[84,86]

Socioeconomic Status

Socioeconomic status (SES) is commonly investigated, with conflicting results depending on where studies were conducted. For example, in a study conducted in South Africa, CVD comorbidity in adults with diabetes was more likely in those with higher education levels.[87] This differs from studies conducted in North American and European countries, which found higher CVD risk in those with lower SES.[82,88,89] Higher levels of material deprivation in a Canadian sample of adolescents with type 1 diabetes were associated with poorer glycemic control, less physical activity, and higher rates of smoking.[82] Similarly, individuals in the two lowest-income quintiles in a study conducted in Sweden had two to three times higher risk of CV events compared with those in the highest-income quartile.[88] The study conducted in South Africa did find a lower likelihood of reporting CVD comorbidities in adults with diabetes who had a high income, which is similar to other countries, and may reflect access to healthcare services and resources for diabetes management.[87] The accumulation of cardiovascular risk over time is hypothesized to result in faster vascular changes, including arterial stiffness.[82] More material deprivation has been associated with increased vascular stiffness, suggesting more vascular dysfunction.[82] While most work to date focuses on objective measures of SES, such as education, employment, and income, one study found differential associations between objective and subjective measures of SES and CVD risk, highlighting the importance of an individual's perspective of their social status.[90] In this study, higher income was associated with lower LDL, and employment was associated with lower HbA_{1c} and higher LDL.[90] Meanwhile, both the lowest and highest levels of subjective social status were significantly associated with higher diastolic blood pressure.[90]

Material deprivation and SES have also been found to influence adherence to medications, a major consideration in ensuring effective care for individuals with diabetes.[91] In a study of 72 primary care clinics in medically underserved neighborhoods of Philadelphia, United States, McClintock and colleagues found that participants with diabetes and CVD were significantly less likely to meet 80% adherence to antidepressant, oral hypoglycemic, or antihypertensive medications.[91] Participants indicated multiple social determinants (social, emotional, and financial) impacted adherence to medications, and paying for medications was difficult given their other basic needs.[91] Forgetting to take medications and a lack of knowledge or insight into the impact of poor adherence were also noted as reasons for nonadherence.[91]

Psychosocial Factors and Trauma

Psychosocial factors, such as anxiety and depression, have also been associated with a higher CVD risk in adults with diabetes.[92] Depression was significantly associated with lower odds of meeting targets for glycemic control, blood pressure, LDL, and smoking in a US registry of patients with diabetes.[13] One study investigated racial/ethnic differences in the prevalence of depression for adults with CVD and diabetes and noted that the prevalence remains significantly lower for African Americans.[45] This difference was suggested to result from discrepancies in the presentation of depression by race, resulting in underreporting and underdiagnosis of depression in African Americans.[45] Based on these results, diagnosis and treatment of depression in adults with diabetes may be an important strategy in not only addressing cardiometabolic targets but reducing cardiovascular risk in adults with diabetes.[45]

Other traumatic experiences have also been associated with an increasing risk for cardiovascular disease. For example, in a study of individuals with type 1 diabetes, childhood trauma was an independent risk factor for a 6-year incidence of CVD after adjusting for age, BMI, blood pressure, proteinuria, and depression.[93]

Social Support and Social Networks

Work has been conducted with racial/ethnic minority groups to identify if social support and social networks can improve outcomes and reduce disparities. Structural social support is defined as social network size and the frequency of personal contacts within the network.[94] In a study conducted with Hispanic adults with diabetes, Hernandez et al. found that individuals with more structural social support, defined as a larger family unit, had higher odds of obesity.[94] However, there was no relationship between structural social support and abdominal obesity, hypertension, hypercholesterolemia, or smoking or between regular contact with family members and any of the CVD risk factors.[94] More work is needed to understand racial/ethnic differences in the use and utility of social support networks in improving CVD risk in individuals with diabetes, with particular attention to how social networks are defined and possible modifiers of the effect.[94] In a post hoc analysis of participants in the ACCORD study, living alone was not associated with a risk of cardiovascular events (cardiac death, nonfatal MI, or nonfatal stroke) in adults with diabetes.[95] This highlights the importance of measuring social support as opposed to using a proxy for measurement such as marital status or living alone.[95]

Peer support interventions are a common strategy to improve diabetes outcomes due to evidence regarding their beneficial impact on glycemic control.[96] In a systematic review of peer support interventions focused on other CVD risk factors, Patil and colleagues also found a small but positive effect on systolic blood pressure in studies where the baseline blood pressure was elevated.[96] However, more studies are needed to investigate additional risk factors. Despite changes in self-management behavior, no reduction in cardiovascular risk was noted in a cluster-randomized controlled trial of a community-based lay peer support intervention in Australia.[97] The authors suggested that the results were explained by over half of the sample already being well controlled at the baseline, highlighting the need to focus the programs on those who may benefit the most.[97]

Neighborhood Characteristics

Neighborhood characteristics, including social cohesion, access to healthy foods, and safe streets, have also been a focus of work specific to improving CVD outcomes for minority populations.[98] In African Americans with type 2 diabetes, social cohesion, violence, and neighborhood problems are hypothesized to influence CVD risk through changes in health behaviors, stress, and limiting social support.[98] A study of adults with diabetes in Kenya found some associations between social cohesion and individual behavioral-based risk factors, such as diet and physical activity, but no influence on the CVD risk score.[99] Results from the Jackson Heart Study indicate that older adults with diabetes are more likely to live in neighborhoods with low social cohesion, more violence, and limited resources.[98] However, more work is needed to understand potential pathways linking neighborhood economic and social conditions and CVD risk and to understand if the neighborhood environment influences specific risk factors more than others in older adults.[98]

Changes in the neighborhood food environment also have the potential to influence disparities in CVD risk for those with diabetes.[4] While dietary quality in the United States has slowly improved over time, this change is greatest in those living at a higher socioeconomic status.[57] This suggests more effort is needed to provide information and access to a higher-quality food supply for individuals living at a lower socioeconomic status.[57] Policies may be effective vehicles for change. For example, more than half the gain in diet quality between 1999 and 2010 was due to a reduction in the consumption of trans fats, which were the target of policy changes during that period.[57] Future work is needed to identify targets for intervention and test the impact on the reduction in CVD risk at an individual and community level.

CONCLUSION

Despite improvements in overall rates of CVD in adults with diabetes, disparities continue in the risk for and complications of CVD. Continued treatment to reduce cardiovascular events and efforts to improve lifestyle change are warranted, particularly through effective tailoring of interventions for high-risk groups. Finally, the coordination between healthcare systems and public health efforts and the incorporation of social determinants of health into treatment efforts will be necessary for long-term sustained improvement in outcomes.

REFERENCES

1. International Diabetes Federation (IDF). IDF Facts & Figures. Available from: https://idf.org/about-diabetes/diabetes-facts-figures/.
2. Centers for Disease Control and Prevention (CDC). National Diabetes Statistics Report website. Available from: https://www.cdc.gov/diabetes/php/data-research/index.html.
3. Centers for Disease Control and Prevention. Diabetes and women. 2022. Accessible from: https://www.cdc.gov/diabetes/risk-factors/diabetes-and-women-1.html?CDC_AAref_Val=https://www.cdc.gov/diabetes/library/features/diabetes-and-women.html.
4. Joseph JJ, Deedwania P, Acharya T, Aguilar D, Bhatt DL, Chyun DA, et al. Comprehensive management of cardiovascular risk factors for adults with type 2 diabetes: a scientific statement from the American Heart Association. Circulation. 2022;145(9):e722–e759.
5. Fan W. Epidemiology in diabetes mellitus and cardiovascular disease. Cardiovasc Endocrinol. 2017;6(1):8–16.
6. Poudel A, Zhou JY, Story D, Li L. Diabetes and Associated Cardiovascular Complications in American Indians/Alaskan Natives: a review of risks and prevention strategies. J Diabetes Res. 2018;2018:2742565.
7. Raghavan S, Vassy JL, Ho YL, Song RJ, Gagnon DR, Cho K, et al. Diabetes mellitus-related all-cause and cardiovascular mortality in a national cohort of adults. J Am Heart Assoc. 2019;8(4):e011295.
8. Dal Canto E, Ceriello A, Ryden L, Ferrini M, Hansen TB, Schnell O, et al. Diabetes as a cardiovascular risk factor: an overview of global trends of macro and micro vascular complications. *Eur J Prev Cardiol*. 2019;26(2_suppl):25–32.
9. Ali MT, Al Suwaidi J. Racial and ethnic differences in cardiovascular disease and outcome in type 1 diabetes patients. *Expert Rev Endocrinol Metab*. 2019;14(4):225–231.
10. Desai JR, Vazquez-Benitez G, Xu Z, Schroeder EB, Karter AJ, Steiner JF, et al. Who must we target now to minimize future cardiovascular events and total mortality?: Lessons from the surveillance, prevention and management of diabetes mellitus (SUPREME-DM) Cohort Study. *Circ Cardiovasc Qual Outcomes*. 2015;8(5):508–516.
11. American Diabetes Association (ADA). Standards of medical care in diabetes – 2024. *Diabetes Care*. 2023;47(Supplement 1).
12. Wong ND, Zhao Y, Patel R, Patao C, Malik S, Bertoni AG, et al. Cardiovascular risk factor targets and cardiovascular disease event risk in diabetes: a pooling project of the atherosclerosis risk in communities study, multi-ethnic study of atherosclerosis, and Jackson Heart Study. *Diabetes Care*. 2016;39(5):668–676.
13. Fan W, Song Y, Inzucchi SE, Sperling L, Cannon CP, Arnold SV, et al. Composite cardiovascular risk factor target achievement and its predictors in US adults with diabetes: the Diabetes Collaborative Registry. *Diabetes Obes Metab*. 2019;21(5):1121–1127.
14. Vargas-Uricoechea H, Caceres-Acosta MF. Control of blood pressure and cardiovascular outcomes in type 2 diabetes. *Open Med (Wars)*. 2018;13:304–323.
15. Gomadam P, Shah A, Qureshi W, Yeboah PN, Freedman BI, Bowden D, et al. Blood pressure indices and cardiovascular disease mortality in persons with or without diabetes mellitus. *J Hypertens*. 2018;36(1):85–92.
16. Coles B, Zaccardi F, Ling S, Davies MJ, Samani NJ, Khunti K. Cardiovascular events and mortality in people with and without type 2 diabetes: an observational study in a contemporary multi-ethnic population. *J Diabetes Investig*. 2021;12(7):1175–1182.
17. de Jong M, Vos RC, de Ritter R, van der Kallen CJ, Sep SJ, Woodward M, Stehouwer CD, Bots ML, Peters SA. Sex differences in cardiovascular risk management for people with diabetes in primary care: a cross-sectional study. *BJGP Open*. 2019;3(2):1–11.
18. Al-Salameh A, Chanson P, Bucher S, Ringa V, Becquemont L. Cardiovascular disease in type 2 diabetes: a review of sex-related differences in predisposition and prevention. *Mayo Clin Proc*. 2019;94(2):287–308.
19. Al-Salameh A, Bucher S, Bauduceau B, Benattar-Zibi L, Berrut G, Bertin P, Corruble E, Danchin N, Derumeaux G, Doucet J, Falissard B, Forette F, Hanon O, Ourabah R, Pasquier F, Pinget M, Ringa V, Becquemont L. Gender-related differences in the control of cardiovascular risk factors in primary care for elderly patients with type 2 diabetes: a cohort study. *Can J Diabetes*. 2018;42(4):365–371. e2.
20. Koutroumpakis E, Aguilar D. Diabetes and cardiovascular disease in women: current challenges and new hope. *Tex Heart Inst J*. 2020;47(2):123–124.
21. Rivellese AA, Riccardi G, Vaccaro O. Cardiovascular risk in women with diabetes. *Nutr Metabol Cardiovasc Dis*. 2010;20:474–480.
22. Madsen TE, Khoury JC, Alwell KA, Moomaw CJ, Demel SL, Flaherty ML, Woo D, Mackey J, De Los Rios La Rosa F, Martini S, Ferioli S, Adeoye O, Khatri P, Kissela BM, Kleindorfer D. Sex differences in cardiovascular risk profiles of ischemic stroke patients with diabetes in the Greater Cincinnati/Northern Kentucky Stroke Study. *J Diabetes*. 2018;10(6):496–501.

23. Bancks MP, Akhabue E, Rana JS, Reis JP, Schreiner PJ, Yano Y, Lewis CE. Sex differences in cardiovascular risk factors before and after the development of type 2 diabetes and risk for incident cardiovascular disease. *Diabetes Res Clin Pract*. 2020;166:108334.
24. Homko CJ, Zamora L, Santamore WP, Kashem A, McConnell T, Bove AA. Gender differences in cardiovascular risk factors and risk perception among individuals with diabetes. *Diab Educ*. 2010;36(3):483–488.
25. de Jong M, Peters SAE, de Ritter R, van der Kallen CJH, Sep SJS, Woodward M, Stehouwer CDA, Bots ML, Vos RC. Sex disparities in cardiovascular risk factor assessment and screening for diabetes-related complications in individuals with diabetes: a systematic review. *Front Endocrinol (Lausanne)*. 2021;12:617902.
26. Galbete A, Cambra K, Foga L, Baquedano FJ, Aizpuru F, Lecea O, Librero J, Ibanez B. Achievement of cardiovascular risk factor targets according to sex and previous history of cardiovascular disease in type 2 diabetes: a population-based study. *J Diabetes Complications*. 2019;33(12):107445.
27. Wang H, Ba Y, Cai R, Xing Q. Association between diabetes mellitus and the risk for major cardiovascular outcomes and all-cause mortality in women compared with men: a meta-analysis of prospective cohort studies. *BMJ Open*. 2019;9(7):e024935.
28. Norhammar A. Schenek-Gustafsson. Type 2 diabetes and cardiovascular disease in women. *Diabetologia*. 2013;56:1–9.
29. Jain RK, Laiteerapong N. Strategies for improving cardiovascular health in women with diabetes mellitus: a review of the literature. *Curr Diab Rep*. 2015;15(11):98.
30. Du T, Fernandez C, Barshop R, Guo Y, Krousel-Wood M, Chen W, Qi L, Harville E, Mauvais-Jarvis F, Fonseca V, Bazzano L. Sex differences in cardiovascular risk profile from childhood to midlife between individuals who did and did not develop diabetes at follow-up: the Bogalusa Heart Study. *Diabetes Care*. 2019;42(4):635–643.
31. Regensteiner JG, Reusch JEB. Sex differences n cardiovascular consequences of hypertension, obesity, and diabetes. JACC Focus Seminar 4/7. *J Am Coll Cardiol*. 2022;79(15):1492–1505.
32. de Ritter R, de Jong M, Vos RC, van der Kallen CJH, Sep SJS, Woodward M, et al. Sex differences in the risk of vascular disease associated with diabetes. *Biol Sex Differ*. 2020;11:1.
33. Millett ERC, Peters SAE, Woodward M. Sex differences in risk factors for myocardial infarction: cohort study of UK Biobank participants. *BMJ*. 2018;363:k4247.
34. de Jong M, Woodward M, Peters SAE. Diabetes, glycated hemoglobin, and the risk of myocardial infarction in women and men: a prospective cohort study of the UK Biobank. *Diabetes Care*. 2020;43(9):2050–2059.
35. Peters SAE, Huxley RR, Woodward M. Diabetes as a risk factor for stroke in women compared with men: a systematic review and meta-analysis of 64 cohorts, including 775,385 individuals and 12,539 strokes. *Lancet (London England)*. 2014;383:1973–1980.
36. Peters SAE, Huxley RR, Woodward M. Diabetes as risk factor for incident coronary heart disease in women compared with men: a systematic review and meta-analysis of 64 cohorts including 858,507 individuals and 28,203 coronary events. *Diabetologia*. 2014;57:1542–1551.
37. Ohkuma T, Komorita Y, Peters SAE, Woodward M. Diabetes as a risk factor for heart failure in women and men: a systematic review and meta-analysis of 47 cohorts including 12 million individuals. *Diabetologia*. 2019;62: 1550–1560.
38. Malmborg M, Schmiegelow MDS, Norgaard CH, Munch A, Gerds T, Schou M, Kistorp C, Torp-Pedersen C, Hlatky MA, Gislason G. Does type 2 diabetes confer higher relative rates of cardiovascular events in women compared with men? *Eur Heart J*. 2020;41:1346–1353.
39. Miller RG, Costacou T. Glucose management and the sex difference in excess cardiovascular disease risk in long-duration type 1 diabetes. *Curr Diab Rep*. 2019;19:139.
40. Chatterjee S, Peters SAE, Woodward M, Arango SM, Batty GD, Beckett N, et al. Type 2 diabetes as a risk factor for dementia in women compared with men: a pooled analysis of 2.3 million people comprising more than 100,000 cases of dementia. *Diabetes Care*. 2016;39:300–307.
41. Hyun KK, Millett ERC, Redfern J, Brieger D, Peters SAE, Woodward M, et al. Sex differences in the assessment of cardiovascular risk in primary health care: a systematic review. *Heart Lung Circ*. 2019;28:1535–1548.
42. Wang Y, O'Neil A, Jiao Y, Wang L, Huang J, Lan Y, Zhu Y, Yu C. Sex differences in the association between diabetes and risk of cardiovascular disease, cancer, and all-cause and cause-specific mortality: a systematic review and meta-analysis of 5,162,654 participants. *BMC Med*. 2019;17(1):36.
43. Harreiter J, Fadl H, Kautzky-Willer A, Simmons D. Do women with diabetes need more intensive action for cardiovascular reduction than men with diabetes. *Curr Diab Rep*. 2020;20:61.
44. Malik MO, Govan L, Petrie JR, Ghouri N, Leese G, Fischbacher C, et al. Ethnicity and risk of cardiovascular disease (CVD): 4.8 year follow-up of patients with type 2 diabetes living in Scotland. *Diabetologia*. 2015;58(4):716–725.
45. Dibato JE, Montvida O, Zaccardi F, Sargeant JA, Davies MJ, Khunti K, et al. Association of cardiometabolic multimorbidity and depression with cardiovascular events in early-onset adult type 2 diabetes: a multiethnic study in the U.S. *Diabetes Care*. 2021;44(1):231–239.
46. Lewis EF, Claggett B, Parfrey PS, Burdmann EA, McMurray JJ, Solomon SD, et al. Race and ethnicity influences on cardiovascular and renal events in patients with diabetes mellitus. *Am Heart J*. 2015;170(2):322–329.
47. Shah BR, Victor JC, Chiu M, Tu JV, Anand SS, Austin PC, et al. Cardiovascular complications and mortality after diabetes diagnosis for South Asian and Chinese patients: a population-based cohort study. *Diabetes Care*. 2013;36(9):2670–2676.
48. Mehta A, Singh S, Saeed A, Mahtta D, Bittner VA, Sperling LS, et al. Pathophysiological mechanisms underlying excess risk for diabetes and cardiovascular disease in South Asians: the perfect storm. *Curr Diabetes Rev*. 2021;17(9):e070320183447.
49. Liu JJ, Lim SC, Yeoh LY, Su C, Tai BC, Low S, et al. Ethnic disparities in risk of cardiovascular disease, end-stage renal disease and all-cause mortality: a prospective study among Asian people with Type 2 diabetes. *Diabet Med*. 2016;33(3):332–339.
50. Bellary S, O'Hare JP, Raymond NT, Mughal S, Hanif WM, Jones A, et al. Premature cardiovascular events and mortality in south Asians with type 2 diabetes in the United Kingdom Asian Diabetes Study - effect of ethnicity on risk. *Curr Med Res Opin*. 2010;26(8):1873–1879.
51. Chee KH, Tan KL, Luqman I, Saiful SS, Chew YY, Chinna K, et al. Prevalence and predictors of left ventricular diastolic dysfunction in Malaysian patients with type 2 diabetes mellitus without prior known cardiovascular disease. *Front Cardiovasc Med*. 2021;8:676862.
52. Kou S, Cao JY, Yeo S, Holmes-Walker DJ, Lau SL, Gunton JE. Ethnicity influences cardiovascular outcomes and complications in patients with type 2 diabetes. *J Diabetes Complications*. 2018;32(2):144–149.
53. Segar MW, Patel KV, Vaduganathan M, Caughey MC, Jaeger BC, Basit M, et al. Development and validation of optimal phenomapping methods to estimate long-term atherosclerotic cardiovascular disease risk in patients with type 2 diabetes. *Diabetologia*. 2021;64(7):1583–1594.
54. Bancks MP, Casanova R, Gregg EW, Bertoni AG. Epidemiology of diabetes phenotypes and prevalent cardiovascular risk factors and diabetes complications in the National Health and Nutrition Examination Survey 2003–2014. *Diabetes Res Clin Pract*. 2019;158:107915.
55. Buljubasic N, Zhao W, Cheng J, et al. Comparison of temporal changes in established cardiovascular biomarkers after acute coronary syndrome between Caucasian and Chinese patients with diabetes mellitus. *Biomarkers*. 2020;25(4):341–348. https://doi.org/10.1080/1354750X.2020.1759692.
56. Owusu Adjah ES, Ray KK, Paul SK. Ethnicity-specific association of BMI levels at diagnosis of type 2 diabetes with cardiovascular disease and all-cause mortality risk. *Acta Diabetol*. 2019;56(1):87–96.
57. Bhupathiraju SN, Hu FB. Epidemiology of obesity and diabetes and their cardiovascular complications. *Circ Res*. 2016;118(11):1723–1735.
58. Aung K, Lorenzo C, Hinojosa MA, Haffner SM. Risk of developing diabetes and cardiovascular disease in metabolically unhealthy normal-weight and metabolically healthy obese individuals. *J Clin Endocrinol Metab*. 2014; 99(2):462–468.
59. Clua-Espuny JL, Gonzalez-Henares MA, Queralt-Tomas MLL, Campo-Tamayo W, Muria-Subirats E, Panisello-Tafalla A, et al. Mortality and cardiovascular complications in older complex chronic patients with type 2 diabetes. *Biomed Res Int*. 2017;2017:6078498.
60. Gobl CS, Brannath W, Bozkurt L, Handisurya A, Anderwalkd C, Luger A, Crebs M, Kautzk-Willer A, Bischof MG. Sex-specific differences in glycemic control and cardiovascular risk factors in older patients with insulin-treated type 2 diabetes mellitus. *Gend Med*. 2010;7(6):593–599.
61. Institute of Medicine (IOM), Committee on Monitoring Access to Personal Health Care Services. *Access to Health Care in America*. Washington, DC: National Academy Press; 1993.
62. Oliver A, Mossialos E. Equity of access to health care: outlining the foundations for action. *J Epidemiol Community Health*. Aug 2004;58(8):655–658.
63. Schroeder EB, Bayliss EA, Daugherty SL, Steiner JF. Gender differences in cardiovascular risk factors in incident diabetes. *Women's Health Issues*. 2014;24(1):e61–e68.
64. Strom Williams JL, Lynch CP, Winchester R, Thomas L, Keith B, Egede LE. Gender differences in composite control of cardiovascular risk factors among patients with type 2 diabetes. *Diabetes Technol Ther*. 2014;16(7): 421–427.
65. de Jong M, Woodward M, Peters SAE. Duration of diabetes and the risk of major cardiovascular events in women and men: a prospective cohort study of UK Biobank participants. *Diabetes Res Clin Pract*. 2022;188: 109899.
66. Salinero-Fort MA, Mostaza-Prieto JM, Lahoz-Rallo C, Diez JIV, Cardenas-Valladolid J. Population-based cross-sectional study of 11 645 Spanish nonagenarians with type 2 diabetes mellitus: cardiovascular profile, cardiovascular preventive therapies, achievement goals and sex differences. *BMJ Open*. 2019;9(9):e030344.
67. Yeo JL, Brady EM, McCann GP, Gulsin GS. Sex and ethnic differences in the cardiovascular complications of type 2 diabetes. *Ther Adv Endocrinol Metab*. 2021;12:1–24.
68. Clemens KK, Woodward M, Neal B, Zinman B. Sex disparitires in cardiovascular outcome trials of populations with diabetes: a systematic review and meta-analysis. *Diabetes Care*. 2020;43:1157–1163.
69. Egede LE, Gebregziabher M, Lynch CP, Gilbert GE, Echols C. Longitudinal ethnic differences in multiple cardiovascular risk factor control in a cohort of US adults with diabetes. *Diabetes Res Clin Pract*. 2011;94(3):385–394.
70. Chatterji P, Joo H, Lahiri K. Racial/ethnic- and education-related disparities in the control of risk factors for cardiovascular disease among individuals with diabetes. *Diabetes Care*. 2012;35(2):305–312.
71. Holland AT, Zhao B, Wong EC, Choi SE, Wong ND, Palaniappan LP. Racial/ethnic differences in control of cardiovascular risk factors among type 2 diabetes patients in an insured, ambulatory care population. *J Diabetes Complications*. 2013;27(1):34–40.

72. Wang Y, Katzmarzyk PT, Horswell R, Zhao W, Li W, Johnson J, et al. Racial disparities in cardiovascular risk factor control in an underinsured population with Type 2 diabetes. *Diabet Med.* 2014;31(10):1230–1236.
73. Joseph JJ, Ortiz R, Acharya T, Golden SH, Lopez L, Deedwania P. Cardiovascular Impact of Race and Ethnicity in Patients With Diabetes and Obesity: JACC Focus Seminar 2/9. *J Am Coll Cardiol.* 2021;78(24):2471–2482.
74. Getaneh A, Light LS, Brillon DJ, Calles Escandon J, Felicetta J, Evans GW, et al. Diabetes control among Hispanics in the action to control cardiovascular risk in diabetes trial. *J Gen Intern Med.* 2012;27(11):1499–1505.
75. Chu A, Han L, Roifman I, Lee DS, Green ME, Jacklin K, et al. Trends in cardiovascular care and event rates among First Nations and other people with diabetes in Ontario, Canada, 1996-2015. *CMAJ.* 2019;191(47):E1291–E8.
76. Davis TM, Hunt K, McAullay D, Chubb SA, Sillars BA, Bruce DG, et al. Continuing disparities in cardiovascular risk factors and complications between aboriginal and Anglo-Celt Australians with type 2 diabetes: the Fremantle Diabetes Study. *Diabetes Care.* 2012;35(10):2005–2011.
77. Harjo TC, Perez A, Lopez V, Wong ND. Prevalence of diabetes and cardiovascular risk factors among California Native American adults compared with other ethnicities: the 2005 California Health Interview Survey. *Metab Syndr Relat Disord.* 2011;9(1):49–54.
78. Anagnostis P, Majeed Z, Johnston DG, Godsland IF. Cardiovascular risk in women with type 2 diabetes mellitus and prediabetes: is it indeed higher than men? Europenal. *Eur J Endocrinol.* 2014;147:R245–R255.
79. Mellbin LG, Anselmino M, Lars R. Diabetes, prediabetes and cardiovascular risk. *Europ J Cardiovasc Prevent Rehab.* 2010;17(1_suppl):s9–s14.
80. Kucera M, Marchewka T, Craib A. Does losing 5–7% of prediabetic body weight from a diabetes prevention program decrease cardiovascular risks? *Spartan Med Res J.* 2021;6(2):27627.
81. Liwo ANN, Howard VJ, Zhu S, Martin MY, Safford MM, Richman JS, et al. Elevated depressive symptoms and risk of all-cause and cardiovascular mortality among adults with and without diabetes: The REasons for Geographic And Racial Differences in Stroke (REGARDS) study. *J Diabetes Complications.* 2020;34(10):107672.
82. Inman M, Daneman D, Curtis J, Sochett E, Clarke A, Dunger DB, et al. Social Determinants of Health Are Associated with Modifiable Risk Factors for Cardiovascular Disease and Vascular Function in Pediatric Type 1 Diabetes. *J Pediatr.* 2016;177:167–172.
83. Powell-Wiley TM, Baumer Y, Baah FO, Baez AS, Farmer N, Mahlobo CT, Pita MA, Potharaju KA, Tamura K, Wallen GR. Social determinants of cardiovascular disease. *Circ Research.* 2022;130(5):782–799.
84. Egede LE, Campbell JA, Walker RJ, Linde S. Structural racism as an upstream social determinant of diabetes outcomes: a scoping review. *Diabetes Care.* 2023;46(4):667–677.
85. Artiga S, Hinton E. *Beyond Health Care: the Role Of Social Determinants In Promoting Health And Health Equity. Issue Brief.* Kaiser Family Foundation; 2018. Available from http://files.kff.org/attachment/issue-brief-beyond-health-care.
86. Egede LE, Walker RJ, Linde S, Campbell JA, Dawson AZ, Williams JS, Ozieh MN. Nonmedical interventions for type 2 diabetes: evidence, actionable strategies, and policy opportunities. *Health Affairs.* 2022;41(7):963–970.
87. Mutyambizi C, Chola L, Groot W, Pavlova M, Labadarios D, Hongoro C. The extent and determinants of diabetes and cardiovascular disease comorbidity in South Africa - results from the South African National Health and Nutrition Examination Survey (SANHANES-1). *BMC Public Health.* 2017;17(1):745.
88. Rawshani A, Svensson AM, Rosengren A, Eliasson B, Gudbjornsdottir S. Impact of socioeconomic status on cardiovascular disease and mortality in 24,947 individuals with type 1 diabetes. *Diabetes Care.* 2015;38(8):1518–1527.
89. Whittaker E, Read SH, Colhoun HM, Lindsay RS, McGurnaghan S, McKnight JA, et al. Socio-economic differences in cardiovascular disease risk factor prevalence in people with type 2 diabetes in Scotland: a cross-sectional study. *Diabet Med.* 2020;37(8):1395–1402.
90. Doshi T, Smalls BL, Williams JS, Wolfman TE, Egede LE. Socioeconomic status and cardiovascular risk control in adults with diabetes. *Am J Med Sci.* 2016;352(1):36–44.
91. McClintock HF, Schatell ET, Bogner HR. Cardiovascular disease and medication adherence among patients with type 2 diabetes mellitus in an underserved community. *Behav Med.* 2022;48(1):31–42.
92. Chu H, Chen L, Yang X, Qiu X, Qiao Z, Song X, et al. Roles of anxiety and depression in predicting cardiovascular disease among patients with type 2 diabetes mellitus: a machine learning approach. *Front Psychol.* 2021;12:645418.
93. Roy A, Janal MN, Roy M. Childhood trauma and prevalence of cardiovascular disease in patients with type 1 diabetes. *Psychosom Med.* 2010;72(8):833–838.
94. Hernandez R, Carnethon M, Giachello AL, Penedo FJ, Wu D, Birnbaum-Weitzman O, et al. Structural social support and cardiovascular disease risk factors in Hispanic/Latino adults with diabetes: results from the Hispanic Community Health Study/Study of Latinos (HCHS/SOL). *Ethn Health.* 2018;23(7):737–751.
95. Zhu Z, Peng Z, Xing Z. Living alone is not associated with cardiovascular events and hypoglycemia in patients with type 2 diabetes mellitus. *Front Public Health.* 2022;10:883383.
96. Patil SJ, Ruppar T, Koopman RJ, Lindbloom EJ, Elliott SG, Mehr DR, et al. Effect of peer support interventions on cardiovascular disease risk factors in adults with diabetes: a systematic review and meta-analysis. *BMC Public Health.* 2018;18(1):398.
97. Riddell MA, Dunbar JA, Absetz P, Wolfe R, Li H, Brand M, et al. Cardiovascular risk outcome and program evaluation of a cluster randomised controlled trial of a community-based, lay peer led program for people with diabetes. *BMC Public Health.* 2016;16(1):864.
98. Leak-Johnson T, Yan F, Daniels P. What the Jackson heart study has taught us about diabetes and cardiovascular disease in the African American community: a 20-year appreciation. *Curr Diab Rep.* 2021;21(10):39.
99. Ruchman SG, Delong AK, Kamano JH, Bloomfield GS, Chrysanthopoulou SA, Fuster V, et al. Egocentric social network characteristics and cardiovascular risk among patients with hypertension or diabetes in western Kenya: a cross-sectional analysis from the BIGPIC trial. *BMJ Open.* 2021;11(9):e049610.

27 The Quality Chasm and the Need for Implementation Science to Reduce Cardiovascular Disease Risk in Type 2 Diabetes

NEHA J. PAGIDIPATI

"A little knowledge that acts is worth infinitely more than much knowledge that is idle."

—Kahlil Gibran

INTRODUCTION

Cardiovascular disease (CVD) has long been the leading cause of death among individuals with type 2 diabetes mellitus (T2DM),[1] who are twice as likely to develop CVD than those without diabetes.[2] Despite the increased CV risk associated with T2DM, much of CVD can be prevented with aggressive risk factor management. Indeed, persons with T2DM who have all five risk factors (glycated hemoglobin [HbA_{1c}], low-density lipoprotein cholesterol [LDL-C], albuminuria, tobacco use, and blood pressure) within the target ranges have minimal excess risk of death, myocardial infarction, or stroke compared with those without T2DM.[3] Beyond traditional risk factor management, we now have increasing therapeutic options with which to combat this increased CV risk. In addition to the significant benefit that high-intensity statins,[4] BP control, ACE inhibitors (ACEi),[5] and angiotensin receptor blockers (ARB)[6] provide in CV risk reduction, glucagon-like peptide-1 receptor agonists (GLP-1RAs) and sodium glucose cotransporter-2 inhibitors (SGLT2i) have more recently been shown to impart significant CV benefit in T2DM, independent of their glycemic effect.[7,8] Thus with appropriate risk factor control and use of effective therapies, we have within our grasp the ability to significantly reduce the burden of CVD among persons with T2DM.

However, the difference between what we know and what we actually do in clinical practice is unfortunately stark. This is the so-called quality chasm, a term coined by the Institute of Medicine in the landmark 2001 report "Crossing the Quality Chasm: A New Health System for the 21st Century."[9] In CV risk reduction in T2DM, this quality chasm manifests as too few persons actually achieving complete risk factor control or being prescribed and taking all evidence-based therapies for which they are eligible. The reasons behind these gaps in care for persons with T2DM are multiple, varied, and as complex as the persons and the healthcare ecosystem itself. To begin to understand and address why persons with T2DM are not receiving optimal care, we must apply the same scientific rigor that we use to develop effective therapies in the first place.

Implementation science provides this backbone for scientific inquiry into the reasons behind and remedies for the quality chasm. The National Institutes of Health defines implementation science as "the study of methods to promote the adoption and integration of evidence-based practices, interventions, and policies into routine health care and public health settings to improve our impact on population health."[10] Indeed, implementation science can been defined in many ways, but at its core, it is the science of systematically getting "what works" to the people who need it.[11] It requires a commitment to producing generalizable knowledge about applying the evidence that can be scaled and used to improve health on a population level.

Here, current challenges facing providers of and persons with T2DM in achieving optimal care will be reviewed, and ways in which implementation science can provide opportunities to improve the management of this high-risk population will be explored.

THE QUALITY CHASM IN CV RISK REDUCTION IN TYPE 2 DIABETES

The quality chasm in CV risk reduction in T2DM exists on multiple levels, including achievement of guideline-recommended risk factor targets and prescription of and adherence to evidence-based therapies. With regard to achieving optimal risk factor levels, data from three diverse US longitudinal cohorts between 1990 and 2004 revealed that only 7.2% of individuals with T2DM were at target for a composite of three risk factors (BP < 130/80 mm Hg, LDL-C < 100 mg/dL, HbA_{1c} < 7%).[12] However, those who did achieve this composite were at significantly decreased risk (HR 0.38 [95% CI 0.25–0.58]) for CVD events compared with those without any risk factors at target. Subsequently, an examination of the US National Health and Nutrition Examination Survey between 1999 and 2010 revealed that even though there were modest improvements over time, only 25% of individuals with T2DM in 2009–2010 had all three of the above risk factors at goal.[13] From a global perspective, within the context of an international trial in 2008–2012, only 29.9% of persons with T2DM and ASCVD achieved five secondary prevention goals (aspirin therapy, LDL-C < 70 mg/dL or statin therapy, BP < 140/90 mm Hg, ACEi or ARB use, nonsmoking status).[14] More recently, a study from the US Diabetes Collaborative Registry found that only 13% of individuals with T2DM achieved a composite of four risk factors at target (HbA_{1c} < 7% or < 8% with ASCVD, LDL-C < 100 mg/dL or < 70 mg/dL with ASCVD, BP < 130/80 mm Hg, and nonsmoking status).[15] Perhaps even more striking were the discrepancies by socioeconomic status and race: individuals with high median household income were 29% more likely to achieve the composite than those with low income, and White individuals were 43% more likely to achieve the composite than non-White individuals.

Contributing to this low level of risk factor control are significant deficiencies in the prescription of evidence-based therapies to reduce CV risk among pesons with T2DM. These gaps persist even with older therapies that are supported by several decades' worth of data. For example, among 155,958 persons with T2DM and ASCVD in a commercially insured population, only 24.7% were on a high-intensity statin, and only 53.1% were on an ACEi or ARB.[16] When SGLT2i and GLP-1RAs were also taken into account, only 2.7% of the eligible population were on all three classes of therapies (Fig. 27.1). An examination of health systems across the United States yields similar findings: among over 320,000 persons with T2DM and ASCVD in 12 large health systems, only 4.6% were on all three classes of therapies; 42.6% were on none.[17]

SGLT2i and GLP-1RA appear to have particularly poor usage in the United States. Despite increasing uptake overall, 80% of clinicians who prescribed metformin to Medicare beneficiaries in 2018 did *not* prescribe SGLT2i, and sulfonylurea prescriptions were three times more frequent than SGLT2i, despite no evidence of CV benefit.[18] Prescription rates are also low in the Veterans Affairs (VA) health system, despite coverage of these agents. In 2020, 11.2% of persons with T2DM and ASCVD in the VA system received an SGLT2i, while 8.0% received a GLP-1RA.[19] These individuals were more likely to be young and White, again highlighting disparities in use. Despite the magnitude of ASCVD and HF benefit from these agents, cardiologists appear to be particularly hesitant to prescribe these medications.[20] This hesitancy is reflected in national prescribing data: in 2020, cardiologists represented only 1.5% of SGLT2i prescriptions and 0.4% of GLP-1RA prescriptions.[21]

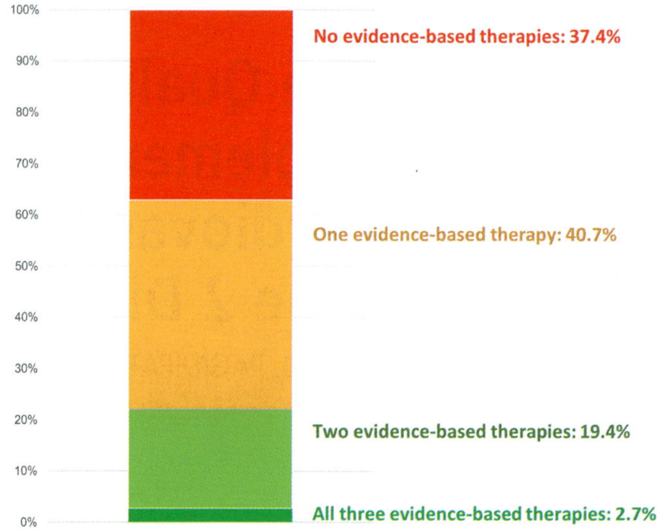

FIG. 27.1 Proportions of persons on all three, two, one, or none of the evidence-based therapies: high-intensity statin, ACEi or ARB, SGLT-2i or GLP-1RA. *ACEI*, Angiotensin-converting enzyme inhibitor; *ARB*, angiotensin receptor blocker; *SGLT2i*, sodium-glucose cotransporter 2 inhibitors; *GLP1-RA*, glucagonlike peptide-1 receptor a gonists. (Nelson AJ, Ardissino M, Haynes K, et al. Gaps in evidence-based therapy use in insured persons in the United States with type 2 diabetes mellitus and atherosclerotic cardiovascular disease. *J Am Heart Assoc.* 2021;10:e016835.)

Adherence to evidence-based therapies in T2DM is also quite low, with significant disparities by race. For example, persistent statin use at 1 year after initiation is significantly lower among younger, Black, and Hispanic persons versus older White persons.[22] With regard to SGLT2i, approximately 55% of persons are not highly adherent (defined as proportion of days covered ≥80%), and those with lower adherence are more likely to be female and/or Black.[23] Rates of adherence to GLP-1RA appear to be similar.[24]

Thus, while new, effective therapies continue to be developed, unacceptably low prescription of and adherence to these therapies persist, and disparities widen.[25] Reasons for this quality chasm are multifactorial and include society-level social determinants of health, as well as health system level, provider level, patient level, and cost barriers.[26] The optimal way to overcome all of these barriers is not clear, but one thing is absolutely certain—what we as a medical community have been doing thus far is not working. It takes approximately 17 years for new evidence from clinical trials to be incorporated into routine clinical practice, and even then application is inequitable, as is supported by the data above.[27] If we are to improve the quality of care for persons with T2DM, we need to apply a rigorous, iterative, scientific process to achieve this goal—such as the one provided by implementation science.

IMPLEMENTATION SCIENCE PRINCIPLES

Implementation science can be thought of as the science of turning what we *know* into what we *do*. By applying research findings to real-world settings, implementation science seeks to integrate knowledge and best practices into practice and policy in a sustainable way.[28] This discipline is distinct from quality improvement, which focuses on a specific problem in a specific healthcare setting; implementation science, in contrast, starts with an

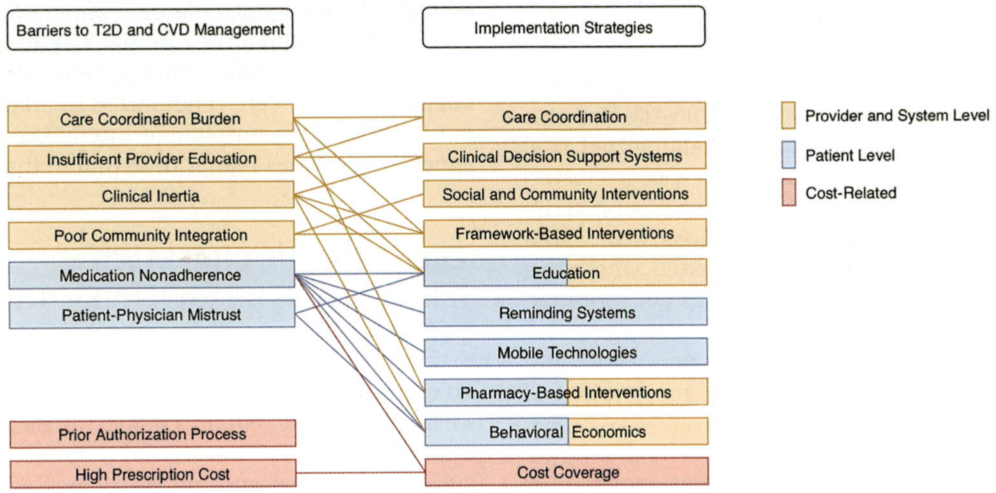

FIG. 27.2 Framework of barriers to optimal management of T2D and CVD and corresponding implementation strategies. *CVD*, Cardiovascular disease; *T2DM*, type 2 diabetes mellitus. (Gao Y, Peterson E, Pagidipati N. Opportunities for improving use of evidence-based therapy in persons with type 2 diabetes and cardiovascular disease. *Clin Cardiol.* 2019;42:1063–1070.)

underutilized evidence-based practice and seeks to create knowledge that can be generalized to other settings.[29]

While clinical studies assess the impact of a therapy or evidence-based practice on health outcomes, implementation studies focus on the rate or quality of use of the therapy or practice.[29] For example, a clinical study may evaluate cardiovascular and renal outcomes of a given SGLT2i, but an implementation study may evaluate the rates of prescription and adherence to SGLT2i across broad populations. As such, outcomes of implementation studies generally focus on process metrics and on the use of the target therapy or practice. As opposed to clinical studies, in which the study teams are often blinded to the outcome during the trial, data in implementation studies can be fed back to the study team to improve the implementation process. This so-called formative evaluation allows for an iterative process that is central to implementation science but must be specified a priori as part of the research plan or study hypothesis.[29] Of note, elements of clinical and implementation studies can be combined in hybrid effectiveness-implementation designs, which both evaluate the effectiveness of a given therapy or practice and evaluate the implementation strategies to increase or improve its use.[30]

An essential component of the implementation science process is early, frequent, and meaningful engagement of all relevant stakeholders.[28] This begins as early as research question formulation. Gaining a deep understanding of the barriers and facilitators that stakeholders face when utilizing a given therapy or practice is a critical first step to the implementation process. In this context, the term *stakeholder* is used broadly to indicate any individual or organization who is relevant to the use of the therapy of interest, including persons, families, caregivers, clinicians of varying types, health systems, payers, policymakers, and others. Importantly, particular thought should be given to those who should be involved in the process but are not because they have been historically marginalized.[28]

Once a gap in care has been identified and stakeholders have been engaged to better understand the barriers and facilitators of the use of the evidence-based therapy or practice, implementation strategies that specifically address those barriers and facilitators must be chosen. Implementation strategies are, quite simply, the "stuff we do" to increase the use of a given therapy or practice.[31] Significant efforts have been made to codify discrete implementation strategies, leading to a compilation of 73 discrete implementation strategies.[32] Examples of implementation strategies as they pertain to patient-, provider-, and system-level barriers to optimal CV care for persons with T2DM are outlined in Fig. 27.2.

Finally, a critically important component of the implementation process is rigorous evaluation of outcomes. Many potential implementation outcomes exist, each with specific measurement tools and metrics available to assess them.[33] Such outcomes include acceptability, adoption, appropriateness, costs, feasibility, fidelity, penetration, and sustainability.[33] Several frameworks have been developed to guide the evaluation process for implementation studies, perhaps the most well-known among them being the RE-AIM framework.[34,35] The RE-AIM framework focuses on concepts that are important for the external validity of a given program: Reach (the proportion or representativeness of individuals who are willing to participate in the program), Effectiveness (the impact of the program on important outcomes), Adoption (the proportion or representativeness of settings and people delivering the intervention who are willing to participate in the program), Implementation (fidelity to the intervention protocol and consistency of delivery), and Maintenance (long-term sustainability).[35] Utilizing a systematic approach to evaluating implementation efforts is critical for the generalizability of this knowledge.

IMPLEMENTATION SCIENCE IN CV RISK REDUCTION IN TYPE 2 DIABETES

Several examples of implementation studies to improve the care of high-risk persons with T2DM can illustrate the principles outlined above.

Provider Level

As outlined above, there are significant deficiencies in the degree to which evidence-based agents are prescribed to persons with T2DM and CVD. The COORDINATE-Diabetes Trial (COOrdinating CaRDIology CliNics RAndomized Trial of Interventions to Improve OutcomEs) was a cluster-randomized implementation trial to increase the prescription of evidence-based therapies in persons with T2DM and CVD (NCT03936660).[36,37] The trial tested whether a multifaceted intervention that incorporates collaboration between cardiologists and diabetes specialists, provider education, site-tailored care pathways, and audit and feedback to providers could increase the prescription of ACEi/ARB, high-intensity statin, and SGLT2i or GLP-1RA. Randomization to this intervention versus standard education occurred at the level of the cardiology clinic. After 6 to 12 months, individuals in the intervention arm were more likely to be prescribed all three therapies (173/457 [37.9%]) versus those in the usual arm (85/588 [14.5%]; absolute difference of 23.4%; adjusted odds ratio [OR], 4.38 [95% CI, 2.49–7.71]; $P<0.001$).[37] This large, randomized trial proved that a coordinated, multifaceted intervention could improve the prescription of evidence-based therapies across cardiology clinics in the United States.

System Level

Several implementation studies targeting system-level aspects of care delivery to high-risk persons with T2DM have been evaluated. A study within the VA health system evaluated the implementation of an intervention that had already been well-proven to prevent T2DM, the Diabetes Prevention Program (DPP).[38] Using the RE-AIM framework to assess outcomes, they found that their method of implementing the DPP, called the VA-DPP, had better fidelity and participant satisfaction than standard of care but experienced significant barriers related to reach. Another study in the Mass General Brigham Network randomly assigned individuals with T2DM and increased CV or kidney risk to simultaneous virtual patient education and prescription of SGLT2i or GLP-1RA versus 2 months of virtual patient education followed by medication prescription.[39] The intervention was innovative because it was completely remotely delivered and was led by nonlicensed navigators and clinical pharmacists. After 6 months, those in the Simultaneous arm were more likely to have a prescription for SGLT2i or GLP-1RA (70%) than those in the Education-First arm (56%). Of note, prescription of either of these therapies was 64% across both arms, indicating a high rate of success of the overall intervention, regardless of whether the prescriptions were given early or later.

Patient Level

Implementation studies at the patient level can focus on increasing adherence to evidence-based therapies. For example, one randomized study found that a comprehensive pharmacy care program can lead to improved medication adherence, persistence, and blood pressure control compared with standard of care among older adults.[40] Another example of a patient-level implementation study examined the optimal way to get persons with uncontrolled T2DM to enroll in a behavioral intervention.[41] Eligible persons were randomized to an opt-in versus opt-out approach; the enrollment rate in the opt-out arm was almost three times higher than that in the opt-in arm.

CROSSING THE CHASM WITH IMPLEMENTATION SCIENCE—THE PATH FORWARD

To cross the quality chasm for CV risk reduction in T2DM, we need to fundamentally change the behavior patterns of health systems, providers, and persons. However, changing organizational and individual behavior is one of the most complex tasks to undertake; without rigorous methods such as those provided by implementation science to guide the process, such an endeavor has little chance of success. The field of implementation science is in its relative infancy, and for persons with T2DM to get the quality of care that they need and deserve, funding for implementation research must be prioritized. Indeed, one could argue that a focus on getting effective therapies used equitably is as important for public health as developing the therapies in the first place. The pharmaceutical industry spent US$83 billion in 2019 on drug research and development.[42] If just a fraction of that funding were put toward implementation science efforts, overall health and quality of life of persons with T2DM would certainly improve.

REFERENCES

1. National Diabetes Statistics Report Website. Centers for Disease Control and Prevention. Available from: https://www.cdc.gov/diabetes/data/statistics-report/index.html.)
2. Emerging Risk Factors C, Sarwar N, Gao P, et al. Diabetes mellitus, fasting blood glucose concentration, and risk of vascular disease: a collaborative meta-analysis of 102 prospective studies. *Lancet*. 2010;375:2215–2222.
3. Rawshani A, Rawshani A, Franzen S, et al. Risk factors, mortality, and cardiovascular outcomes in patients with type 2 diabetes. *N Engl J Med*. 2018;379:633–644.
4. Cholesterol Treatment, Trialists C, Kearney PM, Blackwell L, et al. Efficacy of cholesterol-lowering therapy in 18,686 people with diabetes in 14 randomised trials of statins: a meta-analysis. *Lancet*. 2008;371:117–125.
5. Effects of ramipril on cardiovascular and microvascular outcomes in people with diabetes mellitus: results of the HOPE study and MICRO-HOPE substudy. Heart Outcomes Prevention Evaluation Study Investigators. *Lancet*. 2000;355:253–259.
6. Foulquier S, Bohm M, Schmieder R, et al. Impact of telmisartan on cardiovascular outcome in hypertensive patients at high risk: a Telmisartan Randomised AssessmeNt Study in ACE iNtolerant subjects with cardiovascular Disease subanalysis. *J Hypertens*. 2014;32:1334–1341.
7. Bethel MA, Patel RA, Merrill P, et al. Cardiovascular outcomes with glucagon-like peptide-1 receptor agonists in patients with type 2 diabetes: a meta-analysis. *Lancet Diabetes Endocrinol*. 2018;6:105–113.
8. McGuire DK, Shih WJ, Cosentino F, et al. Association of SGLT2 inhibitors with cardiovascular and kidney outcomes in patients with type 2 diabetes: a meta-analysis. *JAMA Cardiol*. 2021;6:148–158.
9. Institute of Medicine, Committee on Quality of Health Care in America. *Crossing the Quality Chasm: A New Health System for the 21st Century*. Washington (DC): National Academies Press; 2001.
10. *About Implementation Science*. National Institutes of Health, National Cancer Institute. Available from: https://cancercontrol.cancer.gov/is/about.
11. *What is Implementation Science?* University of Washington. Available from: https://impsciuw.org/implementation-science/learn/implementation-science-overview/.
12. Wong ND, Zhao Y, Patel R, et al. Cardiovascular risk factor targets and cardiovascular disease event risk in diabetes: a pooling project of the atherosclerosis risk in communities study, multi-ethnic study of atherosclerosis, and Jackson Heart Study. *Diabetes Care*. 2016;39:668–676.

13. Wong ND, Patao C, Wong K, Malik S, Franklin SS, Iloeje U. Trends in control of cardiovascular risk factors among US adults with type 2 diabetes from 1999 to 2010: comparison by prevalent cardiovascular disease status. *Diab Vasc Dis Res*. 2013;10:505–513.
14. Pagidipati NJ, Navar AM, Pieper KS, et al. Secondary prevention of cardiovascular disease in patients with type 2 diabetes mellitus: international insights from the TECOS Trial (Trial Evaluating Cardiovascular Outcomes With Sitagliptin). *Circulation*. 2017;136:1193–1203.
15. Fan W, Song Y, Inzucchi SE, et al. Composite cardiovascular risk factor target achievement and its predictors in US adults with diabetes: the Diabetes Collaborative Registry. *Diabetes Obes Metab*. 2019;21:1121–1127.
16. Nelson AJ, Ardissino M, Haynes K, et al. Gaps in evidence-based therapy use in insured patients in the United States With Type 2 Diabetes Mellitus and Atherosclerotic Cardiovascular Disease. *J Am Heart Assoc*. 2021;10:e016835.
17. Nelson AJ, O'Brien EC, Kaltenbach LA, et al. Use of lipid-, blood pressure-, and glucose-lowering pharmacotherapy in patients with type 2 diabetes and atherosclerotic cardiovascular disease. *JAMA Netw Open*. 2022;5:e2148030.
18. Sangha V, Lipska K, Lin Z, et al. Patterns of prescribing sodium-glucose cotransporter-2 inhibitors for medicare beneficiaries in the United States. *Circ Cardiovasc Qual Outcomes*. 2021;14:e008381.
19. Mahtta D, Ramsey DJ, Lee MT, et al. Utilization rates of SGLT2 inhibitors and GLP-1 receptor agonists and their facility-level variation among patients with atherosclerotic cardiovascular disease and type 2 diabetes: insights from the department of veterans affairs. *Diabetes Care*. 2022;45:372–380.
20. Gao Y, Peterson E, Pagidipati N. Barriers to prescribing glucose-lowering therapies with cardiometabolic benefits. *Am Heart J*. 2020;224:47–53.
21. Adhikari R, Jha K, Dardari Z, et al. National trends in use of sodium-glucose cotransporter-2 inhibitors and glucagon-like peptide-1 receptor agonists by cardiologists and other specialties, 2015 to 2020. *J Am Heart Assoc*. 2022;11:e023811.
22. Colantonio LD, Rosenson RS, Deng L, et al. Adherence to statin therapy among US adults between 2007 and 2014. *J Am Heart Assoc*. 2019;8:e010376.
23. Hawley CE, Lauffenburger JC, Paik JM, Wexler DJ, Kim SC, Patorno E. Three sides to the story: adherence trajectories during the first year of SGLT2 inhibitor therapy among medicare beneficiaries. *Diabetes Care*. 2022;45:604–613.
24. Weiss T, Carr RD, Pal S, et al. Real-world adherence and discontinuation of glucagon-like peptide-1 receptor agonists therapy in type 2 diabetes mellitus patients in the United States. *Patient Prefer Adherence*. 2020;14:2337–2345.
25. Joseph JJ, Ortiz R, Acharya T, Golden SH, Lopez L, Deedwania P. Cardiovascular impact of race and ethnicity in patients with diabetes and obesity: JACC Focus Seminar 2/9. *J Am Coll Cardiol*. 2021;78:2471–2482.
26. Gao Y, Peterson E, Pagidipati N. Opportunities for improving use of evidence-based therapy in patients with type 2 diabetes and cardiovascular disease. *Clin Cardiol*. 2019;42:1063–1070.
27. Balas EA, Boren SA. Managing clinical knowledge for health care improvement. *Yearb Med Inform*. 2000:65–70.
28. *Fundamentals of Implementation Research*, 2012.
29. Bauer MS, Damschroder L, Hagedorn H, Smith J, Kilbourne AM. An introduction to implementation science for the non-specialist. *BMC Psychol*. 2015;3:32.
30. Curran GM, Bauer M, Mittman B, Pyne JM, Stetler C. Effectiveness-implementation hybrid designs: combining elements of clinical effectiveness and implementation research to enhance public health impact. *Med Care*. 2012;50:217–226.
31. Curran GM. Implementation science made too simple: a teaching tool. *Implement Sci Commun*. 2020;1:27.
32. Powell BJ, Waltz TJ, Chinman MJ, et al. A refined compilation of implementation strategies: results from the Expert Recommendations for Implementing Change (ERIC) project. *Implement Sci*. 2015;10:21.
33. Proctor E, Silmere H, Raghavan R, et al. Outcomes for implementation research: conceptual distinctions, measurement challenges, and research agenda. *Adm Policy Ment Health*. 2011;38:65–76.
34. *RE-AIM: Improving Public Health Relevance and Population Health Impact*. Available from: https://re-aim.org/.
35. Glasgow RE, Vogt TM, Boles SM. Evaluating the public health impact of health promotion interventions: the RE-AIM framework. *Am J Public Health*. 1999;89:1322–1327.
36. Nelson AJ, Pagidipati NJ, Aroda VR, et al. Incorporating SGLT2i and GLP-1RA for cardiovascular and kidney disease risk reduction: call for action to the cardiology community. *Circulation*. 2021;144:74–84.
37. Pagidipati NJ, Nelson AJ, Kaltenbach LA, et al. Coordinated care to optimize cardiovascular preventive therapies in type 2 diabetes: a randomized clinical trial. *JAMA*. 2023;329:1261–1270.
38. Damschroder LJ, Reardon CM, AuYoung M, et al. Implementation findings from a hybrid III implementation-effectiveness trial of the Diabetes Prevention Program (DPP) in the Veterans Health Administration (VHA). *Implement Sci*. 2017;12:94.
39. Blood AJ, Chang LS, Hassan S, et al. Randomized evaluation of a remote management program to improve guideline-directed medical therapy: the DRIVE trial. *Circulation*. 2024;149:1802–1811.
40. Lee JK, Grace KA, Taylor AJ. Effect of a pharmacy care program on medication adherence and persistence, blood pressure, and low-density lipoprotein cholesterol: a randomized controlled trial. *JAMA*. 2006;296:2563–2571.
41. Aysola J, Tahirovic E, Troxel AB, et al. A randomized controlled trial of opt-in versus opt-out enrollment into a diabetes behavioral intervention. *Am J Health Promot*. 2018;32:745–752.
42. *Research and Development in the Pharmaceutical Industry*. Congressional Budget Office. 2021.

Index

Note: Page numbers followed by *b* indicate boxes, *f* indicate figures and *t* indicate tables.

B

C

D

E

F

Preface

A series of reviews and original papers on factorization theory, which were read at the Odessa city seminar on boundary value problems and singular integral equations in 1973-77, served as a source of the present book. Furthermore, lectures given by the authors at the Department of Mechanics and Mathematics of the Odessa University have been incorporated.

The authors are aware that their contribution to factorization theory, although it is very comprehensive (ranging from existence problems of a factorization, questions of estimates and stability of partial indices, to applications to the theory of the generalized Riemann boundary value problem), looks much more modest than the successes of their predecessors. Nevertheless, the necessity of creating a sufficiently complete review of factorization problems of measurable matrix functions explained from a unified point of view seemed so evident to the authors that they decided to write this booklet.

It may be considered complementary to the well-known monographs of N. I. MUSKHELISHVILI and N. P. VEKUA, which are devoted to the classical factorization theory of matrix functions with Hölder elements. We wish to emphasize that the subject matter will be discussed along lines meant not only for specialists familiar with the material, but also for readers who first become acquainted with the topic as well as for persons whose interest focusses, above all, on applications. The reader's judgment will show in how far this attempt has been successful.

The authors

CONTENTS

INTRODUCTION

The notion of factorization is widely used in different branches of mathematics. The term factorization itself simply means the representation of some mathematical object (number, function, matrix, operator, etc.) as a product of objects of the same type, but having certain additional properties. According to the type of the objects and the character of the problem studied (multiplication of numbers, pointwise multiplication of functions, their composition, etc.) this product can be understood in a different manner.
Many mathematical propositions are, in fact, theorems on the existence and properties of a certain factorization. In principle, even the fundamental theorem of arithmetic (on the factorization of natural numbers in prime factors) and the fundamental theorem of algebra (on the polynomial factorization over the complex field) can be considered as examples of factorization theorems. The importance of these theorems needs no comments.

As more special examples we mention the representation of matrices and operators in a Hilbert space in the form of a product of isometric by positively definite ones (so-called polar representation), the representation of functions of Hardy classes as a product of an inner and an outer one and its generalization to the case of matrix and operator functions, but also the representation of entire functions as product of other entire functions.

Many methods for solving equations and boundary value problems of a different kind are based on the idea of factorization. The schema for using factorization in solving equations may be described in the following way: Let some operator A be represented in the form

$$A = A_+^{-1}A_-. \tag{1}$$

Then the equation $y = Ax$ is equivalent to the equation $A_+y = A_-x$. For a suitable choice of representation (1), the latter relation turns out to be more convenient for investigation, and sometimes it can be solved explicitly. Simultaneously, the original equation will also be solved.

For instance, the representation of a square matrix A with principal minors different from zero as the product of non-singular triangular matrices allows us to reduce the solution of a system of linear equations with matrix A to a triangular system. There exists a continuous analogue of the mentioned result for Fredholm integral operators and a more general result on the factorization of an operator acting in a Hilbert space along a chain of projections as well (GOHBERG, KREĬN [5], BARKAR', GOHBERG [1,2]).

The factorization of matrix functions defined on some contour, which is studied in the present book also belongs to factorizations of this type. It appeared in connection with the study of systems of singular integral equations and boundary value problems for analytic functions.

Throughout the book, by a factorization of the matrix function G defined on a closed contour Γ, which divides the closed complex plane into parts $D^+(\ni 0)$ and $D^-(\ni \infty)$, we understand a representation of G in the form

$$G(t) = G_+(t)\Lambda(t)\,G_-(t) \qquad (t \in \Gamma),$$

where $G_\pm$ are boundary values of a matrix function analytic and non-singular in $D^\pm$, and

$$\Lambda(t) = \mathrm{diag}(t^{\varkappa_1},\ldots,t^{\varkappa_n}).$$

Under sufficiently general assumptions, the integers $\varkappa_1,\ldots,\varkappa_n$ are uniquely defined (up to order) by the matrix function G and are called its partial indices[1]).

The factorization of matrix functions is the main part in the theory of vector-valued Riemann boundary value problems. It permits us to reduce the general case of this problem to the so-called jump problem[2]). In this aspect, the problem of factorization has been studied under different restrictions on the smoothness of the contour Γ and the matrix function G, starting from the end of the previous century by several generations of mathematicians. The result of this work for the case of piecewise Hölder matrix functions and piecewise smooth contours are summed up in the well-known monographs of MUSKHELISHVILI [1], VEKUA [4], in the survey of GAKHOV [3] and the paper of KHVEDELIDZE [1].

Since the late fifties, the further development of the theory of the Riemann boundary value problem, systems of singular integral equations with Cauchy kernel and systems of Wiener-Hopf equations has stimulated

---

1) A more complete and exact definition of factorization will be given at the beginning of the second chapter.

2) Incidentally, we note that to vector boundary value problems with a shift (in particular, to the Gazemann problem) there correspond definitions of factorization different from that one given above. In the present book we do not study factorizations of such a type, since in the vector case the theory has not been sufficiently elaborated hitherto. The corresponding factorizations for the scalar case can be found in the monograph of LITVINCHUK [3].

the creation of new directions in the factorization problem. The factorization of matrix functions with elements from the Wiener algebra (GOHBERG, KREĬN [3]), the factorization of continuous (SIMONENKO [2]) and piecewise continuous (GOHBERG, KRUPNIK [1], MANDZHAVIDZE [6]) matrix functions has been studied, and a number of results concerning the factorization of measurable bounded matrix functions was obtained (DANILYUK [4,5], SIMONENKO [4,6], DOUGLAS [1]). At the same time, it became clear that even in case of a continuous non-singular matrix function G a factorization with continuous factors $G_{\pm}$ does not always exist. On the one hand, this gave rise to the search for new classes of matrix functions admitting a factorization with continuous factors (see BUDYANU, GOHBERG [3,4]) and, on the other hand, it led to the creation of the notion of factorization in classes L_p, $1 < p < \infty$. In case of continuous non-singular matrix functions, this factorization does not depend upon the choice of p. However, such a dependence holds already for piecewise continuous matrix functions. In this connection, there arises the task of studying the set of parameter values p, for which a given matrix function G can be factored.

Moreover, in the Riemann boundary value problem theory in L_p spaces, a situation may emerge where the problem has a finite index, but is not normally solvable. Owing to this, we have to impose additional demands upon the factorization in order to guarantee the normal solvability of the boundary value problem. In the following, a factorization satisfying these requirements will be called a Φ-factorization.

There were also studies on the enlargement of the class of contours Γ, for which factorization theorems continue to be valid. The crucial idea of these studies reduces to the development of sufficient conditions for the boundedness of the operator of singular integration on Γ (see e.g. KHVEDELIDZE [4]).

In connection with the problem of calculating defect numbers and the approximate solution of the vector-valued Riemann boundary value problem and singular integral equations, the questions of stability of the factorization factors $G_{\pm}$ and Λ as well as of finding estimates for partial indices are not yet well understood, even under the classic assumptions made in VEKUA [4], GAKHOV [3], MUSKHELISHVILI [1].
In the last 15 years a number of new results has been obtained in this direction (sufficient stability conditions, which can effectively be verified, sign preservation of all partial indices, which is also necessary in some cases (cf. VERBITSKIĬ, KRUPNIK [1,2], SPITKOVSKIĬ [5, 10], POUSSON [2], RABINDRANATHAN [1] and others)).
In obtaining these results, the notion and properties of the numerical

range (or Hausdorff set) of a matrix (MARCUS, MINC [1]) is used, i.e. questions related to the formula for the norm of a Hankel operator (see ADAMYAN, AROV, KREĬN [1]) and the operator of singular integration (VERBITSKIĬ, KRUPNIK [1], KRUPNIK [4]).

We would also like to note that the factorization problem for the spectral density of a stationary random process (ROZANOV [1]) which arose in probability theory, some problems of projection methods for the solution of systems of singular integral and convolution type equations (GOHBERG, FELDMAN [3]) and the theory of canonical systems of linear differential equations (KREĬN, MELIK-ADAMYAN [1,2]) show that the importance of the factorization problem for matrix functions is not limited by its role in the theory of the vector-valued Riemann boundary value problem.
The factorization problem for matrix functions arises also in a natural way in the study of convolution type equations on a finite interval and on systems of intervals (GANIN [1], KARLOVICH, SPITKOVSKIĬ [1], KOMYAK [1-4], NOVOKSHENOV [1], PAL'TSEV [2-6]. SPITKOVSKIĬ [15]). We emphasize that here(in contrast to the classical case of the half-line) even scalar equations yield a matrix problem of factorization.

All this increases interest in the peculiarities of factorization of special type matrix functions (unitary, Hermitian, functionally commutable , etc.), information on which is scattered in various papers (GORDIENKO [1], GOHBERG, KREĬN [3], KREĬN, MELIK-ADAMYAN [1,2], NIKOLAǏCHUK, SPITKOVSKIĬ [1,2], CHEBOTAREV [1,2], SHMUL'YAN [1,2] and others).

At present there do not exist monographs or reviews on the factorization of matrix functions, in which the problems mentioned above would be discussed in a sufficiently complete manner[1]). There are only three papers of a general nature by BOJARSKI [3], GOHBERG, KREǏN [3], KHVEDELIDZE [4] and the monographs of GOHBERG, FELDMAN [3], DANILYUK [6], PRÖSSDORF [1] and PRÖSSDORF, MICHLIN [1], in which some questions on the factorization of matrix functions are explained. The authors hope that the present book will contribute towards filling the gaps existing in the literature concerning this topic.
We now intend to briefly describe the contents of the book. The first chapter is of auxiliary character. It contains propositions from operator theory in Banach spaces and information on different classes of analytic functions (mainly on Smirnov classes) necessary for understanding the material contained in the main part of the book. In Chapter 2 the notions of factorization and the domain of factorability of matrix

[1]) While this manuscript was in preparation for publication, the monograph CLANCEY, GOHBERG [3] came out. Its contents is essentially covered by the present book.

functions are introduced, and their simplest properties are established. Besides, the factorization problem for matrix functions meromorphic in D^+ or D^- (in particular, rational matrix functions) is treated there, and the problem of the change of partial indices when being multiplied by matrix functions of the same kind is studied.
The connection between the factorization problem for matrix functions and the vector-valued Riemann boundary value problem is regarded in Chapter 3. Φ-factorization properties resulting from this connection and corresponding propositions of the theory of Fredholm operators are established.

Chapter 4 is devoted to triangular and functionally commutable matrix functions. In this chapter the criterion of Φ-factorability and estimates for partial indices (but for second-order matrix functions even exact formulae) are derived.

In Chapter 5 necessary and sufficient conditions of Φ-factorability of continuous and piecewise continuous matrix functions, but also for matrix functions of the class $L_\infty^\pm + C$ are established. The factorization problem in decomposing algebras of functions including the factorization problem of Hölder matrix functions on a piecewise smooth contour and matrix functions from the Wiener algebra on the circle will be studied.

The criterion for stability of partial indices, sufficient conditions for their non-positivity, non-negativity, coincidence or equality to zero are explained in Chapter 6. In addition, we shall investigate the behaviour of the factorization factors $G_\pm$ under small perturbations of the matrix function G.

Chapter 7 is dedicated to the factorization problem on the unit circle. Furthermore, the factorization of Hermitian and unitary matrix functions will be studied. The necessity of several sufficient conditions for non-negativity (non-positivity, equality to zero, etc.) of partial indices established in Chapter 6 will be proved.

Chapter 8 is concerned with sufficient conditions for Φ-factorability based on local principle and results of Chapters 5 - 7.

Finally, in Chapter 9 the theory developed in Chapters 3 - 8 is used for the study of the generalized Riemann boundary value problem, which has manifold applications in geometry, mechanics, and physics (see BUDYANU [1], GAKHOV [2]).

The last section of each chapter contains information and comments on results, which were not reflected in the main part of the chapter, but are related to it in certain ways. Some unsolved problems are formulated. The first chapter makes an exception. For the reader's convenience, comments on references accompany every proposition (or a group of closely connected propositions).

Lastly, we want to remark that in the book we do not focus our attention on such problems as the factorization problem relative to a contour lying on a Riemann surface (cf. L.F. ZVEROVICH [2], E.I. ZVEROVICH [1], ZVEROVICH, PANCHENKO [1], KVITKO [1], KRUGLOV [1], PANCHENKO [1], RODIN [1,2], RODIN, TURAKULOV [1], SELEZNEV [2], KOPPELMAN [1], RÖHRL [1]) or with respect to complex (GOHBERG, FELDMAN [1], MANDZHAVIDZE [7,8]) and Jordan non-rectifiable (among them quasiconformal) contours (see KATS [3], SELEZNEV [1-3]). Furthermore, we do not deal with the natural generalization of the factorization problem for matrix functions - the question on factorability of operator functions. Concerning this topic the reader is referred to Chapter 6 in the monograph of CLANCEY and GOHBERG [3] and the literature cited there, but also to the papers of BUDYANU [1], LEITERER [1], SERGEEV [1], GOHBERG, KAASHOEK, van SCHAGEN [1], van der MEE [1,2], MUCKENHOUPT [1], NAKAZI TAKAHIKO [1], SUCIU [1].[1)] We do not dwell on various applications of the factorization problem. We only refer to GUSAK [1,2], DUKHOVNYĬ [1], MALYSHEV [1], ROZANOV [1], where methods and results of the factorization theory are applied to probability-theoretic problems. Applications to mechanics one can find in the monograph of VOROVICH, ALEKSANDROV, BABESHKO [1] as well as the papers BABESHKO [1,2], BELOKOPYTOVA, IVANENKO, FIL'SHTINSKIĬ [1], VOROB'EV [1], KULIEV, SADYKHOV [1], MOSSAKOVSKII, MISHCHISHIN [1], TOLOKONNIKOV, PEN'KOV [1], KHRAPKOV [1], TSITSKISHVILI [3,4], CHEREPANOV [1]. Concerning applications to difraction problems, see the monograph VIROZUB, MATSAEV [1] and the article POPOV [1], CHAKRABARTI [2], HEINS [1,2], IDEMEN [2]. Finally, for applications of the factorization theory to the method of inverse problems and other questions of theoretical physics, the reader is referred to the monograph NOVIKOV (ed.) [1] and the papers of EMETS [1], ZAKHAROV, SHABAT [1], ITS [1], KRICHEVER [1,2], MASKUDOV, VELIEV [1], MEUNARGIYA [1], NOVOSHENOV [2,3], TROITSKIĬ [1], DUVACZ, ZELAZNY [1], IDEMEN [1], MEISTER [1], RAJAMAKI [1], REYMAN, SEMENOV-TIAN-SHANSKY [2], SIEWERT, KELLEY, GARCIA [1].

---

1) see also GOHBERG, LEITERER [1-2].

CHAPTER 1. BACKGROUND INFORMATION

This chapter is of an auxiliary character. Its first section contains facts necessary for the further explanations concerning lineals of finite codimension as well as semi-Fredholm and Fredholm operators in Banach spaces. Most of these statements are well-known and have been published in several recent monographs.[1] However, Theorem 1.12 on the Fredholmness of block operators and the local principle in the theory of Fredholm operators make an exception. The latter was proved in the form we need only in SIMONENKO's paper [5]. Therefore, Theorems 1.12 and 1.14 will be given with detailed proofs. The remaining theorems in Section 1.1 we state without proof, referring the reader in every case to available sources. We do not intend to explain the history of semi-Fredholm and Fredholm operator theory, since this has already been excellently described (see, e.g. KATO [1]).

In the second section of the present chapter, above all, known theorems on analytic functions of Smirnov classes are stated, whereas in Section 1.3 properties of singular integral operators related to the results of Section 1.2 are described. Here as well as in Section 1.1, we give proofs only for those statements, which we did not find in an appropriate form (Theorems 1.26, 1.27, 1.29, 1.31, 1.35) or which are published only in several articles (Theorems 1.20, 1.32, 1.33).

Since the genesis of the formation of many results of the theory of Smirnov classes has received little attention in modern monographic literature, we give some historic information and comments on the material of Sections 1.2 and 1.3.

1.1. SOME FACTS ON THE GEOMETRY OF BANACH SPACES AND OPERATOR THEORY IN THESE SPACES

A linear manifold in a Banach space not necessarily closed we shall call a lineal. For a closed lineal we use the term subspace. The dimension of the factor-space $\mathcal{B}|\mathcal{L}$ is said to be the codimension of the lineal $\mathcal{L}$ being located in a Banach space $\mathcal{B}$:

$$\operatorname{codim}\mathcal{L} = \dim(\mathcal{B}|\mathcal{L}).$$

1) See e.g. GOHBERG, KRUPNIK [4], S.KREIN [1], MICHLIN, PRÖSSDORF [1]

THEOREM 1.1. Suppose $\mathcal{L}_1$ to be a subspace of the Banach space $\mathfrak{B}$, and let $\mathcal{L}_2 \supseteq \mathcal{L}_1$ be a lineal. Then $\dim \mathcal{L}_2|\mathcal{L}_1 < \infty$ implies that $\mathcal{L}_2$ is also a subspace. On the other hand, if $\mathcal{L}_2$ is a subspace and $\mathcal{L}_1 \subseteq \mathcal{L}_2$ is the range of a closed operator, then $\dim \mathcal{L}_2|\mathcal{L}_1 < \infty$ implies that $\mathcal{L}_1$ is a subspace, too.

The first part of the theorem is an elementary fact (we refer to GOHBERG, KRUPNIK [4], p. 50 for its proof). The second part is a consequence of the closed graph theorem (see, e.g., PALAIS [1], Ch. 7, Th. 1).

DEFINITION 1.1. The set of all elements f of the dual space $\mathfrak{B}^*$ with $f(x) = 0$ for all $x \in \mathcal{L}$ is called the orthogonal complement $\mathcal{L}^\perp$ to the lineal $\mathcal{L}$ ($\subseteq \mathfrak{B}$).

Obviously, $\mathcal{L}^\perp$ is a subspace of the space $\mathfrak{B}^*$. The orthogonal complement to the lineal $\mathcal{L}$ coincides with the orthogonal complement to its closure $\overline{\mathcal{L}}$. There is a natural isomorphism between $\mathcal{L}^\perp$ and the space dual to $\mathfrak{B}|\overline{\mathcal{L}}$. As a corollary of this isomorphism, we mention

THEOREM 1.2. For any lineal $\mathcal{L}$ ($\subseteq \mathfrak{B}$), the dimension of the orthogonal complement coincides with the codimension of its closure (in the sense that either both values are infinite or both values are finite, and then they are equal to each other).

DEFINITION 1.2. A subspace $\mathcal{L}_0$ of the Banach space $\mathfrak{B}$ is called complementable, if there exists a subspace $\mathcal{L}_1 (\subseteq \mathfrak{B})$ such that each vector $x \in \mathfrak{B}$ admits a unique representation in the form $x = x_0 + x_1$ ($x_j \in \mathcal{L}_j$, $j = 0,1$). In this case, the subspace $\mathcal{L}_1$ is said to be the direct complement to $\mathcal{L}_0$ (with respect to $\mathfrak{B}$), and the space $\mathfrak{B}$ is said to be decomposed in the direct sum of its subspaces $\mathcal{L}_0$ and $\mathcal{L}_1$ (written $\mathfrak{B} = \mathcal{L}_0 \dotplus \mathcal{L}_1$).

The notion of the direct sum is transferred to the case of an arbitrary finite number of summands in an obvious manner.

Every subspace in a Hilbert space can be complemented; one of its direct complements is the orthogonal complement. In every Banach space not isomorphic to a Hilbert one, there are non-complementable subspaces

(LEE, SARASON [1]). Nevertheless, there holds

THEOREM 1.3 (S. KREĬN [1], p. 31). Let $\mathfrak{B}$ be a Banach space and $\mathfrak{B}_0$ a subspace of finite codimension. Then $\mathfrak{B}_0$ is complementable, and the dimension of all its direct complements is equal to codim $\mathfrak{B}_0$. If, moreover, $\mathcal{L}$ is a lineal dense in $\mathfrak{B}$, then the lineal $\mathcal{L} \cap \mathfrak{B}_0$ is dense in $\mathfrak{B}_0$, and there exists a direct complement to $\mathfrak{B}_0$ with respect to $\mathfrak{B}$ lying in $\mathcal{L}$.

We shall say that a linear (generally speaking, unbounded) operator A acts in the Banach space $\mathfrak{B}$, if its domain dom A and image im A lie in $\mathfrak{B}$ [1)].

The kernel of the operator A, i.e., the solution set of the homogeneous equation $Ax = 0$, will be denoted by ker A.

Owing to the linearity of the operator A, the sets dom A, im A and ker A are lineals in $\mathfrak{B}$. By $[\mathfrak{B}]$ we denote the class of all linear bounded operators acting in $\mathfrak{B}$, the domain of which coincides with $\mathfrak{B}$. This class of operators supplied with the norm $\|A\| = \sup \{\|Ax\| : x \in \mathfrak{B}, \|x\| \leq 1\}$ is itself a Banach space. Furthermore, the class $[\mathfrak{B}]$ is a Banach algebra, i.e. such a Banach space, in which the operation of multiplication is defined (in the case under study, its role plays the composition of operators) consistent with the linear structure and possessing the property $\|AB\| \leq \|A\| \cdot \|B\|$ [2)].

DEFINITION 1.3. The operator B is referred to as a <u>part of the operator</u> A, if dom B $\subseteq$ dom A and $Ax = Bx$ for all $x \in$ dom B.

Under the conditions of Definition 1.3, the operator B is sometimes also said to be the <u>restriction of</u> A on dom B (written $B = A|_{\text{dom } B}$).

DEFINITION 1.4. The values $\alpha(A) = \dim \ker A$ and $\beta(A) = \dim(\mathfrak{B} | \overline{\text{im } A})$ are called <u>defect numbers</u> of the operator A, and their difference

---

1) Most of the definitions and results stated below can be transferred to operators acting from one space into another. However, for our aims it is sufficient to regard operators acting in one space.

2) A short survey of the theory of Banach algebras can be found, for example, in the appendix written by V.M. TIKHOMIROV to the book KOLMOGOROV, FOMIN [1].

$\text{ind } A = \alpha(A) - \beta(A)$ is the <u>index</u> of the operator A.

The index is defined, if at least one of the defect numbers is finite. If both are finite, then A is called an operator with finite index.

In case the image of the operator A is closed, the equation $Ax = y$ is usually said to be normally solvable. For the sake of brevity, in this case the operator A itself is also called <u>normally solvable.</u>

<u>DEFINITION 1.5.</u> A closed normally solvable operator A is called <u>Fredholm</u> iff $\alpha(A)$ and $\beta(A)$ are finite. In case that at least one of these numbers is finite, A is referred to as <u>semi-Fredholm.</u>
If $\alpha(A) < \infty$, A is called a Φ_+- and, if $\beta(A) < \infty$, A is called a Φ_--operator.

It follows from Theorem 1.1 that $A \in [\mathfrak{B}]$ is a Φ_--operator if and only if its image has a finite codimension.

The following five theorems are a collection of fundamental facts on Φ_+-, Φ_-- and Fredholm operators. Their proofs can be found e.g. in GOHBERG, KREĬN [1], KATO [1], S. KREĬN [1]; for the case of bounded operators we also refer to Ch. 4 in GOHBERG, KRUPNIK [4], Ch. 2 in DANILYUK [6] and Section 8 of Ch. 1 of SHUBIN [3].

<u>THEOREM 1.4.</u> For every Φ_+- (Φ_--, Fredholm) operator A acting in $\mathfrak{B}$, there is an $\varepsilon > 0$ such that if $B \in [\mathfrak{B}]$ and $\|B\| < \varepsilon$, then

1) the operator $A + B$ is also a Φ_+- (Φ_--, Fredholm) operator,
2) $\text{ind } (A+B) = \text{ind } A$,
3) $\alpha(A+B) \leq \alpha(A)$, $\beta(A+B) \leq \beta(A)$.

Theorem 1.4 means the stability of semi-Fredholmness or Fredholmness of the index as well as the semi-stability of defect numbers under perturbations of the operator with a sufficiently small norm.

<u>THEOREM 1.5.</u> If the operator A acting in $\mathfrak{B}$ is a Φ_+- (Φ_--, Fredholm) operator and the operator $B \in [\mathfrak{B}]$ is compact, then $A + B$ is also a Φ_+- (Φ_--, Fredholm) operator and $\text{ind } (A+B) = \text{ind } A$.

Theorem 1.5 expresses the stability of semi-Fredholmness and Fredholmness and of the index of the operator A under compact perturbations.

Sometimes Theorems 1.4 and 1.5 are called the first and second stability theorem.

THEOREM 1.6. If the operators A and B acting in $\mathfrak{B}$ are Fredholm and B is densely defined, then the operator BA is also Fredholm and ind BA = ind A + ind B.

DEFINITION 1.6 (see KATO [1], p. 212). The operators A and B acting in $\mathfrak{B}$ and $\mathfrak{B}^*$ respectively, are referred to as adjoint to each other, if for all $x \in \text{dom } A$ and $f \in \text{dom } B$, there holds $(Bf)(x) = f(Ax)$.

Generally speaking, there are many operators acting in $\mathfrak{B}^*$, which are adjoint to A. But if the operator A is densely defined, then all operators adjoint to it are parts of one and the same uniquely defined operator, which will be denoted by A^*. The operator A^* is always closed.

THEOREM 1.7. Let the operator A acting in $\mathfrak{B}$ be closed and densely defined. Then $(\text{im } A)^{\perp} = \ker A^*$ and $(\ker A)^{\perp} \supseteq \text{im } A^*$, where in the last inclusion equality holds if and only if the operator A (or, equivalently, A^*) is normally solvable.

COROLLARY 1.2. The closed and densely defined operator A is a Φ_+- (Φ_--, Fredholm) operator iff the operator A^* is a Φ_-- (Φ_+-, Fredholm) operator. In this case we have $\alpha(A) = \beta(A^*)$, $\beta(A) = \alpha(A^*)$.

DEFINITION 1.7. The operator $M \in [\mathfrak{B}]$ is called a left (right) regularizer of the operator A $(\in [\mathfrak{B}])$, if the operator $MA - I$ $(AM - I)$ is compact. If M is simultaneously a left and right regularizer, then it is called a (two-sided) regularizer.

It follows from the definition that if an operator has left and right regularizers, then all of them are regularizers and differ from each other by compact summands.

THEOREM 1.8. The operator $A \in [\mathfrak{B}]$ admits a regularization from the left (right) if and only if it is a Φ_+- (Φ_--) operator and the subspace im A (ker A) is complementable. Among all operators of class $[\mathfrak{B}]$, the Fredholm operators and only they admit a regularization.

A simple consequence of Theorem 1.8 is

<u>THEOREM 1.9.</u> If the product BA of operators A and B of the class $[\mathfrak{B}]$ is Fredholm, then A is a Φ_+- and B a Φ_--operator. If in this case B is a Φ_+- (A is a Φ_--) operator, then A (respectively B) is Fredholm.

<u>DEFINITION 1.8.</u> The factor algebra of the Banach algebra $[\mathfrak{B}]$ with respect to the ideal $\mathcal{S}$ of compact operators is called <u>Calkin algebra.</u> According to this definition, the elements of the Calkin algebra are classes of equivalent operators, where two operators A and B are said to be equivalent, if $A-B \in \mathcal{S}$. In all what follows, we denote this equivalence by $A \sim B$. The norm of the image $\hat{A}$ of the operator $A \in [\mathfrak{B}]$ in the Calkin algebra is called <u>essential norm</u> of A (written $|A|$). In other words: $|A| = \inf\{\|A+T\| : T \in \mathcal{S}\}$.

Owing to the closedness of the ideal of compact operators, the Calkin algebra provides a Banach algebra.

From Theorem 1.8 we deduce that the operator $A \in [\mathfrak{B}]$ is Fredholm if and only if its image $\hat{A}$ is invertible in the Calkin algebra, and the inverse of $\hat{A}$ is that element of the Calkin algebra, which consists of all regularizers of A (or, what is the same, of any other operator from the class $\hat{A}$).

Next we formulate a simple and well-known result from the theory of Banach algebras, which we need below both in general form, and for the special case of the Calkin algebra.

<u>THEOREM 1.10.</u> Let $\{x_k\}$ be a sequence of invertible elements of the Banach algebra $\mathcal{B}$ converging in $\mathcal{B}$ to x. Then the relation $\sup_k \|x_k^{-1}\| < \infty$ is necessary and sufficient for the invertibility of x.

Applying Theorem 1.10 to the Calkin algebra we obtain

THEOREM 1.11. Let $\{A_k\} \subset [\mathfrak{B}]$ be a sequence of Fredholm operators converging to the operator A. The operator A is Fredholm if and only if there exists a sequence $\{B_k\}$ of regularizers of the operators A_k such that $\sup\|B_k\| < \infty$.

Let the Banach space $\mathfrak{B}$ be represented as the direct sum of its subspaces: $\mathfrak{B} = \mathfrak{B}_1 \dot{+} \mathfrak{B}_2$. Then every operator $A \in [\mathfrak{B}]$ may be written in the form of a block-matrix

$$A = \begin{bmatrix} A_{11} & A_{12} \\ A_{21} & A_{22} \end{bmatrix} \tag{1.1}$$

where A_{ij} is a linear bounded operator from $\mathfrak{B}_j$ into $\mathfrak{B}_i$ $(i,j = 1,2)$. The equation (1.1) must be understood in the sense that the decomposition $x = x_1 + x_2$ $(x_j \in \mathfrak{B}_j)$ corresponds to the decomposition $Ax = y_1 + y_2$ $(y_j \in \mathfrak{B}_j)$, where $y_1 = A_{11}x_1 + A_{12}x_2$, $y_2 = A_{21}x_1 + A_{22}x_2$.

Supposing that in the representation (1.1) one of the blocks A_{ij} is compact we can formulate the criterion of Fredholmness of the operator A in terms of its remaining blocks. For the sake of definiteness, we assume the block A_{12} to be compact.

THEOREM 1.12. Let in the representation (1.1) of the operator $A \in [\mathfrak{B}]$ the block A_{12} be compact. Then for the Fredholmness of the operator A it is necessary and sufficient that the following conditions hold:

1) A_{11} is a Φ_--operator,

2) A_{22} is a Φ_+-operator,

3) $\gamma_1 = \dim \mathcal{L}_1 < \infty$, where $\mathcal{L}_1 = \ker A_{11} \cap (x \in \mathfrak{B}_1 : A_{21}x \in \operatorname{im} A_{22}\}$

4) $\gamma_2 = \operatorname{codim} \mathcal{L}_2 < \infty$, where $\mathcal{L}_2 = \operatorname{im} A_{22} + A_{21} \ker A_{11}$.

If the conditions 1) - 4) are satisfied, then the index of the operator A is calculated by the formula

$$\operatorname{ind} A = \alpha(A_{22}) - \beta(A_{11}) + \gamma_1 - \gamma_2. \tag{1.2}$$

Moreover, if $A_{12} = 0$, then

$$\alpha(A) = \alpha(A_{22}) + \gamma_1 , \quad \beta(A) = \beta(A_{11}) + \gamma_2. \tag{1.3}$$

Proof. Owing to Theorem 1.5 it suffices to study the case $A_{12} = 0$. First let us assume that the conditions 1) – 4) are fulfilled. We show that A is Fredholm and (1.2) holds. Let P_1 denote the projection of $\mathfrak{B}$ onto $\mathfrak{B}_1$ along $\mathfrak{B}_2$ and P_1^0 its restriction on $\ker A$. It is easily verified that

$$\text{im } P_1^0 = \mathcal{L}_1 \quad \text{and} \quad \ker P_1^0 = \ker A_{11}.$$

Since $\ker A|\ker P_1^0$ is isomorphic to $\text{im } P_1^0$, this implies $\alpha(A) < \infty$ and

$$\dim \ker A|\ker P_1^0 = \alpha(A) - \alpha(A_{11}) = \dim \mathcal{L}_1 = \gamma_1.$$

Therefore, the first relation (1.3) is proved.

Next we prove that $\text{im } A$ has finite codimension and (1.3) holds. By assumption, there exist direct complements M_1 to $\text{im } A_{11}$ in $\mathfrak{B}_1$ and M_2 to $\mathcal{L}_2$ in $\mathfrak{B}_2$. We show that $M = M_1 \dotplus M_2$ is a direct complement of $\text{im } A$ in $\mathfrak{B}$. Let $y \in \text{im } A \cap M$. Since $P_1 \text{ im } A = \text{im } A_{11}$, we have $y_1 = P_1 y \in \text{im } A_{11}$ and, on the other hand, $y_1 \in M_1$. Hence $y_1 = 0$. From this we get $y \in \text{im } A \cap M_2$. In view of $\mathcal{L}_2 = \text{im } A \cap \mathfrak{B}_2$ this means $y \in \mathcal{L}_2 \cap M_2$, i.e. $y = 0$. Thus $\text{im } A \cap M = \{0\}$.

Taking now $y = y_1 + y_2$ $(y_j \in \mathfrak{B}_j,\ j = 1,2)$ arbitrarily, we have a decomposition

$$\begin{aligned} y_1 &= A_{11}x_1 && + f_2 \\ y_2 &= A_{21}u_1 + A_{22}x_2 && + f_2, \end{aligned}$$

where $u_1 \in \ker A_{11}$, $f_j \in M_j$, $x_j \in \mathfrak{B}_j$ $(j = 1,2)$.
We have, furthermore, a decomposition

$$A_{21}x_1 = A_{21}u_1' + A_{22}x_2' + f_2'$$

with $u_1' \in \ker A_{11}$, $x_2' \in \mathfrak{B}_2$, $f_2' \in M_2$. Putting $x = x_1+u_1-u_1' + x_2-x_2'$ we obtain

$$Ax = y_1 - f_1 + y_2 - f_2 + f_2',$$

which is $y = Ax + f$, where $f = f_1 + f_2 - f_2' \in M$.
We proved $\mathfrak{B} = \text{im } A \dotplus M$. In particular, this implies that $\text{im } A$ has a finite codimension equal to $\beta(A_{11}) + \gamma_2$. Since by Theorem 1.1 $\text{im } A$ is closed, the second relation (1.3) results. The index formula (1.2) is a consequence of (1.3).

Now let us assume that A is Fredholm and

$$R = \begin{bmatrix} R_{11} & R_{12} \\ R_{21} & R_{22} \end{bmatrix}$$

is a regularizer of A. Then, obviously, R_{11} is a right regulizer of A_{11} and R_{22} a left regularizer of A_{22}. Hence 1) and 2) are fulfilled. Since, as proved above, $\ker A | \ker A_{22}$ is isomorphic to $\mathcal{L}_1$, we have $\gamma_1 < \infty$. Further, the finiteness of $\beta(A)$ implies the finiteness of the codimension of $\mathcal{L}_2 = \operatorname{im} A \cap \mathfrak{B}_2$ in $\mathfrak{B}_2$. Hence 3) and 4) are satisfied, too, and the theorem is proved. ≡

Theorem 1.12 is formulated in SPITKOVSKIĬ [11] (see also SPITKOVSKIĬ [12], where this theorem was presented with proof). Formulae (1.2) allow for obtaining in case $A_{12} = 0$, a criterion of injectivity and surjectivity of the operator A. This result was obtained independently by STOROZH [1]. It is omitted here, since we do not need it. Of course, various special cases of Theorem 1.12 were known previously. One of them important for the following is the case that some of the diagonal blocks of the operator A is Fredholm. This case can be investigated (even without compactness assumption for A_{12}) with the help of Frobenius' formulae (see KIRILLOV, GVISHIANI [1] p. 85 as well as PETROV [1]). However, we need only the case if A_{12} is compact. Thus, we obtain the corresponding result as a consequence of Theorem 1.12.

COROLLARY 1.3. Let in the representation (1.1) of the operator A the block A_{12} be compact, and let one of the diagonal blocks A_{11} and A_{22} be Fredholm. Then for the Fredholmness of the operator A it is necessary and sufficient that the second block is also Fredholm. If this condition is fulfilled, then

$$\operatorname{ind} A = \operatorname{ind} A_{11} + \operatorname{ind} A_{22}.$$

If, in addition, $A_{12} = 0$, then

$$\alpha(A) = \alpha(A_{11}) + \alpha(A_{22}) - m,$$

$$\beta(A) = \beta(A_{11}) + \beta(A_{22}) - m,$$

where $m = \dim(A_{21} \ker A_{11}) | (\operatorname{im} A_{22} \cap A_{21} \ker A_{11})$.

In fact, if e.g. the operator A_{11} is Fredholm, then conditions 1) and 3) of Theorem 1.12 are automatically satisfied, and thanks to the finite dimension of the lineal $A_{21} \ker A_{11}$, condition 4) is equivalent to the condition that A_{22} is a Φ_--operator.

The validity of the formulae for the index and the defect numbers follows from the corresponding formulae of Theorem 1.12, taking into account that for Fredholm A_{11} and A_{22} we have

$$\dim(\ker A_{11} \cap \mathcal{L}_1) = \dim \ker A_{11} - m,$$
$$\dim(\mathfrak{B}_2 | \mathcal{L}_2) = \dim(\mathfrak{B}_2 | \operatorname{im} A_{22}) - m.$$

In view of Corollary 1.3, the condition of Fredholmness of the diagonal blocks of the operator (1.1) with compact blocks outside the diagonal is sufficient for the Fredholmness of the operator A itself. In the general case, this condition is not necessary. A simple example is provided by the operator of two-sided shift of infinite multiplicity acting in a Hilbert space $\mathfrak{H}$. This operator is invertible, but, decomposing $\mathfrak{H}$ in a suitable manner in an orthogonal sum, it can be represented in the form (1.1), where $A_{12} = 0$ and A_{11} is the operator of one-sided shift with an infinite dimensional kernel. In Chapter 4 we shall consider some examples in detail, which illustrate the same situation, but are directly related to the subject of the present book.

COROLLARY 1.4. Let the Banach space $\mathfrak{B}$ be represented as the direct sum of its subspaces $\mathfrak{B}_j$ $(j = 1,\dots,k)$ in such a way that the operator $A \in [\mathfrak{B}]$ commutes up to a compact summand with any operator P_j projecting $\mathfrak{B}$ on $\mathfrak{B}_j$ parallel to the direct sum of the remaining subspaces: $AP_j - P_jA \in \mathcal{S}$. Then for the Fredholmness of A it is necessary and sufficient that the operators $A_{jj} = P_jA|_{\mathfrak{B}_j}$ considered in $\mathfrak{B}_j$ be Fredholm. In this case $\operatorname{ind} A = \sum_{j=1}^{k} \operatorname{ind} A_{jj}$.

Corollary 1.4 can be proved by induction on k with the help of Theorem 1.12. However, we do not intend to verify this assertion, since the result of Corollary 1.4 can be easily obtained directly and is well-known (see e.g. GOHBERG, KREĬN [3]).

As a rule, in the present book the role of the Banach space $\mathfrak{B}$ will be played by the space $L_p^n(\Gamma)$ (briefly L_p^n) of n-dimensional vector functions given on the rectifiable contour Γ, each component of which is summable in the pth power $(1 \leqslant p < \infty)$. In addition to the general theorems given above, we need the following propositions connected with the specific nature of the space L_p^n.

<u>THEOREM 1.13 (M. RIESZ-TORIN).</u> If the operator $A \in [L_{p_1}^n]$ maps the subspace $L_{p_0}^n$ $(1 < p_1 < p_0 < \infty)$ into itself, then, for all $p \in (p_1, p_0]$, the operator $A|_{L_p^n}$ belongs to the class $[L_p^n]$.

The proof of this well-known theorem can be found, for instance, in KRASNOSEL'SKIĬ et al. [1].

Now we are going to explain the local principle of the theory of Fredholm operators by changing the abstract local principle for Banach algebras described in Ch. 12 of the book GOHBERG, KRUPNIK [4] in an appropriate manner. The formulation of the local principle is premised by several definitions.

We denote by $C(\Gamma)$ $(=C)$ the space of continuous functions on Γ, and by R the lineal of rational functions with poles off Γ.

<u>DEFINITION 1.9.</u> The operator $A \in [L_p^n]$ is called an <u>operator of local type</u>, if it commutes up to a compact summand with the operator of multiplication by an arbitrary function of class R.

Since the lineal R is dense in C with respect to the uniform norm (see WALSH [1] p. 67), local type operators possess, for any $a \in C$, the property $aA - AaI \in \mathcal{S}$.

We denote the class of continuous functions on Γ equal to one in some neighbourhood (depending on the function) of the point $t \in \Gamma$ by C_t.

<u>DEFINITION 1.10.</u> The operators $A, B \in [L_p^n]$ are said to be <u>equivalent at the point</u> $t_0 (\in \Gamma)$, if, for every $\varepsilon > 0$, one can find a function $a \in C_{t_0}$ such that $|(A-B)aI| < \varepsilon$, $|a(A-B)| < \varepsilon$.

<u>DEFINITION 1.11.</u> The operator B_l (B_r respectively) $\in [L_p^n]$ is referred to as a <u>left (right) local regularizer</u> of the operator $A \in [L_p^n]$ at the point $t_0 \in \Gamma$, if there exists a function $a \in C_{t_0}$ such that $aI - B_l AaI \in \mathcal{S}$ $(aI - aAB_r \in \mathcal{S})$.

An operator A having a left and a right local regularizer at some point $t_0 \in \Gamma$ will be <u>called locally Fredholm</u> at this point.

<u>THEOREM 1.14 (I.B. SIMONENKO).</u> Let $A \in [L_p^n]$ be a local type operator. If we can, for every $t \in \Gamma$, specify an operator A_t locally Fredholm at the point t and equivalent to the operator A at this point, then the operator A is Fredholm.

<u>Proof.</u> Above all, we show that the existence of a right local regularizer of the operator A_t at the point $t \in \Gamma$ and its equivalence to the operator A at this point imply that the operator A also admits a local regularization from the right at the point t. Here we do not use that the operator A is of local type.

Let B_r be a right local regularizer of the operator A_t at the point t and a_1 be some function from C_t satisfying the condition $a_1 I - a_1 A_t B_r \in \mathcal{S}$. Due to the equivalence of the operators A and A_t at the point t, there exists a function $a_2 \in C_t$ with $|a_2(A-A_t)| < \|B_r\|^{-1}$. In other words, it is possible to choose an operator $T \in \mathcal{S}$ in such a way that $\|a_2(A-A_t) + T\| < \|B_r\|^{-1}$. But then $\|a_2(A-A_t)B_r + TB_r\| < 1$.

The operator $K = I + a_2(A-A_t)B_r + TB_r$ is invertible, and consequently by Theorem 1.5, the operator $I + a_2(A-A_t)B_r$ is Fredholm.

Let B_0 be some regularizer of the operator $I + a_2(A-A_t)B_r$, and suppose a_t to be a non-negative function of class C_t equal to zero at those points $\tau \in \Gamma$ for which either $a_1(\tau) \neq 1$ or $a_2(\tau) \neq 1$.

Then $a_t = a_t a_1 = a_t a_2$ and, therefore, $a_t I - a_t A B_r B_0 =$ $= a_t I - a_t(I + (A-A_t)B_r)B_0 + a_t(I - A_t B_r)B_0 = a_t(I-(I + a_2(A-A_t)B_r)B_0)$ $+ a_t(a_1 I - a_1 A_t B_r)B_0$. Taking into account the compactness of the operators $I - (I + a_2(A-A_t)B_r)B_0$ and $a_1 I - a_1 A_t B_r$, we deduce that the operator $a_t I - a_t A B_r B_0$ is also compact, i.e., the operator $B_t = B_r B_0$ is a right local regularizer of the operator A at the point t.

Using that A is an operator of local type, we show now how to construct a "global" right regularizer from its right local ones.

The neighbourhoods U_t of the points $t \in \Gamma$ in which the functions a_t are positive form an open covering of the contour Γ. We choose a finite subcovering $\{U_{t_j}\}_{j=1}^{N}$ from it. Then the function $a = \sum_{j=1}^{N} a_{t_j}$ is positive at all points of the contour Γ. Hence the operator $B = (\sum_{j=1}^{N} a_{t_j} B_{t_j})a^{-1}I$ is well-defined. It is just the desired regularizer. Indeed, since A is of local type, we have $Aa_{t_j}I \sim a_{t_j}A$ and, therefore, $Aa_{t_j}B_{t_j} \sim a_{t_j}AB_{t_j}$. But we have $a_{t_j}AB_{t_j} \sim a_{t_j}I$, which implies

$$A(\sum a_{t_j}B_{t_j})a^{-1}I = \sum (Aa_{t_j}B_{t_j})a^{-1}I \sim \sum (a_{t_j}I)a^{-1}I = I.$$

The existence of a left regularizer of the operator A is proved in a similar way (of course, from its existence we conclude that the right regularizer constructed above is also a left one). Owing to Theorem 1.8, there results the Fredholmness of A. ≡

We remark that the proof of the local principle described here can be literally transferred to the case of operators acting in $L_p(X)$, where X is a compact Hausdorff space with measure.
This general case was considered in the fundamental work of the theory of local type operators by SIMONENKO [5], where for the first time the notion of such operators was introduced and the local principle was proved.

1.2. SOME INFORMATION ON BOUNDARY PROPERTIES OF FUNCTIONS ANALYTIC AND MEROMORPHIC IN FINITELY CONNECTED DOMAINS

Let us begin with the consideration of functions analytic in the unit disk $\Delta = \{\zeta : |\zeta| < 1\}$. The proofs of the results on such functions formulated here can be found in Ch. 2 of the book of PRIVALOV [2] and in Ch. 5 of HOFFMAN [1].

DEFINITION 1.12. Functions of the form

$$f^{(e)}(z) = \exp(i\nu + \frac{1}{2\pi} \int_{-\pi}^{\pi} \frac{e^{i\theta} + z}{e^{i\theta} - z} \ln k(\theta)d\theta), \tag{1.7}$$

where ν is a real constant and k a non-negative function with summable logarithm, are said to be <u>outer</u>.

Before formulating the theorem about properties of outer functions, we recall that we understand by angular boundary values (or limits) of the function f at the points t of a contour the limit $\lim_{z \to t} f(z)$, when the point z tends to t along paths non-tangent to the contour.

<u>THEOREM 1.15.</u> Functions of the form (1.7) are analytic in Δ and have a.e. on the unit circle angular boundary values $f^{(e)}(e^{i\theta})$ fulfilling the condition $|f^{(e)}(e^{i\theta})| = k(\theta)$. Every analytic function not having zeros in Δ with a continuous bounded logarithm is an outer function.

The class of all functions analytic and bounded in Δ is denoted by H_∞. According to Fatou's theorem, the angular boundary values exist a.e. on the circle for any function from H_∞.

<u>DEFINITION 1.13.</u> A function from H_∞, the angular boundary values of which are a.e. equal to one, taken absolutely, is called inner.

In particular, Blaschke products, i.e. functions of the form

$$B(z) = z^l \prod_{k=1}^{\infty} \frac{\overline{a_k}}{|a_k|} \frac{a_k - z}{1 - \overline{a_k}z},$$

are inner functions, where l is a non-negative integer and $\{a_k\}$ is a sequence of points from Δ with $\sum (1 - |a_k|) < \infty$. A Blaschke product vanishes at the points a_k and, in case $l > 0$, at $z = 0$ and only at these points.

An example of an inner function not having zeros in Δ is provided by the function

$$S(z) = \exp\left(- \frac{1}{2\pi} \int_{-\pi}^{\pi} \frac{e^{i\theta}+z}{e^{i\theta}-z} d\mu(\theta)\right),$$

where μ is a singular (i.e. concentrated on a set of Lebesgue measure zero) measure on $[-\pi,\pi]$. Such a function is referred to as singular.

<u>THEOREM 1.16.</u> Any inner function $f^{(i)}$ can be represented in the form $f^{(i)} = \lambda BS$, where B is a Blaschke product, S is a singular

function and λ is a constant ($|\lambda| = 1$). Such a representation is unique.

DEFINITION 1.14. All functions representable in the form of a quotient of a function from H_∞ to an outer function form the class D.

THEOREM 1.17. A function f not identically zero belongs to the class D if and only if it can be represented in the form of a product of an outer by an inner function. Such a representation is unique. Outer functions and only they belong to the class D together with their reciprocal ones.

It is evident that functions of class D have angular boundary values a.e. on the unit circle.

DEFINITION 1.15. The function f analytic in Δ belongs to the class H_p, $0 < p < \infty$, if

$$\sup_{r<1} \int_{-\pi}^{\pi} |f(re^{i\theta})|^p \, d\theta < \infty . \tag{1.8}$$

We note that, for any function f analytic in Δ, $M_{p,f}(r) = \int_{-\pi}^{\pi} |f(re^{i\theta})|^p \, d\theta$ is a non-decreasing function of r. Consequently, condition (1.8) is equivalent to $\lim_{r\to 1-0} M_{p,f}(r) < \infty$ or, what is the same, $\sup_k M_{p,f}(r_k) < \infty$, where $\{r_k\}$ is an arbitrary sequence of positive scalars tending to one from below.

The classes H_p with $0 < p \leq \infty$ are called Hardy classes. The relation between Hardy classes and the class D is expressed by the following theorem.

THEOREM 1.18 (P.Ya. POLUBARINOVA-KOCHINA). A function f defined in Δ belongs to the class H_p $(0 < p \leq \infty)$ if and only if $f \in D$ and the function $f^{(b)}$ made up of its angular boundary values on the circle belongs to the class L_p.

COROLLARY 1.5 (V.I. SMIRNOV). If $f \in H_p$ and $f^{(b)} \in L_{p_1}$ for some $p_1 > p$, then $f \in H_{p_1}$.

Let $\mathfrak{D}$ be a simply connected domain in the extended complex plane, the boundary of which is a closed rectifiable Jordan curve Γ.

DEFINITION 1.16. We shall say that a function f analytic in $\mathcal{D}$ is an element of the class $E_p(\mathcal{D})$, $0 < p < \infty$, if it is possible to find an expanding sequence of domains $\mathcal{D}_k$ with rectifiable boundaries Γ_k such that:

1) $\mathcal{D}_k \cup \Gamma_k \subseteq \mathcal{D}$,
2) $\bigcup_k \mathcal{D}_k = \mathcal{D}$,
3) $\sup_k \int_{\Gamma_k} |f(t)|^p |dt| < \infty$.

The classes $E_p(\mathcal{D})$ are called Smirnov classes. This definition of Smirnov classes $E_p(\mathcal{D})$ was suggested by M.V. KELDYSH and M.A. LAVRENT'EV. In SMIRNOV's original definition it was required that the curves Γ_k are images of a circle under a conformal mapping of the disk Δ onto the domain $\mathcal{D}$. The definitions of KELDYSH/LAVRENT'EV and SMIRNOV are equivalent (concerning this topic, see DANILYUK [6] p. 91, GOLUZIN [1] p. 423 and PRIVALOV [2] p. 203). Consequently, the following criterion of the membership of functions to Smirnov classes holds.

THEOREM 1.19. The function φ defined in a simply connected domain $\mathcal{D}$ belongs to the class $E_p(\mathcal{D})$ if and only if the function $\psi = \varphi \circ \omega \sqrt[p]{\omega'}$ belongs to the Hardy class H_p. Here by ω a function is denoted, which realizes the conformal mapping of the disk Δ onto the domain $\mathcal{D}$, and $\sqrt[p]{\omega'}$ is an arbitrary branch of the pth root of ω' continuous in Δ.

Below we shall be concerned with functions analytic, generally speaking, in a multiply connected domain $\mathcal{D}^+$. It is assumed that this domain is obtained from a bounded simply connected domain $\mathcal{D}^+(0)$ by removal of pairwise disjoint simply connected domains $\mathcal{D}^+(j)$ $(j = 1,\dots,m-1)$ lying inside it. The boundaries of the domains $\mathcal{D}^+(j)$ $(j = 0,\dots,m-1)$ are supposed to be Jordan rectifiable curves. We denote by $\mathcal{D}^-(j)$ the complement to $\mathcal{D}^+(j) \cup \Gamma(j)$. The contour $\Gamma = \bigcup_{j=0}^{m-1} \Gamma(j)$ is assumed to be oriented in such a manner that at an anticlockwise revolution along it the domain $\mathcal{D}^+$ is on the left.

LEMMA 1.1. Every function f analytic in the domain $\mathcal{D}^+$ admits a unique representation

$$f(z) = \sum_{j=0}^{m-1} f_j(z) , \quad z \in \mathcal{D}^+ , \tag{1.9}$$

where the function f_o is analytic in $\mathcal{D}^+(0)$, and the functions f_j $(j = 1,\dots,m-1)$ are analytic in $\mathcal{D}^-(j)$ and vanish at infinity.

Proof. Set $f_j(z) = \frac{1}{2\pi i} \int_{\gamma_{j,z}} f(\tau) \frac{d\tau}{\tau - z}$, where the contour $\gamma_{j,z}$ $(\subset \mathcal{D}^+)$, which is oriented in the same way as $\Gamma(j)$, is chosen in such a manner that it borders together with $\Gamma(j)$ a doubly connected domain lying in $\mathcal{D}^+$ and not containing the point z. Clearly, $\gamma_{j,z}$ is not unique, but, in view of Cauchy's integral theorem, the value $f_j(z)$ does not depend on the choice of $\gamma_{j,z}$. The equation (1.9) is nothing else than Cauchy's integral formula written in a shortened form.

It is sufficient to prove the uniqueness of the representation (1.9) for the function $f(z) \equiv 0$. If $\sum_{j=0}^{m-1} f_j(z) = 0$, then, for any $k = 1,\dots,m-1$,

$$f_k(z) = - \sum_{j \neq k} f_j(z) , \quad z \in \mathcal{D}^+ .$$

The left-hand side of the equality obtained is analytic in $\mathcal{D}^-(k)$, and the right one in $\mathcal{D}^+ \cup \overline{\mathcal{D}^+(k)}$. Therefore, the function f_k is analytic in $\mathcal{D}^-(k) \cup \mathcal{D}^+ \cup \mathcal{D}^+(k)$, i.e. in the entire complex plane. Since, in addition, $f_k(\infty) = 0$, we can conclude that $f_k \equiv 0$, by Liouville's theorem.

But then we have $f_o(z) = - \sum_{k=1}^{m-1} f_k(z) = 0$ for $z \in \mathcal{D}^+$. Thus, the function f_o is also identically equal to zero in $\mathcal{D}^+(0)$. This proves the uniqueness of the representation in the form (1.9) for $f(z) \equiv 0$. Hence Lemma 1.1 has been proved. ≡

In what follows, we need a generalization of the Smirnov classes to the case of multiply connected domains.

DEFINITION 1.17 (KHAVINSON [1]). The function f analytic in the m-connected domain $\mathcal{D}^+$ belongs to class $E_p(\mathcal{D}^+)$ $(0 < p < \infty)$ if and only if there exists an expanding sequence of m-connected domains $\mathcal{D}_k$ satisfying conditions 1) – 3) of Definition 1.16 and, moreover, the requirement

4) the lengths $|\Gamma_k|$ of the contours Γ_k are equibounded.

THEOREM 1.20 (Decomposition theorem). The function f analytic in the m-connected domain $\mathcal{D}^+$ belongs to the class $E_p(\mathcal{D}^+)$ if and only if the functions f_j from the representation (1.9) fulfil the conditions $f_o \in E_p(\mathcal{D}^+(0))$, $f_j \in E_p(\mathcal{D}^-(j))$, $j = 1,\dots,m-1$.

Proof. Let $f \in E_p(\mathcal{D}^+)$. We represent the boundary Γ_k of the domain $\mathcal{D}_k$ occurring in Definition 1.17 in the form $\Gamma_k = \bigcup_{j=o}^{m-1} \Gamma_k(j)$, where $\Gamma_k(j)$ is a closed curve, which borders together with $\Gamma(j)$ a doubly connected domain lying in $\mathcal{D}^+$. According to equation (1.9) and Minkowski's integral inequality, the following relation holds:

$$\int_{\Gamma_k(j)} |f_j(\tau)|^p |d\tau| \le \Big(\Big(\sum_{l \neq j} \int_{\Gamma_k(j)} |f_l(\tau)|^p |d\tau|\Big)^{\frac{1}{\max(1,p)}} + \Big(\int_{\Gamma_k(j)} |f(\tau)|^p |d\tau|\Big)^{\frac{1}{\max(1,p)}}\Big)^{\max(1,p)} . \tag{1.10}$$

Denoting by M_l the upper bound of the absolute value of the function f_l in the domain $\mathcal{D}_l$, on the strength of the maximum modulus principle, we can claim that it is also an upper bound for $|f(\tau)|$ for $\tau \in \Gamma_k(j)$ $(j \neq l)$. Therefore,

$$\int_{\Gamma_k(j)} |f_l(\tau)|^p |d\tau| \le M_l^p |\Gamma_k(j)| < M_l^p |\Gamma_k| .$$

Moreover, $\int_{\Gamma_k(j)} |f(\tau)|^p |d\tau| \le \int_{\Gamma_k} |f(\tau)|^p |d\tau|$. As the function f belongs to the class $E_p(\mathcal{D}^+)$, we deduce from condition 4) of Definition 1.17 that the right-hand side of the inequality (1.10) is bounded from above by a quantity not depending upon k. This fact as well as Definition 1.16 imply that the functions f_j belong to the Smirnov classes in appropriate domains.

Vice versa, let the conditions $f_o \in E_p(\mathcal{D}^+(0))$, $f_j \in E_p(\mathcal{D}^-(j))$,

$j = 1,\ldots,m-1$ be fulfilled. We introduce curves $\Gamma_k(j)$ which are images of a circle with radius r_k under a conformal mapping of the unit disk on the domain $\mathcal{D}^+(j)$ for $j = 0$, and on $\mathcal{D}^-(j)$ for $j = 1,\ldots,m-1$. Here $\{r_k\}$ is an arbitrary increasing sequence of positive numbers tending to one. Then (at least beginning with some k) the contour $\Gamma = \bigcup_{j=0}^{m-1} \Gamma_k(j)$ is the boundary of a m-connected domain $\mathcal{D}_k$ satisfying conditions 1) and 2) of Definition 1.17. Condition 4) of this definition is fulfilled, since the derivative of the function ω describing a conformal mapping of the disk on a domain with rectifiable boundary, always belongs to the class H_1 (see PRIVALOV [2] p. 173, DANILYUK [6] p. 88, GOLUZIN [1]). Now condition 3) can be readily verified in the same manner as it was done above for the function f_j. Consequently $f \in E_p(\mathcal{D}^+)$, which completes the proof of the theorem. ≡

In TUMARKIN, KHAVINSON [1] it was shown that the omission of condition 4) in Definition 1.17 does not lead to an extension of the notion of classes E_p in finitely connected domains (for a simply connected domain this fact is a consequence of Theorem 1.19 and the relation $\omega' \in H_1$). In other words, Definition 1.16 can be used for arbitrary finitely connected domains[1)].

This allowed for considering Smirnov classes in Jordan domains with non-rectifiable boundary. For such domains the decomposition theorem does not hold as it was clarified in TUMARKIN, KHAVINSON [2,3].

The class of all functions analytic and bounded in some domain $\mathcal{D}$ will be denoted by $E_\infty(\mathcal{D})$.

In what follows, we shall simply write E_p instead of $E_p(\mathcal{D}^+)$, whereas E_p^- denotes the class of functions defined on the set $\mathcal{D}^- = \mathcal{D}^-(0) \cup (\bigcup_{j=1}^{m-1} \mathcal{D}^+(j))$, the restriction of which on $\mathcal{D}^-(0)$ ($\mathcal{D}^+(j)$ respectively) is a function of class $E_p(\mathcal{D}^-(0))$ ($E_p(\mathcal{D}^+(j))$). The class $\overset{\circ}{E}{}_p^-$ consists of functions from E_p^- vanishing at infinity.

It is clear from the proof of Theorem 1.20 that the system of domains $\mathcal{D}_k$

---

1) Note that in the monograph DUREN [1] the problem of description of multiply connected domains for which Definitions 1.16 and 1.17 are equivalent is referred to as an open one.

occurring in Definition 1.17 can be chosen as one and the same for all functions of a Smirnov class. Hence, applying Minkowski's and Hölder's integral inequalities in a standard manner, we can easily derive the following result.

THEOREM 1.21. 1) The classes E_p^+, E_p^- and $\overset{\circ}{E}{}_p^-$ are lineals,
2) for any $p_1, p_2 \in (0,\infty]$, $p_1 < p_2$, the inclusions $E_{p_1}^+ \supseteq E_{p_2}^+$, $E_{p_1}^- \supseteq E_{p_2}^-$ hold,
3) if $f \in E_{p_1}^+ \ (E_{p_1}^-)$, $g \in E_{p_2}^+ \ (E_{p_2}^-)$, then $fg \in E_p^+ \ (E_p^-)$, where $p = (p_1^{-1} + p_2^{-1})^{-1}$.

More profound properties of functions from Smirnov classes are gathered below in Theorems 1.22, 1.24, 1.25. For the case of a simply connected domain $\mathcal{D}^+$, the arguments of these theorems can be found in the monographs GOLUZIN [1], DANILYUK [6], PRIVALOV [2]. With the help of the decomposition theorem 1.20, these theorems can be transferred to the more general case of a finitely connected domain in an obvious manner[1)], which justifies the references to GOLUZIN [1], DANILYUK [6], PRIVALOV [2] before the formulations of Theorems 1.22, 1.24, 1.25.

THEOREM 1.22 (see PRIVALOV [2] p. 204, DANILYUK [6] p. 91, GOLUZIN [1] p. 422). Every function f of the class $E_p^+ \ (E_p^-)$, $p > 0$, has limits $f^+(t) \ (f^-(t))$ along all non-tangent paths at almost all points $t \in \Gamma$. The function $f^+ \ (f^-)$, which is defined on Γ by these limits, belongs to the class L_p.

DEFINITION 1.18. The function f defined a.e. on Γ we assume to belong to the class $L_p^+ \ (L_p^-, \overset{\circ}{L}{}_p^-)$, $0 < p \leq \infty$, if there exists a function of class $E_p^+ \ (E_p^-, \overset{\circ}{E}{}_p^-)$ the boundary values of which coincide with f at almost all $t \in \Gamma$.

We denote by $M_p^{\pm} \ (= L_p^{\pm} + R)$ the class of functions f representable in the form $f = f_1 + f_2$, where $f_1 \in L_p^{\pm}$ and $f_2 \in R$.

---

1) Concerning this topic, see TUMARKIN, KHAVINSON [3], where Theorem 1.24 is formulated (in particular, on p. 73) for the case of a finitely connected domain.

The classes $E_p^{\pm} + R$, $L_p^{\pm} + C$ are introduced in a similar way. Sometimes it will be convenient to use the notations $L^{\pm} = \bigcup_{p>0} L_p^{\pm}$, $M^{\pm} = \bigcup_{p>0} M_p^{\pm}$.

Beginning with Chapter 2, we shall, as a rule, not deal with scalar functions from classes L_p, $L_p^{\pm}$, $M_p^{\pm}$ etc., but with n-dimensional vector functions and $n\times n$ matrix functions, the elements of which belong to these classes. We denote by X^n the space of n-dimensional vector functions, the components of which belong to some function class X (in the case $X = L_p$, this notation was already used in Section 1.1). It would be natural to denote the class of $n\times n$ matrix functions with elements from X by $X^{n\times n}$. However, we renounce this notation, since it is too troublesome. Instead, the class of such matrix functions is simply denoted by X. From the context it will be always clear whether we speak about a scalar or a matrix function.

Vector functions of the class $(E_p^{\pm} + R)^n$ can be reproduced from their limits on Γ in a unique manner. Let us show this. If the vector functions f_1 and f_2 from the class $(E_p^{\pm} + R)^n$ have angular limits coinciding a.e. on Γ, then their difference $f = f_1 - f_2$ is also a vector function from $(E_p^{\pm} + R)^n$ and has angular limits equal to zero a.e. on Γ. But in view of the following uniqueness theorem, this is possible only for $f = 0$.

THEOREM 1.23 (PRIVALOV [2] p. 292, GOLUZIN [1] p. 413). A function meromorphic in a domain with rectifiable boundary, which has angular limits equal to zero on a set of positive linear measure, is identically equal to zero.

Taking into account the injectivity of the correspondence between classes $E_p^{\pm} + R$ and $M_p^{\pm}$ (respectively between $E_p^{\pm}$ and $L_p^{\pm}$), we sometimes shall identify vector functions from $(E_p^{\pm} + R)^n$ with vector functions from $(M_p^{\pm})^n$ formed by their limits.

In particular, if $f \in (M_p^{\pm})^n$, under $f(z)$, $z \in \mathcal{D}^{\pm}$ we shall simply understand the value at the point z of that vector function of class $(E_p^{\pm} + R)^n$, the boundary value of which is f. In connection with this, note that the identification of functions of class H_p with corresponding functions of class L_p^+ on the circle is in general use. For the latter class even the notation H_p (or H_p^+) is preserved (see HOFFMAN [1]). For the sake of uniformity, the class L_p^- on the circle is denoted by H_p^-. Clearly, all the assertions of Theorem 1.21 may be transferred from the classes $E_p^{\pm}$ to classes $(E_p^{\pm} + R)^n$, $(L_p^{\pm})^n$ and $(M_p^{\pm})^n$, if the product fg is defined componentwise.

In the classic case of functions analytic in a domain and continuous up to the boundary, the values in the domain are expressed via boundary ones with the aid of Cauchy's integral. This method cannot be transferred directly to the case of classes $E_p^{\pm}$ for $p < 1$, because a boundary function is not summable. However, for functions from the classes $E_1^{\pm}$, Cauchy's integral remains to be a natural means of continuation from a contour to a domain.

<u>THEOREM 1.24 (PRIVALOV [2] pp. 202, 206, DANILYUK [6] p. 133, GOLUZIN [1] pp. 420–423).</u> The vector function f defined on Γ a.e. belongs to $(L_1^+)^n$ $((\overset{\circ}{L}{}_1^-)^n$, respectively) iff $f \in L_1^n$ and

$$\int_\Gamma f(\tau) \frac{d\tau}{\tau - z} = 0 \quad \text{for} \quad z \in \mathcal{D}^- \ (\mathcal{D}^+) \quad \text{or, equivalently,}$$

$$\int_\Gamma f(\tau)\tau^k d\tau = 0 \tag{1.11}$$

for all non-negative (negative) integers k.

If this condition is fulfilled, then the function Φ from $(E_1^+)^n$ $((\overset{\circ}{E}{}_1^-)^n)$, whose boundary value is f, can be determined by the formula

$$\Phi(z) = \frac{\varepsilon}{2\pi i} \int_\Gamma f(\tau) \frac{d\tau}{\tau - z}, \quad z \in \mathcal{D}^+ \ (\mathcal{D}^-),$$

where $\varepsilon = 1$ if $z \in \mathcal{D}^+$ and $\varepsilon = -1$ if $z \in \mathcal{D}^-$.

In accordance with Theorems 1.24 and 1.22, any vector function f of the class $(L_p^+)^n$ $((\overset{\circ}{L}{}_p^-)^n)$, $p \geq 1$ lies in the subspace of L_p^n consisting of all functions satisfying (1.11) and, for $p = 1$, coincides with it. Corollary 1.5 shows that for the circle the coincidence holds for

$p > 1$, too. To characterize the situation in general, we introduce another definition.

DEFINITION 1.19 (see PRIVALOV [2] p. 250, DANILYUK [6] p. 90).

A simply connected domain $\mathcal{D}$ is called Smirnov, if the derivative of the function ω , which maps Δ conformally on $\mathcal{D}$, is an outer function.

A closed Jordan curve Γ will be called Smirnov (curve of class $\mathfrak{C}$), if each of the domains in which Γ decomposes the extended complex plane is Smirnov.

The class of Smirnov curves is so wide that it is rather difficult to construct examples of curves not belonging to this class. For the first time, such an example was built by M.V. KELDYSH and M.A. LAVRENT'EV. Their construction, with some simplifications, is described in PRIVALOV [2] pp. 229-250. An analytic description of all non-Smirnov curves the interested reader can find in DUREN, SHAPIRO, SHIELDS [1]. Various sufficient conditions of membership of curves to the Smirnov class are established in PRIVALOV [2] pp. 250-257. In particular, one can find there LAVRENT'EV's result that a curve is Smirnov as soon as

$$\operatorname{ess\,sup}\left\{\frac{s(t_1,t_2)}{|t_1 - t_2|} : t_1,t_2 \in \Gamma\right\} < \infty . \tag{1.12}$$

Here $s(t_1,t_2)$ is the distance between points t_1 and t_2 measured along Γ .

THEOREM 1.25 (PRIVALOV [2] pp. 264-266, DANILYUK [6] pp. 92-95).

If the contour Γ consists only of Smirnov curves, then, for $0 < p_1 < p_2 \leq \infty$, the equalities $(L^+_{p_2})^n = (L^+_{p_1})^n \cap L^n_{p_2}$ and $(L^-_{p_2})^n = (L^-_{p_1})^n \cap L^n_{p_2}$ are valid. Especially, in case that $p \geq 1$ we have $f \in (L^+_p)^n$ $((\mathring{L}^-_p)^n$ respectively) if and only if $f \in L^n_p$ and condition (1.11) is fulfilled. If at least one component of the contour Γ is not a Smirnov curve, then there exists a function $f \in L_\infty$ such that $f \in L^+_1$ $(\mathring{L}^-_1)$, but $f \notin L^+_p$ $(\mathring{L}^-_p)$ for all $p > 1$.

Due to Theorem 1.25, in the case of a contour Γ consisting of Smirnov curves, the lineals $(L^+_p)^n$ and $(L^-_p)^n$ are subspaces in L^n_p . In fact, this assertion is true for every rectifiable contour Γ , however, the corresponding argument requires some preliminary constructions, which we are now going to deal with.

We shall identify the space L_q^n with the dual to L_p^n $(1 \leq p < \infty$, $q = p/(p-1))$ via the bilinear form

$$\langle f,g\rangle = \sum_{j=1}^{n} \int_{\Gamma} f_j(t)g_j(t)dt \ , \tag{1.13}$$

where $f = \sum_{j=1}^{n} f_j e_j \in L_p^n$, $g = \sum_{j=1}^{n} g_j e_j \in L_q^n$.

It goes without saying that in this case L_p^n and L_q^n have to be regarded as real Banach spaces. The norm in L_p^n consistent with the form (1.13) (i.e. satisfying the condition $\|f\|_{L_p^n} = \sup\{\langle f,g\rangle : g \in L_q^n, \|g\|_{L_q^n} = 1\})$ looks as

$$\|f\|_{L_p^n} = \left(\int_{\Gamma} \left(\sum_{j=1}^{n} |f_j(t)|^2\right)^{p/2} |dt|\right)^{1/p} ,$$

where $f = \sum_{j=1}^{n} f_j e_j$ and e_j denotes the j th unit vector.

<u>THEOREM 1.26.</u> The orthogonal (in the sense of the form (1.13)) complement to $(L_p^+)^n$ $((\overset{\circ}{L}{}_p^-)^n)$ coincides with $(L_q^+)^n$ $((\overset{\circ}{L}{}_q^-)^n)$.

<u>Proof.</u> Obviously, it is sufficient to prove the statement for $n = 1$. If $f \in L_q^+$, $g \in L_p^+$, then we deduce $fg \in L_1^+$ and $\langle f,g\rangle = 0$ by Theorem 1.24. The same theorem enables us to conclude that $\langle f,g\rangle = 0$, if $f \in \overset{\circ}{L}{}_q^-$, $g \in \overset{\circ}{L}{}_p^-$, since in this case the function $tf(t)g(t)$ belongs to the class $\overset{\circ}{L}{}_1^-$.

Conversely, let the function $f \in L_q$ be such that $\langle f,g\rangle = 0$ for all $g \in L_p^+$ $(\overset{\circ}{L}{}_p^-)$. Setting $g(t) = t^k$, where k is a non-negative (negative) integer, we obtain $\int_{\Gamma} f(t)t^k dt = 0$. According to Theorem 1.24, this means that $f \in L_1^+$ $(\overset{\circ}{L}{}_1^-)$.

The following considerations are first made for the case of a simply connected domain $\mathcal{D}^+$. Suppose that the function ω realizes a conformal mapping of the unit disk onto $\mathcal{D}^+$. After substituting $\tau = \omega(\zeta)$ the condition $\int_{\Gamma} f(\tau)g(\tau)d\tau = 0$ can be rewritten as

$$\int_{\mathbb{T}} f(\omega(\zeta)) \sqrt[q]{\omega'(\zeta)}\, g(\omega(\zeta)) \sqrt[p]{\omega'(\zeta)}\, d\zeta = 0 \tag{1.14}$$

(for $p = 1$, i.e. $q = \infty$, we put $\sqrt[q]{\omega'} = 1$) where $\mathbb{T}$ is the unit circle.

The function $\varphi = (f \circ \omega)\sqrt[q]{\omega'}$ belongs to the class L_q ($\subset L_1$) simultaneously with f. If g ranges over the whole class L_p^+, then in view of Theorem 1.19, $(g \circ \omega)\sqrt[p]{\omega'}$ ranges over the whole class H_p. By what was proved above, relation (1.14) implies $\varphi \in H_1$. From this relation and the condition $\varphi \in L_q$, in virtue of Corollary 1.5, one can conclude $\varphi \in H_q$. Applying Theorem 1.19 once more, we observe $f \in L_q^+$.

Considering a conformal mapping of the disk onto the domain $\mathcal{D}^-$, it can be shown in a similar way that the orthogonal complement to $\mathring{L}_p^-$ consists of functions of the class $\mathring{L}_q^-$.

Now we return to the general case of a m-connected domain $\mathcal{D}^+$. A function $f \in L_q$ orthogonal to L_p^+ lies in L_1^+ as was already shown. Applying the decomposition theorem 1.20 to that function from E_1^+ the boundary value of which is f, we get the representation $f = \sum_{j=0}^{m-1} f_j$, where f_0 (f_j) is the boundary value on Γ of a function from $E_1(\mathcal{D}^+(0))$ $(\mathring{E}_1(\mathcal{D}^-(j))$, $j = 1,\ldots,m-1)$. Let us choose as g the boundary value on Γ of a function from $E_q(\mathcal{D}^+(0))$. Then, of course, $g \in L_q^+$ and thus

$$\int_\Gamma f(t)g(t)dt = \sum_{j=0}^{m-1} \int_\Gamma f_j(t)g(t)dt = 0 .$$

Directly by definition we check that, for $j = 1,\ldots,m-1$, the functions $f_j g$ belong to the class L_1^+. As a result of this we obtain that in the last sum all summands are equal to zero, with the exception of the first one. Hence,

$$\int_\Gamma f_0(t)g(t) = 0 . \tag{1.15}$$

Furthermore, the product $f_0 g$ can be continued to a function analytic in the closure of the domains $\mathcal{D}^+(j)$ $(j = 1,\ldots,m-1)$. Owing to

Cauchy's classical integral theorem, $\int_{\Gamma(j)} f_o(t)g(t)dt = 0 \quad (j=1,\dots,m-1)$.
Thus, condition (1.15) can be rewritten as

$$\int_{\Gamma(0)} f_o(\tau)g(\tau)d\tau = 0 \text{ .}$$

In summary, it has been shown that the boundary value on $\Gamma(0)$ of the function f_o analytic in $\mathcal{D}^+(0)$ belongs to the orthogonal complement of the set of boundary values of functions from $E_p(\mathcal{D}^+(0))$. Due to the result established above for simply connected domains, f_o is the boundary value of a function from $E_q(\mathcal{D}^+(0))$.
Taking as g the boundary value on Γ of functions from the class $E_p(\mathcal{D}^-(j))$ and acting by the scheme described, we can state that f_j is in fact the boundary value of a function from $E_q(\mathcal{D}^-(j))$.
By Theorem 1.20, this just means that $f \in L_q^+$. Thus, also in case of a multiply connected domain the orthogonal complement to L_p^+ is the class L_q^+. Analogously, the assertion concerning the classes $\overset{\circ}{L}{}_p^-$, $\overset{\circ}{L}{}_q^-$ allow to be transferred to the case of multiply connected domains. ≡

<u>COROLLARY 1.6.</u> For any $p \in [1,\infty]$, the sets $(L_p^+)^n$, $(\overset{\circ}{L}{}_q^-)^n$ are subspaces in L_p^n.

Indeed, for $p \in (1,\infty]$, $(L_p^+)^n$ $((\overset{\circ}{L}{}_p^-)^n)$ is the orthogonal complement to some lineal and is therefore a subspace. The closedness of the classes $(L_1^+)^n$ and $(\overset{\circ}{L}{}_1^-)^n$ was already mentioned.

<u>THEOREM 1.27.</u> Let the vector functions $\Phi^+ \in (M_1^+)^n$ and $\Phi^- \in (M_1^-)^n$ coincide a.e. on some arc $\gamma \subseteq \Gamma$. Then each of these vector functions is the analytical continuation of the other through γ.

<u>Proof.</u> By definition of the classes $(M_1^{\pm})^n$, there exist representations $\Phi^+ = \varphi^+ + r_1$, $\Phi^- = \varphi^- + r_2$ with $\varphi^{\pm} \in (L_1^{\pm})^n$ and $r_j \in R^n$.
In its turn, $r_j = r_j^+ - r_j^-$, where $r_j^{\pm}$ is a rational vector function with poles concentrated in $\mathcal{D}^{\mp}$, $j = 1,2$. The coincidence of the functions Φ^+ and Φ^- a.e. on γ, obviously, implies that the vector functions $\Psi^+ = \varphi^+ + r_1^+ - r_2^+$ and $\Psi^- = \varphi^- + r_1^- - r_2^-$ belonging to the classes $(L_1^+)^n$ and $(L_1^-)^n$, respectively, coincide a.e. on γ.
Changing the vector functions $r_2^{\pm}$ by one and the same constant, one

may always obtain $\Psi^- \in (\overset{\circ}{L}{}_1^-)^n$. In view of Theorem 1.24, for $z \in \mathcal{D}^+$, the following equalities hold:

$$\Psi^+(z) = \frac{1}{2\pi i} \int_{\Gamma\setminus\gamma} \Psi^+(\tau) \frac{d\tau}{\tau-z} + \frac{1}{2\pi i} \int_{\gamma} \Psi^+(\tau) \frac{d\tau}{\tau-z} ,$$

$$0 = \frac{1}{2\pi i} \int_{\Gamma\setminus\gamma} \Psi^-(\tau) \frac{d\tau}{\tau-z} + \frac{1}{2\pi i} \int_{\gamma} \Psi^-(\tau) \frac{d\tau}{\tau-z} .$$

Having regard to the relation $\int_{\gamma} \Psi^+(\tau) \frac{d\tau}{\tau-z} = \int_{\gamma} \Psi^-(\tau) \frac{d\tau}{\tau-z}$, we come to the representation

$$\Psi^+(z) = \frac{1}{2\pi i} \int_{\Gamma\setminus\gamma} \Psi^+(\tau) \frac{d\tau}{\tau-z} - \frac{1}{2\pi i} \int_{\Gamma\setminus\gamma} \Psi^-(\tau) \frac{d\tau}{\tau-z} . \tag{1.16}$$

Consequently, the vector function Ψ^+ is analytically continuable from the domain $\mathcal{D}^+$ through the arc γ . But then, in some neighbourhood of γ , the vector function $\Psi^+ - r_1^- + r_2^+$ coinciding a.e. on γ with Φ^+ (and Φ^-) is also analytic. Thus Theorem 1.27 is proved. ≡

If, in particular, $\gamma = \Gamma$, then we can conclude from formula (1.16) that $\Psi^+ = 0$, i.e. $\Phi^+ \in R^n$. Taking into account that a rational function that has no poles is a constant, we get the following uniqueness theorem.

<u>THEOREM 1.28.</u> The intersection of the classes $(M_1^+)^n$ and $(M_1^-)^n$ consists precisely of vector functions of class R^n , the intersection of the classes $(L_1^+)^n$ and $(L_1^-)^n$ consists of constants, and the intersection of $(L_1^+)^n$ and $(\overset{\circ}{L}{}_1^-)^n$ contains the zero function only.

Finally, we want to insert some remarks on the notion of the index of a function.

<u>DEFINITION 1.20.</u> Suppose f is a function continuous and nonvanishing on Γ . Then the integer

$$\text{ind } f = \frac{1}{2\pi} \{\arg f(t)\}_\Gamma$$

is called the (Cauchy) <u>index</u> of f . Here $\{\arg f(t)\}_\Gamma$ denotes the sum of the argument increments of the function f , when the variable t ranges over all closed curves $\Gamma_{(j)}$ which form the contour Γ, once in each case in positive direction.

If the function f admits a continuation to a function F, which is continuous in $\mathcal{D}^+ \cup \Gamma$ and analytic in $\mathcal{D}^+$ with the exception of a finite number of poles, then, due to the argument principle,

$$\text{ind } f = N - P, \tag{1.17}$$

where N and P are the numbers of zeros and poles of the function F in $\mathcal{D}^+$ calculated with regard to their multiplicity.

Starting from this result, we take equation (1.17) as the definition of the index for functions f belonging to the class M^+ together with their inverses. This definition is correct, since the condition $f \in M^+$ guarantees the finiteness of the number of poles, and the condition $f^{-1} \in M^+$ the finiteness of zeros of the meromorphic continuation of f from the contour Γ into $\mathcal{D}^+$.

The index of invertible elements of class M^+ defined in this way will be denoted by the symbol ind_+.

Analogously, for functions f satisfying the condition $f^{\pm 1} \in M^-$ we introduce the index via the formula

$$\text{ind}_- f = P - N, \tag{1.17'}$$

where P and N are the numbers of poles and zeros in $\mathcal{D}^-$ of f.

THEOREM 1.29.

1) If i is one of the functions ind_+, ind_-, ind defined on the invertible elements of M^+, M^-, C, respectively, then

$$i(f_1 f_2) = i(f_1) + i(f_2),$$

2) $\text{ind}_+ f \geq 0$ if $f \in L^+$, $\text{ind}_- f \leq 0$ if $f \in L^-$,

3) for a rational function f the value $\text{ind}_- f - \text{ind}_+ f$ coincides with the difference of the number of poles and zeros of this function that lies on Γ taking into account their multiplicity,

4) if $f^{\pm 1} \in M_1^+$ and $f^{\pm 1} \in M_1^-$, then $\text{ind}_+ f = \text{ind}_- f$ (= ind f).

Proof. Assertions 1) and 2) result directly from the definition. Assertion 3) follows from the fact that $\text{ind}_- f - \text{ind}_+ f$ is the difference of the number of poles and zeros (with regard to their multiplicity) of the function f in $\mathcal{D}^+ \cup \mathcal{D}^-$, i.e. in the complement to the contour Γ with respect to the complete plane, and the corresponding difference in the complete plane is equal to zero. Finally, under the condition $f \in M_1^+ \cap M_1^-$, the function f is rational by Theorem 1.28 and does not have poles on Γ. Moreover, since $f^{-1} \in M_1^{\pm}$, the function f does not have any zeros on Γ either. According to assertion 3), we have $\operatorname{ind}_- f = \operatorname{ind}_+ f$, which proves the theorem. ≡

Immediately from the definition of classes M we deduce that, for each matrix function $G \in M^+$ (M^-), one can choose a scalar function $f \in R$ not vanishing on Γ and such that

$$fG \in L^+ \quad (L^-) \, . \tag{1.18}$$

Applying assertion 2) of Theorem 1.29 to the function $\det(fG)$, we find by the equality $\operatorname{ind}_{\pm}(\det fG) = n \cdot \operatorname{ind} f + \operatorname{ind}_{\pm} \det G$ that the value $\operatorname{ind} f$ is bounded from below, if $G \in M^+$, and from above, if $G \in M^-$. The corresponding exact bound of the value $\operatorname{ind} f$, when f ranges over the set of all non-degenerating functions from R satisfying condition (1.18), we shall denote by $\mathcal{P}_+(G)$ $(-\mathcal{P}_-(G))$. Clearly, $\mathcal{P}_{\pm}(G)$ is less or equal than the total number of poles of the entries of G in $\mathcal{D}^{\pm}$.

1.3. ON THE OPERATOR OF SINGULAR INTEGRATION IN SPACES OF SUMMABLE FUNCTIONS

In the previous section it was shown that the classes $(L_1^+)^n$ and $(\overset{\circ}{L}{}_1^-)^n$ are subspaces in L_1^n, the only common element of which is 0. This allows for correctly defining the operator S of the lineal $\mathcal{L}_1^n = (L_1^+ \dotplus \overset{\circ}{L}{}_1^-)^n$ as follows: if $\varphi^+ \in (L_1^+)^n$, $\varphi^- \in (L_1^-)^n$, then $S(\varphi^+ + \varphi^-) = \varphi^+ - \varphi^-$.

Furthermore, we define operators in $\mathcal{L}_1^n$ by $P = \frac{1}{2}(I + S)$ and $Q = \frac{1}{2}(I - S)$. Obviously, P projects $\mathcal{L}_1^n$ onto $(L_1^+)^n$ along $(\overset{\circ}{L}{}_1^-)^n$, and Q projects $\mathcal{L}_1^n$ onto $(\overset{\circ}{L}{}_1^-)^n$ along $(L_1^+)^n$.

In view of Theorem 1.24, we can write that with $\varphi = \varphi^+ + \varphi^-$ $(\varphi^+ \in (L_1^+)^n$, $\varphi^- \in (\overset{\circ}{L}{}_1^-)^n)$ for the analytic continuations $\Phi^{\pm}$ of the vector functions $\varphi^{\pm}$ in $\mathcal{D}^{\pm}$ the following formulae are valid:

$$\Phi^+(z) = \frac{1}{2\pi i} \int_\Gamma \varphi(\tau)\frac{d\tau}{\tau - z}, \quad z \in \mathcal{D}^+,$$
$$\Phi^-(z) = -\frac{1}{2\pi i} \int_\Gamma \varphi(\tau)\frac{d\tau}{\tau - z}, \quad z \in \mathcal{D}^-. \tag{1.19}$$

But for angular limits on Γ of a Cauchy type integral with summable density φ, the following formula holds a.e. on Γ (see PRIVALOV [2] p. 194, DANILYUK [6] p. 125):

$$\lim_{z \to t} \frac{1}{2\pi i} \int_\Gamma \varphi(\tau)\frac{d\tau}{\tau - z} = \pm \frac{1}{2}\varphi(t) + \frac{1}{2\pi i}\int_\Gamma \varphi(\tau)\frac{d\tau}{\tau - t},$$

where the sign is chosen depending on whether the point z lies in $\mathcal{D}^+$ or $\mathcal{D}^-$, and the integral is to be understood in the sense of the principal value.

Passing in formulae (1.19) to the limit for $z \to t$ along non-tangent paths, we get the following result.

THEOREM 1.30. If $\varphi \in \mathcal{L}_1^n$ a.e. on Γ, then the formulae

$$(P\varphi)(t) = \frac{1}{2}\varphi(t) + \frac{1}{2\pi i}\int_\Gamma \varphi(\tau)\frac{d\tau}{\tau - t},$$
$$(Q\varphi)(t) = \frac{1}{2}\varphi(t) - \frac{1}{2\pi i}\int_\Gamma \varphi(\tau)\frac{d\tau}{\tau - t}$$

are valid.

These formulae were obtained for the first time by Yu.V. SOKHOTSKIǏ and are called after him[1]. Subtracting the second Sokhotskiǐ formula from the first one, we find that the relation

$$(S\varphi)(t) = \frac{1}{\pi i}\int_\Gamma \varphi(\tau)\frac{d\tau}{\tau - t}$$

holds a.e. on Γ.

In view of the latter equality, the operator S is called the operator of singular integration along the contour Γ.

It is evident that the conditions $\varphi \in L_p^n$ and $S\varphi \in L_p^n$ $(p \geq 1)$ are fulfilled simultaneously iff $\varphi = \varphi^+ + \varphi^-$, where $\varphi^+ \in L_p^n \cap (L_1^+)^n$ and $\varphi^- \in L_p^n \cap (\mathcal{L}_1^-)^n$. Therefore, the natural domain of the operators S, P and Q in the space L_p^n coincides with the lineal

1) In the English literature these formulae are usually called after PLEMELJ.

$(L_p \cap L_1^+)^n \dotplus (L_p \cap \overset{\circ}{L}{}_1^-)^n$. According to Theorems 1.24 and 1.25, in case of a Smirnov contour Γ this lineal agrees with $\mathcal{L}_p^n = (L_p^+ \dotplus \overset{\circ}{L}{}_p^-)^n$. If Γ is not Smirnov and $p > 1$ then it contains $\mathcal{L}_p^n$ as a proper part. However, for our purposes it is convenient to consider the operators S , P and Q in the spaces L_p^n , assuming their domains of definition to be the lineal $\mathcal{L}_p^n$, irrespective of the nature of the contour Γ . Henceforth we shall do so.

THEOREM 1.31.

1) The operators S, P and Q studied in L_p^n $(1 \le p \le \infty)$ are closed and, for $p < \infty$, densely defined,

2) the operators S (P, Q) and $-S$ (Q, P) considered in the spaces L_p^n and L_q^n $(1 < p < \infty,\ q = p/(p-1))$, respectively are adjoint to each other in the sense of Definition 1.6,

3) the operator S is involutory, and P as well as Q are idempotent: $S^2 = I|_{\mathcal{L}_p^n}$, $P^2 = P$, $Q^2 = Q$,

4) for the function $\varphi \in \mathcal{L}_{2p}$ the equality

$$(S\varphi)^2 = 2S(\varphi S\varphi) - \varphi^2 \tag{1.20}$$

is true.

Proof. Since $P = \frac{1}{2}(I + S)$ and $Q = \frac{1}{2}(I - S)$, it suffices to verify the assertions concerning the operator S .

1) Let $\{\varphi_k\}$ be a sequence from the domain of the operator S considered in L_p^n , $\varphi_k \to \varphi$ and $S\varphi_k \to \Psi$. Then $\varphi_k \in \mathcal{L}_p^n$, i.e. $\varphi_k = \varphi_k^+ + \varphi_k^-$ $(\varphi_k^+ \in (L_p^+)^n$, $\varphi_k^- \in (\overset{\circ}{L}{}_p^-)^n)$, and $S\varphi_k = \varphi_k^+ - \varphi_k^-$. Consequently, each of the sequences $\{\varphi_k^+ + \varphi_k^-\}$ and $\{\varphi_k^+ - \varphi_k^-\}$ and, thus, also each of the sequences $\{\varphi_k^+\}$ and $\{\varphi_k^-\}$ converges in L_p^n . Denoting the limits of the latter two sequences by φ^+ and φ^- respectively, we obtain $\varphi = \varphi^+ + \varphi^-$ and $\Psi = \varphi^+ - \varphi^-$. In view of Corollary 1.6, we have $\varphi^+ \in (L_p^+)^n$, $\varphi^- \in (\overset{\circ}{L}{}_p^-)^n$. Hence $\varphi \in \mathcal{L}_p^n$ and $S\varphi = \Psi$, which proves the closedness of the operator S .

For $p < \infty$ the lineal R^n being located in $\mathcal{L}_p^n$ is dense in L_p^n , therefore, for $p < \infty$, the operator S is densely defined.

2) Suppose $f \in \mathcal{L}_p^n$, $g \in \mathcal{L}_q^n$ and $f = f^+ + f^-$, $g = g^+ + g^-$, where $f^+ \in (L_p^+)^n$, $g^+ \in (L_q^+)^n$, $f^- \in (\overset{\circ}{L}{}_p^-)^n$, $g^- \in (\overset{\circ}{L}{}_q^-)^n$, then we obtain, taking into account Theorem 1.26,

$$\langle Sf,g\rangle = \langle f^+-f^-, g^++g^-\rangle = \langle f^+,g^+\rangle - \langle f^-,g^+\rangle +$$

$$\langle f^+,g^-\rangle - \langle f^-,g^-\rangle = \langle f^+,g^-\rangle - \langle f^-,g^+\rangle$$

and

$$\langle f, -Sg\rangle = \langle f^++f^-, g^--g^+\rangle = \langle f^+,g^-\rangle + \langle f^-,g^-\rangle -$$

$$\langle f^+,g^+\rangle - \langle f^-,g^+\rangle = \langle f^+,g^-\rangle - \langle f^-,g^+\rangle .$$

Thus $\langle Sf,g\rangle = \langle f,-Sg\rangle$ for arbitrary f, g from the corresponding domains of definition.

Assertion 3) is obvious.

Now we are going to prove assertion 4). If $\varphi = \varphi^+ + \varphi^-$ with $\varphi^+ \in L_{2p}^+$, $\varphi^- \in L_{2p}^-$, then $S\varphi = \varphi^+ - \varphi^-$, $\varphi S\varphi = (\varphi^+)^2 - (\varphi^-)^2$. But in virtue of assertion 3) from Theorem 1.21, $(\varphi^+)^2 \in L_p^+$, $(\varphi^-)^2 \in \overset{\circ}{L}{}_p^-$. Consequently, the function $\varphi S\varphi$ belongs to the domain of S, where $S(\varphi S\varphi) = (\varphi^+)^2 + (\varphi^-)^2$. Hence $2S(\varphi S\varphi) - \varphi^2 = 2(\varphi^+)^2 + 2(\varphi^-)^2 - (\varphi^+)^2 - 2\varphi^+\varphi^- - (\varphi^-)^2 = (\varphi^+-\varphi^-)^2 = (S\varphi)^2$. Theorem 1.31 has completely been proved. ≡

Now we turn to the question on the boundedness of the operator S in the spaces L_p^n, $1 < p < \infty$. Above all, we note that the operator S is defined componentwise. In other words, the vector function $f = \sum_{j=1}^n f_j e_j$ belongs to the domain of S iff the scalar functions f_j belong to this domain. If this condition is fulfilled, then we have $Sf = \sum_{j=1}^n (Sf_j)e_j$.

In particular, the operator S is bounded in L_p^n for any natural n if and only if it is bounded in L_p.

Further, since the operator S is densely defined and closed, it is bounded if and only if its domain of definition is the whole space. Consequently, the boundedness of the operator S in L_p, $1 < p < \infty$, is equivalent to the fact that the space L_p is the direct sum of its subspaces L_p^+ and $\overset{\circ}{L}{}_p^-$.

THEOREM 1.32. In the case of a fixed contour Γ the operator S is either bounded in all L_p, $1 < p < \infty$, or is not bounded in any one of these spaces.

Proof. Let the operator S be bounded in some space L_p. Due to equation (1.20), we can conclude that, for $\varphi \in \mathcal{L}_{2p}$,

$$\|(S\varphi)^2\|_{L_p} \leq 2\|S(\varphi S\varphi)\|_{L_p} + \|\varphi\|^2_{L_p} .$$

But

$$\|(S\varphi)^2\|_{L_p} = \|S\varphi\|^2_{L_{2p}} , \quad \|\varphi^2\|_{L_p} = \|\varphi\|^2_{L_{2p}}$$

and

$$\|S(\varphi S\varphi)\|_{L_p} \leq \|S\|_{L_p} \cdot \|\varphi(S\varphi)\|_{L_p} \leq \|S\|_{L_p} \cdot \|\varphi\|_{L_{2p}} \|S\varphi\|_{L_{2p}} .$$

Consequently,

$$\|S\varphi\|^2_{L_{2p}} \leq 2\|S\|_{L_p} \|\varphi\|_{L_{2p}} \cdot \|S\varphi\|_{L_{2p}} + \|\varphi\|^2_{L_{2p}} .$$

Solving this quadratic inequality relative to $\|S\varphi\|_{L_{2p}}$, we get

$$\|S\varphi\|_{L_{2p}} \leq (\|S\|_{L_p} + \sqrt{1+\|S\|^2_{L_p}}) \cdot \|\varphi\|_{L_{2p}} .$$

The last inequality means that the operator S regarded in L_{2p} is bounded on its natural domain. Moreover, the following estimation is valid:

$$\|S\|_{L_{2p}} \leq \|S\|_{L_p} + \sqrt{1+\|S\|^2_{L_p}} .$$

Repeating this reasoning, we deduce that the operator S is bounded in the spaces L_r with $r = 2^k p$ $(k = 0,1,\dots)$. With the help of the interpolation theorem 1.13 we conclude that the operator S is bounded in all spaces L_r with $p \leq r < \infty$.

Now we utilize assertion 2) of Theorem 1.31. Taking into account that S is densely defined, this assertion implies that the operator S is bounded in L_p iff it is bounded in L_q.

In this way, the operator S is bounded in spaces L_r not only for

$r \in [p,\infty)$, but also for $r \in (1,p/(p-1)]$. If $p \leq 2$, then there remains nothing to show. If $p > 2$, it is still necessary to establish the boundedness of S in L_r for $r \in (q,p)$, using the boundedness of S in L_p and L_q and again applying Theorem 1.13. ≡

Theorem 1.32 was proved in PAATASHVILI [1] (see also COTLAR [1]), where relation (1.20) occurs for the first time. The proof described here is borrowed from KHVEDELIDZE [4].

Acting as in KHVEDELIDZE [4], we introduce the following

<u>DEFINITION 1.21.</u> We say that the contour Γ belongs to the <u>class</u> $\mathcal{R}$ if the operator S of singular integration along Γ is bounded in the spaces L_p, $1 < p < \infty$.

<u>THEOREM 1.33 (KHAVIN [1]).</u> A contour of class $\mathcal{R}$ consists only of Smirnov curves.

<u>Proof.</u> Let $\Gamma \in \mathcal{R}$, and let the function f $(\in L_1^+)$ be summable with some power $p > 1$. Then, due to the boundedness of S in L_p , one has $L_p = L_p^+ \dot{+} \overset{\circ}{L}{}_p^-$, thus $f = f^+ + f^-$, where $f^+ \in L_p^+$, $f^- \in \overset{\circ}{L}{}_p^-$. Hence $f - f^+ = f^-$. The left-hand side of the equality obtained is a function of class L_1^+ and the right-hand side of class $\overset{\bullet}{L}{}_1^-$. Owing to Theorem 1.28, we therefore conclude that $f = f^+$, i.e. $f \in L_p^+$. Hence, for a contour of class $\mathcal{R}$ the correctness of the equality $L_1^+ \cap L_p = L_p^+$ has been shown. According to Theorem 1.25, we can conclude that each component of the contour Γ is a Smirnov curve. ≡

Note that Theorem 1.33 cannot be converted: In that very article of KHAVIN [1] there was constructed a Smirnov curve Γ such that not all functions continuous on Γ are elements of the lineal $\mathcal{L}_1$. By PAATASHVILI, KHUSKIVADZE [1] another necessary condition for the membership of a curve Γ to the class $\mathcal{R}$ was discovered. It consists in the requirement

$$\operatorname*{ess\,sup}_{\xi \in \Gamma} \operatorname*{ess\,sup}_{\varrho > 0} \varrho^{-1} l_\xi(\varrho) < \infty ,$$

where $l_\xi(\varrho)$ is the length of that part of Γ , which lies in the disk with centre at ξ and radius ϱ . In this paper it was suspected that this condition is sufficient, too.

Obviously, the contour Γ belongs to the class $\mathcal{R}$ if and only if every of its components has this property.

<u>THEOREM 1.34.</u> Each of the following conditions is sufficient for the curve Γ to belong to class $\mathcal{R}$:

1) Γ is a curve of bounded rotation,
2) Γ is a piecewise smooth curve.

Recall that Γ is called a curve of bounded rotation (or a Radon curve), if the function $t'(s)$ is of bounded variation, where s is a natural parameter on Γ.

Assertion 1) of Theorem 1.34 for curves without recurrence points is proved in DANILYUK, SHELEPOV [1] (a detailed explanation can be found in the monograph of DANILYUK [6] pp. 133-139); to Radon curves with recurrence points it was generalized in GORDADZE [6]. The membership of all smooth curves to the class $\mathcal{R}$ was shown in CALDERON [1]. The last assertion can be transferred to the case of piecewise smooth curves with the aid of results from GORDADZE [3], where it is established that each contour consisting of smooth arcs of class $\mathcal{R}$ belongs also to the class $\mathcal{R}$.

Let us remark that assertion 2) of Theorem 1.34 preceded chronologically some weaker sufficient conditions of membership to class $\mathcal{R}$. These conditions are special cases of the criterion 2) (Lyapunov or piecewise Lyapunov[1]) contours etc.) They can be found (with names of their authors and corresponding references) in KHVEDELIDZE [4], p. 62ff. After the article of CALDERON [1] there appeared papers, in which further weakenings of sufficient conditions for the membership of curves to class $\mathcal{R}$ were derived (e.g. KOKILASHVILI, PAATASHVILI [3]). Nevertheless, sufficient and necessary conditions for $\Gamma \in \mathcal{R}$ which can be checked effectively have not been found yet.

Here we introduce one subclass of class $\mathcal{R}$ which we shall deal with,

---

1) Recall that the curve $t=t(s)$ is said to be a Lyapunov curve, if the function $t'(s)$ satisfies a Hölder condition.

investigating the factorization of piecewise continuous functions.

DEFINITION 1.22 (KHVEDELIDZE [4]). To the class $\widetilde{\mathcal{R}}$ we shall ascribe contours $\Gamma \in \mathcal{R}$, which are representable as the union of a finite number of arcs satisfying condition (1.12), do not have pairwise common inner points, and are smooth in a neighbourhood of their common points t_j.

Let us clarify that condition (1.12) may or may not be fulfilled for the whole contour Γ $(\in \widetilde{\mathcal{R}})$, since the points t_j can be recurrence points for Γ.

Each piecewise smooth contour belongs to class $\widetilde{\mathcal{R}}$.

We have to examine operators of the type AQFPB and APFQB in the space L_p^n, where A, B and F are n×n matrix functions. In the general case, the domain of definition of these operators consists of vector functions $\varphi \in L_p^n$ satisfying

$$\varphi_1 = B\varphi \in \mathcal{L}_1^n, \quad \varphi_2 = FP\varphi_1 \ (FQ\varphi_1) \in \mathcal{L}_1^n, \qquad \varphi_3 = AQ\varphi_2 \ (AP\varphi_2) \in L_p^n. \tag{1.21}$$

THEOREM 1.35. Let A and B be n×n matrix functions of classes L_p and L_q respectively, and let one of the following conditions be fulfilled:

1) $F \in M_\infty^+$ (M_∞^-),

2) $F \in M^+$ (M^-), and the contour Γ consists of Smirnov curves.

Then the operator $T = AQFPB$ (APFQB) is finite dimensional and bounded in L_p^n. To the domain of definition of this operator belong, under condition 1), all vector functions $\varphi \in L_p^n$ satisfying relation (1.21), and in case of condition 2), only those of them for which $FP\varphi_1$ $(FQ\varphi_1) \in L_1^n$.

Proof. Consider the case of operator $T = AQFPB$. The matrix function F can be represented as $F = F_0 + F_1$, where F_0 is a rational matrix function with poles concentrated in $\mathcal{D}^+$, and $F_1 \in L_\infty^+$ under condition 1), $F_1 \in L^+$ under condition 2). Regard vector functions $\varphi \in L_p^n$ satisfying condition (1.21), which is necessary for φ to belong to the domain of the operator T. For such vector functions the relation $PB\varphi \in (L_1^+)^n$ is valid. Assuming condition 1) to be fulfilled, we have in this case $F_1PB\varphi \in (L_1^+)^n$ and $QF_1PB\varphi = 0$. If condition 2) is satisfied, generally speaking, we can only claim that $F_1PB\varphi \in (L^+)^n$. If we, in addition, suppose that $F_1PB\varphi \in (L_1^+)^n$, we get $F_1PB\varphi = FPB\varphi - F_0PB\varphi \in L_1^n$. According to Theorem 1.25, $F_1PB\varphi \in (L^+ \cap L_1)^n = (L_1^+)^n$. Therefore, under such suppositions we obtain $QF_1PB\varphi = 0$. It remains to verify the assertion of the theorem for the operator AQF_0PB. First, suppose that $F_0 = f_{-k}H_{ij}$, where $f_{-k}(t) = (t-z_0)^{-k}$, $z_0 \in \mathcal{D}^+$, k is an integer, H_{ij} is a matrix the (i,j) th entry of which is equal to one and the others are identically equal to zero. Then, for each vector function $\psi \in (\mathcal{L}_1^+)^n$,

$$QFP\psi = QF_0\psi^+ = Q((t-z_0)^{-k}\psi_j^+)e_i = \sum_{l=0}^{k} c_l f_{l-k} e_i ,$$

where c_l are the coefficients of the Taylor series expansion of the function ψ_j^+ $(= P\psi_j)$ at the point z_0. Using the formulae

$$c_l = \frac{1}{2\pi i} \int_\Gamma \psi_j^+(\tau) \frac{d\tau}{(\tau-z_0)^{l+1}} = \frac{1}{2\pi i} \int_\Gamma \psi_j(\tau) \frac{d\tau}{(\tau-z_0)^{l+1}} =$$

$$= \frac{1}{2\pi i} \langle \psi, f_{-l-1}e_j \rangle ,$$

we get

$$QF_0P\psi = \sum_{l=0}^{k-1} \frac{1}{2\pi i} \langle \psi, f_{-l-1}e_j \rangle f_{l-k}e_i .$$

Denoting by A_i and B_j the i th column and the j th row of the matrix function A and B, respectively, we obtain for vector functions φ satisfying relation (1.21) that $AQF_0PB\varphi = T_0\varphi$, where

$$T_0\varphi = \sum_{l=0}^{k-1} \frac{1}{2\pi i} \langle \varphi, f_{-l-1}B_j' \rangle f_{l-k}A_i .$$

Since, for an arbitrary integer s, $f_sB_j' \in L_q^n$ and $f_sA_i \in L_p^n$, then the operator T_0 defined by the last equation is bounded, defined on the whole space L_p^n and maps it into the linear hull of the vector functions f_sA_i $(s = -k,\dots,-1)$. Consequently, this operator is finite dimensional. Moreover, $f_s \in \overset{\circ}{L}^-_\infty$ for $s < 0$. Thus, the image of the operator T_0 lies in $(\overset{\bullet}{L}^-_p)^n$ as soon as $A \in L^-_p$.

In summary, for $F_0 = f_{-k}H_{ij}$ the operator AQF_0PB is the restriction of the operator T_0 on the lineal of vector functions φ satisfying condition (1.21). From this fact, for the case $F_0 = f_{-k}H_{ij}$, the assertion to be proved results.

Taking into account that each rational matrix function with poles concentrated in $\mathcal{D}^+$ can be represented as the linear combination of special type matrix functions considered above, we find that in the general case the operator AQF_0PB is also finite dimensional and bounded in L^n_p, defined on all vector functions $\varphi \in L^n_p$ satisfying condition (1.21) and, for $A \in L^-_p$, the image of this operator lies in $(\overset{\circ}{L}^-_p)^n$. Theorem 1.35 is completely proved. ≡

CHAPTER 2. GENERAL PROPERTIES OF FACTORIZATION

In Section 2.1 the notion of factorization in L_p , which is fundamental to the present book, will be introduced. As a rule, in the current literature the factorization problem is considered in connection with the study of the Riemann boundary value problem. The definition of factorization of a matrix function proposed below is more general than those previously introduced for the aims of solvability theory for the problem considered.

In the present chapter we study only those properties of factorization which can be formulated and proved regardless of the Riemann boundary value problem. In the next chapter we shall discuss the question concerning the role which is played by the factorability in L_p of the matrix coefficient of a Riemann problem for the solvability theory of this problem.

We do not make any a priori suppositions about the matrix function G except the requirement of measurability. However, it turns out that, for fixed p , the diagonal factor of factorization is defined uniquely (which justifies the notion of partial p-indices), and the left and right factor are defined with the same degree of arbitrariness that holds in the classical case. This will be demonstrated in Section 2.2. In the same section the monotonic dependence of partial p-indices on p is established as well as the fact that if different values of p correspond to equal total p-indices, then we can say that the corresponding families of factorizations also coincide. In connection with the study of the factorization dependence on p , in Section 2.3 the notion of the domain of factorability will be introduced, and its explicit description in case of the power function will be given. The latter result plays an important role in Chapter 5, where we shall study the question of factorability of arbitrary piecewise continuous functions.

Section 2.4 includes the factorability criterion for meromorphic (in particular, rational) matrix functions as well as estimates for their

partial indices. These results are basic to all the following theorems on the existence of a factorization including the theorem on the factorability of continuous matrix functions in Chapter 5. As a consequence of the factorability criterion of meromorphic matrix functions, the factorability of matrix functions, which can be represented as the product of meromorphic functions, will be demonstrated in the same section. In turn, with the help of the latter result, we shall prove the theorem on the preservation of the factorability property under multiplication from the left (right) by matrix functions belonging together with their inverses to the class M_∞^+ (M_∞^-). The study of the connection between factorizations of one and the same matrix function G in different spaces L_p will be led to the very end.
Finally, Section 2.5 contains comments on further reading.

2.1. THE DEFINITION OF FACTORIZATION

DEFINITION 2.1. A factorization in L_p $(1 < p < \infty)$ of a matrix function G relative to the contour Γ is, by definition, a representation

$$G(t) = G_+(t)\Lambda(t)G_-(t), \tag{2.1}$$

where $G_+ \in L_p^+$, $G_- \in L_q^-$, $G_+^{-1} \in L_q^+$, $G_-^{-1} \in L_p^-$ $(q = p/(p-1))$,

$$\Lambda(t) = \mathrm{diag}[t^{\varkappa_1},\dots,t^{\varkappa_n}], \tag{2.2}$$

and $\varkappa_1 \geq \dots \geq \varkappa_n$ are integers.

As will be shown in Section 2.2, the integers $\varkappa_j$ are uniquely defined by G and p. We shall call them partial p-indices of G.
Their sum $\varkappa = \varkappa_1 + \dots + \varkappa_n$ will be called its total p-index.

If it is convenient to emphasize groups of coinciding partial p-indices, we shall write the diagonal factor in the form

$$\Lambda(t) = \mathrm{diag}[t^{\tilde{\varkappa}_1}I_{l_1},\dots,t^{\tilde{\varkappa}_k}I_{l_k}],$$

where $\tilde{\varkappa}_1 > \dots > \tilde{\varkappa}_k$. The number l_j is said to be the multiplicity of the partial p-index $\tilde{\varkappa}_j$ $(j=1,\dots,k)$.

The partial p-indices and the total p-index will be simply called partial and total indices, if it is clear from the context what a value of the parameter is meant.

In the scalar case ($n = 1$) there exists only one partial p-index, which, consequently, coincides with the total one. In the following, we simply call it p-index (index).

Immediately from the definition we deduce that for the matrix function G to be factorable in some L_p it is necessary that G and its inverse be summable. In Sections 2.3 and 2.4 we shall obtain factorability criteria for some special classes of matrix functions. From these criteria it will be clear that the mentioned necessary condition is far from be sufficient. A necessary and sufficient factorability condition applicable to arbitrary measurable matrix functions fails to be known at present.

Besides the factorization (2.1) one can consider representations of the matrix function G in the form

$$G(t) = G_-(t)\Lambda(t)G_+(t) , \tag{2.1'}$$

where $G_- \in L_p^-$, $G_+ \in L_q^+$, $G_-^{-1} \in L_q^-$, $G_+^{-1} \in L_p^+$, and the matrix function Λ is defined by formula (2.2).

If it is necessary to consider both representations (2.1) and (2.1') simultaneously, we call the first of them a left, and the second a right factorization. In doing so, the partial indices will be called left, unlike the right ones, which occur in the representation (2.1'). The following example shows that the tuples of left and right indices, generally speaking, do not coincide.

<u>Example.</u> Let $G(t) = \begin{bmatrix} t & 1 \\ 0 & t^{-1} \end{bmatrix}$. The equations

$$G(t) = \begin{bmatrix} 1 & 0 \\ 0 & 1 \end{bmatrix} \begin{bmatrix} t & 0 \\ 0 & t^{-1} \end{bmatrix} \begin{bmatrix} 1 & t^{-1} \\ 0 & 1 \end{bmatrix}$$

and

$$G(t) = \begin{bmatrix} 1 & 0 \\ t^{-1} & -1 \end{bmatrix} \begin{bmatrix} 1 & 0 \\ 0 & 1 \end{bmatrix} \begin{bmatrix} t & 1 \\ 1 & 0 \end{bmatrix}$$

provide a left and right factorization of the matrix function G, respectively. Consequently, its left indices are equal to ± 1, and the right ones are equal to zero.

Clearly, from a left factorization in L_p of G one may obtain a right factorization in L_q of G', transposing both parts of (2.1), and a right factorization of G^{-1} in L_p, taking the inverse to both parts of (2.1).

Analogously, from a right factorization of the matrix function G one can get a left factorization of G' and G^{-1}. In particular, the tuple of left (right) p-indices of G coincides with the tuple of right (left) q-indices of G' and differs only by the sign from the tuple of right (left) p-indices of G^{-1}. Therefore, all the assertions about a right factorization can be obtained by restating the corresponding assertions for a left one.

Thanks to the latter remark, in the following we focus our attention on the study of a left factorization and left (partial) indices.

2.2. PROPERTIES OF FACTORIZATION FACTORS

Leaving for a moment the questions of existence we clarify in the present section that degree of arbitrariness with which the factorization factors $G_{\pm}$ and Λ are defined. First of all, we study the middle factor.

THEOREM 2.1. Let the matrix function G admit a factorization in L_{p_1} and L_{p_2} $(p_1 \leq p_2)$. Then $\varkappa_i^{(1)} \geq \varkappa_i^{(2)}$, $i = 1,\ldots,n$, where $\varkappa_i^{(j)}$ $(j = 1,2)$ denotes the p_j-indices of G.

Proof. Starting from equation $G_+^{(1)}\Lambda^{(1)} G_-^{(1)} = G_+^{(2)} \Lambda^{(2)} G_-^{(2)}$ [1], we find

$$\Lambda^{(1)}H_- = H_+ \Lambda^{(2)}, \tag{2.3}$$

[1] Here and further on, the superscript specifies the factorization we deal with.

where

$$H_- = G_-^{(1)}(G_-^{(2)})^{-1}\ ,\quad H_+ = (G_+^{(1)})^{-1}G_+^{(2)}\ . \tag{2.4}$$

If we write equation (2.3) componentwise, it takes the form

$$t^{\varkappa_i^{(1)}-\varkappa_j^{(2)}}\ h_{ij}^-(t) = h_{ij}^+(t)\ ,\quad i,j = 1,\dots,n. \tag{2.3'}$$

Since $G_-^{(1)} \in L_{q_1}^-$ and $G_-^{(2)} \in L_{p_2}^-$, then $H_- \in L_p^-$, where $p = (p_2^{-1} + q_1^{-1})^{-1} = (1+p_2^{-1} - p_1^{-1})^{-1} \geq 1$. Similarly $H_+ \in L_p^+$. Applying Theorem 1.28 to equality (2.3') we deduce that h_{ij}^+ is a polynomial of degree less than or equal to $\varkappa_i^{(1)} - \varkappa_j^{(2)}$, if $\varkappa_i^{(1)} \geq \varkappa_j^{(2)}$, and identically equal to zero otherwise.

In spite of the assertion of the theorem, assume, for some r , $\varkappa_r^{(1)} < \varkappa_r^{(2)}$. Then, for $j \leq r \leq i$, $\varkappa_i^{(1)} \leq \varkappa_r^{(1)}$, $\varkappa_j^{(2)} \geq \varkappa_r^{(2)}$ and hence $\varkappa_i^{(1)} < \varkappa_j^{(2)}$. Consequently, $h_{ij}^+ = 0$ for $i = r,\dots,n;$ $j = 1,\dots,r$, and each minor of rth order lying in the first r columns of the matrix function H_+ is equal to zero. Due to Laplace's theorem, in this case the determinant of H_+ is equal to zero a.e. on Γ , which contradicts the non-singularity of the factorization factors. Thus Theorem 2.1 has been proved. ≡

COROLLARY 2.1. The factor Λ is uniquely defined by the matrix function G and the parameter p .

Now we turn to the factorization factors $G_\pm$. According to Theorem 2.1, for increasing p , the total index does not increase, thus $\varkappa^{(1)} \geq \varkappa^{(2)}$. From formulae (2.3) and (2.4) obtained in the proof of Theorem 2.1 we conclude that

$$G_+^{(2)} = G_+^{(1)}H_+\ ,\quad G_-^{(2)} = \Lambda^{(2)-1}H_+^{-1}\ \Lambda^{(1)}G_-^{(1)}\ , \tag{2.5}$$

where H_+ is a matrix function, the (i,j) th entry of which is a polynomial of degree not higher than $\varkappa_i^{(1)} - \varkappa_j^{(2)}$ if $\varkappa_i^{(1)} \geq \varkappa_j^{(2)}$, and identically zero otherwise.

Formulae (2.5) mean, in particular, that

$$\det H_+(z) = \frac{\det G_+^{(2)}(z)}{\det G_+^{(1)}(z)}, \quad z \in \mathcal{D}^+$$

and

$$\det H_+(z) = z^{\varkappa^{(1)}-\varkappa^{(2)}} \cdot \frac{\det G_-^{(1)}(z)}{\det G_-^{(2)}(z)}, \quad z \in \mathcal{D}^-,$$

so that $\det H_+$ does not vanish in $\mathcal{D}^+$ and at finite points of $\mathcal{D}^-$. At the point $z = \infty$ it has a pole of order $\varkappa^{(1)} - \varkappa^{(2)}$. As $\det H_+$ is a polynomial, we deduce that its degree is $\varkappa^{(1)} - \varkappa^{(2)}$, and the zeros(if they exist, i.e. in the case $\varkappa^{(1)} \neq \varkappa^{(2)}$) are located on Γ. A somewhat more exact result for the case $\varkappa^{(1)} \neq \varkappa^{(2)}$ will be obtained in Section 2.4. Here we study the case $\varkappa^{(1)} = \varkappa^{(2)}$.

THEOREM 2.2. Let the matrix function G be factorable in the spaces L_{p_1} and L_{p_2} $(p_1 \leq p_2)$ with one and the same total index. Then

a) the transition from a factorization in L_{p_1} to a factorization in L_{p_2} is accomplished according to formulae (2.5), where

1) $\Lambda^{(1)}(t) = \Lambda^{(2)}(t)$ $(= \Lambda(t) = \operatorname{diag}[t^{\tilde{\varkappa}_1} I_{l_1}, \ldots, t^{\tilde{\varkappa}_k} I_{l_k}])$;

2) if $H_+ = (H_{ij})_{i,j=1}^k$ provides a splitting of the matrix H into blocks for which the order of the j th diagonal block is equal to l_j, then the diagonal blocks are constant matrices, and the blocks outside the diagonal are equal to zero, if $i > j$, and consist of polynomials of degree not exceeding $\tilde{\varkappa}_i - \tilde{\varkappa}_j$, if $i < j$;

b) the representation (2.1) with

$$G_+ = G_+^{(1)} H_+, \quad G_- = \Lambda^{-1} H_+^{-1} \Lambda\, G_-^{(1)}, \tag{2.6}$$

where H is an arbitrary matrix function satisfying condition 2), is a factorization of G in the space L_{p_1}.

Proof.

a) Due to Theorem 2.1, $\varkappa_i^{(1)} \geq \varkappa_i^{(2)}$. By assumption we have $\sum_{i=1}^n \varkappa_i^{(1)} = \sum_{i=1}^n \varkappa_i^{(2)}$. Hence $\varkappa_i^{(1)} = \varkappa_i^{(2)}$ $(= \varkappa_i)$ for $i = 1, \ldots, n$, i.e., condition 1) is fulfilled. Condition 2) results from the properties of the matrix function H_+ established above and the equation $\det H_+ = \prod_{j=1}^{n} \det H_{jj}$, which holds in view of Laplace's theorem.

b) If H_+ is a matrix function fulfilling condition 2), then $H_+^{\pm 1} \in L_\infty^+$, $(\Lambda^{-1}H_+\Lambda)^{\pm 1} \in L_\infty^-$, so that the relations $G_+^{(1)} \in L_{p_1}^+$, $G_-^{(1)} \in L_{q_1}^-$, $G_+^{(1)-1} \in L_{q_1}^+$, $G_-^{(1)-1} \in L_{p_1}^-$ imply that $G_+ \in L_{p_1}^+$, $G_+^{-1} \in L_{q_1}^+$, $G_- \in L_{q_1}^-$, $G_-^{-1} \in L_{p_1}^-$, where the matrix functions $G_\pm$ are defined via formulae (2.6). Thus, the representation $G_+\Lambda G_-$ is a factorization of G in L_{p_1}, which proves Theorem 2.2. ≡

If $p_1 = p_2$, the condition of equality of partial indices is fulfilled in view of Corollary 2.1. Therefore, Theorem 2.2 yields the description of all factorizations in the space L_p, if at least one of them is known. If all partial indices are pairwise equal, then H_+ is a constant non-degenerate matrix, and the factorization is uniquely defined by giving one of the matrices $G_\pm$ at some point of $\mathcal{D}^\pm$; commonly, the value $G_-(\infty)$ is fixed.

COROLLARY 2.2. A factorization of the matrix function G in one of the spaces L_p is a factorization in all L_p-spaces in which G admits a factorization with the same total index.

Indeed, if G is factorable in L_{p_1} and L_{p_2} $(p_1 \le p_2)$ with the same total index, then, as it is clear from the proof of Theorem 2.2, there exists a representation $G = G_+^{(1)}\Lambda G_-^{(1)}$ which is a factorization of G simultaneously in L_{p_1} and L_{p_2}. But then all factorizations of the matrix function G both in L_{p_1} and in L_{p_2} can be obtained by formulae (2.6). In this case, on the matrix function H_+ there are imposed one and the same restrictions. Thus, the sets of factorizations of G in L_{p_1} and L_{p_2} coincide.

THEOREM 2.3 (Interpolation theorem). If the matrix function G admits a factorization with one and the same total index in L_{p_1} and L_{p_2}, then it admits a factorization (with the same total index) in all L_p, $p \in [p_1, p_2]$.

Proof. First of all, let us note that if $p_1 \leq p \leq p_2$, then $q_2 \leq q \leq q_1$. If (2.1) is a factorization of G in L_{p_1}, then $G_+^{-1} \in L_{q_1}^+$, $G_- \in L_{q_1}^-$ and, therefore, $G_+^{-1} \in L_q^+$, $G_- \in L_q^-$. According to Corollary 2.2, the representation (2.1) is also a factorization of G in L_{p_2}. Consequently $G_+ \in L_{p_2}^+$, $G_-^{-1} \in L_{p_2}^-$ and, finally, $G_+ \in L_p^+$, $G_-^{-1} \in L_p^-$. Theorem 2.3 is proved. ≡

The following result often proves to be useful in the study of properties of the factorization factors $G_\pm$.

THEOREM 2.4. Let the matrix functions G_1 and G_2 admit a factorization in the space L_p and coincide (a.e.) on some open arc $\gamma \subseteq \Gamma$. Then the factorization factors $G_\pm^{(j)}$ $(j = 1,2)$ are connected via the relations

$$G_+^{(1)}(t) = G_+^{(2)}(t)V(t), \quad G_-^{(1)}(t) = W(t)G_-^{(2)}(t), \quad t \in \gamma, \tag{2.7}$$

where V and W are matrix functions analytic and non-degenerating on γ.

Proof. Arguing as in Theorem 2.1, we get the equation (2.3), however, not on the whole contour Γ, but only on the arc γ. Matrix functions $H_\pm$ determined by formulae (2.4) belong together with their inverses to the classes $L_1^\pm$, since in the case under study $p_1 = p_2$. With the help of Theorem 1.27, we deduce from here that the matrix functions $\Lambda^{(1)}H_-$ and $H_+\Lambda^{(2)}$ and their inverses are analytic on the arc γ. Consequently, either of the matrix functions H_+ and H_- is analytic and non-degenerate on γ. From here and from formula (2.4) relations (2.7) follow, which proves Theorem 2.4. ≡

Formulae (2.7) allow us to make conclusions about the smoothness and integrability of the matrix functions $G_\pm^{(1)}$ and their inverses, if the corresponding properties of $G_\pm^{(2)}$ are known. Theorem 2.4 shows that the behaviour of the factorization factors $G_\pm$ is determined by the local behaviour of the matrix function G itself.

2.3. THE DOMAIN OF FACTORABILITY

<u>DEFINITION 2.2.</u> The set $\mathfrak{F}(G)$ of those values of the parameter $p \in (1,\infty)$ for which the matrix function G can be factored in L_p is said to be the <u>domain of factorability of G</u>.

All results of the present chapter obtained till now, in principle, were related to general laws of the structure of $\mathfrak{F}(G)$. Now they can be formulated more compactly: $\mathfrak{F}(G)$ is the union of disjoint connected (may be, empty) sets $\mathfrak{F}_k(G) = \{p : G$ admits a factorization in L_p with total index $k\}$. If $k_1 < k_2$, then the set $\mathfrak{F}_{k_1}(G)$ is located on the real line more to the right than $\mathfrak{F}_{k_2}(G)$. If $p_0 \in \mathfrak{F}_k(G)$, then a factorization of G in L_{p_0} is a factorization of G in all spaces L_p with $p \in \mathfrak{F}_k(G)$. The partial p-indices of the matrix function G are non-increasing functions with the domain of definition $\mathfrak{F}(G)$ constant on any of the sets $\mathfrak{F}_k(G)$.

For the sake of illustration of the notions introduced, we consider the factorization problem for the power function. As not to complicate matters, we assume the contour Γ to be a simple closed curve dividing the plane into an inner domain $\mathfrak{D}^+$ and an outer $\mathfrak{D}^-$. Let us take a fixed branch $\psi(z)$ of the power function z^α defined on the plane with a cut connecting the point 0 with ∞ and intersecting Γ at the only point t_0. The parts of the cut connecting 0 with t_0 and t_0 with ∞ will be denoted by l_0 and l_∞, respectively. Clearly, only the case of a non-integer α is of interest.

Suppose that

1) Γ is a curve of the Smirnov class;

2) $$\sup \left\{\frac{s(t,t_0)}{|t - t_0|} : t \in \Gamma\right\} < \infty , \tag{2.8}$$

where $s(t,t_0)$ is the distance between the points t and t_0 along the curve Γ;

3) there is a bounded and continuous function $\arg(t - t_0)$ on $\Gamma \setminus \{t_0\}$.

Conditions 2) and 3) are of local character; they are fulfilled, for example, if a certain neighbourhood of the point t_0 on Γ is a piecewise smooth curve without recurrence points.

The function $\psi(t)$ is continuous on the contour Γ with the exception of the point t_0. At the point t_0 it has limits from the left and right (recall that the contour is oriented anticlockwise) satisfying the relation

$$\psi(t_0 - 0) = e^{2\pi i\alpha}\,\psi(t_0 + 0)\,.$$

Thus, the function ψ is piecewise continuous. In Chapter 5 we shall see that the factorization problem for an arbitrary piecewise continuous matrix function (under some additional restrictions on the contour) can be reduced to the factorization of power functions.

<u>THEOREM 2.5.</u> The function $\psi(t) = t^\alpha$ can be factored in L_p if and only if $\{\mathrm{Re}\,\alpha\} \neq 1 - \frac{1}{p}$. [1]

<u>Proof.</u> Denote by $\psi_+(z)$ that (uniquely determined) branch of the power function $(z - t_0)^\alpha$ defined on the plane with the cut l_∞ and by $\psi_-(z)$ that branch of $(1 - t_0/z)^{-\alpha}$ defined on the plane with the cut l_0 such that $\psi_-(\infty) = 1$ and

$$\psi(t) = \psi_+(t)\psi_-(t)\,, \quad t \in \Gamma\setminus\{t_0\}\,. \tag{2.9}$$

For any integer k we have

$$\psi(t) = \psi_{+,k}(t)t^k\,\psi_{-,k}(t)\,, \quad t \in \Gamma\setminus\{t_0\}\,, \tag{2.10}$$

where $\psi_{+,k}(z) = \psi_+(z)(z-t_0)^{-k}$, $\psi_{-,k}(z) = \psi_-(z)(1-t_0/z)^k$.

Evidently, the functions $\psi_{+,k}^{\pm 1}$ and $\psi_{-,k}^{\pm 1}$ are analytic in the domains $\mathfrak{D}^+$ and $\mathfrak{D}^-$, respectively, where $\psi_{+,k}(z) = (z-t_0)^{\mathrm{Re}\alpha-k}(z-t_0)^{i\,\mathrm{Im}\alpha}$, under a suitable choice of the branches of the factors defined on the plane with cut l_∞. Denoting $(z-t_0)^{k-\mathrm{Re}\alpha}$ by $\varphi(z)$, we get $|\varphi(z)| = |z-t_0|^{k-\mathrm{Re}\alpha}$. Hence, for $\mathrm{Re}\,\alpha \geq k$, there is $\varphi^{-1} \in L_\infty^+$. Furthermore, we denote by $t_1(s)$ and $t_2(s)$ $(0 \leq s \leq d$, where $2d$ is the length of the curve $\Gamma)$ the begin and the end of the anticlock-

---

[1] By $\{x\}$ we denote the fractional part of x : $\{x\} = x - [x]$.

wise oriented arc of the contour Γ with the length $2s$ the centre of which is the point t_0. Then, for real λ,

$$\int_\Gamma |t-t_0|^\lambda |dt| = \int_0^d |t_1(s)-t_0|^\lambda ds + \int_0^d |t_2(s)-t_0|^\lambda ds .$$

Due to condition (2.8), the integrals on the right-hand side of the last equation converge only simultaneously with $\int_0^d s^\lambda ds$, i.e., if and only if $\lambda > -1$. Hence $\varphi \in L_p$ if $p < 1/(\mathrm{Re}\,\alpha - k)$ and $\varphi \notin L_{1/(\mathrm{Re}\alpha-k)}$. Moreover, $\varphi \notin L^+_{1/(\mathrm{Re}\alpha-k)}$. Now we intend to show that $\varphi \in L^+_p$, if $p < 1/(\mathrm{Re}\alpha-k)$. For this purpose, we consider the function $\chi = (\varphi \circ \omega)\sqrt{\omega'}$, where ω conformally maps the unit disk Δ onto the domain $\mathcal{D}^+$. In view of condition 3) imposed upon Γ as well as Theorem 1.15, the function $\varphi \circ \omega$ is outer. With regard to condition 1) imposed on Γ, the function $\sqrt[p]{\omega'}$ is also outer. Together with $\varphi \circ \omega$ and $\sqrt[p]{\omega'}$, their product χ is outer, too. But then, in view of Theorem 1.18, from the relation $\chi \in L_p$ (which is equivalent to the condition $\varphi \in L_p$) we deduce that $\chi \in H_p$. From here and from Theorem 1.19 the assertion to be proved results.

In summary, if $\mathrm{Re}\,\alpha \geq k$, then $\varphi \in L^+_p$ for $p < 1/(\mathrm{Re}\alpha-k)$, and $\varphi^{-1} \in L^+_\infty$. Since $|(z - t_0)^{i\mathrm{Im}\alpha}| = \exp(-\mathrm{Im}\alpha \arg(t-t_0))$, condition 3) guarantees the membership of the function $(z - t_0)^{i\mathrm{Im}\alpha}$ together with its inverse to the class L^+_∞. Consequently, the statements proved above concerning the function φ can be transferred to the function $\psi^{-1}_{+,k}$ without any changes. Analogously, we can argue that $\psi^{-1}_{-,k} \in L^-_{1/(\mathrm{Re}\alpha-k)}$, $\psi^{-1}_{-,k} \in L^-_p$ for $p < 1/(\mathrm{Re}\alpha-k)$.

Thus, if $k \leq \mathrm{Re}\,\alpha$, the representation (2.10) is a factorization of the function $\psi(t)$ in L_p if and only if $q < 1/(\mathrm{Re}\,\alpha - k)$, i.e. $k > \mathrm{Re}\,\alpha + 1/p - 1$. But this is only possible if there exists an integer in the interval $(\mathrm{Re}\,\alpha + 1/p - 1, \mathrm{Re}\,\alpha]$, i.e. if $\{\mathrm{Re}\,\alpha\} < 1 - 1/p$. In this case, the p-index of the function ψ coincides with k and is equal to $[\mathrm{Re}\,\alpha]$.

Supposing that $k > \mathrm{Re}\,\alpha$, we observe that $\psi^{-1}_{+,k} \in L^+_\infty$, $\psi_{-,k} \in L^-_\infty$, $\psi_{+,k} \in L^+_p$, $\psi^{-1}_{-,k} \in L^-_p$ for $p < 1/(k - \mathrm{Re}\,\alpha)$, $\psi_{+,k} \notin L^+_{1/(k - \mathrm{Re}\,\alpha)}$,

$\psi^{-1}_{-,k} \notin L^{-}_{1/(k - \mathrm{Re}\,\alpha)}$. **Therefore**, the representation (2.10) is a factorization of ψ in L_p if and only if $p < 1/(k - \mathrm{Re}\,\alpha)$, i.e. $k < \mathrm{Re}\,\alpha + 1/p$. But this is only possible when $\{\mathrm{Re}\,\alpha\} > 1 - 1/p$ and $k = [\mathrm{Re}\,\alpha] + 1$.

Summarizing, for $p \in (1, 1/(1 - \{\mathrm{Re}\,\alpha\}))$, the function $\psi(t) = t^{\alpha}$ can be factored in L_p , and its index is equal to $[\mathrm{Re}\,\alpha] + 1$. For $p \in (1/(1- \{\mathrm{Re}\,\alpha\}), \infty)$, it is factorable in L_p with the index $[\mathrm{Re}\,\alpha]$.

It remains to show that the function ψ is not factorable in L_{p_0} , where $p_0 = 1/(1 - \{\mathrm{Re}\,\alpha\})$. Assuming the contrary, on the strength of the p-index monotonicity proved in Theorem 2.1, we find that the p_0-index of the function ψ lies between $[\mathrm{Re}\,\alpha]$ and $[\mathrm{Re}\,\alpha] + 1$ and, therefore, coincides either with the first or with the second of these numbers. According to Corollary 2.2, a factorization of the function ψ for $p > p_0$ would be also suitable for $p = p_0$ in the first case. In the second case, the role of a factorization in L_{p_0} could play any factorization of ψ for $p < p_0$. However, as was shown above, neither of these holds.

Thus, the factorability domain of the function $\psi(t) = t^{\alpha}$, for non-integer α , consists of two components: $\mathfrak{F}_{[\mathrm{Re}\,\alpha]+1} = (1, 1/(1-\{\mathrm{Re}\,\alpha\}))$ and $\mathfrak{F}_{[\mathrm{Re}\,\alpha]} = (1/(1-\{\mathrm{Re}\,\alpha\}), \infty)$, which proves Theorem 2.5. ≡

Consider, in particular, the function $\psi(e^{i\theta}) = e^{i\theta/2}$ defined on the unit circle $= \{e^{i\theta} : -\pi < \theta < \pi\}$. This is the function $t^{1/2}$ with a discontinuity at the point -1 . The representation $t^{1/2} = (t + 1)^{-1/2} t (t^{-1} + 1)^{1/2}$ provides its factorization for $p \in (1,2)$, and the representation $t^{1/2} = (t + 1)^{1/2} (t^{-1} + 1)^{-1/2}$ yields a factorization for $p \in (2, \infty)$. For $p = 2$, the function $t^{1/2}$ fails to be factorable.

An example of a matrix function, all components of the factorability domain of which are non-empty, will be given in Section 5.4.

2.4. FACTORIZATION OF MEROMORPHIC MATRIX FUNCTIONS AND THEIR PRODUCTS

In this section we are concerned with the question of the connection between the factorization of a matrix function G and its representations in the form

$$G = A_+ A_- , \tag{2.11}$$

where

$$A_+ \in M_p^+ , \quad A_+^{-1} \in M_q^+ , \quad A_- \in M_q^- , \quad A_-^{-1} \in M_p^- . \tag{2.12}$$

Formally, the representation (2.11) is more general than the factorization (2.1). Indeed, from a factorization (2.1) of the matrix function G one can obtain the equation (2.11), setting, for example, $A_+ = G_+ \Lambda$, $A_- = G_-$. However, it turns out that the existence of a representation (2.11) implies the factorability of the matrix function G in L_p. Moreover, a factorization of G in L_p can be built effectively, as soon as its representation (2.11) is known. To verify this statement, we shall prove the factorability of A_+ and A_- individually. Then it will be checked that the factorability will remain on multiplication.

Incidentally, estimates for the partial p-indices of the matrix functions A_+, A_- and G will be obtained. Furthermore, in the case $G \in M_p^+$ (M_q^-), the necessity of the condition $G^{-1} \in M_q^+$ (M_p^-) for the factorability of G will be proved.

The following result plays an important role in the proof.

<u>LEMMA 2.1.</u> Let the matrix function B be analytic in the domain $\mathcal{O}$ and $\det B(z_0) = 0$ for some $z_0 \in \mathcal{O}$. Then

$$B = CU , \tag{2.13}$$

where the matrix function C is analytic in $\mathcal{O}$ and has the same zeros of the determinant with the same multiplicities as B except z_0, where the multiplicity of the zero of $\det C$ is smaller than that of $\det B$ by one;

$$U(z) = \begin{bmatrix} 1 & & & \lambda_1 & & & \\ & \ddots & & \vdots & & & \\ & & 1 & \lambda_{k-1} & & & \\ & & & z-z_o & & & \\ & & & & 1 & & \\ & & & & & \ddots & \\ & & & & & & 1 \end{bmatrix}, \tag{2.14}$$

where $\lambda_1, \ldots, \lambda_{k-1}$ are certain numbers standing in the k th column of U .

Proof. For $z \neq z_o$, the matrix $U(z)$ is invertible, and the inverse is of the form

$$V(z) = \begin{bmatrix} 1 & & & -\lambda_1/(z-z_o) & & & \\ & \ddots & & \vdots & & & \\ & & 1 & -\lambda_{k-1}/(z-z_o) & & & \\ & & & 1/(z-z_o) & & & \\ & & & & 1 & & \\ & & & & & \ddots & \\ & & & & & & 1 \end{bmatrix}.$$

Set $C(z) = B(z)V(z)$ for $z \neq z_o$. As $\det C(z) = (\det B(z))/(z-z_o)$ and the matrix function V is analytic in the plane except the point z_o, it remains only to make sure that the matrix function C is analytic at the point z_o . Denoting the j th columns of C and B by c_j and b_j , $(j = 1,\ldots,n)$, respectively, we obtain that $c_j = b_j$ for $j \neq k$, $c_k(z) = \frac{1}{z - z_o} (b_k(z) - \sum_{i=1}^{k-1} \lambda_i b_i(z))$.

Hence, it is clear that for the matrix function C to be analytic at the point z_o , it is necessary and sufficient that column $b_k(z_o)$ be a linear combination of the columns $b_i(z_o)$ $(i = 1,\ldots,k-1)$ and the scalars λ_i be the coefficients of this linear combination. The existence of such k and $\{\lambda_i\}_{i=1}^{k-1}$ results from the condition $\det B(z_o) = 0$, which proves the lemma. ≡

Remark. In the proof of Lemma 2.1 we choose a column of the matrix $B(z_o)$ which is the linear combination of the previous ones. One can also choose a column being the linear combination of the next ones and, owing to this, obtain a representation (2.13) with a right factor of the kind

$$\begin{bmatrix} 1 & & & & & & \\ & \ddots & & & & & \\ & & 1 & & & & \\ & & & z-z_o & & & \\ & & & \lambda_{k+1} & 1 & & \\ & & & \vdots & & \ddots & \\ & & & \lambda_n & & & 1 \end{bmatrix} . \qquad (2.14')$$

Considering the rows of $B(z_o)$, one may "split off" a left factor of the kind (2.14) or (2.14').

THEOREM 2.6. The matrix function $G \in M_p^+$ can be factored in L_p if and only if $G^{-1} \in M_q^+$. If this condition is fulfilled, then the partial indices of G are included between $-\mathcal{P}_+(G)$ [1] and $\operatorname{ind}_+ \det G + (n-1)\,\mathcal{P}_+(G)$, the total index is equal to $\operatorname{ind}_+ \det G$, and the right factorization factor G_- is a rational matrix function.

Proof. If the matrix function $G (\in M_p^+)$ is factorable in L_p, then, proceeding from equation (2.1), we observe

$$G_+^{-1} G = \Lambda G_- \quad (= F) . \qquad (2.15)$$

Since $G_+^{-1} G \in M_1^+$ and $\Lambda G_- \in M_q^-$, Theorem 1.28 is applicable, thanks to which the matrix function F defined via equation (2.15) is rational and has no poles on Γ. Moreover, this matrix function is non-degenerating on Γ, since otherwise the matrix function F^{-1} would have poles on Γ, which contradicts the relation $F^{-1} = G_-^{-1} \Lambda^{-1} \in M_p^-$.
Consequently, $F^{-1} \in M_\infty^+$ and, therefore, $G^{-1} \, (= F^{-1} G_+^{-1}) \in M_q^+$.
The necessity of the condition $G^{-1} \in M_q^+$ for the factorability of $G \in M_p^+$ has been proved.
Now we are going to verify its sufficiency.
We shall study representation of G in the form

---

[1] $\mathcal{P}_\pm(G)$ denotes the number of poles (counting multiplicities) of G in $\mathcal{D}_\pm$

$$G = G_+^{(j)} \Lambda^{(j)} G_-^{(j)} , \qquad (2.16)$$

where $G_-^{(j)}$ are rational matrix functions with poles and zeros of the determinant concentrated in $\mathfrak{D}^+$, and $\Lambda^{(j)}$ are matrix functions of the type (2.2), i.e.,

$$\Lambda^{(j)}(t) = \mathrm{diag}[t^{\varkappa_1^{(j)}}, \dots, t^{\varkappa_n^{(j)}}] , \quad \varkappa_1^{(j)} \geq \dots \geq \varkappa_n^{(j)} ,$$

$G_+^{(j)} \in L_p^+$, $(G_+^{(j)})^{-1} \in M_q^+$, and the number of zeros of $\det G_+^{(j)}$ calculated with regard to their multiplicity is equal to j .

Obviously, such representations exist. We shall obtain one of them by introducing the scalar rational function f of index $\mathcal{P}_+(G)$ the zeros and poles of which are concentrated in $\mathfrak{D}^+$, where we suppose that $fG \in L_p^+$. Furthermore, we set

$$G_+^{(N)} = fG , \quad \Lambda^{(N)}(t) = t^{-\mathcal{P}_+(G)} I , \quad G_-^{(N)}(z) = \frac{z^{\mathcal{P}_+(G)}}{f(z)} I , \qquad (2.17)$$

where N is the number of zeros of the function $\det(fG)$ in $\mathfrak{D}^+$. In virtue of the fact that this function has no poles in $\mathfrak{D}^+$, N may be calculated as follows:

$$N = \mathrm{ind}_+ \det (fG) = n \;\mathrm{ind}\, f + \mathrm{ind}_+ \det G = n\,\mathcal{P}_+(G) + \mathrm{ind}_+ \det G .$$

Now we describe the procedure of "zero separation" of $\det G_+^{(j)}$, which permits, for a given representation (2.16) of the matrix function G , a representation of precisely this type but with an index j smaller by one. Starting from the representation (2.16) of G defined by formulae (2.17) for $j = N$ and applying this procedure N times, we get a representation (2.16) of G for $j = 0$, i.e., a factorization of this matrix function in L_p .

The procedure mentioned consists in the following: For a given matrix function $G_+^{(j)}$ from the representation (2.16) and an arbitrarily chosen zero z_0 of the function $\det G_+^{(j)}$ in $\mathfrak{D}^+$, we construct a matrix function U as indicated in Lemma 2.1.

By $\varkappa_1^{(j-1)}, \dots, \varkappa_n^{(j-1)}$ we denote the tuple obtained by ordering the sequence $\varkappa_1^{(j)}, \ldots, \varkappa_{k-1}^{(j)}, \varkappa_k^{(j)}+1, \varkappa_{k+1}^{(j)}, \ldots, \varkappa_n^{(j)}$ in a non-increasing manner. It is clear that such an ordering can be carried out with the help of one transposition permuting the k th element of the sequence with the l th one ($l \le k$). By $T^{(j)}$ we denote the matrix obtained from the unit matrix after permutation of the columns with the same numbers. Then, setting $\Lambda^{(j-1)}(t) = \operatorname{diag}[t^{\varkappa_1^{(j-1)}}, \ldots, t^{\varkappa_n^{(j-1)}}] = T^{(j)} \operatorname{diag}[t^{\varkappa_1^{(j)}}, \ldots, t^{\varkappa_k^{(j)}+1}, \ldots, t^{\varkappa_n^{(j)}}]T^{(j)}$, $G_+^{(j-1)} = G_+^{(j)}U^{-1}T^{(j)}$, $G_-^{(j-1)} = T^{(j)}W^{(j)}G_-^{(j)}$, where

$$W^{(j)}(z) = T^{(j)}(\Lambda^{(j-1)}(z))^{-1}T^{(j)}U(z)\Lambda^{(j)}(z) =$$

$$\begin{bmatrix} 1 & & & \lambda_1 z^{\varkappa_k^{(j)}-\varkappa_1^{(j)}} & & & \\ & \ddots & & \vdots & & & \\ & & 1 & \lambda_{k-1} z^{\varkappa_k^{(j)}-\varkappa_{k-1}^{(j)}} & & & \\ & & & 1-\dfrac{z_0}{z} & & & \\ & & & & 1 & & \\ & & & & & \ddots & \\ & & & & & & 1 \end{bmatrix},$$

we obtain the desired representation of the matrix function G.

In fact, the matrix function $G_-^{(j-1)}$ is rational with poles and zeros of its determinant concentrated in $\mathcal{D}^+$, since $G_-^{(j)}$ and $W^{(j)}$ possess these properties. The matrix function $G_+^{(j-1)}$ is analytic in $\mathcal{D}^+$ and, according to Lemma 2.1, its determinant has one zero less than the determinant of $G_+^{(j)}$. At the same time, $G_+^{(j-1)} \in M_p^+$, because $G_+^{(j)} \in L_p^+$ and $U^{-1} \in M_\infty^+$. Consequently, $G_+^{(j-1)} \in L_p^+$. The validity of the condition $G_+^{(j-1)} \in M_q^+$ is evident, and to verify the equation

$$G = G_+^{(j-1)}\Lambda^{(j-1)}G_-^{(j-1)} \tag{2.18}$$

itself is a straightforward matter.

Thus, a procedure for changing the representation (2.16) by (2.18) has been constructed. At the same time, under the condition $G^{-1} \in M_q^+$, the existence of a factorization of G ($\in M_p^+$) in L_p with a rational factor G_- has been proved. In view of Theorem 2.2, the factor G_- is rational for every factorization of G, but not only for the one built by means of the procedure described above.

It remains to prove the estimates for the partial and the formula for the total index of the matrix function G. To this end, note that the diagonal factor $\Lambda^{(0)}$ $(= \Lambda)$ from the factorization of G is obtained from the matrix function $\Lambda^{(N)}$ as the result of N operations, each of which increases one of the exponents by one and leaves the others (up to a permutation) without changes. As the initial values of all exponents are equal to $-\mathcal{P}_+(G)$, we can claim that the partial indices of G are included between $-\mathcal{P}_+(G)$ and $-\mathcal{P}_+(G) + N = -\mathcal{P}_+(G) + n\mathcal{P}_+(G) + \mathrm{ind}_+\det G = \mathrm{ind}_+\det G + (n-1)\mathcal{P}_+(G)$, and its total index is equal to $-n\mathcal{P}_+(G) + N = \mathrm{ind}_+\det G$. Thus Theorem 2.6 has been proved. $\equiv$

The following statement about the matrix function $G \in M_q^-$ can be proved in a similar way.

THEOREM 2.7. The matrix function $G \in M_q^-$ is factorable in L_p if and only if $G^{-1} \in M_p^-$. If this condition is fulfilled, then the partial indices of G are included between $-(n-1)\mathcal{P}_-(G) + \mathrm{ind}_-\det G$ and $\mathcal{P}_-(G)$, the total index is equal to $\mathrm{ind}_-\det G$, and the left factorization factor G_+ is a rational matrix function.

Remark that the property of the right (left) factorization factor established in Theorem 2.6 (2.7) is characteristic. In fact, if the matrix function G can be factored in L_p and the factor G_- (G_+) is rational, then, obviously, $G \in M_p^+$ (M_q^-).

The estimates for the partial indices from Theorems 2.6 and 2.7 are exact, although they are not necessarily attained. This can be easily seen by simplest examples of diagonal matrix functions.

In the case of a Smirnov contour Γ, Theorems 2.6 and 2.7 can be made more precise.

THEOREM 2.8. A matrix function G of class M^+ (M^-) defined on a Smirnov contour Γ can be factored in L_p if and only if $G \in L_p$ (L_q) and $G^{-1} \in M_q^+$ (M_p^-). In this case the formulae for the total index and the estimates for the partial indices formulated in Theorems 2.6 and 2.7 continue to be valid.

Proof. If the matrix function $G \in M^+$ belongs to the class L_p, then according to Theorem 1.25, $G \in M_p^+$. Consequently, under these conditions, Theorem 2.6 may be applied to G. It remains only to prove that the requirement $G \in L_p$ is necessary for the factorability in L_p of the matrix function G of class M^+. For this purpose, as in the proof of Theorem 2.6, we proceed from the factorization (2.1) of G to equation (2.15), the left-hand side $(G_+^{-1}G)$ of which belongs to the class M^+, and the right-hand side (ΛG_-) to M_q^-. But in case of a Smirnov contour $M^+ \cap M_q^- = (M^+ \cap L_q) \cap M_q^- = M_q^+ \cap M_q^- = R$. Therefore, the matrix function $F = G_+^{-1}G$ is rational. Hence $G\ (= G_+F) \in M_p^+ \subset L_p$. The case $G \in M^-$ can be treated analogously. ≡

With regard to Theorem 2.8, in case of a Smirnov contour, the total index of $G \in M^{\pm}$ is one and the same for all possible factorizations. Consequently, the factorability domain of such matrix functions consists of no more than one component, which (in view of the general properties of the factorability domain) is a connected subset of the ray $(1, \infty)$.

It appears that every connected subset of the ray $(1, \infty)$ may be the factorability domain of a matrix function $G \in M^{\pm}$. Appropriate examples can be built even in case of scalar functions defined on the unit circle. To this end, we state a corollary from Theorem 2.8 related to the indicated special case.

COROLLARY 2.3. The function $f \in D$ can be factored in L_p if and only if in its inner-outer decomposition $f = f^{(i)}f^{(e)}$ the inner function $f^{(i)}$ is a finite Blaschke product and the outer function $f^{(e)}$ satisfies the conditions $f^{(e)} \in L_p$, $(f^{(e)})^{-1} \in L_q$.

Proof. If the function f is factorable in L_p, then, in particular, it is summable and, according to Theorem 1.18, belongs to the class H_1. Consequently, Theorem 2.8 can be applied, in view of which $f \in L_p$

and $f^{-1} \in M_q^+$. The first of the relations obtained is equivalent to $f^{(e)} \in L_p$, and the second implies the finiteness of the Blaschke product B belonging to the factor $f^{(i)}$ as well as the membership of $(f^{(e)})^{-1}$ to the class L_q. Furthermore, the function $\varphi = B^{-1}f$ is an invertible element of H_1 ($\varphi^{-1} = Bf^{-1} \in H_q$, because Bf^{-1} belongs to M_q^+ and does not have poles in the unit disk). Consequently, φ is an outer function. In this way, it has been proved that $f^{(i)} = B$.

Vice versa, if $f = Bf^{(e)}$, where B is a finite Blaschke product and $f^{(e)}$ an outer function with $f^{(e)} \in L_p$, $f^{(e)-1} \in L_q$, then $f \in H_p$, $f^{-1} \in M_q^+$. It remains to utilize the sufficiency part of Theorem 2.6 to prove Corollary 2.3. ≡

Due to Theorem 1.15 and Corollary 2.3, the function $f = f^{(e)}$ defined by formula (1.7) is factorable in L_p if and only if $k \in L_p$ and $k^{-1} \in L_q$. Thus, an example of a function G ($\in H_1$) with a given connected subset σ of the ray $(1, \infty)$ as factorability domain can be built as soon as a non-negative function k defined on the interval $(-\pi,\pi)$ will be found, for which $k \in L_p$, $k^{-1} \in L_q$ for all $p \in \sigma$, $k \notin L_p$ for p lying to the right of σ, and $k^{-1} \notin L_q$ for p to the left of σ. A function k satisfying the conditions enumerated can be found, for instance, among the continuous and non-vanishing functions on $(-\pi,\pi)$ converging to zero if $\theta \to -\pi$ and to infinity if $\theta \to \pi$.

Actually, let $p_1 = \inf\{p : p \in \sigma\}$, $p_2 = \sup\{p : p \in \sigma\}$.
We impose the following requirements on the asymptotic behaviour of the function k at the right end of the domain of definition:

$$k(\theta) \sim \begin{cases} \ln(\pi - \theta) & , \text{ if } p_2 = \infty , \\ (\pi - \theta)^{-1/p_2} & , \text{ if } p_2 < \infty , \ p_2 \notin \sigma , \\ (\pi - \theta)^{-1/p_2} \ln^{\varepsilon}(\pi-\theta) \ (0 < \varepsilon < 1/p_2), & \text{ if } p_2 \in \sigma . \end{cases}$$

Then it is easy to verify that $k \in L_p$ for $p \in \sigma$, and $k \notin L_p$ for $p \notin \sigma$, $p \geq p_2$. The demands on the function k^{-1} can be satisfied due to the asymptotic behaviour of the function k at the left end chosen in a similar way.

We still mention that, owing to Corollary 2.3, an inner function f different from a finite Blaschke product yields an example of a function belonging to class L_∞ together with its inverse, which cannot be factored in any L_p.

On the strenght of either Theorem 2.6 or 2.7, it is possible to obtain the following result on factorization of rational matrix functions.

THEOREM 2.9. Let X be a rational matrix function. If the poles and the zeros of the determinant of X do not lie on Γ, then it admits a representation

$$X(t) = X_+(t)\Lambda(t)\,X_-(t) \tag{2.19}$$

where X_+ (X_-) is a rational matrix function with poles and zeros of the determinant concentrated in $\mathcal{D}^-$ ($\mathcal{D}^+$), and Λ is a matrix function of the kind (2.2). This representation provides a factorization of X in all L_p, $1 < p < \infty$. On the other hand, if at least one pole or a zero of the determinant of X is placed on Γ, then the set $F(X)$ is empty.

Proof. If the poles and the zeros of the determinant of X do not lie on Γ, then X and X^{-1} can be viewed as elements of the class M_∞^+. Hence, by Theorem 2.6, there follows the existence of a representation (2.19) in which the X_--factor is rational and X_+ is analytic and non-degenerate in $\mathcal{D}^+$. Since the matrix function X itself is rational, the factor X_+ is also a rational matrix function. Consequently, $X_+^{\pm 1} \in L_\infty^+$, $X_-^{\pm 1} \in L_\infty^-$, so that the representation (2.19) is a factorization of X in all L_p, $1 < p < \infty$.

We could obtain the same conclusion, considering X as an element of M_∞^- and applying Theorem 2.7. If one pole of the matrix function X lies on Γ, then $X \notin L_1$, and if X degenerates on Γ, then X^{-1} has poles on Γ and, therefore, $X^{-1} \notin L_1$. Thus, the necessary condition that $F(X)$ is non-empty indicated in Theorem 2.6 is violated, which proves Theorem 2.9. ≡

Evidently, the estimates for the partial indices both from Theorem 2.6 and from Theorem 2.7 can be applied to rational matrix functions.

Now we are prepared to prove the factorability of matrix functions of the type (2.11).

<u>THEOREM 2.10.</u> Let the matrix function G be representable in the form (2.11), where $A_\pm$ are matrix functions satisfying conditions (2.12). Then this matrix function can be factored in L_p, and its factorization may be obtained from the representation (2.11) with the help of a finite number of algebraic operations. The total p-index $\varkappa$ of G is equal to $\operatorname{ind}_+\det A_+ + \operatorname{ind}_-\det A_-$, and the partial p-indices are included between $-P_+(A_+) - (n-1)P_-(A_-) + \operatorname{ind}_-\det A_-$ and $P_-(A_-) + (n-1)P_+(A_+) + \operatorname{ind}_+\det A_+$.

<u>Proof.</u> According to Theorems 2.6 and 2.7, the matrix functions A_+ and A_- admit a factorization in L_p:

$$A_+ = G_+^{(1)} \Lambda^{(1)} G_-^{(1)}, \tag{2.20}$$

$$A_- = G_+^{(2)} \Lambda^{(2)} G_-^{(2)}, \tag{2.21}$$

where $G_-^{(1)}$ and $G_+^{(2)}$ are rational, have no poles and do not degenerate on Γ. Consequently, the matrix function $X = \Lambda^{(1)} G_-^{(1)} G_+^{(2)} \Lambda^{(2)}$ has the same properties. Therefore, the representation (2.19) holds. Setting $G_+ = G_+^{(1)} X_+$, $G_- = X_- G_-^{(2)}$, we obtain a factorization (2.1) of G in L_p, since $G_+^{(1)} \in L_p^+$, $(G_+^{(1)})^{-1} \in L_q^+$, $G_-^{(2)} \in L_q^-$, $(G_-^{(2)})^{-1} \in L_p^-$ and $X_+^{\pm 1} \in L_\infty^+$, $X_-^{\pm 1} \in L_\infty^-$.

Each of the factorizations (2.20), (2.21) and (2.19) is realized with the help of a finite number of algebraic operations. Hence, a factorization of G can be derived with the same degree of effectiveness. The partial p-indices of the matrix function G coincide with the partial p-indices of X. To get lower bounds of the latter, we represent X in the form

$$X = G_+^{(1)-1} A_+ G_+^{(2)} \Lambda^{(2)}. \tag{2.22}$$

From the non-degeneracy and analyticity of $G_+^{(1)}$ and $G_+^{(2)}$ in $\mathfrak{D}^+$ it follows that $P_+(X) \le P_+(A_+) - \varkappa_n^{(2)}$, where $\varkappa_n^{(2)}$ is the smallest of the partial indices of A_-. According to Theorem 2.7, for the value $\varkappa_n^{(2)}$, the estimate from below

$$\varkappa_n^{(2)} \geq -(n-1)P_-(A_-) + \mathrm{ind}_- \det A_-$$

holds, owing to which we have

$$P_+(X) \leq P_+(A_+) + (n-1)P_-(A_-) - \mathrm{ind}_-\det A_- .$$

Since, by Theorem 2.6, the value $-P_+(X)$ serves as a lower bound for the partial indices of X, the desired lower bound for the partial indices of G has been derived. An upper bound of the partial indices may be established analogously, and the formula for the total index results from equation (2.22), taking into account that $\mathrm{ind}_+\det G_+^{(j)} = 0$ $(j = 1,2)$ and $\mathrm{ind}\det \Lambda^{(2)} = \mathrm{ind}_-\det A_-$. Thus Theorem 2.10 is completely proved. ≡

It is of interest that the factorization factors $G_\pm$ of a matrix function G of the type (2.11) differ from $A_\pm$ by a rational factor.
In fact,

$$G_+ = A_+(G_-^{(1)})^{-1}(\Lambda^{(1)})^{-1}X_+ \quad (= A_+G_+^{(2)}\Lambda^{(2)}X_-^{-1}\Lambda) ,$$

$$G_- = X_-(\Lambda^{(2)})^{-1}(G_+^{(2)})^{-1}A_- \quad (=\Lambda^{-1}X_+^{-1}\Lambda^{(1)}G_-^{(1)}A_-) .$$

This implies, in particular, that if some of the matrix functions $A_+^{\pm 1}$, $A_-^{\pm 1}$ is summable with larger exponent that it is caused by relations (2.12), or if it is smooth on some arc $\gamma \subset \Gamma$, then this property is acquired by the corresponding matrix functions $G_+^{\pm 1}$, $G_-^{\pm 1}$.

<u>THEOREM 2.11.</u> Let the matrix function G be factorable in L_p , let $\{\varkappa_j\}_{j=1}^n$ be the set of its partial p-indices, and suppose B_+ (B_-) to be a matrix function belonging to class M_∞^+ (M_∞^-) together with its inverse. Then the matrix function B_+GB_- is also factorable in L_p , its partial p-indices are included between $\varkappa_n - P_+(B_+) - (n-1)P_-(B_-) + \mathrm{ind}_-\det B_-$ and $\varkappa_1 + P_-(B_-) + (n-1)P_+(B_+) + \mathrm{ind}_+\det B_+$, and the total p-index is equal to $\varkappa + \mathrm{ind}_+\det B_+ + \mathrm{ind}_-\det B_-$.

<u>Proof.</u> If (2.1) is a factorization of G in L_p, then, setting e.g.

$$A_+ = B_+G_+ , \quad A_- = \Lambda G_-B_- , \tag{2.23}$$

we obtain a representation of the matrix function $\hat{G} = B_+GB_-$ in the form (2.11). Consequently, $\hat{G}$ satisfies the conditions of Theorem 2.10 and, according to this theorem, it is factorable in L_p. The upper estimate for the partial indices and the formula for the total p-index of $\hat{G}$ can be also deduced from Theorem 2.10, taking into account that $P_+(A_+) = P_+(B_+)$, $P_-(A_-) \leq P_-(B_-) + \varkappa_1$, $\mathrm{ind}_+\det A_+ = \mathrm{ind}_+\det B_+$, and $\mathrm{ind}_-\det A_- = \varkappa + \mathrm{ind}_-\det B_-$. In order to derive the lower estimate for the partial indices stated in the theorem, we have to choose $A_+ = B_+G_+\Lambda$, $A_- = G_-B_-$.

Theorem 2.10 allows us to solve the question of the connection between the factorizations of one and the same matrix function G in different L_p to the very end.

<u>THEOREM 2.12.</u> Let $G = G_+^{(1)}\Lambda^{(1)}G_-^{(1)}$ be a factorization of the matrix function G in L_{p_1}. If the rational matrix function X is such that

$$G_+^{(1)} X \in M_{p_2}^+ , \quad X^{-1}(G_+^{(1)})^{-1} \in M_{q_2}^+ ,$$
$$X^{-1} \Lambda^{(1)}G_-^{(1)} \in M_{q_2}^- , \quad G_-^{(1)}(\Lambda^{(1)})^{-1} X \in M_{p_2}^- , \tag{2.24}$$

then G can be factored in L_{p_2}, and the total indices $\varkappa^{(1)}$ and $\varkappa^{(2)}$ of G in L_{p_1} and L_{p_2} are connected via the relation

$$\varkappa^{(1)} - \varkappa^{(2)} = N - P , \tag{2.25}$$

where N (P) is the number of zeros (poles) of the function $\det X$ on Γ.

Conversely, if G is factorable in L_{p_1} and L_{p_2} with the total indices $\varkappa^{(1)}$ and $\varkappa^{(2)}$ respectively, then there exists a triangular polynomial matrix function Y, the degree of whose determinant is equal to $|\varkappa^{(1)} - \varkappa^{(2)}|$ such that relations (2.24) are satisfied for $X = Y$, if $\varkappa^{(1)} \geq \varkappa^{(2)}$, and for $X = Y^{-1}$, if $\varkappa^{(1)} < \varkappa^{(2)}$.

<u>Proof.</u> If the requirements (2.24) are fulfilled, then the matrix function G satisfies the conditions of Theorem 2.10 for $p = p_2$, $A_+ = G_+^{(1)}X$, $A_- = X^{-1}\Lambda^{(1)}G_-^{(1)}$. Consequently, this matrix function

can be factored in L_{p_2}, where its total p_2-index is equal to $\mathrm{ind}_+\det(G_+^{(1)}X) + \mathrm{ind}_-(X^{-1}\Lambda^{(1)}G_-^{(1)}) = \mathrm{ind}_+\det X + \mathrm{ind}_-\det X^{-1} + \mathrm{ind}\det\Lambda^{(1)} = \mathrm{ind}_+\det X - \mathrm{ind}_-\det X + \varkappa^{(1)}$.
This implies $\varkappa^{(1)} - \varkappa^{(2)} = \mathrm{ind}_-\det X - \mathrm{ind}_+\det X$. Applying statement 2) of Theorem 1.29 to the function $f = \det X$, we therefore get the relation (2.25).

For the sake of definiteness, in the following it is assumed that $\varkappa^{(1)} \geq \varkappa^{(2)}$.

In order to prove the converse statement, we study the matrix function H_+ occurring in the formulae (2.5) of transfer from a factorization in L_{p_1} to a factorization in L_{p_2}. Splitting off left factors of the type (2.14) as indicated in the remark to Lemma 2.1, we obtain the representation $H_+ = XH_1$, where H_1 is a polynomial matrix function with constant determinant different from zero, and X is the product of $\varkappa^{(1)} - \varkappa^{(2)}$ factors of the kind (2.14). Hence, it is a polynomial upper-triangular matrix and $\deg\det X = \deg\det H = \varkappa^{(1)} - \varkappa^{(2)}$.
As was shown in Section 2.2, all the zeros of $\det H$ and, thus, of the diagonal elements of X lie on the contour Γ.
Since $G_+^{(1)}X = G_+^{(2)}H_1^{-1}$, $X^{-1}\Lambda^{(1)}G_-^{(1)} = H_1\Lambda^{(2)}G_-^{(2)}$ and H_1 is analytic and non-degenerate at all finite points, the relations (2.24) are valid. Separating from H left factors of the type (2.14'), but not of type (2.14), we could obtain a lower-triangular matrix function.
Theorem 2.12 has been proved. ≡
From Theorem 1.21 we deduce that a matrix function X satisfying conditions (2.24) belongs to the class $M^+_{p_2q_1/(p_2+q_1)}$ and its inverse X^{-1} to $M^+_{p_1q_2/(p_1+q_2)}$. Hence, for $p_2 \geq p_1$, the entries of X must be summable on Γ, therefore, $P = 0$. Similarly, for $p_2 \leq p_1$, we have $N = 0$. Furthermore, $p_2q_1/(p_2+q_1) > 1/2$ and $p_1q_2/(p_1+q_2) > 1/2$, thus, the elements of the matrix functions $X^{\pm 1}$ are summable with exponent $1/2$. Consequently, their poles lying on Γ must be simple.

If, in particular, Y is the triangular polynomial matrix function occurring in the converse statement, then all roots of its diagonal elements must be simple. The number of different roots of det Y lies, therefore, between $-[-|\varkappa^{(1)} - \varkappa^{(2)}|/n]$ (i.e. the smallest integer greater than or equal to $|\varkappa^{(1)} - \varkappa^{(2)}|/n$) and $|\varkappa^{(1)} - \varkappa^{(2)}|$. For $n = 1$, the first value is precisely equal to $|\varkappa^{(1)} - \varkappa^{(2)}|$.

2.5. COMMENTS

The factorization of the type (2.1) as well as the notions of partial and total indices, under classical assumptions concerning the matrix function G and the contour Γ, where introduced in the paper of MUSKHELISHVILI and VEKUA [1] (see also the monographs N. VEKUA [4], MUSKHELISHVILI [1]).

Factorization in L_p was first studied by PRIVALOV [1], for a review of subsequent results, see KHVEDELIDZE [1]. The right-factorization was presented for the first time in GOHBERG, KREǏN [3].

It would seem that the first detailed study of the relations between the factorization of one and the same matrix function for different values of the parameter p is accomplished in the present book.

Theorems 2.1 and 2.3 were formulated in SPITKOVSKIǏ [2].

At the same place the notion of the factorability domain was introduced.

Corollary 2.1 is usually called the invariance theorem for partial indices (see N. VEKUA [4], GAKHOV [3], MUSKHELISHVILI [1], SIMONENKO [4]).

Theorem 2.2 on the connections between factorizations with one and the same total index was actually proved in MUSKHELISHVILI, VEKUA [1] (see also GOHBERG [4]).

For the factorization of power functions, see VEKUA [4], GAKHOV [3], GOHBERG, KRUPNIK [4].

The method of "splitting off zeros" was first applied to the factorization problem by GAKHOV [1-3]. The factorization problem for rational matrix functions (Theorem 2.9) was solved by N.P. VEKUA [1] (see also N. VEKUA [4]), and for matrix functions of the type (2.11) with Hölder factors $A_{\pm}$ (up to Γ) by GAKHOV. In a spezial case, the latter problem was studied by N. VEKUA, KVESELAVA [1,2] and SHERMAN [1]. The general

Theorem 2.10 has been proved here, in principle, by the same method as was used by GAKHOV for the result mentioned above.
Note that a somewhat different procedure of constructing a factorization based on the preceding transition to a matrix function with constant determinant and with trigonometric polynomials as elements, has been recently proposed in JONCKHEERE, DELSARTE [1].
This applies, in particular, to rational matrix functions with zero partial indices.

In Ch. 1 of CLANCEY, GOHBERG [3] formulae are presented which express the partial indices of rational matrix functions by spectral data of the matrix polynomial corresponding to it. For more results in this direction we refer to BART, GOHBERG, KAASHOEK [1-3]. The factorization of a matrix function of the kind (2.11), if the contour Γ is the real line and det $A_{\pm}$ are entire functions, was considered in HURD [1] in connection with applications to problems of determining a stationary temperature regime.

Theorems 2.6 - 2.8 and 2.11 are proved in SPITKOVSKIǏ [13] (see also SPITKOVSKIǏ [2]). The estimates of the partial indices established in these theorems generalize results of NIKOLAǏCHUK [1] obtained by him for the classical case by the same method of "separating zeros". The formulae for the total index stated in these theorems are analogues of the classical formula of MUSKHELISHVILI (see VEKUA [4], MUSKHELISHVILI [1]), according to which the total index of a non-degenerate Hölder matrix function is equal to the index of its determinant. For Muskhelishvili's formula and its extensions to other classes, we refer to Chapter 5.

Remark that the formula for the total index and the non-negativity of the partial indices of a matrix function analytic in $\mathcal{D}^+$ (and continuous in $\mathcal{D}^+ \cup \Gamma$) are also presented in the article of CHEBOTAREV and GAKHOV [1].
Theorem 2.12 is published for the first time.

CHAPTER 3. THE CRITERION OF FACTORABILITY.

Φ-FACTORIZATION AND ITS BASIC PROPERTIES

In this chapter we shall study relationships between properties of the Riemann boundary value problem for a piecewise analytic vector function and the factorability of its coefficient, i.e. the matrix function G. It is well-known that in the classical case, if we seek for a solution of the Riemann problem with a Hölder matrix G, the factorability of G is equivalent to the Fredholmness of the boundary value problem. The transition to the solution of the Riemann problem with measurable matrix function G in the Smirnov classes $E_p^{\pm}$ leads to a new quality. It turns out that the factorability of G, generally speaking, does not imply the Fredholmness of the corresponding boundary value problem. In fact, the vector-valued Riemann boundary value problem with a factorable matrix function G and the associate problem considered in the classes L_p and L_q, respectively, have finite defect numbers, and the indices of the problems are opposite. However, these problems are, in general, not normally solvable, i.e. their images can be not closed. Nevertheless, these images are in a sense well-situated. More strictly speaking, the following weakened closedness condition is fulfilled: the image of the Riemann boundary value problem (and of the problem associate to it) contains all those rational vector functions belonging to its closure. Moreover, the factorability of the matrix coefficient of a Riemann problem in L_p is equivalent to the property described above, a property intermediate between finiteness of the defect numbers and Fredholmness. This fact is the main result of Sections 3.1 and 3.2. In Section 3.3 it will be further stated that to guarantee the normal solvability and, thus, the Fredholmness of the Riemann problem with factorable coefficient G, certain two operators K and K_1 composed with the help of the factorization factors of G in a certain way as well as the projectors P and Q have to be bounded in L_p^n. In order to make the notions of Fredholmness of a boundary value problem and factorability of its coefficient equivalent, it is natural to confine the definition of factorization given in Ch. 2 by adding the requirement of boundedness of the mentioned operators K and K_1 in the space L_p^n. This special type of factorization ensuring the Fredholmness of the corresponding Riemann problem will be introduced in Section 3.4 and called Φ-factorization. In what follows we shall almost always have to deal with just Φ-factorization.

The results of Sections 3.1 - 3.4 will be formulated and proved under the only suppositions that the contour is rectifiable. The matrix function G is unbounded in general. In Section 3.5, the contour Γ is, in addition, assumed to belong to the class $\mathfrak{R}$, on which, by the very definition, the operator of singular integration S is bounded in the spaces L_p, $1 < p < \infty$. The condition $\Gamma \in \mathfrak{R}$ permits us to consider the closed operator $P + GQ$ [1] instead of the Riemann problem with matrix coefficient G. This enables us to utilize the powerful apparatus of operator theory for investigation.

Here we shall demonstrate the necessity of the condition $G^{-1} \in L_\infty$ for $P + GQ$ to be a Φ_--operator and the criterion of Φ-factorability resulting from this fact.

Finally, under the condition $G \in L_\infty$, in Section 3.6 we change over from the examination of closed, generally speaking, unbounded operators to the study of bounded ones. It will be established that the problem of Φ-factorability of a matrix function G defined on a composite contour can be reduced to the corresponding problem for its restrictions on the connected components of the contour. Φ-factorability is preserved and of local character if the images of the contours are smooth enough.

In 3.7 comments for further reading will be given.

---

[1] Incidentally, note that the equation $(P+GQ)\varphi = f$ is, in principle, the characteristic system of singular integral equations with Cauchy kernels. In the classical case (if G is a matrix with Hölder elements and Γ a piecewise smooth contour) it was studied in the monographs MUSKHELISHVILI [1] and VEKUA [4].

3.1. ON SOLVABILITY OF THE RIEMANN BOUNDARY VALUE PROBLEM WITH FACTORABLE MATRIX COEFFICIENT

Let G be a matrix function of n th order and g a n-dimensional vector function both defined on Γ. The <u>vector-valued Riemann boundary value problem</u> is stated in the following way:

Find n-dimensional vector functions φ^+ and φ^- analytic in $\mathcal{D}^+$ and $\mathcal{D}^-$, respectively, satisfying the condition

$$\varphi^+(t) + G(t)\varphi^-(t) = g(t) \tag{3.1}$$

imposed on their boundary values on the contour Γ.

Problem (3.1) is viewed in the class L_p. This means that the vector function g is defined in L_p^n, and the components of the desired vector functions $\varphi^{\pm}$ must belong to the classes E_p^+ and $\overset{\circ}{E}{}_p^-$ respectively. Equation (3.1) must hold a.e. on the contour Γ, which henceforth (up to Section 3.5) is assumed to be merely rectifiable.

Together with problem (3.1) we consider the problem

$$\psi^-(t) + G'(t)\psi^+(t) = h(t) \tag{3.2}$$

in the class L_q. Problem (3.2) is called <u>associate</u> [1] <u>to problem (3.1)</u>.

The pair $\{\varphi^+, \varphi^-\}$ is referred to as the solution of problem (3.1). We shall call φ^+ the "+"-component of the solution, and φ^- the "-"-component. Borrowing the terminology from operator theory (for which we have serious reasons, as will become clear later on), the solution set of the homogeneous problem (3.1) is called its <u>kernel</u>, and the set of vector-functions $g(t)$, for which the inhomogeneous problem is solvable, is said to be its <u>image</u>.

Clearly, the kernel and the image of problem (3.1) are lineals. The dimension α_1 of the first of them and the codimension (in L_p^n) β_1 of the closure of the second are called <u>defect numbers</u> of problem (3.1).

---

[1] Sometimes the problem $\psi^+ + (G')^{-1}\psi^- = h$ related to (3.2) in an obvious manner is called associate to (3.1).

The difference $\alpha_1 - \beta_1$, which makes sense if at least one of the numbers α_1 and β_1 is finite, is referred to as its <u>index.</u> Problem (3.1) is said to be normally solvable, if its image is closed; it is called Fredholm, if it is normally solvable and has a finite index.

Analogous terms and notations are introduced for problem (3.2). In particular, the defect numbers α_2 and β_2 of problem (3.2) are the dimension of its kernel and the codimension in L_q^n of the closure of its image, respectively.

<u>THEOREM 3.1.</u>

1) The orthogonal complement [1] to the image of problem (3.1) contains the set of "+"-components of the kernel of problem (3.2) and, for $G \in L_\infty$, coincides with it.
2) The orthogonal complement to the image of problem (3.2) contains the set of "−"-components of the kernel of problem (3.1) and, provided that $G \in L_\infty$, coincides with it.
3) In the case of a scalar function G different from zero on a subset of positive measure of each of the components of the contour Γ, at least one of the defect numbers α_1 and α_2 is equal to zero.

<u>Proof.</u>

1) The image of problem (3.1) consists precisely of all vector functions of the form $\varphi^+ + G\varphi^-$, where $\varphi^+ \in (L_p^+)^n$, and the vector function $\varphi^- \in (\overset{\circ}{L}{}_p^-)^n$ is such that $G\varphi^- \in L_p^n$. Therefore, the vector function $\psi \in L_q^n$ is orthogonal to the image of problem (3.1) if and only if it is orthogonal to $(L_p^+)^n$ (in view of Theorem 1.26, this condition means that $\psi = \psi^+ \in (L_q^+)^n$), and

$$\langle G\varphi^- , \psi^+ \rangle = 0 \qquad (3.3)$$

for all $\varphi^- \in (\overset{\circ}{L}{}_p^-)^n$ with $G\varphi^- \in L_p^n$.

If ψ^+ is the "+"-component of a vector function from the kernel

[1] Here orthogonality is understood in the sense of the bilinear form (1.13).

of problem (3.2), then $G'\psi^+ \ (= -\psi^-) \in (\overset{\circ}{L}{}_q^-)^n$, and $\langle G\varphi^-,\psi^+\rangle = \langle \varphi^-,G'\psi^+\rangle = \langle \varphi^-,-\psi^-\rangle = 0$. Thus, condition (3.3) is fulfilled. Hence, the "+"-components of the kernel of problem (3.2) are orthogonal to the image of problem (3.1).

If $G \in L_\infty$, condition (3.3) simply means that $\langle \varphi', G'\psi^+\rangle = 0$ for all $\varphi^- \in (\overset{\circ}{L}{}_p^-)^n$, i.e. $G'\psi^+ \in (\overset{\circ}{L}{}_q^-)^n$ (here Theorem 1.26 is used again). Consequently, for $G \in L_\infty$, the orthogonal complement to the image of problem (3.1) does not contain vector functions different from "+"-components of the kernel of problem (3.2).

The argument for statement 2) is similar.

3) Let $n = 1$, and let $\{\varphi^+,\varphi^-\}$ and $\{\psi^+,\psi^-\}$ be solutions of the homogeneous problems (3.1) and (3.2), respectively. Consider the function $f = \psi^+G\varphi^-$. On the one hand, $\psi^+ \in L_q^+$ and $G\varphi^- = -\varphi^+ \in L_p^+$, so that $f \in L_1^+$. On the other hand, $G\psi^+ = -\psi^-$, and $\varphi^- \in \overset{\circ}{L}{}_p^-$, hence $f \in \overset{\circ}{L}{}_1^-$. According to Theorem 1.28, $f(t) = 0$ a.e. on Γ . Denoting by γ_j those subsets of the curves $\Gamma(j)$ of positive linear measure on which $G(t) \not\equiv 0$, we get $\psi^+(t)\varphi^-(t) = 0$ a.e. on γ_j $(j = 0,\dots,m-1)$. Owing to Theorem 1.23, we thus deduce that either $\psi^+ = 0$ or $\varphi^- = 0$. In the first case we have $\psi^- = -G'\psi^+ = 0$, i.e. the homogeneous problem (3.2) has only the trivial solution and, hence $\alpha_2 = 0$. In the second case we have $\alpha_1 = 0$. Theorem 3.1 is completely proved. ≡

By Theorem 1.2, the codimension of the closure of the image of problem (3.1) (and 3.2)) coincides with the dimension of its orthogonal complement. On the strength of Theorem 3.1, we conclude from this that the defect numbers of (3.1) and (3.2) are connected by the inequalities

$$\alpha_1 \le \beta_2 , \quad \alpha_2 \le \beta_1 . \tag{3.4}$$

In virtue of the same Theorem 3.1, for $G \in L_\infty$, inequalities (3.4) turn into equalities. However, in the general case, the equality sign in relations (3.4) fails to be true.

EXAMPLE. Assume the contour Γ to be a circle and $G(t) = t\, f(t)$, where f is an outer function with the properties $f \notin L_p$, $f^{-1} \in L_q$, $f \in L_r$ for some $r > 0$. The kernel of the corresponding problem (3.1) is trivial. Actually, if $\varphi^+ \in L_p^+$, $\varphi^- \in \overset{\circ}{L}{}_p^-$ and $\varphi^+ + G\varphi^- = 0$, then $f^{-1}(t)\varphi^+(t) = -\, t\, \varphi^-(t)$. The right-hand side of the equation obtained lies in the class L_p^-, and the left one in L^+. Since a circle is a Smirnov curve, in accordance with Theorems 1.25 and 1.28, we conclude that either of the functions $f^{-1}(t)\varphi^+(t)$ and $t\,\varphi^-(t)$ is equal to a certain constant c a.e. on Γ. Hence $\varphi^+(t) = c\, f(t)$. Taking into consideration that $\varphi^+ \in L_p^+$ and $f \notin L_p$, we find that $c = 0$. Consequently, $\varphi^+ = \varphi^- = 0$, i.e., the homogeneous problem (3.1) does not have nontrivial solutions. At the same time, the orthogonal complement of the image of the corresponding problem (3.2) is nontrivial: it contains, in any case, the function f^{-1}, as for $\psi^+ \in L_q^+$, $\psi^- \in \overset{\circ}{L}{}_q^-$, we have $\langle f^{-1}, \psi^- + G\psi^+ \rangle = \langle f^{-1}, G\psi^+ \rangle = \langle f^{-1}, tf\,\psi^+ \rangle = \langle 1, t\,\psi^+ \rangle = 0$. Thus, for the considered scalar function G, $\alpha_1 = 0$ and $\beta_2 > 0$.

Below in this section we will be concerned with matrix functions G which can be factored in L_p. A criterion of solvability and formulae for the defect numbers of problems (3.1) and (3.2) will be obtained, meaning, in particular, that the equality sign in the inequalities (3.4) is attained for all factorable matrix functions G irrespective of whether they are bounded or not.

THEOREM 3.2. Let the matrix function G admit a factorization (2.1) in L_p. Then

1) problem (3.1) with the right-hand side g is solvable if and only if

$$G_+^{-1} g \in \mathcal{L}_1^n \text{ [1]}, \quad \varphi_0^+ = G_+ P G_+^{-1} g \in (L_p^+)^n, \tag{3.5}$$
$$\varphi_0^- = G_-^{-1} \Lambda^{-1} Q G_+^{-1} g \in (\overset{\circ}{L}{}_p^-)^n;$$

[1] Concerning the definition of $\mathcal{L}_1^n$ see p.47.

2) if the conditions (3.5) are fulfilled, then the general solution of problem (3.1) is of the form

$$\varphi^+ = \varphi_0^+ + G_+\varrho \ , \quad \varphi^- = \varphi_0^- + G_-^{-1}\Lambda^{-1}\varrho \ , \tag{3.6}$$

where ϱ is a vector function, the j th element of which is a polynomial of degree less than or equal to $\varkappa_j - 1$, if $\varkappa_j > 0$, and equal to zero, if $\varkappa_j \leq 0$.

Proof. Assume that $\{\varphi^+,\varphi^-\}$ is a solution of problem (3.1). Substituting the representation (2.1) of the matrix function G into the boundary condition (3.1), we obtain

$$f^+ + \Lambda f^- = G_+^{-1}g \ , \tag{3.7}$$

where $f^+ = G_+^{-1}\varphi^+$ and $f^- = G_-\varphi^-$. Since $G_+^{-1} \in L_q^+$, $\varphi^+ \in (L_p^+)^n$, we have $f^+ \in (L_1^+)^n$. Analogously, $f^- \in (\mathring{L}_1^-)^n$. Therefore, equation (3.7) means that $G_+^{-1}g \in \mathcal{L}_1^n$, so that $PG_+^{-1}g \ (\in (L_1^+)^n)$ and $QG_+^{-1}g \ (\in (\mathring{L}_1^-)^n)$ are well-defined.

Rewriting equation (3.7) componentwise, we get

$$f_j^+ - P(G_+^{-1}g)_j = -t^{\varkappa_j} f_j^- + Q(G_+^{-1}g)_j \quad (=: \varrho_j) \ , \quad j = 1,\dots,n \ .$$

Applying Theorem 1.28 to the latter equation and taking into account that the functions f_j^- and $Q(G_+^{-1}g)_j$ vanish at infinity, we find that ϱ_j is identically zero, if $\varkappa_j \leq 0$, and a polynomial of degree not higher than $\varkappa_j - 1$ otherwise.

Thus, $f_j^+ = P(G_+^{-1}g)_j + \varrho_j$, $f_j^- = t^{-\varkappa_j} Q(G_+^{-1}g)_j - t^{-\varkappa_j}\varrho_j$.

Returning to the vector functions $\varphi^\pm$, we obtain formulae (3.6).

According to the assumption, $\{\varphi^+,\varphi^-\}$ is the solution of problem (3.1), thus $\varphi^+ \in (L_p^+)^n$, $\varphi^- \in (\mathring{L}_p^-)^n$. Since $\varrho \in (L_\infty^+)^n$, $\Lambda^{-1}\varrho \in (\mathring{L}_\infty^-)^n$, the conditions $G_+\varrho \in (L_p^+)^n$ and $G_-^{-1}\Lambda^{-1}\varrho \in (\mathring{L}_p^-)^n$ are satisfied and, therefore, $\varphi_0^+ \in (L_p^+)^n$, $\varphi_0^- \in (\mathring{L}_p^-)^n$.

In this way, the necessity of conditions (3.5) for the solvability of problem (3.1) has been proved as well as the fact that every solution of the problem is of the form (3.6).

It is not hard to see that conditions (3.5) imply that every pair $\{\varphi^+,\varphi^-\}$ defined by formulae (3.6) is a solution of problem (3.1), which proves Theorem 3.2. ≡

The following result on the solvability of the associate problem can be proved in a similar way.

THEOREM 3.2'. Let the matrix function G admit a factorization (2.1) in L_p. Then

1) problem (3.2) with the right-hand side h is solvable if and only if

$$(G'_-)^{-1}h \in \mathcal{L}_1^n , \quad \psi_0^- = G'_- Q(G'_-)^{-1}h \in (\mathring{L}_q^-)^n , \quad \psi_0^+ = (G'_+)^{-1} \Lambda^{-1} P(G'_-)^{-1}h \in (L_q^+)^n ; \qquad (3.5')$$

2) if the conditions (3.5') are fulfilled, then the general solution of problem (3.2') has the form

$$\psi^+ = \psi_0^+ + (G'_+)^{-1}\sigma , \quad \psi^- = \psi_0^- - G'_- \Lambda \sigma , \qquad (3.6')$$

where σ is a vector function, the j th component σ_j of which is identically zero, if $\varkappa_j \geq 0$, and a polynomial of order less than or equal to $-\varkappa_j - 1$ otherwise.

The general solution of the homogeneous problem (3.1) is determined by formula (3.6) with $\varphi_0^+ = \varphi_0^- = 0$. In other words, the "+"-component of the solution of the homogeneous problem (3.1) is a linear combination (with polynomial coefficients of a certain degree) of the columns of the matrix function G_+, and its "−"-component is the combination (with opposite coefficients) of the columns of $G_-^{-1}\Lambda^{-1}$. In connection with this, the matrix function taking the values $G_+(z)$ for $z \in \mathcal{D}^+$ and $G_-^{-1}(z)\Lambda^{-1}(z)$ for $z \in \mathcal{D}^-$ is called a canonical matrix of the problem (3.1).

Analogously, the general solution of the homogeneous problem (3.2) is determined by formula (3.6') in which $\psi_0^+ = \psi_0^- = 0$.

It is easy to see that the pairs of vector functions

$$\{G_+(z)\, z^k e_j , \; - G_-^{-1}(z)\Lambda^{-1}(z)\, z^k e_j\} \quad (k = 0,\dots,-1+\varkappa_j,$$

where j ranges over those indices for which $\varkappa_j > 0$) form a basis in the space of solutions of the homogeneous problem (3.1). In the space of solutions of the homogeneous problem (3.2) a basis is generated by pairs of the form $\{(G'_+)^{-1}(z)z^k e_j \, , \, -G'_-(z)\Lambda(z)z^k e_j\}$ $(k = 0,\ldots,-1-\varkappa_j$ where j ranges over those indices for which $\varkappa_j < 0$).
From this and Theorem 3.1 we deduce the following result.

COROLLARY 3.1. Let the matrix function G admit a factorization (2.1) in L_p. Then

1) the dimensions of the kernels of problems (3.1) and (3.2) can be calculated via the formulae

$$\alpha_1 = \sum_{j=1}^{n} \max\{\varkappa_j, 0\} \, , \qquad \alpha_2 = \sum_{j=1}^{n} \max\{-\varkappa_j, 0\} \, ; \tag{3.8}$$

2) for the solvability of problem (3.1) it is necessary that, for all $j = 1,\ldots,n$ with $\varkappa_j < 0$, the conditions

$$\int_\Gamma (G_+^{-1}(t)g(t))_j \, t^k dt = 0 \, , \quad k = 0,\ldots,-\varkappa_j-1 \tag{3.9}$$

are satisfied;

3) for the solvability of problem (3.2) it is necessary that, for all $j = 1,\ldots,n$ with $\varkappa_j > 0$, the conditions

$$\int_\Gamma ((G'_-)^{-1}(t)h(t))_j \, t^k dt = 0 \, , \quad k = -\varkappa_j,\ldots,-1 \tag{3.9'}$$

are valid.

According to formulae (3.8), for $n > 1$, both defect numbers α_1 and α_2 may be different from zero, so that assertion 3) of Theorem 3.1 cannot be transferred to the vector case (for $n = 1$, formula (3.8) in close agreement with assertion 3) of Theorem 3.1 shows that $\alpha_1\alpha_2 = 0$). If the vector function $G_+^{-1}g$ lies in $\mathcal{L}_1^n$ (in view of assertion 1) of Theorem 3.2 only this case is of interest), then condition (3.9) may be rewritten as follows: for those j for which $\varkappa_j < 0$, the j th component of the vector function $Q(G_+^{-1}g)$ has a zero of order not less than $1 - \varkappa_j$ at infinity.

The equivalence of the latter condition with condition (3.9) is an immediate consequence of the following proposition.

<u>LEMMA 3.1.</u> For a function $\varphi \in \mathcal{L}_1^n$, the condition

$$\int_\Gamma \varphi(t)t^k dt = 0 , \quad k = 0,\dots,l \tag{3.10}$$

is fulfilled if and only if the function $Q\varphi$ has a zero of order not less than $l + 2$ at infinity.

<u>Proof.</u> In virtue of Theorem 1.24, for $k \geq 0$, we have

$$\int_\Gamma (P\varphi)(t)t^k dt = 0 , \quad \text{hence} \quad \int_\Gamma \varphi(t)t^k dt = \int_\Gamma (Q\varphi)(t)t^k dt .$$

The restrictions of the function $Q\varphi$ on $\mathfrak{D}^+(j)$ are of classes $E_1(\mathfrak{D}^+(j))$, $j = 1,\dots,m-1$. Consequently,

$$\int_{\Gamma(j)} (Q\varphi)(t)t^k dt = 0 \quad (j = 1,\dots,m-1; \quad k \geq 0)$$

and therefore,

$$\int_\Gamma (Q\varphi)(t)t^k dt = \int_{\Gamma(0)} (Q\varphi)(t)t^k dt .$$

Let us represent the function $Q\varphi$ in the form $(Q\varphi)(z) = \psi(z) + \sum_{s=1}^{l+1} a_s z^s$, where a_s $(s = 1,\dots,l+1)$ are constants, and ψ is a function having a zero of order equal or greater than $l + 2$ at infinity. Then, for $k = 0,\dots,l$,

$$\int_{\Gamma(0)} (Q\varphi)(t)t^k dt = \int_{\Gamma(0)} \psi(t)t^k dt + \sum_{s=1}^{l+1} a_s \int_{\Gamma(0)} t^{k-s} dt = 2\pi i a_{k+1} .$$

In this way, condition (3.10) is fulfilled if and only if $a_{k+1} = 0$ for $k = 0,\dots,l$, i.e. function $(Q\varphi)(z)$ coincides with $\psi(z)$. Thus Lemma 3.1 is proved. ≡

From this lemma we also deduce that, under the condition $(G'_-)^{-1}h \in \mathcal{L}_1^n$ (which is by Theorem 3.2' necessary for the solvability of problem (3.2)), relations (3.9') are equivalent to the following: if $\varkappa_j > 0$, then the j th component of the vector function $P(G'_-)^{-1}h$ has a zero of order not less than $\varkappa_j$ at the point $z = 0$.

THEOREM 3.3. Let the matrix function G be factorable in L_p. Then the image of problem (3.1) ((3.2), respectively) contains all rational vector functions satisfying conditions (3.9) ((3.9')).

Proof. Above all, note that if $g(z) = (z - z_o)^{-k} e_j$, where $z_o \in \mathfrak{D}^+$ and k is a natural number, then, denoting the j th column of the matrix function G_+^{-1} by φ, we get successively:

$$(G_+^{-1}g)(z) = (z-z_o)^{-k}\varphi(z) \in (M_q^+)^n ,$$

$$(QG_+^{-1}g)(z) = \sum_{s=o}^{k-1} \frac{1}{s!} \varphi^{(s)}(z_o)(z-z_o)^{s-k} ,$$

$$(PG_+^{-1}g)(z) = (z-z_o)^{-k} \left(\varphi(z) - \sum_{s=o}^{k-1} \frac{(z-z_o)^s}{s!} \varphi^{(s)}(z_o)\right) ,$$

$$(G_+PG_+^{-1}g)(z) = (z-z_o)^{-k}\left(e_j - \sum_{s=o}^{k-1} \frac{(z-z_o)^s}{s!} G_+(z) \varphi^{(s)}(z_o)\right) .$$

Therefore,

$$G_+^{-1}g \in \mathcal{L}_1^n , \quad G_+PG_+^{-1}g \in (L_p^+)^n , \quad QG_+^{-1}g \in (\overset{\circ}{L}{}_\infty^-)^n . \tag{3.11}$$

Since any rational function vanishing at infinity the poles of which lie in $\mathfrak{D}^+$ may be represented as the linear combination of functions of the form $(z - z_o)^{-k}$, and any vector function - as the sum of vector functions each of which has only one non-zero component, conditions (3.11) are satisfied for all rational vector functions vanishing at infinity with poles in $\mathfrak{D}^+$.[1)]

If $g \in (L_p^+)^n$, then $G_+^{-1}g \in (L_1^+)^n$, $PG_+^{-1}g = G_+^{-1}g$, hence $G_+PG_+^{-1}g = g$, and conditions (3.11) are also fulfilled. Consequently, the conditions (3.11) are fulfilled for all vector functions from R^n regardless of where their poles are located.

If, for the vector function $g \in R^n$, conditions (3.9) are satisfied, then according to Lemma 3.1, the j th component of $QG_+^{-1}g$ has a zero of order not less than $1 - \varkappa_j$ (if $\varkappa_j < 0$) at infinity. Therefore,

---

1) Compare with analogous arguments in the proof of Theorem 1.35.

from relations $QG_+^{-1}g \in (\overset{\circ}{L}{}_\infty^-)^n$ and (3.9) we conclude that $\Lambda^{-1}QG_+^{-1}g \in (\overset{\circ}{L}{}_\infty^-)^n$ and, thus, $G_-^{-1}\Lambda^{-1}QG_+^{-1}g \in (\overset{\circ}{L}{}_p^-)^n$.

Consequently, for a vector function from R^n satisfying conditions (3.9), the requirements (3.5) are fulfilled. Owing to Theorem 3.2, such a vector function belongs to the image of problem (3.1).

It can be verified in a similar way that any vector function from R^n satisfying conditions (3.9') belongs to the image of problem (3.2). ≡

COROLLARY 3.2. In the case of a matrix function G which can be factored in L_p, a vector function from L_p^n (L_q^n) belongs to the closure of the image of problem (3.1) ((3.2) respectively) iff conditions (3.9) ((3.9')) are satisfied.

Proof. Conditions (3.9) generate a lineal $\mathcal{L}$ of finite codimension in L_p^n, which is closed in view of Corollary 1.1. Since R^n is dense in L_p^n; we deduce by Theorem 1.3 that rational vector functions satisfying conditions (3.9) form a dense lineal in $\mathcal{L}$. In summary, the image of problem (3.1) lies in the closed set $\mathcal{L}$ (due to Corollary 3.1), but contains a subset dense in it (by Theorem 3.3). Consequently, the closure of the image of problem (3.1) coincides with $\mathcal{L}$. The argument for the statement related to problem (3.2) is similar. ≡

3.2. A CRITERION OF FACTORABILITY

According to Theorem 3.3, from the factorability of the matrix function G in L_p with partial indices equal to zero it follows that the lineal R^n belongs to the image of the problems (3.1) and (3.2). The converse assertion proves also to be true. Moreover, this converse assertion may be strengthened.

THEOREM 3.4. Let there exist linearly independent systems $\{a_j\}_{j=1}^n$ and $\{b_j\}_{j=1}^n$ of constant vectors such that the vector functions $t^{-1}a_j$ lie in the image of problem (3.1) and b_j in the image of problem (3.2). Then the matrix function G can be factored in L_p and all its partial indices are equal to zero.

Proof. By assumption, there exist vector functions $\varphi_j^+ \in (E_p^+)^n$,

$\varphi_j^- \in (\overset{\circ}{E}{}_p^-)^n$ for the boundary values of which the equation $\varphi_j^+(t) + G(t)\varphi_j^-(t) = t^{-1}a_j$ holds a.e. on Γ. Denote by X that matrix function the j th column of which is $z\varphi_j^-(z)$. Obviously $X \in E_p^-$. Since $tG(t)\varphi_j^-(t) = a_j - t\varphi_j^+(t)$, the matrix function $F = GX$ is an element of class L_p^+ and $F(0) = (a_1,\dots,a_n)$, so that $\det F(0) \neq 0$. Furthermore, there are vector function $\psi_j^+ \in (E_q^+)^n$, $\psi_j^- \in (\overset{\circ}{E}{}_q^-)^n$ such that $\psi_j^-(t) + G'(t)\psi_j^+(t) = b_j$ $(j = 1,\dots,n)$. Therefore, the matrix function $Y = (\psi_1^+,\dots,\psi_n^+)$ belongs to the class E_q^+, and $H = G'Y = (b_1 - \psi_1^-,\dots,b_n - \psi_n^-)$ belongs to E_q^-. Besides, $H(\infty) = (b_1,\dots,b_n)$, thus $\det H(\infty) \neq 0$.

Now we consider the matrix function $Z = Y'GX$. On the one hand, $Y'GX = H'X$, where $H \in L_q^-$, $X \in L_p^-$, so that $Z \in L_1^-$. On the other hand, $Z = Y'F$, where $Y \in L_q^+$, $F \in L_p^+$, thus $Z \in L_1^+$. According to Theorem 1.28, Z is a constant matrix. We now intend to show that it is non-degenerating. If $\det Z = 0$, then $\det H \cdot \det X = 0$ in the domain $\mathcal{D}^-$. Because $\det H(\infty) \neq 0$ and the function $\det H(z)$ is analytic in $\mathcal{D}^-(0)$, the set of its zeros in $\mathcal{D}^-(0)$ is at most countable and has points of condensation only on Γ. Consequently, $\det X$ vanishes on a subset of $\mathcal{D}^-(0)$ having a non-empty interior. Owing to the analyticity, $\det X = 0$ in the domain $\mathcal{D}^-(0)$ and, thus, a.e. on Γ. This implies, in particular, that the function $\det F$, which is analytic in $\mathcal{D}^+(0)$, has angular limits equal to zero a.e. on the boundary. From Theorem 1.23 we conclude that $\det F = 0$ in $\mathcal{D}^+$. At the same time $\det F(0) \neq 0$. The contradiction obtained proves the non-degeneracy of the matrix Z.

Setting $G_+ = F$, $G_- = Z^{-1}H'$, we obtain $G_+ \in L_p^+$, $G_- \in L_q^-$, $G_+^{-1} = Z^{-1}Y' \in L_q^+$, $G_-^{-1} = X \in L_p^-$ and $G_+G_- = FZ^{-1}H' = GXZ^{-1}Y'G = G$.

In this way, the matrix function G is factorable in L_p and all its partial indices are equal to zero. Theorem 3.4 is proved. ≡

Consequently, we have obtained a criterion of factorability in case of zero partial indices. Before formulating the corresponding criterion in the general case, we state another auxiliary proposition.

LEMMA 3.2.

1) Let the kernel of problem (3.1) be finite dimensional, and assume all "−"-components of a vector function from R^n orthogonal to it (in the sense of the form (1.13)) to lie in the image of problem (3.2). Then there is a rational matrix function F not having poles and non-degenerating on Γ such that the problem

$$\varphi^+(t) + G(t)F(t)\varphi^-(t) = g(t) \qquad (3.12)$$

has the same image as problem (3.1), and the problem

$$\psi^-(t) + (G(t)F(t))'\psi^+(t) = h(t) \qquad (3.13)$$

associate to it has the same set of "+"-components of the kernel as problem (3.2) and an image containing R^n.

2) Let the kernel of problem (3.2) be finite dimensional. Furthermore, all "+"-components of a vector function from R^n orthogonal to it are assumed to belong to the image of problem (3.1). Then there exists a rational matrix function H not having poles and non-degenerating on Γ such that the Riemann problem with matrix coefficient HG has the same set of "−"-components of the kernel as problem (3.1) and an image containing R^n. The problem associate to it has the same image as problem (3.2).

Proof. We shall verify only assertion 1); the argument for assertion 2) is similar.

If the kernel of the initial proolem (3.1) is trivial, then it is sufficient to set $F = I$. However, if problem (3.1) has a nontrivial kernel, then there exist a point $z_0 \in \mathcal{D}^-$ and a number j $(1 \leq j \leq n)$ such that the j th coordinate of the "−"-component of some solution $\{\varphi_0^+, \varphi_0^-\}$ of the homogeneous problem (3.1) does not vanish at the point z_0. Consider the problems (3.12) and (3.13), choosing as F the matrix function

$$F_{j,z_0}(z) = \operatorname{diag}[1,\dots,1,\ \ 1 - z_0/z,\ \ 1,\dots,1],$$

where the element $1 - z_0/z$ stands at the j th place. The multiplication by such a matrix function is a linear injective mapping of $(\overset{\circ}{L}{}_p^-)^n$

onto the class $(L_p^-)_j^n$ of those vector functions from $(\mathring{L}_p^-)^n$ the j th component of which vanishes at the point z_0. Therefore, after substituting $F\varphi^- = \varphi_1^-$, problem (3.12) may be rewritten in the form

$$\varphi^+ + G\varphi_1^- = g \quad (\varphi^+ \in (L_p^+)^n, \quad \varphi_1^- \in (L_p^-)_j^n) . \tag{3.14}$$

Since the class $(L_p^-)_j^n$ is narrower than $(\mathring{L}_p^-)^n$, the kernel and the image of problem (3.14) are contained in the kernel and the image, respectively, of problem (3.1). Now we are going to show that, in fact, the images of problems (3.1) and (3.14) coincide and the dimension of the kernel of problem (3.14) is smaller than the dimension of the kernel of problem (3.1) by exactly one. For this purpose, starting from the representation $g = \varphi^+ + G\varphi^-$ $(\varphi^+ \in (L_p^+)^n, \varphi^- \in (L_p^-)^n)$ of an arbitrary element from the image of problem (3.1), we write $g = (\varphi^+ - \lambda\varphi_0^+) + G(\varphi^- - \lambda\varphi_0^-)$, where λ is the relation between the j th coordinates of the vectors $\varphi^-(z_0)$ and $\varphi_0^-(z_0)$. Clearly, $\varphi^+ - \lambda\varphi_0^+ \in (L_p^+)^n$, $\varphi^- - \lambda\varphi_0^- \in (L_p^-)_j^n$, hence the vector function g belongs to the image of problem (3.14). The assertion on the dimension of the kernel of problem (3.14) results from the fact that the pair $\{\varphi_0^+, \varphi_0^-\}$ belongs to the kernel of problem (3.1), but not of problem (3.14), and any other pair $\{\varphi^+, \varphi^-\}$ from the kernel of problem (3.1) may be represented as the sum of an element of the kernel of problem (3.14) and a scalar multiple of the pair $\{\varphi_0^+, \varphi_0^-\}$.

Now we proceed to problem (3.13), rewriting it in the form

$$\psi_1^- - \lambda h_0 + G'\psi^+ = h_1 . \tag{3.15}$$

Here $h_1 = F_{j,z_0}^{-1} h$, $h_0(z) = (z-z_0)^{-1} e_j$, $\psi_1^- = F_{j,z_0}^{-1}\psi^- + \lambda h_0$ and, in addition to the vector functions $\psi^+ \in (L_q^+)^n$ and $\psi_1^- \in (\mathring{L}_q^-)^n$, we seek also for the scalar λ.

Evidently, the image of problem (3.15) is a lineal generated by the image of problem (3.2) and the vector funktion h_0. The latter does not belong to the image of problem (3.2), as

$$\int_\Gamma (h_0(t))'\varphi_0^-(t)dt = \int_\Gamma \varphi_0^-(t)e_j \frac{d\tau}{t-z_0} = -2\pi i(\varphi_0^-(z_0))_j \neq 0 .$$

That means, the necessary solvability condition for the associate problem stated in assertion 2) of Theorem 3.1 is not fulfilled for h_o. By assumption, the codimension in R^n of the intersection of R^n with the image of problem (3.2) is equal to the dimension α of the kernel of problem (3.1) and, consequently, finite. Therefore, the codimension in R^n of the intersection of R^n with the image of problem (3.15) is equal to $\alpha - 1$. Since the multiplication by F_{j,z_o} is a linear isomorphism of the lineal R^n onto itself, the intersection of R^n with the image of problem (3.13) has the same codimension in R^n.

The homogeneous problem (3.13) leads to the homogeneous problem (3.15), i.e. to the problem (3.2) with right-hand side λh_o. Because the vector function h_o does not belong to the image of problem (3.2) as mentioned above, we have $\lambda = 0$. Consequently, the sets of "+"-components of the kernels of problems (3.2) and (3.13) coincide.
The above reasonings guarantee the validity of assertion 1) of Lemma 3.2 in case $\alpha = 1$. In the general case they may be considered as the first step of an induction showing that the desired matrix function F always exists and may be constructed in the form of a product of α multipliers of the kind F_{j,z_o}. ≡

THEOREM 3.5. The following statements are equivalent:

1) the matrix function G can be factored in L_p,
2) the indices of problems (3.1) and (3.2) are finite and opposite, and the image of either of them contains all rational vector functions belonging to its closure.

In this case the index of problem (3.1) coincides with the total index of G.

Proof. If condition 2) is satisfied, then in inequalities (3.4) the equality sign is attained. Therefore, the closure of the image of problem (3.2) coincides with the orthogonal (in the sense of form (1.13)) complement to the "-"-components of the kernel of problem (3.1). Moreover, the image of problem (3.2) contains all vector functions from R^n belonging to its closure. Thus, all the conditions of asser-

tion 1) of Lemma 3.2 are fulfilled.
Let F be the rational function, the existence of which is guaranteed by this assertion. Then the image of problem (3.12) contains all those vector functions from R^n which are orthogonal to the "−"-components of the kernel of problem (3.13) (because problems (3.1) and (3.2) have this property), and the image of problem (3.13) contains R^n. The kernel of problem (3.13) as well as the kernel of problem (3.2) are finite dimensional. Consequently, the conditions of assertion 2) of Lemma 3.2 are satisfied. Therefore, there exists a rational matrix function H with poles and the zeros of the determinant off Γ and, moreover, such that the image of the Riemann problem with matrix coefficient HGF contains R^n, and the image of the associate problem coincides with the image of problem (3.13) and, therefore, contains also R^n. According to Theorem 3.4, the matrix function HGF can be factored in L_p. But then, by Theorem 2.11, the initial matrix function G is also factorable in L_p. Consequently, 2) implies 1).

Vise versa, let G be factorable in L_p. Owing to Corollary 3.2, the closure of the image of problem (3.1) coincides with the subspace $\mathfrak{L}$ generated in L_p^n by conditions (3.9). All rational vector functions from this subspace belong, by Theorem 3.3, to the image of problem (3.1). Moreover, since the conditions (3.9) are linearly independent, the codimension of the subset $\mathfrak{L}$ coincides with the number of these conditions, i.e. with the dimension of the kernel of problem (3.2).
Hence $\beta_1 = \alpha_2$. Analogously, it can be deduced that all rational vector functions lying in the closure of the image of problem (3.2) lie in the image itself, and $\beta_2 = \alpha_1$. From here and from formulae (3.8) we obtain for the defect numbers α_1 and α_2:

$$\alpha_1 - \beta_1 = -(\alpha_2 - \beta_2) = \alpha_1 - \alpha_2 = \sum_{j=1}^{n} \max\{\varkappa_j, 0\},$$

$$-\sum_{j=1}^{n} \max\{-\varkappa_j, 0\} = \sum_{j=1}^{n} (\max\{\varkappa_j, 0\} + \min\{\varkappa_j, 0\}) = \sum_{j=1}^{n} \varkappa_j .$$

In this way, the implication 1) ==> 2), the formula for the indices of problem (3.1) and, together with them, the complete Theorem 3.5 have been proved. ≡

Notice that for the factorability of a matrix function G, it does not suffice to assume only finiteness and opposite indices in problems (3.1) and (3.2). Any matrix function $G \in L_\infty$ which is not factorable in L_p, but in L_{p_1} and L_{p_2} for some $p_1 < p$ and $p_2 > p$ yields an example for this. As a matter of fact, the factorability of G in L_p implies that the kernel of problem (3.1) is finite dimensional in $L^n_{p_1}$ and, therefore, also in the narrower space L^n_p. Similarly, finite dimension of the kernel of problem (3.2) in L^n_q is a consequence of factorability of G in L_{p_2}. Consequently, the ddfect numbers α_1 and α_2 are finite. From the condition $G \in L_\infty$ and by Theorem 3.1 it follows that the indices of problems (3.1) and (3.2) are finite and opposite, in spite of the absence of a factorization of G in L_p. As a concrete example we may cite the power function $\psi(t) = t^{1/q}$. According to Theorem 2.5, under sufficiently general assumptions on the contour Γ, this function can be factored in L_r for $r \in (1,p)$ and $r \in (p,\infty)$, but it cannot be factored in L_p.

3.3. ON THE NORMAL SOLVABILITY OF THE VECTOR-VALUED RIEMANN BOUNDARY VALUE PROBLEM AND THE PROBLEM ASSOCIATE TO IT

As in Section 3.1, we assume the matrix function G to be factorable in L_p. Under this condition, the index of problem (3.1) and of (3.2) is finite. Therefore, the normal solvability of any of them is equivalent to its Fredholmness. Moreover, in view of Corollary 3.2, to say that problem (3.1) (or (3.2)) is normally solvable amounts to saying that conditions (3.9) (or (3.9') respectively), which are necessary for its solvability, are also sufficient.

In the present section we shall obtain a criterion of normal solvability of problems (3.1) and (3.2) formulated in terms of the factorization factors of G. We have to consider operators of the form ATB in L^n_p, where A and B are measurable matrix functions of n th order and T is one of the operators P, Q or S. We assume that the domain of definition of these operators is the lineal of vector functions $\varphi \in L_p^n$ for which $\chi = B\varphi \in \mathcal{L}_1^n$ (so that the vector function $T\chi$ is well-defined) and $AT\chi \in L_p^n$. Simple properties of operators of the form ATB, but which are of some significance to what follows, are gathered in the following lemma.

LEMMA 3.3.

1) If the operator ATB is defined on the whole space L_p^n, then $B \in L_q$; if, in addition, the matrix function B is non-degenerate a.e., then $A \in L_p$,
2) if A, $B^{-1} \in L_p$, then the operator ATB is densely defined,
3) if A^{-1}, $B \in L_q$, then the operator ATB is closed,
4) if the operator ATB is defined and bounded on L_p^n, then the matrix function B is non-degenerate a.e., and if X is a rational $n\times n$ matrix function with poles off Γ and non-degenerating on Γ, then the operator $AXTX^{-1}B$ is also defined and bounded on L_p^n.

Proof. 1) If the operator ATB is defined on L_p^n, then, in particular, $B\varphi \in \mathcal{L}_1^n$ for all $\varphi \in L_p^n$. Since $\mathcal{L}_1^n \subseteq L_1^n$, we deduce from here that $B \in L_q$. Furthermore, if the matrix function B^{-1} is defined a.e., we set $\varphi = B^{-1}\chi e_j$, where χ is a scalar function of class L_∞ different from zero, for which $B^{-1}\chi \in L_p$ (one may take, for instance $\chi(t) = \|B^{-1}(t)\|^{-1}$, if $\|B^{-1}(t)\| \geq 1$, and $\chi(t) = 1$ otherwise). Then we have $\varphi \in L_p^n$ and, by assumption, $\chi e_j = B\varphi \in \mathcal{L}_1^n$. We choose an integer k in such a way that the function $Q(z^k\chi)$ has a simple zero at infinity. One can easily verify that in this case $T(z^{k+1}\chi e_j) - zT(z^k\chi e_j) = ce_j$, where c is a constant different from zero.

Thus, $ATB(z^{k+1}\varphi) - zATB(z^k\varphi) = cAe_j$. Since the left-hand side of the latter equation is the difference of two vector functions from L_p^n, we conclude from this that $Ae_j \in L_p^n$. The relation obtained is valid for $j = 1,\ldots,n$, which means $A \in L_p$.

2) Under the conditions $A, B^{-1} \in L_p$, all vector functions of the form $\varphi = B^{-1}\chi$ belong to the domain of definition of the operator ATB, where $\chi \in R^n$. Indeed, for such vector functions the condition $B\varphi \in \mathcal{L}_1^n$ is obviously fulfilled. Moreover, $ATB\varphi \in L_p^n$, since $TB\varphi = T\chi \in R^n$ and $A \in L_p$. With regard to the condition $B^{-1} \in L_p$, the lineal $B^{-1}R^n$ is contained in L_p^n. Now we are going to show that it is a dense subset of L_p^n. If the vector function ψ $(\in L_q^n)$ is orthogonal to all vector functions from $B^{-1}R^n$, i.e.

$$\int_\Gamma \psi'(t)B^{-1}(t)\chi(t)dt = 0, \quad \chi \in R^n,$$

then the vector function $(B')^{-1}\psi$ $(\in L_1^n)$ is orthogonal to R^n and, thus, equal to zero a.e. Along with this, the vector function ψ is also equal to zero a.e. Consequently, there are no nontrivial elements in L_q^n orthogonal to the lineal $B^{-1}R^n$, which proves the density of this lineal in L_p^n.

3) Let $\{\varphi_k\}_{k=1}^\infty$ be a sequence of vector functions from the domain of the operator ATB, and let $\psi_k = ATB\varphi_k$, where the sequences $\{\varphi_k\}$ and $\{\psi_k\}$ converge in L_p^n to the vector functions φ and ψ, respectively. Then $f_k = B\varphi_k \in \mathcal{L}_1^n$ and, provided that $B \in L_q$, we may claim that the sequence $\{f_k\}$ converges in L_1^n to the vector function $f = B\varphi$. Analogously, under the condition $A^{-1} \in L_q$, the sequence $\{g_k\}$ of vector functions $g_k = A^{-1}\psi_k$ converges in L_1^n to the vector function $g = A^{-1}\psi$.

But $g_k = Tf_k$. This and the closedness of the operator T in L_1^n, which holds by Theorem 1.31, imply that $f \in \mathcal{L}_1^n$ and $Tf = g$. Consequently, for the limit φ of the sequence $\{\varphi_k\}$, we have $B\varphi \in \mathcal{L}_1^n$, $ATB\varphi = ATf = Ag = \psi \in L_p^n$. In other words, the vector function φ belongs to the domain of the operator ATB. Furthermore, $ATB\varphi = \psi$, which proves the closedness of operator ATB.

We verify assertion 4), say, for the case $T = P$. Since the operator ATB is defined on the whole space, condition (1.22) is satisfied for all $\varphi \in L_p^n$. But then, evidently, $X^{-1}B\varphi \in \mathcal{L}_1^n$ for all $\varphi \in L_p^n$.

In addition, by assertion 1) of the present lemma, $A \in L_p$ and $B \in L_q$, because the operator ATB is defined everywhere. Applying Theorem 1.35 to the case $F = X$ (replacing the matrix function B by $X^{-1}B$), we observe that the operators $APXQX^{-1}B$ and $AQXPX^{-1}B$ are finite dimensional and bounded on the whole of L_p^n. At the same time, equation

$$AXPX^{-1}B = APB - APXQX^{-1}B + AQXPX^{-1}B$$

is valid, which can be directly verified. Consequently, the operator $AXPX^{-1}B$ is also defined and bounded on L_p^n. Lemma 3.3 is completely proved. ≡

<u>THEOREM 3.6.</u> Let the matrix function G be factorable in L_p. For the normal solvability (and, thus, the Fredholmness) of problem (3.1), it is necessary and sufficient that the operators

$$K = G_-^{-1} \Lambda^{-1} Q G_+^{-1} \quad \text{and} \quad K_1 = G_+ P G_+^{-1} \tag{3.16}$$

be bounded in the space L_p^n.

<u>Proof.</u> According to assertions 2) and 3) of Lemma 3.3, the operators K and K_1 are densely defined and closed. Consequently, they are bounded if and only if they are defined on the whole space, i.e., if and only if, for all $g \in L_p^n$, the conditions $G_+^{-1} g \in \mathcal{L}_1^n$, $G_+ P G_+^{-1} g \in L_p^n$ and $G_-^{-1} \Lambda^{-1} Q G_+^{-1} g \in L_p^n$ are fulfilled. Furthermore, for rational vector functions g, relations (3.11) hold, as established in the proof of Theorem 3.3. With regard to the condition $t^{\varkappa_n} G_-^{-1} \Lambda^{-1} \in L_p^-$, we deduce from this theorem that

$$\begin{gathered} G_+^{-1} g \in \mathcal{L}_1^n, \quad G_+ P G_+^{-1} g \in (L_p^+)^n, \\ t^{\varkappa_n} G_-^{-1} \Lambda^{-1} Q G_+^{-1} g \in (\mathring{L}_p^-)^n . \end{gathered} \tag{3.17}$$

In case of bounded operators K and K_1, relations (3.17) allow for transferring to arbitrary vector functions g from L_p^n by passing to the limit. In this way, the operators K and K_1 are bounded in L_p^n if and only if conditions (3.17) are satisfied for all $g \in L_p^n$. In view of assertion 1) of Theorem 3.2, conditions (3.17), at any rate, are fulfilled for all vector functions g from the image of problem (3.1). Therefore, if problem (3.1) is normally solvable, then conditions (3.17) are fulfilled on the subspace of finite codimension generated by relations (3.9). Owing to Theorem 1.3, we may choose a direct complement to this subspace lying in R^n, i.e. in the set of such vector functions which also satisfy conditions (3.17). In virtue of the linearity of conditions (3.17), we may assert that they are fulfilled for all vector functions from L_p^n.

Conversely, if conditions (3.17) are satisfied for all vector functions from L_p^n, then by Lemma 3.1, we may claim that for those $g \in L_p^n$ which satisfy the requirements (3.9) the more rigorous relations (3.5) hold. In accordance with Theorem 3.2, such vector functions belong to the image of problem (3.1). Consequently, problem (3.1) is normally solvable, and Theorem 3.6 is proved. ≡

<u>Remark.</u> The requirement of boundedness of the operator $G_+PG_+^{-1}$ amounts to demanding that either of the operators $G_+QG_+^{-1}$ and $G_+SG_+^{-1}$ is bounded.

<u>COROLLARY 3.3.</u> Let $G \in L_\infty$ be a matrix function factorable in L_p. Problem (3.1) is Fredholm if and only if the operator K is bounded in the space L_p^n.

<u>Proof.</u> The necessity of the mentioned condition follows from Theorem 3.6. To prove the sufficiency, we note that, under the condition $G \in L_\infty$, the operator GK is a part of operator $G_+QG_+^{-1}$. Therefore, if $K \in [L_p^n]$, then we have also $G_+QG_+^{-1} \in [L_p^n]$. ≡

The next theorem related to the normal solvability of the associate problem can be proved by similar arguments as Theorem 3.6.

<u>THEOREM 3.6'.</u> Let the matrix function G be factorable in L_p. For the normal solvability (and, thus, for the Fredholmness) of problem (3.2) in the space L_q^n, it is necessary and sufficient that the operators

$$K' = (G'_+)^{-1} \Lambda^{-1} P(G'_-)^{-1} \quad \text{and} \quad K'_1 = G'_-Q(G'_-)^{-1}$$

be bounded in the space L_q^n. Instead of the operator K_1' we may consider any of the operators $G_-'P(G_-')^{-1}$ and $G_-'S(G_-')^{-1}$.

COROLLARY 3.3'. Let $G \in L_\infty$ be a matrix function factorable in L_p. Problem (3.2) is Fredholm if and only if the operator K' is bounded in the space L_q^n.

In the following, we are interested in relationships between the normal solvability of problem (3.1) and (3.2).

In order to compare the criteria of normal solvability of these problems in a more convenient manner, we need the following result.

LEMMA 3.4. The operator K' is bounded in the space L_q^n iff the operator K is bounded in L_p^n. The boundedness of the operator K_1' in L_q^n is equivalent to the boundedness of the operator $G_-^{-1}SG_-$ in L_p^n.

Proof. Consider the operators K' and $G_-^{-1}Q\Lambda^{-1}G_+^{-1}$ acting in the spaces L_q^n and L_p^n, respectively. For arbitrary vector functions f from the domain of K', and g from the domain of $G_-^{-1}Q\Lambda^{-1}G_+^{-1}$, we have $\langle K'f,g\rangle = \langle (G_+')^{-1}\Lambda^{-1}P(G_-')^{-1}f,g\rangle = \langle P(G_-')^{-1}f,\Lambda^{-1}G_+^{-1}g\rangle =$ $\langle (G_-')^{-1}f, Q\Lambda^{-1}G_+^{-1}g\rangle = \langle f,G_-^{-1}Q\Lambda^{-1}G_+^{-1}g\rangle$ (in this calculation assertion 2) of Theorem 1.31 has been used).
In this way, the operators K' and $G_-^{-1}Q\Lambda^{-1}G_+^{-1}$ are adjoint to each other in the sense of Definition 1.6. Being densely defined by assertion 2) of Lemma 3.3, these operators are bounded only simultaneously. Furthermore, due to assertion 3) of the same lemma, the operator $G_-^{-1}Q\Lambda^{-1}G_+^{-1}$ is closed and therefore bounded if and only if it is defined on the whole space. Applying now assertion 4) of Lemma 3.3 for $A = G_-^{-1}$, $B = \Lambda^{-1}G_+^{-1}$ and $X = \Lambda^{-1}$, we find that the operator $G_-^{-1}Q\Lambda^{-1}G_+^{-1}$ is bounded only together with the operator $G_-^{-1}\Lambda^{-1}QG_+^{-1} = K$.
The second statement of the lemma results from the fact that the operators $G_-'S(G_-')^{-1}$ and $G_-^{-1}SG_-^{-1}$ considered in L_q^n and L_p^n, respectively, are densely defined and adjoint to each other. ≡

From Corollaries 3.3, 3.3' and the first assertion of Lemma 3.4 we derive following result.

THEOREM 3.7. Assume G to be a bounded measurable matrix function factorable in L_p. Then problems (3.1) and (3.2) are normally solvable (Fredholm) only simultaneously.

At the end of Section 3.5 we shall construct examples of factorable (of course, unbounded) functions for which the operators $G_+SG_+^{-1}$ and K are bounded, but the operator $G_-SG_-^{-1}$ is unbounded. In doing so, the existence of a matrix function G will be proved for which problem (3.1) is Fredholm, but problem (3.2) fails to be normally solvable.

3.4. LEFT AND RIGHT Φ-FACTORIZATION. A CRITERION OF SIMULTANEOUS FREDHOLMNESS OF THE RIEMANN BOUNDARY VALUE PROBLEM AND THE ASSOCIATE PROBLEM TO IT

It is clear from Theorem 3.6 that among all matrix functions which can be factored in L_p a special role is played by those functions for which the operators (3.16) are bounded in the space L_p^n. Therefore, it is convenient to introduce a shortened notation for factorizations satisfying the additional condition just mentioned.

DEFINITION 3.1. A factorization (2.1) of a certain matrix function G in L_p will be called a Φ-factorization, if the operators $K = G_-^{-1}\Lambda^{-1}QG_+^{-1}$ and $K_1 = G_+PG_+^{-1}$ associated with it are bounded in L_p^n.

Above all, we intend to show that Φ-factorability is a property depending only on the matrix function itself as well as the value of the parameter p, but not on the concrete choice of the factorization.

THEOREM 3.8. Two different factorizations of a matrix function G in L_p are either both Φ-factorizations or neither of them is a such one.

Proof. According to Theorem 3.6, a factorization of G in L_p is a Φ-factorization if and only if problem (3.1) with the matrix coefficient G is normally solvable, i.e. irrespective of which factorization from all possible ones has been chosen. ≡

We may also give a direct proof based upon Theorem 2.2 on the general form of a factorization and assertion 4) of Lemma 3.3. However, it is omitted here.

The domain of Φ-factorability $\Phi(G)$ may be defined in a similar manner as it was done for the factorability domain $\mathfrak{F}(G)$. Obviously $\Phi(G) \subseteq \mathfrak{F}(G)$. More exactly, $\Phi(G) = \bigcup_k \Phi_k(G)$, where $\Phi_k(G)$ $(\subseteq \mathfrak{F}_k(G))$ is the set of such values p for which the matrix function G admits a Φ-factorization in the space L_p with total index k. The next theorem shows that $\Phi_k(G)$ is a connected subset of $\mathfrak{F}_k(G)$.

THEOREM 3.9 (Interpolation theorem). Assume that the matrix function G admits a Φ-factorization with one and the same total index in L_{p_1} and L_{p_2} $(p_1 \leq p_2)$. Then G admits a Φ-factorization in all L_p, where $p \in [p_1,p_2]$.

Proof. Suppose that equation (2.1) provides a Φ-factorization of G in L_p. As in the proof of Corollary 2.2, we establish that (2.1) is a factorization of G in L_p $(p_1 \leq p \leq p_2)$, which is, due to Theorem 3.8, a Φ-factorization of G in L_{p_2}. Thus, the operators (3.16) are bounded in the spaces $L^n_{p_1}$ and $L^n_{p_2}$. By Theorem 1.13, they are bounded in L^n_p, $p \in [p_1,p_2]$, either. Consequently, (2.1) is a Φ-factorization of G in L_p for any $p \in [p_1,p_2]$. Theorem 3.9 is proved. ≡

The class of transformations preserving the factorability of a matrix function, which was considered in Theorem 2.11, preserves, actually, also the Φ-factorability. Now we are going to show this.

THEOREM 3.10. Let G be a matrix function admiting a Φ-factorization in L_p, and suppose B_+ and B_- to be matrix functions belonging together with their inverses to classes M^+_∞ and M^-_∞, respectively. Then the matrix function $\hat{G} = B_+GB_-$ admits a Φ-factorization in L_p, too.

Proof. On the strength of formulae (2.23) and the remark after Theorem 2.10, we may claim that the factorization factors of G and $\hat{G}$ are connected by the relations

$$\hat{G}_+ = B_+G_+X , \quad \hat{G}_- = \hat{\Lambda}^{-1}X^{-1}\Lambda\, G_-B_- ,$$

where X is some rational matrix function not having poles and non-degenerating on Γ. In accordance with this, the operators constructed analogously to formulae (3.16) are, for $\hat{G}$, of the form

$$\hat{K} = \hat{G}_-^{-1}\hat{\Lambda}^{-1}Q\hat{G}_+^{-1} = B_-^{-1}G_-^{-1}\Lambda^{-1}XQX^{-1}G_+^{-1}B_+^{-1},$$

$$\hat{K}_1 = \hat{G}_+P\hat{G}_+^{-1} = B_+G_+XPX^{-1}G_+^{-1}B_+^{-1}.$$

Due to assertion 4) of Lemma 3.3, the boundedness of the operators $K = G_-^{-1}\Lambda^{-1}QG_+^{-1}$ and $K_1 = G_+PG_+^{-1}$ implies the boundedness of operators $G_-^{-1}\Lambda^{-1}XQX^{-1}G_+^{-1}$ and $G_+XPX^{-1}G_+^{-1}$. Multiplying the first of them from the left by B_-^{-1} and the second one by B_+, and both from the right by B_+^{-1}, in view of the condition $B_\pm^{\pm 1} \in L_\infty$, we do not go beyond the class of bounded operators. Moreover, it is easy to see, that we just obtain the operators $\hat{K}$ and $\hat{K}_1$, which proves Theorem 3.10. ≡

Above problem (3.1) was viewed as the main subject and problem (3.2) as an auxiliary one. As a matter of fact, they are completely equivalent. If we assume

$$\varphi^-(t) + G(t)\varphi^+(t) = g(t) \qquad (3.18)$$

to be the initial problem and $\psi^+(t) + G'(t)\psi^-(t) = h(t)$ the problem constructed by it, then the right-factorization of G will be the natural means of investigation. On the condition that G admits a right factorization in L_q, the normal solvability (and Fredholmness) of problem (3.18) in L_q^n is equivalent to the boundedness of the operators $G_-QG_-^{-1}$ and $G_+^{-1}\Lambda^{-1}PG_-^{-1}$ in L_q^n (after obvious transformations this result is a direct consequence of Theorem 3.6').

In accordance with this, representation (2.1') of the matrix function G is said to be its right Φ-factorization (in L_q), as soon as the operators $G_-QG_-^{-1}$ and $G_+\Lambda^{-1}PG_-^{-1}$ are bounded in L_q^n. For the sake of uniformity, a Φ-factorization of the form (2.1), when it occures besides a right Φ-factorization, is referred to as a left Φ-factorization. With the help of the notions introduced we formulate the crucial result of the present chapter.

THEOREM 3.11. The following assertions are equivalent:

1) problems (3.1) and (3.2) are Fredholm and their indices are opposite,

2) the matrix function G is Φ-factorable from the left in L_p, and the matrix function G' is Φ-factorable from the right in L_q.

<u>Proof.</u> Suppose assertion 1) to be fulfilled. Then, in particular, the indices of Problems (3.1) and (3.2) are finite and opposite, and the images of these problems involve all vector functions from R^n belonging to their closure. According to Theorem 3.5, G is factorable in L_p (and, thus, G' is factorable from the right in L_q). Since, in addition, problems (3.1) and (3.2) are normally solvable, with regard to Theorems 3.6 and 3.6', we deduce that a (left) factorization of G in L_p and a (right) factorization of G' in L_q are Φ-factorizations. Consequently, 1) implies 2).
Vice versa, if 2) applies, then, thanks to Theorems 3.6 and 3.6' respectively, problems (3.1) and (3.2) are Fredholm and their indices are opposite by Theorem 3.5. Thus Theorem 3.11 is proved. ≡

In case $G \in L_\infty$, the indices of problems (3.1) and (3.2) are automatically opposite, in virtue of Theorem 3.1. Moreover, by restating Theorem 3.7, with regard to the definition of a right Φ-factorization, we obtain the following result.

<u>THEOREM 3.7'.</u> The matrix function $G \in L_\infty$ admits a left Φ-factorization in L_p if and only if the matrix function G' admits a right Φ-factorization.

Therefore, for bounded matrix functions, Theorem 3.11 admits the following simplification.

<u>COROLLARY 3.4.</u> If the matrix function G belongs to the class L_∞, then for the simultaneous Fredholmness of problems (3.1) and (3.2), it is necessary and sufficient for G to be Φ-factorable in L_p.

3.5. Φ-FACTORIZATION OF UNBOUNDED MATRIX FUNCTIONS ON CONTOURS OF CLASS $\mathfrak{R}$

Beginning with this section, we shall assume that the contour Γ belongs to class $\mathfrak{R}$. As noted in Section 1.1, under this condition, the spaces L_p^n $(1 < p < \infty)$ split into the direct sum of the subspaces $(L_p^+)^n$ and $(\overset{\circ}{L}{}_p^-)^n$, and P and Q are bounded projections related to the mentioned decomposition.

It is quite natural to emphasize the contours of class $\mathfrak{R}$ for the study of questions associated with Φ-factorization, as can be seen from the following theorem.

THEOREM 3.12. Let $G = A_+A_-$, where $A_+^{\pm 1} \in M_\infty^+$, $A_-^{\pm 1} \in M_\infty^-$. The condition $\Gamma \in \mathfrak{R}$ is necessary for the Φ-factorability of G in L_p for at least one value $p \in (1,\infty)$ and sufficient for its Φ-factorability for all such p .

Proof. According to Theorem 2.10 and the remark after it, the matrix function G admits a factorization (2.1) in which $G_+^{\pm 1} \in L_\infty^+$, $G_-^{\pm 1} \in L_\infty^-$. Therefore, the condition of boundedness of the operator $K = G_-^{-1}\Lambda^{-1}QG_+^{-1}$, which is necessary and sufficient (due to Corollary 3.3) for the Φ-factorability of G , is equivalent to the boundedness of the operator $Q = \frac{1}{2}(I-S)$. ≡

In this way, condition $\Gamma \in \mathfrak{R}$ is necessary for the Φ-factorability of rational and even constant non-degenerate matrix functions.

To the measurable matrix function G we assign the operator of multiplication by this matrix function in the space L_p^n , denoting it by the same letter G . We shall consider this operator on the lineal $\mathrm{dom}_p G$ of such vector functions $\varphi \in L_p^n$ for which $G\varphi \in L_p^n$. Apparently, the operator of multiplication defined in this fashion is closed. It is bounded if and only if $G \in L_\infty$. In the latter case, the norm of the operator of multiplication does not depend upon p for the norm in L_p^n introduced by us. Moreover, it can be calculated via the formula

$$\|G\| = \operatorname*{ess\,sup}_{t\in\Gamma} \|G(t)\|^{1)}. \tag{3.19}$$

In what follows, the operators $P + GQ$ and $Q + G'P$ defined on the lineals $(L_p^+)^n \dotplus ((\mathring{L}_p^-)^n \cap \mathrm{dom}_p G)$ and $((L_q^+)^n \cap \mathrm{dom}_q G') \dotplus (\mathring{L}_q^-)^n$, respectively, will play an important role. Obviously, these operators are closed. Problems (3.1) and (3.2) may be rewritten in the form $(P+GQ)\varphi = g$ and $(Q+G'P)\psi = h$, where the vector functions $\varphi \in L_p^n$ and $\psi \in L_q^n$ are taken from the domain of definition of the corresponding operator. Consequently, the image of the operator $P + GQ$ coincides with the image of problem (3.1), and $\varphi \in \ker(P+GQ)$ if and only if the pair $\{P\varphi, Q\varphi\}$ is the solution of the homogeneous problem (3.1). Therefore, the defect numbers of the operator $P + GQ$ coincide with the corresponding defect numbers of problem (3.1).
Besides, this operator is normally solvable, Fredholm etc. iff problem (3.1) possesses the corresponding property. The operator $Q + G'P$ is associated with problem (3.2) in an analogous manner.

Summarizing, in case $\Gamma \in \mathbf{R}$, Theorems 3.5 - 3.7 and 3.9 - 3.11 may be interpreted as conditions (necessary or sufficient) of finiteness of the index and Fredholmness of the operators $P + GQ$ and $Q + G'P$.
In the present section we shall obtain a necessary condition for $P + GQ$ and $Q + G'P$ to be Φ_--operators (of course, it will be also necessary for the Φ-factorability of the matrix function G). To this end, we need the following auxiliary result.

<u>LEMMA 3.4.</u> Let G be a measurable matrix function, such that G^{-1} does not belong to L_∞. Then, for all $\varepsilon > 0$, we may find a matrix function $G_1 \in L_\infty$ such that $\|G_1\| < \varepsilon$ and the matrix function $G - G_1$ degenerates on a set of positive measure.

---

1) We identify the matrix A with the operator of multiplication by A in the space $\mathbb{C}^n$ supplied with the scalar product $(x,y) = \sum x_j\bar{y}_j$, where $x = \sum x_j e_j$, $y = \sum y_j e_j$, and the norm $\|x\| = (x,x)^{1/2}$. In this case, the norm of A is the largest eigenvalue of its left modulus $(AA^*)^{1/2}$ (or, equivalently, of its right modulus $(A^*A)^{1/2}$).

Proof. Unboundedness of the matrix function G^{-1} means that, for all $\varepsilon > 0$, the set $\Gamma_\varepsilon = \{t \in \Gamma : \inf_{\|x\|=1} \|G(t)x\| < \varepsilon/3,\ x \in \mathbb{C}^n\}$ has positive measure. We represent the matrix function G as the limit of an almost everywhere converging sequence of matrix functions $G^{(k)}$ the elements of which are step functions. Due to Egorov's theorem, there exists a set Δ_ε of positive measure lying in Γ_ε on which the sequence $\{G^{(k)}\}$ converges uniformly. Now we choose a number k so large that $\|G^{(k)}(t)-G(t)\| < \varepsilon/3$ for all $t \in \Delta_\varepsilon$. Then $\inf_{\|x\|=1} \|G^{(k)}(t)x\| < 2\varepsilon/3$ for all $t \in \Delta_\varepsilon$. Therefore, we may choose a vector function $x(t)$ defined on Δ_ε with $\|x(t)\| = 1$ such that $\|G^{(k)}(t)x(t)\| < 2\varepsilon/3$. Since the elements of the matrix function $G^{(k)}$ are step functions, the elements of $x(t)$ can also be chosen as step functions. In doing so, we have $\|G(t)x(t)\| \leq \|G^{(k)}(t)x(t)\| + \|G(t)-G^{(k)}(t)\| < \varepsilon$. As G_1 we choose a matrix function equal to zero outside Δ_ε and defined by the equation $G_1(t)y = (y,x(t))G(t)x(t)$ on Δ_ε. The matrix function G_1 is measurable, because G and x are measurable.

Apparently, $\|G_1(t)\| = \begin{cases} 0, & t \notin \Delta_\varepsilon, \\ \|G(t)x(t)\|, & t \in \Delta_\varepsilon \end{cases}$ and, therefore, $\|G_1\| < \varepsilon$.

Further, $G_1(t)x(t) = G(t)x(t)$ for $t \in \Delta_\varepsilon$, so that the matrix function $G - G_1$ degenerates on the set Δ_ε. The proof of Lemma 3.4 is complete. ≡

Notice that in case $n = 1$ the assertion of the lemma is evident.

THEOREM 3.13. If at least one of the operators $P + GQ$ and $Q + G'P$ is a Φ_--operator, then $G^{-1} \in L_\infty$.

Proof. For the sake of definiteness, we consider the operator $P + GQ$. If it is a Φ_--operator, then by Theorem 1.4, there exists an $\varepsilon > 0$ such that the operator $P + G_1Q$ is also a Φ_--operator, as soon as $\|G-G_1\| < \varepsilon$. If, in addition, $G^{-1} \notin L_\infty$, then in view of Lemma 3.4, we may assume that G_1 degenerates on a set of positive measure.

Since the image of the operator $P + GQ$ is a subspace of finite codimension in L_p, it has a nontrivial intersection with any infinite-dimensional lineal contained in L_p^n, in particular, with the lineals M_j $(j = 1,\ldots,n)$ of those vector functions the j th component of which is a polynomial of t^{-1} vanishing at infinity, and the remaining components are identically equal to zero. In other words, there are vector functions $\varphi_j \in (L_p^+)^n$, $\varphi_j^- \in (\overset{\circ}{L}{}_p^-)^n$ and $h_j \in M_j$, $h_j(t) \not\equiv 0$ such that $\varphi_j^+ + G_1\varphi_j^- = h_j$. Composing the matrix functions Φ_+, Φ_- and H from the vector functions φ_j^+, φ_j^- and h_j respectively, taken as columns, we obtain $\Phi_+ + G_1\Phi_- = H$ or $H - \Phi_+ = G_1\Phi_-$, from which we conclude that $\det(H - \Phi_+) = \det(G_1\Phi_-)$ (a.e. on Γ). The left-hand side of the latter equation is a function of class $M_{p/n}^+$ having a pole at zero of at least n th order. Therefore, it is not identically zero. At the same time, its angular limits on Γ are equal to zero at almost all points at which the matrix function G_1 degenerates, i.e. on a set of positive measure. This contradicts Theorem 1.23, therefore, the supposition $G^{-1} \notin L_\infty$ is not consistent with the requirement that $P + GQ$ is a Φ_--operator. Theorem 3.13 is proved. ≡

COROLLARY 3.5. For the Φ-factorability of the matrix function G in some L_p, it is necessary that $G^{-1} \in L_\infty$ and $G \in L_1$.

Proof. The condition $G \in L_1$ is necessary for factorability, all the more, it is necessary for Φ-factorability. According to Theorem 3.6, Φ-factorability of G implies Fredholmness of the operator $P + GQ$, from which the inclusion $G^{-1} \in L_\infty$ follows, by Theorem 3.13. ≡

THEOREM 3.14. A left factorization of the matrix function G in L_p is its Φ-factorization if and only if $G^{-1} \in L_\infty$ and the operator $G_+SG_+^{-1}$ is bounded in the space L_p^n. A right factorization of G in L_p is its Φ-factorization iff $G^{-1} \in L_\infty$ and the operator $G_-SG_-^{-1}$ is bounded in L_p^n.

Proof. We intend to prove the first part of the theorem. The necessity of the condition $G^{-1} \in L_\infty$ for Φ-factorability of G is precisely Corollary 3.5; the boundedness of the operator $G_+SG_+^{-1}$ is equivalent to the boundedness of operator $G_+PG_+^{-1}$. The latter demand is involved in the definition of Φ-factorization. Conversely, if $G^{-1} \in L_\infty$ and the operator $G_+SG_+^{-1}$ (and, thus, also $G_+QG_+^{-1}$) is bounded, then the operator $G^{-1}G_+QG_+^{-1}$, a part of which is the first operator K from (3.16), is bounded. The argument concerning the second assertion is similar, thus the proof of Theorem 3.14 is complete. ≡

<u>COROLLARY 3.6.</u> The matrix function $G \in L_\infty$ is left (right) Φ-factorable in L_p if and only if the matrix function G^{-1} is right (left) Φ-factorable in L_p.

<u>Proof.</u> Assume the representation (2.1) to be a left Φ-factorization of $G \in L_\infty$ in L_p. By Theorem 3.14, $G^{-1} \in L_\infty$ and the operator $G_+SG_+^{-1}$ is bounded in L_p^n. In this case, the operator $G^{-1}(G_+SG_+^{-1})G = G_-^{-1}\Lambda^{-1}S\Lambda G_-$ and, consequently, also the operator $G_-^{-1}SG_-$ differing from it by a finite-dimensional bounded summand are bounded. Due to Theorem 3.14, the representation $G^{-1} = G_-^{-1}\Lambda^{-1}G_+^{-1}$ is a right Φ-factorization of G^{-1} in L_p. Hence, the right Φ-factorability of G^{-1} follows from the left Φ-factorability of the matrix function $G \in L_\infty$. The remaining assertions can be verified analogously. ≡

<u>COROLLARY 3.7.</u> The factorization

$$G(t) = G_+(t)t^{\varkappa}G_-(t) \tag{3.20}$$

of the scalar function G in L_p is a Φ-factorization if and only if $G^{-1} \in L_\infty$ and the operator S is bounded in the space L_p with weight $|G_+|^p$.

This result follows from Theorem 3.14 and the fact (verifiable by the very definition) that the boundedness of the operator fSf^{-1} in L_p is equivalent to the boundedness of S in the space L_p with weight $|f|^p$.

For a fairly wide class of contours (including, in particular, piecewise Lyapunov and smooth curves), a necessary and sufficient condition for the operator S to be bounded in the space L_p with weight ϱ is the following one:

$$\sup\{|\gamma|^{-1}(\int_\gamma \varrho(t)|dt|)^{1/p}(\int_\gamma \varrho(t)^{-q/p}|dt|)^{1/q}\} < \infty . \tag{3.21}$$

The supremum in (3.21) is taken over all arcs $\gamma \subseteq \Gamma$, and $|\gamma|$ denotes the length of arc γ.

In this way, the factorization (3.20) in L_p of the scalar function G defined on a contour from the class under study is its Φ-factorization if and only if $G^{-1} \in L_\infty$ and

$$\sup\{|\gamma|^{-1}(\int_\gamma |G_+(t)|^p|dt|)^{1/p}(\int_\gamma |G_+(t)|^{-q}|dt|)^{1/q}\} < \infty .$$

With the help of Theorem 3.14 one may obtain necessary and sufficient conditions of Φ-factorability of matrix functions from classes $M^{\pm}$.

<u>THEOREM 3.15.</u> The matrix function $G \in M^+$ is left Φ-factorable in L_p if and only if $G^{-1} \in M^+_\infty$ and the operator GSG^{-1} is defined on the whole space L_p^n. It is right Φ-factorable in L_p iff $G^{-1} \in M^+_\infty$ and $G \in L_q$.

<u>Proof.</u> Since the contour Γ belongs to class $\mathfrak{R}$ and is, specifically, a Smirnov curve, Theorem 2.8 can be applied, thanks to which the conditions $G \in L_p$, $G^{-1} \in M_q^+$ are necessary for G to be left factorable in L_p. According to Theorem 3.14, for the Φ-factorability of G it is necessary that $G^{-1} \in L_\infty$. Consequently, if the considered matrix function G $(\in M^+)$ is Φ-factorable in L_p, then $G^{-1} \in L_\infty \cap M_q^+ = M_\infty^+$.

Furthermore, if the relations $G \in L_p$, $G^{-1} \in M_\infty^+$ are fulfilled, then the matrix function $G \in M^+$ admits a factorization (2.1) with a rational matrix function G_- with poles and the zeros of the determinant only in $\mathfrak{D}^+$. In accordance with assertion 4) of Lemma 3.3, the operators $GSG^{-1} = G_+(\Lambda G_-)S(\Lambda G_-)^{-1}$ and $G_+SG_+^{-1}$ are bounded only simultaneously. Therefore, the condition of boundedness (or, equivalently, the condition to be defined everywhere) of the operator GSG^{-1} is also necessary for the Φ-factorability of G. Conversely, if this condition is satisfied, then by statement 1) of Lemma 3.3, we have $G \in L_p$. If, in addition, the condition $G^{-1} \in M_\infty^+$ applies, then, because of Theorem 2.8, G can be factored in L_p and the operator $G_+SG_+^{-1}$ is bounded (in view of the boundedness of GSG^{-1}).

The necessity of conditions $G \in L_q$ and $G^{-1} \in L_\infty$ for G to be right Φ-factorable in L_p can be verified analogously. However, they **prove** to be also sufficient, as the factorization factor G_- is a rational matrix function not having poles and non-degenerating on Γ and the operator $G_-SG_-^{-1}$ is bounded in L_p^n along with S. The proof of Theorem 3.15 is complete. $\equiv$

The argument for the following result differs only in detail from that given above, hence, it is omitted.

THEOREM 3.15'. The matrix function $G \in M^-$ is left Φ-factorable in L_p if and only if $G \in L_q$, $G^{-1} \in M_\infty^-$; it is right Φ-factorable in L_p iff $G^{-1} \in M_\infty^-$ and the operator GSG^{-1} is bounded in L_p^n.

Consider the outer function defined via formula (1.7). Let us assume that $k \in L_p$, $k^{-1} \in L_\infty$ and condition (3.21) is not fulfilled for any $p \in (1,\infty)$ substituting $\varrho = k^p$. Then, in view of Theorem 3.15, the function $f^{(e)}$ fails to be left Φ-factorable in L_p for any $p \in (1,\infty)$, although it is right Φ-factorable in L_p for all $p \in (1,\infty)$. Problem (3.1) with $G = f^{(e)}$ is not Fredholm, although the associate problem (3.2) is Fredholm.

It remains to specify a function k having the desired properties. Set $k(\theta) = s$ for $2^{1-2s}-1 \le \frac{\theta}{\pi} < 2^{2-2s}-1$ and $k(\theta) = 1$ for $2^{2-2s}-1 \le \frac{\theta}{\pi} < 2^{3-2s}-1$ $(s = 1,2,\dots)$. Then $\int_{-\pi}^{\pi} k(\theta)^p d\theta =$ $\pi\left(\sum_{s=1}^{\infty} \frac{s^p}{2^{2s-1}} + \frac{4}{3}\right)$, so that $k \in L_p$ for all $p < \infty$, and $|k(\theta)| \ge 1$, thus $k^{-1} \in L_\infty$. Now we choose the interval $\gamma = \{e^{i\theta} : 2^{1-2s}-1 \le \frac{\theta}{\pi} < 2^{3-2s}-1\}$. Then

$$\int_\gamma k(\theta)^p d\theta = \pi(2^{2-2s} + s^p \cdot 2^{1-2s}), \quad \int_\gamma k(\theta)^{-q} d\theta = \pi(2^{2-2s} + s^{-q} \cdot 2^{1-2s})$$

and

$$\frac{1}{|\gamma|}\left(\int_\gamma k(\theta)^p d\theta\right)^{1/p}\left(\int_\gamma k(\theta)^{-q} d\theta\right)^{1/q} =$$

$$= \frac{2^{2s-1}}{3} \cdot (2^{2-2s} + s^p \cdot 2^{1-2s})^{1/p}(2^{2-2s} + s^{-q} \cdot 2^{1-2s})^{1/q} =$$

$$= \frac{1}{3}(2+s^p)^{1/p}(2+s^{-q})^{1/q}.$$

Passing to the limit $s \to \infty$, the expression obtained increases infinitely. Consequently, condition (3.21) is not fulfilled.

Utilizing Theorem 3.15', one may quote examples in which problem (3.1) is Fredholm, but the associate problem (3.2) is not Fredholm. Choosing a function $k \in L_\infty$ in such a way that $k^{-1} \notin L_\infty$, but $k^{-1} \in L_p$ for all $p < \infty$, we obtain, by Corollary 2.3, a function $f^{(e)}$ which is factorable in all spaces L_p, $p \in (1,\infty)$, but in none of them it is Φ-factorable, because the necessary condition for Φ-factorability $(f^{(e)})^{-1} \in L_\infty$ fails to be fulfilled.

3.6. Φ-FACTORIZATION OF BOUNDED MEASURABLE MATRIX FUNCTIONS ON CONTOURS OF CLASS $\mathfrak{R}$

Under the conditions $G \in L_\infty$ and $\Gamma \in \mathfrak{R}$, the operators $P + GQ$ and $Q + G'P$ are, obviously, defined and bounded on the whole of the space L_p^n, $1 < p < \infty$. We now introduce auxiliary operators

$$T_Q(G) = QG|_{\operatorname{im} Q} \text{ and } T_P(G') = PG'|_{\operatorname{im} P}, \qquad (3.22)$$

which will be considered in the spaces $(\overset{\circ}{L}{}_p^-)^n$ and $(L_q^+)^n$, respectively. These operators are also bounded and defined everywhere.

LEMMA 3.5.

1) The operator $P + GQ$ $(Q + G'P)$ considered in the space L_p^n (L_q^n) is normally solvable if and only if the operator $T_Q(G)$ $(T_P(G'))$ is normally solvable, and the corresponding defect numbers of these operators coincide;
2) the operators $T_Q(G)$ and $T_P(G')$ are normally solvable only simultaneously.

Proof. It is easily shown that $\operatorname{im}(P + GQ) = (L_p^+)^n \dotplus \operatorname{im} T_Q(G)$ and that $\varphi \in \ker(P + GQ)$ if and only if $\varphi^- = Q\varphi \in \ker T_Q(G)$, $P\varphi = -PG\varphi^-$. Assertion 1) for the pair of operators $P + GQ$ and $T_Q(G)$ follows from here immediately. Incidentally, this assertion may be proved by Corollary 1.2, representing the space L_p^n in the form of the direct sum $(\overset{\circ}{L}{}_p^-)^n \dotplus (L_p^+)^n$. In fact, for such a decomposition, the blocks of the operator $A = P + GQ$ in the representation (1.1) are $A_{11} = T_Q(G)$,

$A_{12} = 0$, $A_{22} = I|_{(L_p^+)^n}$, $A_{21} = PG|_{(\overset{\circ}{L}_p^-)^n}$ and the assumptions of Corollary 1.2 are satisfied, where m $(= \dim A_{21} \ker A_{11} / (\operatorname{im} A_{22} \cap A_{21} \ker A_{11})) = 0$.
The part of assertion 1) related to the operators $Q + G'P$ and $T_P(G')$ can be proved analogously. This is left to the reader.

Proceeding to the proof of assertion 2), first of all, note that the images of operators $T_Q(G)$ and $T_P(G')$ coincide with the images of operators QGQ (considered in L_p^n) and $PG'P$ (considered in L_q^n), respectively. Besides, the operators QGQ and $PG'P$ are adjoint to each other: if $f \in L_p^n$, $g \in L_q^n$, then by Theorem 1.31,

$$\langle QGQf, g \rangle = \langle QGQf, Pg \rangle = \langle GQf, Pg \rangle = \langle Qf, G'Pg \rangle = \langle Qf, PG'Pg \rangle = \langle f, PG'Pg \rangle .$$

According to Theorem 1.7, the images of operators QGQ (in L_p^n) and $PG'P$ (in L_q^n) are closed only simultaneously. Consequently, the operators $T_Q(G)$ and $T_P(G')$ have the same property, which proves Lemma 3.5. ≡

THEOREM 3.16. The matrix function $G \in L_\infty$ defined on a contour of class $\mathfrak{R}$ is Φ-factorable in L_p if and only if the operator $P + GQ$ is Fredholm in the space L_p^n . In this case, the dimension of the kernel of operator $P + GQ$ coincides with the sum of positive partial indices of G , the codimension of the image is opposite to the sum of negative partial indices, and the index is equal to the total index of G . The operator $K + K_1$ (where K and K_1 are defined by formulae (3.16)) is a two-sided regularizer for the operator $P + GQ$.

Proof. Comparing assertions 1) and 2) of Lemma 3.5, we find that the images of the operators $P + GQ$ (in L_p^n) and $Q + G'P$ (in L_q^n) are closed only simultaneously. Due to Theorem 3.1, the indices of these operators are also finite only simultaneously. Consequently, the Fredholmness of one of these operators is equivalent to the Fredholmness of the other. With regard to Corollary 3.4, this enables us to derive the criterion of Φ-factorability mentioned in the theorem. Taking Theorem 3.1 into consideration, the formulae for the defect numbers of the operator $P + GQ$ are obtained from relations (3.8).

Now we evaluate the product $K + K_1$ by $P + GQ$:

$$(K+K_1)(P+GQ) = (G_-^{-1}\Lambda^{-1}QG_+^{-1} + G_+PG_+^{-1})(P + G_+\Lambda G_-Q)$$
$$= G_-^{-1}\Lambda^{-1}QG_+^{-1}P + G_+PG_+^{-1}P + G_-^{-1}\Lambda^{-1}Q\Lambda G_-Q + G_+P\Lambda G_-Q$$
$$= G_-^{-1}\Lambda^{-1}QG_+^{-1}P + P - G_+QG_+^{-1}P + Q - G_-^{-1}\Lambda^{-1}P\Lambda G_-Q$$
$$+ G_+P\Lambda G_-Q = I + (G_-^{-1}\Lambda^{-1} - G_+)(QG_+^{-1}P - P\Lambda G_-Q) .$$

Taking into account that $QG_+^{-1}P = 0$ and that the operator $(G_-^{-1}\Lambda^{-1} - G_+)P\Lambda G_-Q$ is finite dimensional by Theorem 1.35, we recognize that $K + K_1$ is a left regularizer for $P + GQ$. Now we may either analogously check that the product $(P + GQ)(K + K_1)$ also differs from I by a finite-dimensional summand, or we may use that general fact that a left regularizer of a Fredholm operator is also its right regularizer. ≡

In the formulation of Theorem 3.16 the operator $P + GQ$ can be replaced by $T_Q(G)$; then the restriction of the operator K on $\operatorname{im} Q$ serves as a regularizer of this operator.

<u>COROLLARY 3.8.</u> The matrix function $G \in L_\infty$ is Φ-factorable in L_p with a non-negative (non-positive, zero) tuple of partial indices if and only if the operator $P + GQ$ is Fredholm and right-invertible (left-invertible, two-sided invertible) in the space L_p^n. In case of Φ-factorability of G with a non-positive (zero) tuple of partial indices, the operator $K + K_1$ is left (two-sided) inverse to the operator $P + GQ$. If the partial indices are non-negative, the operator $G_-^{-1}Q\Lambda^{-1}G_+^{-1} + K_1$, which differs from $K + K_1$ by a finite-dimensional summand, serves as a right inverse.

<u>Proof.</u> We have merely to verify the statement concerning the operators inverse to $P + GQ$. If all partial indices are non-positive, then in the transformations of the product $(K + K_1)(P + GQ)$ carried out above,

we have $\Lambda \in L_\infty^-$. Thus, the operator $P\Lambda G_-Q$ and along with it also $(G_-^{-1}\Lambda^{-1} - G_+)P\Lambda G_-Q$ is equal to zero. Consequently, in case of non-positive partial indices, we have $(K + K_1)(P + GQ) = I$, i.e., the operator $K + K_1$ is a left inverse for $P + GQ$. The remaining cases can be treated similarly. ≡

Now we intend to state several results without proof related to right Φ-factorization.

<u>THEOREM 3.16'.</u> The matrix function G admits a right Φ-factorization in L_p iff the operator $Q + GP$ is Fredholm in the space L_p^n. In this case the kernel dimension of $Q + GP$ is opposite to the sum of negative right indices of G, and the codimension of the image is equal to the sum of positive right indices.

<u>COROLLARY 3.8'.</u> The matrix function $G \in L$ admits a right Φ-factorization in L_p with a non-negative (non-positive, zero) tuple of partial indices if and only if the operator $Q + GP$ is Fredholm and left-invertible (right-invertible, two-sided invertible).

In Theorem 3.16' and Corollary 3.8' the operator $Q + GP$ can be replaced by $T_p(G)$.

As an example of some importance we take up the power functions regarded in Section 2.3. Suppose that the contour Γ belongs to class $\mathfrak{R}$ and condition (2.8) is fulfilled. The branch $\arg(t - t_0)$ continuous on $\Gamma \setminus \{t_0\}$ is assumed to be bounded (here t_0 is the chosen point of discontinuity of the function $\psi(t) = t^\alpha$). Then, in particular, the assumptions on the contour Γ stipulated in Theorem 2.5 are satisfied. The statement of this theorem can now be made more precise.

<u>THEOREM 3.17.</u> The domain of Φ-factorability of the function $\psi(t) = t^\alpha$ consists of one component filling the whole ray $(1,\infty)$ if $\operatorname{Re}\alpha$ is an integer, and consists of the two components $\left(1, \frac{1}{1-\{\operatorname{Re}\alpha\}}\right)$ and $\left(\frac{1}{1-\{\operatorname{Re}\alpha\}}, \infty\right)$ otherwise.

<u>Proof.</u> Let $p \in \left(\frac{1}{1-\{\operatorname{Re}\alpha\}}, \infty\right)$. In Theorem 2.5 it was proved that the representation (2.10), where $k = [\operatorname{Re}\alpha]$ and $\psi_{+,k}$ is a fixed branch

of the function $(z - t_o)^{\alpha-k}$, $t_o \in \Gamma$, is a factorization of ψ in L_p. Since $\psi^{-1} \in L_\infty$ and in view of Corollary 3.7, it suffices to prove the boundedness of the operator S in the space L_p with weight

$$|\psi_{+,k}(t)|^p = |t-t_o|^{p\{Re\ \alpha\}}\exp(-p\ Im\ \alpha\ \arg(t-t_o)) .$$

The boundedness condition for the function $\arg(t - t_o)$ allows us to substitute the considered weight by $|t - t_o|^{p\{Re\ \alpha\}}$. The boundedness of the operator S on a contour of class $\tilde{\mathfrak{R}}$ in the space L_p with such a weight results from a theorem of B.V. KHVEDELIDZE (see. e.g. NIKOLAĬCHUK [1], p.81).

If $\{Re\ \alpha\} = 0$, then there is nothing to prove. Otherwise, we still have to examine the case $p \in (1, \frac{1}{1-\{Re\ \alpha\}})$, which can be done analogously. The non-existence of a factorization and, thus, also of a Φ-factorization for $p = \frac{1}{1 - \{Re\ \alpha\}}$ $(\{Re\ \alpha\} \neq 0)$ was shown in Theorem 2.5. ≡

<u>Remark.</u> Theorem 3.17 remains true even without assumption (2.8). In fact, in verifying the existence of a factorization in L_p for the function t^α with $p \neq (1 - \{Re\ \alpha\})^{-1}$ (see Theorem 2.5) and the boundedness of the operator S in the space L_p with appropriate weight, we did not take advantage of condition (2.8). This condition plays an essential role only in the argument concerning the non-existence of a factorization in L_p with $p = \frac{1}{1 - \{Re\ \alpha\}}$. However, it appears that the non-existence of a Φ-factorization may be proved without using condition (2.8), too. The corresponding proof for arbitrary piecewise continuous functions will be given in Section 5.3. Therefore, it is omitted here.

Besides the operator $P + GQ$, we sometimes have to study operators of more general type, namely $AP + BQ$, where $A, B \in L_\infty$. In order to derive a criterion of Fredholmness for such an operator, we need the following auxiliary proposition.

LEMMA 3.6. If $G \in L_\infty$, then, for all $\varepsilon > 0$, there exists a matrix function $\hat{G} \in L_\infty$ such that $\|G - \hat{G}\| < \varepsilon$, $\hat{G}^{-1} \in L_\infty$.

Proof. The lemma will be proved by induction on the order k of G. For $k = 1$, the assertion to be proved is obvious. Assuming that it is true for $k = n-1$, we consider a $n \times n$ matrix function $G \in L_\infty$. Taking $\varepsilon > 0$, we choose a matrix function $(\hat{G}_{ij})_{i,j=1}^{n-1}$ differing from $(G_{ij})_{i,j=1}^{n-1}$ by less than $\varepsilon/2$ with respect to the norm, the determinant $a(t)$ of which satisfies the relation $a^{-1} \in L_\infty$ (by the induction hypothesis, this can always be done).

Setting $\hat{G}_{in} = G_{in}$, $\hat{G}_{nj} = G_{nj}$ $(i,j = 1,\ldots,n-1)$, $\hat{G}_{nn}(t) = \varepsilon(t) + G_{nn}(t)$, where $|\varepsilon(t)| = \varepsilon/2$, $\arg \varepsilon(t) = \arg(\det G(t)/a(t))$, we have

$$|\det \hat{G}(t)| = |\det G(t)+a(t)\varepsilon(t)| = |\det G(t)|+|a(t)\varepsilon(t)| \geq \frac{\varepsilon}{2}|a(t)|.$$

Since $a^{-1} \in L_\infty$, the matrix function $\hat{G}$ also belongs to class L_∞. At the same time, $\|G - \hat{G}\| < \varepsilon$, which proves Lemma 3.6. $\equiv$

THEOREM 3.18. If A, $B \in L_\infty$ and $AP + BQ$ is a Φ_+- or Φ_--operator, then A^{-1}, $B^{-1} \in L_\infty$.

Proof. Let $AP + BQ$ be a Φ_--operator. Due to Theorem 1.4, there exists an $\varepsilon > 0$ such that if $\|A - A_1\| < \varepsilon$, then $A_1P + BQ$ is also a Φ_--operator. In accordance with Lemma 3.6, we may assume that $A_1^{-1} \in L_\infty$. But then, along with operator $A_1P + BQ$, the operator $A_1^{-1}(A_1P + BQ) = P + A_1^{-1}BQ$ is also Fredholm. In view of Theorem 3.13, the matrix function $B^{-1}A_1$ inverse to $A_1^{-1}B$ belongs to the class L_∞. Therefore, B^{-1} $(= B^{-1}A_1A_1^{-1})$ also belongs to L_∞.

Furthermore, for $B \in L_\infty$, $Q + B^{-1}AP$ is a Φ_--operator together with $AP + BQ$. Using Theorem 3.13 again (that part related to operators of the kind $Q + GP$), we observe that $A^{-1}B \in L_\infty$. From this we get $A^{-1} \in L_\infty$.

If $AP + BQ$ is a Φ_+-operator, then arguing as above, we conclude that $P + A_1^{-1}BQ$ is a Φ_+-operator. In virtue of Lemma 3.5 and Theorem 3.1, $Q + (A_1^{-1}B)'P$ is then a Φ_--operator.

The further argument is trivial. $\equiv$

THEOREM 3.19. Let A and B be $n \times n$ matrix function of class L_∞. The operator $AP + BQ$ is Fredholm in L_p^n if and only if $A^{-1} \in L_\infty$ and the matrix function $G = A^{-1}B$ is Φ-factorable in L_p. In this case the kernel dimension of the operator $AP + BQ$ is equal to the sum of positive partial indices of G, and the codimension of the image is opposite to the sum of negative partial indices.

Proof. The necessity of the condition $A^{-1} \in L_\infty$ follows from the preceding theorem. If this condition applies, then in view of the equality $AP + BQ = A(P + GQ)$, the operators $AP + BQ$ and $P + GQ$ are Fredholm only simultaneously and have the same defect numbers. To complete the proof, we have to apply Theorem 3.16. ≡

Notice that the following condition will also be necessary and sufficient for the Fredholmness of the operator $AP + BQ$ in the space L_p^n : $B^{-1} \in L_\infty$ and the matrix function $B^{-1}A$ is Φ-factorable from the right in L_p.

Theorems 3.16 and 3.16' serve as a chain link, with the help of which results and methods of the theory of linear bounded operators can be used for the study of problems related to Φ-factorization. In particular, the stability property of Fredholmness under small perturbations (Theorem 1.4) leads to the next result.

THEOREM 3.20. If the matrix function $G \in L_\infty$ is Φ-factorable from the left (right) in L_p, then, for some $\varepsilon > 0$, the matrix function F is also Φ-factorable from the left (right) in L_p, as soon as $\|F - G\| < \varepsilon$, where the total indices of F and G coincide.

THEOREM 3.21.

1) Let Γ and L be two simple smooth closed contours, and assume β to be a diffeomorphism of the contour L onto Γ. The matrix function $G \in L_\infty$ defined on Γ is Φ-factorable from the left (right) in L_p iff $G_0 = G \circ \beta$ defined on L is Φ-factorable in L_p from the left (right), if β remains the orientation, and from the right (left), if β changes the orientation. In the first case the total index of G_0 is equal to the total index

of G, and in the second case it is opposite to it.

2) Assume Γ to be a closed contour consisting of m connected curves Γ_j, and let G be a measurable bounded matrix function defined on Γ. By G_j, $j = 0,\ldots,m-1$ we denote the matrix function defined on Γ_j and coinciding on it with G. The matrix function G is Φ-factorable from the left (right) in L_p if and only if the matrix function G_0 is Φ-factorable from the left (right) in L_p and G_j, $j = 1,\ldots,m-1$, are Φ-factorable from the right (left) in L_p. In this case the total index of G is equal to the left (right) total index of G_0 minus the right (left) total indices of G_j, $j = 1,\ldots,m-1$.

Proof. 1) We introduce the operator W mapping from $L_p^n(\Gamma)$ onto $L_p^n(L)$ by the rule $(W\varphi)(t) = \varphi(\beta(t))$. Clearly, W provides an isomorphism of the spaces $L_p^n(L)$ and $L_p^n(\Gamma)$. Therefore, $P + GQ$ is Fredholm iff the operator $W(P + GQ)W^{-1} = WPW^{-1} + WGQW^{-1} = WPW^{-1} + (WGW^{-1})(WQW^{-1}) = WPW^{-1} + G_0(WQW^{-1})$ is Fredholm.

If S_0 is the operator of singular integration along the contour L, then

$$((WSW^{-1} - S_0)\varphi)(t) = (WSW^{-1}\varphi)(t) - (S_0\varphi)(t) =$$

$$\frac{1}{\pi i}\int_\Gamma \varphi(\beta^{-1}(\zeta))\frac{d\zeta}{\zeta-\beta(t)} - \frac{1}{\pi i}\int_L \varphi(\tau)\frac{d\tau}{\tau-t}.$$

Now we assume that the mapping β preserves the orientation. Substituting $\zeta = \beta(\tau)$, $\tau \in L$ in the first integral, we get

$$((WSW^{-1}-S_0)\varphi)(t) = \frac{1}{\pi i}\int_L \varphi(\tau)\frac{\beta'(\tau)}{\beta(\tau)-\beta(t)}d\tau - \frac{1}{\pi i}\int_L \varphi(\tau)\frac{d\tau}{\tau-t}. \quad (3.22)$$

In this way, $WSW^{-1}-S_0$ is an integral operator with the kernel $\frac{1}{\pi i}\left(\frac{\beta'(\tau)}{\beta(\tau)-\beta(t)} - \frac{1}{\tau-t}\right)$. The compactness of such an operator was established in GRUDSKIǏ [1], GRUDSKIǏ, DYBIN [1][1] using a result of CALDERON [1]. Then the operators $WPW^{-1}-P_0$ and $WQW^{-1}-Q_0$ are also

[1] Note that if β' satisfies a Hölder condition, then the compactness of $WSW^{-1}-S_0$ simply results from the weak polarity of the kernel of this integral operator (cf. LITVINCHUK [3]).

compact, where $P_0 = \frac{1}{2}(I + S_0)$, $Q_0 = \frac{1}{2}(I - S_0)$. Therefore, the operators $WPW^{-1} + G_0WQW^{-1}$ and $P_0 + G_0Q_0$ differ from each other by a compact summand, thus, they are Fredholm only simultaneously and their indices coincide (Theorem 1.5).

In case the mapping β changes the orientation, the substitution $\zeta = \beta(\tau)$ leads to the change of sign preceding the first integral into equality (3.22). Consequently, already the operator $WSW^{-1}-S_0$ will be compact. From this we deduce the compactness of the operators $WPW^{-1}-Q_0$ and $WQW^{-1}-P_0$ in $L_p^n(L)$. Thus, the operators $WPW^{-1} + G_0WQW^{-1}$ and $Q_0 + G_0P_0$ are equivalent in the sense of Fredholmness. In view of Corollary 3.6, the Fredholmness of the last operator is equivalent to the Φ-factorability of the matrix function G_0 from the right, and the index of this operator is opposite to the (right) total index of G_0. To prove that part of assertion 1) which is related to the left Φ-factorization of G, it remains to apply Theorem 3.16 to the operator $P + GQ$. The case of right Φ-factorization can be treated analogously.

Proving assertion 2), we restrict ourselves to the case of left Φ-factorization of G. In the space $L_p^n(\Gamma)$ we introduce the operators Π_j $(j = 0,\ldots,m-1)$ of multiplication by a function equal to 1 on $\Gamma_{(j)}$ and to zero on the other components of the contour Γ. Evidently, Π_j is the projector of $L_p^n(\Gamma)$ on the subspace of vector functions equal to zero on all components of Γ with the exception of $\Gamma_{(j)}$. The space $L_p^n(\Gamma)$ is the direct sum of the images of operators Π_j. The projectors Π_j commute with the operator of multiplication by the matrix function G and, for $i \neq j$, $\Pi_i S \Pi_j$ is an integral operator with continuous kernel and therefore compact. Thus, Corollary 1.4 can be applied, owing to which the Fredholmness of the operator $P + GQ$ is equivalent to the Fredholmness of all operators $(\Pi_j P + G_j \Pi_j Q)|_{\mathrm{im}\,\Pi_j}$, and the index of the operator $P + GQ$ equals the sum of indices of these operators.

Since the contour Γ_0 is oriented anticlockwise, but the other $\Gamma_{(j)}$'s clockwise, $\Pi_j P|_{\text{im}\,\Pi_j}$ and $\Pi_j Q|_{\text{im}\,\Pi_j}$ are just the operators P and Q for the contour $\Gamma_{(0)}$ in case $j = 0$ and the operators Q and P, respectively, for the contours $\Gamma_{(j)}$ $(j = 1,\ldots,m-1)$. In order to complete the proof of Theorem 3.21, it remains to apply Theorem 3.16 to the operator $P + G_0Q$ and Theorem 3.16' to the operators $Q + G_jP$ $(j = 1,\ldots,m-1)$. ≡

For arbitrary $G \in L_\infty$, $P + GQ$ is an operator of local type. Indeed, for an arbitrary scalar function a, we have $(P + GQ)aI - a(P + GQ)$ $= (Pa - aP) + G(Qa - aQ) = (PaQ - QaP) + G(QaP - PaQ) = (I-G)(PaQ-QaP)$. In the function a is rational and has no poles on Γ, then from Theorem 1.35 we obtain the compactness (and even the finite rank property) of the operators PaQ and QaP and, along with them, of the difference $(P + GQ)aI - a(P + GQ)$.

Summarizing, the local principle can be applied to operators of type $P + GQ$. In order to formulate the result corresponding to Theorem 1.14 exclusively in terms of G, we introduce the following definition.

DEFINITION 3.2. The matrix functions G_1 and G_2 will be called *ε-locally equivalent* at the point $t_0 \in \Gamma$, if for all $\varepsilon > 0$, there exists an arc $\gamma(\ni t_0)$ such that $\|G_1(t) - G_2(t)\| < \varepsilon$ a.e. on γ.

THEOREM 3.22 (ε-local principle). Let G be a matrix function defined on Γ such that for all points $t \in \Gamma$ there exists a matrix function $G_t \in L_\infty$ which is Φ-factorable in L_p and ε-locally equivalent to G at the point t. Then G admits a Φ-factorization in L_p.

Proof. Obviously, under the conditions imposed on G, the relation $G \in L_\infty$ holds. We now introduce the operators $A = P + GQ$ and $A_t = P + G_tQ$. By assumption and according to Theorem 3.16, the operators A_t are Fredholm (and, thus, also locally Fredholm at the point t) for all $t \in \Gamma$. As $P + GQ$ is an operator of local type, its Fredholmness and, thus, the Φ-factorability of the matrix function G will be proved, as soon as we clarify that the operators A and A_t are equivalent at the point $t(\in \Gamma)$.

Taking a number $\varepsilon > 0$ arbitrarily, we choose an arc $\gamma(\ni t)$ in such a way that $\|G(\tau) - G_t(\tau)\| < \varepsilon\|Q\|^{-1}$ a.e. on γ (this is possible owing to the ε-local equivalence of G and G_t at t). By a we denote a function continuous on Γ which is equal to zero outside γ, takes values from the interval $[0,1]$ on γ, and equals 1 in some neighbourhood of the point t. Then we have

$$|a(A-A_t)| \leq \|a(A-A_t)\| = \|a(G-G_t)Q\| \leq \|a(G-G_t)\|\cdot\|Q\|$$

$$= \|Q\| \operatorname*{ess\,sup}_{\tau\in\gamma}\|a(\tau)(G(\tau)-G_t(\tau))\| \leq \|Q\|\cdot\operatorname*{ess\,sup}_{\tau\in\Gamma}\|G(\tau)-G_t(\tau)\| < \varepsilon .$$

Together with A and A_t, the operator $A - A_t$ is of local type. As mentioned in Section 1.1, for any function f continuous on Γ, the operator $f(A-A_t) - (A-A_t)fI$ is compact, In particular, we have $|a(A-A_t)| = |(A-A_t)aI|$ and, thus, $|(A-A_t)aI| < \varepsilon$.

Due to Definition 1.10, the operators A and A_t are equivalent at the point t, which proves Theorem 3.22. $\equiv$

A simple example of matrix functions ε-locally equivalent at a certain point t yield those matrix functions which coincide a.e. in a neighbourhood of this point. Now we mention the ε-local principle corresponding to this special case.

<u>COROLLARY 3.9.</u> Let the contour Γ be covered by the system $\{\gamma_j\}$ of open arcs. If one can, for given G, specify a collection of matrix functions $G_j \in L_\infty$ which are Φ-factorable in L_p such that $G_j(\tau) = G(\tau)$ a.e. on γ_j, then G is also Φ-factorable in L_p.

Sufficient conditions of Φ-factorability obtained via the ε-local principle will be derived in Chapter 8.

3.7. COMMENTS

The material explained in Section 3.1 - 3.5 is, in principle, taken from SPITKOVSKIĬ [13,14]. The results of Section 3.1 generalize the classical solution scheme for the Riemann boundary value problem based on factorization of its matrix coefficient (VEKUA [4], GAKHOV [3], MUSKHELISHVILI [1], KHVEDELIDZE [4]).

Assertion 3) of Theorem 3.1, under different assumptions on G ensuring, however, its factorability, was mentioned in GOHBERG [1], SIMONENKO [1,4]. Its validity for an arbitrary function of class L_∞ defined on the circle was, for $p = 2$, proved in COBURN [1] and, for arbitrary $p \in (1,\infty)$, in GOHBERG, KRUPNIK [3]. The proof conducted here is essentially that of COBURN [1].

In connection with Theorem 3.2 we still refer to MEUNARGIYA [3], where the general solution of problem (3.1) is obtained in a form containing the values of the unknown vector function and its derivatives explicitly.

Arguments close to those used in the proof of Theorem 3.4 the reader can find in GOHBERG, FELDMAN [3] as well as in IDEMEN [2], where the case of rational matrix functions given on the circle is examined, but also in HEINIG [1], where a similar approach was used for the inversion of operators $A = a + \sum_{j=1}^{N} b_j S c_j$ generalizing (from case $N = 1$) operators of the type $AP + BG$ (see also HEINIG/ROST [1]).

Theorems 3.5, 3.15, 3.15' are explained in SPITKOVSKIĬ [6]. The original variant of Theorems 3.15 and 3.15' can be found in SPITKOVSKIĬ [2]. In the same paper the interpolation property of Φ-factorability (Theorem 3.9) was mentioned. In connection with this, we refer to the article KUCHMENT [1], in which the interpolation property of Fredholmness with the same index for an arbitrary linear operator acting and bounded in an interpolation family of Banach spaces was proved.

The notion of Φ-factorization of a bounded measurable matrix function in L_p is due to I.B. SIMONENKO (for $p = 2$, in SIMONENKO [3,4], for the general case, in SIMONENKO [6]. Lemma 3.5 and Theorems 3.16, 3.21, 3.22 are also due to him.

In the case $n = 1$, the notion of Φ-factorization, in principle can be found also in DANILYUK [1,2] and WIDOM [1].

The term "Φ-factorization" was proposed in SPITKOVSKIǏ [2,13] and motivated by Theorem 3.16, according to which the operator $P + GQ$ is Fredholm, i.e., it is a Φ-operator if and only if the matrix function G is Φ-factorable.

Notice that operators of the type $T_P(F)$ and $T_Q(F)$ introduced at the beginning of Section 3.6 are known in the literature as Toeplitz operators, and the matrix function F is usually called the symbol of the corresponding operator. In this way, Lemma 3.5 allows us to reformulate all the assertions about operators of the kind $P + GQ$ and $Q + G'P$ in terms of Toeplitz operators and vice versa. The results of some authors are formulated for Toeplitz operators. Henceforth, we shall refer to such results having in mind their analogues for the operators $P + GQ$ and $Q + G'P$.

Theorems 3.6, 3.6' and 3.11 formulated in SPITKOVSKIǏ [6] are a natural extension of Theorem 3.16 to the case of a rectifiable contour and a matrix function not necessarily bounded, whereas Theorems 3.13 and 3.14 are generalizations of corresponding results of SIMONENKO [4,6] from the case $G \in L_\infty$, $\Gamma \in \mathcal{R}$ renouncing the restriction $G \in L_\infty$. Note that the requirement $\Gamma \in \mathcal{R}$ can here also be omitted (see SPITKOVSKIǏ [14]). Actually, Theorem 3.13 in the scalar case with $p = 2$ was proved in WIDOM [1] and, for real-valued functions, in HARTMAN, WINTNER[1].

The boundedness criterion (3.21) for the operator S in the space L_p with weight ϱ has been derived for the circle in HUNT, MUCKENHOUPT, WHEEDEN [1] and, for a smooth contour, in KOKILASHVILI [1]. In the same paper the sufficiency of condition (3.21) in case of piecewise smooth curves was mentioned, whereas the necessity in case of piecewise Lyapunov curves was established in KRUPNIK [5].

Theorem 3.17 (on the Φ-factorability of power functions) is an auxiliary result for the theory of Φ-factorization of piecewise continuous functions, with which we shall be concerned in Chapter 5. Appropriate references will also be given there.

Lemmas 3.4, 3.6 and Theorems 3.18, 3.19 are borrowed from KRUPNIK [3]. Finally, we insert some remarks on results not mentioned in the present chapter, but being directly related to it.

First of all, we refer to NYAGA [1] and DZHVARSHEĬSHVILI [1], where the study of the scalar Riemann boundary value problem on a rectifiable contour Γ in wider classes than $L_1^{\pm}$ has been initiated (in particular, in classes of functions which can be represented as a differentiated Cauchy integral). Under sufficiently general assumptions on the coefficient G, the scalar Riemann boundary value problem in classes different from L_p was studied in ANTONTSEV [1], KATS [1-3]. The papers of DANILOV [1], ZAPUSKALOVA, KATS [1], KATS [3] and SEIFULLAEV [1] are devoted to the investigation of new effects occurring in the theory of the scalar Riemann boundary value problem under weakened conditions on the contour Γ.
Operators of the type $T_{\mathcal{P}}(F) = \mathcal{P}F|_{\mathrm{im}\,\mathcal{P}}$, where $\mathcal{P}$ is an arbitrary (bounded) projector in some Banach space $\mathfrak{B}$ and F is an arbitrary operator from $[\mathfrak{B}]$, are an abstract analogue of Toeplitz operators. In particular, Wiener-Hopf operators, i.e. integral operators on the half-line with a kernel depending on the difference of the arguments can be represented in the form $T_{\mathcal{P}}(F)$. Therefore, the operators $T_{\mathcal{P}}(F)$ are referred to as generalized Toeplitz operators or generalized Wiener-Hopf operators. The general theory of such operators was created in DEVINATZ, SHINBROT [1]. Especially, (under some additional restrictions) the validity of the abstract analogue of Theorem 3.13 is shown there, namely, the necessity of the invertibility condition of the operator F for $T_{\mathcal{P}}(F)$ to be a Φ_+- or a Φ_--operator. For more results in this direction we refer to the recent monograph of SPECK [1]. Incidentally, note that the theory of systems of Wiener-Hopf equations is equivalent to the theory of operators $P + GQ$ and $Q + G'P$. This equivalence can be established with the help of the Fourier transform; for more detail concerning this topic, see GOHBERG, KREĬN [3], GOHBERG, FELDMAN [3].

In Ch. 8 of the book GOHBERG, FELDMAN [3] also other types of systems of integral equations are enumerated, the theory of which may be erected with the aid of results related to operators studied in the present chapter. In particular, the examination of operators of the form $AP + BQ$ has been suggested by the study of systems of so-called paired integral equations. A variety of types of integral eqations and problems of mathematical physics reducible to the Riemann boundary value problem were discussed in the monograph by GAKHOV and CHERSKIĬ [1] (see also Chapters 1-7 in GOHBERG, FELDMAN [3]).

Variants of the local principle (Theorem 3.22) can be found in CLANCEY, GOHBERG [1] and CLANCEY, GOSSELIN [1]. In CLANCEY, GOHBERG [1] the notion of local factorability of matrix functions was introduced (a matrix function $G \in L_\infty$ defined on Γ is called locally factorable at the point $t_0 \in \Gamma$, if there exist an open arc $\gamma \subseteq \Gamma$ containing this point, domains $\Omega^{\pm} \subseteq \mathcal{D}^{\pm}$ the boundary of which contains γ, and matrix functions $A_{\pm} \in E_p(\Omega^{\pm})$ such that $A_{\pm}^{-1} \in E_q(\Omega^{\pm})$, the operator $A_+SA_+^{-1}$ is bounded in $L_p^n(\gamma)$, and $G(t) = A_+(t)A_-(T)$ a.e. on γ). Furthermore, there was proved that the Φ-factorability of $G \in L_\infty$ is equivalent to its local factorability at every point of the contour. In CLANCEY, GOHBERG [2] it is established that in the scalar case for a Lyapunov contour Γ, the local factorability of the function G at the point t_0 implies the local Fredholmness of the operator $P + GQ$ at this point. For $p = 2$, the converse assertion is also true.

In CLANCEY, GOHBERG [2] it was mentioned that for $p \neq 2$ the question of validity of the converse assertion is still open. This problem has been solved by I.B. SIMONENKO, who in a series of papers (SIMONENKO [7-11]) successively renounced the restrictions on p, n and Γ and, finally, proved the equivalence of local Fredholmness of the operator $P + GQ$ and local factorability of the $n\times n$ -matrix function G (at the same point) for arbitrary $p \in (1,\infty)$, natural n and $\Gamma \in \mathfrak{R}$.

By SHNEĬBERG [1,2] it was recognized that the Fredholmness of an operator A in one space of an analytical scale implies its Fredholmness with the same index in any sufficiently close space of this scale in which the operator **A** is bounded. An immediate consequence of this result is that all components of the domain of Φ-factorability of a matrix function $G \in L_\infty$ defined on a contour of class $\mathcal{R}$ are open, which was proved in SPITKOVSKIǏ [9]. For a scalar function defined on a smooth or piecewise Lyapunov contour, the corresponding result follows from Corollary 3.7 as well as the properties of condition (3.21) discussed in MIAMEE, SALEHI [1]. In this case it appears that for an unbounded function G the set $\Phi(G)$ is not necessarily open (but $\Phi_k(G)$ is open in $\mathfrak{F}_k(G)$, $k \in \mathbb{Z}$).

CHAPTER 4. Φ-FACTORIZATION OF TRIANGULAR MATRIX FUNCTIONS AND REDUCIBLE TO THEM

If it is known that the scalar function G can be factored in L_p with index $\varkappa$, then its factorization may be constructed effectively. Let us explain this in more detail, assuming for the sake of simplicity the contour Γ to be connected. From the representation (3.20) with suitable selection of $\arg G(t)$, we obtain

$$\ln t^{-\varkappa}G(t) = \ln G_+(t) + \ln G_-(t) , \tag{4.1}$$

where the functions $\ln G_\pm$ are determined up to a constant summand.

Starting from the obvious inequality $\ln x < x$ $(x > 0)$, it is easy to deduce the relations

$$-\left(\frac{r}{q}\right)^r |G_+(z)|^{-q} < (\ln|G_+(z)|)^r < \left(\frac{r}{p}\right)^r |G_+(z)|^p$$

for all finite r.

Since $G_+ \in E_p^+$ and $G_+^{-1} \in E_q^+$, the last inequality implies that for the function $f(z) = \ln|G_+(z)|$, for all finite r, condition 3) of Definition 1.16 is fulfilled. Under sufficiently general assumptions on the contour Γ one can conclude that this condition is also fulfilled for the analytic function $\ln G_+$, the real part of which is $\ln|G_+|$. In other words, the function $\ln G_+$ belongs to the classes E_r^+, $r < \infty$.

By analogy, it can be established that $\ln G_- \in E_r^-$, $r < \infty$. Therefore, with regard to Theorem 1.28 and equation (1.19), from equation (4.1) we conclude that

$$\begin{aligned} G_+(z) &= C^{-1} \exp\left(\frac{1}{2\pi i} \int_\Gamma \ln \tau^{-\varkappa}G(\tau) \frac{d\tau}{\tau - z}\right), \quad z \in \mathcal{D}^+, \\ G_-(z) &= C \exp\left(-\frac{1}{2\pi i} \int_\Gamma \ln \tau^{-\varkappa}G(\tau) \frac{d\tau}{\tau - z}\right), \quad z \in \mathcal{D}^-, \end{aligned} \tag{4.2}$$

where C is a constant different from zero. The existence of a multiplier C is caused by that degree of arbitrariness with which, according to Theorem 2.2, the factorization is determined. Obviously, $C = G_-(\infty)$.

Our considerations essentially use the commutativity of multiplication. Thus, they fail to be true when turning to the matrix case. Indeed, trying to use formulae (4.2) for $n > 1$ (at least in case of partial indices and $C = I$, we obtain $G_+G_- = \exp(P \ln G) \exp(Q \ln G)$. Thus, the equation $G_+G_- = G$ is valid under the following necessary and sufficient condition:

$$\exp(P \ln G) \exp(Q \ln G) = \exp(P \ln G + Q \ln G) , \quad (4.3)$$

which is satisfied only in some isolated cases.

Up to now only a comparatively small number of examples is known, in which the factorization problem for a matrix function is solved with the same degree of effectiveness as in the scalar case, i.e., with the help of a finite number of algebraic operations and using the operators P and Q. Diagonal matrix functions yield a trivial example. For their factorization it suffices to factorize every diagonal element.

In this chapter we shall examine the factorization problem for triangular matrix functions. It turns out that this task may be solved effectively in the sense pointed out above. We also study some cases reducible to this problem. The contour Γ is assumed to belong to the class $\mathfrak{R}$, and the matrix function G defined on it is supposed to be an element of class L_∞.

In Section 4.1 a criterion of Φ-factorability of block-triangular matrix functions, for which the defect numbers of the corresponding Riemann problem are finite, will be established. From the mentioned criterion we deduce that the condition of Φ-factorability of the diagonal elements of a triangular matrix function is sufficient for Φ-factorability of the matrix function itself. It is shown that this condition is, generally speaking, not necessary. However, we succeed in specifying not too hard restrictions on the diagonal elements, under which their Φ-factorability is equivalent to the Φ-factorability of the triangular matrix function. In particular, these restrictions are fulfilled for arbitrary piecewise continuous functions, a fact which will permit us in Chapter 5 to deduce the criterion of Φ-factorability of piecewise continuous functions from the corresponding criterion for the scalar case.

In Section 4.2 we shall deal with triangular matrix functions with Φ-factorable diagonal elements. Here we investigate relationships between the partial indices of their diagonal elements. Moreover, an algorithm for constructing the factorization will be presented. It appears that in the special case when the indices of the diagonal elements of a triangular matrix function are equal to zero, its partial indices are also equal to zero and, therefore, they do not depend on the elements outside the diagonal. In the general case this is not so. For the study of the general case, a partial ordering over the set of tuples of n integers is introduced, and it is established that the set of partial indices of a triangular matrix function is majorized by the set of indices k_j of the diagonal elements in the sense of the ordering introduced. In doing so, the factorization itself is constructed effectively. Incidentally, remark that the partial ordering introduced here will also be used in Chapter 6 in connection with the study of the stability of partial indices of arbitrary matrix functions belonging to the class L_∞.

Furthermore, in Section 4.2 we shall formulate the criterion for coincidence of the partial indices with the numbers k_j, the indices of the diagonal elements. Such a coincidence holds, in particular, if the numbers k_j $(j = 1,\dots,n)$ differ from each other at most by one.

In Section 4.3 it will be shown that for second-order triangular matrix functions the problem of calculating the partial indices may be solved to the very end.

In Section 4.4 it will be established that functionally commutable matrix functions can be reduced to block-diagonal form with triangular blocks by a constant similarity transformation. In this case, Φ-factorability of the initial matrix function G is equivalent to Φ-factorability of all diagonal elements of the obtained matrix function F, and the partial indices of G are equal to the indices of the diagonal elements of F. For second-order matrix functions, a simple criterion of functional commutativity will be presented, which permits us to reduce the question of Φ-factorability of such matrix functions to the corresponding question for a pair of scalar functions which are effectively constructed by G.

As usually, the last section contains comments.

4.1. EXISTENCE PROBLEMS OF A Φ-FACTORIZATION OF TRIANGULAR MATRIX FUNCTIONS

We shall be interested in Φ-factorability both of lower and upper triangular matrix functions, where the factorization itself may also be left and right. In connection with this, mention that the multiplication from the left and from the right by the counteridentity matrix $[\delta_{i,n-j}]_1^n$ transforms upper (lower) triangular matrix functions into lower (upper) ones taking no influence on the left and right Φ-factorability and on the values of the partial indices. Moreover, the transposition operation also transfers upper (lower) triangular matrix functions into lower (upper) ones and, according to Theorem 3.7', a left (right) Φ-factorization in L_p changes into a right (left) Φ-factorization in L_q. These considerations allow us to transfer results obtained for a left Φ-factorization of lower triangular matrix functions to the remaining cases.

As an auxiliary step, examine a block-triangular matrix function G of the form

$$G = \begin{pmatrix} G_1 & 0 \\ H & G_2 \end{pmatrix}. \tag{4.4}$$

By n_j we denote the orders of the diagonal blocks G_j of this matrix function. Let $\mathfrak{B}_1$ ($\mathfrak{B}_2$, respectively) be the subspace of vector functions $f = \sum_{k=1}^{n} f_k e_k$ from the space $\mathfrak{B} = (\overset{\circ}{L}{}_p^-)^n$ such that $f_k = 0$ for $k = n_1+1,\dots,n$ ($k = 1,\dots,n_1$, respectively). Then of course, $\mathfrak{B} = \mathfrak{B}_1 \dotplus \mathfrak{B}_2$, and in the representation (1.1) of the operator $A = T_Q(G)$

we have: $A_{jj} = T_Q(G_j)$ $(j = 1,2)$, $A_{12} = 0$, $A_{21} = QH$.

Consequently, Theorem 1.12 may be used, due to which we obtain the following criterion of Fredholmness of the operator $T_Q(G)$, i.e. of Φ-factorability of the matrix function G .

THEOREM 4.1. A matrix function G of the form (4.4) is Φ-factorable in L_p if and only if the following conditions are satisfied:

1) the codimension β_1 of the lineal $\operatorname{im} T_Q(G_1)$ in $(\overset{\circ}{L}{}_p^-)^{n_1}$ is finite,
2) the dimension α_2 of the kernel of the operator $T_Q(G_2)$ is finite,
3) the dimension γ_1 of the lineal $\{\varphi \in \ker T_Q(G_1) : QH\varphi \in \operatorname{im} T_Q(G_2)\}$ is finite,
4) the codimension γ_2 of the lineal $\operatorname{im} T_Q(G_2) + QH \ker T_Q(G_1)$ in $(\overset{\circ}{L}{}_p^-)^{n_2}$ is finite.

If conditions 1) - 4) are satisfied, then for the defect numbers of problem (3.1) with the matrix coefficient G the formulae

$$\alpha = \alpha_2 + \gamma_1 , \qquad \beta = \beta_1 + \gamma_2 \tag{4.5}$$

are valid. Applying Corollaries 1.3 and 1.4 to the operator $T_Q(G)$, from Theorem 1.12 we obtain the following results.

COROLLARY 4.1. If one of the diagonal blocks G_1 and G_2 of the matrix function G of the form (4.4) is Φ-factorable, then the Φ-factorability of its second diagonal block is a necessary and sufficient condition for the Φ-factorability of the matrix function G itself. The defect numbers α , β and α_j , β_j of problems (3.1) with matrix coefficients G and G_j $(j = 1,2)$ respectively, are connected by the relations

$$\alpha = \alpha_1 + \alpha_2 - \gamma , \qquad \beta = \beta_1 + \beta_2 - \gamma , \tag{4.6}$$

where γ is the dimension of the direct complement to $\operatorname{im} T_Q(G_2) \cap QH \ker T_Q(G_1)$ in $QH \ker T_Q(G_1)$.

COROLLARY 4.2. A block-diagonal matrix function G is Φ-factorable iff all its diagonal blocks are Φ-factorable.

The necessary and sufficient condition of Φ-factorability of block-diagonal matrix functions formulated in Corollary 4.2 remains sufficient also in the general case of block-triangular matrix functions. To be more exact, the following result is valid.

THEOREM 4.2. Let the matrix function G be block-triangular, and let G_{jj} $(j = 1,\dots,k)$ be its diagonal blocks. Then the Φ-factorability of all matrix functions G_{jj} implies the Φ-factorability of G. Moreover, for the defect numbers α and β of problem (3.1) with matrix coefficient G, the following estimations are true:

$$\alpha \leq \sum_{j=1}^{k} \alpha_j , \quad \beta \leq \sum_{j=1}^{k} \beta_j ,$$

where α_j and β_j are the defect numbers of problem (3.1) with the matrix coefficient G_{jj} $(j = 1,\dots,k)$.

Proof. In view of the remarks made at the beginning of the present section, it suffices to examine the case of a lower block-triangular matrix function G. We prove the assertion for this case by induction on the number k of diagonal blocks of G. For $k = 1$, the statement to be proved is obvious. Supposing the statement to be correct for $k \leq k_0$, we shall study a block-triangular matrix function G for which $k = k_0 + 1$ and the diagonal blocks of which are Φ-factorable. We represent this matrix function in the form (4.4), setting $G_1 = G_{11}$. Then the matrix function G_2 is also block-triangular and we have for it $k = k_0$. By induction hypothesis, we can assert that G_2 is Φ-factorable and the defect numbers α' and β' of the corresponding Riemann problem satisfy the inequalities $\alpha' \leq \sum_{j=2}^{k} \alpha_j$ and $\beta' \leq \sum_{j=2}^{k} \beta_j$. Since, by assumption, the block G_1 is Φ-factorable, on the strength of Corollary 4.1, one can claim that the complete matrix function G is Φ-factorable and, moreover, $\alpha = \alpha_1 + \alpha' - \gamma \leq \alpha_1 + \alpha' \leq \sum_{j=1}^{k} \alpha_j$,

$\beta = \beta_1 + \beta' - \gamma \leq \beta_1 + \beta' \leq \sum_{j=1}^{k} \beta_j$.

Thus Theorem 4.2 has been proved. ≡

The next result is an immediate consequence of Theorem 4.2 in the case of one-dimensional diagonal blocks.

THEOREM 4.3. If all diagonal elements of the triangular matrix function G are Φ-factorable in L_p, then the matrix function G itself is Φ-factorable in L_p, too.

The sufficient conditions of Φ-factorability indicated in Theorem 4.3 are not necessary. To verify that, we study the question of Φ-factorability of triangular matrix functions of a special form given on the circle.

THEOREM 4.4. Let G be a matrix function of the form $\begin{pmatrix} \omega & 0 \\ 1 & \overline{\omega} \end{pmatrix}$ defined on T, where $\omega \in L_\infty$. Then for the Φ-factorability of G in L_2 it is necessary and sufficient for $T_Q(\omega)$ to be a Φ_--operator. In this case the partial indices are equal to $\pm\beta(T_Q(\omega))$.

Proof. Condition 1) of Theorem 4.1 shows that for the Φ-factorability of the matrix function under study, it is necessary for $T_Q(\omega)$ to be a Φ_--operator. Introducing in the space L_2^- a scalar product by the formula $(f,g) = \int_{-\pi}^{\pi} f(e^{i\theta})\overline{g(e^{i\theta})}d\theta$, we may regard the operator $T_Q(\omega)$ as the adjoint to $T_Q(\omega)$.[1] According to Theorem 1.7 and Corollary 1.2, to say that $T_Q(\omega)$ is a Φ_--operator amounts to saying that $T_Q(\overline{\omega})$ is a Φ_+-operator. Besides, the subspaces $\ker T_Q(\omega)$ and $\operatorname{im} T_Q(\overline{\omega})$ are orthogonal complements to each other. Taking into consideration that, for the considered matrix function, we have $H = I$, we find that in case of a Φ_--operator $T_Q(\omega)$ the conditions 1) - 4) of Theorem 4.1 are fulfilled, where $\gamma_1 = \gamma_2 = 0$ and $\alpha_2 = \beta_1 = \beta(T_Q(\omega))$. Consequently, the matrix function G is Φ-factorable in L_2 and, according to formulae (4.5), both defect numbers of the corresponding problem (3.1) coincide with the number $\beta(T_Q(\omega))$. Thus, the total index of G is equal to zero and, therefore, $\varkappa_1 = -\varkappa_2 = \alpha = \beta(T_Q(\omega))$. Theorem 4.4 is completely proved. ≡

If, in particular, the function ω belongs to the class H_∞, then $T_Q(\overline{\omega})$ coincides with the operator of multiplication by the function $\overline{\omega}$

---

[1] This can be established in the same way as the corresponding result for the operators QGQ and $PG'P$ from the proof of Lemma 3.5.

in the space L_2^-. Consequently, $\ker T_Q(\overline{\omega}) = \{0\}$ and $\operatorname{im} T_Q(\overline{\omega}) = \overline{\omega}L_2^-$. Hence, $T_Q(\overline{\omega})$ is a Φ_+-operator iff $\omega^{-1} \in L_\infty$. This condition, which is equivalent to the requirement concerning $T_Q(\omega)$ to be a Φ_--operator (and, thus, equivalent to the Φ-factorability of G), means only that the outer multiplier of the function ω is separated from zero, and does not impose any restrictions upon its inner multiplier. At the same time, for the factorability of the function ω (and $\overline{\omega}$) it is necessary (in view of Corollary 2.3) that its inner multiplier can be reduced to a finite Blaschke product. Choosing, for instance, the infinite Blaschke product as the function ω, we therefore obtain a triangular matrix function with non-factorable diagonal elements, which is Φ-factorable in L_2.

The example considered is based on the existence of such functions $\omega \in L_\infty$ for which $T_Q(\omega)$ is a Φ_-- or Φ_+-operator but not Fredholm. However, for a wide class of measurable bounded functions (including all piecewise continuous functions, as will be demonstrated in Chapter 5) such a situation is impossible. Let Φ denote the class of functions $\omega \in L_\infty$ for which $T_Q(\omega)$ is Fredholm. Then we have the following result

THEOREM 4.5. Let G be a triangular matrix function the diagonal elements of which (with the possible exception of one) belong to the class Φ. Then for the Φ-factorability of G in L_p it is necessary and sufficient that its diagonal elements be Φ-factorable in L_p.

Proof. The sufficiency follows from Theorem 4.3. In proving the necessity, we restrict ourselves to the case of a lower triangular matrix function G and use induction on its dimension n. In case $n = 1$, the statement is obvious. Supposing that it is true for $n = k$, we examine a lower triangular matrix function of $(k+1)$th order which is Φ-factorable in L_p. If at least k of its diagonal elements belong to the class Φ, then at least one of its left upper and right lower diagonal element is a member of this class. For the sake of definiteness, let the left upper element G_1 of the studied matrix function G be in class Φ.

Using Theorem 4.1 for $n_1 = 1$ and $n_2 = n-1$, we see that $T_Q(G_1)$ is a Φ_--operator. Because of the condition $G_1 \in \Phi$, we conclude from this that the operator is Fredholm, i.e., the function G_1 is Φ-factorable in L_p. With regard to Corollary 4.1, we thus obtain that the matrix function G_2 which is obtained from G by cancelling the first column and row can be factored in L_p. But G_2 is lower triangular, its order is equal to k and at least $k-1$ diagonal elements belong to the class Φ. Due to the induction hypothesis, the diagonal elements of the matrix function G_2 are Φ-factorable in L_p.
Therefore, the Φ-factorability of all diagonal elements of the matrix function G has been verified and, thus, Theorem 4.5 has been completely proved. Ξ

4.2. EFFECTIVE CONSTRUCTION OF A Φ-FACTORIZATION AND ESTIMATES FOR THE PARTIAL INDICES OF TRIANGULAR MATRIX FUNCTIONS WITH Φ-FACTORABLE DIAGONAL ELEMENTS

In accordance with Theorem 4.5, triangular matrix functions with Φ-factorable diagonal elements are Φ-factorable themselves. In this section we shall study the questions of calculating the partial indices of such matrix functions, their relationships with the indices of the diagonal elements and the effective construction of a factorization.

THEOREM 4.6. Let the diagonal elements of the upper (lower) triangular matrix function G be Φ-factorable in L_p, and let their indices be equal to zero. Then G is Φ-factorable in L_p, the partial indices of G are equal to zero, and the factorization factors $G_\pm$ may be chosen as upper (lower) triangular. The determination of the elements of the matrix functions $G_\pm$ leads to the solution of a finite number of scalar Riemann problems the coefficients of which are the diagonal elements of G.

Proof. Let us examine the case of a lower triangular matrix function. We try to find lower triangular matrix functions $F_\pm \in L_p^\pm$ satisfying the relation $F_+ = GF_-$, which may be elementwise rewritten in the form

$$f_{ij}^{+} - G_{ii}f_{ij}^{-} = \sum_{k=j}^{i-1} G_{ik}f_{kj}^{-} , \quad i \geq j . \tag{4.7}$$

We divide the equations of system (4.7) into groups, assigning to the l th group those of them for which $i-j = l$ $(l=0,\ldots,n-1)$. Equations of the zero group are of the form $f_{ii}^{+} = G_{ii}f_{ii}^{-}$ $(i=1,\ldots,n)$ and, under the condition $f_{ii}(\infty) = 1$, they possess a unique solution in view of the condition of factorability of the functions G_{ii} and since their indices are equal to zero.

If the solutions of all groups of equations (4.7) with numbers k less than the given l are already found, then the right-hand sides of the equations of the l th group are known (since condition $j \leq k < i$ means that $k-j < i-j = l$), moreover, they belong to L_p (because $G_{ik} \in L_\infty$ and $f_{kj}^{-} \in L_p$).

Considering, for $l > 0$, the equations of the l th group as scalar Riemann problems with respect to $f_{ij}^{+} \in L_p^{+}$ and $f_{ij}^{-} \in \overset{\circ}{L}{}_p^{-}$, we recognize, with regard to the conditions imposed upon G_{ii}, that all of them also may be solved and even in a unique manner. Consequently, with the help of mathematical induction, the solvability of system (4.7) has been proved, where on condition that $F_-(\infty) = I$, the solution is unique.

Analogously, one can prove the existence (and uniqueness) of upper triangular matrix functions $\Phi_\pm \in L_q^{\pm}$ such that $G'\Phi_+ = \Phi_-$, $\Phi_-(\infty) = I$. We consider the matrix function $Z = \Phi_+'F_+$. On the one hand, $\Phi_+ \in L_q^{+}$ and $F_+ \in L_p^{+}$, so that $Z \in L_1^{+}$. On the other hand, $\Phi_+'F_+ = \Phi_+'GF_- = \Phi_-'F_- \in L_1^{-}$, since $\Phi_- \in L_q^{-}$ and $F_- \in L_p^{-}$.

According to Theorem 1.28, the matrix function Z is constant. Moreover, $F_-(\infty) = \Phi_-(\infty) = I$, thus $Z = I$. Consequently, $F_-^{-1} = \Phi_-' \in L_q^{-}$, $F_+^{-1} = \Phi_+' \in L_q^{+}$. Hence it is clear that the representation $G = G_+G_-$ with $G_+ = F_+ = (\Phi_+')^{-1}$, $G_- = F_-^{-1} = \Phi_-'$ is a factorization of G in L_p with zero partial indices. According to Theorem 4.3, G is Φ-factorable in L_p, so that every factorization of it, including the factorization we have constructed, is a Φ-factorization (Theorem 3.8). Thus the proof is complete. ≡

Therefore, if the indices of the diagonal elements of a triangular matrix function are equal to zero, then its partial indices do not depend on the elements outside the diagonal. As we shall see later on, in the general case this is not true. In order to study the question of possible values of partial indices of a triangular matrix function with fixed diagonal elements, we must introduce a partial ordering on the set $\mathbb{Z}^n$ of tuples (k_j) of n integers.

DEFINITION 4.1. Let us say that the tuple (k_j) majorizes the tuple (k'_j) (written $(k_j) \succ (k'_j)$), iff for all integers k, the relations

$$\sum_{j=1}^{n} \max\{k_j-k,0\} \geq \sum_{j=1}^{n} \max\{k'_j-k,0\} , \tag{4.8}$$

$$\sum_{j=1}^{n} \min\{k_j-k,0\} \leq \sum_{j=1}^{n} \min\{k'_j-k,0\} , \tag{4.8'}$$

are satisfied.

It is obvious that the relation $\succ$ is reflexive and transitive, i.e., it is indeed a partial ordering. We intend to note some more properties of the relation $\succ$, which are important in what follows.

LEMMA 4.1. 1) If $(k_j) \succ (k'_j)$, then the inequalities

$$\max_j k_j \geq \max_j k'_j , \quad \min_j k_j \leq \min_j k'_j , \tag{4.9}$$

$\sum_{j=1}^{n} k_j = \sum_{j=1}^{n} k'_j$ are valid.

2) If the tuples (k_j) , $(k'_j) \in \mathbb{Z}^n$ have the property that (4.8), (4.8') are satisfied for all integer k from the interval $[\min_j k_j , \max_j k_j]$, then $(k_j) \succ (k'_j)$.

3) The relations $(k_j) \succ (k'_j)$ and $(k'_j) \succ (k_j)$ hold simultaneously iff the tuple (k'_j) is some permutation of the tuple (k_j) .

Proof. First of all, we intend to explain what do conditions (4.8) and (4.8') mean for some concrete values of k . If $k = \max k_j$, then $\max\{k_j-k,0\} = 0$ for all $j=1,\dots,n$. Consequently, inequality (4.8) with this choice of k is equivalent to $\sum_{j=1}^{n} \max\{k'_j-k,0\} \leq 0$. In turn, the latter inequality is satisfied if and only if $\max\{k'_j-k,0\} = 0$ $(j=1,\dots,n)$, i.e. if $\max_j k'_j \leq \max_j k_j$. In this way, condition (4.8) with $k = \max_j k_j$ is equivalent to $\max_j k'_j \le \max_j k_j$.

If the latter inequality is fulfilled, then for $k \ge \max k_j$, the equalities

$$\min\{k_j-k,0\} = k_j-k\ ,\quad \min\{k'_j-k,0\} = k'_j-k$$

are true and, therefore, to say that condition (4.8') is valid amounts to saying that $\sum_{j=1}^{n}(k_j-k) \le \sum_{j=1}^{n}(k'_j-k)$. Obviously, the inequality obtained is satisfied iff

$$\sum_{j=1}^{n} k_j \le \sum_{j=1}^{n} k'_j .$$

Analogously, one can readily verify that, for $k = \min k_j$, condition (4.8') is satisfied iff $\min k_j \le \min k'_j$. When the latter inequality is fulfilled, then, for $k \le \min k_j$, condition (4.8) is equivalent to $\sum_{j=1}^{n} k_j \ge \sum_{j=1}^{n} k'_j$.

Thus, if the conditions (4.8) and (4.8') are fulfilled for $k = \min k_j$ and $k = \max k_j$, then relations (4.9) are true, which proves statement 1) of the lemma.

Furthermore, if the relations (4.9) are valid, it follows from what was proved above that conditions (4.8) and (4.8') are satisfied for $k \le \min k_j$ and $k \ge \max k_j$. From this we conclude the correctness of assertion 2).

Now we proceed to the last statement of the lemma. Clearly, a change of order of the elements in the tuples (k_j), (k'_j) does not influence on the values of the sums occurring in inequalities (4.8) and (4.8'). Consequently, every tuple $(k_j) \in \mathbb{Z}^n$ majorizes any of its permutations and is majorized by it. The converse statement we shall prove by induction on n. For $n = 1$, the statement results from relations (4.9). Supposing that the statement has been proved for $n = l$, we now consider the tuples $(k_j)_{j=1}^{l+1}$ and $(k'_j)_{j=1}^{l+1}$. Without loss of generality, we may assume that $k_1 \ge k_2 \ge \dots \ge k_{l+1}$, $k'_1 \ge k'_2 \ge \dots \ge k'_{l+1}$. In this case, $k_{l+1} = \min k_j$, $k'_{l+1} = \min k'_j$, and if $(k_j)_{j=1}^{l+1} \succ (k'_j)_{j=1}^{l+1}$, $(k'_j)_{j=1}^{l+1} \succ (k_j)_{j=1}^{l+1}$, then in view of relations (4.9), $k_{l+1} = k'_{l+1}$. But then, obviously, $(k_j)_{j=1}^{l} \succ (k'_j)_{j=1}^{l}$ and $(k'_j)_{j=1}^{l} \succ (k_j)_{j=1}^{l}$.

Due to the induction hypothesis, the tuple $(k'_j)_{j=1}^{l}$ provides a permutation of the tuple $(k_j)_{j=1}^{l}$. Reordering these tuples in a non-increasing manner, we thus deduce that they coincide. Consequently, the initial tuples $(k_j)_{j=1}^{l+1}$ and $(k'_j)_{j=1}^{l+1}$ coincide, too. Lemma 4.1 is proved. ≡

THEOREM 4.7. Let the diagonal elements of the matrix function G be Φ-factorable in L_p, and assume the index of the j th diagonal element to be equal to k_j. Then the tuple $(\varkappa_j)$ of partial indices of G is majorized by the tuple (k_j). The factorization factors $G_{\pm}$ and Λ can be obtained with the help of a finite number of algebraic operations and solutions of scalar Riemann problems.

Proof. According to Corollary 3.1, the dimension of the kernel of problem (3.1) with matrix coefficient G is equal to $\alpha = \sum_{j=1}^{n} \max\{\varkappa_j, 0\}$, and the dimension of the kernel of the scalar problem with the coefficient G_{jj} is equal to $\alpha_j = \max\{k_j, 0\}$. On the strength of Theorem 4.2, we conclude that $\sum_{j=1}^{n} \max\{\varkappa_j, 0\} \leq \sum_{j=1}^{n} \max\{k_j, 0\}$.

Analogously, $-\sum_{j=1}^{n} \min\{\varkappa_j, 0\} \leq -\sum_{j=1}^{n} \min\{k_j, 0\}$, i.e. $\sum_{j=1}^{n} \min\{\varkappa_j, 0\} \geq$ $\geq \sum_{j=1}^{n} \min\{k_j, 0\}$. Multiplying G by t^{-k}, its partial indices and the indices of the diagonal elements decrease by k. Consequently, the inequalities proved continue to be valid, substituting in them $\varkappa_j$ by $\varkappa_j - k$ and k_j by $k_j - k$. Thus $(k_j) \succ (\varkappa_j)$.

Now we introduce the matrix function $D(t) = \operatorname{diag}[t^{k_1}, \ldots, t^{k_n}]$. The matrix function $G_1 = GD^{-1}$ is triangular along with G, its diagonal elements are Φ-factorable in L_p, and their indices are equal to zero. According to Theorem 4.6, the partial indices of the matrix function G_1 are equal to zero and its factorization factors $G_+^{(1)}$ and $G_-^{(1)}$ are constructed with the help of a finite number of algebraic operations and the solutions of scalar Riemann problems. Using Theorem 2.7, we see that the matrix function G can be factored with the same degree of effectiveness. The proof of Theorem 4.7 is complete. ≡

From Theorem 4.7 and statement 1) of Lemma 4.1 we obtain the following result.

COROLLARY 4.3. The partial indices of a triangular matrix function G with Φ-factorable diagonal elements are situated between the smallest and largest index of the diagonal elements, and the total index is equal to the sum of the diagonal elements indices.

We denote by μ_{ij} the order of the zero of the (i,j) th entry of the matrix function $(G_-^{(1)})^{-1}$ (introduced in the proof of Theorem 4.7) at infinity. Note that all entries outside the diagonal of $G_-^{(1)}$ vanish at ∞, so that $\mu_{ij} \geq 1$ for $i \neq j$.

We shall write $\mu_{ij} = \infty$, if the (i,j) th entry of $(G_-^{(1)})^{-1}$ is identically zero.

THEOREM 4.8. The tuple of partial indices of a lower (upper) triangular matrix function coincides (up to a permutation) with the tuple of indices of its diagonal elements if and only if

$$k_j - k_i \leq \mu_{ij} \quad \text{for} \quad i > j \quad (i < j) . \tag{4.10}$$

Proof. We focus our attention on the case of a lower triangular matrix function. If condition (4.10) is fulfilled, then, setting $G_+ = G_+^{(1)}$, $\Lambda = D$, $G_- = D^{-1}G_-^{(1)}D$, we get a factorization of G. Thus we have only to verify the analyticity of the entries outside the diagonals of the matrix functions G_- and G_-^{-1} at the point $z = \infty$. It is guaranteed by the fact that the (i,j) th entry of the matrix function $(G_-^{(1)})^{-1}$ is equal to zero, if $i < j$, and has a zero of order μ_{ij} at the point $z = \infty$, if $i > j$, and the (i,j) th entry of G_-^{-1} is obtained from it via multiplication by $z^{k_j - k_i}$.

Now, let condition (4.10) fail to be fulfilled. Suppose, at first, that $k_1 - k_i \leq \mu_{i1}$ $(i=1,\ldots,n-1)$, $k_1 > 0$ and $k_n + \mu_{n1} \leq 0$.

Setting $n_1 = n-1$, $n_2 = 1$, we represent the matrix function G in the form (4.4). In this case G_2 is the right lower entry G_{nn} of G, the factorization of which in L_p we write down in the following way:

$$G_{nn}(t) = G_{nn}^+(t)t^{k_n}G_{nn}^-(t) .$$

By φ we denote that vector function which is obtained from the first column of the matrix function $D^{-1}(G_-^{(1)})^{-1}$ by cancelling its last element φ_n. Now we are going to show that the vector function φ lies in the kernel of the operator $T_Q(G_1)$ and that, at the same time, the relation $H\varphi \notin \mathrm{im}(P+G_{nn}Q)$ holds. In fact, the i th component of the vector function φ has a zero of order $k_i + \mu_{i1} \geq k_1 > 0$ $(i=1,\dots,n-1)$ at infinity. Consequently, $\varphi \in (\overset{\circ}{L}{}_p^-)^{n-1}$. Moreover, the equation $GD^{-1}(G_-^{(1)})^{-1} = G_+^{(1)}$ is satisfied, in view of which all the elements of $GD^{-1}(G_-^{(1)})^{-1}$ lie in L_p^+. But the first column of this matrix function is of the form

$$\begin{pmatrix} G_1 \varphi \\ G_{nn}\varphi_n + H\varphi \end{pmatrix},$$

so that $G_{nn}\varphi_n + H\varphi \in L_p^+$ and $G_1\varphi \in (L_p^+)^{n-1}$. The first of the relations obtained allows us to claim that $\varphi \in \ker T_Q(G_1)$. After multiplication by $(G_{nn}^+)^{-1}$, from the second relation we conclude

$$f = G_{nn}^- t^{k_n}\varphi_n + (G_{nn}^+)^{-1}H\varphi \in L_1^+ .$$

Making use of the relation (1.11), we find that, for $j \geq 0$, the equation

$$\int_\Gamma (G_{nn}^+)^{-1}(\tau)H(\tau)\varphi(\tau)\tau^j d\tau = -\int_\Gamma G_{nn}^-(\tau)\tau^{k_n+j}\varphi_n(\tau)d\tau$$

holds. Setting $j = \mu_{n1}-1$, in the right part of the last equation we get a quantity different from zero, since the order of the zero of φ_n (and, thus, also of $G_{nn} - \varphi_n$) at infinity is precisely equal to $\mu_{n1} + k_n$. But $\mu_{n1}-1 \leq -k_n-1$. Consequently, for the function $H\varphi$, the necessary condition of membership to the image of the operator $P+G_{nn}Q$ is not fulfilled.

In summary, we have found a nontrivial vector function $\varphi \in \ker T_Q(G_1)$ for which $H\varphi \notin \mathrm{im}\,(P+G_2Q)$ or, equivalently, $QH\varphi \notin \mathrm{im}\, T_Q(G_2)$. Therefore, the value γ arising in formulae (4.6) is positive, so that the number α of linearly independent solutions of the homogeneous problem (3.1) with matrix coefficient G is strictly smaller than the sum of the corresponding numbers α_1 and α_2 of problems (3.1) with matrices G_1 and G_2. However, owing to Theorem 4.2, $\alpha_1 \leq \sum_{j=1}^{n-1} \max\{k_j, 0\}$ and, with regard to Corollary 3.1, $\alpha_2 = \max\{k_n, 0\}$. Hence,

$$\alpha < \sum_{j=1}^{n} \max\{k_j, 0\} .$$

Proceeding to the general case, we remark that element G_{kl} nearest to the main diagonal for which $k_k - k_l > \mu_{lk}$ (if such an element is not unique, we choose an arbitrary of them). Now we specify an integer k with $k_k > k$, $k_l + \mu_{lk} \leq k$ and partition the matrix function $t^{-k}G(t)$ into blocks in such a way that one of the diagonal blocks, say G_0, be placed in the rows and columns with numbers from l till k, and the remaining blocks be one-dimensional. Taking into account that on multiplication by t^{-k} the numbers k_j and $\varkappa_j$ decrease by k and the values μ_{ij} remain unchanged, we see that the matrix function G_0 satisfies the conditions of the special case considered above. Therefore, $\alpha_0 < \sum_{j=l}^{k} \max\{k_j - k, 0\}$. Here α_0 is the number of linearly independent solutions of the homogeneous Riemann problem with matrix coefficient G_0. Moreover, in virtue of Theorem 4.2,

$$\sum_{j=1}^{n} \max\{\varkappa_j - k, 0\} \leq \sum_{j=1}^{l-1} \max\{k_j - k, 0\} + \alpha_0 + \sum_{j=k+1}^{n} \max\{k_j - k, 0\} .$$

Comparing the last two inequalities, we obtain,

$$\sum_{j=1}^{n} \max\{\varkappa_j - k, 0\} < \sum_{j=1}^{n} \max\{k_j - k, 0\} .$$

Thus, if condition (4.10) is not fulfilled, the tuple (k_j) is not majorized by the tuple $(\varkappa_j)$ and, in view of statement 3) of Lemma 4.1, none of these tuples may be obtained from another one with the help of a permutation. In that way Theorem 4.8 is completely proved. ≡

COROLLARY 4.4. If the indices of the diagonal elements of a lower (upper) triangular matrix function satisfy the condition $k_i > k_j$ for $i > j$ $(i < j)$, then the partial indices coincide with the indices of the diagonal elements.

In order to prove this proposition, we have to use Theorem 4.8 and the fact that $\mu_{ij} \geq 1$ for $i \neq j$. ≡

4.3. CALCULATION OF PARTIAL INDICES OF SECOND-ORDER TRIANGULAR MATRIX FUNCTIONS

In case of second-order triangular matrix functions, the question of calculating the partial indices admits a complete solution. For the sake

of definiteness, we study lower triangular matrix functions, i.e. matrix functions of the form (4.4) with $n_1 = n_2 = 1$.
First of all, consider the case of Φ-factorable diagonal elements (in accordance with Theorem 4.3, in this case the matrix function G is Φ-factorable). Denoting the indices of the functions G_1 and G_2 by k_1 and k_2 respectively, in view of Theorem 4.7 and Corollary 4.4, we may only claim the following: the partial indices of G coincide with k_1 and k_2, if $k_1-k_2 \leq 1$, and are equal to $k_1-\lambda$ and $k_2+\lambda$, if $k_1-k_2 > 1$, where λ is an integer situated between 0 and $[\frac{1}{2}(k_1-k_2)]$.

For the exact calculation of the partial indices of a matrix function G of the form (4.4), we propose the following algorithm.

As in the proof of Theorem 4.7, we construct matrix functions

$$G_+^{(1)} = \begin{pmatrix} \xi_1^+ & 0 \\ a^+ & \xi_2^+ \end{pmatrix}, \quad G_-^{(1)} = \begin{pmatrix} \xi_1^- & 0 \\ a^- & \xi_2^- \end{pmatrix}, \quad \text{and} \quad D(t) = \begin{pmatrix} t^{k_1} & 0 \\ 0 & t^{k_2} \end{pmatrix}$$

such that $G = G_+^{(1)} G_-^{(1)} D$.

The function $\Phi(z) = a^-(z)/\xi_1^-(z)$ lies in the class $\dot{E}_1^-$. Denote the order of the zero of function Φ at ∞ by μ_0.
Then $\Phi^{-1}(z) = Q_0(z) + R_1(z)/\Phi(z)$, where Q_0 is a polynomial of degree $q_0 = \mu_0$, $R_1 \in E_1^-$ and R_1 has at ∞ a zero of order $\mu_1 > \mu_0$.
Furthermore, $\Phi R_1^{-1} = Q_1 + R_2 R_1^{-1}$, where Q_1 is a polynomial of degree $q_1 = \mu_1 - \mu_0$, $R_2 \in E_1^-$ and R_2 has at ∞ a zero of order $\mu_2 > \mu_1$.
Acting in this way, we get a sequence of polynomials $Q_0, Q_1, Q_2, \dots$ of degrees $q_0 = \mu_0$, $q_1 = \mu_1 - \mu_0$, $Q_2 = \mu_2 - \mu_1, \dots$. If the process stops at some stage, i.e. $R_k \equiv 0$, we put $\mu_k = \infty$.

<u>THEOREM 4.9.</u> If $k_1 - k_2 \leq \mu_0$, then the partial indices of the matrix function G are equal to k_1 and k_2. If $\mu_0, \mu_0+\mu_1, \dots, \mu_{i-1}+\mu_i < k_1-k_2$, but $\mu_i + \mu_{i+1} \geq k_1 - k_2$, then the partial indices of G are $k_1 - \mu_i$ and $k_2 + \mu_i$.

<u>Proof.</u> The first statement of the theorem follows from Theorem 4.8, since Φ has the same order at ∞ as the lower left element of the

matrix function $(G_-^{(1)})^{-1}$. If $\mu_0 < k_1-k_2$, but $\mu_0+\mu_1 \geq k_1-k_2$, then we obtain a factorization of G by setting [1])

$$G_-(t) = \begin{pmatrix} \xi_1^-(t)R_1(t)^{k_1-k_2-\mu_0} & \xi_2^-(t)Q_0(t)t^{-\mu_0} \\ a^-(t)t^{\mu_0} & \xi_2^-(t)t^{-k_1+k_2+\mu_0} \end{pmatrix},$$

$$G_+ = G_+^{(1)}\begin{pmatrix} 1 & Q_0 \\ 0 & 1 \end{pmatrix}, \quad \Lambda(t) = \begin{pmatrix} t^{k_2+\mu_0} & 0 \\ 0 & t^{k_1-\mu_0} \end{pmatrix}.$$

In case that $\mu_0+\mu_1 < k_1-k_2$, but $\mu_1+\mu_2 \geq k_1-k_2$, we put

$$G_+ = G_+^{(1)}\begin{pmatrix} 1 & Q_0 \\ 0 & 1 \end{pmatrix}\begin{pmatrix} 1 & 0 \\ Q_1 & 1 \end{pmatrix}, \quad \Lambda(t) = \begin{pmatrix} t^{k_1-\mu_1} & 0 \\ 0 & t^{k_2+\mu_1} \end{pmatrix},$$

$$G_-(t) = \begin{pmatrix} \xi_1^-(t)R_1(t)t^{\mu_1} & \xi_2^-(t)^{k_1+k_2+\mu_1}Q_0(t) \\ \xi_1^-(t)R_2(t)t^{k_1-k_2-\mu_1} & \xi_2^-(t)t^{-\mu_1}(1-Q_0(t)Q_1(t)) \end{pmatrix}$$

etc. ⊣

COROLLARY 4.5. Let G_1, G_2 $(\in L_\infty)$ be Φ-factorable functions with indices k_1 and k_2 respectively, and suppose $k_1 > k_2$. Then for every integer $\lambda \in (0,[\frac{1}{2}(k_1-k_2)])$, one can choose a function $H \in L_\infty$ in such a manner that the partial indices of the matrix function (4.4) are equal to $k_1-\lambda$ and $k_2+\lambda$.

Proof. We intend to look for functions H of the form $H = \xi_1^-\xi_2^+t^{k_1}\Phi$, where $\Phi \in E_1^-$ and has a zero of order $\mu_0 = k_1-k_2-\lambda$ at the point $z = \infty$. The condition $H \in L_\infty$ is equivalent to $\xi_1^-\Phi/\xi_2^- \in L_\infty$ and is, obviously, fulfilled iff $\Phi = \xi_2^-\varphi/\xi_1^-$ with $\varphi \in E_\infty^-$. If this requirement is satisfied, then (in notations of Theorem 4.9) $a^+ = 0$, $a^- = \Phi\xi_1^-$. Hence, function Φ coincides with the function occurring in the proof

[1]) Exactly speaking, the representation obtained will be a factorization only in case if the index of the right lower element of the matrix function Λ does not exceed the index of its left upper element. Otherwise, it is still necessary to rearrange the rows of the matrix function G_-, the columns of the matrix function G_+ and the diagonal elements of Λ.

of Theorem 4.9. Since $\mu_0 \leq k_1-k_2$ and $\mu_1+\mu_0 > 2\mu_0 \geq k_1-k_2$, then, owing to Theorem 4.9, the partial indices of the matrix function (4.4) are equal to $k_1-\mu_0 = k_2+\lambda$ and $k_2+\mu_0 = k_1-\lambda$. ≡

Now we proceed to the case of a Φ-factorable matrix function (4.4) the diagonal elements of which are not Φ-factorable.

THEOREM 4.10. Let the diagonal elements G_1 and G_2 of the matrix function (4.4) be not Φ-factorable in L_p. Then for the Φ-factorability in L_p of the matrix function G it is necessary and sufficient that the image of the operator $T_Q(G_1)$ coincides with $\mathring{L}_p^-$, the kernel of the operator $T_Q(G_2)$ is trivial, and the codimension γ_1 of the sum $\operatorname{im} T_Q(G_2) + T_Q(H)\ker T_Q(G_1)$ as well as the dimension γ_2 of the lineal $M = \{\varphi \in \ker T_Q(G_1) : T_Q(H)\varphi \in \operatorname{im} T_Q(G_2)\}$ are finite. If these conditions are fulfilled, then the partial indices of G are determined by the formulae

$$\varkappa_1 = \gamma_2 , \quad \varkappa_2 = -\gamma_1 \tag{4.11}$$

if $\gamma_1\gamma_2 \neq 0$ or $\gamma_1+\gamma_2 \leq 1$, and by the formulae

$$\varkappa_1 = [\gamma_2/2] + r , \quad \varkappa_2 = \gamma_2 - [\gamma_2/2] - r \tag{4.12}$$

if $\gamma_1 = 0$, $\gamma_2 > 1$ [1].

Here r is the dimension of the subspace consisting of those functions $\varphi \in M$ for which

$$\begin{aligned} &\int_\Gamma [H(\tau)\varphi(\tau) - G_2(\tau)(T_Q(G_2)^{-1}GH\varphi)(\tau)]\tau^{-j}d\tau = \\ &\int_\Gamma G_1(\tau)\varphi(\tau)\tau^{-j}d\tau = 0 , \quad j=1,\ldots,[\gamma_2/2] . \end{aligned} \tag{4.13}$$

Proof. The sufficiency of the conditions for Φ-factorability of the matrix function G stated in the formulation of the theorem follows immediately from Theorem 4.1.

In order to prove their necessity, according to the same Theorem 4.1, we have only to verify that the numbers $\beta_1 = \beta(T_Q(G_1))$ and $\alpha_2 = \alpha(T_Q(G_2))$ are equal to zero. Assuming $\beta_1 > 0$, owing to statement 3) of Theorem 3.1, we may conclude that $\alpha(T_Q(G_1)) = 0$. This and the

---

[1] Analogous formulae are valid for $\gamma_2 = 0$, $\gamma_1 > 1$.

finiteness of the value β_1 imply that the operator $T_Q(G_1)$ is Fredholm, i.e., function G_1 is Φ-factorable in L_p, which contradicts the assumption of the theorem. Thus $\beta_1 = 0$. The equality $\alpha_2 = 0$ may be proved analogously.

In this way, the conditions described in the formulation of Theorem 4.10 are actually necessary and sufficient for the Φ-factorability of G. In addition, from the equalities $\beta_1 = \alpha_2 = 0$ and the relations (4.5), the following formulae for the defect numbers of the Riemann boundary value problem with matrix coefficient G result:

$$\alpha = \gamma_2 , \qquad \beta = \gamma_1 .$$

Comparing these formulae with the expressions of the defect numbers via partial indices established in Theorem 3.16, we see that the following cases are possible:

1) $\varkappa_1 \geq 0$, $\varkappa_2 \leq 0$.

Then $\gamma_1 = -\varkappa_2$, $\gamma_2 = \varkappa_1$, i.e., formulae (4.11) are fulfilled regardless of the values $\gamma_1\gamma_2$ and $\gamma_1 + \gamma_2$.

2) $\varkappa_1 > 0$, $\varkappa_2 \leq 0$.

Then $\gamma_1 = 0$, $\gamma_2 = \varkappa_1 + \varkappa_2 \geq 1$, where $\varkappa_2 \leq \frac{1}{2}(\varkappa_1+\varkappa_2) = \gamma_2/2$.

Since $\varkappa_2$ is an integer, we obtain that $\varkappa_2 \leq [\gamma_2/2]$ and, if $\gamma_2 = 1$, then $\varkappa_2 = 0$, which means $\varkappa_1 = \gamma_2$.

3) $\varkappa_1 \leq 0$, $\varkappa_2 < 0$.

Then $\gamma_2 = 0$, $\gamma_1 = -(\varkappa_1+\varkappa_2) \geq 1$. As in case 2), we can establish that, for $\gamma_1 = 1$, the equalities $\varkappa_2 = -1$ and $\varkappa_1 = 0$ hold.

In summary, if either of the conditions $\gamma_1\gamma_2 \neq 0$ and $\gamma_1+\gamma_2 \leq 1$ is fulfilled, then formulae (4.11) are true. Therefore, only one situation remains to be examined, namely, when $\gamma_1 = 0$, $\gamma_2 > 1$.

To this end, we introduce the matrix function $G_0(t) = t^{-k}G(t)$ with $k = [\gamma_2/2]$. The partial indices $\varkappa_1^{(0)} = \varkappa_1 - k$ and $\varkappa_2^{(0)} = \varkappa_2 - k$ of this matrix function meet the conditions of case 1). In fact, the inequality $\varkappa_2 \leq k$ was proved above, and $\varkappa_1 \geq \frac{1}{2}(\varkappa_1+\varkappa_2) = \gamma_2/2 \geq k$. Consequently $\varkappa_1^{(0)} = \dim M_0$, where

$$M_0 = \{\varphi \in \ker T_Q(t^{-k}G_1) : Qt^{-k}H\varphi \in \operatorname{im} T_Q(t^{-k}G_2)\} .$$

In this way, $\varkappa_1 = k + \dim M_0$, $\varkappa_2 = \gamma_2 - k - \dim M_0$, and the proof of the theorem will be perfected as soon as we establish that M_o coincides with the subspace generated in M by conditions (4.13).

The relation $\varphi \in \ker T_Q(t^{-k}G_1)$ may be rewritten in the form $t^{-k}G_1\varphi \in L_p^+$. If the latter condition applies, then $G_1\varphi \in L_p^+$, so that $QG_1\varphi = 0$ and $\varphi \in \ker T_Q(G_1)$. In turn, if $\varphi \in \ker T_Q(G_1)$, then $Qt^{-k}G_1\varphi = Qt^{-k}PG_1\varphi$. Consequently, $\varphi \in \ker T_Q(t^{-k}G_1)$ iff $\varphi \in \ker T_Q(G_1)$ and $Qt^{-k}PG_1\varphi = 0$. If further, $Qt^{-k}H\varphi \in \operatorname{im} T_Q(t^{-k}G_2)$, i.e. $Qt^{-k}H\varphi = Qt^{-k}G_2f$, where $f \in \overset{\circ}{L}{}_p^-$, then $t^kQt^{-k}H\varphi = t^kQt^{-k}G_2f$. Hence $H\varphi - t^kPt^{-k}H\varphi = G_2f - t^kPt^{-k}G_2f$. Applying the projections Q and P to the last equation successively, we obtain

$$QH\varphi = QG_2f \,,$$
$$(P - t^kPt^{-k})H\varphi = (P - t^kPt^{-k})G_2f \,. \tag{4.14}$$

The first of the relations obtained means that

$$QH\varphi \in \operatorname{im} T_Q(G_2) \,. \tag{4.15}$$

According to what was proved above, the kernel of the operator $T_Q(G_2)$ is trivial and, thus, the pre-image f of the function $QH\varphi$ may be written in the form $f = T_Q(G_2)^{-1}QH\varphi$. With regard to this fact and the equation $P - t^kPt^{-k} = t^kQt^{-k}P$, we rewrite relation (4.14) in the following manner:

$$Qt^{-k}P(H\varphi - G_2T_Q(G_2)^{-1}QH\varphi) = 0 \,. \tag{4.16}$$

The transformations of the condition $Qt^{-k}H\varphi \in \operatorname{im} T_Q(t^{-k}G_2)$ carried out above are reversible. Consequently, this condition is equivalent to the requirements (4.15) and (4.16).

Summarizing, the inclusion $\varphi \in M_o$ holds if and only if $\varphi \in M$ and the functions $G_1\varphi$ and $H\varphi - G_2T_Q(G_2)^{-1}QH\varphi$ lie in the kernel of the operator $Qt^{-k}P$.

Since to the kernel of the operator $Qt^{-k}P$ there belong those and only those functions ψ from L_p the component $P\psi$ of which has the first k coefficients of the power series expansion equal to zero, it follows from the above considerations that conditions (4.13) are necessary and sufficient for the function $\varphi \in M$ to lie in the subspace M_o. Therefore, the equality $\dim M_o = r$ has been proved and, along with it, also Theorem 4.10. $\equiv$

Example. Let us discuss the problem of calculating the partial 2-indices of the matrix function

$$G_m = \begin{pmatrix} t^m\omega & 0 \\ 1 & \overline{\omega} \end{pmatrix}$$

given on the unit circle, where ω is an inner function not reducible to a finite Blaschke product, and m is a non-negative integer.

For $m = 0$, this matrix function meets the conditions of Theorem 4.4. According to this theorem, it is Φ-factorable in L_2. Moreover, in the proof of Theorem 4.4 it was established that, in this case we have $\gamma_1 = \gamma_2 = 0$. In virtue of Theorem 4.10, we are able to claim that the partial 2-indices of G_0 are equal to zero.
Representing the function G_m in the form

$$G_m = \begin{pmatrix} t^m & 0 \\ 0 & 1 \end{pmatrix} G_0 ,$$

from Theorem 2.11 we obtain that G_m is Φ-factorable in L_2 together with G_0, its partial 2-indices are non-negative, and the total 2-index is equal to m.

Thus, for the matrix function G_m, the relations $\gamma_1 = 0$ and $\gamma_2 = \gamma$ are valid and, consequently, for $m = 1$, we have $\varkappa_1 = 1$, $\varkappa_2 = 0$. In case $m > 1$, formulae (4.12) can be applied for calculating the partial 2-indices of G_m.

In the considered case, we have $H = 1$ and the operator $T_Q(G_2)$ coincides with the operator of multiplication by $\overline{\omega}$, therefore, $H\varphi - G_2 T_Q(G_2)^{-1} QH\varphi = P\varphi$, and the first group of conditions (4.13) is automatically fulfilled.

Furthermore, in the case under study, the subspace M coincides with $\ker T_Q(t^m\omega) \cap \overline{\omega}\, \mathring{L}_p^-$, i.e. with the set of functions of the form $\varphi = \overline{\omega} f$, where $f \in \mathring{L}_p^-$ and $t^m \omega\, \overline{\omega} f \in L_p^+$. Since $\omega\overline{\omega} = 1$, the requirements enumerated are fulfilled iff

$$f(t) = \sum_{s=-m}^{-1} c_s t^s .$$

Substituting the obtained representation of the functions $\varphi \in M$ into the second group of conditions (4.13), we get

$$0 = \int_{\mathbf{T}} \tau^m \omega(\tau)\overline{\omega(\tau)} f(\tau)\tau^{-j} d\tau =$$

$$\int_{\mathbf{T}} \sum_{s=-m}^{-1} c_s t^{m+s-j} dt = 2\pi i\, c_{j-1-m} ,$$

where $j=1,\dots,[m/2]$.

Therefore, conditions (4.13) are fulfilled for those and only those functions $\varphi \in M$ for which $c_s = 0$ for $s = -m,\dots,[m/2]-1-m$. For that reason, the subspace M_0 consists exactly of functions $\varphi \in M$ of the form

$$\varphi(t) = \overline{\omega}(t) \sum_{s=[\frac{m}{2}]-m}^{-1} c_s t^s .$$

Hence $r = \dim M_0 = m-[m/2]$.

On the strength of formulae (4.12), we thus obtain $\varkappa_1 = m$, $\varkappa_2 = 0$. In this way, for every non-negative integer m , we have constructed examples of second-order lower triangular matrix functions the diagonal elements of which are not Φ-factorable and whose partial indices are m and 0 . Multiplying these matrix functions by scalar factorable functions with suitable index (for instance, simply by t^j), one can easily obtain examples of second-order triangular matrix functions with an arbitrary tuple of partial indices and non-Φ-factorable diagonal elements.

4.4. Φ-FACTORIZATION OF FUNCTIONALLY COMMUTABLE MATRIX FUNCTIONS

All the suggestions made in Sections 4.1 – 4.3 can, with obvious modifications, be transferred to the case when the matrix function G is not triangular, but becomes a such one after multiplication from the left and the right by a constant non-degenerating matrix. In the present section a class of matrix functions possessing such a property will be investigated.

DEFINITION 4.2. A measurable matrix function G defined on a contour Γ is said to be functionally commutable if

$$G(t_1)G(t_2) = G(t_2)G(t_1) \quad (t_1,t_2 \in \Gamma) . \tag{4.17}$$

LEMMA 4.2. The matrix function G is functionally commutable if and only if

$$G(t) = \sum_{j=1}^{m} \varphi_j(t) G_j , \qquad (4.18)$$

where $m \leq n^2$, G_j $(j=1,\dots,m)$ are pairwise commuting constant matrices and φ_j are measurable scalar functions.

Proof. The sufficiency of the conditions of the lemma is evident. We are going to prove their necessity. For this purpose, we form the linear hull $\mathcal{L}$ of the set of all matrices of the form $G(t)$, $t \in \Gamma$ in the space of all constant matrices of n th order and choose in it a basis $G_1,\dots,G_m$. Since the space of $n \times n$ matrices has the dimension n^2, then $m \leq n^2$. Furthermore, condition (4.17) implies that any two matrices from $\mathcal{L}$ commute. Consequently, all matrices $G_1,\dots,G_m$ commute pairwise. Finally, as $G(t) \in \mathcal{L}$ for all $t \in \Gamma$ and $\{G_j\}_{j=1}^m$ is a basis in $\mathcal{L}$, then there exists a unique representation $G(t)$ in the form of a linear combination of the G_j's. Supposing $\varphi_j(t)$ to be equal to the j th coefficient of this linear combination, we have $G(t) = \sum \varphi_j(t) G_j$. The measurability of functions φ_j follows from the measurability of G as well as the linear independence of $G_1,\dots,G_m$, which proves Lemma 4.2. ≡

LEMMA 4.3. If the matrices $G_1,\dots,G_m$ commute pairwise, then there exists a non-degenerating constant matrix S such that all matrices $S^{-1}G_jS$, $j=1,\dots,m$ are lower triangular.

Proof. Above all, we show by induction on m that the matrices $G_1,\dots,G_m$ have a common eigensubspace. For $m = 1$, this is obvious. Supposing that the statement is correct for $m = k-1$, we consider the pairwise commutating matrices $G_1,\dots,G_k$. By assumption, for a certain choice of scalars λ_j, $j=1,\dots,k-1$, the subspace $M = \{x: G_jx = \lambda_jx, j=1,\dots,k-1\}$ is nontrivial. Owing to the commutativity, we have, for all $x \in M$, $G_jG_kx = G_kG_jx = G_k\lambda_jx = \lambda_jG_kx$, i.e. $G_kx \in M$. Thus, the subspace M is invariant with respect to G_k and, therefore, it contains some eigensubspace.

This will just be the common eigensubspace for $G_1,\dots,G_k$.

From what was proved above we conclude that, by all means, the matrices $G_1,\dots,G_k$, which commute pairwise, have a common eigenvector x . Let S_1 be a non-degenerate matrix the last column of which is x . As can be easily seen, in this case

$$S_1^{-1}G_jS_1 = \left(\begin{array}{ccc|c} & G_j^{(1)} & & 0 \\ \hline G_{n_1}^{(j)} & \dots & G_{n,n-1}^{(j)} & \lambda_j \end{array}\right),$$

where $G_j^{(1)}$ is a matrix of (n-1) th order. The matrices $S_1^{-1}G_jS_1$ commute pairwise and, along with them, the matrices $G_j^{(1)}$ also commute. If we succeed in finding a non-degenerate matrix $S^{(1)}$ of (n-1) th order such that all matrices $(S^{(1)})^{-1}G_j^{(1)}S^{(1)}$ are lower triangular, then, setting $S_2 = \mathrm{diag}[S^{(1)},1]$ and $S = S_1S_2$, we obtain the desired matrix S .

In this way, if the statement to be proved is true for matrices of (n-1) th order, then it is also correct for matrices of n th order. Since, for $n = 1$, the assertion is trivial, then it is valid for every natural n . Thus Lemma 4.3 is proved. ≡

On the strength of Lemmas 4.2 and 4.3, we can assert that if the matrix function G is functionally commutable, then there exists such a constant non-degenerating matrix S that the matrix function $F = S^{-1}GS$ is lower triangular, and if $G \in L_\infty$, then we have also $F \in L_\infty$. According to Theorem 4.3, the Φ-factorability of the diagonal elements of F is sufficient for the Φ-factorability of G , and its partial indices can be estimated with the aid of Theorem 4.7. However, it turns out that the matrix S may be chosen in such a way that the matrix function G is Φ-factorable only simultaneously with the diagonal elements of the matrix function F , and its partial indices coincide with the indices of the diagonal elements of F .

THEOREM 4.11. Let $G\ (\in L_\infty)$ be a functionally commutable matrix function. Assume that there exists a constant non-degenerating matrix S such that the matrix function $F = S^{-1}GS$ is block-diagonal and every diagonal block is a lower triangular matrix function all the diagonal elements of which are equal to each other. The matrix function G is Φ-factorable if and only if the diagonal elements of F are Φ-factorable, and the partial indices of G are equal to the indices of the diagonal elements of F.

Proof. In the linear hull $\mathfrak{L}$ of the set of all values of G we choose the matrix with the largest number of different eigenvalues (if such a matrix is not unique, then we take an arbitrary of them) and denote it by G_o. As well-known (GANTMAKHER [1], MAL'TSEV [1]), there exists a constant non-degenerating matrix T such that

$$T^{-1}G_oT = \operatorname{diag}[A_1^{(o)},\dots,A_k^{(o)}] ,$$

where the block $A_i^{(o)}$ is a matrix with the unique point of the spectrum λ_i, $\lambda_{i_1} \neq \lambda_{i_2}$ for $i_1 \neq i_2$, $i_1,i_2 = 1,\dots,k$.

In view of Lemma 4.2, $G(t) = \sum_{j=1}^{m} \varphi_j(t)G_j$ with $G_j \in \mathfrak{L}$. Therefore, the matrices G_j commute with G_o. But in this case the matrices $T^{-1}G_jT$ and $T^{-1}G_oT$ commute, too. With regard to the description of all matrices permutable with a given one (see GANTMAKHER [1], p. 204 or MAL'TSEV [1], p. 192), every matrix $T^{-1}G_jT$ is also block-diagonal:

$$T^{-1}G_jT = \operatorname{diag}[A_1^{(j)},\dots,A_k^{(j)}] ,$$

where the matrices $A_i^{(o)},\dots,A_i^{(m)}$, $i=1,\dots,k$, commute pairwise. Applying Lemma 4.3 to these matrices, we establish that there exists a matrix S_i (of the same order as all matrices $A_i^{(j)}$, $j=0,\dots,m$) such that $S_i^{-1}A_i^{(j)}S_i$ are lower triangular matrices $(i=1,\dots,k;\ j=0,\dots,m)$. Setting $S = T\operatorname{diag}[S_1,\dots,S_k]$, we recognize that the matrices $S^{-1}G_jS$ are block-diagonal, and every diagonal block is triangular $(j=0,\dots,m)$. Consequently, on the diagonal of any of the blocks there are located its eigenvalues. Therefore, in the matrix $S^{-1}G_oS$, the diagonal elements of one and the same block agree. Now, assume that for some of the matrices $S^{-1}G_jS$, say, for $S^{-1}G_1S$, this is not true. Then, for ε small enough, the matrix $S^{-1}(G_o+\varepsilon G_1)S$ and, along with it, also the matrix $G_o+\varepsilon G_1$ has more different eigenvalues than G_o. But this contradicts the way of choosing G_o . Thus, $S^{-1}G_jS = \mathrm{diag}[G_1^{(j)},\dots,G_k^{(j)}]$, where every block $G_i^{(j)}$ is a lower triangular matrix with equal elements on the main diagonal.

Utilizing formula (4.18), we see that

$$S^{-1}G(t)S = F(t) = \mathrm{diag}[F_1(t),\dots,F_k(t)] ,$$

the blocks $F_i(t)$ are lower triangular, and the elements standing on the diagonal of one and the same block are equal to each other. Therewith, the first statement of the theorem is proved.

Furthermore, the matrix functions G and F are Φ-factorable only simultaneously and, in accordance with Corollary 4.2, the matrix function F is Φ-factorable if and only if every block $F_1,\dots,F_k$ is Φ-factorable. Let us consider one of these blocks, say F_i , denoting its diagonal element by a_i .

Applying Theorem 4.1 for $n_1 = 1$, we obtain that, if the matrix function F_i is Φ-factorable, then, in view of assertion 1), the image of the operator $P + a_iQ$ must have finite codimension. For $n_2 = 1$, due to assertion 2) of the same theorem, we conclude that the kernel of this operator must be finite dimensional. Consequently, from the Φ-factorability of F_i , the Fredholmness of the operator $P + a_iQ$ results, i.e. the Φ-factorability of its diagonal elements. The validity of the opposite statement can be seen from Theorem 4.3.

In summary, the matrix function G is Φ-factorable iff all diagonal elements of the matrix function F are Φ-factorable.

Finally, the partial indices of G and F coincide, the set of partial indices of F is obtained by uniting the tuples of partial indices of its diagonal blocks, and all partial indices of the block F_i are equal to the index of the element a_i , because for the blocks F_i the conditions of Corollary 4.4 are fulfilled. Hence the last statement of the theorem is also proved. $\equiv$

Note that the diagonal elements of the matrix $F(t)$ are its eigenvalues and, thus, also eigenvalues of the matrix $G(t)$. Roughly speaking, we may therefore say that the partial indices of the functionally commutable matrix function G coincide with the indices of its eigenvalues.

Example. Recall that a matrix of the form

$$C = \begin{pmatrix} c_0 & c_1 & \cdots & c_{n-1} \\ c_{n-1} & c_0 & \cdots & c_{n-2} \\ \cdots & \cdot & \cdot & \cdot \\ c_1 & c_2 & \cdots & c_0 \end{pmatrix} \tag{4.19}$$

is called a circulant (see e.g. MARCUS, MINC [1], p. 96). The product of two circulants is again a circulant as can be readily verified, where the product does not depend on the order of the factors. Consequently, a matrix function G all values of which are circulants is functionally commutable, and Theorem 4.11 is applicable. We shall get an explicit formula for the matrix S . Using this formula, F turns out to be diagonal.

Setting

$$S = n^{-1/2}\left(e^{\frac{2\pi i}{n}(k-1)(j-1)}\right)_{k,j=1}^{n},$$

we consider the product $D = S^*CS$, where C is the matrix defined by formula (4.19). Its (r,s) th entry is determined by the formula

$$d_{rs} = n^{-1}\Big(\sum_{l\geq k} c_{l-k}\, e^{\frac{2\pi i}{n}[(l-1)(s-1)-(r-1)(k-1)]} +$$

$$\sum_{l<k} c_{n+l-k}\, e^{\frac{2\pi i}{n}[(l-1)(s-1)-(r-1)(k-1)]}\Big).$$

Denoting $l-k = j$ in the first sum and $n+l-k = j$ in the second one, we obtain

$$d_{rs} = n^{-1}\Big(\sum_{j=o}^{n-1}\sum_{k=1}^{n-j} c_j\, e^{\frac{2\pi i}{n}[(j+k-1)(s-1)-(r-1)(k-1)]} +$$

$$\sum_{j=1}^{n-1}\sum_{k=n-j+1}^{n} c_j\, e^{\frac{2\pi i}{n}[(j+k-m-1)(s-1)-(r-1)(k-1)]}\Big).$$

Taking into account that $e^{\frac{2\pi i}{n}(j+k-n-1)(s-1)} = e^{\frac{2\pi i}{n}(j+k-1)(s-1)}$, we are able to unite the two sums into one:

$$d_{rs} = n^{-1} \sum_{j=0}^{n-1} \sum_{k=1}^{n} c_j \, e^{\frac{2\pi i}{n}[(j+k-1)(s-1)-(r-1)(k-1)]} =$$

$$n^{-1} \sum_{j=0}^{n-1} \Big(\sum_{k=1}^{n} e^{\frac{2\pi i}{n}(k-1)(s-r)} \Big) e^{\frac{2\pi i}{n}j(s-1)} c_j \, .$$

If $s = r$, the inner sum is equal to n and, for $s \neq r$, it is equal to zero. Thus, D is a diagonal matrix and

$$d_{rr} = \sum_{j=0}^{n-1} e^{\frac{2\pi i}{n}j(r-1)} c_j \, .$$

In particular, choosing $C = I$, we get $d_{rr} = 1$, i.e. $S^*S = I$, and the matrix S is unitary and therefore non-degenerating.

Now let G be a matrix function all values of which are circulants. Denote the elements of the first row of G by $g_0,\dots,g_{n-1}$ and introduce the functions

$$f_r(t) = \sum_{j=0}^{n-1} e^{\frac{2\pi i}{n}jr} g_j(t) \, , \quad r=0,\dots,n-1 \, . \tag{4.20}$$

According to the above considerations, the matrix function $F = S^*GS$ $(= S^{-1}GS)$ is of the form $F = \mathrm{diag}[f_0,\dots,f_{n-1}]$.

From here we obtain the final conclusion: a matrix function G all values of which are circulants is Φ-factorable if and only if all functions f_j determined via formulae (4.20) are Φ-factorable, where the partial indices of G are equal to the indices of the functions f_j. A factorization of the matrix function G will be known as soon as these functions are factored.

At the end of this section we focus our attention on second-order matrix functions.

<u>LEMMA 4.4.</u> The matrix function $G = \begin{pmatrix} g_{11} & g_{12} \\ g_{21} & g_{22} \end{pmatrix}$ is functionally commutable iff $g_{11}-g_{22}$, g_{12} and g_{21} are scalar multiples of one and the same function φ, i.e.

$$g_{12}(t) = \alpha\varphi(t) \, , \; g_{21}(t) = \beta\varphi(t), \; g_{11}(t)-g_{22}(t) = \gamma\varphi(t), \tag{4.21}$$

where α, β, γ are numbers.

Proof. If the conditions (4.21) are fulfilled, then

$$G(t) = \begin{pmatrix} g_{22}(t)+\gamma\varphi(t) & \alpha g(t) \\ \beta\varphi(t) & g_{22}(t) \end{pmatrix}.$$

A direct verification shows that, for any $t_1, t_2 \in \Gamma$, $G(t_1)G(t_2) = G(t_2)G(t_1)$.

Vice versa, let the matrix function G be functionally commutable. At first, suppose that $g_{11}(t) \equiv g_{22}(t)$. If in addition, $g_{12} = g_{21} = 0$, then the conditions (4.21) are satisfied for $\alpha = \beta = \gamma = 0$. In the opposite case, a point $t_0 \in \Gamma$ can be found at which at least one of the functions g_{12} or g_{21} is different from zero. Equating the diagonal elements of the matrices $G(t)G(t_0)$ and $G(t_0)G(t)$, we get $g_{12}(t)g_{21}(t_0) = g_{12}(t_0)g_{21}(t)$. If $g_{21}(t_0) \neq 0$, we may take $\varphi = g_{21}$, $\beta = 1$, $\gamma = 0$, $\alpha = g_{12}(t_0)/g_{21}(t_0)$, and if $g_{12}(t_0) \neq 0$, then we can choose $\varphi = g_{12}$, $\alpha = 1$, $\gamma = 0$, $\beta = g_{21}(t_0)/g_{12}(t_0)$.

Now let the functions g_{11} and g_{22} be different. Then there exists a point $t_0 \in \Gamma$ such that $g_{11}(t_0) \neq g_{22}(t_0)$. Equating the elements outside the diagonals of the matrices $G(t)G(t_0)$ and $G(t_0)G(t)$, we obtain

$$(g_{11}(t)-g_{22}(t))\, g_{12}(t_0) = (g_{11}(t_0)-g_{22}(t_0))\, g_{12}(t),$$

$$(g_{11}(t)-g_{22}(t))\, g_{21}(t_0) = (g_{11}(t_0)-g_{22}(t_0))\, g_{21}(t),$$

so that we may set $\varphi = g_{11}-g_{22}$, $\gamma = 1$, $\alpha = g_{12}(t_0)/(g_{11}(t_0)-g_{22}(t_0))$, $\beta = g_{21}(t_0)/(g_{11}(t_0)-g_{22}(t_0))$, and Lemma 4.4 has been proved. ≡

THEOREM 4.12. Let the measurable bounded matrix function

$$G = \begin{pmatrix} g_{11} & g_{12} \\ g_{21} & g_{22} \end{pmatrix}$$

be functionally commutable. It is Φ-factorable in L_p iff the functions

$$\lambda_1 = \tfrac{1}{2}(g_{11}+g_{22}) + \nu\varphi \quad \text{and} \quad \lambda_2 = \tfrac{1}{2}(g_{11}+g_{22}) - \nu\varphi$$

are Φ-factorable in L_p, where ν is an arbitrary value of the square root of $\alpha\beta + \frac{1}{4}\gamma^2$, and α, β, γ and φ are defined by formulae (4.21).

In this case the partial indices of G coincide with the indices of the functions λ_1 and λ_2.

Proof. In accordance with Theorem 4.11, the matrix function G can be converted into a diagonal or a triangular form with equal elements on the diagonal by means of a constant similarity transformation. Now we intend to describe the concrete form of these transformations depending on the parameter values involved in formulae (4.21).

a) $\nu \neq 0, \alpha \neq 0$:

$$G(t) = -\frac{1}{2\alpha\nu}\begin{pmatrix} \alpha & \alpha \\ -\frac{\gamma}{2}+\nu & -\frac{\gamma}{2}-\nu \end{pmatrix}\begin{pmatrix} \lambda_1 & 0 \\ 0 & \lambda_2 \end{pmatrix}\begin{pmatrix} -\frac{\gamma}{2}-\nu & -\alpha \\ \frac{\gamma}{2}-\nu & \alpha \end{pmatrix};$$

b) $\nu \neq 0, \alpha = 0$:

$$G(t) = \begin{pmatrix} 1 & 0 \\ \frac{\beta}{2\nu} & 1 \end{pmatrix}\begin{pmatrix} \lambda_1 & 0 \\ 0 & \lambda_2 \end{pmatrix}\begin{pmatrix} 1 & 0 \\ -\frac{\beta}{2\nu} & 1 \end{pmatrix};$$

c) $\nu = 0, \alpha \neq 0$:

$$G(t) = \frac{1}{2\sqrt{\alpha}}\begin{pmatrix} 0 & \sqrt{\alpha} \\ 1 & i\sqrt{\beta} \end{pmatrix}\begin{pmatrix} g_{11}+g_{22} & 0 \\ 2\sqrt{\alpha}\,\varphi & g_{11}+g_{22} \end{pmatrix}\begin{pmatrix} -i\sqrt{\beta} & \sqrt{\alpha} \\ 1 & 0 \end{pmatrix};$$

d) $\nu = \alpha = 0$:

$$G(t) = \begin{pmatrix} g_{22} & 0 \\ \beta\varphi & g_{22} \end{pmatrix}.$$

Since, for $\nu = 0$, $\lambda_1 = \lambda_2 = \frac{1}{2}(g_{11}+g_{22})$ and, for $\nu = \alpha = 0$, the relation $g_{11} = g_{22}$ is valid, the assertion to be proved follows now from Theorem 4.11. Thus, Theorem 4.12 is proved. ≡

As an example we want to consider a second-order orthogonal[1)] matrix with determinant equal to 1. As can be easily verified, its general form is given by the formula

$$\begin{pmatrix} \sqrt{1-\varphi^2} & \varphi \\ -\varphi & \sqrt{1-\varphi^2} \end{pmatrix},$$

[1)] A matrix A is called orthogonal if $AA' = I$. For an orthogonal matrix one has $\det A = \pm 1$.

where one has to choose one and the same value of the root. Consequently, a second-order matrix function all values of which are orthogonal matrices with determinant equal to 1 satisfies the conditions (4.21) for $\gamma = 0$, $\alpha = 1$, $\beta = -1$ and is therefore functionally commutable. Using the formula of case a) from the proof of Theorem 4.12, we obtain

$$G(t) = \frac{1}{2i} \begin{pmatrix} 1 & 1 \\ i & -i \end{pmatrix} \begin{pmatrix} \sqrt{1-\varphi^2} + i\varphi & 0 \\ 0 & \sqrt{1-\varphi^2} - i\varphi \end{pmatrix} \begin{pmatrix} i & 1 \\ i & -1 \end{pmatrix}.$$

Hence, the matrix function under study is Φ-factorable only simultaneously with the functions $\sqrt{1-\varphi^2} + i\varphi$ and $\sqrt{1-\varphi^2} - i\varphi$, and its partial indices coincide with the indices of these functions.

A second-order orthogonal matrix function with determinant -1 is, generally speaking, not functionally commutable. However, after multiplication by the matrix $\begin{pmatrix} 1 & 0 \\ 0 & -1 \end{pmatrix}$ from an arbitrary side, it changes over into an orthogonal matrix function with determinant 1 and, consequently, becomes functionally commutable.

In this way, if G is a second-order orthogonal matrix function with determinant equal to -1, then

$$G = \begin{pmatrix} \sqrt{1-\varphi^2} & \varphi \\ \varphi & -\sqrt{1-\varphi^2} \end{pmatrix} = \frac{1}{2i} \begin{pmatrix} 1 & 1 \\ -i & i \end{pmatrix} \begin{pmatrix} \sqrt{1-\varphi^2} + i\varphi & 0 \\ 0 & \sqrt{1-\varphi^2} - i\varphi \end{pmatrix} \begin{pmatrix} i & 1 \\ i & -1 \end{pmatrix}.$$

Consequently, for an orthogonal matrix function with negative determinant, the result obtained above for an orthogonal matrix function with positive determinant continues to be valid.

4.5. COMMENTS

The criterion of Φ-factorability of a block-triangular matrix function in L_p (Theorem 4.1) and the Theorems 4.2, 4.3, 4.5 resulting from it are due to one of the authors (SPITKOVSKIĬ [11,12]).

In Section 1 of the next chapter it will be shown that, for matrix functions from the classes $L_\infty^{\pm} + C$, the Φ-factorability is equivalent to the invertibility in these classes. Therefore, Theorem 4.1 is obvious for such matrix functions.

Theorem 4.4 is a special case (for $p = 2$) of a result from SPITKOVSKII [8]. In connection with this theorem, note that, for $p = 2$, the decision when operators of the form $T_Q(\omega)$ are Φ_--operators, is well-known (DOUGLAS, SARASON [1]); the criterion consists in the fact that there must exist a function $\varphi \in H_\infty + C$ such that $\operatorname{ess\,sup}|1-\varphi\omega^{-1}| < 1$. The proof of Theorem 4.6 is borrowed from the article of GOHBERG and KREĬN [3]. In the same article the order relation $\succ$ was introduced with the aim to study the question of stability of partial indices (concerning this topic, see Chapter 6). Furthermore, in this paper those properties of the relation $\succ$ were demonstrated which are gathered in Lemma 4.1. Theorem 4.7 based on this lemma was proved in SPITKOVSKIĬ [11,12]. The approach of "shifting" by k used in the proof of the mentioned theorem may also be applied in other cases. For instance, with the help of this approach, from results of MANDZHAVIDZE [7], it is derived in MANDZHAVIDZE [8,9] that the tuple of partial indices of the Riemann boundary value problem with shift depending on a parameter is constant. Moreover, it is majorized (for all values of the parameter with the possible exception of a finite number of points) in the sense of the relation $\succ$ by the tuple of partial indices of the corresponding problem without shift.

Theorem 4.8 and Corollary 4.3 (for $n = 2$) were established by CHEBOTAREV [2]. For $n > 2$, Corollary 4.3 was proved in GOHBERG, KREĬN [3], and Theorem 4.8 is due to NIKOLAĬCHUK [1] and PRIMACHUK [2]. Here a new proof of the necessity has been presented.
We refer also to another result from LITVINCHUK, SPITKOVSKIĬ [2] according to which the partial indices of a triangular matrix function coincide with the indices of the diagonal elements if and only if this matrix function admits a factorization with factors $G_\pm$ of the same triangularity. In the paper GAVDZINSKIĬ, SPITKOVSKIĬ [1] (see also ISKENDEROV [1]) the reduction of the factorization problem of a second-order matrix function to the corresponding problem for a triangular matrix function is discussed.
The factorization of second-order matrix functions given on a contour

$\Gamma = \Gamma_1 \cup \Gamma_2$ bounding a doubly connected domain which are upper triangular on Γ_1 and lower triangular on Γ_2 was considered in Section 4.3 of CLANCEY, GOHBERG [3].

Corollary 4.4 was presented in NIKOLAǏCHUK [1], PRIMACHUK [2] and, in a somewhat weaker variant, in GOHBERG, KREǏN [3].

Theorem 4.9 and Corollary 4.5 resulting from it have been proved in NIKOLENKO [2]; in the present book a proof of Corollary 4.5 is described that is adapted to the factorization in L_p (in NIKOLAǏCHUK [1], PRIMACHUK [2], CHEBOTAREV [2] the factorization of Hölder matrix functions was considered). Theorem 4.10 was published in SPITKOVSKIǏ [11,12]. The question of an effective factorization of triangular matrix functions with non-factorable diagonal elements has not been solved yet even for $n = 2$. This question is very important (and difficult), since the consideration of convolution type equations on a finite interval leads to the factorization of exactly such matrix functions (cf. GLAZMAN, LYUBICH [1], KARLOVICH, SPITKOVSKIǏ [1], NOVOKSHENOV [1], PAL'TSEV [5], SPITKOVSKIǏ [15]). In the papers GLAZMAN, LYUBICH [1], KOMYAK [1-4], in principle, a way of effectively factorizing matrix functions of the kind

$$\begin{pmatrix} e^{iax} & 0 \\ h(x) & e^{-iax} \end{pmatrix}$$

defined on the real line was proposed, where $a \in \mathbb{R}$, $h^{\pm 1} \in M_\infty^{+}$ or $h^{\pm 1} \in M_\infty^{-}$.

In his review [3] F.D. GAKHOV formulated the problem of finding a matrix function possessing such algebraic properties which allows us to solve the factorization problem effectively. In particular, in this paper the possibility of an effective factorization of functionally commutable matrix functions was discussed. The corresponding investigations based on the algebraic properties of functionally commutable matrix functions proved in MOROZOV [1] (Lemmas 4.2 and 4.3) were accomplished by CHEBOTAREV [1]. The Theorem 4.11 formulated here is a slight modification of results of CHEBOTAREV [1] (see also CHEBOTAREV [3]), where he considered some classes of matrix functions not functionally commutable for which condition (4.3) is valid and, consequently, a factorization may be constructed effectively. Note that these classes contain, for example, the matrix function

$$G(w) = \begin{pmatrix} 1 & -i\sqrt{k^2-w^2} \\ -\dfrac{i}{\sqrt{k^2-w^2}} & 1 \end{pmatrix}, \quad w \in \mathbb{R}$$

given on the real line, the factorization of which was built in HEINS [1] in connection with the study of the diffraction problem on the half-plane.

The factorization of triangular matrix functions was employed in TSITSKISHVILI [4] in solving some problems from filtration theory, and the factorization of functionally commutable matrix functions was used in MEISTER [1], where by its help questions of solvability of integral equations of the first kind with a generalized power kernel were examined.

The factorization of a circulant was studied in the paper GORDIENKO [1]. In GOHBERG, FELDMAN [1] the factorization of matrix functions was discussed which differ from the circulant (4.19) by the presence of the factor t^{-1} at the elements located below the main diagonal.

The paper GOHBERG, FELDMAN [2] is devoted to the generalization of these results to the case when $c_0, c_1, \ldots, c_{n-1}$ are quadratic blocks. Note that the matrix functions considered in GOHBERG, FELDMAN [1,2], generally speaking, fail to be functionally commutable. A detailed explanation of the results from GOHBERG, FELDMAN [1,2] can be found in Section 6.1 of the monograph CLANCEY, GOHBERG [3].

Lemma 4.4 is due to LAPPO-DANILEVSKIĬ [1], p. 82, and Theorem 4.12 to CHEBOTAREV [1].

The factorization of complex orthogonal matrix functions was considered by DIDENKO and CHERNETSKIĬ [1].

CHEBOTAREV's results [1,2] were applied in LE-DINZON [1] in order to obtain sufficient conditions for the effective solution of the Hilbert problem and in VOROB'EV [1] for the factorization of 3×3 matrix functions of a special kind occurring in problems of elasticity theory.

In VOROB'EV [1] the method of separating zeros was also employed for solving the factorization problem. Furthermore, this method was used in TROITSKIǏ [1], where the problem of finding the Jost matrix for the mixture of partial waves in case of a rational dependence of the mixture angle tangent on the squared impulse module was reduced to the factorization problem for a special matrix function.

There is a close connection between the factorization problem for functionally commutable matrix functions and matrix functions of permutation type, i.e. such matrix functions G for which, for every $t \in \Gamma$, exactly one element from any row and column of $G(t)$ is different from zero. If this nontrivial element is equal to one, then $G(t)$ provides a matrix of some permutation, where G is functionally commutable iff the permutations associated with the values of the matrix function G generate an Abelian group. Basing on this fact and making use of well-known results on the structure of finite Abelian groups, KRUGLOV [2,3] succeeded in constructing a factorization of such functionally commutable matrix functions of permutation type and calculated their partial indices. He also studied in [3-6] the factorization of some classes of permutation type matrix functions which are not functionally commutable. In his investigations he used profound connections between the Riemann problem for a pair of functions on a Riemann surface and the corresponding problem for n pairs of functions on the plane with matrix coefficient of permutation type established in È.I. ZVEROVICH [1] (see also ZVEROVICH, POMERANTSEVA [1]). In turn, the results concerning the solution of the factorization problem are applied in KRUGLOV [2-6] to the constructive determination of a field of algebraic functions defined by a monodromy group.

The factorization problem for permutation type matrix functions that are not functionally commutable was considered by PRIMACHUK [3,4] either. Let us point out that the factorization problem for permutation type matrix functions appeared first in CHEREPANOV's papers [1-3] related to certain problems of elasticity theory.

In connection with the question of an effective solution of the factorization problem for matrix functions we would still like to mention the article of KRAVCHENKO, NIKOLAǏCHUK [1], where it was shown that, if some (n-1) th order minor of the nxn matrix function G is factored, then the factorization problem of the matrix function G itself can be reduced to the solution of a special type integral equation with respect to one unknown function.

In PAL'TSEV [2,6], POPOV [1], KHRAPKOV [1], HURD [1], RAWLINS, WILLIAMS [1] one can find several approaches different from the ones pursued here, which allow for effectively factorizing some new classes of matrix functions occurring in applied problems. The search for such approaches is still an actual task because of the non-existence of general methods for constructing factorizations.

Finally, let us focus our attention on another unsolved problem. We have in mind the problem of describing all possible tuples $(\varkappa_j)$ of partial indices of a triangular matrix function with fixed diagonal elements. According to Theorem 4.7, in case of factorable diagonal elements the relation $(k_j) \succ (\varkappa_j)$ necessarily holds, where k_j are the diagonal element indices. For $n = 2$, it follows from Corollary 4.5 that, thanks to the choice of an element outside the diagonal, we succeed in obtaining an arbitrary tuple $(\varkappa_j)$ satisfying this condition. However, it is not clear whether this property preserves for $n > 2$. In case of given non-factorable diagonal elements, the question of the description of all possible tuples $(\varkappa_j)$ remains open even for $n = 2$.

CHAPTER 5. SOME CLASSES OF FACTORABLE MATRIX FUNCTIONS

In this chapter we consider the factorization problem for some special classes of matrix functions with specific analytic properties. In Section 5.1 the criterion of Φ-factorability in L_p of matrix functions of the classes $L_\infty^\pm + C$ will be derived. Section 5.2 is dedicated to the factorization in some Banach algebras of functions, and in Section 5.3 we shall study the Φ-factorization of piecewise continuous matrix functions. The consideration of classes of special matrix functions is useful by making general factorability and Φ-factorability criteria proved in the previous more precise. Moreover, via this approach we are able to clarify some principal facts of factorization theory.

In Section 3.6 we have established that the Φ-factorability of a bounded measurable matrix function G on a contour of the class $\mathfrak{R}$ is equivalent to the Fredholmness of the singu ar integral operator $P + GQ$. Naturally, there arises the question of existence of closed subclasses of L_∞ such that the Φ-factorability criterion of matrix functions from these subclasses can be immediately expressed in terms of the matrix function G itself. It appeared (see Section 3.1) that $L_\infty^\pm + C$ are just subclasses in L_∞ of such a type: for any p, the Φ-factorability of a matrix function $G \in L_\infty^\pm + C$ is equivalent to the membership of the inverse matrix G^{-1} to the same class. For continuous matrix functions, this criterion looks quite simple: the Φ-factorability in L_p of the matrix function $G \in C$ is, for any p, equivalent to the non-singularity of G.

In Chapter 3 it was also shown that the condition $G^{-1} \in L_\infty$ is a necessary condition for Φ-factorability of the matrix function $G \in L_\infty$ in L_p and the gap between this condition and the exact condition of Φ-factorability is rather large. In Section 5.1 below we shall prove that, for a matrix function $G \in L_\infty^\pm + C$, the condition $G^{-1} \in L_\infty$ is equivalent to the demand that $P + GQ$ is a Φ_+- or Φ_--operator. Thus, the consideration of classes $L_\infty^\pm + C$ allowed for more precisely characterizing the gap between necessary and exact condition of Φ-factorability mentioned above: in case $G \in L_\infty^+ + C$ $(L_\infty^- + C)$, the operator $P + GQ$

is a Φ_-- (Φ_+-) operator, but not Fredholm if and only if $G^{-1} \in L_\infty$ and $G^{-1} \notin L_\infty^+ + C$ ($L_\infty^- + C$) .

The following principal fact is connected with the statement proved below (in 5.1): for matrix functions $G \in L_\infty^\pm + C$ Φ-factorable in L_p, the factorization factors are summable with arbitrary power p. The weakness of this result strikes the eye, however, it turns out that it cannot be improved.

In Section 5.2 it will be established that the factorization factors really go beyond the initial class $L_\infty^\pm + C$. From here, in particular, it follows that it is inevitable for the factorization factors of continuous matrix functions to go beyond the "natural" classes $C^\pm$ of matrix functions analytic in $\mathfrak{D}^\pm$ and continuous in $\mathfrak{D}^\pm \cup \Gamma$. In connection with this, it is necessary to find such classes (narrower than L_∞ or C), which, along with every matrix function, contain also its factorization factors.

In Section 5.2 we shall clarify the conditions under which the role of such classes may be played by the classes of matrix functions with entries from Banach algebras of functions containing R and belonging to L_∞ or C (in what follows they are called (L_∞,R)- and (C,R)-algebras, respectively). Furthermore, the connection between factorability in such algebras and the Fredholmness of the operators $P + GQ$ and $Q + G'P$ in the corresponding spaces will be investigated, where we shall essentially use the analogy with results of Chapter 3.

A special case of a (C,R)-algebra are R-algebras, which are, by definition, Banach algebras of functions containing R as a dense subset. It appears that all non-singular matrix functions with entries from some R-algebra $\mathfrak{C}$ admit a factorization with factors of the same class iff the algebra is decomposing, that means, it consists only of elements analytically continuable in $\mathfrak{D}^+$ and $\mathfrak{D}^-$ as well as sums of such elements. For a more general case of a (C,R)-algebra $\mathfrak{A}$, decomposition continues to be a necessary condition of factorability in $\mathfrak{A}$ for all non-singular matrix functions with entries from $\mathfrak{A}$. Unfortunately, a necessary and sufficient condition can be formulated only in a more complicated way. This condition will be discussed in the comments 5.4. In the main text of the chapter only one sufficient condition will be proved, and various corollaries will be obtained from it.

A concrete example of a decomposing R-algebra important for application is the algebra W of functions defined on the unit circle and representable in the form of absolutely convergent Fourier series. The algebra H^{α} of functions satisfying a Hölder condition with exponent $0<\alpha \leq 1$ provides an example of a (C,R)-algebra which is not an R-algebra.

In Section 5.2 we present also a local principle which allows for constructing new classes of matrix functions, which admit a factorization with continuous factors, by sticking together matrix functions from the classes indicated.

The results of Section 5.3 on Φ-factorability of piecewise continuous matrix functions rest essentially upon the factorization of the power function (considered in Chapter 2) and enlarge our knowledge on the structure of the domain of Φ-factorability.

Unlike the case of matrix functions from $L_{\infty}^{\pm} + C$, the domain of Φ-factorability of piecewise continuous matrix functions may be not only an empty set or the ray $(1,\infty)$, but may consist of a finite number of connected components. Correspondingly, the complement to a non-empty domain of Φ-factorability of piecewise continuous matrix functions with respect to the ray $(1,\infty)$ consists of a finite number of isolated values of the parameter p.

The characterization of the results of the present chapter would be incomplete, if we did not indicate that for Φ-factorable continuous and piecewise continuous matrix functions effective formulae will be presented with the aid of which the total index can be evaluated.

In addition to comments on references, in Section 5.4 we shall discuss the question of relationships between Φ-factorization in L_p of piecewise Hölder matrix functions and the classical factorization problem for these matrix functions in special classes introduced by N. I. MUSKHELISHVILI and named after him as well as the Φ-factorization problem in weighted L_p spaces.

5.1. Φ-FACTORIZATION OF MATRIX FUNCTIONS FROM CLASSES $L_\infty^{\pm} + C$

In this section as well as in the whole previous chapter, the contour Γ is assumed to belong to the class $\mathcal{R}$. Under this condition, for any matrix function G belonging together with its inverse to L_∞, the following relations are satisfied:

$$T_Q(G^{-1})T_Q(G) = (I - QG^{-1}PGQ)|_{\operatorname{im} Q} , \tag{5.1}$$

$$T_Q(G)T_Q(G^{-1}) = (I - QGPG^{-1}Q)|_{\operatorname{im} Q} . \tag{5.2}$$

Employing formulae (3.22), these equations can be immediately verified.

The key to the investigation of Φ-factorization of matrix functions from $L_\infty^{\pm} + C$ is, in addition to relations(5.1) and (5.2), the following simple statement.

LEMMA 5.1. If $G \in L_\infty^{+} + C$ $(L_\infty^{-} + C)$, then the operator QGP (PGQ) is compact in all spaces L_p, $1 < p < \infty$.

Proof. According to the definition of $L_\infty^{+} + C$, a matrix function G from this class can be represented in the form $G = G_0 + G_+$, where $G_0 \in C$, $G_+ \in L_\infty^{+}$. Now we introduce a sequence of rational matrix functions F_k uniformly converging to G_0. Its poles are assumed to lie off Γ. Moreover, we set $G_k = F_k + G_+$. Obviously $G_k \in M_\infty^{+}$, thus, according to Theorem 1.35, the operators QG_kP defined on the whole space L_p^n are bounded and finite dimensional. Furthermore, the sequence $\{QG_kP\}$ converges to QGP in the operator topology. Consequently, the operator QGP is the limit of a uniformly convergent sequence of finite-dimensional bounded operators and therefore compact. The case $G \in L_\infty^{-} + C$ can be treated analogously. ∎

THEOREM 5.1. Let $G \in L_\infty^{+} + C$ $(L_\infty^{-} + C)$. Then $P + GQ$ is a Φ_-- (Φ_+-) operator iff $G^{-1} \in L_\infty$.

Proof. The necessity of the condition $G^{-1} \in L_\infty$ for $P + GQ$ to be a Φ_-- (Φ_+-) operator results from Theorem 3.18 (for $A = I$, $B = G$) and holds regardless of the validity of the requirement $G \in L_\infty^{\pm} + C$.

If $G \in L_\infty^+ + C$, then, owing to Lemma 5.1, the operator QGP is compact. If in this case $G^{-1} \in L_\infty$, then the operator $QGPG^{-1}Q$ is also compact. Therefore, in view of relation (5.2), the operator $T_Q(G^{-1})$ is a right regularizer for $T_Q(G)$. With regard to Theorem 1.8, we conclude from this that $T_Q(G)$ is a Φ_--operator. Due to assertion 1) of Lemma 3.5, $P + GQ$ is a Φ_--operator, too.

Analogously, making use of (5.1), we establish that, for $G \in L_\infty^- + C$, $P + GQ$ is a Φ_+-operator if $G^{-1} \in L_\infty$. This proves Theorem 5.1. ≡

<u>COROLLARY 5.1.</u> If $G \in L_\infty^+ + C$ $(L_\infty^- + C)$, then the property of the operator $P + GQ$ to be a Φ_+- (Φ_--) operator is equivalent to its Fredholmness.

In fact, if $P + GQ$ is a Φ_+- (Φ_--) operator, then it follows that $G^{-1} \in L_\infty$. If, in addition, $G \in L_\infty^+ + C$ $(L_\infty^- + C)$, then, in view of Theorem 5.1, the operator $P + GQ$ is a Φ_-- (Φ_+-) operator, and, consequently, Fredholm. ≡

However, from the fact that $P + GQ$ is a Φ_-- (Φ_+-) operator and $G \in L_\infty^+ + C$ $(L_\infty^- + C)$ does not follow the Fredholmness. A class of examples of this kind was presented in the previous chapter after Theorem 4.4.

In order to get a criterion of Fredholmness of the operator $P + GQ$ in case $G \in L_\infty^\pm + C$, we need, in addition to Lemma 5.1, some more properties of the classes $L_\infty^\pm + C$ formulated below as Lemmas 5.2 and 5.3. As in Theorem 3.21, we denote by G_j the restriction of the matrix function G on the contour $\Gamma(j)$, $j = 0,\ldots,m-1$.

<u>LEMMA 5.2.</u> The inclusion $G \in L_\infty^+ + C$ holds if and only if $G_0 \in (L_\infty^+ + C)(\Gamma(0))$ and $G_j \in (L_\infty^- + C)(\Gamma(j))$, $j=1,\ldots,m-1$. The inclusion $G \in L_\infty^- + C$ is valid iff $G_0 \in (L_\infty^- + C)(\Gamma(0))$ and $G_j \in (L_\infty^+ + C)(\Gamma(j))$, $j=1,\ldots,m-1$.

<u>Proof.</u> Let $G \in L_\infty^+ + C$, i.e. $G = \Psi + F$, where $\Psi \in L_\infty^+$ and $F \in C$. Set $\Psi_j(z) = \frac{1}{2\pi i} \int_{\Gamma(j)} \Psi(\tau) \frac{d\tau}{\tau - z}$, $j=0,\ldots,m-1$.

Then $\Psi_j \in E(\mathfrak{D}^-(j))$, $j=1,\ldots,m-1$, $\Psi_0 \in E(\mathfrak{D}^+(0))$, and $\Psi = \sum_{j=0}^{m-1} \Psi_j$.

Each of the matrix functions Ψ_j is continuous on Γ with the exception of the curve $\Gamma(j)$. From here and $\Psi \in L^+_\infty$ it follows that $\Psi_j \in L_\infty$. With regard to Theorems 1.25 and 1.33, we have $\Psi_j \in E_\infty(\mathfrak{D}^-(j))$, $j=1,\dots,m-1$, $\Psi_o \in E_\infty(\mathfrak{D}^+(0))$.

Now we define a continuous matrix function H on the contour Γ by setting $H_j = F_j + \sum_{s \neq j} \Psi_s$. Then $G_j = \Psi_j + H_j$ and, therefore $G_o \in (L^+_\infty + C)(\Gamma(0))$, $G_j \in (L^-_\infty + C)(\Gamma(j))$, $j=1,\dots,m-1$.

Conversely, if $G_j = \Psi_j + H_j$, where H_j is a matrix function continuous on $\Gamma(j)$, $\Psi_j \in E_\infty(\mathfrak{D}^-(j))$ for $j=1,\dots,m-1$, and $\Psi_o \in E_\infty(\mathfrak{D}^+(0))$, then $G = \Psi + F$ for $\Psi = \sum_{j=o}^{m-1} \Psi_j$ and $F_j = H_j - \sum_{s \neq j} \Psi_s$. Hence $G \in L^+_\infty + C$. The assertion related to a matrix function $G \in L^-_\infty + C$ may be proved in an analogous manner. $\equiv$

<u>LEMMA 5.3.</u> The classes $L^\pm_\infty + C$ are closed in L_∞.

<u>Proof.</u> Lemma 5.2 enables us to restrict ourselves to the case of a connected contour Γ. Since a conformal mapping of a simply connected domain with Jordan boundary onto the circle may be extended to a continuous mapping of the closure of this domain onto the closed disk (VLADIMIROV, VOLOVICH [1], p.46), it is sufficient to verify the closedness of the classes $H^\pm_\infty + C$. Denote by C^+ the subspace of C consisting of boundary values of functions analytic in the unit disk, and consider the mapping i of the factor space $C|C^+$ into the factor space $L_\infty|H_\infty$ defined by the equation

$$i(f + C^+) = f + H_\infty , \quad f \in C .$$

For any function $f \in L_\infty$, we have $\inf_{h \in H_\infty}\|f-h\| \leq \inf_{h \in C^+}\|f-h\|$, thus, the mapping i is a contraction. Now we intend to show that, of course, it is isometric, i.e., $\inf_{h \in H_\infty}\|f-h\| = \inf_{h \in C^+}\|f-h\|$ holds for every $f \in C$.

For this purpose, we choose $h \in H_\infty$ arbitrarily and consider the k th Cesaro means f_k and h_k of the functions f and h, respectively. Clearly, $\|f-h_k\| \leq \|f-f_k\| + \|f_k-h_k\| \leq \|f-f_k\| + \|f-h\|$.

Since $\lim_{k\to\infty} \|f-f_k\| = 0 \quad h_k \in C^+$, from the latter inequality we obtain the assertion to be proved. Therefore, the image $\mathfrak{C}$ of the whole subspace $C|C^+$ under the mapping i must be closed. But then the pre-image of the subspace $\mathfrak{C}$ under the natural projection of L_∞ onto $L_\infty|H_\infty$ is also closed. In order to prove the closedness of $H_\infty + C$ in L_∞, it remains to note that $H_\infty + C$ is just this pre-image. The class $H_\infty^- + C$ is obtained from $H_\infty + C$ by applying conjugation. Consequently, it is closed along with the class $H_\infty + C$, and the proof of Lemma 5.3 is complete. ≡

COROLLARY 5.2. The classes $L_\infty^+ + C$ and $L_\infty^- + C$ are subalgebras of L_∞.

Proof. It is easy to check that the product of a rational function by a function from L_∞^+ may be represented as the sum of a rational function and a function from L_∞^+. Hence, it follows that the multiplication does not go beyond the class M_∞^+. Therefore, M_∞^+ is a subalgebra of L_∞. Since M_∞^+ is dense in $L_\infty^+ + C$, and $L_\infty^+ + C$ is a closed subset of L_∞ (in view of the previous lemma), $L_\infty^+ + C$ is just the closure of M_∞^+. Thus, it is a subalgebra simultaneously with M_∞^+. The class $L_\infty^- + C$ can be considered in the same way. ≡

THEOREM 5.2. Let $G \in L_\infty^+ + C$ $(L_\infty^- + C)$. Then the condition $G^{-1} \in L_\infty^+ + C$ $(L_\infty^- + C)$ is necessary for Φ-factorability of the matrix function G for at least one $p \in (1,\infty)$ and sufficient for its Φ-factorability for all $p \in (1,\infty)$. If this condition is satisfied, then each factorization of G has the properties

$$G_+^{\pm 1} \in \bigcap_{p<\infty} L_p^+ \ , \quad G_-^{\pm 1} \in \bigcap_{p<\infty} L_p^- \tag{5.3}$$

and is a Φ-factorization in all spaces L_p, $1 < p < \infty$.

Proof. Assume $G \in L_\infty^+ + C$. We choose a sequence $G_k \in M_\infty^+$ uniformly converging to G. If, for some $p \in (1,\infty)$, the matrix function G is Φ-factorable in L_p, then, according to Corollary 3.4, $G^{-1} \in L_\infty$. Therefore, for k large enough, the matrix functions G_k are invertible and $G_k^{-1} \to G^{-1}$. Moreover, since the property of Φ-factorability is stable (Theorem 3.20), we conclude the Φ-factorability of G_k

(again for sufficiently large k). Owing to Theorem 3.15, $G_k^{-1} \in M_\infty^+$. From here and the closedness of the class $L_\infty^+ + C$, it follows that $G^{-1} \in L_\infty^+ + C$.

Conversely, if $G^{\pm 1} \in L_\infty^+ + C$, then formulae (5.1) and (5.2) show that the operator $T_Q(G^{-1})$ is a two-sided regularizer of the operator $T_Q(G)$ in all subspaces $(\mathring{L}_p^-)^n$, $1 < p < \infty$. Consequently, the operator $T_Q(G)$ (and, thus, also $P + GQ$) is Fredholm. By Theorem 3.16, the matrix function G is Φ-factorable in all spaces L_p, $1 < p < \infty$. Now we are going to show that its factorization does not depend upon p. Since the regularizer of the operator $T_Q(G)$ constructed above is one and the same in all spaces $(\mathring{L}_p^-)^n$, $1 < p < \infty$, then its index also does not depend upon p and, therefore, the total index of G does not depend upon p, too. According to Corollary 2.2 and Theorem 3.8, any factorization of G is its Φ-factorization in all L_p, $1 < p < \infty$. From this fact we get, in particular, the property (5.3). Thus Theorem 5.2 has been proved. ≡

<u>COROLLARY 5.3.</u> Suppose $G \in M_\infty^+$ (M_∞^-). Then the conditions $G^{-1} \in M_\infty^+$ (M_∞^-) and $G^{-1} \in L_\infty^+ + C$ $(L_\infty^- + C)$ are equivalent.

In fact, with regard to Theorem 3.15 (3.15'), the condition $G^{-1} \in M_\infty^+$ (M_∞^-) is necessary and sufficient for the Φ-factorability of the matrix function $G \in M_\infty^+$ (M_∞^-). At the same time, Φ-factorability of G is, thanks to Theorem 5.2, equivalent to the requirement $G^{-1} \in L_\infty^+ + C$ $(L_\infty^- + C)$. ≡

<u>COROLLARY 5.4.</u> Suppose $G \in L_\infty^+ + C$ $(L_\infty^- + C)$. Then $P + GQ$ is a Φ_-- $(\Phi_+$-$)$ operator but not Fredholm if and only if $G^{-1} \in L_\infty$ but $G^{-1} \notin L_\infty^+ + C$ $(L_\infty^- + C)$.

<u>COROLLARY 5.5.</u> The domain of Φ-factorability of the matrix function $G \in L_\infty^{\pm} + C$ is either empty (in case $G^{-1} \notin L_\infty^{\pm} + C$) or consists of a single component occupying the whole ray $(1,\infty)$ (in case $G^{-1} \in L_\infty^{\pm} + C$).

<u>COROLLARY 5.6.</u> The matrix function $G \in L_\infty^{\pm} + C$ admits or does not admit a right Φ-factorization only simultaneously with a left one,

and its left total index coincides with its right total index.

Proof. In virtue of Theorem 3.7', the matrix function $G \in L_\infty$ is right Φ-factorable in L_p iff the matrix function G' is left Φ-factorable in L_q. But if $G \in \overset{\pm}{L}_\infty + C$, then also $G' \in \overset{\pm}{L}_\infty + C$, and by Theorem 5.2, the left Φ-factorability of G' in L_q is equivalent to the requirement $(G')^{-1} \in \overset{\pm}{L}_\infty + C$ or, what is the same, $G^{-1} \in \overset{\pm}{L}_\infty + C$. The latter demand is, again by Theorem 5.2, equivalent to the left Φ-factorability of G in L_p. With regard to Theorem 3.20, it suffices to prove the coincidence of the left total index with the right one for matrix functions from the class $\overset{\pm}{M}_\infty$, which is dense in $\overset{\pm}{L}_\infty + C$. For matrix functions of this class, the assertion to be proved is valid by Theorems 2.6 and 2.7. ≡

Let us consider in more detail that important case when the matrix function under study is continuous.

THEOREM 5.3. Let the matrix function G be continuous. Its non--singularity on Γ is necessary for the Φ-factorability of G in at least one L_p and sufficient for its Φ-factorability in all L_p, $1 < p < \infty$. Furthermore, the total index of a non-singular continuous matrix function G can be calculated by the formula

$$\varkappa = \frac{1}{2\pi}\{\arg \det G(t)\}_\Gamma . \tag{5.4}$$

Proof. If the matrix function G is Φ-factorable for at least one value $p \in (1,\infty)$, then, by Corollary 3.5, $G^{-1} \in L_\infty$. Hence the function $\det G^{-1}$ is bounded and, consequently, the continuous function $\det G$ is separated from zero. Therefore, G is non-singular on Γ.
Vice versa, if the continuous matrix function G is non-singular on Γ, then the inverse matrix function G^{-1} is also continuous.
By Theorem 5.2, G is Φ-factorable in all L_p, $1 < p < \infty$.

Now we intend to prove formula (5.4). Both parts of this formula are continuous functions, if we consider them on the set $\hat{C}$ of continuous non-degenerating matrix functions with the topology of uniform convergence. According to Theorem 2.6 and statement 4) of Theorem 1.29, formula (5.4) holds on the set of rational matrix functions not having poles and being non-singular on Γ . Since this set is dense in $\hat{C}$, formula (5.4) is true for all continuous non-singular matrix functions. Thus Theorem 5.3 is proved. ≡

COROLLARY 5.7. Assume G to be a continuous non-degenerating matrix function. Its partial indices are equal to zero (non-positive, non-negative) if and only if the operator $P + GQ$ is invertible (right invertible, left invertible) in the space L_p^n for at least one $p \in (1,\infty)$.

Corollary 5.7 is a reformulation of Corollary 3.8, taking into account that the Fredholmness of the operator $P + GQ$ is guaranteed by the continuity and non-singularity of G .

COROLLARY 5.8. A continuous non-singular matrix function admits a right Φ-factorization in any space L_p , $1 < p < \infty$, where the total right index coincides with the total left one.

Proof. In order to prove the existence of a right Φ-factorization, it is necessary to apply Theorem 5.3 to the matrix function G' and, after this, to use Theorem 3.7. The sum of right indices of the matrix function G coincides with the sum of left indices of G' . Consequently, it is equal to $\frac{1}{2\pi}\{\arg\det G'(t)\}_\Gamma = \frac{1}{2\pi}\{\arg\det G(t)\}_\Gamma$, i.e., it coincides with the sum of left indices of G . ≡

In connection with Theorem 5.3, note that the sufficiency of the non-singularity condition of a continuous matrix function G for its Φ-factorability can be easily proved by means of the local principle, i.e., with the aid of Theorem 3.2. Indeed, the continuous matrix function G is, at each point $t_0 \in \Gamma$, ε-locally equivalent to its value at this point. The Φ-factorability of a constant non-singular matrix $G(t_0)$ is evident.

The factorization factors $G_\pm$ of G belonging together with its inverse to the class $L_\infty^+ + C$ $(L_\infty^- + C)$ possess the property (5.3). Therefore, they themselves and their inverses are summable with any finite power. With the help of Theorem 2.4 we are able to prove a local variant of this assertion.

THEOREM 5.4. Let the matrix function G be factorable in L_p and G_1 be such that $G_1^{\pm 1} \in L_\infty^+ + C$ or $G_1^{\pm 1} \in L_\infty^- + C$, and G coincides with G_1 on some open arc γ of the contour Γ. Then the factorization factors $G_\pm$ of the matrix function G as well as their inverses are summable with any finite power on each arc $\tilde{\gamma}$ whose closure lies in γ.

COROLLARY 5.9. If the matrix function G is factorable in L_p, continuous and non-degenerating on the open arc $\gamma \subset \Gamma$, then the factorization factors $G_\pm$ of G and their inverses are summable with any finite power on every arc whose closure lies in γ.

THEOREM 5.5. Let $G_1^{\pm 1} \in L_\infty^+ + C$, $G_2^{\pm 1} \in L_\infty^- + C$. If the matrix function G is Φ-factorable in L_p, then G_1GG_2 is also Φ-factorable in L_p, where the total indices of the matrix functions G, G_1, G_2 and G_1GG_2 are connected by the relation $\varkappa(G_1GG_2) = \varkappa(G_1)+\varkappa(G)+\varkappa(G_2)$.

Proof. For arbitrary matrix functions $G_1, G, G_2 \in L_\infty$, the equation

$$T_Q(G_1GG_2) = QG_1GG_2|_{\text{im } Q} = QG_1QGQG_2|_{\text{im } Q} + QG_1PGQG_2|_{\text{im } Q} + QG_1GPG_2Q|_{\text{im } Q}$$

holds. By Lemma 5.1, the operators QG_1P and PG_2Q are compact if $G_1 \in L_\infty^+ + C$, $G_2 \in L_\infty^- + C$. Hence, the operators $T_Q(G_1GG_2)$ and $QG_1QGQG_2Q|_{\text{im } Q} = T_Q(G_1)T_Q(G)T_Q(G_2)$ are Fredholm only simultaneously and have the same index. It remains to note that, in view of Theorem 5.2, the condition $G_1^{\pm 1} \in L_\infty^+ + C$ implies the Fredholmness of the operator $T_Q(G_1)$ and the condition $G_2^{\pm 1} \in L_\infty^- + C$ the Fredholmness of $T_Q(G_2)$. Due to Theorems 1.6 and 1.9, the product $T_Q(G_1)T_Q(G)T_Q(G_2)$ is Fredholm only simultaneously with the operator $T_Q(G)$ and has an index equal to the sum of the indices of the factors. Thus Theorem 5.5 is completely proved. ≡

COROLLARY 5.10. If the matrix functions G_1 and G_2 are continuous and non-singular on Γ, then the matrix functions G and G_1GG_2 are Φ-factorable only simultaneously, and their total indices are connected via the relation

$$\varkappa(G_1GG_2) = \varkappa(G) + \frac{1}{2\pi}\{\arg \det G_1(t)G_2(t)\}_\Gamma .$$

Owing to the inclusion $M_\infty^\pm \in L_\infty^\pm + C$, Theorem 5.5 is a generalization of Theorem 3.10. Theorem 5.5 and Corollary 5.10 are often useful, even if one of the matrix functions G_1 and G_2 is chosen equal to I.

5.2. FACTORIZATION IN BANACH ALGEBRAS OF MATRIX FUNCTIONS

Theorem 5.2 answers the question of Φ-factorability of continuous matrix functions completely. However, the boundary properties of the factorization factors established in this theorem (inclusion (5.3)) seem to be too weak. Consequently, we wish to strengthen them. The following example shows that it is impossible to do this without additional restrictions, even for continuous G and $n = 1$.

<u>EXAMPLE.</u> Let Γ be the unit circle $\mathbb{T}$ and

$$G(t) = \exp\left[\sum_{k=2}^{\infty} \frac{1}{k \ln k}(t^k - t^{-k})\right].$$

G is a continuous and non-vanishing function. Setting

$$G_+(z) = \exp\left(\sum_{k=2}^{\infty} \frac{1}{k \ln k} z^k\right), \quad G_-(z) = \exp\left(-\sum_{k=2}^{\infty} \frac{1}{k \ln k} z^{-k}\right),$$

$\Lambda(t) = 1$, we obtain its factorization (and, thus, also its Φ-factorization). Since the series $\sum_{k=2}^{\infty} \frac{1}{k \ln k}$ diverges, the function $\sum_{k=2}^{\infty} \frac{1}{k \ln k} z^k$ is not bounded from above on the interval $(0,1)$ and, consequently, its absolute value is not bounded from above in the open unit disk. Therefore $G_+ \notin H_\infty^+$. Hence, the relation $|G_+G_-| = |G| = 1$ implies $G_-^{-1} \notin H_\infty^-$.

In this way, it is actually necessary to go beyond the classes $L_\infty^\pm$ (and, moreover, the classes $C^\pm$ of functions analytic in $\mathcal{D}^\pm$ and continuous in $\mathcal{D}^\pm \cup \Gamma$) if we look for the factorization of all continuous matrix functions. Nevertheless, there exist continuous matrix functions the factorization factors $G_\pm$ of which satisfy the condition

$$G_+^{\pm 1} \in L_\infty^+, \quad G_-^{\pm 1} \in L_\infty^-. \tag{5.5}$$

According to Theorem 2.9, all rational matrix functions not possessing poles and non-degenerating on Γ are of this type. The following problem arises in a natural way: find classes of matrix functions (as wide as possible) which admit a factorization with property (5.5). Going towards the solution of this problem, we come to the notion of factorization in a Banach algebra of functions.

In what follows, we shall consider algebras $\mathcal{A}$ intermediate between R and L_∞ :

$$R \subseteq \mathcal{A} \subseteq L_\infty .$$

In doing so, it is clear that 1 (the function identically equal to 1) is the unit element in $\mathcal{A}$. The algebra $\mathcal{A}$ is assumed to be supplied with a norm $\|\cdot\|_{\mathcal{A}}$ with respect to which it is complete. A Banach algebra of functions defined on Γ having the properties enumerated is called a (L_∞, R)-algebra.

A trivial example of such an algebra provides $\mathcal{A} = L_\infty$ with the natural norm

$$\|a\|_\infty = \text{ess sup}\{|a(t)| : t \in \Gamma\} .$$

The role of $\mathcal{A}$ can also be played by any subalgebra of L_∞ , e.g. by $L_\infty^\pm + C$ or C . Other examples, in which $\|\cdot\|_{\mathcal{A}}$ is not equivalent to $\|\cdot\|_\infty$, will be given below.

LEMMA 5.4. Let $\mathcal{A}$ be a (L_∞, R)-algebra. Then we have:

1) for the invertibility of $a \in \mathcal{A}$ it is necessary that $a^{-1} \in L_\infty$,

2) for all $a \in \mathcal{A}$, the relation

$$\|a\|_{\mathcal{A}} \geq \|a\|_\infty \qquad (5.6)$$

holds.

Proof. Assertion 1) is an obvious consequence of the inclusion $\mathcal{A} \subseteq L_\infty$. To prove 2), let us consider an arbitrary element $a \in \mathcal{A}$. One can specify a number ζ_0 such that $|\zeta_0| = \|a\|_\infty$ and $a - \zeta_0$ is not invertible in L_∞ . In fact, in the opposite case we could, for every point ζ of the circle $C_0 = \{\zeta : |\zeta| = \|a\|_\infty\}$, indicate a neighbourhood the values of which are attained by the function a only on a set of measure zero [1]. Choosing from the obtained covering of C_0 a finite subcovering, we would get that a.e. the function a attains values which have a positive distance from C_0 . But this contradicts the

---

[1] We assume $\zeta_0 \neq 0$, since otherwise $a \equiv 0$ and $\|a\|_{\mathcal{A}} = \|a\|_{L_\infty} = 0$.

definition of $\|a\|_\infty$. Thus, the existence of the desired ζ_0 has been proved. According to assertion 1) just proved, the non-invertibility of $a - \zeta_0$ in L_∞ implies its non-invertibility in $\mathfrak{A}$. Along with $a - \zeta_0$, the element $a\zeta_0^{-1} - 1$ is also non-invertible in $\mathfrak{A}$. But then $\|a\zeta_0^{-1}\|_{\mathfrak{A}} \geq 1$, because otherwise from the contracting mapping principle we would obtain the invertibility of $a\zeta_0^{-1} - 1$.
Thus, $\|a\|_{\mathfrak{A}} = \|a\zeta_0^{-1}\|_{\mathfrak{A}}|\zeta_0| \geq |\zeta_0| = \|a\|_\infty$, which proves Lemma 5.4. ≡

The necessary invertibility condition stated in assertion 1) of Lemma 5.4 is, generally speaking, not sufficient. A suitable example yield the algebras $L_\infty^{\pm} + C$. The invertibility criteria in these algebras will be presented in Section 5.4. Nevertheless, in a number of important cases (for instance, for the algebra C) an assertion converse to 1) is true. With this in mind, the following definition is of interest.

DEFINITION 5.1. The (L_∞,R)-algebra $\mathfrak{A}$ is said to have the *invertibility property* if the conditions $a \in \mathfrak{A}$ and $a^{-1} \in L_\infty$ imply $a^{-1} \in \mathfrak{A}$.

From assertion 2) of Lemma 5.4 there results now the following proposition.

COROLLARY 5.11. The convergence in a (L_∞,R)-algebra $\mathfrak{A}$ implies the uniform convergence.

Setting $\mathfrak{A}^{\pm} = \mathfrak{A} \cap L_\infty^{\pm}$ and $\overset{\circ}{\mathfrak{A}}{}^{-} = \mathfrak{A} \cap \overset{\circ}{L}{}_\infty^{-}$, we observe that $\mathfrak{A}^{\pm}$ and $\overset{\circ}{\mathfrak{A}}{}^{-}$ are subalgebras of $\mathfrak{A}$ closed in virtue of Corollary 5.11.

DEFINITION 5.2. The representation (2.1) with

$$G_+^{\pm 1} \in \mathfrak{A}^+ , \quad G_-^{\pm 1} \in \mathfrak{A}^- , \tag{5.7}$$

where the matrix function Λ is defined by formula (2.2), is called a *factorization of the matrix function* G *in the* (L_∞,R)-*algebra* $\mathfrak{A}$.

It is clear from this definition that only matrix functions belonging together with their inverses to the algebra $\mathfrak{A}$ may admit a factorization in $\mathfrak{A}$. With this in mind, remark that for a matrix function $G \in \mathfrak{A}$ the condition $G^{-1} \in \mathfrak{A}$ is fulfilled if and only if $(\det G)^{-1} \in \mathfrak{A}$. If the algebra $\mathfrak{A}$ has the invertibility property, then, for a matrix function $G \in \mathcal{A}$, the conditions $G^{-1} \in \mathcal{A}$ and $G^{-1} \in L_\infty$ are equivalent to each other.

Clearly, a factorization in an arbitrary (L_∞, R)-algebra $\mathcal{A}$ is simultaneously a factorization of G in all L_p , $1 < p < \infty$. A simple calculation of the argument increment of the determinants on the left- and right-hand sides in equation (2.1) shows that, for a factorization in $\mathcal{A}$, the rule (5.4) for calculating the total index is valid. According to formulae (2.6) related to the passage from one factorization to another (with the same total index), from the relation $R \subseteq \mathcal{A}$ we conclude that either every factorization of a matrix function in L_p is its factorization in $\mathcal{A}$ or there does not exist any factorization in $\mathcal{A}$.

DEFINITION 5.3. The (L_∞, R)-algebra $\mathcal{A}$ is said to be <u>decomposing</u> if every element $a \in \mathcal{A}$ admits a representation in the form $a = a_+ + a_-$, where $a_+ \in \mathcal{A}^+$ and $a_- \in \mathring{\mathcal{A}}^-$.

LEMMA 5.5. The following assertions are equivalent:

1) the (L_∞, R)-algebra $\mathcal{A}$ is decomposing,

2) $\mathcal{A} = \mathcal{A}^+ \dot{+} \mathring{\mathcal{A}}^-$,

3) $P\mathcal{A} = \mathcal{A}^+$, $Q\mathcal{A} = \mathring{\mathcal{A}}^-$,

4) the operator S maps $\mathcal{A}$ into itself,

5) the operator S is bounded in $\mathcal{A}$.

Proof. The equivalence of assertions 1) and 2) follows from the relation $\mathcal{A}^+ \cap \mathring{\mathcal{A}}^- \subseteq L_\infty^+ \cap \mathring{L}_\infty^- = \{0\}$. If 2) is fulfilled, then $P\mathcal{A} = P(\mathcal{A}^+ \dot{+} \mathring{\mathcal{A}}^-) = P\mathcal{A}^+ = \mathcal{A}^+$. Analogously, $Q\mathcal{A} = \mathring{\mathcal{A}}^-$. Therefore, 2) implies 3).

If 3) holds, then, for every $\varphi \in \mathcal{A}$, the inclusion $S\varphi = P\varphi - Q\varphi \in \mathcal{A}^+ \dot{+} \mathring{\mathcal{A}}^- = \mathcal{A}$ is valid. Thus, 3) ==> 4).

Vice versa, if $S\mathcal{A} \subseteq \mathcal{A}$, then also $P\mathcal{A} \subseteq \mathcal{A}$. Since $\mathcal{A} \subseteq L_\infty$, we have in this case $P\mathcal{A} \subseteq L_p^+$ for any $p < \infty$. Hence $P\mathcal{A} \subseteq \mathcal{A} \cap L_p^+$. Taking into consideration that Γ is a Smirnov contour, we obtain from Theorem 1.25 that $\mathcal{A} \cap L_p^+ = \mathcal{A} \cap L_\infty^+ = \mathcal{A}^+$. In other words, $P\mathcal{A} \subseteq \mathcal{A}^+$. Analogously, $Q\mathcal{A} \subseteq \mathring{\mathcal{A}}^-$. Since the converse inclusions are obvious, the implication 4) ==> 3) is valid. If 3) is satisfied, then, for every $a \in \mathcal{A}$, we have $a = Pa + Qa \in \mathcal{A}^+ \dot{+} \mathring{\mathcal{A}}^-$, i.e. 3) ==> 1). Implication 5) ==> 4) is evident, thus, it remains to prove the implication 4) ==> 5). In view of 4), the operator S is defined everywhere on $\mathfrak{A}$. Now we want to show that it is closed: if $a_k \to a$, $Sa_k \to b$ $(a_k, a, b \in \mathfrak{A})$, then $Pa_k = \frac{1}{2}(I + S)a_k \to \frac{1}{2}(a+b)$, $Qa_k = \frac{1}{2}(I - S)a_k \to \frac{1}{2}(a-b)$. Since, for all $k=1,2,\ldots$, the inclusions $Pa_k \in \mathfrak{A}^+$, $Qa_k \in \mathring{\mathfrak{A}}^-$ hold (here we use the implication 4) ==> 3) proved above) and $\mathfrak{A}^+$, $\mathring{\mathfrak{A}}^-$ are closed in $\mathfrak{A}$, then $a+b \in \mathfrak{A}^+$, $a-b \in \mathring{\mathfrak{A}}^-$.

Hence, $S(a+b) = a+b$, $S(a-b) = b-a$ and $Sa = S(\frac{1}{2}(a+b) + \frac{1}{2}(a-b))$ $= \frac{1}{2}(a+b) + \frac{1}{2}(b-a) = b$. Due to the closed graph theorem, the operator S is bounded in $\mathfrak{A}$. Thus Lemma 5.5 is completely proved. ≡

In the space $\mathfrak{A}^n$ of n-dimensional vector functions with components from $\mathfrak{A}$ we introduce a norm, setting $\|f\|_{\mathfrak{A}^n} = \sum_{j=1}^{n} \|f_j\|_{\mathfrak{A}}$, where $f = \sum_{j=1}^{n} f_j e_j$. To any matrix function $A \in \mathfrak{A}$ we assign the operator of multiplication by this matrix function in $\mathfrak{A}^n$.

As it can be easily verified, the norm of this operator is determined by the formula

$$\|A\| = \max_j \sum_{i=1}^{n} \|a_{ij}\|_{\mathfrak{A}} \tag{5.8}$$

with $A = (a_{ij})_{i,j=1}^n$.

In the sequel we suppose that the (L_∞, R)-algebra $\mathfrak{A}$ is decomposing. According to Lemma 5.5, this supposition is equivalent to the boundedness of S viewed as an operator in $\mathfrak{A}$ and, thus, also in $\mathfrak{A}^n$.

Consequently, it plays here the same role as the assumption $\Gamma \in \mathfrak{R}$ in Section 3.5 and 3.6. Up to the end of the present section (with the exception of Theorems 5.12 and 5.13), the latter condition (i.e. $\Gamma \in \mathfrak{R}$) can be replaced by the weaker requirement $\Gamma \in \mathfrak{C}$ used in the proof of the previous lemma.

Every $n \times n$ matrix function $G \in \mathfrak{A}$ can be associated with the linear bounded operators $P + GQ$ and $Q + G'P$ acting in $\mathfrak{A}^n$. The defect numbers of these operators are connected by the relations

$$\alpha(P+GQ) \le \beta(Q+G'P), \quad \beta(P+GQ) \ge \alpha(Q+G'P) \tag{5.9}$$

as in case when the operators $P + GQ$ and $Q + G'P$ are studied in the spaces L_p^n and L_q^n, respectively.

The relations (5.9) are a simple consequence of the fact that the kernel of the operator $P + GQ$ $(Q + G'P)$ exactly coincides with the set of vector functions on $\mathfrak{A}^n$ orthogonal (in the sense of the bilinear form (1.13)) to the image of the operator $Q + G'P$ $(P + GQ)$. In its turn, this assertion can be proved in the same way as the corresponding result from Theorem 3.1.

As in Chapter 3, in addition to the operators $P + GQ$ and $Q + G'P$, it is convenient to introduce the operators $T_Q(G)$ and $T_P(G')$ defined via formulae (3.22). Since in the case in question $\operatorname{im} P = (\mathfrak{A}^+)^n$ and $\operatorname{im} Q = (\mathring{\mathfrak{A}}^-)^n$, these operators act in $(\mathfrak{A}^+)^n$ and $(\mathring{\mathfrak{A}}^-)^n$, respectively. Assertion 1) of Lemma 3.5 on the relationships between defect numbers of the operators $P + GQ$ and $T_Q(G)$ as well as $Q + G'P$ and $T_P(G')$ can be transferred (together with its proof) without any changes to the situation under study. However, assertion 2) of this lemma is no longer valid, since the operators QGQ and $PG'P$ do not act in spaces dual to each other (as it was the case in Chapter 3), rather in one and the same space $\mathfrak{A}^n$. Therefore, nothwithstanding that formulae (5.9) are available, we cannot a priori assert that the operators $P + GQ$ and $Q + G'P$ are Fredholm only simultaneously.

<u>THEOREM 5.6.</u> Let $\mathfrak{A}$ be a decomposing (L_∞, R)-algebra, and let G be a matrix function of n th order with entries from $\mathfrak{A}$. The matrix function G is factorable in $\mathfrak{A}$ if and only if the operators $P + GQ$ and $Q + G'P$ regarded in $\mathfrak{A}^n$ are Fredholm and their indices are opposite. In addition, the value $\alpha(P + GQ)$ coincides with the sum of positive partial indices and $\beta(P + GQ)$ is opposite to the sum of negative partial indices of G.

<u>Proof.</u> Let G be factorable in $\mathfrak{A}$. Due to conditions (5.7), the operators $G_+PG_+^{-1}$, $G'_-Q(G'_-)^{-1}$, $G_-^{-1}\Lambda^{-1}QG_+^{-1}$ and $(G'_+)^{-1}\Lambda^{-1}P(G'_-)^{-1}$ are bounded in $\mathfrak{A}^n$. The same calculations which where carried out in the proof of Theorem 3.16 show that the operator $G_-^{-1}\Lambda^{-1}QG_+^{-1}+G_+PG_+^{-1}$ is a two-sided regularizer of the operator $P + GQ$. In the same way one can deduce that $(G'_+)^{-1}\Lambda^{-1}P(G'_-)^{-1} + G'_-Q(G'_-)^{-1}$ is a two-sided regularizer for $Q + G'P$. Therefore, according to Theorem 1.8, the

Fredholmness of the operators $P + GQ$ and $Q + G'P$ acting in $\mathfrak{A}^n$ will be proved on condition that G can be factored in $\mathfrak{A}$. Furthermore, in case of a matrix function G factorable in $\mathfrak{A}$, all solutions of the homogeneous equation $(P+GQ)\varphi = 0$ determined by formulae (3.6)(for $\varphi_0^{\pm} = 0$), clearly belong to the space $\mathfrak{A}^n$. Consequently, the dimension of the kernel of the operator $P + GQ$ remains the same as in class L_p^n, i.e., it is equal to the sum of positive partial indices of G. As in Chapter 3, the conditions (3.9) continue to be necessary for the solvability of the equation $(P+GQ)\varphi=g$. If they are fulfilled, then the vector functions φ_0^+ and φ_0^- defined by formulae (3.5) belong to the classes $\mathfrak{A}^+$ and $\overset{\bullet}{\mathfrak{A}}{}^-$, respectively. Hence, conditions (3.9) are necessary and sufficient solvability conditions as in case when G is Φ-factorable. Therefore, $\beta(P+GQ)$ is opposite to the sum of negative partial indices of G.

Similar considerations related to the equation $(Q+G'P)\psi = h$ show that in relations (5.9) equality holds. Hence, the indices of the operators $P + GQ$ and $Q + G'P$ are opposite, which finishes the proof of the direct assertion of the theorem.

Vice versa, let the operators $P + GQ$ and $Q + G'P$ be Fredholm in the space $\mathfrak{A}^n$, and assume their indices to be opposite. Then there exist [1] matrix functions F and H belonging to class R together with their inverses such that $\operatorname{im} T_Q(G) = \operatorname{im} T_Q(GF)$, $\operatorname{im} T_P((GF)') = \operatorname{im} T_P((HGF)')$, $\ker T_Q(HGF) = \ker T_Q(GF) = \{0\}$, $\ker T_P((GF)') = \ker T_P(G')$, $\ker T_P((HGF)') = \{0\}$. According to Theorem 2.9, the matrix functions F and H admit factorizations with factors from R being, consequently, factorizations in $\mathfrak{A}$. Owing to what was proved above, the operators $T_Q(F)$, $T_Q(H)$, $T_P(F')$ and $T_P(H')$ are Fredholm, where $\operatorname{ind} T_Q(F) = -\operatorname{ind} T_P(F')$, $\operatorname{ind} T_Q(H) = -\operatorname{ind} T_P(H')$. But the operators $T_Q(G_1)$ and $T_P(G_1')$ with $G_1 = HGF$ differ only by a finite-dimensional summand from the products $T_Q(H)T_Q(G)T_Q(F)$ and $T_P(F')T_P(G')T_P(H')$, respectively. In view of Theorems 1.5 and 1.6, from this we obtain that the

---

[1] This can be proved in precisely the same way as the existence of matrix functions F and H in Lemma 3.2.

operators $T_Q(G_1)$ and $T_P(G_1')$ are Fredholm either, moreover,

$$\operatorname{ind} T_Q(G_1) = \operatorname{ind} T_Q(H) + \operatorname{ind} T_Q(G) + \operatorname{ind} T_Q(F)$$
$$= -\operatorname{ind} T_P(H') - \operatorname{ind} T_P(G') - \operatorname{ind} T_P(F') .$$

At the same time, the kernels of the operators $T_Q(G)$ and $T_P(G')$ are trivial, so that their indices are non-positive. Consequently, these indices are equal to zero. But then the codimensions of the images of operators $T_Q(G_1)$ and $T_P(G_1')$ are also equal to zero. In other words, $T_Q(G_1)$ and $T_P(G_1')$ are invertible (in $(\mathfrak{A}^-)^n$ and $(\mathfrak{A}^+)^n$, respectively). From here it follows that the operators $P + G_1Q$ and $G + G_1'P$ are invertible in $\mathfrak{A}^n$. Acting now as in the proof of Theorem 3.4, we recognize that the matrix function G_1 is factorable in $\mathfrak{A}$ and thus also in all L_p (moreover, its partial indices are equal to zero; however, in the sequel we shall not make use of this fact). According to Theorem 2.11, this implies the factorability of G in L_p. In addition, the factorization factors of G are obtained from the factorization factors of G_1 by multiplication by a matrix function from R as it is clear from the proof of Theorem 2.11. The multiplication by such matrix functions does not go beyond the algebra $\mathfrak{A}$.
Hence, the matrix function G is factorable in $\mathfrak{A}$ simultaneously with G_1, and the proof of Theorem 5.6 is complete. ≡

COROLLARY 5.12. If the operators $T_Q(G)$ and $T_P(G')$ are Fredholm and their indices are opposite, then the matrix function G is invertible in $\mathfrak{A}$.

The (L_∞,R)-algebra $\mathfrak{A}$ is said to be a (C,R)-algebra if all its elements are continuous functions, i.e. if $\mathfrak{A} \subseteq C$. For (C,R)-algebras, Theorem 5.6 allows the following strengthening.

THEOREM 5.7. Let the (C,R)-algebra $\mathfrak{A}$ possess the invertibility property, and assume, for every non-degenerating matrix function G, the operators $T_Q(G)$ and $T_P(G)$ to be Fredholm. Then any non-degenerating matrix function from $\mathfrak{A}$ is factorable in $\mathfrak{A}$.

Proof. Consider an arbitrary non-degenerating matrix function $G \in \mathfrak{A}$. Since $\mathfrak{A} \subseteq C$, G can be approximated in the metric of L_∞ with

arbitrary accuracy by rational matrix functions. Now we choose $F \in R$ close to G in such a way that, for all $\lambda \in [0,1]$, the matrix function $G_\lambda = \lambda F + (1-\lambda)G$ does not degenerate on Γ.
Owing to the conditions of the theorem, the operators $A_\lambda = T_Q(G_\lambda)$ and $B_\lambda = T_P(G'_\lambda)$ are then Fredholm for any $\lambda \in [0,1]$. Since A_0 and A_1 as well as B_0 and B_1 are homotopic, we get $\text{ind } A_0 = \text{ind } A_1$ and $\text{ind } B_0 = \text{ind } B_1$. At the same time, the matrix function G_1 $(=F)$ can be factored in $\mathcal{A}$. Thus, by Theorem 5.6, $\text{ind } A_1 = -\text{ind } B_1$. Hence $\text{ind } A_0 = -\text{ind } B_0$, i.e., the indices of the operators $T_Q(G)$ and $T_P(G')$ are opposite. Now the factorability of G in $\mathcal{A}$ results from Theorem 5.6. ≡

In some cases the Fredholmness condition for the operators $T_Q(G)$ and $T_P(G')$ can be replaced by another one more suitable for checking.

<u>THEOREM 5.7'.</u> Let the decomposing (C,R)-algebra $\mathcal{A}$ possess the invertibility property, and let, for all $a \in \mathcal{A}$, the operator QaP (PaQ) be compact in $\mathcal{A}$. Then every invertible matrix function from $\mathcal{A}$ admits a factorization in $\mathcal{A}$.

<u>Proof.</u> Consider, e.g., the case of compactness of QaP for all $a \in \mathcal{A}$. From the hypothesis of the theorem it is not hard to conclude that the operator QGP is compact in $\mathcal{A}^n$ for arbitrary $G \in \mathcal{A}$. Formulae (5.1) and (5.2), which continue to be valid in the situation under study, show that the operator $T_Q(G^{-1})$ is a regularizer for $T_Q(G)$. Hence, the operator $T_Q(G)$ is Fredholm. The Fredholmness of the operator $T_P(G')$ may be verified in a similar way. According to Theorem 5.7, G can be factored in $\mathcal{A}$, which proves Theorem 5.7'. ≡

<u>COROLLARY 5.13.</u> If the decomposing (C,R)-algebra $\mathcal{A}$ has the property that the closure of R in $\mathcal{A}$ contains $\mathcal{A}^+$ or $\mathcal{A}^-$, then any invertible matrix function from $\mathcal{A}$ admits a factorization in $\mathcal{A}$.

<u>Proof.</u> Let, for instance, $\text{clos}_{\mathcal{A}} R \supseteq \mathcal{A}^+$. Taking an arbitrary $a \in \mathcal{A}$, we can write (since $\mathcal{A}$ is decomposing): $a = a_+ + a_-$, where $a_+ \in \mathcal{A}^+$, $a_- \in \mathring{\mathcal{A}}^-$. Now we take a sequence $r_n \in R$ such that $\|r_n - a_+\|_{\mathcal{A}} \to 0$. Then the sequence of operators $P(r_n + a_-)Q$ converges in the norm to PaQ.

At the same time, $P(r_n+a_-)Q = Pr_nQ$ is a finite-dimensional operator. Consequently, the operator PaQ is compact in $\mathfrak{R}$. It remains to use Theorem 5.7'. ≡

Now we intend to illustrate Theorem 5.7' by the following examples, which are of some significance for applications.

1°. To H^α, the space of Hölder (or H-continuous) functions with exponent α $(0 < \alpha \leq 1)$, there belong such functions defined on Γ for which the quantity

$$\sup_{\tau, t \in \Gamma} \frac{|a(\tau)-a(t)|}{|\tau-t|^\alpha}$$

is finite (Hölder condition). Setting

$$\|a\|_{H^\alpha} = \|a\|_C + \sup_{\tau, t \in \Gamma} \frac{|a(\tau)-a(t)|}{|\tau-t|^\alpha},$$

H^α becomes a Banach algebra. Obviously $R \subset H^\alpha \subset C$, thus, H^α is a (C,R)-algebra. If the contour Γ is piecewise smooth and $\alpha < 1$, then the operator S is bounded in H^α (GOHBERG, KRUPNIK [4], MUSKHELISHVILI [1]) and the operator $aS-SaI$ is compact for all $a \in H^\alpha$ (see GOHBERG, KRUPNIK [4]). Since $aS-Sa = 2(QaP-PaQ)$, we deduce from this the compactness of operators PaQ and QaP. Moreover, H^α has the invertibility property (see e.g. MUSKHELISHVILI [1]). Owing to Theorem 5.7', we thus obtain the following result.

<u>THEOREM 5.8.</u> If the contour Γ is piecewise smooth and G is a non-degenerating matrix function all entries of which fulfil a Hölder condition of order α $(0 < \alpha < 1)$, then the representation (2.1) is valid, where $G_\pm$ are matrix functions analytic in $\mathfrak{D}^\pm$, continuous and non-degenerating in $\mathfrak{D}^\pm \cup \Gamma$ and fulfilling on Γ a Hölder condition of the same order α.

2°. Let $H^{\alpha,k}$ denote the set of k times continuously differentiable functions defined on Γ the k th derivative of which belongs to the class H^α. Furthermore, we introduce the norm

$$\|a\|_{H^{\alpha,k}} = \sum_{j=0}^{k} \frac{1}{j!} \max_{\tau \in \Gamma} |a^{(j)}(\tau)| + \sup_{\tau, t \in \Gamma} \frac{|a^{(k)}(\tau)-a^{(k)}(t)|}{|\tau - t|^\alpha}$$

in $H^{\alpha,k}$.

In GOHBERG, KRUPNIK [4] it is shown that, if the contour Γ is piecewise smooth, then $H^{\alpha,k}$ is a decomposing (C,R)-algebra which meets the assumptions of Corollary 5.13. As in the case of the algebra H^{α}, all functions from $H^{\alpha,k}$ non-vanishing on Γ are invertible elements in $H^{\alpha,k}$. Therefore, the following statement holds.

THEOREM 5.9. Let Γ be a piecewise smooth contour. A non-degenerating matrix function all entries of which are functions of class $H^{\alpha,k}$ $(0 < \alpha < 1)$ admits a factorization (2.1) in which $G_{\pm}$ are matrix functions analytic in $\mathfrak{D}^{\pm}$, continuous and non-degenerating in $\mathfrak{D}^{\pm} \cup \Gamma$ and belonging to class $H^{\alpha,k}$ on Γ.

Obviously, $H^{\alpha,k}$ is, for $k > 0$, a proper subclass of H^{α}, thus, the H-continuity of $G_{\pm}$ in Theorem 5.9 is not a new result (in comparison with Theorem 5.8). The crucial fact of Theorem 5.9 is that differential properties of G are acquired by its factorization factors to a certain extent.

3°. In 1° and 2° two concrete examples of (C,R)-algebras have been described which possess the invertibility property and fulfil the conditions of Corollary 5.13. Here we focus our attention on one subclass of the class of (C,R)-algebras for which the invertibility property is automatically fulfilled and which, under the additional supposition of decomposition, satisfies also the condition of compactness of operators of the type $aS-SaI$.

DEFINITION 5.4. A (C,R)-algebra $\mathfrak{C}$ is called a R-algebra, if the lineal R is dense in $\mathfrak{C}$ with respect to the norm of $\mathfrak{C}$.

LEMMA 5.6. 1) A R-algebra possesses the invertibility property. 2) If the R-algebra $\mathfrak{C}$ is decomposing, then $\mathfrak{C}^{+}$, $\mathfrak{C}^{-}$ and $\mathring{\mathfrak{C}}^{-}$ coincide with the closure in $\mathfrak{C}$ of the lineals R^{+}, R^{-} and $\mathring{R}^{-}$, respectively.

Proof. 1) We use the well-known fact from the theory of commutative Banach algebras according to which an element $a \in \mathfrak{C}$ is invertible in $\mathfrak{C}$ if and only if $\varphi(a) \neq 0$ for any multiplicative linear functional φ. After choosing such a functional φ arbitrarily, we denote its value on the function $u(t) = t$ by t_o. Then

$$\varphi(u-t_oe) = \varphi(u) - t_o\varphi(e) = t_o - t_o = 0 .$$

Therefore, the function $t-t_o$ is not invertible in $\mathfrak{C}$. If $t_o \notin \Gamma$, the function $(t-t_o)^{-1}$ belongs to $\mathfrak{C}$. Consequently, the non-invertibility of $t-t_o$ in $\mathfrak{C}$ means that $t_o \in \Gamma$. Now, let r be a rational function not having poles on Γ, and assume $r(t) = \sum_{k=o}^{N_1} c_k t^k / \sum_{k=o}^{N_2} b_k t^k$. Then

$$\varphi(r) = \frac{\varphi(\sum_{k=o}^{N_1} c_k u^k)}{\varphi(\sum_{k=o}^{N_2} b_k u^k)} = \frac{\sum_{k=o}^{N_1} c_k \varphi(u)^k}{\sum_{k=o}^{N_2} b_k \varphi(u)^k} = \frac{\sum_{k=o}^{N_1} c_k t_o^k}{\sum_{k=o}^{N_2} b_k t_o^k} = r(t_o) .$$

Using the density of R in $\mathfrak{C}$, we choose, for arbitrary $a \in \mathfrak{C}$, a sequence $\{r_k\}$ in R converging to a in $\mathfrak{C}$. Then $\varphi(a) = \lim_{k\to\infty} \varphi(r_k) = \lim_{k\to\infty} r_k(t_o) = a(t_o)$ (the last equation holds in view of Corollary 5.11). Thus, every multiplicative linear functional is of the form $\varphi(a) = a(t_o)$, where $t_o \in \Gamma$.

Hence, $a(t) \neq 0$ for any $t \in \Gamma$ is a necessary and sufficient condition for the invertibility of the element a in $\mathfrak{C}$, which proves statement 1).

2) The inclusions $\mathfrak{C}^{\pm} \supseteq \operatorname{clos}_{\mathfrak{C}} R^{\pm}$, $\mathring{\mathfrak{C}}^{-} \supseteq \operatorname{clos}_{\mathfrak{C}} \mathring{R}^{-}$ [1] result from the closedness of the classes $\mathfrak{C}^{\pm}$ and $\mathring{\mathfrak{C}}^{-}$ in $\mathfrak{C}$ and hold irrespective of whether the algebra $\mathfrak{C}$ is decomposing or not. In order to prove the inclusion $\mathfrak{C}^{+} \subseteq \operatorname{clos}_{\mathfrak{C}} R^{+}$ in case of a decomposing R-algebra $\mathfrak{C}$, we choose an arbitrary element $a \in \mathfrak{C}^{+}$ and consider the sequence $\{r_k\} \subset R$ converging in $\mathfrak{C}$ to a. According to Lemma 5.5, the operators S and P are bounded in $\mathfrak{C}$ and, therefore, $\{Pr_k\}$ converges in $\mathfrak{C}$ to Pa. But $Pa = a$ and $Pr_k \in R^{+}$. Hence, $a \in \operatorname{clos}_{\mathfrak{C}} R^{+}$, i.e. $\mathfrak{C}^{+} \subseteq \operatorname{clos}_{\mathfrak{C}} R^{+}$. The inclusions $\mathfrak{C}^{-} \subseteq \operatorname{clos}_{\mathfrak{C}} R^{-}$ and $\mathring{\mathfrak{C}}^{-} \subseteq \operatorname{clos}_{\mathfrak{C}} \mathring{R}^{-}$ can be verified analogously. Lemma 5.6 is proved. $\equiv$

Notice that the (C,R)-algebras H^{α} and $H^{\alpha,k}$ are not R-algebras (cf. BOJARSKI [2]), although statements 1) and 2) of Lemma 5.6 are correct

---

[1] By clos we denote the closure of a set: the index indicates, in which space the closure is taken.

for them. Every (C,R)-algebra $\mathfrak{A}$ contains some R-algebra $\mathfrak{C}$ as a subalgebra. This algebra is the closure of the lineal R in the norm of $\mathfrak{C}$. Thus, it is defined uniquely. The R-algebra $\mathfrak{C}$ coincides with $\mathfrak{A}$ if and only if the initial (C,R)-algebra $\mathfrak{A}$ is itself a R-algebra.

From Corollary 5.13 and statements 1) and 2) of Lemma 5.6 we obtain the following result.

THEOREM 5.10. Assume $\mathfrak{C}$ to be a decomposing R-algebra. The matrix function $G \in \mathfrak{C}$ admits a factorization in $\mathfrak{C}$ if and only if it is non-singular on Γ.

An obvious example of a R-algebra provides C. Theorem 5.10, along with the example given at the beginning of this section, show that the R-algebra of functions continuous on the circle fails to be decomposing.

As an example of a decomposing R-algebra we quote the class $C^+ \dot{+} \overset{\circ}{C}{}^-$ supplied with the direct sum norm

$$\|a_+ + a_-\|_{C^+ \dot{+} \overset{\circ}{C}{}^-} = \|a_+\|_C + \|a_-\|_C .$$

This class coincides with the closure of R with respect to the norm $\|\cdot\|_{C^+ \dot{+} \overset{\circ}{C}{}^-}$ and is therefore a R-algebra. Clearly, every other decomposing R-algebra is contained in $C^+ \dot{+} \overset{\circ}{C}{}^-$.

A less trivial example of a decomposing R-algebra provides the Wiener algebra W, whose elements are functions defined on the unit circle representable in the form of absolutely convergent series

$$a(t) = \sum_{k=-\infty}^{+\infty} a_k t^k \quad (|t|=1), \quad \sum_{k=-\infty}^{+\infty} |a_k| < \infty .$$

The norm in W is introduced by the formula $\|a\|_W = \sum_{k=-\infty}^{+\infty} |a_k|$.

Apparently, functions of the kind $\sum_{k=-N_1}^{N_2} a_k t^k$ form a dense lineal in W.

Furthermore, W contains all twice continuously differentiable functions, because for them an estimate $|a_k| \le \text{const}/k^2$ holds.

Especially $R \subset W$. Hence W is a R-algebra. If $a \in W$ and

$$a(t) = \sum_{k=-\infty}^{+\infty} a_k t^k ,$$

then

$$a_+(t) = \sum_{k=0}^{\infty} a_k t^k \in W^+ , \quad a_-(t) = \sum_{k=-\infty}^{-1} a_k t^k \in W^- \text{ and } a = a_+ + a_- .$$

Thus, the R-algebra W is decomposing [1] and, therefore, the following proposition is true.

<u>THEOREM 5.11.</u> A non-degenerating matrix function defined on the unit circle $\mathbb{T}$ with elements from W admits a factorization in W.

In summary, we have constructed some classes of matrix functions admitting a factorization in C. The following local principle enables us to "stick together" new classes from already known ones.

<u>THEOREM 5.12.</u> Let the contour Γ belong to class $\mathcal{R}$, and assume the matrix function G to have the property that, for all points $t \in \Gamma$, there exists a matrix function G_t coinciding with G on some open arc γ_t $(\ni t)$ and admitting a factorization in C. Then G also admits a factorization in C.

<u>Proof.</u> Every matrix function G_t is continuous and non-degenerating on Γ. Hence, for all $t \in \Gamma$, the matrix function G is continuous on γ_t and, thus, also on the whole contour Γ. Therefore (Theorem 5.3), G admits a factorization in the spaces L_p, $1 < p < \infty$. Applying Theorem 2.4 to matrix functions G and G_t, we recognize that the factorization factors $G_{\pm}$ are continuous and non-degenerating in $\mathcal{D}^{\pm} \cup \gamma_t$ for all $t \in \Gamma$. Hence, the matrix functions $G_{\pm}$ are continuous and non-degenerating in $\mathcal{D}^{\pm} \cup \Gamma$, which proves Theorem 5.12. ≡

<u>COROLLARY 5.14.</u> Suppose $\{\gamma_j\}_{j=1}^{N}$ to be a system of open arcs covering the unit circle $\mathbb{T}$. If on every arc γ_j the elements of the matrix function G possess one of the properties

1) they fulfil a Hölder condition of order α $(0 < \alpha < 1)$,
2) they are restrictions of certain functions possessing a absolutely convergent Fourier series,

then the matrix function G admits a factorization in C.

In order to apply Theorem 5.12 to some matrix function G, it is necessary to cover the contour Γ with a system of arcs $\{\gamma_j\}$ and to find

---

[1] It is obvious that $\|P\|_W = \|Q\|_W = 1$.

the extension of G from every of these arcs γ_j to such a matrix function G_j which is factorable in C. In doing so, it is clear from the proof of Theorem 5.12 that the continuity of the factorization factors for G_j is essential not on the entire contour Γ, but only on the arc γ_j. This way of reasoning leads to a modification of Theorem 5.12 more convenient for applications.

<u>DEFINITION 5.5.</u> The matrix function G is said to admit a <u>local factorization in</u> C with respect to the arc γ of the contour Γ, if there exists a neighbourhood (on the plane) U_γ of this arc as well as a pair of matrix functions $G_\gamma^{\pm}$ analytic in $\mathcal{D}^{\pm} \cap U_\gamma$, continuous and non-degenerate in $(\mathcal{D}^{\pm} \cup \Gamma) \cap U_\gamma$ such that $G(t) = G_\gamma^{+}(t)G_\gamma^{-}(t)$ for $t \in \Gamma \cap U_\gamma$.

<u>LEMMA 5.7.</u> If the matrix function G admits a factorization in L_p with respect to the contour Γ and a local factorization in C with respect to some arc γ, then the factorization factors $G_{\pm}$ are continuously extendable from $\mathcal{D}^{\pm}$ onto γ. Moreover, these extensions do not degenerate on γ.

The proof differs only in detail from the proof of Theorem 2.4.

In Lemma 5.7 and the definition preceding it, the class C may be replaced by H^α or $H^{\alpha,k}$. In this case, in Definition 5.5 we have to demand that the matrix functions $G_\gamma^{\pm}$ fulfil the condition in H^α ($H^{\alpha,k}$, respectively) on the arc γ, and in Lemma 5.7 we may claim that the extensions of the matrix functions $G_{\pm}$ onto γ satisfy the condition in H^α ($H^{\alpha,k}$, respectively).

<u>COROLLARY 5.15.</u> Suppose the matrix function G to be factorable in L_p with respect to the contour Γ, and assume that G fulfils a Hölder condition of order α on the piecewise smooth arc γ. Then the factorization factors $G_{\pm}$ are continuously extendable from $\mathcal{D}^{\pm}$ onto the arc γ, and these extensions are non-degenerating and fulfil a Hölder condition of the same order α on every arc $\tilde{\gamma}$ whose closure lies in γ.

THEOREM 5.13. If the matrix function G admits a local factorization in C with respect to the system of open arcs $\{\gamma_j\}$ covering the contour Γ which belongs to class $\mathcal{R}$, then it admits a factorization in C with respect to the contour Γ.

Proof. From the local factorability in C of a certain matrix function with respect to the arc γ there results its continuity and non-degeneracy on this arc. Therefore, the studied matrix function G is continuous and non-degenerating on the whole contour Γ and, according to Theorem 5.3, it is factorable with respect to this contour. Hence Lemma 5.7 is applicable, in virtue of which the factorization factors $G_\pm$ are continuously extendable on every arc γ_j and therefore also on the whole contour Γ. Moreover, these extensions are non-degenerating matrix functions. In this way, the factorization of the matrix function G, existing in view of Theorem 5.3, is, actually, its factorization in C. Thus Theorem 5.13 is proved. ≡

Finally, note that Theorems 5.7 - 5.13 may be transferred to the case of right-factorization, since the matrix function G admits a right-factorization in $\mathcal{A}$ (or C) if and only if G' admits a left-factorization in $\mathcal{A}$ (or C).

5.3. Φ-FACTORIZATION OF PIECEWISE CONTINUOUS MATRIX FUNCTIONS

We are going to discuss the case of a piecewise continuous matrix function G, which is important for applications. First of all, recall that a matrix function G is said to be piecewise continuous if it is continuous on the contour Γ with the exception of a finite number of points t_j, $j=1,\dots,N$ at every of which there exists the limit from the left $G(t_j-0)$ and from the right $G(t_j+0)$ [1)]

From Corollaries 5.9 and 5.15 we get the following result.

THEOREM 5.14. Assume G to be a piecewise continuous matrix function non-degenerating at continuity points and factorable in L_p.

1) "From the left" and "from the right" one has to understand in the sense of the orientation of the contour Γ as it was explained in Chapter 1.

Furthermore, γ is assumed to be an arc of the contour Γ not containing discontinuity points of G. Then

1) if the operator of singular integration along the arc γ is bounded, then the factorization factors $G_{\pm}$ and the inverse to them are summable with any finite power on every arc $\tilde{\gamma}$ the closure of which lies in γ,

2) if γ is a piecewise smooth arc and the matrix function G fulfils on γ a Hölder condition with exponent α, then the matrix functions $G_{\pm}$ are continuously extendable from $\mathcal{D}^{\pm}$ onto Γ, and these extensions are non-degenerating and fulfil a Hölder condition with the same exponent α on every arc $\tilde{\gamma}$ the closure of which lies in γ.

Up to the very end of the present chapter we shall assume (by tacit agreement) that the contour Γ belongs to class $\tilde{\mathcal{R}}$ and that for the discontinuity points t_j of G the boundedness requirement for branches of the functions $\operatorname{Arg}(t-t_j)$, which are continuous on $\Gamma \setminus \{t_j\}$, is fulfilled. In any case, this requirement is satisfied, if there are tangents to Γ at the points t_j.

Above all, we intend to prove a result which is related to the factorization problem for scalar piecewise continuous functions.

THEOREM 5.15. Let G be a piecewise continuous function and $\{t_j\}_{j=1}^{N}$ be the set of its discontinuity points. The function G is Φ-factorable in L_p if and only if

1) G does not vanish at continuity points and $G(t_j \pm 0) \neq 0$ and

2) $\arg G(t_j+0)/G(t_j-0) \neq 2\pi/p$, $j=1,\dots,N$ [1].

If conditions 1) and 2) are fulfilled, the p-index of G is calculable with the aid of the formula

$$\varkappa = \frac{1}{2\pi}\Big(\sum_{j=1}^{N} \{\operatorname{Arg} G(t)\}_{\gamma_j} + \sum_{j=1}^{N} \arg \frac{G(t_j+0)}{G(t_j-0)}\Big) - l\,, \tag{5.10}$$

where l is the number of discontinuities at which $\arg G(t_j+0)/G(t_j-0) > 2\pi/p$, and $\{\gamma_j\}$ is the set of arcs into which the contour Γ

[1] Here and below in this section the value arg is taken from the interval $[0,2\pi)$.

is divided by the discontinuity points of the function G .

If at least one of the conditions 1) and 2) is violated, then $P + GQ$ is neither a Φ_+- nor a Φ_--operator in L_p .

<u>Proof.</u> The necessity of condition 1) for $P + GQ$ to be a semi-Fredholm operator results from Theorem 3.10. Therefore, it will be assumed that the first condition is fulfilled. In view of statement 2) of Theorem 3.21, it is possible to restrict oneself to the case of a connected contour Γ . Setting

$$\alpha_j = \frac{1}{2\pi}(\arg[G(t_j-0)/G(t_j+0)] - i \log|G(t_j-0)/G(t_j+0)|) , \quad j = 1,\ldots,N ,$$

we define functions $\psi_j(t) = t^{\alpha_j}$ with a discontinuity at the point t_j as it was done in Theorem 2.5. We further introduce the family of functions $\{G_\tau\}_{\tau\in\Gamma}$ as follows:

$$G_\tau(t) = \begin{cases} G(\tau) & \text{if} \quad \tau \neq t_j , \\ \dfrac{G(t_j-0)}{\psi_j(t_j-0)}\psi_j(t) & \text{if} \quad \tau = t_j . \end{cases} \qquad j=1,\ldots,N$$

The function G_τ is ε-locally equivalent to the function G at the point τ . For $\tau \neq t_j$ $(j=1,\ldots,N)$, this is evident and, for $\tau = t_j$, it follows from the relation $G_{t_j}(t_j \pm 0) = G(t_j \pm 0)$.

According to Theorem 3.17 and the remark after it, condition 2) guarantees Φ-factorability in L_p of the functions ψ_j and, thus, also of G_{t_j}. The functions G_τ are constant if $\tau \neq t_j$ and, therefore, Φ-factorable in L_p either. Taking this into account, we are able to apply Theorem 3.22, due to which function G is Φ-factorable in L_p . In this way, the sufficiency of conditions 1) and 2) for the Φ-factorability of G in L_p has been proved.

Now we are going to verify formula (5.10). First of all, the equation $G(t) = f(t) \prod_{j=1}^{N} \psi_j(t)$ holds, where f is continuous and non-degenerating on Γ . Utilizing the factorization $f(t) = f^+(t)t^k f^-(t)$ of the function f existing by Theorem 5.3 as well as the factorization (2.10) of functions of the form t^α , we obtain

$$G(t) = (f^+(t)\prod_{j=1}^{N}(t-t_j)^{\alpha_j-k_j})\, t^{k+\sum_{j=1}^{N}k_j}(f^-(t)\prod_{j=1}^{N}(1-\frac{t_j}{t})^{k_j-\alpha_j}) , \quad (5.11)$$

where $k = \frac{1}{2\pi}\{\mathrm{Arg}\ f(t)\}_\Gamma$ and $k_j = \begin{cases} 0 & \text{if } \operatorname{Re}\alpha_j < 1 - \frac{1}{p} \\ 1 & \text{if } \operatorname{Re}\alpha_j > 1 - \frac{1}{p} . \end{cases}$

With regard to the boundary properties of the functions $f^{\pm}$ stated in Theorem 5.3 and of the functions $(t-t_j)^{\alpha_j-k_j}$ and $(1-\frac{t_j}{t})^{k_j-\alpha_j}$ described in Theorem 2.5, we find that the representation (5.11) is a factorization and, therefore, also a Φ-factorization of the function G. Hence the p-index of G is equal to $k + \sum_{j=1}^{N} k_j$. It remains to note that

$$\frac{1}{2\pi}\sum_{j=1}^{N}\{\mathrm{Arg}\ G(t)\}_{\gamma_j} = \frac{1}{2\pi}\sum_{j=1}^{N}\{\mathrm{Arg}\ f(t)\}_{\gamma_j} + \sum_{j=1}^{N}\operatorname{Re}\alpha_j = k + \sum_{j=1}^{N}\operatorname{Re}\alpha_j ,$$

$$\frac{1}{2\pi}\sum_{j=1}^{N}\arg\frac{G(t_j+0)}{G(t_j-0)} = \sum_{j=1}^{N}(1-\operatorname{Re}\alpha_j) = N - \sum_{j=1}^{N}\operatorname{Re}\alpha_j \quad\text{and}\quad \sum_{j=1}^{N}k_j = N-1 .$$

Finally, we want to prove the last statement of the theorem. If condition 1) is fulfilled, but condition 2) is violated, then there exist piecewise continuous functions arbitrarily close (in the sense of the norm in L_∞) to the given function G such that for them conditions 1) and 2) are satisfied, but the quantity (5.10) takes different values. In other words, in any neighbourhood of the operator P + GQ there exist Fredholm operators with different indices, which means that P + GQ can be neither a Φ_+- nor a Φ_--operator. Thus, the proof of Theorem 5.15 is complete. ≡

Applying the notation introduced in Section 4.1, one may claim that piecewise continuous functions are contained in the class Φ .

THEOREM 5.16. Let G be a piecewise continuous matrix function, let, further, $\{t_j\}_{j=1}^{N}$ be the set of its discontinuities and $\{\gamma_j\}$ the set of arcs into which the contour Γ is divided by these discontinuity points. The matrix function G is Φ-factorable in L_p if and only if

1) for all $t \in \Gamma$, the relation

$$\det G(t \pm 0) \neq 0 \tag{5.12}$$

holds and

2) all eigenvalues of the matrix $G^{-1}(t_j-0)G(t_j+0)$, $j=1,\dots,N$ are outside the ray l_p drawn from the origin at an angle of $2\pi/p$ with the positive x-axis.

If conditions 1) and 2) apply, then the total index of G is defined by the formula

$$\varkappa = \frac{1}{2\pi}\left(\sum_{j=1}^{N} \{\operatorname{Arg} \det G(t)\}_{\gamma_j} + \sum_{j=1}^{N}\sum_{k=1}^{n} \arg \lambda_{jk}\right) - l\ , \tag{5.13}$$

where $\{\lambda_{jk}\}_{k=1}^{n}$ is the set of eigenvalues of the matrix $G^{-1}(t_j-0)G(t_j+0)$, and l is the number of such scalars λ_{jk} ($j=1,\dots,N$; $k=1,\dots,n$) for which $\arg \lambda_{jk} > 2\pi/p$.

Proof. The necessity of condition 1) for the Φ-factorability of the matrix function G results from Theorem 3.13. Assuming condition 1) to be fulfilled, we denote by A_j some constant non-singular matrix transforming $G^{-1}(t_j-0)G(t_j+0)$ into upper triangular form, i.e. such that the matrix $A_jG^{-1}(t_j-0)G(t_j+0)A_j^{-1}$ is upper triangular, $j=1,\dots,N$ [1].

Let A be a continuous matrix function non-singular on Γ such that $A(t_j) = A_j$ ($j=1,\dots,N$), and assume X to be an upper triangular non-singular matrix function continuous on Γ with the possible exception of those points t_j at which $X(t_j-0) = I$, $X(t_j+0) = A_jG^{-1}(t_j-0)G(t_j+0)A_j^{-1}$.

Set $B(t) = G(t)A^{-1}(t)X^{-1}(t)$. Clearly, the matrix function B is continuous on Γ with the possible exception of the points t_j.

Since $B(t_j-0) = G(t_j-0)A_j^{-1}$,

$$B(t_j+0) = G(t_j+0)A_j^{-1}A_jG^{-1}(t_j+0)G(t_j-0)A_j^{-1} = B(t_j-0)\ ,$$

the matrix function B is continuous (and non-singular) on the contour Γ. Thus $G = BXA$, where the matrix functions A and B are continuous and non-singular, and X is upper triangular and piecewise continuous.

[1] The existence of matrices A_j having this property follows for example, from the reduction theorem to Jordan's normal form.

Owing to Corollary 5.10, the matrix function G is Φ-factorable only simultaneously with X. Since the diagonal elements of the matrix function X are piecewise continuous and therefore belong to the class Φ, Theorem 4.5 can be applied, according to which the Φ-factorability of the matrix function X is equivalent to the Φ-factorability of its diagonal elements. Denoting the k th diagonal element of the matrix $X(t)$ by $x_k(t)$ and using Theorem 5.15, we see that the matrix function X (and, thus, also G) is Φ-factorable in L_p if and only if

$$\arg x_k(t_j+0) \neq 2\pi/p \quad (j=1,\dots,N;\ k=1,\dots,n)\ . \tag{5.14}$$

Furthermore, $\{x_k(t)\}_{k=1}^{n}$ is the set of eigenvalues of the matrix $X(t)$, and the matrices $X(t_j+0)$ and $G^{-1}(t_j-0)G(t_j+0)$ are similar. Therefore, their eigenvalues coincide. Consequently, condition (5.14) is equivalent to condition 2) of the theorem. In this way, the necessity of condition 2) as well as the sufficiency of both conditions 1) and 2) for the Φ-factorability of G in L_p have been proved. According to Corollary 4.4, the total p-index $\varkappa(X)$ of the matrix function X is equal to the sum of p-indices of the functions x_k, $k=1,\dots,n$. Applying formula (5.10) for calculating them, we get

$$\varkappa(X) = \sum_{k=1}^{n}\Big(\frac{1}{2\pi}\Big(\sum_{j=1}^{N}\{\mathrm{Arg}\ x_k(t)\}_{\gamma_j} + \sum_{j=1}^{N} \arg \lambda_{jk}\Big) - l_k\Big)\ ,$$

where l_k is the number of such scalars λ_{jk} for which $\arg \lambda_{jk} > 2\pi/p$. Since

$$\begin{aligned}\sum_{k=1}^{n}\ \sum_{j=1}^{N}\{\mathrm{Arg}\ x_k(t)\}_{\gamma_j} &= \sum_{j=1}^{N}\{\mathrm{Arg} \prod_{k=1}^{n} x_k(t)\}_{\gamma_j}\\ &= \sum_{j=1}^{N}\{\mathrm{Arg}\ \det X(t)\}_{\gamma_j}\end{aligned}$$

and $\sum_{k=1}^{n} l_k = l$, we may write:

$$\varkappa(X) = \frac{1}{2\pi}\Big(\sum_{j=1}^{N}\{\mathrm{Arg}\ \det X(t)\}_{\gamma_j} + \sum_{j=1}^{N}\ \sum_{k=1}^{n} \arg \lambda_{jk}\Big) - l\ .$$

To prove formula (5.13), it remains to remark that

$$\varkappa(G) = \varkappa(X) + \frac{1}{2\pi}\{\mathrm{Arg}\ \det A(t)B(t)\}_{\Gamma}$$

(in view of Corollary 5.10) and

$$\sum_{j=1}^{N}\{\text{Arg}\det X(t)\}_{\gamma_j} + \{\text{Arg}\det A(t)B(t)\}_{\Gamma} = \sum_{j=1}^{N}\{\text{Arg}\det G(t)\}_{\gamma_j}.$$

Theorem 5.16 is proved. ≡

Let us note that formula (5.13) may be rewritten in the form

$$\varkappa = \frac{1}{2\pi}\Big(\sum_{j=1}^{N}\{\text{Arg}\det G(t)\}_{\gamma_j} + \sum_{j=1}^{N}\sum_{k=1}^{n}\arg_p \lambda_{jk}\Big), \tag{5.13'}$$

where $\arg_p$ is the branch of Arg with values from the interval $(\frac{2\pi}{p} - 2\pi, \frac{2\pi}{p})$.

COROLLARY 5.16. The domain of Φ-factorability of a piecewise continuous matrix function is either empty (if condition (5.12) is violated at least at one point $t \in \Gamma$) or consists of a finite number of components $(1,p_1)$, $(p_1,p_2),\dots,(p_{r-1},p_r)$, (p_r,∞), where $\{p_s\}_{s=1}^{r}$ is the sequence of all different numbers of the form $2\pi/\arg \lambda_{jk}$ $(j=1,\dots,N;\ k=1,\dots,n;\ \arg\lambda_{jk} \neq 0)$ arranged in increasing order. Passing from the s th component to the (s+1) th one, the total index decreases by the number of scalars λ_{jk} the argument of which is equal to $2\pi/p_s$.
In particular, if condition (5.12) is fulfilled and all numbers λ_{jk} are positive, then the domain of Φ-factorability of the matrix function G consists of one component occupying the whole ray $(1,\infty)$.

The criterion of Φ-factorability stated in Theorem 5.16 may be expressed in a somewhat different form which is sometimes more convenient. Denote by Δ_p the locus from which the interval $[0,1]$ of the x-axis is visible at the angle of $2\pi/p$ [1]. It is well-known that Δ_p is an arc of a certain circle connecting the points 0 and 1. Suppose that $0,1 \in \Delta_p$.

THEOREM 5.16'. The piecewise continuous matrix function G is Φ-factorable in L_p if and only if, for all $t \in \Gamma$ and $\mu \in \Delta_p$, the relation

$$\det((1-\mu)G(t-0) + \mu G(t+0)) \neq 0 \tag{5.15}$$

is valid.

[1] Assume that the interval $[0,1]$ is visible from the upper semi-plane at an angle smaller than π, and from the lower at an angle greater than π.

Proof. For $\mu = 0$ and $\mu = 1$, condition (5.15) changes over into condition (5.12); for $\mu \neq 0$, it is equivalent to the fact that $1-\mu^{-1}$ does not provide an eigenvalue of the matrix $G^{-1}(t-0)G(t+0)$.
It remains to point out that, when μ ranges over $\Delta_p \setminus \{0\}$, the point $\lambda = 1-\mu^{-1}$ ranges over the ray l_p. ≡

COROLLARY 5.17. The piecewise continuous matrix function G is right Φ-factorable in L_p iff the matrix $\mu G(t-0) + (1-\mu)G(t+0)$ is non-degenerating for all $t \in \Gamma$ and $\mu \in \Delta_p$.

Proof. Due to Theorem 3.7', the matrix function G is right Φ-factorable in L_p if and only if the matrix function G' is left Φ-factorable in L_q. It remains to remark that the matrix function G' is piecewise continuous along with G and to apply Theorem 5.16' taking into account that the transformation $\mu \to 1-\mu$ maps Δ_p onto Δ_q.
In the scalar case, for fixed t and μ ranging over Δ_p, the set of points of the form $(1-\mu)G(t-0) + \mu G(t+0)$ forms an arc such that from its points the interval with the ends $G(t-0)$ and $G(t+0)$ is visible at the angle $2\pi/p$. In the general case one can also imagine the set $\{(1-\mu)G(t-0) + \mu G(t+0) : \mu \in \Delta_p\}$ as an arc connecting $G(t-0)$ and $G(t+0)$. For $p = 2$, we have $\Delta_2 = [0,1]$, and this arc reduces to an interval. ≡

5.4. COMMENTS

The sufficient condition of compactness of the operators QGP and PGQ in case of a Lyapunov contour given in Lemma 5.1 is also necessary.
For $p = 2$ and the unit circle, this has been proved in ADAMYAN, AROV, KREĬN [1], JONCKHEERE, DELSARTE [1].

Theorem 5.1 in the scalar case on the circle was proved by LEE and SARASON [1], as well as by AMBARTSUMYAN [2]; concerning the general case, see SPITKOVSKIĬ [10]. The closedness of the class $H_\infty + C$ was observed by SARASON [1]; the proof of Lemma 5.3 presented here is based on results of ZALCMAN [1] and is borrowed from SARASON [2].
The Φ-factorization of matrix functions of the class $H_\infty + C$ was con-

sidered by DOUGLAS [1] and AMBARTSUMYAN [1]. In the latter paper the sufficiency of the condition $G^{-1} \in H_\infty + C$ for the Φ-factorability of a matrix function G ($\in H_\infty + C$) was verified for all $p \in (1,\infty)$, and in the former its necessity and sufficiency was proved for $p = 2$.
In addition, in DOUGLAS [1] it is proved that the matrix function $G \in H_\infty + C$ is invertible in $H_\infty + C$ if and only if the harmonic extension of the function $\det G$ into the unit disk Δ is separated from zero in a certain annulus $\{z: r \leq |z| < 1\}$, and its total index can be calculated by the formula $\varkappa = \frac{1}{2\pi}\{\arg \det G(\varrho e^{i\theta})\}_{\theta=-\pi}^{\pi}$, where ϱ is an arbitrary number of the interval $(r,1)$.

After some modification this result can be transferred to the general case considered in Theorem 5.2. This theorem is contained in SPITKOVSKIĬ [10]; for the case of a Lyapunov contour, see also SPITKOVSKIĬ [2].
In Ch. 7 of DOUGLAS [2] problems related to Φ-factorization in L_2 of functions of the class $H_\infty + C$ are explained in full detail. One of the authors has obtained the criterion of Φ-factorability of unbounded matrix functions of classes $L^{\pm} + C$ (SPITKOVSKIĬ [6,14]).

Corollary 5.6 becomes false without the assumption $G \in L_\infty^{\pm} + C$: there exist matrix functions $G \in L_\infty$ which are left Φ-factorable, but not right factorable (and vice versa) (SPITKOVSKIĬ [4]).

The Φ-factorization problem of a continuous function in terms of singular integral equations was studied by MIKHLIN [1]. His results were later completed by GOHBERG [1]. Theorem 5.3 in the scalar case has been established by IVANOV [1], SIMONENKO [1] and KHVEDELIDZE [2], and in the matrix case by MANDZHAVIDZE, KHVEDELIDZE [1,2] and SIMONENKO [2]. Formula (5.4) for calculating the total index in case of a Hölder matrix function G was presented by MUSKHELISHVILI [1] (see also MUSKHELISHVILI, VEKUA [1]).
Corollary 5.10, whose generalization is Theorem 5.5 from SPITKOVSKIĬ [10], is, in principle, contained in SIMONENKO [4]. The example on page 180 is taken from GOHBERG, FELDMAN [3].

Theorem 5.10 on the factorization in a decomposing R-algebra (and the notion of the R-algebra itself) is due to GOHBERG [3,4]. The factorization of functions from the Wiener algebra W was studied by KREǏN [1] and of matrix functions with elements from W (Theorem 5.11) by GOHBERG and KREǏN [3].

The factorization of certain singular matrix functions with elements from the Wiener algebra on the real line has been studied in ENGIBARYAN [1]. The factorization in a (C,R)-algebra with the invertibility property was considered by BUDYANU and GOHBERG [3,4], who have proved Theorems 5.7 and 5.7'. The way of proving Theorems 5.8 - 5.10 described here is also borrowed from BUDYANU, GOHBERG [3,4]. The passage to (L_∞,R)-algebras was accomplished in HEINIG, SILBERMANN [1], where Theorem 5.6 was established. Remark that in the latter paper the condition $R \subseteq \mathfrak{A}$ was replaced by a weaker one: $1, t, t^{-1} \in \mathfrak{A}$. This condition, of course, means that $\mathfrak{A}$ contains all rational functions with poles located outside the annulus $\{\zeta : \min_{\tau\in\Gamma}|\tau| < |\zeta| < \max_{\tau\in\Gamma}|\tau|\}$. We leave to the reader to verify that, in virtue of the mentioned circumstance, the argument of Theorem 5.6, in principle, remains unchanged under such a weakening of the condition $R \subseteq \mathfrak{A}$.

Theorem 5.8 is a classical result of the factorization theory of matrix functions (see VEKUA [4], MUSKHELISHVILI [1]). Theorem 5.9 was independently obtained by ISAKHANOV [1] (see also VEKUA [4], p. 336). In the paper of LAGVILAVA [1] the proof of Theorems 5.8 and 5.11 based on the theory of Banach algebras is outlined but somewhat differing from the one given here. Direct proofs of Theorem 5.10, which are not founded on the factorization theory in (C,R)-algebras, the reader can find in Ch. 8 of GOHBERG, FELDMAN [3] and in LEITERER [1].

Notice that the decomposability condition of the (C,R)-algebra $\mathfrak{A}$ stipulated here is necessary for any non-singular matrix (and even scalar) function $G \in \mathfrak{A}$ to admit a factorization in $\mathfrak{A}$ (BUDYANU, GOHBERG [3,4]). As it is clear from Theorem 5.10, for R-algebras, this condition is also sufficient. It turns out that in the scalar case it remains sufficient for arbitrary (C,R)-algebras with the invertibility

property (concerning this topic, see GOHBERG, KRUPNIK [4]). In case that $n > 1$, necessary and sufficient conditions of factorability of all non-singular $n\times n$ matrix functions from a (C,R)-algebra possessing the invertibility property were obtained in BUDYANU, GOHBERG [3,4]. Besides the demand of decomposability of $\mathfrak{A}$, these conditions include the requirement of boundedness of the quantities $\operatorname{spr} U_G/\|G\|_C$ and $\operatorname{spr} V_G/\|G\|_C$ by a certain constant independent of G.
Here U_G and V_G are operators defined in the space $\mathfrak{A}^{n\times n}$ of $n\times n$ matrix functions with elements from $\mathfrak{A}$ via the formulae $U_G X = PGX$, $V_G X = QXG$; the symbol spr denotes the spectral radius, and G ranges over the class $\mathfrak{A}^{n\times n}$.
An abstract analogue of the established result as well as other aspects of the factorization problem in abstract algebras was studied in BUDYANU [1] and BUDYANU, GOHBERG [2]. Factorization in Banach algebras and its applications to the factorization problem of operators along a chain of projectors are subjects of Ch. 4 of the book GOHBERG, KREĬN [5]. This chapter also containes a detailed bibliography concerning this topic.

Classes of matrix functions different from those described in the main text of the present book and admitting a factorization in C were described in BABAEV, SALAEV [1], BELARMINO [1], GERUS [1], MAGNARADZE [1], PAL'TSEV [1], YANDAROV [1]. In particular, as stated in MAGNARADZE [1] (see also PAL'TSEV [1]), the condition that the modulus of continuity $\omega(\tau)$ for the elements of the considered matrix function be of order $\log^{-p}(|\tau|^{-1})$ for some $p > 1$ is sufficient.

In HEINIG, SILBERMANN [1], from where the study of factorization in (L_∞,R)-algebras originates, one can find concrete examples of algebras in which each matrix function invertible in them is factorable. Algebras with elements from the following classes are of this type:
1) $H^\alpha + E^\pm_\infty$ and $h^\alpha + E^\pm_\alpha$ (h^α denotes the closure of R with respect to the norm in H^α),
2) $B^1_1 + H_\infty$ and $K^{\alpha,\beta}_{p,q} = \{f \in L_\infty\text{: } Pf \in B^\beta_q,\ Qf \in B^\alpha_p\}$ for $\alpha p > 1$, $p \geq 1$,

$\beta > 0$, $q < \infty$ (here B^{ν}_{r} denotes the Besov classes defined as follows:

$$B^{\nu}_{r} = \{f \in L_r(\mathbb{T}) : \int_{-\pi}^{\pi} \|\Delta^n_t f\|_{L_r} |t|^{-1-r\nu} dt < \infty\} ,$$

where $n > \nu$ is integer, $\Delta^n_t = \Delta_t \Delta^{n-1}_t$, $(\Delta_t f)(e^{ix}) = f(e^{i(x+t)}) - f(e^{ix})$).

Remark that results of VERBITSKIǏ [1] were essentially employed in the proof of factorability in case 1), whereas in case 2) ideas of PELLER [1] were used.

The search for new classes of matrix functions admitting a factorization in C or in L_{∞} is of great interest.

THEOREM 5.13 was proved by SHUBIN [2] with the aid of a local principle of RÖHRL [1], which rests upon the theory of holomorphic fibre bundles.

In SHUBIN [2] Theorem 5.12 was obtained as a consequence of the more general Theorem 5.13. The proof of the latter one given here is, in principle, involved in GOHBERG, KRUPNIK [4]. Note that the Definition 5.5 of local factorization in C borrowed here from SHUBIN [2] has chronologically preceded the definition of factorization mentioned in the final section of Chapter 3.

The factorization of piecewise Hölder functions was studied by GAKHOV [4] and MUSKHELISHVILI [1] and of matrix functions by VEKUA [4]. The factorization of piecewise continuous functions in L_p , under different assumptions on the contour Γ , was considered in KHVEDELIDZE [3,5], SHAMIR [1], GORDADZE [1,2,4–6], GORDADZE and KHVEDELIDZE [1], KHVEDELIDZE and ISHCHENKO [1,2], ISHCHENKO [1], GOHBERG and KRUPNIK [4], and of matrix functions by GOHBERG, KRUPNIK [1], MANDZHAVIDZE [6], ISHCHENKO [2,3], SOLDATOV [2]. Let us remark that the two latter authors studied problems of the asymptotic behaviour of the factorization factors $G_{\pm}$ in a neighbourhood of discontinuities of a piecewise continuous matrix function G , which have not been considered here (concerning this topic, see VEKUA [4] for results under additional restrictions on G). Theorems 5.15 and 5.16 are explained here supporting mainly on GOHBERG, KRUPNIK [1,4]. For the formula of the total index we chose a form found by KARAPETYANTS and SAMKO [1]. In our view, it is more convenient for calculations than the formula contained in GOHBERG, KRUPNIK [1,4].

The study of convolution type equations on an interval with a kernel being of a quite general type of a generalized function can also be reduced to the factorization problem of piecewise continuous matrix functions (see KARLOVICH, SPITKOVSKIĬ [1], NOVOKSHENOV [1], PAL'TSEV [3,4], SPITKOVSKIĬ [15]). Studying systems of generalized Abel equations, the factorization of piecewise continuous matrix functions also appears in a natural way (see VASIL'EV [1,2], LOWENGRUB, WALTON [1], WALTON [1]).

The Riemann problem with a piecewise Hölder matrix function in special classes of piecewise Hölder functions $h(c_1,\dots,c_q)$ (Muskhelishvili classes) was considered in VEKUA [4]. The classes $h(c_1,\dots,c_q)$ include functions φ satisfying a Hölder condition on any closed arc which does not contain a certain fixed set of points $c_1,\dots,c_m$ $(m \geq q)$ and allowing the estimation $|\varphi(t)| \leq \text{const}|t-c_j|^{-\lambda}$ in a neighbourhood of these points, where λ (> 0) is arbitrarily small for $j=q+1,\dots,m$, and $\lambda < 1$, if $j=1,\dots,q$. The factorization of a piecewise Hölder matrix function G corresponding to the study of a Riemann problem in the class $h(c_1,\dots,c_q)$, where the set $\{c_j\}_{j=1}^q$ covers the discontinuities of G, coincides with its factorization in L_p corresponding to the most left component of the domain of Φ-factorability. If $\{c_j\}_{j=1}^q$ does not intersect the set of discontinuities of the matrix funtion G, then we get a factorization corresponding to the most right component. Intermediate cases of location of $\{c_j\}_{j=1}^q$ and of the set of discontinuities of G are not comprehended by factorization in L_p. Incidentally, the factorization of piecewise Hölder matrix functions associated with the study of a Riemann problem in the Muskhelishvili classes, conversely, does not comprehend the Φ-factorization, when p lies in intermediate components of the Φ-factorability domain.

As a rule, singular integral operators with discontinuous (and, in particular, with piecewise continuous) coefficients are regarded in the spaces $L_p(\varrho)$ of functions summable in the p th power with weight $\varrho(t) = \prod |t-t_k|^{\beta_k}$, $-1 < \beta_k < p-1$ (see e.g. GORDADZE [2,5], ZVEROVICH [1], MISHCHISHIN [1], NIKOLAǏCHUK [1]). Analogously, piecewise continuous matrix functions can also be factored in $L_p(\varrho)$. The results thus obtained generalize the statements of Theorems 5.15 and 5.16, however, qualitative differences do not occur. As a matter of fact, for given weight ϱ, one can always choose a piecewise continuous function h such that Φ-factorability of the matrix function G in $L_p(\varrho)$ is equivalent to Φ-factorability of the matrix function hG in L_p (concerning this topic, see e.g. NYAGA [3]). Therefore, in particular, the structure of the domain of Φ-factorability of piecewise continuous matrix functions described in Corollary 5.16 is preserved: a change of weight causes only a shift (with a possible splitting or confluence) of exceptional points $p_1,\dots,p_r$. Any factorization of a piecewise Hölder matrix function in the classes $h(c_1,\dots,c_q)$ can be viewed as its factorization in $L_p(\varrho)$ with specially chosen p and β_k. In NYAGA [2] it is shown that, if Γ is an unbounded closed contour (i.e. a closed curve on a Riemann sphere passing through ∞) and

$$\varrho(t) = |t|^{\beta_0} \prod_{k=1}^{N} \left|\frac{t-t_k}{t}\right|^{\beta_k},$$

then the Fredholmness of $AP_\Gamma + BQ_\Gamma$ in $L_p(\Gamma,\varrho)$ is equivalent to the Fredholmness of $\tilde{A}P_{\tilde{\Gamma}} + \tilde{B}Q_{\tilde{\Gamma}}$ in $L_p(\tilde{\Gamma},\tilde{\varrho})$. Here $\tilde{f}(z) = f(1/(z-z_0))$ (z_0 is an arbitrarily chosen fixed point lying beyond the domain bounded by Γ, $\tilde{\Gamma}$ is the image of Γ under the mapping $z \to \frac{1}{z-z_0}$ and

$$\tilde{\varrho}(t) = |t|^{p-\beta_0-2} \prod_{k=1}^{N} \left|t - \frac{1}{t_k-z_0}\right|^{\beta_k}).$$

This result allows us to transfer all statements concerning Φ-factorization of matrix functions defined on bounded contours to the case of unbounded contours (in particular, to the real line).

The papers MISHCHISHIN [1,2], MOSSAKOVSKIǏ, MISHCHISHIN [1], KHVOSHCHINSKAYA [1], TSITSKISHVILI [1-4], CHAKRABARTI [1] are dedicated to the construction of a factorization of piecewise continuous matrix functions and its applications. In these papers methods of analytical theory of differential equations are employed.

A natural generalization of piecewise continuous matrix functions is the case of matrix functions $G(t)$ for which, at each point $t \in \Gamma$, there exists the (finite) limit from the left $G(t-0)$ and from the right $G(t+0)$. The set of discontinuities of such a matrix function is at most countable, and the class of these matrix functions coincides with the closure $\overline{PC}$ of the class of piecewise continuous matrix functions PC in L_∞ (BOURBAKI [1]). Theorem 5.16' and Corollary 5.17 can be transferred to $\overline{PC}$-matrix functions without any changes.

The Φ-factorization of $\overline{PC}$-matrix functions was considered in GOHBERG, KRUPNIK [2], concerning the scalar case, see also GOHBERG, KRUPNIK [4], DANILYUK [1,3,6], FROLOV [1], SHELEPOV [1].

Note (cf. SPITKOVSKIǏ [2]) that the domain of Φ-factorability of a $\overline{PC}$-matrix function is either empty or the ray $(1,\infty)$ with exceptional points $\{p_s\}$ condensing at most at 1 and ∞. Vice versa, any set of this kind is the domain of Φ-factorability of a certain $\overline{PC}$-matrix function (and even of a scalar $\overline{PC}$-function). An appropriate example (for the case of the single condensation point ∞) yields the function G equal to $\exp \frac{2\pi i\lambda_s(t)}{p_s}$ on the arc (t_s, t_{s+1}), $s=0,1,\ldots,$ where $\{t_s\}_{s=1}^{\infty}$ is an increasing (in the sense of the orientation of the contour) sequence of points of the contour Γ converging to a fixed point t_0, and λ_s is a function continuous on (t_s, t_{s+1}) and monotonically decreasing from 1 to 0.

In the case of a Lyapunov contour and $p = 2$, Theorem 5.16 has been transferred to all matrix functions that have no more than two limits $G_1(t)$ and $G_2(t)$ at each point $t \in \Gamma$. In this case in (5.15) one has to substitute $G(t \pm 0)$ by $G_{1,2}(t)$ (CLANCEY [1]). The corresponding result for $p \neq 2$ is no longer a literal analogue of Theorem 5.16, but runs as follows:

For Φ-factorability of the matrix function G in L_p it is necessary and sufficient that

1) $\det G_1(t)G_2(t) \neq 0$ for all $t \in \Gamma$,

2) $\omega_j(t) \neq 2\pi/p$ at those points $t \in \Gamma$ where $G_1(t)$ is the right-side limit for G and $G_2(t)$ is the left-side limit,

3) $\omega_j(t)$ is not located on the interval with ends $2\pi/p$ and $2\pi/q$ at those points $t \in \Gamma$ for which the matrix function G has two essential limits at least from one side.

Here $\omega_1(t),\dots,\omega_n(t)$ is the collection of arguments of all eigenvalues of the matrix $G_2^{-1}(t)G_1(t)$.

This result has been derived by one of the authors (SPITKOVSKIĬ [11]); its complete proof can be found in SPITKOVSKIĬ [16].

CHAPTER 6. ON THE STABILITY OF FACTORIZATION FACTORS

The present chapter is devoted to the study of the behaviour of the factorization factors under small perturbations of the matrix function G. Here we encounter another qualitative difference between the matrix case $(n > 1)$ and the scalar one $(n = 1)$. It appears that the partial indices of a matrix function and the factorization factors $G_{\pm}$ are unstable, in general. This fact gives rise to principle difficulties in the solution of the two most important problems in the factorization theory of a matrix function G and the solvability theory of the vector-valued Riemann boundary value problem with this matrix:

1) the problems of calculating the partial indices (of calculating the defect numbers of the Riemann problem) and

2) the problems of constructing an approximate factorization of a matrix function (of finding an approximate solution of the Riemann boundary value problem).

Till now, an effective solution has not been found yet for both problems in the general case. Therefore, it is still actual to look for effectively verifiable estimates for the partial indices.

In the framework of the latter problem, those cases when the partial indices preserve one and the same sign and, especially, are stable are of particular interest. The equality of sign of all partial indices is necessary and sufficient for the stability of the defect numbers α and β of the Riemann boundary value problem. In this and only this case they can be determined by the total index $\varkappa$ of the matrix function G via the formulae $\alpha = \max\{0,\varkappa\}$, $\beta = \max\{0,-\varkappa\}$. As we shall see later on, the stability of partial indices is necessary and sufficient for the stability of the solutions of the Riemann problem, which is important for an effective application of approximate solution methods.

Now as ever, the theory of Fredholm operators will be an important means of research in the present chapter. Thus, we shall be concerned with one of the following two situations:

1) Φ-factorization of a matrix function $G \in L_\infty$ given on a contour of class $\mathfrak{R}$;

2) factorization of a matrix function $G \in \mathfrak{A}$ in a decomposing (C,R)-algebra $\mathfrak{A}$.

In considerations of Sections 6.1, 6.2 which apply to both situations just mentioned we shall simply write "factorization" instaed of "Φ-factorization" or "factorization in $\mathfrak{A}$". Perturbations of the matrix function G we shall estimate in the operator norm, i.e., in the norm (3.19) in situation 1) and by means of (5.8) in situation 2).

Let us clarify that a certain characteristic $f(G)$ of the matrix function G is called stable, if it is a continuous function of G, i.e., small (in the sense of the indicated norm) perturbations of G correspond to small variations of $f(G)$. In particular, to say that integer characteristics (partial indices) are stable amounts to saying that they remain unchanged under sufficiently small variations of G.

The crucial result of Section 6.1 is the stability criterion for the partial indices of a matrix function G consisting in the fact that the largest of the partial indices of G differs from the smallest one by at most one. The proof of this criterion is preceded by the proof of the stability of the partial indices $\varkappa_1,\ldots,\varkappa_n$ written in a non-increasing order to remain in the interval $[\varkappa_n,\varkappa_1]$ and, in particular, the stability of the property of partial indices to preserve one and the same sign. As mentioned above, the latter statements are very important and without doubt of independent interest, thus, we emphasized them in separate theorems, departing from the traditional method of presenting the stability criterion for partial indices.

The statements of Section 6.1 are based on the stability property of the defect numbers of one-sided invertible Fredholm operators. These assertions show, especially, that the change of partial indices of the matrix function G obeys certain laws in case they are unstable. Applying the more sophisticated theorem on the semi-stability of the defect numbers of Fredholm operators, one can obtain an exhaustive description of the character of change of partial indices under perturbations of G. This description is contained in Section 6.2. It is formulated in terms of the ordering $\succ$ introduced in Chapter 4, which is defined over tuples of n integers ordered in a special way.

The main disadvantage of the stability criterion for partial indices and the other theorems from Section 6.1 consists in their non-effectivity: for checking the assumptions of these theorems, first of all, one has to evaluate the largest and the smallest index $\varkappa_1$ and $\varkappa_n$ or at least to determine their signs. Therefore, we are interested in sufficient conditions of stability, non-negativity or non-positivity of partial indices which enable a more effective method of checking to be applied than the direct calculation of $\varkappa_1$ and $\varkappa_n$ or the determination of their signs. This topic is pursued in Section 6.3 and 6.4. The method, with the help of which sufficient conditions will be derived in 6.1, is based on the application of the contracting mapping principle. As will be clarified in the next chapter, if the contour is a circle and the factorization is considered in L_2, then the conditions of Section 6.3 are exact. Another way of obtaining conditions of sign definiteness and stability of partial indices is presented in 6.4. It rests upon the utilization of certain algebraic properties and notions. For instance, such a property is the normality of the matrix function in question a.e. on the contour Γ. The main result of Section 6.4 related to normal matrices consists in the factorability with equal partial indices of a matrix function whose eigenvalues are located in some disk. A natural generalization of this fact is provided by an analogous result (factorability with equal partial indices) for matrix functions $G \in L_\infty$ not necessarily normal, but such that its numerical domain is separated from zero for all points of Γ.

For matrix functions of classes $L_\infty^{\pm} + C$ as well as for continuous matrix functions, the results of 6.3 and 6.4 will be made more precise in Section 6.5.

Section 6.6 is devoted to the stability of the factorization factors $G_\pm$.

It will be shown that for matrix functions close to the original one which have different tuples of partial indices, the factorization factors $G_{\pm}$ cannot be too close. The opposite assertion is particularly important: the closeness of matrix functions whose tuples of partial indices coincide implies the closeness of the factorization factors $G_{\pm}$. This means the stability of factorization with a stable tuple of partial indices.

Section 6.7 contains comments on published papers.

6.1. STABILITY CRITERION FOR PARTIAL INDICES

In Chapter 3 the stability of the factorability property and the stability of the total index (Theorem 3.20) have been proved. Thus, in the scalar case the diagonal factorization factor Λ is stable. Passing to the matrix case, the situation essentially changes. This will be demonstrated by the following example.

Example. Suppose $\Lambda_{\varepsilon}(t) = \begin{pmatrix} t^{\nu} & 0 \\ \varepsilon t^{\mu+1} & t^{\mu} \end{pmatrix}$, where ε is a constant, ν and μ are integers and $\nu-\mu \geq 2$. If $\varepsilon \neq 0$, then the matrix function Λ_{ε} admits the factorization

$$\Lambda_{\varepsilon}(t) = \begin{pmatrix} 1 & \varepsilon^{-1}t^{\nu-\mu-1} \\ 0 & 1 \end{pmatrix} \begin{pmatrix} t^{\nu-1} & 0 \\ 0 & t^{\mu+1} \end{pmatrix} \begin{pmatrix} 0 & -\varepsilon^{-1} \\ \varepsilon & t^{-1} \end{pmatrix}$$

and, thus, its partial indices are $\nu-1$ and $\mu+1$. Clearly, the matrix function Λ_{ε} depends continuously on the parameter ε. At the same time, the matrix function Λ_0 is diagonal and its partial indices are equal to λ and μ. Therefore, in any neighbourhood of Λ_0 there exists a matrix function the tuple of partial indices of which does not coincide with the tuple of partial indices of Λ_0. In other words, the system of partial indices of the matrix function is unstable.

However, in some cases the tuple of partial indices can be stable. For instance, the equality of all partial indices to zero is, in view of Corollary 3.8 (or Theorem 5.6), equivalent to the invertibility of the operator $P + GQ$ (and $Q + \overline{G'}P$). Therefore, it is a stable characteristic of factorization. This assertion is a special case of the following proposition,

THEOREM 6.1. Let the matrix function G admit a factorization with non-negative (non-positive) partial indices. Then there exists a $\delta > 0$ such that every matrix function G_1 from the δ-neighbourhood of G is factorable with the same total index and its partial indices are also non-negative (non-positive).

Proof. We study the case of non-negative partial indices. According to Corollary 3.8, the operator $T_Q(G)$ is invertible from the right and its kernel is of dimension $\varkappa$. In view of the stability of one-sided invertibility, all operators from a certain ε-neighbourhood of $T_Q(G)$ are also invertible from the right. Since the kernel dimension of a one-sided invertible operator does not change under small perturbations, it is constant on connected sets consisting of operators invertible from the right and, particularly, on an ε-neighbourhood of $T_Q(G)$. Setting $\delta = \varepsilon\|Q\|^{-1}$, we find that $\|T_Q(G_1) - T_Q(G)\| < \varepsilon$ as soon as $\|G - G_1\| < \delta$. Thus, the operator $T_Q(G_1)$ is invertible from the right and its kernel dimension is $\varkappa$. In other words, the matrix function G_1 can be factored, its partial indices are non-negative and the total index is equal to $\varkappa$. ≡

Let us note how one can specify an estimate for δ. Since ε can be taken as $\varepsilon = \|T_Q(G)^{-1}\|^{-1}$, where $T_Q(G)^{-1}$ denotes an arbitrary one-sided inverse of $T_Q(G)$, one may choose

$$\delta = \|Q\|^{-1}\|G_-^{-1}Q\Lambda^{-1}G_+^{-1}|_{\mathrm{im}\ Q}\|^{-1} \tag{6.1}$$

in the case of non-negative and

$$\delta = \|Q\|^{-1}\|G_-^{-1}\ \Lambda^{-1}QG_+^{-1}|_{\mathrm{im}\ Q}\|^{-1} \tag{6.1'}$$

in the case of non-positive partial indices. For $G_\pm^{-1} \in L_\infty^\pm$, one can take

$$\delta = \|Q\|^{-2}\|G_+^{-1}\|\|G_-^{-1}\|\|\Lambda^{-1}\| . \tag{6.1''}$$

THEOREM 6.2. Let the matrix function G admit a factorization with partial indices $\varkappa_1 \geq \ldots \geq \varkappa_n$. Then there exists a $\delta > 0$ such that every matrix function G_1 from the δ-neighbourhood of G can be factored with the same total index and partial indices lying in $[\varkappa_n, \varkappa_1]$.

Proof. Consider the matrix function $t^{-\varkappa_n}G(t)$. Its partial indices are non-negative. Due to the previous theorem, there exists a $\delta_n > 0$ such that all matrix functions from the δ_n-neighbourhood of $t^{-\varkappa_n}G(t)$ are factorable with the same total index and have non-negative partial indices. Analogously, all matrix functions from a certain δ-neighbourhood of $t^{-\varkappa_1}G(t)$ have non-positive partial indices. Set $\delta = \min\{\delta_n \|t^{-\varkappa_n}\|, \delta_1\|t^{-\varkappa_1}\|\}$. Then, provided that $\|G - G_1\| < \delta$, we have $\|t^{-\varkappa_1}G_1 - t^{-\varkappa_1}G\| < \delta_1$ and $\|t^{-\varkappa_n}G_1 - t^{-\varkappa_n}G\| < \delta_n$, which means that the matrix function $t^{-\varkappa_n}G_1$ has non-negative and $t^{-\varkappa_1}G_1$ has non-positive partial indices. Consequently, the partial indices of G_1 are included between $\varkappa_n$ and $\varkappa_1$. The equality of total indices of the matrix functions $t^{-\varkappa_1}G$ and $t^{-\varkappa_1}G_1$ implies the equality of total indices of G and G_1. Theorem 6.2 is proved. ≡

Now we proceed to the main result of the present section.

THEOREM 6.3 (Stability criterion for partial indices). The system $\varkappa_1 \geq \ldots \geq \varkappa_n$ of partial indices is stable if and only if

$$\varkappa_1 - \varkappa_n \leq 1. \tag{6.2}$$

Proof. Note that the partial indices are defined uniquely by condition (6.2) and the value of the total index $\varkappa$. Namely,

$$\begin{aligned} \varkappa_n &= \varkappa_{n-1} = \ldots = \varkappa_{r+1} = [\varkappa/n], \\ \varkappa_r &= \ldots = \varkappa_1 = [\varkappa/n] + 1, \end{aligned} \tag{6.3}$$

where r $(0 \leq r < n)$ is the remainder from the division of $\varkappa$ by n. If condition (6.2) is fulfilled, then, in accordance with Theorem 6.2, it remains valid for all matrix functions from some neighbourhood of G. The value of the total index is also preserved and, consequently, formulae (6.3) either. Thus, the sufficiency of the condition (6.2) for the stability of the system of partial indices is proved.
Now, let (2.1) be a factorization of the matrix function G, and assume the condition (6.2) to be not fulfilled. Denote by A that matrix of

n th order the only non-zero element of which is equal to one and situated in the left lower corner. By φ we denote some function from E_∞^- which has a zero of order $\varkappa_1 - \varkappa_n - 2$ at infinity and satisfies the condition $|\varphi(t)g_{in}^+(t)g_{1j}^-(t)| \leq 1$ $(i,j=1,\dots,n)$ a.e. on Γ. Here g_{in}^+ and g_{1j}^- are entries of the last column and the first row of the matrix functions G_+ and G_- respectively.

Such a function φ can always be constructed. To this end, we assume $\varphi \equiv 0$ in the domains $\mathfrak{D}^+(j)$, $j=1,\dots,m-1$, and reduce the construction of φ in $\mathfrak{D}^+(0)$ with the help of a conformal mapping to the problem of the reconstruction of a function analytic in a disk by the values of its absolute value on its boundary. If $g_{in}^+, g_{1j}^- \in L_\infty$ $(i,j=1,\dots,n)$, but also in case of factorization in a (C,R)-algebra $\mathfrak{R}$, it suffices to set $\varphi(z) = cz^{-\varkappa_1+\varkappa_n+2}$, where c is a constant sufficiently small. The matrix function $F_\varepsilon(t) = \Lambda(t) + \varepsilon\varphi(t)At^{\varkappa_1-1}$ is lower triangular. By a method similar to the one used in Theorem 4.9, for $\varepsilon \neq 0$, we may get its factorization

$$F_\varepsilon(t) = F_{+,\varepsilon}(t)\ \Lambda^{(1)}(t)F_{-,\varepsilon}(t),$$

where

$$F_{+,\varepsilon}(t) = I + \varepsilon^{-1}Q_0(t)A',$$

$$\Lambda^{(1)}(t) = \operatorname{diag}[t^{\varkappa_1-1}, t^{\varkappa_2},\dots,t^{\varkappa_{n-1}}, t^{\varkappa_n+1}],$$

$$F_{-,\varepsilon}(t) = \begin{pmatrix} t-Q_0(t)\varphi(t) & & & & -\varepsilon^{-1}Q_0(t)t^{1-\varkappa_1+\varkappa_n} \\ & 1 & & & \\ & & \ddots & & \\ & & & 1 & \\ \varepsilon\varphi(t)t^{\varkappa_1-\varkappa_n-2} & & & & t^{-1} \end{pmatrix}$$

$$Q_0(z) = c_1 z^{\varkappa_1-\varkappa_n-1} + c_2 z^{\varkappa_1-\varkappa_n-2},$$

and the numbers c_1 and c_2 are chosen in such a way that the function $z - Q_0(z)\varphi(z)$ vanishes at infinity.

Apparently, the representation

$$G_+F_\varepsilon G_- = (G_+F_{+,\varepsilon})\Lambda^{(1)}(F_{-,\varepsilon}G_-)$$

is a factorization of the matrix function $G_+F_\varepsilon G_-$. At the same time,

$$G_+F_\varepsilon G_- - G = \varepsilon\varphi t^{\varkappa_1-1}\ G_+AG_- = \varepsilon\varphi t^{\varkappa_1-1}(g^+_{in}g^-_{1j})^n_{i,j=1} .$$

In this way, arbitrarily close to the matrix function G we may indicate a factorable matrix function the tuple of partial indices of which $-\varkappa_1-1, \varkappa_2,\ldots,\varkappa_{n-1}, \varkappa_n+1$ does not coincide with the tuple of partial indices of G (the equation $\varkappa_1-1 = \varkappa_n$ is impossible, because $\varkappa_1-\varkappa_n \geq 2$) . This implies the necessity of condition (6.2) for the stability of the tuple of partial indices. The proof of Theorem 6.3 is complete. ≡

6.2. ON THE BEHAVIOUR OF PARTIAL INDICES UNDER SMALL PERTURBATIONS. THE STRUCTURE OF THE FAMILY OF Φ-FACTORABLE MATRIX FUNCTIONS

In the previous section it was shown that, if the system of partial indices is of the form (6.3), then it remains unchanged under small perturbations of the matrix function. From Theorem 6.2 it is clear that in the general case the changes of partial indices are also not of arbitrary nature. In the proof of Theorem 6.2 the stability of the defect numbers of one-sided invertible operators was used. Taking advantage of the semistability of the defect numbers of Fredholm operators (Theorem 1.4), one can obtain a more precise result. It will be formulated in terms of the ordering $\succ$ introduced in Chapter 4 (Definition 4.1).

<u>THEOREM 6.4.</u> Assume the matrix function G to admit a factorization with the tuple of partial indices $(\varkappa_j)^n_{j=1}$. Then there exists a neighbourhood of this matrix function consisting only of such factorable matrix functions whose tuple of partial indices is majorized (in the sense of the ordering $\succ$) by the tuple $(\varkappa_j)^n_{j=1}$.

Note that, by assertion 1) of Lemma 4.1, the partial indices of all matrix functions from the indicated neighbourhood are concentrated in the interval $[\varkappa_n,\varkappa_1]$ and the total index coincides with the total index of G. Thus, Theorem 6.4 makes Theorem 6.2 more precise.

<u>Proof.</u> Choosing an integer k from the interval $[\varkappa_n,\varkappa_1]$, we consider

the operator $P + t^{-k}G(t)Q$. It is Fredholm, since the matrix function $t^{-k}G(t)$ is factorable along with $G(t)$. Consequently, all operators from some neighbourhood of it are Fredholm and, due to Theorem 1.2, their defect numbers do not exceed the corresponding defect numbers of the operator $P + t^{-k}G(t)$.

We can find a number $\delta_k > 0$ such that the operator $P + t^{-k}F(t)Q$ belongs to the mentioned neighbourhood of the operator $P + t^{-k}G(t)Q$ as soon as $\|F-G\| < \delta_k$. Utilizing the formulae stated in Theorem 3.16 for the defect numbers of such operators, we obtain

$$\begin{aligned} \sum_{j=1}^{n} \max\{\varkappa'_j - k, 0\} &\leq \sum_{j=1}^{n} \max\{\varkappa_j - k, 0\}, \\ \sum_{j=1}^{n} \min\{\varkappa'_j - k, 0\} &\geq \sum_{j=1}^{n} \min\{\varkappa_j - k, 0\}, \end{aligned} \tag{6.4}$$

where $(\varkappa'_j)_{j=1}^{n}$ is the tuple of partial indices of the matrix function F. Setting $\delta = \min\{\delta_k\}_{k=\varkappa_n}^{\varkappa_1}$, we observe that, for all matrix functions F from the δ-neighbourhood of G, the inequalities (6.4) are fulfilled for $k = \varkappa_n, \ldots, \varkappa_1$. According to assertion 2) of Lemma 4.1, this implies that the tuple $\{\varkappa'_j)$ is majorized by the tuple $(\varkappa_j)$, which proves Theorem 6.4. ≡

The result of Theorem 6.4 is of final nature. In order to support this, we must describe the relation $\succ$ in a somewhat different way. To this end, we first introduce some definitions and notations.

Let σ_n be the collection of tuples $(k_j)_{j=1}^{n}$ of integers satisfying $k_1 \geq \ldots \geq k_n$.

DEFINITION 6.1. Let us say that (k'_j) $(\in \sigma_n)$ is obtained from the tuple (k_j) $(\in \sigma_n)$ with the aid of an elementary operation, if for some integers r and s $(1 \leq r < s \leq n)$,

$$k'_r = k_r - 1, \quad k'_s = k_s + 1, \quad k'_j = k_j \quad (j \neq r, s). \tag{6.5}$$

We shall write $(k_j) \to (k'_j)$, if the tuple $\{k'_j\}$ $(\in \sigma_n)$ either coincides with (k_j) $(\in \sigma_n)$ or is obtained from it as a result of a finite number of elementary operations.

Obviously, $\to$ is a partial order relation on the set σ_n. For comparability of the tuples (k'_j) and (k_j), it is necessary (and, for n=2, also sufficient) that $\sum_{j=1}^{n} k'_j = \sum_{j=1}^{n} k_j$. Minimal elements in the sense of the relation $\to$ are those and only those tuples $(\varkappa_j)_{j=1}^{n}$ which satisfy the condition (6.2).

<u>LEMMA 6.1.</u> Let $(k_j)_{j=1}^{n}, (k'_j)_{j=1}^{n} \in \sigma_n$. Then the relation $(k_j) \underset{..}{\to} (k'_j)$ holds if and only if $(k_j) \succ (k'_j)$.

<u>Proof.</u> Suppose $(k_j) \underset{..}{\to} (k'_j)$. By the very definition, either $(k_j) = (k'_j)$ (and then, clearly $(k_j) \succ (k'_j)$) or (k'_j) is obtained from (k_j) as the result of a certain number of elementary operations. If we succeed in proving that as the result of an arbitrary elementary operation there will be obtained a tuple which is majorized (in the sense of the relation $\succ$) by the initial one, then, in view of the transitivity of the ordering $\succ$, $(k_j) \succ (k'_j)$.

Thus, it is sufficient to examine tuples connected via relations (6.5). It is easily checked that in this case the inequalities (4.8) and (4.8') are true.

Now we are going to show that, if $(k_j), (k'_j) \in \sigma_n$ and $(k_j) \succ (k'_j)$, then $(k_j) \underset{..}{\to} (k'_j)$. For this purpose, we use induction on n. For $n = 2$, the condition $(k_j) \succ (k'_j)$ means that $k'_1 = k_1 - k$, $k'_2 = k_2 + k$, where $0 \le k \le (k_1-k_2)/2$. Apparently, the tuple (k'_j) is obtained from (k_j) by means of k elementary operations. Therefore, $(k_j) \underset{..}{\to} (k'_j)$.

Supposing that the assertion to be proved is true for $n \neq 1$, we consider two tuples of length n. The condition $(k_j)_{j=1}^{n} \succ (k'_j)_{j=1}^{n}$ means, in particular, that $k_1 \ge k'_1$, $k_n \le k'_n$. If, for instance, $k_n = k'_n$, then $(k_j)_{j=1}^{n} \succ (k'_j)_{j=1}^{n}$ implies $(k_j)_{j=1}^{n-1} \succ (k'_j)_{j=1}^{n-1}$. By induction hypothesis, $(k_j)_{j=1}^{n-1} \underset{..}{\to} (k'_j)_{j=1}^{n-1}$. But in this case we have also $(k_j)_{j=1}^{n} \underset{..}{\to} (k'_j)_{j=1}^{n}$. Analogous reasonings are applicable for $k_1 = k'_1$. Consequently, we shall assume that $k_1 > k'_1$ and $k_n < k'_n$. Then $k_1 - k_n \ge (k'_1+1) - (k'_n-1) \ge 2$. Therefore, there exist numbers l and $m, l < m$, such that $k_1 = \ldots = k_l > k_{l+1}$, $k_1 - k_{m-1} \le 1$, $k_1 - k_m \ge 2$,

Consider the tuple $(k_j^{(1)})_{j=1}^n$ obtained from $(k_j)_{j=1}^n$ with the aid of the elementary operation for $r = l$, $s = m$ and show that $(k_j^{(1)})_{j=1}^n \succ (k'_j)_{j=1}^n$. We restrict ourselves to the verification of inequality (4.8) in which k_j is replaced by $k_j^{(1)}$.

For $k \geq k'_1$, we have $\sum_{j=1}^n \max\{k'_j-k,0\} = 0$, for $k \leq k_m$, $\sum_{j=1}^n \max\{k_j^{(1)}-k,0\} \geq \sum_{j=1}^n \max\{k'_j-k,0\}$. Finally, if $k_m < k < k'_1$, $k_j > k$, then $k_j \geq k_{m-1} \geq k_l-1 \geq k'_j$, where $k_j > k'_j$ for $j=1,\ldots,l$, so that $\sum_{j=1}^n \max\{k'_j-k,0\} \leq \sum_{j=1}^n \max\{k_j-k,0\} -l \leq \sum_{j=1}^n \max\{k_j-k,0\} -1 = \sum_{j=1}^n \max\{k_j^{(1)}-k,0\}$.

Repeating these considerations, after d $(\leq l)$ steps we come to the tuple $(k_j^{(d)})_{j=1}^n \succ (k'_j)_{j=1}^n$, where either $k_n^{(d)} > k_n$ (if $d < l$) or $k_1^{(d)} < k_1$ (if $d = l$) . From this we conclude that after the application of a finite number N of elementary operations one can obtain a tuple $(k_j^{(N)})_{j=1}^n \succ (k'_j)_{j=1}^n$ for which either $k_n^{(N)} = k'_n$ or $k_1^{(N)} = k'_1$. In any case, as shown above, $(k_j^{(N)})_{j=1}^n \to (k'_j)_{j=1}^n$. But then $(k_j)_{j=1}^n \ddot{\to} (k'_j)_{j=1}^n$, because $(k_j)_{j=1}^n \ddot{\to} (k_j^{(N)})_{j=1}^n$.

Lemma 6.1 is proved. ≡

<u>THEOREM 6.5.</u> Let the matrix function G be factorable, and assume the tuple of its partial indices to be $(\varkappa_j)_{j=1}^n$. If $(\varkappa_j)_{j=1}^n \succ (\varkappa'_j)_{j=1}^n$, then in an arbitrary neighbourhood of G there exists a matrix function the tuple of partial indices of which is $(\varkappa'_j)_{j=1}^n$.

<u>Proof.</u> The assertion is evident if $(\varkappa'_j) = (\varkappa_j)$. If $(\varkappa'_j) \neq (\varkappa_j)$, then, according to Lemma 6.1, there exist tuples $(\varkappa_j^{(k)})_{j=1}^n$, $k=0,\ldots,N$, such that $\varkappa_j^{(o)} = \varkappa_j$, $\varkappa_j^{(N)} = \varkappa'_j$ and the (k+1) th tuple is obtained from the k th one with the aid of one elementary operation. Arguing as in the proof of the necessity in Theorem 6.3, we conclude that in any neighbourhood of the given (factorable) matrix function there exists a matrix function whose tuple of partial indices is obtained from the tuple of partial indices of the initial one with the help of one elementary operation previously chosen. Specifying $\varepsilon > 0$, we choose in the $\varepsilon/2$-neighbourhood of G a matrix function G_1 with the tuple of partial

indices $(\varkappa_j^{(1)})_{j=1}^n$, in the ε/4-neighbourhood of G_1 a matrix function G_2 the tuple of partial indices of which is $(\varkappa_j^{(2)})_{j=1}^n$ and so on. After all, we obtain a matrix function G_N from the ε-neighbourhood of G with the tuple of partial indices $(\varkappa_j')_{j=1}^n$, which proves Theorem 6.5. ≡

COROLLARY 6.1. In any neighbourhood of a factorable matrix function there exists a matrix function with a stable tuple of partial indices.

With the help of Theorem 3.7' all results derived in the present section can be transferred to the case of right-factorization.

COROLLARY 6.2. In any neighbourhood of a matrix function factorable from the left and the right there exists a matrix function with a stable tuple of left as well as right indices.

Proof. For given $\varepsilon > 0$, we take in the ε/2-neighbourhood of the original matrix function G a matrix function G_1 with a stable tuple of partial indices (due to Corollary 6.1, this is always possible). If ε is sufficiently small, then the matrix function G_1 will be factorable not only from the left but also from the right. In view of the stability of its left indices there is a δ-neighbourhood of G_1 to which belong only matrix functions with the same tuple of partial indices. Setting $\delta_1 = \min\{\delta, \varepsilon/2\}$ and using an analogue of Corollary 6.1 related to right-factorization, we find in the δ_1-neighbourhood of G_1 a matrix function G_2 with a stable tuple of right indices. This is just the desired one. ≡

The results of the present section admit a topological interpretation. Denote by $\Phi_{(\varkappa_j)}$ the set of factorable matrix functions[1)] the tuple of partial indices of which is $(\varkappa_j)$. The representation $\Phi = \bigcup_{(\varkappa_j)\in\sigma_n} \Phi_{(\varkappa_j)}$ yields a decomposition of the class of all factorable matrix functions into disjoint non-empty sets, where:

1) if $(\varkappa_j) \succ (\varkappa_j')$, then $\Phi_{(\varkappa_j)} \subseteq \operatorname{clos} \Phi_{(\varkappa_j')}$,

2) if $(\varkappa_j) \not\succ (\varkappa_j')$, then $\Phi_{(\varkappa_j)} \cap \operatorname{clos} \Phi_{(\varkappa_j')} = \emptyset$.

---

1) Recall that in this section the factorization is always understood as Φ-factorization.

Properties 1) and 2) are reformulations of Theorem 6.5 and 6.4, respectively. Theorem 6.3 means that

3) the set $\Phi_{(\varkappa_j)}$ is open if and only if the tuple $(\varkappa_j)$ satisfies condition (6.2).

Since a tuple $(\varkappa_j)$ having the property (6.2) is comparable with all tuples with the same sum and is minimal (in the sense of the ordering $\succ$), then property 1) means, especially, that

4) under the condition (6.2), the set $\Phi_{(\varkappa_j)}$ is dense in

$$\Phi_\varkappa = \cup\{\Phi_{(k_j)} : (k_j) \in \sigma_n , \sum_{j=1}^{n} k_j = \sum_{j=1}^{n} \varkappa_j \ (= \varkappa)\} .$$

If the tuple $(\varkappa_j)$ fails to have property (6.2), then the set $\Phi_{(\varkappa_j)}$ lies in the complement (with respect to $\Phi_\varkappa$) of an open dense set. Therefore, it is nowhere dense. Because, for different $\varkappa$, the sets $\Phi_\varkappa$ are open and disjoint, $\Phi_{(\varkappa_j)}$ is nowhere dense in their union either. Thus:

5) if $\varkappa_1 - \varkappa_n \geq 2$, then $\Phi_{(\varkappa_j)}$ is a nowhere dense subset of Φ.

Finally, from property 2) we can conclude that

6) the sets $\Phi_{(\varkappa_j)}$ and $\Phi_{(\varkappa'_j)}$ are separated iff the tuples $(\varkappa_j)$ and $(\varkappa'_j)$ are not comparable.

With Theorem 3.20 in mind we can imagine the set Φ as the union of a countable number of separated open sets $\Phi_\varkappa$. Now we can every of the $\Phi_\varkappa$'s divide into an open set $\Phi_{(\varkappa_j)}$ $(\sum_{j=1}^{n} \varkappa_j = \varkappa , \ \varkappa_1 - \varkappa_n \leq 1)$ and a nowhere dense set $\Phi_{(\varkappa'_j)}$ $(\sum_{j=1}^{n} \varkappa'_j = \varkappa , \ \varkappa'_1 - \varkappa'_n \geq 2)$.

6.3. ESTIMATES FOR THE PARTIAL INDICES OF MEASURABLE BOUNDED MATRIX FUNCTIONS

In Section 6.1 it was shown that inequality (6.2) is a necessary and sufficient condition of stability of partial indices. However, if we want to use this criterion, we must know the value of the largest and smallest partial index. Therefore, we are interested in assertions in which besides Φ-factorability of a certain matrix function also estimates of its partial indices are established.

Sufficient criteria of non-negativity and non-positivity of partial indices are also of some significance, since the defect numbers of the vector-valued Riemann boundary value problem with matrix coefficient G are stable if and only if all its partial indices have the same sign. The present section is devoted to a result of precisely such a type. Owing to Theorem 6.2, every $n \times n$ matrix function which is Φ-factorable in L_p with zero partial indices has a neighbourhood entirely consisting of matrix functions which have the same property. In particular, the matrix function identically equal to I possesses such a neighbourhood. Denote by $\delta_{p,n}(\Gamma)$ the largest possible value of the radius of such a neighbourhood. In other words, $\delta_{p,n}(\Gamma)$ is a number such that, for

$$\|I - G_0\| < \delta_{p,n}(\Gamma) , \tag{6.6}$$

the operator $P + G_0Q$ is invertible and there exists an $n \times n$ matrix function F for which $\|I - F\| = \delta_{p,n}(\Gamma)$ and the operator $P + FQ$ is non-invertible.

We denote by A_p the interval with ends p and $q = p/(p-1)$.

LEMMA 6.2. The following assertions related to $\delta_{p,n}(\Gamma)$ are true:

1) the numbers $\|Q\|^{-1}_{L^n_p}$ and $\dfrac{2\|S\|_{L^n_p}}{1 + \|S\|^2_{L^n_p}}$ are estimates from below for $\delta_{p,n}(\Gamma)$; if $\Gamma \in \widetilde{\mathfrak{R}}$, then $\delta_{p,n}(\Gamma) \leq \sin \pi/\max\{p,q\}$;

2) $\delta_{p,n}(\Gamma) = \delta_{q,n}(\Gamma)$;

3) $\delta_{r,n}(\Gamma) \geq \delta_{p,n}(\Gamma)$ for $r \in A_p$; in particular, $\delta_{2,n}(\Gamma) = \max\{\delta_{p,n}(\Gamma): 1 < p < \infty\}$.

Proof. 1) The estimate $\delta_{p,n}(\Gamma) \geq \|Q\|^{-1}_{L^n_p}$ follows from the contracting mapping principle, since, for $\|I - G\| < \|Q\|^{-1}_{L^n_p}$, the operator $P + GQ = I + (G - I)Q$ differs from the unity operator by a summand with norm smaller than one. To prove the second estimate from below for $\delta_{p,n}(\Gamma)$, we consider an arbitrary matrix function G from the $2\|S\|/(1+\|S\|^2)$-neighbourhood of the identity matrix function. Then

$$\|I - G\| \leq \frac{2\sigma}{1 + \sigma^2} \tag{6.7}$$

for some $\sigma > \|S\|_{L_p^n}$ (≥ 1). We introduce the matrix functions

$G_1 = \frac{\sigma^2 + 1}{\sigma^2 - 1} G$ and $\hat{G} = (I-G_1)(I+G_1)^{-1}$. Obviously, G and G_1 are Φ-factorable only simultaneously and the tuple of their partial indices coincide. Moreover, due to condition (6.7) and the identity

$$I + G_1 = \frac{2\sigma^2}{\sigma^2 - 1} \left(I + \frac{\sigma^2+1}{2\sigma^2} (G-I)\right),$$

the matrix function $I + G_1$ is invertible in L_∞. Consequently, the invertibility if the operator $P + G_1Q = \frac{1}{2}(I+\hat{G}S)(I+G_1)$ is equivalent to the invertibility of the operator $I + \hat{G}S$. In this way, the desired estimate will be obtained, if we clarify that the inequality $\|\hat{G}\| \leq \sigma^{-1}$ holds, provided that condition (6.7) is valid. In other words, we have to show that the matrix function $Y = \sigma\hat{G}$ will be contracting as soon as the matrix function $X = \frac{1 + \sigma^2}{2\sigma}(I-G)$ is contracting. But X and Y are connected via the relation

$$Y = (I - \varepsilon X)^{-1}(X - \varepsilon I), \tag{6.8}$$

where $\varepsilon = \sigma^{-1}$. It remains to use the well-known fact from matrix theory that, for any $\varepsilon \in [0,1]$, transformation (6.8) maps a contraction into a contraction. The latter can easily been checked by showing that the spectrum of Y lies inside the unit disk.

Finally, let the condition $\Gamma \in \widetilde{R}$ be fulfilled. Consider a piecewise continuous function f given on Γ which takes only the two values $\cos^2\pi/\bar{p} + \frac{i}{2} \sin 2\pi/\bar{p}$ and $\cos^2\pi/\bar{p} - \frac{i}{2} \sin 2\pi/\bar{p}$ with $\bar{p} = \max\{p,q\}$. Clearly, $\|f - 1\| = \sin \pi/\bar{p}$. Furthermore, at the half of the points of discontinuity of the function f the argument jump is equal to $2\pi/\bar{p}$ and at the other half it equals $2\pi - 2\pi/\bar{p} = 2\pi/\min\{p,q\}$. If at the discontinuities of f there exist the tangents to the contour Γ (which can always be effected), then we are able to use Theorem 5.15, according to which this function is not Φ-factorable in L_p (and L_q). Hence $\delta_{p,1}(\Gamma) \leq \sin \pi/\bar{p}$. From here and the obvious relation $\delta_{p,n}(\Gamma) \leq \delta_{p,1}(\Gamma)$ we deduce the inequality to be proved.

2) It is not hard to see that the inverse transformation to (6.8) is this transformation itself. Therefore, it maps the 1-neighbourhood of the zero matrix function onto itself (and not only into itself as mentioned above). Moreover, it is a one-to-one mapping. Setting $Y_1 = I + \varepsilon Y$, $X_1 = (I - \varepsilon X)'$, from (6.8) we observe that, for arbitrary $\varepsilon < 1$, the transformation

$$Y_1 = (1 - \varepsilon^2)(X_1')^{-1}$$

maps the ε-neighbourhood of the identity matrix function one-to-one onto itself. At the same time, Theorem 3.7' and Corollary 3.6 imply that the matrix function X_1 is Φ-factorable in L_p with zero partial indices if and only if the matrix function Y_1 is Φ-factorable in L_q with zero partial indices. Thus, for some $\varepsilon < 1$, the ε-neighbourhood of the identity matrix function consists completely of matrix functions which are Φ-factorable in L_r with zero partial indices for $r = p$ if and only if they possess this property for $r = q$. This as well as the evident relation $\delta_{r,n}(\Gamma) \leq 1$ (which is true for all $r \in (1,\infty)$) imply assertion 2) of the lemma.

3) Now we consider the $\delta_{p,n}(\Gamma)$-neighbourhood of the identity matrix function I . According to assertion 2), every matrix function G from this neighbourhood is Φ-factorable with zero partial indices not only in L_p but also in L_q . Owing to Theorem 3.9 and 2.2, the matrix function G is Φ-factorable with zero partial indices in all L_r with $r \in \Lambda_p$. Hence, the $\delta_{p,n}(\Gamma)$-neighbourhood of the identity matrix function is a part of its $\delta_{r,n}(\Gamma)$-neighbourhood, i.e. $\delta_{p,n}(\Gamma) \leq \delta_{r,n}(\Gamma)$ $(r \in \Lambda_p)$. Since, for all $p \in (1,\infty)$, the interval Λ_p contains the point $r = 2$, we deduce that the last of the relations to be proved is also correct. ≡

<u>THEOREM 6.6.</u> Let the matrix functions G and $X_{\pm} \in L_\infty$ be such that

$$\|I - X_+ G X_-\|_{L_p^n} < \delta_{p,n}(\Gamma) . \tag{6.9}$$

Then:

1) if $X_+ \in M_\infty^+$, $X_+^{-1} \in L_\infty^+$, $X_- \in L_\infty^-$, $X_-^{-1} \in M_\infty^-$, then $\Lambda_p \subseteq \Phi(G)$ and, for all $r \in \Lambda_p$, the partial r-indices of G are non-negative,

2) if $X_+ \in L^+_\infty$, $X_+^{-1} \in M^+_\infty$, $X_- \in M^-_\infty$, $X_-^{-1} \in L^-_\infty$, then $A_p \subseteq \Phi(G)$ and, for all $r \in A_p$, the partial r-indices of G are non-positive.

<u>Proof.</u> Under the condition (6.9), the matrix function $G_0 = X_+GX_-$ satisfies relation (6.6). Therefore, from assertion 3) of Lemma 6.2 we conclude that the matrix function G_0 is Φ-factorable in L_r for all $r \in A_p$ and its partial r-indices are equal to zero. With regard to Theorem 3.10 we can claim that not only in case 1) but also in case 2) the matrix function G. is Φ-factorable in L_r $(r \in A_p)$ simultaneously with G_0, i.e. $A_p \subseteq \Phi(G)$. The non-negativity of the partial r-indices of G in case 1) and their non-positivity in case 2) follow from Theorem 2.11 by setting $B_\pm = X_\pm^{-1}$. Let us check this, say, in case 2). Taking into consideration that the partial indices of G_0 are equal to zero, we find that, in view of Theorem 2.11, the value $\mathfrak{P}(B_-) + (n-1) \times \mathfrak{P}(B_+) + \text{ind}_+\det B_+$ serves as an upper bound of the partial indices of G. But $B_- = X_-^{-1} \in L^-_\infty$, so that $\mathfrak{P}(B_-) \leq 0$. We represent the matrix function B_+ in the form $B_+ = f^{-1}A_+$, where $A_+ \in L^+_\infty$ and f is a rational function with index equal to $\mathfrak{P}(B_+)$. Then $\text{ind}_+\det B_+ = \text{ind}_+\det A_+ - n\mathfrak{P}(B_+)$, thus, $\text{ind}_+\det B_+ + (n-1)\mathfrak{P}(B_+) = \text{ind}_+\det A_+ - \mathfrak{P}(B_+)$. The value standing on the right-hand side of the last equation is opposite to the number $\text{ind}_+ B_+^{-1}$ and, with regard to the condition $B_+^{-1} \in L^+_\infty$, non-positive. Consequently, the upper estimate of the partial indices of the matrix function G is non-positive and, therefore, also the partial indices themselves. The proof of Theorem 6.6 is complete. ≡

On the strenght of Theorem 6.6 we can get sufficient conditions under which the partial indices are contained in a given interval.

In particular, we may obtain stability criteria for partial indices.

<u>THEOREM 6.7.</u> Let the matrix functions $G \in L_\infty$ and $X_{1,2} \in L^+_\infty$, $Y_{1,2} \in L^-_\infty$ be such that $X_{1,2}^{-1} \in M^+_\infty$, $Y_{1,2}^{-1} \in M^-_\infty$ and

$$\begin{aligned} &\|I - t^{-a}X_1^{-1}GY_1\| < \delta_{p,n}(\Gamma), \\ &\|I - t^{-b}X_2GY_2^{-1}\| < \delta_{p,n}(\Gamma), \end{aligned} \tag{6.9'}$$

where a and b $(a \leq b)$ are integers. Then for all $r \in A_p$, we have $r \in \Phi(G)$ and the partial r-indices of G are included between a and b.

Proof. The first of the inequalities (6.9') ensures that assertion 1) of Theorem 6.6 can be applied to the matrix function $t^{-a}G(t)$. The second one enables us to apply assertion 2) of the same theorem to the matrix function $t^{-b}G(t)$. Hence it follows that the matrix function G is Φ-factorable in L_r for $r \in A_p$, the partial r-indices of the matrix function $t^{-a}G(t)$ are non-negative and the partial r-indices of $t^{-b}G(t)$ are non-positive, which is equivalent to the assertion of the theorem. ≡

THEOREM 6.8. Suppose $G \in L_\infty$. For the matrix function G to be Φ-factorable in L_p and for its partial p-indices to be stable, it is sufficient that there exist an integer k as well as matrix functions $X_{1,2} \in L_\infty^+$ and $Y_{1,2} \in L_\infty^-$ such that $X_{1,2}^{-1} \in M_\infty^+$, $Y_{1,2}^{-1} \in M_\infty^-$ and $\|I - t^{-k}X_1^{-1}GY_1\| < \delta_{p,n}(\Gamma)$, $\|I-t^{-k-1}X_2GY_2^{-1}\| < \delta_{p,n}(\Gamma)$.

Proof. Setting $a = k$, $b = k+1$, we meet the conditions of Theorem 6.7, according to which $p \in \Phi(G)$ and the partial p-indices of G can only attain the values k and $k+1$. In virtue of Theorem 6.3, the partial p-indices of G are stable, which proves Theorem 6.8. ≡

The obtained stability criterion for partial indices can be simplified, if the total index $\varkappa$ is assumed to be known. This supposition is justified, for example, for piecewise continuous matrix functions (under the additional restrictions on the contour Γ mentioned in Section 5.3), but also for matrix functions of class $L_\infty^\pm + C$. In the general case $G \in L_\infty$, too, the calculation of the total index is, in virtue of its stability, a simpler problem than the determination of all partial indices.

THEOREM 6.9. Let the matrix function $G \in L_\infty$ admit a factorization in L_p with total index $\varkappa$. If

1) $\varkappa \equiv 0 \pmod n$ or $\varkappa \equiv 1 \pmod n$ and

a) there exist matrix functions $X_\pm \in L_\infty^\pm$ such that $X_\pm^{-1} \in M_\infty^\pm$ and $\|I - t^{-[\varkappa/n]}X_+^{-1}GX_-\| < \delta_{n,p}(\Gamma)$ or

2) $\varkappa \equiv 0 \pmod n$ or $\varkappa \equiv -1 \pmod n$ and

b) there exist matrix functions $X_\pm \in L_\infty^\pm$ such that $X_\pm^{-1} \in M_\infty^\pm$ and $\|I - t^{-[\varkappa/n]-1} X_+ G X_-^{-1}\| < \delta_{p,n}(\Gamma)$,

then the tuple of partial p-indices of G is stable.

Proof. In the first case, $\varkappa = kn + r$, where $r = 0$ or $r = 1$, and k is an integer. Due to Theorem 6.6, $p \in \Phi(G)$, so that a factorization of G is, properly, a Φ-factorization. Moreover, the inequalities $\varkappa_j \geq k$, $j=1,\ldots,n$ are fulfilled. Since in this case $\sum_{j=1}^{n} \varkappa_j \leq kn+1$, we have, actually, $\varkappa_j = k$ $(j=2,\ldots,n)$, $\varkappa_1 = k$ for $r = 0$ and $\varkappa_1 = k+1$ if $r = 1$. Consequently, the tuple of partial indices of the matrix function G is stable. The second case may be considered analogously. Theorem 6.9. has been proved. ≡

COROLLARY 6.3. If $n = 2$, then either of the conditions a) and b) mentioned in Theorem 6.9 is sufficient for the stability of the partial indices. If $n = 3$, then at least one of these conditions is sufficient.

6.4. SUFFICIENT CONDITIONS FOR COINCIDENCE OF PARTIAL INDICES OF MATRIX FUNCTIONS WHOSE NUMERICAL DOMAIN IS SEPARATED FROM ZERO

Theorems 6.6 - 6.9 are based on Φ-factorability in L_p and equality to zero of partial p-indices of a matrix function G_0 satisfying condition (6.6). Now we are going to obtain another sufficient conditions of coincidence of partial indices which rest upon some additional suppositions on algebraic properties of the matrix function G. Using them and acting as in Theorems 6.6 - 6.9, one can get criteria of non-negativity, non-positivity and stability of partial indices. This is left to the reader.

Below we shall need the following result on the behaviour of partial indices of a matrix function on multiplication by a scalar continuous function.

LEMMA 6.3. Let the matrix functions F and G $(\in L_\infty)$ be connected by the equation $F = \chi G$, where χ is a continuous non-vanishing function. Then F and G are Φ-factorable in some L_p only simultaneously and the tuple $(\hat{\varkappa}_j)$ of partial p-indices of F is obtained from the tuple $(\varkappa_j)$ of partial p-indices of G by the formula $\hat{\varkappa}_j = \varkappa_j + k$, $j=1,\dots,n$, where k is the index of the function χ .

Proof. The assertion concerning the simultaneous Φ-factorability of the matrix functions F and G results from Corollary 5.10. Since any function continuous on Γ may be uniformly approximated by rational ones with arbitrary accuracy, then, for every $\varepsilon > 0$, there exists a representation of F of the form $F = \chi_1 G_1$, where $\|\chi-\chi_1\| < \varepsilon$, $\|G-G_1\| < \varepsilon$ and the function χ_1 is rational. For sufficiently small ε, the function χ_1 does not vanish, its index coincides with the index of the function χ , the matrix function G_1 is Φ-factorable in L_p and its tuple of partial p-indices $(\varkappa_j^{(1)})$ is majorized by the tuple $(\varkappa_j)$ in the sense of the ordering $\succ$ (Theorem 6.4).

If $G_1 = G_+^{(1)}\Lambda^{(1)}G_-^{(1)}$ provides a Φ-factorization of the matrix function G_1 in L_p and $\chi_1 = \chi_+^{(1)}t^k\chi_-^{(1)}$ is a factorization of the rational function χ_1 in which, by Theorem 2.9, $(\chi_+^{(1)})^{\pm1} \in L_\infty^+$, $(\chi_-^{(1)})^{\pm1} \in L_\infty^-$, then, setting $F_+ = \chi_+^{(1)}G_+^{(1)}$, $F_- = \chi_-^{(1)}G_-^{(1)}$ and $\Lambda(t) = t^k\Lambda^{(1)}(t)$, we get the Φ-factorization $F = F_+\Lambda F_-$ of F in L_p . Consequently, $\hat{\varkappa}_j = \varkappa_j^{(1)} + k$, $j=1,\dots,n$ and, due to what was proved above, $(\varkappa_j) \succ (\hat{\varkappa}_j-k)$. Applying similar arguments to the equation $G = \chi^{-1}F$, we can show that $(\hat{\varkappa}_j-k) \succ (\varkappa_j)$. Owing to assertion 3) of Lemma 4.1, we thus deduce that $\hat{\varkappa}_j = \varkappa_j+k$, $j=1,\dots,n$, which proves Lemma 6.3. ≡

Recall that the matrix A is said to be normal, if it commutes with its adjoint: $AA^* = A^*A$. The norm of a normal matrix coincides with the largest absolute value of its eigenvalues (GANTMAKHER [1]).

THEOREM 6.10. Let F be a measurable $n\times n$ matrix function taking normal values a.e. on Γ and having the following properties: for every point $t \in \Gamma$, there are an arc γ_t $(\ni t)$ on Γ and a disk Δ_t which is visible from the origin at an angle of $\alpha_t < \arcsin \delta_{p,n}(\Gamma)$

such that the eigenvalues of almost all matrices $F(\tau)$, $\tau \in \gamma_t$ lie in the disk Δ_t.

Then the interval A_p is completely contained in some component of the domain of Φ-factorability of F and all partial r-indices of F are equal to each other $(r \in A_p)$.

Proof. Without loss of generality, the arcs γ_t may be assumed to be open. From the covering $\{\gamma_t\}_{t\in\Gamma}$ we choose a finite subcovering $\{\gamma_{t_j}\}_{j=1}^{N}$. Cancelling, if necessary, some of the arcs γ_{t_j}, we may assume that every point $t \in \Gamma$ is contained in at most two elements of the covering. Furthermore, we take the largest (say, α) of the numbers α_{t_j}, $j=1,\dots,N$, and set $\delta = \sin \alpha/2$. Evidently $\delta < \delta_{p,n}(\Gamma)$.

By z_j we denote the centre of the disk Δ_{t_j} and by l_{kj} the interval connecting the points z_k^{-1} and z_j^{-1} $(k,j=1,\dots,N)$. Finally, on the contour Γ we define a continuous function ψ with the following properties:

1) if $t \in \gamma_{t_j}$, $t \notin \gamma_{t_k}$ for $k \neq j$, then $\psi(t) = z_j^{-1}$,

2) if $t \in \gamma_{t_j} \cap \gamma_{t_k}$, $j \neq k$, then $\psi(t) \in l_{kj}$.

The function ψ does not vanish on Γ. Indeed, if $\gamma_{t_j} \cap \gamma_{t_k} \neq \emptyset$, then, by assumption, the eigenvalues of $F(\tau)$ lie in the intersection of Δ_{t_j} and Δ_{t_k} a.e. on $\gamma_{t_j} \cap \gamma_{t_k}$.

Therefore, $\Delta_{t_j} \cap \Delta_{t_k} \neq \emptyset$. Since neither of the disks Δ_{t_j} and Δ_{t_k} contains zero, then the interval connecting their centres z_j and z_k does not contain zero either. Consequently, zero does not belong to the interval l_{kj}.

Now we are going to show that the matrix function $G_0 = \psi F$ satisfies the condition (6.6). For this purpose, note that, if the eigenvalues of $F(t)$ lie in the disk Δ_{t_j}, then the eigenvalues of the matrix $z_j^{-1}F(t)$ lie in the disk Δ_0 with centre at the point 1 and radius $\delta = \sin \alpha/2$ $(\geq \sin \alpha_j/2)$. If the eigenvalues of $F(t)$ lie both in Δ_{t_j} and Δ_{t_k}, then we recognize that the eigenvalues of both the matrices $z_j^{-1}F(t)$ and $z_k^{-1}F(t)$ lie in Δ_0 and, therefore, also of all matrices of the form $\zeta F(t)$ with $\zeta \in l_{kj}$. Hence, the eigenvalues of the matrix $G_o(t)$ lie in Δ_o a.e. on Γ , and those of $I - G_o(t)$ in the disk $\{z:|z| \leq \delta\}$. Taking into account that $\delta < \delta_{p,n}(\Gamma)$ and the matrices $I - G_o(t)$ are normal together with $F(t)$, we find that condition (6.6) is fulfilled.

In view of statement 3) of Lemma 6.2, the matrix function G_o is Φ-factorable in L_r for all $r \in A_p$ and its partial indices are equal to zero. Applying now Lemma 6.3 with $\chi = \psi^{-1}$, we conclude that the matrix function F is also Φ-factorable in L_r , $r \in A_p$ and its partial indices are equal to each other and to the index of the function χ . Thus Theorem 6.10 is proved. ≡

<u>COROLLARY 6.4.</u> Let the matrix $U(t)$ be unitary a.e. on Γ . Furthermore, suppose that, for any point $t \in \Gamma$, we are able to indicate an arc γ_t $(\ni t)$ of the contour Γ and a sector S_t with vertex at the origin of apex angle $\alpha_t < 2 \arcsin \delta_{p,n}(\Gamma)$ such that all eigenvalues of the matrices $U(\tau)$ lie in S_t for almost all $\tau \in \gamma_t$. Then the interval A_p is entirely contained in some component of the domain of Φ-factorability of the matrix function U and all partial p-indices of U are equal to each other.

In fact, a unitary matrix is a normal matrix the eigenvalues of which have absolute value 1. Therefore, the fact that the eigenvalues of the matrices $U(\tau)$, $\tau \in \gamma_t$ lie in the sector S_t implies that they lie in the intersection l_t of this sector with the unit circle. It remains to note that the arc l_t may be included into a disk Δ_t inscribed in the sector S_t . After that, Theorem 6.10 will be applied. ≡

The normality condition occurring in Theorem 6.10 is very incisive. Thus, we try to find an analogue of these propositions related to matrix functions which do not necessarily take normal values. In looking for such an analogue, the following considerations are useful.

The eigenvalues of the normal matrix $G(t)$ belong to some disk if and only if the convex hull of the set of eigenvalues of $G(t)$ belongs to this disk. It is well-known that the convex hull of the set of eigenvalues of the normal matrix $A = (a_{ij})_{i,j=1}^n$ coincides with the set

$$H(A) = \{ \sum_{i,j=1}^{n} a_{ij}\xi_i\bar{\xi}_j : \sum_{j=1}^{n} |\xi_j|^2 = 1\} . \tag{6.10}$$

However, formula (6.10) continues to make sense for a matrix A not necessarily normal.

DEFINITION 6.2. The set $H(A)$ is called the numerical domain (or Hausdorff set) of the matrix A.

For any matrix A, $H(A)$ is a convex compact subset of the complex plane containing all eigenvalues of the matrix A (GLAZMAN, LYUBICH [1], MARCUS, MINC [1]).

It is quite natural to suspect that there exist sufficient conditions of Φ-factorability of the matrix function G and estimates for its partial indices formulated in terms of $H(G)$.

DEFINITION 6.3. By $d(A)$ we denote the smallest value of the real part of points from $H(A)$.

It is well-known (cf. MARCUS, MINC [1]) that $d(A)$ is the smallest eigenvalue of the Hermitian matrix $\operatorname{Re} A = \frac{1}{2}(A+A^*)$.

LEMMA 6.4. Assume the matrix function $G \in L_\infty$ to satisfy the condition

$$\operatorname*{ess\,inf}_{t\in\Gamma} d(G(t)) > \sqrt{1-\delta_{p,n}^2(\Gamma)}\ \|G\| . \tag{6.11}$$

Then $A_p \subseteq \Phi(G)$ and all partial r-indices of G are equal to zero for $r \in A_p$.

Proof. We shall show that the matrix function G differs from the matrix function G_0 satisfying inequality (6.6) only by a constant multiplier $\mu > 0$. For this purpose, using the equation $\|A\|^2 = \|AA^*\|$ and choosing the point $t \in \Gamma$ arbitrarily, we write $\|I-\mu G(t)\|^2 =$
$= \|(I-\mu G(t))(I-\mu G(t))^*\| = \|I+\mu^2 G(t)G(t)^* - 2\mu \operatorname{Re} G(t)\|$.
Inside the norm sign we have obtained a Hermitian non-negative matrix N the norm of which, as well-known, is the maximum of the quantity (Nx,x) taken over all vectors x of the unit sphere. Since $(Ix,x) = \|x\|^2 = 1$, $(\mu^2 G(t)G(t)^*x,x) = \mu^2\|G(t)^*x\|^2 \le \mu^2\|G(t)^*\|^2 = \mu^2\|G(t)\|^2$ and

$(-2\mu \operatorname{Re} G(t)x,x) = -2\mu(\operatorname{Re} G(t)x,x) \leq -2\mu d(G(t))$, we deduce $\|I-\mu G(t)\|^2 \leq 1 + \mu^2\|G(t)\|^2 - 2\mu d(G(t))$. Therefore, the inequality $\|I-\mu G(t)\|^2 \leq 1 + \mu^2\|G\|^2 - 2\mu \operatorname{ess\,inf}_{t\in\Gamma} d(G(t))$ holds a.e. on Γ . Choosing $\mu = \|G\|^{-2} \operatorname{ess\,inf}_{t\in\Gamma} d(G(t))$, we obtain that $\|I-\mu G(t)\|^2 \leq 1 - \|G\|^{-2} \operatorname{ess\,inf}_{t\in\Gamma} d(g(t))$ a.e. on Γ. Thus, due to condition (6.11), $\|I-\mu G\| < \delta_{p,n}(\Gamma)$. From this and assertion 3) of Lemma 6.2 we conclude the Φ-factorability in L_r , $r \in A_p$, of the matrix function μG . Moreover, we see that its partial r-indices are equal to zero. Clearly, the initial matrix function G is, together with μG , also Φ-factorable and the tuples of partial indices of these matrix functions coincide. ≡

Acting as in the proof of Theorem 6.10, from Lemma 6.4 one can get the following result.

THEOREM 6.11. Let the matrix function $G \in L_\infty$ be such that, for every point $t \in \Gamma$, there exist an arc γ_t ($\ni t$) and a straight line l_t whose distance from zero is greater than $\|G\| \sqrt{1-\delta^2_{p,n}(\Gamma)}$ and which has the property: for almost all $\tau \in \gamma_t$, the set $H(G(\tau))$ is separated from zero by the straight line l_t . Then the matrix function G is Φ-factorable in L_r for $r \in A_p$ and all its partial indices coincide.

Supposing, in addition, that the contour Γ satisfies the Lyapunov condition, we are able to strengthen Lemma 6.4. To this end, we need the following result related to factorization of positive functions.

LEMMA 6.5. Let α be a function given on the Lyapunov contour Γ which takes only non-negative values and for which $\alpha^{\pm 1} \in L_\infty$. Then there exists a representation $\alpha = \alpha_+\alpha_-$ with $\alpha_+^{\pm 1} \in L_\infty^+$, $\alpha_-^{\pm 1} \in L_\infty^-$.

Proof. We set $\alpha_+ = \exp(P \ln \alpha)$, $\alpha_- = \exp(Q \ln \alpha)$. Evidently, $\alpha = \alpha_+\alpha_-$ and the function α_+ (α_- , respectively) is analytic and non-degenerate in $\mathcal{D}^+$ ($\mathcal{D}^-$) . Also, $|\alpha_+^{\pm 1}(z)| = \exp(\pm \operatorname{Re}(P \ln \alpha)(z))$. Furthermore, if we prove that $\operatorname{Re}(P \ln \alpha)$ is a function bounded in $\mathcal{D}^+$, then the inclusion $\alpha_+^{\pm 1} \in L_\infty^+$ will be proved.

We have

$$(P \ln \alpha)(z) = \frac{1}{2\pi i} \int_\Gamma \ln \alpha(\tau) \frac{d\tau}{\tau - z} ,$$

so that

$$|\mathrm{Re}(P \ln \alpha)(z)| = \left|\frac{1}{2\pi} \int_\Gamma \ln \alpha(\tau) \,\mathrm{Im} \frac{d\tau}{\tau-z}\right| \leq \frac{M}{2\pi} \int_\Gamma \left|\mathrm{Im} \frac{d\tau}{\tau-z}\right|,$$

where $M = \operatorname{ess\,sup}_{t\in\Gamma} |\ln \alpha(\tau)|$ ($< \infty$, because $\alpha^{\pm 1} \in L_\infty$) . In this way, the crucial fact to be verified is the finiteness of $\sup_{z\in \mathfrak{D}^+} \int_\Gamma |\mathrm{Im} \frac{d\tau}{\tau-z}|$. Obviously, it is sufficient to conduct the proof for a connected contour. By ω we denote a function realizing a conformal mapping of the open unit disk onto the domain $\mathfrak{D}^+$. Setting $\tau = \omega(e^{i\theta})$, $z = \omega(\zeta)$, we obtain

$$\left|\int_\Gamma \mathrm{Im} \frac{d\tau}{\tau-z}\right| = \int_{\mathbf{T}} \left|\mathrm{Im} \frac{\omega'(e^{i\theta})de^{i\theta}}{\omega(e^{i\theta})-\omega(\zeta)}\right| = \int_{-\pi}^{\pi} \left|\mathrm{Re} \frac{\omega'(e^{i\theta})e^{i\theta}}{\omega(e^{i\theta})-\omega(\zeta)}\right| d\theta$$

$$\leq \int_{-\pi}^{\pi} \left|\frac{\omega'(e^{i\theta})}{\omega(e^{i\theta})-\omega(\zeta)} - \frac{e^{i\theta}}{e^{i\theta}-\zeta}\right| d\theta + \int_{-\pi}^{\pi} \left|\mathrm{Re} \frac{e^{i\theta}}{e^{i\theta}-\zeta}\right| d\theta .$$

Since the contour Γ is Lyapunov, the function ω' satisfies a Hölder condition (GOLUZIN [1]). Thus, the kernel of the first integral obtained is weakly polar (see e.g. LITVINCHUK [3], p.35). From this we deduce the boundedness of this integral by a certain quantity not depending on ζ. The second integral is an integral with Poisson kernel and therefore equal to 2π . Consequently, we have proved the boundedness of the function $\mathrm{Re}(P \ln \alpha)$ and, thus, also the condition $\alpha_+^{\pm 1} \in L_\infty^+$. The inclusion $\alpha_-^{\pm 1} \in L_\infty^-$ can be verified in a similar way. ≡

<u>LEMMA 6.4'.</u> Assume that Γ is a Lyapunov contour. If, for some $\varepsilon > 0$, the matrix function $G_0 \in L_\infty$ satisfies the inequality

$$d(G_0(t)) \geq \sqrt{1-\delta^2_{p,n}(\Gamma)}\, \|G_0(t)\| + \varepsilon \qquad (6.11')$$

a.e. on Γ , then G_0 is Φ-factorable in L_r $(r \in A_p)$ and all its partial r-indices are equal to zero.

<u>Proof.</u> The inequality (6.11') means, in particular, that $d(G_0(t)) \geq \varepsilon$ a.e. on Γ . Consequently, $\|G_0(t)^{-1}\| \leq \varepsilon^{-1}$ a.e. on Γ [1)], so that

$G_0^{-1} \in L_\infty$. Since $\|G_0(t)\|^{-1} \leq \|G_0(t)^{-1}\|$, then the function $\alpha(t) = \|G_0(t)\|^{-1}$ meets the assumptions of Lemma 6.5. Therefore, the matrix functions G_0 and αG_0 are Φ-factorable only simultaneously and the tuples of their partial indices coincide.

Multiplying inequality (6.11') termwise by $\alpha(t)$, we get $d(G(t)) \geq \sqrt{1-\delta^2_{p,n}(\Gamma)}\,\|G\| + \varepsilon\|G_0\|^{-1}$, so that G fulfils the assumptions of Lemma 6.4. Now the assertion to be proved follows immediately. ≡

Lemma 6.4' enables us to strengthen Theorem 6.11 in the following manner:

<u>THEOREM 6.11'.</u> Let the contour Γ be Lyapunov, and assume the matrix function G to belong to L_∞. Moreover, let, for all $t \in \Gamma$, exist an arc γ_t ($\ni t$) of the contour Γ and a straight line l_t with distance to zero greater than $\sqrt{1-\delta^2_{p,n}(\Gamma)}$ such that, for almost all $\tau \in \gamma_t$, the set $\|G(\tau)\|^{-1}H(G(\tau))$ is separated from zero by the straight line l_t. Then G is Φ-factorable in L_r for $r \in A_p$ and all its partial indices are equal to each other.

Finally, note that the conditions of all the theorems in the present section are insensitive to transposition of the matrix function under study. Consequently, a matrix function satisfying these theorems is Φ-factorable not anly from the left but also from the right. Furthermore, its right partial indices coincide with the left ones (and are also equal to each other).

6.5. ON PARTIAL INDICES OF MATRIX FUNCTIONS OF CLASSES $L_\infty^{\pm} + C$

The results obtained in Sections 6.3 and 6.4 provided information both about the existence of a Φ-factorization and about the values of the partial indices. In case when the matrix function G belongs to one of the classes considered in Chapter 5, the question of existence of a

---

[1] Here we used the fact from matrix theory that, if $d(A) > 0$, then $\|A^{-1}\| \leq d(A)^{-1}$. It is a straightforward matter to prove this: on the one hand, $|(Ax,x)| \geq \mathrm{Re}(Ax,x) \geq d(A)\|x\|^2$, on the other hand, $|(Ax,x)| \leq \|Ax\|\cdot\|x\|$, which implies $\|Ax\| \geq d(A)\|x\|$. Hence A is invertible and $\|A^{-1}\| \leq d(A)^{-1}$.

Φ-factorization is already well understood. This allows for making more precise the results on the values of partial indices.

First of all, suppose that $G \in L_\infty^+ + C$ $(L_\infty^- + C)$. According to Theorem 5.2, from the Φ-factorability of such a matrix function in some L_p we deduce the Φ-factorability in all L_p, $1 < p < \infty$, moreover, with the same tuple of partial indices. Hence, in the formulations of Theorems 6.6 - 6.11' and Lemmas 6.4, 6.4' we may replace $\delta_{p,n}(\Gamma)$ by its maximal value $\delta_{2,n}(\Gamma)$, which will be denoted by $\delta_n(\Gamma)$, and claim the existence of a Φ-factorization with non-negative (non-positive, coinciding, etc.) partial indices irrespective of the parameter value p. In addition, Theorems 6.6 - 6.9 can be simplified as follows: if $G \in L_\infty^+ + C$, then in assertion 2) of Theorems 6.6 and 6.9 the requirement $X_+^{-1} \in M_\infty^+$ can be omitted, and in Theorems 6.7 and 6.8 - the demand that $X_2^{-1} \in M_\infty^+$. If $G \in L_\infty^- + C$, then in assertion 1) of Theorems 6.6 and 6.9 we may cancel the requirement $X_-^{-1} \in M_\infty^-$, but in Theorems 6.7 and 6.8 - the demand $Y_1^{-1} \in M_\infty^-$.

Now we are going to state the exact formulation and to conduct the proof of the restated assertion 1) of Theorem 6.6 in the case $G \in L_\infty^- + C$. The other variants can be considered analogously, which is left to the interested reader.

<u>THEOREM 6.12.</u> Suppose that $G \in L_\infty^- + C$, $X_+ \in M_\infty^+$, $X_- \in L_\infty^-$ satisfy the conditions: 1) $\|I - X_+GX_-\| < \delta_n(\Gamma)$, 2) $X_+^{-1} \in L_\infty^+$.
Then (i) $X_-^{-1} \in M_\infty^-$, (ii) the matrix function G admits a Φ-factorization in all spaces L_p $(1 < p < \infty)$ with a non-negative tuple of partial indices.

<u>Proof.</u> The relation $X_- \in L_\infty^-$ implies that $PX_-Q = 0$. Moreover, the operator PGQ is compact by Lemma 5.1. Consequently,

$$P + X_+GX_-Q = (P+X_+Q)(P+GQ)(P+X_-G) + T, \qquad (6.12)$$

where T is compact.
From condition 1) of the theorem we conclude the invertibility of the operator $P+X_+GX_-Q$ in the space L_2^n, and from condition 2) and Theorem 5.2 we get the Fredholmness of the operator $P+X_+Q$ (in all spaces L_p^n).

Therefore, equation (6.12) and Theorem 1.9 imply the Fredholmness of the product $(P+GQ)(P+X_-Q)$ in the space L_2^n. In turn, from the Fredholmness of this product and the same Theorem 1.9 there follows that $P+GQ$ is a Φ_--operator.

Due to Corollary 5.1, if $P+GQ$ is a Φ_--operator and $G \in L_\infty^- + C$, then the operator $P+GQ$ is Fredholm. In this case the second factor $P+X_-Q$ of the product $(P+GQ)(P+X_-Q)$ will also be Fredholm. Since $X_- \in L_\infty^-$, then, in virtue of Theorem 3.15', we may conclude that $X_-^{-1} \in M_\infty^-$. In this way, assertion (i) has been proved. As soon as this condition is fulfilled, we can apply assertion 1) of Theorem 6.6, according to which the partial 2-indices of the matrix function G are non-negative (the Φ-factorability of this matrix function in L_2 results from the Fredholmness of the operator $P+GQ$ just proved). The result obtained can be transferred to all parameter values p, as was mentioned at the beginning of the section. $\equiv$

If the considered matrix function G is continuous, then we can apply the strengthenings of Theorems 6.6 - 6.11 for the case $G \in L_\infty^+ + C$ as well as for the case $G \in L_\infty^- + C$ mentioned at the beginning of the section. In the case of a continuous matrix function G, a particularly clear form can be given to Theorem 6.11.

<u>DEFINITION 6.3.</u> By $h(A)$ we denote the distance from the numerical domain of matrix A to zero. The matrix A will be called strictly non-degenerate, if $h(A) > 0$, i.e. if $H(A)$ does not contain zero.

This definition is justified by the fact that a strictly non-degenerate matrix is clearly non-degenerate.

<u>THEOREM 6.13.</u> If the matrix function G is continuous and, for all $t \in \Gamma$,

$$h(G(t)) > \sqrt{1-\delta_n^2(\Gamma)}\ \|G(t)\| , \tag{6.13}$$

then all the partial indices of G are equal to each other.

<u>Proof.</u> The continuity of G implies the continuity of the function $\alpha(t) = \|G(t)\|$. In accordance with inequality (6.13) this function does not vanish.

From relation (6.13) we deduce an analogous relation for the matrix function $F = \alpha^{-1}G$. In addition, for all $t \in \Gamma$, we have $\|F(t)\| = 1$. Consequently, for all $t \in \Gamma$,

$$h(F(t)) > \sqrt{1-\delta_n^2(\Gamma)}\, \|F\| . \tag{6.14}$$

The closed convex set $H(F(t))$ contains a unique point nearest to zero, which we denote by $z(t)$. Due to inequality (6.14), $z(t) \neq 0$. Let l_t be the straight line passing through the point $\frac{1}{2}(h(F(t)) + \sqrt{1-\delta_n^2(\Gamma)}\,\|F\|)z(t)$ and orthogonal to the radius vector of this point. Utilizing inequality (6.14) again, we find that l_t has a distance to zero greater than $\sqrt{1-\delta_n^2(\Gamma)}\,\|F\|$ and separates the set $H(F(t))$ from zero. Since the matrix functions F and G are continuous, the straight line l_t separates from zero all sets $H(F(\tau))$, where τ is sufficiently close to t.

Summarizing, for the matrix function F, the assumptions of Theorem 6.11 are fulfilled (for $p = 2$). In view of this theorem, the partial indices of F are equal to each other. Applying Lemma 6.3 for $\chi = \alpha^{-1}$, we observe that the partial indices of G are also equal to each other, which proves Theorem 6.13. ≡

For the total index of a continuous matrix function, Muskhelishvili's formula is true. Therefore, it is not hard to evaluate the partial indices of a matrix function G which meets the assumptions of Theorem 6.13: each of them is equal to $\frac{1}{2\pi n}\{\arg \det G(t)\}_\Gamma$ (thus, the value $\frac{1}{2\pi}\{\arg \det G(t)\}_\Gamma$ automatically proves to be divisible by n). Notice, however, that in the suppositions of Theorem 6.13 the values of the partial indices of G are closely connected with the behaviour of its numerical domain. To illuminate this connection, we first remark that the index of a function ψ continuous on Γ is uniquely defined by the condition

$$\psi(t) \in H(G(t)) . \tag{6.15}$$

In fact, if ψ_0 is any other function continuous on Γ and satisfying this condition, then, for every $\lambda \in [0,1]$, the function $\psi_\lambda(t) = \lambda\psi(t) + (1-\lambda)\psi_0(t)$ is continuous and fulfils condition (6.15), therefore, it does not vanish on Γ. The mapping $\lambda \to \psi_\lambda$ maps the interval $[0,1]$ continuously into the functional space $C(\Gamma)$. Consequently, the indices of all functions ψ_λ coincide. Especially, the indices of ψ_0 and $\psi_1 = \psi$ are the same.

It is quite natural to call the common value of the indices of all functions ψ continuous on Γ and satisfying condition (6.15) the winding number of the numerical domain around zero. The partial indices of G coincide with precisely this number as soon as Theorem 6.13 applies. Indeed, the function ψ may be chosen in such a way that the matrix function $\psi^{-1}(t)\|G(t)\|^{-1}$ satisfies the hypothesis of Lemma 6.4 (it suffices to set, e.g., $\psi(t) = z(t)$). But then the partial indices of F are equal to zero, and, as follows from Lemma 6.3, the partial indices of G coincide with the index of the function ψ, i.e., with the winding number of rotations of the numerical domain around zero.

Clearly, the remark made at the end of the previous section can be applied to Theorem 6.13 in full. Thus, not only the left but also the right indices of an arbitrary matrix function G satisfying the conditions of this theorem coincide with the winding number of the numerical domain around zero.

6.6. ON THE STABILITY OF THE FACTORIZATION FACTORS $G_\pm$

Up to now, the question of stability of the factors $G_\pm$ from the Φ-factorization (2.1) of the matrix function G in L_p has not been studied in full detail. Hence, we restrict ourselves to the explanation of results associated with the factorization problem in a (C,R)-algebra $\mathfrak{A}$. Following the agreement at the beginning of the chapter, instead of "factorization in $\mathfrak{A}$" we shall simply write "factorization", under "norm" we shall understand the norm in $\mathfrak{A}$, etc.

Closeness of the factorization factors $G_\pm$ of the matrix function G and $F_\pm$ of the matrix function

$$F(t) = F_+(t)\Lambda_1(t)F_-(t) \tag{6.16}$$

is characterized by the quantities

$$\|G_+-F_+\|,\ \|G_--F_-\|,\ \|G_+^{-1}-F_+^{-1}\|,\ \|G_-^{-1}-F_-^{-1}\|. \tag{6.17}$$

THEOREM 6.14. Let G be a certain matrix function admitting a factorization (2.1). Then there exists a $\delta > 0$ such that, if $\|G-F\| < \delta$, (6.16) is a factorization of the matrix function F and at least one of the values (6.17) is smaller than δ, then $\Lambda_1 = \Lambda$.

Proof. For the sake of definiteness, let $\|G-F\| < \delta$ and $\|G_-^{-1}-F_-^{-1}\| < \delta$. Since $G_+\Lambda - F_+\Lambda_1 = GG_-^{-1} - FF_-^{-1} = G(G_-^{-1}-F_-^{-1}) + (G-F)F_-^{-1}$, then

$$\begin{aligned}\|G_+\Lambda - F_+\Lambda_1\| &\leq \|G\|\|G_-^{-1}-F_-^{-1}\| + \|G-F\|\|F_-^{-1}\| \\ &\leq \delta(\|G\| + \|F_-^{-1}\|) \\ &\leq \delta(\|G\| + \|G_-^{-1}-F_-^{-1}\| + \|G_-^{-1}\|) \\ &\leq \delta(\|G\| + \|G_-^{-1}\| + \delta)\end{aligned}$$

so that the difference of corresponding columns of the matrix functions $G_+\Lambda$ and $F_+\Lambda_1$ can be made arbitrarily small, if δ is chosen in a suitable manner.

Consequently, if we choose δ small enough, then the norm of the vector function $g_j - f_j t^{\varkappa_j^{(1)}-\varkappa_j}$ can also be made arbitrarily small, where g_j and f_j, $j=1,\dots,n$ are the j th columns of the matrix functions G_+ and F_+, respectively. Assume that, for some j, $\varkappa_j^{(1)} > \varkappa_j$. Then $g_j(0) = \frac{1}{2\pi i}\int_\Gamma (g_j(\tau) - f_j(\tau)\tau^{\varkappa_j^{(1)}-\varkappa_j})\,\tau^{-1}d\tau$. Letting $\delta \to 0$, the right-hand side becomes arbitrarily small and the left one does not depend on δ. Consequently, $g_j(0) = 0$, which is impossible, as the matrix function G_+ is non-degenerate in $\mathfrak{D}^+$. The contradiction obtained shows that, for sufficiently small δ, $\varkappa_j^{(1)} \leq \varkappa_j$, $j=1,\dots,n$. Since, for δ small enough, the total indices of G and F agree, we conclude that $\varkappa_j^{(1)} = \varkappa_j$, $j=1,\dots,n$, which proves Theorem 6.14. ≡

In this way, for close matrix functions with different tuples of partial indices, the factorization factors $G_\pm$ cannot be too close. It turns out that the converse statement, the formulation of which must somewhat be strengthened because of the lack of uniqueness of the factors $G_\pm$, is also true.

THEOREM 6.15. Let G be a factorable matrix function. For any $\varepsilon > 0$, we can specify a $\delta > 0$ such that, if $\|F-G\| < \delta$ and the partial indices of the matrix function F coincide with the partial indices of the matrix function G, then, for every factorization of G, there can be found a factorization of F for which any of the values in (6.17) are smaller than ε.

In order to prove this theorem, first of all remark that $\|F_+-G_+\| = \|F(F_-^{-1}-G_-^{-1})\Lambda^{-1} + (F-G)G_-^{-1}\Lambda^{-1}\| \leq (\|F\|\|F_-^{-1}-G_-^{-1}\|+\|G_-^{-1}\|\|F-G\|)\|\Lambda^{-1}\|$. Thus, it can be guaranteed that the quantity $\|F_+-G_+\|$ is small as soon as $\|F-G\|$ and $\|F_-^{-1}-G_-^{-1}\|$ are small. Since in every Banach algebra the operation of taking the inverse element is continuous for fixed G, $\|F_+^{-1}-G_+^{-1}\|$ will be small, if $\|F_+-G_+\|$ is small. Analogously, the smallness of $\|F_--G_-\|$ results form the smallness of $\|F_-^{-1}-G_-^{-1}\|$.

In summary, it suffices to prove a simplified form of Theorem 6.15 in which it is only stated that $\|G_-^{-1}-F_-^{-1}\| < \varepsilon$. We shall show that the columns of the matrix function G_-^{-1} may be interpreted as vectors from the kernel of an operator of the form $P+Qt^{-k}G$. The Fredholmness of such operators results from the following proposition.

<u>LEMMA 6.6.</u> The kernels of the operators $P+GQ$ and $T_Q(G)$ have equal dimensions and the images are closed only simultaneously and have equal codimensions.

Lemma 6.6 is close to assertion 1) of Lemma 3.5 with respect to its formulation and way of proving. Thus, its proof is omitted here. We only wish to explain that $\ker(P+GQ) = 0 \dotplus \ker T_Q(G)$, i.e., $x \in \ker(P+GQ)$ if and only if x^+ $(= Px) = 0$ and $x^- \in \ker T_Q(G)$.

<u>LEMMA 6.7.</u> Let G be a factorable matrix function the partial indices of which are $\varkappa_1 \geq \dots \geq \varkappa_n$. Then

1) the j th column of the matrix function G_-^{-1} is a solution of the equation

$$(Pt^{-1} + Qt^{-\varkappa_j}G)x = 0 \, ; \tag{6.18}$$

2) if X is a matrix function which is non-degenerate at least at one point of Γ and the j th column of which solves the equation (6.18), then X^{-1} may play the role of a right factor in some factorization of G.

Proof. Relation (6.18) is equivalent to both equations $Pt^{-1}x = 0$ and $Qt^{-\varkappa_j}Gx = 0$. The first of the latter two equations means that $t^{-1}x \in (\mathring{R}^-)^n$ or, what is the same, $x \in (R^-)^n$; the second amounts to saying that $t^{-\varkappa_j}Gx \in (R^+)^n$. If we take $x = x_j$, where x_j is the j th column of the matrix function G_-^{-1}, then obviously $x_j \in (R^-)^n$. Moreover, $t^{-\varkappa_j}Gx_j = t^{-\varkappa_j}G_+\Lambda G_-x_j$ is the j th column of the matrix function G_+. Thus, assertion 1) has been proved. Now we proceed to the proof of 2). If the vector function x_j is the solution of equation (6.18), then, as mentioned above, $x_j \in (R^-)^n$ and $t^{-\varkappa_j}G_+\Lambda G_-x_j \in (R^+)^n$, therefore, we deduce that $G_-x_j \in (R^-)^n$ and $t^{-\varkappa_j}\Lambda G_-x_j \in (R^+)^n$. Hence, for the regarded matrix function X, we have $G_-X \in R^-$, $H = \Lambda G_-X\Lambda^{-1} \in R^+$. From this we obtain (compare with the considerations in Section 2.2) that the matrix function H is block-lower triangular, its (i,j) th element is equal to zero for $\varkappa_i < \varkappa_j$, constant for $\varkappa_i = \varkappa_j$, and a polynomial of degree not higher than $\varkappa_i - \varkappa_j$, if $\varkappa_i > \varkappa_j$. In particular, $\det H$ is constant. Since $\det H = \det G_- \cdot \det X$, then $\det G_-$ is different from zero everywhere on Γ, and because $\det X$ is non-zero at least at one point of Γ, then H is non-degenerate. Thus, H satisfies the condition 2) of Theorem 2.2. According to this theorem, setting $\hat{G}_+ = G_+H$, $\hat{G}_- = X^{-1} = \Lambda^{-1}H^{-1}\Lambda G_-$, we get the factorization $\hat{G}_+\Lambda\hat{G}_-$ of the matrix function G, which proves Lemma 6.7. ≡

A similar result holds for the left factorization factor, too.

Now we are able to prove Theorem 6.15.

Proof of Theorem 6.15. Due to Lemma 6.7, the j th column x_j of the matrix function G_-^{-1} is a solution of equation (6.18), i.e., it belongs to the kernel of the operator $A = Pt^{-1}+Qt^{-\varkappa_j}G = (P+Qt^{1-\varkappa_j}G)t^{-1}$. Besides of A we consider the operator $B = (P+Qt^{1-\varkappa_j}F)t^{-1}$, where F is a matrix function with the same tuple of partial indices as G. Since the operator of multiplication by t^{-1} is invertible, the operator A is Fredholm simultaneously with $P+Qt^{1-\varkappa_j}G$ and has the same defect numbers. In virtue of Lemma 6.6 the dimension of the kernel of the operator $P-Qt^{1-\varkappa_j}G$ $(P+Qt^{1-\varkappa_j}F)$ is equal to the sum of positive partial indices of $t^{1-\varkappa_j}G$ ($t^{1-\varkappa_j}F$) . Consequently, the dimensions of the kernels of the operators $P+Qt^{1-\varkappa_j}G$ and $P+Qt^{1-\varkappa_j}F$ (and, together with them, also of the operators A and B) are equal. Due to a theorem from GOHBERG, KRUPNIK [4], p. 170, for any vector x from $\ker A$ there exists a vector $y \in \ker B$ such that $\|x-y\| < c\,\|A-B\|$, where the constant c is determined only by the operator A . Since $\|A-B\| \leq \|Q\|\cdot\|t^{1-\varkappa_j}\|\cdot\|G-F\|$, for any $\varepsilon_j > 0$, one can find a $\delta_j > 0$ such that, for $\|G-F\| < \delta_j$, there exists a vector $y_j \in \ker B$ with $\|y_j-x_j\| < \varepsilon_j$. Now we form the matrix function $Y = (y_1 \ldots y_n)$. Since the matrix function $(x_1 \ldots x_n)$ $(=G_-^{-1})$ is non-singular, for sufficiently small ε_j , the matrix Y will also be non-singular at least at one point of Γ . Owing to assertion 2) of Lemma 6.7, there exists a factorization of the matrix function F such that $F_- = Y^{-1}$. Clearly, for given $\varepsilon > 0$, one can choose ε_j , $j=1,\ldots,n$ such that the inequalities $\|y_j-x_j\| < \varepsilon_j$ $(j=1,\ldots,n)$ imply $\|X-Y\| < \varepsilon$, i.e., $\|F_-^{-1}-G_-^{-1}\| < \varepsilon$.

In order to finish the proof of the simplified form of Theorem 6.15, it remains only to set $\delta = \min\{\delta_j : j=1,\ldots,n\}$. At the same time. we have proved Theorem 6.15 in full. ≡

COROLLARY 6.5. Assume the matrix function G to be factorable and the tuple of its partial indices to be stable. Then, for every $\varepsilon > 0$, there exists a $\delta > 0$ such that, for $\|F-G\| < \delta$, the matrix function F admits a factorization in which each of the quantities (6.17) is less then ε .

In fact, if the tuple of partial indices of the matrix function G is stable, then, for $\delta > 0$ small enough, the condition $\|F-G\| < \delta$ implies the coincidence of the tuples of partial indices of F and G. Thus, Theorem 6.15 can be applied. ≡

In brief, the latter result can be formulated in the following way: If the middle factorization factor Λ is stable, then the factors $G_\pm$ are also stable.

Now we intend to formulate Theorem 6.15 in terms of sequences.

THEOREM 6.15'. Let $\{G^{(k)}\}_{k=1}^{\infty}$ be a sequence of matrix functions admitting a factorization with one and the same tuple of partial indices and converging to the matrix function G which is also assumed to be factorable and to have the same tuple of partial indices. Then one may choose factorizations $G^{(k)} = G_+^{(k)} \Lambda G_-^{(k)}$ in such a manner that $G_{\pm}^{(k)} \to G_{\pm}$, $(G_{\pm}^{(k)})^{-1} \to G_{\pm}^{-1}$ (in the norm (5.8), where $G_{\pm}$ are factorization factors of G.

COROLLARY 6.5'. Let $\{G^{(k)}\}_{k=1}^{\infty}$ be a sequence of matrix functions which converge to the factorable matrix function G with a stable tuple of partial indices. Then, beginning with some element of the sequence, the conclusion of Corollary 6.5 is valid.

For a factorable matrix function all partial indices of which are equal to each other, Corollary 6.5 can be made more precise. This refinement amounts for stating that the closeness of the factorization factors of close matrix functions F and G may be ensured by the requirement $G_-(\infty) = F_-(\infty)$.

Up to now, in the present chapter we have been concerned with the following problem: knowing the properties of a given matrix function, determine the properties of matrix functions sufficiently close to it. Now we turn to the "inverse" problem consisting in the determination of the factorization properties for the limit of a sequence of matrix functions, if we know the factorization properties of the terms of this sequence.

Theorem 6.5 shows that any factorable matrix function G with the tuple of partial indices $(\varkappa_j)_{j=1}^{n}$ may be represented as the limit of a sequence $\{G^{(k)}\}_{k=1}^{\infty}$ of factorable matrix functions the tuples of partial indices $(\varkappa_j^{(k)})_{j=1}^{n}$ of which obey the condition $(\varkappa_j) \succ (\varkappa_j^{(k)})$, but, in other respect, they are not interconnected or joined with the tuple $(\varkappa_j)$. Vice versa, if the sequence of factorable matrix functions $\{G^{(k)}\}_{k=1}^{\infty}$ converges to the factorable matrix function G, then, according to Theorem 6.4, for sufficiently large k, the condition $(\varkappa_j)_{j=1}^{n} \succ (\varkappa_j^{(k)})_{j=1}^{n}$ is fulfilled. Finally, the limit of a sequence of factorable matrix functions may not permit any factorization at all.

However, we are able to indicate conditions under which the passage to the limit does not go beyond the class of factorable matrix functions and does not influence on the values of partial indices.

THEOREM 6.16. Let $\{G^{(k)}\}_{k=1}^{\infty}$ be a sequence of factorable matrix functions converging to the matrix function G. Then the following assertions are equivalent:

1) the factorization factors of the matrix functions $G^{(k)}$ may be chosen in such a way that $\|(G_{\pm}^{(k)})^{-1}\| \leq M$, where the constant $M < \infty$ does not depend on k;

2) the matrix function G can be factored and all matrix functions $G^{(k)}$, beginning with some number k, have one and the same tuple of partial indices which agrees with that of the matrix function G.

Proof. Suppose that 2) is fulfilled. Due to Theorem 6.15', the factorizations of $G^{(k)}$ can be chosen in such a fashion that the sequences $\{(G_+^{(k)})^{-1}\}$ and $\{(G_-^{(k)})^{-1}\}$ converge (to G_+^{-1} and G_-^{-1}, respectively). In this case these sequences will be bounded either. Thus, 1) follows from 2).

Conversely, let 1) be valid. As it was mentioned in the proof of Theorem 5.6, the operator $(G_-^{(k)})^{-1}\Lambda_k^{-1}Q(G_+^{(k)})^{-1}$ considered in $(\mathring{R}^-)^n$ is a regularizer for $T_Q(G^{(k)})$. Hence, there exists an equibounded sequence of regularizers of the operators $T_Q(G^{(k)})$. In accordance with Theorem 1.11 this means that the limit of the sequence $T_Q(G^{(k)})$, i.e., the operator $T_Q(G)$, is also Fredholm. The Fredholmness of the operator $T_P(G')$ can be shown in a similar way. With regard to Theorem 5.6, the matrix function G can be factored. Its tuple of partial indices will be denoted by $(\varkappa_j)_{j=1}^n$. In virtue of Theorem 6.4, in a certain neighbourhood of G we encounter only such matrix functions whose tuples of partial indices $(\varkappa_j')$ fulfil the condition $(\varkappa_j) \succ (\varkappa_j')$. Since there exists only a finite number of such tuples, one of the following two situations always applies: a) there is a neighbourhood of G such that all matrix functions $G^{(k)}$ contained in it have one and the same tuple of partial indices $(\varkappa_j)$; b) it is possible to choose a sequence $\{G^{(k_s)}\}_{s=1}^{\infty}$ all terms of which have one and the same tuple of partial indices $(\hat{\varkappa}_j)$, where $(\hat{\varkappa}_j) \neq (\varkappa_j)$.

Assume that situation b) applies. As the sequence $G^{(k_s)} = G_+^{(k_s)} \hat{\Lambda} G_-^{(k_s)}$ converges to G and $\| \hat{\Lambda} - (G_+^{(k_s)})^{-1} \Lambda (G_-^{(k_s)})^{-1} \| =$ $= \| (G_+^{(k_s)})^{-1} (G^{(k_s)} - G)(G_-^{(k_s)})^{-1} \| \leq M^2 \| G^{(k_s)} - G \|$, then the sequence $F_s = (G_+^{(k_s)})^{-1} \Lambda (G_-^{(k_s)})^{-1}$ converges to $\hat{\Lambda}$. Consequently, in any neighbourhood of the matrix function $\hat{\Lambda}$ there exists a matrix function the tuple of partial indices of which is just the same as that of the matrix function G . According to Theorem 6.4, $(\hat{\varkappa}_j) \succ (\varkappa_j)$, and this is a contradiction to the conditions $(\varkappa_j) \succ (\hat{\varkappa}_j)$ and $(\varkappa_j) \neq (\hat{\varkappa}_j)$.

Summarizing, situation a) holds by all means, i.e., assertion 2) is true. The proof of Theorem 6.16 is complete. ≡

6.7. COMMENTS

The question of stability of partial indices was first considered in MANDZHAVIDZE [2] in connection with the problem of the approximate solution of the Riemann boundary value problem. Theorems 6.1 and 6.2 as well as the criterion of stability of partial indices (Theorem 6.3) were obtained by GOHBERG and KREĬN [2,3] and BOJARSKI [1]. The proof of Theorems 6.1 and 6.2 conducted here is close to the one suggested in MANDZHAVIDZE [5]. The same applies to the proof of the sufficiency in Theorem 6.3. The proof of the necessity in Theorem 6.3 given above generalizes correspondent arguments from BOJARSKI [1], GOHBERG, KREĬN [3] to the case of matrix functions with unbounded factorization factors. In Section 10.2 of the book CLANCEY, GOHBERG [3] another way of proving the necessity is explained, which is based on the following general result of WIDOM [3] related to perturbations of Fredholm operators: Let T be a Fredholm operator in the Banach space X , and let S be a subspace of $[X]$ such that, for every non-zero $x \in X$, $f \in X^*$, there exists an $A \in S$ such that $f(Ax) \neq 0$. Then there exist $B \in S$ and a number $r > 0$ such that, for any $\varepsilon \in (0,r)$, at least one of the defect numbers of the operator $T + \varepsilon B$ is equal to zero. The application of this result to the case $T = P+t^{-s}GQ$, $S = \{AP+BQ: A,B \in \in L_\infty\}$, where s is an integer strictly included between the smallest and largest partial index of the matrix function G , proves the necessity of condition (6.2) for the stability of partial indices.

Theorems 6.4 and 6.5 and Lemma 6.1 are due to GOHBERG and KREĬN [3]. The topological interpretation of Theorems 6.3 - 6.5 is given by the authors under the influence of BOJARSKI's paper [3].
Remark, incidentally, that in this paper there was proved the connectedness of the intersection of the sets $\Phi_\varkappa$ with the class of matrix functions continuous on Γ and of the sets $\Phi_{(\varkappa_j)}$ with the class of matrix functions continuous on Γ and factorable in $C(\Gamma)$. The connectedness of the intersection of $\Phi_\varkappa$ and the class of piecewise continuous matrix function was studied in GLEBOV, DEUNDYAK [1]. Furthermore, the question of connectedness of the sets $\Phi_\varkappa$ themselves as also of the density in L_∞ of the set Φ of all Φ-factorable matrix functions remains to be solved.

Theorems 6.6 - 6.13 are obtained by one of the authors (SPITKOVSKIĬ [2,3,5,10]). The idea of transition from the matrix function G_1 to its Cayley transform used in the proof of Lemma 6.2 is borrowed from KRUPNIK, NYAGA [1], where this device was applied to the study of unitary matrix functions.

In connection with Lemma 6.3, note that in the article of SPITKOVSKIĬ [9] one can find the description of the class $\mathfrak{M}$ consisting of all those functions the multiplication by which does not violate the Φ-factorability in L_p . It appeared that this class does not depend on p and, being multiplied by a function $\chi \in \mathfrak{M}$, the partial indices of an arbitrary Φ-factorable matrix function G behave precisely as in case of a continuous function χ , i.e., they are shifted by its index.

Lemma 6.4 is due to DANILYUK [4,5], its precising for the case of a Lyapunov contour (Lemma 6.4') was obtained by one of the authors (SPITKOVSKIĬ [2]). Lemma 6.5, with the help of which the latter lemma was derived, is well-known for a long time and was already used in SIMONENKO [4]. The proof of Lemma 6.5 is borrowed from the book GOHBERG, KRUPNIK [4].

In SHELEPOV [1] it was mentioned that, with regard to RADON's [1] results, Lemma 6.5 may be transferred to the case when Γ is a Radon curve without cusps. Therefore, Theorem 6.11' can also be transferred to this case. Concerning the considerations after Theorem 6.13 related to the values of the partial indices, let us still mention the following.

Generally speaking, starting from a matrix function G continuous on Γ, it is not always possible to construct a tuple of n functions $\lambda_j(t)$, $j=1,\dots,n$ continuous on Γ and coinciding, for all $t \in \Gamma$, with the tuple of its eigenvalues counted with regard to their algebraic multiplicity (as a matter of fact, in moving along the components of the contour Γ, the continuous branches of the solutions of the equation $\det(G(t)-\lambda I) = 0$ move into another, not necessarily coinciding with the original ones). But if we do succeed in doing so, then it makes sense to speak about indices of eigenvalues of the matrix funktion G.

In GAKHOV's review article [3] among others there was posed the problem of describing all those matrix functions the partial indices of which coincide with the indices of eigenvalues. The complete solution of this problem has not been found yet [1]. The relations $\lambda_j(t) \in H(G(t))$, however, imply that, under the conditions of Theorem 6.13, the indices of eigenvalues coincide with the winding number of the numerical domain of the matrix function G around zero and, thus, with the partial indices of G. In this way, matrix functions satisfying the conditions of Theorem 6.13 form a certain subclass of the desired set.

The application of Theorems 6.6 - 6.13 is impossible without the knowledge of lower estimates for the values $\delta_{p,n}(\Gamma)$. Assertion 1) of Lemma 6.2 allows for replacing the problem of finding such estimates by the problem of evaluating (or obtaining upper estimates for) the norms

[1] The problem of the description of all triangular matrix functions - whose partial indices coincide with the indices of the diagonal elements solved in Chapter 4 is a special case of this problem.

of operators Q and S. In case when the contour Γ is a circle, the norm of the operator S has been calculated in all spaces L_p^n, $1 < p < \infty$ (VERBITSKIǏ, KRUPNIK [1,2], KRUPNIK [4]). This fact will be used in the next chapter. With our definition of the norm in L_p^n (see Section 1.2) the norms of the operators S and Q, generally speaking, depend on n. However, for $p = 2$, such a dependence fails to exist. In SPITKOVSKIǏ [3] it was shown that the norms of the operators S and Q in L_2 are connected via the relation $\|Q\| = \frac{1}{2}(\|S\|+\|S\|^{-1})$. Therefore, the estimates for $\delta_{2,n}(\Gamma)$ mentioned in assertion 1) of Lemma 6.2 coincide. Unfortunately, we do not know whether these estimates are exact or not. It is also unknown, which of these estimates is the most exact one for $p \neq 2$ and a contour Γ different from the circle.

Theorem 6.15 (on the continuity of the factorization factors for fixed partial indices) is due to SHUBIN [1]. He has also proved there that, if the matrix function G is a k times continuously differentiable (analytic) function of some parameter ω and the partial indices do not depend on ω, then the factorization factors $G_{\pm}$ are also k times continuously differentiable (analytic) functions of ω. The factorization of matrix functions depending on a parameter was also examined by NIKOLENKO [1,2]. In NIKOLENKO [1] he derived the stability criterion for partial indices in case when the parameter ranges over even-dimensional spheres or triangulations. In this paper it was further shown that the triple $(T_+ \times T_-, p_{\bar{\varkappa}}, \mathcal{L}_{\bar{\varkappa}})$ forms a locally trivial fibre bundle, where $T_{\pm}$ is the class of $n\times n$ matrix functions non-singular and satisfying a Hölder condition in $\mathcal{D}^{\pm} \cup \Gamma$ and analytic in $\mathcal{D}^{\pm}$, $\mathcal{L}_{\bar{\varkappa}}$ is the class of Hölder continuous matrix functions with the tuple of partial indices $\bar{\varkappa}$ $(=(\varkappa_1,\dots,\varkappa_n))$, and $p_{\bar{\varkappa}}$ is the mapping from $T_+ \times T_-$ into $\mathcal{L}_{\bar{\varkappa}}$ acting according to formula $p_{\bar{\varkappa}}(F_+,F_-) = F_+\Lambda F_-$. In NIKOLENKO [2] it is shown that this fibre bundle is trivial if and only if $\varkappa_1 = \dots = \varkappa_n$.

Theorem 6.16 was first formulated in LITVINCHUK, NIKOLAǏCHUK, SPITKOVSKIǏ [1].

A series of papers is devoted to the approximate solution of singular integral equations (and, especially, to the vector-valued Riemann boundary value problem). A systematic explanation of the state of the arts (up to 1978) related to methods of their approximate solution the reader can find in the last chapter of the monograph PRÖSSDORF [1]. Concerning later results, see BABESHKO [3], DIDENKO [1-3], DIDENKO, TIKHONENKO [1,2], ZOLOTAREVSKIĬ [1], PRÖSSDORF, SCHMIDT [1], SILBERMANN [1].

In MEUNARGIYA [1,2] several cases are examined in which the solution of the vector-valued Riemann boundary value problem with matrix $G_0 + \lambda G_1$ may be found as a series $\sum_{k=0}^{\infty} \lambda^k F^{(k)}$, where $F_\lambda^{(k)}$ are successively determined as solutions of Riemann problems with matrix G_0 and a free term depending on $F^{(j)}$ $(j=0,\dots,k-1)$.

Now we focus our attention on another results associated with the stability problem and estimates of partial indices. KRAVCHENKO and NIKOLAĬCHUK [1] have obtained formulae for partial indices of second-order matrix functions such that at least one element of them does not degenerate on Γ. These formulae involve the dimension of the kernel of an integral operator which can be effectively constructed by a given matrix function.

CHORIEV [1-3] has studied the relationships between stability of partial indices of sufficiently smooth matrix functions G and the validity of Liouville's theorem for the equation

$$\bar{\partial} U = BU \ ,$$

where $B(z) = \mathcal{G}(z)^{-1}\bar{\partial}\mathcal{G}(z)$ for $z \in \mathcal{D}^+$, $B(z) = 0$ for $z \in \mathcal{D}^-$, and $\mathcal{G}$ is an extension of the matrix function GD^{-1} into the domain $\mathcal{D}^+$ differentiable in L_p $(p > 2)$ in the generalized sense.

Here $D(t) = \mathrm{diag}[t^{k+1},\dots,t^{k+1},t^k,\dots,t^k]$ is a matrix function annulling the total index of G.

In LAX [1] it was established that the property of the partial indices of a matrix function G given on the circle to be equal to zero is equivalent to the solvability of the Dirichlet problem for the differential equation $G_{z\bar{z}} = G_z G^{-1} G_{\bar{z}}$.

In the author's opinion, the problem of finding estimates for the partial indices and of obtaining effectively verifiable conditions of their stability or non-negativity is still far from being completely solved and any new result towards its solution is of considerable interest.

CHAPTER 7. FACTORIZATION ON THE CIRCLE

The results of this chapter may be divided into two groups, which are associated with each other in a natural way. The first of them is formed by problems of factorization and Φ-factorization on the circle $\mathbb{T}$ of Hermitian (in particular, of definite) and unitary matrix functions. The properties in which these matrix functions are peculiar enable for obtaining more complete and exact theorems on factorization. Some of these theorems are useful, especially, for the study of relationships between necessary and exact conditions of factorability, a problem, which was already stated in Chapters 2 and 3.

The second group represents essential strengthenings for the space $L_2(\mathbb{T})$ of a series of important results from the preceding chapter related to Φ-factorization with non-negative, non-positive, stable, in particular, with equal partial indices of arbitrary matrix functions from the classes L_∞, $L_\infty^{\pm} + C$ and C. This group of results is based on the utilization of exact estimates for the norms of the operators S, P, Q, PGQ, QGP, which hold in $L_2(\mathbb{T})$, but also on the application of results of the first group concerning Φ-factorization of matrix functions with the algebraic properties mentioned above.

In Section 7.1 a definition of factorization specific for the circle $\mathbb{T}$ will be introduced, from which we immediately shall obtain the connection between factorizations of the matrix function G in $L_p(\mathbb{T})$ and the matrix function G^* in $L_q(\mathbb{T})$, $q = p/(p-1)$, which is of some significance to what follows.

In Section 7.2 we shall be concerned with factorization and Φ-factorization of Hermitian matrix functions, where the structure of the factorability domain will be revealed, relations for partial indices will be derived and a necessary condition for the domain of factorability to be non-empty will be established. A representation for a Hermitian matrix function factorable in $L_2(\mathbb{T})$ the total index of which is equal to zero will be described. This representation enables us to estimate the number of zero partial indices of a given matrix function G with the aid of the absolute value of the signature of G.

Section 7.3 is dedicated to the factorization problem in L_2 of those Hermitian matrix functions for which the corresponding quadratic form preserves the sign. The main result of this section is a theorem which asserts that, for a positively definite matrix function G, the necessary condition $G^{\pm} \in L_1$ of its factorability is also sufficient. The proof of this theorem rests upon the claim on the existence of a representation of a positively definite matrix function G as the product of a certain outer matrix function A and its adjoint A^*. This proposition is of independent interest and significance for applications.

The aim of Section 7.4 consists in making more precise various results of 6.3 and 6.4. The most general result of this section is the theorem on the existence of a Φ-factorization in L_p with coinciding partial indices for those matrix functions the numerical domain of which may be locally (i.e., for any sufficiently small arc of the contour $\mathbb{T}$) included into a sector whose apex angle is less than $2\pi/\max(p,q)$. A special case of this theorem is provided by the assertion that every uniformly positively definite matrix function admits a Φ-factorization with zero partial indices. It appears that the factorization factors of such matrix functions are necessarily bounded. This assertion, which is of independent interest (cf. Theorem 5.2 from Section 5.1), allows for reducing in Section 7.5 the problem of Φ-factorability of an arbitrary matrix function $G \in L_\infty$ to the same problem for a certain unitary matrix function. Moreover, this assertion permits us with the help of this reduction to obtain criteria of Φ-factorability in L_2 with non-negative, non-positive and stable (in particular, zero) partial indices. These criteria are the conversions (and that even in a stronger form) of corresponding sufficient conditions from 6.3. Thus, for the problem of Φ-factorization in $L_2(\mathbb{T})$ they are also necessary. Note that for unitary matrix functions the criterion of existence of a Φ-factorization in L_2 with definite partial indices will be derived from the sophisticated result on the calculation of the norms of the Hankel operators PGQ and QGP, which has important applications beyond the factorization theory for matrix functions either.

Furthermore, we intend to specify the results of 7.4 and 7.5 for the case of a matrix function G which satisfies certain analytic conditions, mainly for the case of a continuous matrix function G. This topic is pursued in Section 7.6. Here, in particular, it is established that the partial indices of a continuous strictly non-singular (i.e., satisfying the condition $0 \notin H(G(t))$) matrix function G are equal to each other. This result is a strengthening but also a simplification of Theorem 6.13 for the case when the contour Γ is a circle.

Section 7.7 contains information on the history of the subject and comments related to current literature.

7.1. DEFINITION OF FACTORIZATION ON THE CIRCLE

In the present chapter we deal with the factorization problem in case when the contour Γ is a circle. Without loss of generality, we may suppose that Γ is the unit circle $\mathbb{T} = \{\zeta : |\zeta| = 1\}$.
In this case complex conjugation realizes a one-to-one correspondence between the classes L_p^- and L_p^+ $(= H_p)$. Indeed, the function f defined in the unit disk belongs to the Hardy class H_p if and only if the function $\tilde{f}$ defined outside the unit disk by the equation $\tilde{f}(\zeta) = \overline{f(\bar{\zeta}^{-1})}$ lies in the class E_p^-, where the boundary values of the functions f and $\tilde{f}$ are connected via the relation $\tilde{f}(t) = \overline{f(t)}$.

Redenoting the matrix function G_+ from the representation (2.1) by A and the matrix function G_- by B^*, in view of the remark made above, we may claim that, in the case $\Gamma = \mathbb{T}$, Definition 2.1 is equivalent to the following one.

DEFINITION 7.1. A representation

$$G = A\Lambda B^* \tag{7.1}$$

will be called a factorization in L_p of the matrix function G defined on the unit circle, if the matrix functions A and B^{-1}

(A^{-1} and B) belong to the class H_p (H_q, $q = p/(p-1)$) and Λ is a diagonal matrix function of the form (2.2).

From Theorems 1.17 and 1.18 it is clear that the requirements $A \in H_p$, $A^{-1} \in H_q$ are fulfilled if and only if A is an outer matrix function[1], $A \in L_p$ and $A^{-1} \in L_q$. A similar assertion is true for the matrix function B.

THEOREM 7.1. The matrix function G defined on $\mathbb{T}$ can be factored in L_p if and only if the matrix function G^* can be factored in L_q. In this case the tuple $(\varkappa_j^*)$ of partial q-indices of G^* and the tuple $(\varkappa_j)$ of partial p-indices of G are connected via the relations

$$\varkappa_j^* = -\varkappa_{n-j+1}, \quad j = 1,2,\dots,n. \tag{7.2}$$

In particular, the total q-index of G^* is opposite to the total p-index of G.

Proof. We introduce the constant matrix

$$T = \begin{pmatrix} 0 & \dots & 1 \\ & \cdot^{\cdot^{\cdot}} & \\ 1 & \dots & 0 \end{pmatrix}. \tag{7.3}$$

The matrix T is both Hermitian and unitary, i.e. $T = T^* = T^{-1}$. Taking these properties into consideration, the expression $G^* = B\Lambda^*A^*$, which is obtained from (7.1), may be rewritten in the equivalent form

$$G^* = BT(T\Lambda^*T)(AT)^*. \tag{7.4}$$

Since $T\Lambda^*T = T\Lambda^{-1}T = \operatorname{diag}[t^{-\varkappa_n},\dots,t^{-\varkappa_1}]$, the representation (7.1) is a factorization of the matrix function G in L_p if and only if equation (7.4) provides a factorization of G^* in L_q (therefore, the factorizations exist only simultaneously) and the corresponding partial indices of G and G^* are connected by the relations (7.2), which proves the theorem.

THEOREM 7.1'. A matrix function G of class L_∞ defined on $\mathbb{T}$ is Φ-factorable in L_p if and only if the matrix function G^* is Φ-fac-

---

[1] A nxn matrix function A is called outer, if its entries belong to the class D and det A is an outer function.

torable in L_q. Moreover, the assertions concerning the values of total and partial indices formulated in Theorem 7.1 continue to be valid.

<u>Proof.</u> If the matrix function G is not factorable in L_p, then, owing to the previous theorem, the matrix function G^* is not factorable in L_q, which is consistent with the assertion to be proved. It remains to consider the case of a matrix function G which can be factored in L_p. According to Corollary 3.3 and the definition of Φ-factorization, the representation (7.1) is a Φ-factorization of G in L_p if and only if the operator $K_G = (B^*)^{-1}\Lambda^{-1}QA^{-1}$ is bounded in L_p^n, and the representation (7.4) is a Φ-factorization of G^* in L_q iff the operator $K_{G^*} = [(AT)^*]^{-1}(T\Lambda^*T)^{-1}Q(BT)^{-1}$ is bounded in L_q^n.

But the operator $K_{G^*} = (A^*)^{-1}\Lambda TQTB^{-1} = (A^*)^{-1}\Lambda QB^{-1}$ may be viewed as adjoint (in the sense of Definition 1.6) to the operator $(B^*)^{-1}Q\Lambda^{-1}A^{-1}$, if we identify L_q^n with the dual of the space L_p^n with the aid of the bilinear form

$$(f,g) = \int_{\mathbf{T}} g(t)^*f(t)|dt| .$$ [1]

In virtue of assertions 2) and 3) of Lemma 3.3 the operators K_G and $(B^*)^{-1}Q\Lambda^{-1}A^{-1}$ are densely defined and closed. Therefore, assertion 4) of the same lemma may be applied, owing to which these operators are bounded only simultaneously.

Thus, the operators K_G and K_{G^*} considered in L_p^n and L_q^n, respectively, are bounded only simultaneously. From here and Theorem 3.8 we deduce the assertion to be proved. ≡

<u>COROLLARY 7.1.</u> The matrix functions G and G^* are factorable (and, provided that $G \in L_\infty$, also Φ-factorable) in L_2 only simultaneously. In addition, their total 2-indices are opposite and the partial indices are connected by relation (7.2).

Corollary 3.6 taken together with Theorem 7.1' leads to the following conclusion.

---

[1] This can be established just as the corresponding part from the proof of Lemma 3.4.

COROLLARY 7.2. The matrix function $G \in L_\infty$ is left Φ-factorable in L_p if and only if the matrix function $(G^*)^{-1}$ is right Φ-factorable in L_q, where the corresponding tuples of partial indices coincide.

Due to Corollary 7.2, a unitary matrix function G (i.e., a function for which $G(t)^* = G(t)^{-1}$ a.e. on $\mathbb{T}$) is left Φ-factorable in L_p if and only if it is right Φ-factorable in L_q.

7.2. FACTORIZATION OF HERMITIAN MATRIX FUNCTIONS

From Theorems 7.1 and 7.1' it is clear that Hermitian matrix functions (i.e. such that $G(t) = G(t)^*$ a.e. on $\mathbb{T}$) play a special role in the factorization problem with respect to $\mathbb{T}$.

THEOREM 7.2. Under the mapping $p \to p/(p-1)$, the domain of factorability (and, if $G \in L_\infty$, then also the domain of Φ-factorability) of a Hermitian matrix function G is transformed into itself. In addition, for its partial p-indices, the relations

$$\begin{aligned} \varkappa_j + \varkappa_{n-j+1} &\le 0 \quad \text{if} \quad p > 2, \\ \varkappa_j + \varkappa_{n-j+1} &= 0 \quad \text{if} \quad p = 2, \\ \varkappa_j + \varkappa_{n-j+1} &\ge 0 \quad \text{if} \quad p < 2 \end{aligned} \tag{7.5}$$

are valid.

The assertion of Theorem 7.2 follows from Corollary 7.1 and Theorem 2.1 (on the monotony of partial p-indices).

COROLLARY 7.3. The components of the factorability domain of a Hermitian matrix function which correspond to positive (negative) values of the total index are situated strictly to the left (right) of the point $p = 2$. The component $\mathfrak{F}_0(G)$, provided that it is not empty, necessarily contains the point $p = 2$.

Consider the Hermitian matrix function G with non-empty factorability domain. In accordance with Theorem 7.2 G can be factored in L_p for some $p \ge 2$. If (7.1) provides a factorization of G in L_p, then, since G is Hermitian, equation (7.4) yields a factorization of this matrix function in L_q. According to formulae (2.5), which express the connection between factorization factors from different factorizations of one and the same matrix function, we have

$$A = BTH \, , \tag{7.6}$$

where H is a polynomial matrix function the structure of which is described in Chapter 2 immediately after formulae (2.5). In particular, there was also shown that det H is a polynomial whose degree is equal to the difference of the total indices of G in the considered factorizations. In the case under study, thanks to Theorem 7.1 and Corollary 7.3, we may assert that this degree is equal to $-2\varkappa$, where $\varkappa\ (\le 0)$ is the total p-index of G.

Utilizing equations (7.1) and (7.6), we may represent the matrix function G in the form

$$G = BTH\Lambda B^* \, . \tag{7.7}$$

Consequently, for almost all $t \in \mathbb{T}$, the quadratic forms associated with the matrices $G(t)$ and $TH(t)\Lambda(t)$ are congruent. Hence, the signatures (i.e. the differences of the numbers of positive and negative squares of the corresponding quadratic forms) of these matrices also coincide a.e. on $\mathbb{T}$. Since the matrix function $TH\Lambda$ is continuous on $\mathbb{T}$, its signature is a piecewise constant function of t the discontinuities of which are contained in the set of zeros of the function $\det(TH\Lambda) = (-1)^n t^{\varkappa} \det H$, i.e. in the set of zeros of the polynomial det H. However, the latter vanishes at no more than $2|\varkappa|$ points of the circle $\mathbb{T}$. In this way, the following statement has been proved.

THEOREM 7.3. Let G be a Hermitian matrix function. For the set $\mathfrak{F}_{\varkappa}(G)$ to be non-empty, it is necessary that there exist points $t_j \in \mathbb{T}$, $j = 1,\dots,N$ which partition $\mathbb{T}$ into $N \le 2|\varkappa|$ arcs such that the signature of the matrix $G(t)$ is constant on a each of them a.e..

COROLLARY 7.4. For $\mathfrak{F}_0(G)$ to be non-empty, it is necessary that the signature of the matrix $G(t)$ is constant a.e..

COROLLARY 7.5. For $\mathfrak{F}(G)$ to be non-empty, it is necessary that there exists a partition of $\mathbb{T}$ into a finite number of arcs such that on each of them the signature of the matrix $G(t)$ is constant a.e..

With the help of Corollary 7.5 one can easily construct an example of a scalar function taking the values 1 and -1 which does not admit a factorization in any of the spaces L_p. In particular, one may set $f(t) = 1$ if $[1/|t-1|]$ is even, and $f(t) = -1$ otherwise.

The conditions found in Theorem 7.3 are not sufficient for the domain of factorability of the matrix function G to be non-empty, even in case we require $G^{\pm 1} \in L_\infty$ and $N = 0$. As an example we consider the matrix function $G(t) = \operatorname{diag}[f(t),-f(t)]$, where the function f is real-valued, changes its sign infinitely many times and $f^{\pm 1} \in L_\infty$. For all $t \in \mathbb{T}$, the matrix $G(t)$ is Hermitian and its signature is equal to zero. At the same time, the matrix function in question differs from the Hermitian matrix function $\operatorname{diag}[f,f]$, the signature of which changes infinitely many times, by the constant multiplier $\begin{pmatrix} 1 & 0 \\ 0 & -1 \end{pmatrix}$. Consequently, the factorability domain of G is empty.

Now we intend to consider in more detail an Hermitian matrix function G for which the component $\mathfrak{F}_0(G)$ is not empty. According to Corollary 7.3, in this case the inclusion $2 \in \mathfrak{F}_0(G)$ necessarily holds and the partial indices of G are connected by relations (7.5). Thus, the tuple of partial indices of G is uniquely determined by the numbers $k_m > \dots > k_1 > 0$ $(m \geq 0)$ of different positive indices and their multiplicities $l_m, \dots, l_1$.

<u>THEOREM 7.4.</u> Assume that for the Hermitian matrix function G the set $\mathfrak{F}_0(G)$ is non-empty. Then G admits a representation in the form

$$G = A_0 \Lambda_0 A_0^* , \tag{7.8}$$

where $A_0^{\pm 1} \in H_2$,

$$\Lambda_0(t) = \begin{pmatrix} &&&&&& t^{k_m} I_{l_m} \\ &&&&& \cdot^{\cdot^{\cdot}} & \\ &&&& t^{k_1} I_{l_1} && \\ &&& J &&& \\ && t^{-k_1} I_{l_1} &&&& \\ & \cdot^{\cdot^{\cdot}} &&&&& \\ t^{-k_m} I_{l_m} &&&&&& \end{pmatrix} , \tag{7.9}$$

$$J = \begin{pmatrix} I_{l_+} & \\ & -I_{l_-} \end{pmatrix},$$ and l_+ and l_- are integers such that their sum is equal to $l_0 = n-2\sum_{j=1}^{m} l_j$ and their difference equals the signature σ of G.

Before proving the theorem, let us remark that by σ one has to understand that value of the signature which is taken by the matrix function G a.e. on $\mathbb{T}$. Because of Corollary 7.4, such a value exists.

Proof. Starting with an arbitrary factorization (7.1) of the matrix function G in L_2 and arguing as in the proof of Theorem 7.3, we obtain equation (7.7) in which $B^{\pm 1} \in H_2$ and H is a transition matrix from one factorization of G in L_2 to another. Consequently, the structure of H is described by assertion 2) of Theorem 2.2. With regard to relations (7.5), we deduce the following description of the structure of the matrix function $W = TH$.

Let the matrix function W be partitioned into blocks in the same way as the matrix function Λ_0 defined by equation (7.9), and let these blocks be numbered in lines and columns by the indices from $-m$ to m from bottom to top and from the left to the right, respectively. Then:

1) if $r < s$, then $W_{r,s} = 0$,

2) $W_{r,r}$ is a constant non-singular matrix,

3) if $r > s$, then $W_{r,s}$ is a polynomial matrix function such that the degrees of its elements do not exceed k_r-k_s (for the sake of uniformity, set $k_s = -k_{-s}$ for $s < 0$, and $k_0 = 0$).

Now we want to show that there exists a polynomial matrix function Ψ with a constant non-zero determinant such that the equation

$$W(t)\Lambda(t) = \Psi(t)\Lambda_0(t)\Psi(t)^* \tag{7.10}$$

is valid.

Partitioning the matrix function Ψ into blocks in the same manner as W and imposing on it the additional condition

$$\Psi_{r,s} = 0 \quad \text{for} \quad r+s < 0, \tag{7.11}$$

we get a system which is equivalent to (7.10):

$$t^{-k_s} W_{r,-s}(t) = \sum_{\nu} \Psi_{r,-\nu}(t)\, J_\nu \Psi_{s,\nu}(t)^* t^{k_\nu} , \tag{7.12}$$

where the summation on the right-hand side is carried out for ν lying between $-s$ and r, $J_\nu = I$ for $\nu \neq 0$ and $J_0 = J$.

Since the matrix function $W\Lambda$ is Hermitian, the system (7.12) is transformed into itself after conjugation and changing r and s with each other. Consequently, those equations with $r < s$ may be omitted. The remaining equations of the system (7.12) are partitioned into $2m+1$ groups, assigning to the j th group those of the equations for which $r+s = j$ $(j=0,\ldots,2m)$. The zero group consists of the equations

$$\begin{aligned} W_{r,r}(t) &= \Psi_{r,-r}(t)\Psi_{-r,r}(t)^* , \quad r=1,\ldots,m , \\ W_{o,o} &= \Psi_{o,o}\, J\Psi^*_{o,o} . \end{aligned} \tag{7.13}$$

For the solvability of the last equation, it is necessary and sufficient to equate the integers l_+ and l_- to the number of positive and negative squares, respectively, of the matrix $W_{o,o}$. The remaining equations are always solvable. The solutions of all the equations (7.13) may be chosen in the class of constant matrices.

Now we take advantage of the fact that the equations of the j th group involve only those unknown matrices $\Psi_{r,s}$ for which $0 \le r+s \le j$. Suppose that, for $j \le j_0$ $(< 2m+1)$, the equations of the j th group are solved, where the matrix functions $\Psi_{r,s}$ already obtained are polynomial with degree of its elements not exceeding k_r+k_s. Each equation of the (j_0+1) th group may be rewritten in the form

$$\begin{aligned} &\Psi_{r,s}(t)J_s\Psi^*_{s,-s} + \Psi_{r,-r}J_r\Psi_{s,r}(t)^* t^{k_r+k_s} = \\ &W_{r,-s}(t) - \sum_{\nu} \Psi_{r,-\nu}(t)J_\nu\Psi_{s,\nu}(t)^* t^{k_\nu+k_s} . \end{aligned} \tag{7.14}$$

The summation on the right-hand side is carried out for ν lying between $-s+1$ and $r-1$.

In view of the assumption stipulated the right-hand side of (7.14) is a polynomial matrix function the degrees of the entries of which are not

greater than k_r+k_s. Setting $\Psi_{s,r}=0$ for $s \neq r$, from (7.14) we get $\Psi_{r,s}$ in the form of a polynomial matrix function the degrees of the entries of which are also less than or equal to k_r+k_s.
For $s=r$, equation (7.14) reads as follows:

$$2\,\mathrm{Re}(t^{-k_r}\Psi_{r,r}(t)\Psi^*_{r,-r}) =$$

$$t^{-k_r}W_{r,-r}(t) - \sum_{|\nu|\leq r-1}\Psi_{r,-\nu}(t)J_\nu\Psi_{r,\nu}(t)^*t^{k_\nu}\,.$$

Starting from the fact that $W\Lambda$ is a Hermitian matrix function and changing the summation index ν by $-\nu$, it is not hard to verify that the right-hand side of the latter relation is a Hermitian matrix function and its elements are of the form $\sum_{|j|\leq k_r} c_j t^j$. Therefore, it can be represented in the form $2\,\mathrm{Re}\,Z(t)$, where Z is a polynomial matrix function such that the degrees of its entries are not greater than k_r. It remains to set $\Psi_{r,r}(t)=t^{k_r}Z(t)(\Psi^*_{r,-r})^{-1}$.
Concequently, under the assumption made above, all the equations of the (j_0+1) th group can be solved and the obtained solutions $\Psi_{r,s}$ $(r+s=j_0+1)$ are polynomial matrix functions of degree less than or equal to k_r+k_s.

We obtained that there exists a polynomial matrix function Ψ satisfying equation (7.10). Its non-degeneracy results from condition (7.11) and the non-degeneracy of the diagonal blocks $\Psi_{r,-r}$.

The constructed matrix function Ψ satisfies the requirements $\Psi^{\pm 1}\in H_\infty$. Hence, the matrix function $A_0=B\Psi$ belongs, together with its inverse, to the class H_2. At the same time, successively applying equations (7.10) and (7.7), we get $A_0\Lambda_0A_0^*=B(\Psi\Lambda_0\Psi^*)B=BW\Lambda B^*=BTH\Lambda B^*=G$. Thus, the existence of the desired representation (7.8) has been proved. Equation (7.8) implies that the signature of the matrices $G(t)$ and $\Lambda_0(t)$ coincide a.e. on $\mathbb{T}$. Since the signature of the latter is equal to l_+-l_-, we obtain the equation $l_+-l_-=\sigma$, whereas the equation $l_++l_-=l_0$ is evident. The proof of Theorem 7.4 is complete. ≡

As a consequence from the relations for the numbers $l_{\pm}$ established in Theorem 7.4 and the obvious inequality $l_+ + l_- \geq |l_+ - l_-|$ we derive the following statement.

COROLLARY 7.6. The number of zero 2-indices of a Hermitian matrix function is not less than the absolute value of its signature (to be more precise, of that value of the signature which is attained on a set of complete measure).

COROLLARY 7.7. Let G be a Hermitian matrix function defined on $\mathbb{T}$ which admits a factorization in a certain (L_∞, R)-algebra $\mathfrak{A}$. Then this matrix function admits also a representation (7.8) with $A_0^{\pm 1} \in \mathfrak{A}^+$.

Proof. A factorization of the matrix function G in $\mathfrak{A}$ may be chosen as the factorization (7.1) being the initial one in the argument of Theorem 7.4. Then we have $B^{\pm 1} \in \mathfrak{A}$. Taking into account that the multiplication by polynomial matrix functions does not go beyond the class $\mathfrak{A}$, we see that along with B the matrix function $A_0 = B\Psi$ is an invertible element of $\mathfrak{A}^+$. $\equiv$

COROLLARY 7.8. A second-order Hermitian matrix function G which can be factored in L_2 and has a negative determinant admits a representation

$$G(t) = A(t) \begin{pmatrix} 0 & t^{\varkappa_1} \\ t^{-\varkappa_1} & 0 \end{pmatrix} A(t)^* ,$$

where $A^{\pm 1} \in H_2$, $\varkappa_1$ (≥ 0) and $-\varkappa_1$ $(= \varkappa_2)$ are its partial 2-indices.

In fact, if $\varkappa_1 > 0$, then the mentioned representation exists by Theorem 7.4. If $\varkappa_1 = 0$, then Theorem 7.4 ensures the existence of the representation $G = A_0 \begin{pmatrix} 1 & 0 \\ 0 & -1 \end{pmatrix} A_0^*$. It remains only to remark that

$$\begin{pmatrix} 1 & 0 \\ 0 & -1 \end{pmatrix} = \frac{1}{2} \begin{pmatrix} 1 & 1 \\ -1 & 1 \end{pmatrix} \begin{pmatrix} 0 & 1 \\ 1 & 0 \end{pmatrix} \begin{pmatrix} 1 & -1 \\ 1 & 1 \end{pmatrix}$$

and to set

$$A = \frac{1}{\sqrt{2}} A_0 \begin{pmatrix} 1 & 1 \\ -1 & 1 \end{pmatrix} .$$

7.3. FACTORIZATION OF DEFINITE MATRIX FUNCTIONS

An important subclass of Hermitian matrix functions are positively (negatively) definite matrix functions, i.e. such that the signature of the matrix $G(t)$ is equal to n $(-n)$ a.e. on $\mathbb{T}$. Since negatively definite matrix functions become positively definite after multiplication by -1, it is sufficient to study only positively definite matrix functions.

If a positively definite matrix function is factorable in L_2, then, by Corollary 7.6, all its partial 2-indices are equal to zero. Moreover, $l_+ = n$ and $l_- = 0$, since only in this case the equation $l_+ - l_- = n$ may be guaranteed. Thus, for positively definite matrix functions, the factor Λ_0 is the unit matrix. Consequently, if a positively definite matrix function can be factored in L_2, then it admits also a representation

$$G = AA^* \tag{7.15}$$

with $A^{\pm 1} \in H_2$.

The necessary condition for $\mathfrak{F}_0(G)$ to be non-empty established in Corollary 7.4 (i.e. of factorability in L_2) is fulfilled for a positively definite matrix function. If we complete this condition by the requirements $G^{\pm 1} \in L_1$, which are obviously necessary for factorability, then the obtained collection of conditions proves already to be sufficient. In other words, the following result holds.

THEOREM 7.5. A positively definite matrix function G defined on $\mathbb{T}$ can be factored in L_2 if and only if $G^{\pm 1} \in L_1$.

Theorem 7.5 may be derived as a consequence of a more general result on the representation of a positively definite matrix function G in the form of the product (7.15) of an outer matrix function and its adjoint[1]. Let us begin with the scalar case.

[1] The reader who is only interested in the problem of Φ-factorization of matrix functions from the class L_∞ may omit all the material up to the end of the present section. The question of Φ-factorability of positively definite matrix functions of the mentioned class will be solved in 7.4 irrespective of Theorem 7.5.

LEMMA 7.1. Let g be a non-negative function defined on $\mathbb{T}$. The representation $g(t) = |f(t)|^2$, where f is a certain outer function, is possible if and only if $\log g \in L_1$. If the desired function f exists, then it is defined up to a constant multiplier with absolute value 1.

Proof. From Definition 1.12 of an outer function and Theorem 1.15 it is clear that the relation $g = |f|^2$ holds if and only if $g(t) = k(t)^2$ a.e. on $\mathbb{T}$. Since the role of the function k in (1.7) may be played by any non-negative function with summable logarithm, it follows that the condition $\log g \in L_1$ is necessary and sufficient for the existence of the desired representation.

If this condition is fulfilled, then the corresponding function f is defined up to the constant ν from relation (1.7), which proves Lemma 7.1. ≡

In particular, Lemma 7.1 allows for solving the question of factorability in L_2 of a real-valued function to the very end.

THEOREM 7.6. Let G be a real-valued scalar function. The inclusion $2 \in \mathfrak{F}(G)$ holds if and only if

1) $G^{\pm} \in L_1$ and

2) G takes values of one and the same sign a.e.

Proof. The necessity of condition 1) is obvious; the necessity of condition 2) results from Corollary 7.4. If condition 1) and 2) are satisfied, then $G = \varepsilon g$, where g is a non-negative (a.e.) function such that $g^{\pm 1} \in L_1$ and ε is a constant equal to 1 or -1. Due to Lemma 7.1, $g = |f|^2$, where f is an outer function belonging with its inverse to the class H_2. Setting $A = f$, $B = \varepsilon f$, we get a factorization of G in L_2. Thus Theorem 7.6 is proved. ≡

Now let $G \in L_1$ be a positively definite matrix function of n th order. We introduce the Hilbert space $\mathfrak{h}$ of n-dimensional vector functions (rows) f defined on $\mathbb{T}$ for which the value $\frac{1}{2\pi} \int f(e^{i\theta})G(e^{i\theta})f(e^{i\theta})^* d\theta$[1]

[1] All the integrals in the present section are taken over the interval $[-\pi,\pi]$.

makes sense and is finite. The scalar product in $\mathfrak{H}$ is defined by the formula $(f,g) = \frac{1}{2\pi} \int f(e^{i\theta})G(e^{i\theta})g(e^{i\theta})^* d\theta$. We denote by $\mathcal{L}$ the closure (with respect to the norm in $\mathfrak{H}$) of the space L consisting of all vector functions of the form

$$f(e^{i\theta}) = \sum_{k=0}^{N} e^{ik\theta} f^{(k)} , \tag{7.16}$$

where $f^{(k)}$ $(k=0,\ldots,N;\ N=0,1,\ldots)$ are constant row vectors.

Let $\mathcal{L}_0$ be the closure (again with respect to the norm in $\mathfrak{H}$) of the space L_0 of those vector functions $f \in L$ for which $f^{(0)} = 0$. Clearly, $\mathcal{L} \supset \mathcal{L}_0$ and $\dim \mathcal{L} | \mathcal{L}_0 \le n$.

LEMMA 7.2. Let $G \in L_1$ be a positively definite matrix function of n th order such that $\log \det G \in L_1$. Then $\dim \mathcal{L} | \mathcal{L}_0 = n$.

Proof. Suppose at first $n = 1$. According to Lemma 7.1, the condition $\log G \in L_1$ implies that $G = |G_+|^2$, where G_+ is an outer function. Since $G \in L_1$, then $G_+ \in H_2$. For an arbitrary function f, instead of $\int f(e^{i\theta})G(e^{i\theta})\overline{f(e^{i\theta})}d\theta$ we may write $\int |G_+(e^{i\theta})f(e^{i\theta})|^2 d\theta$. From this it is clear that, for all $f \in L$, $(f,f) = \frac{1}{2\pi} \int |G_+(e^{i\theta})f(e^{i\theta})|^2 d\theta \ge |G_+(0)f(0)|^2$. Setting $f = 1-g$ with $g \in L_0$, we thus obtain $\|1-g\|_{\mathfrak{H}} = (1-g,1-g)^{1/2} \ge |G_+(0)|$. Consequently, the distance from 1 to L_0 (and, therefore, also to the subspace $\mathcal{L}_0$) is not less than $|G_+(0)|$. Thus, $\mathcal{L}_0 \neq \mathcal{L}$ and $\dim(\mathcal{L} | \mathcal{L}_0) = 1$. Returning to the general case, we denote by $\lambda_1(e^{i\theta}) \ge \ldots \ge \lambda_n(e^{i\theta})$ the collection of all eigenvalues of the matrix $G(e^{i\theta})$. Since

$$\log \lambda_n(e^{i\theta}) \le \frac{1}{n} \sum_{j=1}^{n} \log \lambda_j(e^{i\theta}) =$$

$$\frac{1}{n} \log \prod_{j=1}^{n} \lambda_j(e^{i\theta}) = \frac{1}{n} \log \det G(e^{i\theta})$$

and

$$\log \det G(e^{i\theta}) = \sum_{j=1}^{n} \log \lambda_j(e^{i\theta}) \le \log \lambda_n(e^{i\theta}) + (n-1)\log \lambda_1(e^{i\theta})$$

$$< \log \lambda_n(e^{i\theta}) + (n-1)\lambda_1(e^{i\theta}) < \log \lambda_n(e^{i\theta}) + (n-1) \sum_{j=1}^{n} \lambda_j(e^{i\theta})$$

$$= \log \lambda_n(e^{i\theta}) + (n-1)\operatorname{tr} G(e^{i\theta}) ,$$

the conditions $\log \det G \in L_1$ and $\log \lambda_n \in L_1$ are equivalent for a positively definite matrix function $G \in L_1$. By $\operatorname{tr} G(e^{i\theta})$ we denote the trace of the matrix $G(e^{i\theta})$[1]. We shall make use of its summability. Choosing a vector function $f \in L$ and denoting its j th component by f_j, we have

$$(f,f) = \frac{1}{2\pi} \int f(e^{i\theta})G(e^{i\theta})f(e^{i\theta})^* d\theta$$

$$\geq \frac{1}{2\pi} \int f(e^{i\theta})\lambda_n(e^{i\theta})f(e^{i\theta})^* \, d\theta = \sum_{j=1}^{n} \frac{1}{2\pi} \int \lambda_n(e^{i\theta})|f_j(e^{i\theta})| d\theta .$$

The inclusion $\log \lambda_n \in L_1$ established above permits us to assert that $\lambda_n = |\lambda_+|^2$, where λ_+ is an outer function. In addition, due to the inequality $0 \leq \lambda_n(e^{i\theta}) \leq \operatorname{tr} G(e^{i\theta})$, the function λ_n is summable and, thus, $\lambda_+ \in L_2$. By what was proved in the first part of the lemma,

$$\frac{1}{2\pi} \int \lambda_n(e^{i\theta})|f_j(e^{i\theta})|^2 d\theta \geq |\lambda_+(0)f_j(0)|^2 .$$

Hence

$$(f,f) \geq \sum_{j=1}^{n} |\lambda_+(0)f_j(0)|^2 = |\lambda_+(0)|^2 \|f(0)\|^2 .$$

Setting $f = a - g$, where a is a fixed constant vector and g ranges over L_0, we find that the distance from a to g is not less than $|\lambda_+(0)| \|a\|$. Since L_0 is dense in $\mathcal{L}_0$, every constant non-zero vector does not belong to $\mathcal{L}_0$. Consequently, $\dim(\mathcal{L} | \mathcal{L}_0) = n$, which proves Lemma 7.2. ≡

<u>THEOREM 7.7.</u> The matrix function G defined on $\mathbb{T}$ admits a representation $G = AA^*$ with an outer matrix function A if and only if

1) G is positively definite,
2) $\log \det G \in L_1$,
3) $\log \|G\| \in L_1$.

If the indicated representation exists, then the matrix function A is defined up to a constant right unitary multiplier.

<u>Proof.</u> Assume that $G = AA^*$, where $A = (a_{jk})_{j,k=1}^{n}$ is an outer matrix function. Then, for an arbitrary n-dimensional vector x, $(G(t)x,x) = (A(t)A(t)^*x,x) = \|A(t)^*x\|^2 \geq 0$ holds a.e. on $\mathbb{T}$, i.e.,

---

[1] $\operatorname{tr} G(e^{i\theta})$ is the sum of the diagonal elements of $G(e^{i\theta})$, where $G \in L_1$.

the matrix function G is positively definite and condition 1) is fulfilled. Moreover, from Lemma 7.15 and the relation $\det G = |\det A|^2$ we deduce that condition 2) is also satisfied.

Furthermore, we denote by $\lambda_1(t) \geq \dots \geq \lambda_n(t)$ the collection of eigenvalues of the matrix $G(t)$ at those points $t \in \mathbb{T}$ where this matrix is positively definite. Then $\|G(t)\| = (\lambda_{max}(G(t)G(t)^*))^{1/2} = \lambda_{max}(G(t)) = \lambda_1(t)$. We have, on the one hand, $\lambda_1(t) \geq (\lambda_1(t)\dots\lambda_n(t))^{1/n} = (\det G(t))^{1/n}$. On the other hand, $\lambda_1(t) \leq \lambda_1(t)+\dots+\lambda_n(t) = \operatorname{tr} G(t) = \sum_{j=1}^{n} g_{jj}(t) = \sum_{j,k=1}^{n} |a_{jk}(t)|^2 \leq n^2 \max_{j,k}|a_{jk}(t)|$. Thus

$$\frac{1}{n}\log\det G(t) \leq \log\|G(t)\| \leq 2\log n + \max_{j,k}\log|a_{jk}(t)| \quad \text{a.e. on } \mathbb{T}.$$

With regard to the definition of an outer function each of the functions a_{jk} belongs to the class D. Therefore, it is either identically equal to zero or, taken absolutely, coincides with a certain outer function. In any case, $\int \log|a_{jk}(e^{i\theta})|\,d\theta < +\infty$ and, consequently, $\int \max_{j,k}\log|a_{jk}(e^{i\theta})|\,d\theta < +\infty$. From the inequalities obtained for $\log\|G(t)\|$ and the summability of the function $\log\det G$, we thus conclude that $\log\|G\| \in L_1$. In this way, condition 3) is also necessary for the existence of a representation (7.15).

It is obvious that, replacing in (7.15) the matrix function A by AU, where U is a constant unitary multiplier, we do not violate equation (7.15) and do not go beyond the class of outer matrix functions. Vice versa, assume that, besides of the representation (7.15), the equation $G = BB^*$ with an outer matrix function B is valid. Then

$$A^{-1}(t)B(t) = (B^{-1}(t)A(t))^*$$

a.e. on $\mathbb{T}$.

The latter equation means that the matrix function $U = A^{-1}B$ is unitary and, in particular, belongs to the class L_∞. Moreover, this matrix function is outer along with A and B. Therefore, on the basis of Theorem 1.18, from the condition $U \in L_\infty$ we can conclude that $U \in H_\infty$. To verify that the matrix function U^* $(= B^{-1}A)$ lies in the class H_∞ can be done in a similar way. But then $U \in H_\infty \cap L^-$, so that, by Theorem 1.28, the matrix function U is constant. Thus $B = AU$, where U is a constant unitary matrix.

It remains to prove the existence of a representation (7.15) in case the conditions 1) – 3) are fulfilled. Replacing the matrix function G by $f^{-1}G$, where $f(t) = \|G(t)\|$, we get a summable positively definite matrix function with summable logarithm of the determinant. If the existence of a representation $f^{-1}G = BB^*$ with an outer matrix function B will be proved, then setting $A = Bf_+$ (where f_+ is an outer function with the property $|f_+|^2 = f$ existing in view of Lemma 7.1), we shall obtain a representation (7.15) of the original matrix function G. Hence, without loss of generality, we may assume the matrix function G to be summable.

If we stipulate the mentioned assumption and use the notations introduced before Lemma 7.2, we observe that, due to this lemma, the orthogonal complement of $\mathcal{L}_0$ with respect to $\mathcal{L}$ is n-dimensional. Now we choose an orthonormal basis $\{\varphi_j\}_{j=1}^n$ in $\mathcal{L} \ominus \mathcal{L}_0$ [1]. Since, for arbitrary $f \in \mathcal{L}$ and $k = 1,2,\ldots$, $e^{ik}f \in \mathcal{L}_0$, then for all $f \in \mathcal{L}$:

$$\int f(e^{i\theta})G(e^{i\theta})\varphi_j(e^{i\theta})^* e^{ik\theta}d\theta = 0 , \qquad (7.17)$$
$$j = 1,\ldots,n;\ k = 1,2,\ldots .$$

In particular, taking $f = \varphi_l$, we have

$$\int \varphi_l(e^{i\theta})G(e^{i\theta})\varphi_j(e^{i\theta})^* e^{ik\theta}d\theta = 0 ,$$
$$j,l = 1,\ldots,n;\ k = 1,2,\ldots .$$

Changing in the last equation j and l with each other and passing to the adjoint, we find that this equation continues to be true also for $k = -1,-2,\ldots$. But this means that the measure $\varphi_l(e^{i\theta})G(e^{i\theta})\varphi_j(e^{i\theta})^*d\theta$ is orthogonal to all trigonometric polynomials vanishing at zero. In its turn, this allows for concluding that the function $\varphi_l(e^{i\theta})G(e^{i\theta})\varphi_j(e^{i\theta})^*$ is equal to a certain constant c_{lj} $(l,j = 1,\ldots,n)$ a.e. .

Furthermore, $c_{lj} = \frac{1}{2\pi}\int \varphi_l(e^{i\theta})G(e^{i\theta})\varphi_j(e^{i\theta})^*d\theta = (\varphi_l,\varphi_j) = \delta_{lj}$ (here the orthonormality of the system has been used).

---

[1] $\mathcal{L} \ominus \mathcal{L}_0$ denotes the orthogonal complement of $\mathcal{L}_0$ in $\mathcal{L}$.

In this way, if we denote by Φ that matrix function the j th row of which is φ_j, then $\Phi(e^{i\theta})G(e^{i\theta})\Phi(e^{i\theta})^* = I$ a.e. on $\mathbf{T}$. From here we conclude that equation (7.15) holds, for instance, for $A = G\Phi^*$ $(= \Phi^{-1})$. It only remains to show that the matrix function A defined in this manner is outer.

Relation (7.15) and condition 2) of the theorem imply the inclusion $A \in L_2$. Equation (7.17) means (if we choose in it the rows $(0,\dots,0,1,0,\dots,0)$ as f, where the 1 stands on the l th place) that the Fourier coefficients with negative numbers of the (l,j) th element of A $(= G\Phi^*)$ are equal to zero and, thus, $A \in H_2$. Furthermore, the rows of the matrix function A^{-1} $(= \Phi)$ are elements of $\mathfrak{L}$. Consequently, they can be approximated (in the metric of $\mathfrak{H}$) by vector functions of the form (7.16). In other words, there exists a sequence of polynomial matrix functions $\{P_k\}_{k=1}^{\infty}$ such that

$$\int (P_k(e^{i\theta})-(A(e^{i\theta}))^{-1})G(e^{i\theta})\,(P_k(e^{i\theta})-(A(e^{i\theta}))^{-1})^*d\theta =$$

$$\int (P_k(e^{i\theta})A(e^{i\theta})-I)(P_k(e^{i\theta})A(e^{i\theta})-I)^*d\theta \to 0\,.$$

This means that the sequence $\{P_kA\}_{k=1}^{\infty}$ converges to I in L_2. But then the sequence $\{\det A \det P_k\}_{k=1}^{\infty}$ converges to 1 in the metric of the space $L_{2/n}$ [1]. If $\det A = f^{(i)}f^{(e)}$ is a representation of $\det A$ in the form of the product of an inner function and an outer one, then the sequence $\{f^{(e)}\det P_k\}_{k=1}^{\infty}$ lying in $H_{2/n}$ converges to the function $(f^{(i)})^{-1}$ in the metric of the space $L_{2/n}$. Consequently, $(f^{(i)})^{-1}$ belongs to the class $H_{2/n}$, i.e., $f^{(i)}$ is an invertible element of $H_{2/n}$ and thus an outer function. Since $f^{(i)}$ is an outer and inner function simultaneously, it reduces to a constant. Hence, the function $\det A$ and, by definition, also the matrix function A is outer. The proof of Theorem 7.7 is complete. $\equiv$

Now we are prepared to prove Theorem 7.5.

---

[1] Notice that, for $p\in(0,1)$, L_p is a complete metric space with the metric $\varrho(f,g) = \int |f(e^{i\theta})-g(e^{i\theta})|^p d\theta$, and H_p is its closed subspace (see, for example, DUREN [1], p. 37).

<u>Proof of Theorem 7.5.</u> The inequality $-nx^{-1/n} < \log x < nx^{1/n}$, which is true for all $x > 0$, shows that the condition $G^{\pm 1} \in L_1$ implies the summability of $\log \det G$. Therefore, Theorem 7.7 can be applied to the matrix function G, which consequently, admits a representation (7.15) with an outer matrix function A. In virtue of equation (7.15), the condition $G \in L_1$ $(G^{-1} \in L_1)$ is equivalent to $A \in L_2$ $(A^{-1} \in L_2)$ Thus, the representation (7.15) yields a factorization of G in L_2. ∎

<u>COROLLARY 7.9.</u> The positively definite matrix function G defined on $\mathbb{T}$ can be factored in L_{p_0} with a zero total index if and only if $G^{\pm 1} \in L_r$, where $r = \frac{1}{2} \max\{p_0, p_0/(p_0-1)\}$.

<u>Proof.</u> If $G^{\pm 1} \in L_r$, then in any case $G^{\pm 1} \in L_1$ and the matrix function G admits a representation (7.15) with $A^{\pm 1} \in H_2$. The inclusion $G \in L_r$ implies that $A \in L_{2r}$ and, consequently, $A \in H_{2r}$. Analogously, it can be verified that $A^{-1} \in H_{2r}$, i.e., (7.15) is also a factorization of G for all $p \in [2r/(2r-1), 2r]$ and, in particular, for $p = p_0$.

Conversely, let the matrix function G be factorable in L_{p_0} with a zero total index. Then $\mathfrak{F}_0(G)$ is not empty and, thus, $2 \in \mathfrak{F}_0(G)$ as mentioned in Corollary 7.3. Owing to Theorem 7.2, the component $\mathfrak{F}_0(G)$ contains along with the point p_0 the point $q_0 = p_0/(p_0-1)$. As was shown at the beginning of the present section, a factorization of the matrix function G in L_2 may be chosen in the form (7.15). Thanks to Corollary 2.2, it will also be a factorization of G in all L_p for $p \in \mathfrak{F}_0(G)$, especially, for $p = p_0$ and $p = q_0$. From this the inclusion $A^{\pm 1} \in H_{2r}$ and thus $G^{\pm 1} \in L_r$ results. ∎

Corollary 7.9 illustrates that every connected subset of the ray $(1,\infty)$ which, under the mapping $p \to p/(p-1)$, is transferred into itself, is a component of the factorability domain corresponding to the zero total index of a certain positively definite matrix function defined on $\mathbb{T}$.

7.4. CRITERIA FOR EXISTENCE OF Φ-FACTORIZATION AND COINCIDENCE OF PARTIAL INDICES ASSOCIATED WITH THE BEHAVIOUR OF THE NUMERICAL DOMAIN

For the factorization problem on the circle the results of Sections 6.3 - 6.5 enable for being made more precise. One of the reasons guaranteeing these strengthenings is the exact equation

$$\|S\|_{L_p^n} = \operatorname{ctg} \frac{\pi}{2 \max(p,q)} \tag{7.18}$$

for the norm of the operator S in the space L_p^n proved in VERBITSKIĬ, KRUPNIK [1], KRUPNIK [4]. In view of relation (7.18), the lower estimate $2\|S\|/(1+\|S\|^2)$ for the quantity $\delta_{p,n}(\Gamma)$ from assertion 1) of Lemma 6.2 coincides, for $\Gamma = \mathbb{T}$, with its upper estimate $\sin(\pi/\max(p,q))$. Consequently, the equations

$$\delta_{p,n}(\mathbb{T}) = \sin \frac{\pi}{\max(p,q)}, \quad \delta_n(\mathbb{T}) = 1 \tag{7.19}$$

are true, which allows us to give the formulations of the statements from 6.3 - 6.5 a more concrete form.

In particular, Lemma 6.4 (and its strengthening, Lemma 6.4') can, for $p = 2$, be reformulated in the following manner.

THEOREM 7.8. Let G ($\in L_\infty$) be a matrix function with a uniformly positive real part, i.e., the value $d(G(t))$ in Definition 6.3 is bounded from below a.e. on $\mathbb{T}$ by a positive constant which does not depend on t. Then G is Φ-factorable in L_2 and all its partial 2-indices are equal to zero.

From Theorem 7.8 we can easily derive the analogue of Theorem 7.5 related to the special case when $G^{\pm 1} \in L_\infty$, which is of particular interest. To be more exact, the following result is true.

THEOREM 7.9. Let $G \in L_\infty$ be a positively definite matrix function. The domain of Φ-factorability of G is either empty (if $G^{-1} \notin L_\infty$) or consists of the only component $\Phi_0(G)$ filling up the whole ray $(1,\infty)$ (if $G^{-1} \in L_\infty$). In the latter case the matrix function G admits a representation (7.15) in which $A^{\pm 1} \in H_\infty$.

Proof. The necessity of the condition $G^{-1} \in L_\infty$ for the set $\Phi(G)$ to be non-empty is of a general character and has already been proved in Chapter 3 (Corollary 3.5). Now we assume that this condition is fulfilled. For a positively definite matrix function G, the value $d(G(t))$ is the smallest eigenvalue of the matrix $G(t)$. Hence, it coincides with $\|G(t)^{-1}\|^{-1}$. Consequently, the condition $G^{-1} \in L_\infty$ allows us to apply Theorem 7.8 to the matrix function G. According to this theorem, there exists a factorization of G in L_2. But then, as was pointed out at the beginning of Section 7.3, there exists also a representation of G in the form (7.15) with an outer matrix function A. From the relations $G^{\pm 1} \in L_\infty$ we deduce that $A^{\pm 1} \in H_\infty$. Therefore, the representation (7.15) is a Φ-factorization of the matrix function G in all L_p, $1 < p < \infty$ and, thus, $\Phi_0(G) = (1,\infty)$, which completes the proof of Theorem 7.9. ≡

Theorem 7.9, which is specific for the circle, is the second circumstance (after equations (7.19)) which permits us to make the results of the preceding chapter more precise. Now we are going to show how the assertion of Corollary 6.4 (after substitution of the set of eigenvalues by the numerical domain) can be transferred from unitary matrix functions to arbitrary ones with the aid of this theorem as well as Theorem 6.10.

THEOREM 7.10. Let the matrix function $F \in L_\infty$ defined on $\mathbf{T}$ have the property: for every point $t \in \mathbf{T}$ there exists an arc γ_t ($\ni t$) of the contour $\mathbf{T}$, a scalar $\varepsilon_t > 0$ and a sector S_t with vertex at the origin of apex angle $\alpha_t < 2\pi/\max(p,q)$ $(q=p/(p-1))$ such that $h(F(\tau)) \geq \varepsilon_t$ and $H(F(\tau)) \subseteq S_t$ a.e. on γ_t. Then the interval with the end points p and q lies entirely inside a certain component of the Φ-factorability domain of the matrix function F and all partial p-indices of F are equal to each other.

Proof. Arguing as in the proof of Theorem 6.10, we establish the existence of a continuous and non-vanishing function χ such that $F = \chi G$, where G is a matrix function the numerical domain of which is contained in the sector $S_\alpha = \{z : |\arg z| \leq \alpha/2\}$ a.e. on $\mathbf{T}$, $\alpha < 2\pi/\max(p,q)$ and $h(G(\tau)) \geq \varepsilon > 0$ a.e. on $\mathbf{T}$. Since $H(G(\tau))$ lies outside the disk of radius ε with centre at 0 and in the sector S_α, we conclude that $H(G(\tau))$ is located to the right of the vertical line passing through the point $(\varepsilon \cos \frac{\alpha}{2}, 0)$. Consequently, a.e. on $\mathbb{T}$ we have $d(G(\tau)) \geq \varepsilon \cos \alpha/2$, so that Theorem 7.9 may be applied to the matrix function $M = \mathrm{Re}\, G$. Owing to this theorem, $M = M_+ M_+^*$, where $M_+^{\pm 1} \in H_\infty$. Denoting $K = \mathrm{im}\, G$, we obtain $G = M + iK = M_+ M_+^* + iK = M_+(I + iM_+^{-1} K (M_+^*)^{-1}) M_+^* = M_+(I+iN)M_+^*$, where $N = M_+^{-1} K (M_+^*)^{-1}$. The matrix function N is Hermitian together with K. Since $H(G(\tau)) \subseteq S_\alpha$, then $|(K(\tau)x,x)| \leq \mathrm{tg} \frac{\alpha}{2} \|M_+^*(\tau)x\|^2$. Denoting $M_+^*(\tau)x$ by y and using the equation $(K(\tau)x,x) = (M_+(\tau)N(\tau)M_+^*(\tau)x,x) = (N(\tau)y,y)$, we find that $|(N(\tau)y,y)| \leq \mathrm{tg} \frac{\alpha}{2} \|y\|^2$. This means that the numerical domain of the matrix $N(\tau)$ is situated on the interval $[-\mathrm{tg} \frac{\alpha}{2}, \mathrm{tg} \frac{\alpha}{2}]$ a.e. on $\mathbb{T}$. Consequently, the numerical domain of the matrix $I + iN(\tau)$ is located on the interval which connects the points $1 - i \cdot \mathrm{tg} \frac{\alpha}{2}$ and $1 + i \cdot \mathrm{tg} \frac{\alpha}{2}$. This interval lies in the disk with centre at the point $(\sec^2 \frac{\alpha}{2}, 0)$ of radius $\sin(\alpha/2)/(\cos^2(\alpha/2))$, which is visible from the origin at the angle α. In addition, the matrix $I + iN(\tau)$ is obviously normal. Therefore, Theorem 6.10 can be applied to the matrix function $I + iN$. Due to this theorem, the interval A_p with the end points p and q lies entirely in a certain component of the domain of Φ-factorability and all partial indices are equal to each other. Since the interval A_p passes through the point 2 and the matrix function $I + iN$ has a uniformly positive real part, we may claim that, according to Theorem 7.8, all its partial 2-indices are equal to zero. Consequently $A_p \subseteq \Phi_0(I+iN)$. Apparently, this implies that $A_p \subseteq \Phi_0(G)$ and all partial r-indices of G, $r \in A_p$, are equal to zero. Utilizing Lemma 6.3, we conclude that the interval A_p lies inside a certain component of the domain of Φ-factorability of the matrix function F and all partial r-indices $(r \in A_p)$ of F are equal to each other. ≡

Theorem 7.10 is an essential generalization of Theorem 6.10, because the sector S_t contains the disk Δ_t and the rigorous requirement of normality is no longer imposed upon the matrix $F(t)$ in Theorem 7.10. Moreover, Theorem 7.10 generalizes Theorem 6.11', too. In fact, under the condition of Theorem 6.11', the sets $\|F(\tau)\|^{-1} H(F(\tau))$, $\tau \in \gamma_t$ are separated from zero by the straight line l_t which is distant from zero by more than $\cos(\pi/2\max(p,q))$. At the same time, these sets are concentrated in the unit disk, as the numerical domain of an arbitrary matrix A lies in the disk with centre at zero and radius $\|A\|$. Thus, the sets $\|F(\tau)\|^{-1}H(F(\tau))$ are located in the circular segment which is cut off from the unit disk by the line l_t, and this segment may be inscribed into a sector S_t the apex angle of which satisfies the restrictions of Theorem 7.10. Consequently, the numerical domain of all matrices $F(\tau)$, $\tau \in \gamma_t$ lie in the same sector, i.e., the conditions of Theorem 7.10 are fulfilled for the matrix function F.

For $p = 2$, however, Theorem 7.10 is equivalent to Theorem 6.11' reformulated with regard to equations (7.19). This reformulation looks as follows.

<u>THEOREM 7.11.</u> Assume the matrix function F of class L_∞ defined on $\mathbb{T}$ to be such that, for every point $t \in \mathbb{T}$, there exist an arc γ_t ($\ni t$) and a straight line l_t which does not pass through zero and has the following property: for almost all $\tau \in \gamma_t$, the set $H(F(\tau))$ is separated from zero by l_t. Then the matrix function G is Φ-factorable in L_2 and all its partial 2-indices are equal to each other.

Finally, note that, as also in Section 6.4, under the conditions of Theorem 7.8 - 7.11, there exists not only a left but also a right Φ-factorization of the matric function G (and F), where the right partial indices coincide with the left ones and with each other.

7.5. DEFINITENESS CRITERIA AND STABILITY OF PARTIAL INDICES OF BOUNDED MEASURABLE MATRIX FUNCTIONS

One more circumstance (besides equations (7.19) and Theorem 7.9) thanks to which, ultimately, we succeed in proving assertions converse to Theorems 6.6 - 6.9 for $p = 2$, is the existence of exact formulae for the norms of the operators QGP and PGQ in the case $\Gamma = \mathbb{T}$.

<u>LEMMA 7.3.</u> Let G be a matrix function from L_∞ defined on $\mathbb{T}$. The norms of the operators QGP and PGQ in the space L_2^n are calculated by the formulae

$$\|QGP\| = \min_{X\in H_\infty^+} \|G-X\| , \quad \|PGQ\| = \min_{Y\in H_\infty^-} \|G-Y\| . \tag{7.20}$$

<u>Proof.</u> We shall consider the spaces L_1 and L_2 of $n\times n$ matrix functions as Banach spaces the norm in which is defined by the formulae

$$\|A\|_1 = \frac{1}{2\pi} \int \operatorname{tr}(A(e^{i\theta})A(e^{i\theta})^*)^{1/2}d\theta$$

and

$$\|A\|_2 = (\frac{1}{2\pi} \int \operatorname{tr} A(e^{i\theta})A(e^{i\theta})^* d\theta)^{1/2} ,$$

respectively.

The space dual to L_1 may be identified with the space of measurable essentially bounded matrix functions (supplied with the norm (3.19)) by assigning to the matrix function $G \in L_\infty$ the functional

$$\psi_G(A) = \frac{1}{2\pi} \int \operatorname{tr} A(e^{i\theta})G(e^{i\theta})^* d\theta . \tag{7.21}$$

With regard to the mentioned correspondence the subspace H_∞^- is an orthogonal complement to the subspace $\overset{\circ}{H}{}_1^+$ of those $n\times n$ matrix functions from H_1^+ which vanish at zero.

The space L_2 supplied with the scalar product

$$(A,B) = \frac{1}{2\pi} \int \operatorname{tr}(A(e^{i\theta})B(e^{i\theta})^*)d\theta$$

becomes a Hilbert space, where for all $A,B \in L_2$, $\|AB\|_1 \le \|A\|_2\|B\|_2$.

In this way, the set of matrix functions of the form

$$F = AB \tag{7.22}$$

with $A,B\in H_2^+$, $\|A\|_2$, $\|B\|_2 < 1$ lies in the open unit ball of the subspace H_1^+ of the space L_1 . Let us show that it is dense in this ball.

For this purpose, above all, note that an arbitrary matrix function $F \in H_1^+$, $\|F\|_1 < 1$ for which $\log|\det F| \in L_1$ admits a representation (7.22). Indeed, in this case the matrix function $(FF^*)^{1/2}$ satisfies the conditions of Theorem 7.7. Thus, $(FF^*)^{1/2} = AA^*$, where $A \in H_2^+$ is an outer matrix function. Besides,

$$\|A\|_2^2 = \frac{1}{2\pi} \int \operatorname{tr} A(e^{i\theta})A(e^{i\theta})^* d\theta = \frac{1}{2\pi} \int \operatorname{tr}(F(e^{i\theta})F(e^{i\theta})^*)^{1/2}d\theta$$

$$= \|F\|_1 < 1 .$$

In order to satisfy (7.22), we set $B = A^{-1}F$. Since

$$\|B\|_2^2 = \frac{1}{2\pi} \int tr(B(e^{i\theta})B(e^{i\theta})^*)d\theta$$

$$= \frac{1}{2\pi} \int tr(A(e^{i\theta})^{-1}F(e^{i\theta})F(e^{i\theta})^*(A(e^{i\theta})^*)^{-1})d\theta$$

$$= \frac{1}{2\pi} \int tr(A(e^{i\theta})^*A(e^{i\theta}))d\theta$$

$$= \frac{1}{2\pi} \int tr(A(e^{i\theta})A(e^{i\theta})^*)d\theta$$

$$= \|F\|_1 < 1 ,$$

the matrix function B is situated in the open unit ball of the space L_2 . Furthermore, since B is of class D , then it also lies in the open unit ball of the space H_2^+ . Hence the desired representation has been constructed.

In turn, the set of matrix functions $F \in H_1^+$, $\|F\|_1 < 1$ for which $\log|\det F| < L_1$ is dense in the unit ball of H_1^+ . In fact, with the aid of an arbitrarily small perturbation of the matrix function F we may guarantee that $\det F(0) \neq 0$. Applying now Jensen's inequality (GOLUZIN [1], PRIVALOV [2]) to the function $\det F(\in H_{1/n}^+)$, we get

$$\frac{1}{2\pi} \int \log|\det F(e^{i\theta})|\,d\theta \geq \log|\det F(0)| > -\infty .$$

Multiplying the matrix functions F and B by $e^{i\theta}$, it can easily be seen that the set of matrix functions of the form AB with $A \in H_2^+$, $B \in \overset{\circ}{H}{}_2^+$, $\|A\|_2$, $\|B\|_2 < 1$ is dense in the ball $\{F \in \overset{\circ}{H}{}_1^+ : \|F\|_1 < 1\}$.

Now we intend to show that the norm of the operator PGQ in L_2^n coincides with the norm of the functional ψ_G defined by formula (7.21) on $\overset{\circ}{H}{}_1^+$.

By the very definition,

$$\|\psi_G|_{\overset{\circ}{H}{}_1^+}\| = \sup\{\frac{1}{2\pi} \int tr(F(e^{i\theta})G(e^{i\theta})^*)d\theta : \|F\|_1 < 1 , F \in \overset{\circ}{H}{}_1^+\} ,$$

where sup may be taken not over the whole of the unit ball, but only over its dense subset consisting of matrix functions of the form $F_1F_2^*$ with $\|F_j\|_2 < 1$ $(j=1,2)$, $F_1 \in H_2^+$, $F_2 \in \overset{\circ}{H}{}_2^-$. At the same time,

$$\frac{1}{2\pi}\int \operatorname{tr}(F_1(e^{i\theta})F_2(e^{i\theta})^*G(e^{i\theta})^*)d\theta$$

$$= \frac{1}{2\pi}\int \operatorname{tr}(F_2(e^{i\theta})^*G(e^{i\theta})^*F_1(e^{i\theta}))d\theta$$

$$= \frac{1}{2\pi}\int \operatorname{tr}((G(e^{i\theta})F_2(e^{i\theta}))^*F_1(e^{i\theta}))d\theta$$

$$= \frac{1}{2\pi} \operatorname{tr}\int (G(e^{i\theta})F_2(e^{i\theta}))^*F_1(e^{i\theta})d\theta .$$

Denoting the columns of the matrix functions F_j by $f_1^{(j)},\dots,f_n^{(j)}$ $(j=1,2)$, instead of $\int (G(e^{i\theta})F_2(e^{i\theta}))^*F_1(e^{i\theta})d\theta$ we may write the matrix the (i,k) th entry of which is the scalar product (in L_2^n) of $f_k^{(1)}$ and $Gf_i^{(2)}$. Therefore

$$\frac{1}{2\pi} \operatorname{tr}\int (G(e^{i\theta})F_2(e^{i\theta}))^*F_1(e^{i\theta})d\theta = \frac{1}{2\pi}\sum_{k=1}^{n}(f_k^{(1)},Gf_k^{(2)})$$

$$= \frac{1}{2\pi}\sum_{k=1}^{n}(f_k^{(1)},PGQf_k^{(2)}) .$$

The condition $\|F_j\|_2 < 1$ is equivalent to the inequality

$\frac{1}{2\pi}\sum_{k=1}^{n}\|f_k^{(j)}\|^2 < 1 \quad (j=1,2).$

Thus, it only remains to note that, under the conditions

$\frac{1}{2\pi}\sum_{k=1}^{n}\|f_k^{(j)}\|^2 < 1 \quad (j=1,2)$, $f_k^{(1)}\in(H_2^+)^n$, $f_k^{(2)}\in(\overset{\circ}{H}{}_2^-)^n$, the value

$\frac{1}{2\pi}\sup\sum_{k=1}^{n}(f_k^{(1)}, PGQf_k^{(2)})$ is equal to $\|PGQ\|$.

Summarizing, $\|PGQ\| = \|\psi_G|_{\overset{\circ}{H}{}_1^+}\|$. An arbitrary extension of the functional $\psi_G|_{H_1^+}$ to the whole space L_1 is of the form ψ_{G_1} . Besides, since $\psi_G(F) = \psi_{G_1}(F)$ for all $F \in \overset{\circ}{H}{}_1^+$, then $G-G_1 \in H_\infty^-$, i.e., $G_1 = G-Y$ with $Y \in H_\infty^-$. Conversely, for any $Y \in H_\infty^-$, the functional ψ_{G-Y} is an extension of the functional $\psi_G|_{\overset{\circ}{H}{}_1^+}$. Using the fact that in extending a functional the norm does not decrease, we recognize that $\|PGQ\| \le \|\psi_{G-Y}\| = \|G-Y\|$ for all $Y \in H_\infty^-$. At the same time, due to the Hahn-Banach theorem, there exists a[illegible]nsion which preserves the norm. This proves the second of the formu[illegible] (7.20).

[U]tilizing the fact that QGP is an operator adjoint to PG^*Q , so that

$$\|QGP\| = \|PG^*G\| = \min_{Y\in H_\infty^-}\|G^*-Y\| = \min_{X\in H_\infty^+}\|G^*-X^*\| = \min_{X\in H_\infty^+}\|G-X\| ,$$

the first formula may be readily derived from the second one. Thus, the proof of Lemma 7.3 is complete. ≡

The criterion of non-negativity (non-positivity) of partial 2-indices, first of all, will be proved for unitary matrix functions. Above all, this is caused by the fact that the proof of the corresponding criterion for arbitrary matrix functions employs the statement related to unitary matrix functions as an auxiliary result. However, there are, in addition, two more important reasons: 1) for unitary matrix functions the definiteness criterion for partial indices can be formulated in the most transparent form, revealing the relationships between the structure of the set of partial indices and the approximation properties of matrix functions, and 2) matrix functions occurring in applied problems are often unitary (see, for instance, KREĬN, MELIK-ADAMYAN [1], TROITSKIĬ [1]).

THEOREM 7.12. Let U be a unitary matrix function defined on $\mathbf{T}$. The operator $P+UQ$ is invertible from the right (left) in L_2^n if and only if there exists a matrix function $X \in H_\infty^+$ (H_∞^-) such that

$$\|U - X\| < 1 . \tag{7.23}$$

Proof. Owing to assertion 1) of Lemma 3.5, the operator $P+UQ$ is invertible from the right only simultaneously with the operator $T_Q(U)$, which, in turn, is invertible from the right only simultaneously with the operator $P+QUQ$. The latter is invertible from the right if and only if the operator

$$\begin{aligned}(P+QUQ)(P+QUQ)^* &= (P+QUQ)(P+QU^*Q) = P+QUQU^*Q = P+QUU^*Q-QUPU^*Q \\ &= P+Q-(QUP)(PU^*Q) = I-(QUP)(QUP)^*\end{aligned}$$

is invertible [1]. Since $\|QUP\| \le \|U\| = 1$, then for the invertibility of this operator, it is necessary and sufficient that $\|QUP\| < 1$. It remains to apply the first of the formulae (7.20). The case of invertibility from the left can be regarded analogously. Thus Theorem 7.12 is proved. ≡

[1] Here we used the fact that a linear bounded operator T acting in a Hilbert space is invertible from the right if and only if the operator TT^* is invertible.

THEOREM 7.13. Assume that U is a unitary matrix function defined on $\mathbb{T}$. Then the following assertions are equivalent:

1) U is Φ-factorable in L_2 and all its partial indices are non-negative (non-positive),

2) there exists a matrix function $X \in H_\infty^+$ (H_∞^-) such that $X^{-1} \in M_\infty^+$ (M_∞^-) and $\|U-X\| < 1$,

3) there exists a matrix function $Y \in M_\infty^-$ (M_∞^+) such that $Y^{-1} \in H_\infty^-$ (H_∞^+) and $\|U-Y\| < 1$.

In this case the total index of U coincides with the number of zeros of $\det X$ inside the unit disk and with the number of poles of $\det Y$ outside it.

Proof. We shall conduct the proof for the case of non-negative partial indices. Since, for any matrix function $X \in L_\infty$,

$$\|U - X\| = \|I - XU^*\| , \tag{7.24}$$

then the inequality (7.23) guarantees the applicability of assertion 2) from Theorem 6.6 to the matrix function U^* (with $X_+ = X$, $X_- = I$), according to which this matrix function is Φ-factorable in L_2 and its partial indices are non-positive. In view of Corollary 7.1, from here we deduce the Φ-factorability in L_2 of the matrix function U as well as the non-negativity of its partial indices. Thus, 2) implies 1).

Now we are going to prove that 1) implies 2). From the Φ-factorability of the matrix function U and the non-negativity of its partial indices we conclude that the operator $P + UQ$ is invertible from the right (Corollary 3.8). By Theorem 7.12, there exists a matrix function $X \in H_\infty^+$ satisfying the inequality (7.23). We want to show that $X^{-1} \in M_\infty^+$ and calculate the total index of U. To this end, we shall employ the equation $T_Q(XU^*) = QXU^*|_{(\mathring{H}_2^-)^n} = QXQU^*|_{(\mathring{H}_2^-)^n} + QXPU^*|_{(\mathring{H}_2^-)^n} = T_Q(X)T_Q(U^*)$, which holds because of $QXP = 0$. As follows from relations (7.23) and (7.24), the operator $T_Q(XU)$ is invertible. Due to Corollary 1.2, the operator $T_Q(U^*) = T_Q(U)^*$ is Fredholm simultaneously with the operator $T_Q(U)$. Consequently (see Theorem 1.9), the operator $T_Q(X)$ is also Fredholm and its index is opposite to the index of $T_Q(U^*)$ and, thus, coincides with the index of the operator $T_Q(U)$. On the strength of Theorem 3.15 we conclude from the Φ-factorability of the matrix function $X \in H_\infty^+$ that $X^{-1} \in M_\infty^+$ and, due to Theorem 2.6, the total index of X (i.e., the index of the operator $T_Q(X)$) coincides with the number of zeros of $\det X$ in the unit disk. Thus, the equivalence of assertions 1) and 2) as well as the validity of one of the formulae for the total index U have been proved. The equivalence of assertions 1) and 3) and the second formula for the total index can be established in a similar way. ≡

<u>COROLLARY 7.10.</u> Assume U to be a unitary matrix function defined on $\mathbb{T}$. The following assertions are equivalent:

1) U is Φ-factorable in L_2 and all its partial indices are equal to zero,

2) there exists a matrix function $X \in H_\infty^+$ such that $X^{-1} \in H_\infty^+$ and $\|X-U\| < 1$,

3) there exists a matrix function $X \in H_\infty^-$ such that $X^{-1} \in H_\infty^-$ and $\|X-U\| < 1$.

The transition from unitary matrix functions to arbitrary matrix functions of class L_∞ may be accomplished with the aid of the following auxiliary result.

<u>LEMMA 7.4.</u> Let the matrix function G given on $\mathbb{T}$ satisfy the condition $G^{\pm 1} \in L_\infty$. Then it can be represented in the form

$$G = AU\,, \tag{7.25}$$

but also as

$$G = VB^*\,, \tag{7.25'}$$

where $A^{\pm 1}, B^{\pm 1} \in H_\infty$ and the matrix functions U and V are unitary.

<u>Proof.</u> The matrix functions GG^* and G^*G meet the conditions of Theorem 7.9. Therefore, the equations $GG^* = AA^*$, $G^*G = BB^*$ with $A^{\pm 1}, B^{\pm 1} \in H_\infty$ are valid. Setting $U = A^{-1}G$, $V = G(B^*)^{-1}$, we may guarantee that relations (7.25) and (7.25') are fulfilled. Thus we are only obliged to check that the matrix functions U and V are unitary:

$$U(t)U(t)^* = A(t)^{-1}G(t)G(t)^*(A(t)^*)^{-1} = A(t)^{-1}A(t)A(t)^*(A(t)^*)^{-1} = I$$

a.e. on $\mathbb{T}$. The unitarity of the matrix $V(t)$ can analogously be verified. ≡

Equations (7.25) and (7.25') mean that the matrix functions G, U and V are factorable (Φ-factorable) only simultaneously, where the tuples of their partial indices coincide.

Now, finally, we are prepared for proving the existence criterion for a Φ-factorization in L_2 with definite partial indices.

THEOREM 7.14. For a matrix function $G \in L_\infty$ defined on $\mathbb{T}$, the following statements are equivalent:

1) $2 \in \Phi(G)$ and all partial indices of G are non-negative,
2) there exists a matrix function $X_- \in H_\infty^-$ such that $X_-^{-1} \in M_\infty^-$ and $\|I-GX_-\| < 1$,
3) there exists a matrix function $X_+ \in M_\infty^+$ such that $X_+^{-1} \in H_\infty^+$ and $\|I-X_+G\| < 1$,
4) $G = Y_+G_0$, where $Y_+ \in H_\infty^+$, $Y_+^{-1} \in M_\infty^+$, $d(G_0(t)) \geq d > 0$ a.e. on $\mathbb{T}$,
5) $G = G_0Y_-$, where $Y_- \in M_\infty^-$, $Y_-^{-1} \in H_\infty^-$, $d(G_0(t)) \geq d > 0$ a.e. on $\mathbb{T}$.

If these conditions hold, then the total index of the matrix function G coincides with the number of poles of $\det X_+$ and with the number of zeros of $\det Y_+$ in the unit disk, but also with the number auf zeros of $\det X_-$ and the number of poles of $\det Y_-$ outside the unit disk.

Proof. The implications 2) ==> 1) and 3) ==> 1) are special cases of statement 1) from Theorem 6.6. If 1) is fulfilled, then due to Corollary 3.4, $G^{-1} \in L_\infty$. Thus, Lemma 7.4 can be applied. The unitary matrix function V defined in this lemma is Φ-factorable in L_2 together with G and its partial indices are non-negative. According to Theorem 7.13, there exists a matrix function $X \in H_\infty^+$ such that $X^{-1} \in M_\infty^+$ and $\|V-X\| < 1$. Setting $X_- = (XB^{-1})^*$, where B is the matrix function

from representation (7.25'), we get $X_- \in H_\infty^-$, $X_-^{-1} \in M_\infty^-$ and
$\|I-GX_-\| = \|I-VB^*(B^*)^{-1}X^*\| = \|I-VX^*\| = \|V^*-X^*\| = \|V-X\|$.
Therefore, 1) ==> 2).
In order to verify the implication 1) ==> 3), we introduce the matrix function U from representation (7.25) and a matrix function $Y \in M_\infty^-$ such that $Y^{-1} \in H_\infty^-$, $\|U-Y\| < 1$ existing by Theorem 7.13. Furthermore, we set $X_+ = Y^*A^{-1}$. Then $X_+ \in M_\infty^+$, $X_+^{-1} = A(Y^*)^{-1} \in H_\infty^+$ and
$\|I-X_+G\| = \|I-Y^*A^{-1}AU\| = \|I-Y^*U\| = \|U^*-Y^*\| = \|U-Y\| < 1$.

In this way, we have checked that statements 1), 2) and 3) are equivalent. Now we want to show the equivalence of assertions 2) and 5).
If 2) is true, then the matrix function GX_- has a uniformly positive real part, because $\operatorname{Re}(GX_-x,x) = (x,x) - \operatorname{Re}((I-GX_-)x,x) \geq (1-\|I-GX_-\|)\|x\|^2$.
Setting $Y_- = X_-^{-1}$, we conclude that 2) ==> 5). Conversely, if 5) is fulfilled, then the condition $\|I-GX_-\| < 1$ is satisfied for $X_- = \mu Y_-^{-1}$, where μ is some positive constant (concerning the choice of μ, see the proof of Lemma 6.4). Thus, 2) ==> 5). The implication 3) ==> 4) can be verified analogously.

The formulae for the total index established in the theorem can be proved in just the same way as in Theorem 7.13. Thus, the proof of Theorem 7.14 is complete. ≡

COROLLARY 7.11. For the matrix function $G \in L_\infty$ given on $\mathbb{T}$, the following statements are equivalent:

1) $2 \in \Phi(G)$ and all partial indices of G are equal to zero,
2) there is a matrix function $X_+ \in H_\infty^+$ such that $X_+^{-1} \in H_\infty^+$ and $\|I-X_+G\| < 1$,
3) there is a matrix function $X_- \in H_\infty^-$ such that $X_-^{-1} \in H_\infty^-$ and $\|I-GX_-\| < 1$,
4) $G = Y_+G_0$, where $Y_+^{\pm 1} \in H_\infty^+$, $d(G_0(t)) \geq d > 0$ a.e. on $\mathbb{T}$,
5) $G = G_0Y_-$, where $Y_-^{\pm 1} \in H_\infty^-$, $d(G_0(t)) \geq d > 0$ a.e. on $\mathbb{T}$.

In this way, statements 1) and 3) of Theorem 6.6 as well as Lemma 6.4 admit an inversion for the factorization problem in L_2 on $\mathbb{T}$.

Apparently, the correctness of the inversion of Theorem 6.7 - 6.9 and of the remaining statements of Theorem 6.6 may be proved in a similar manner. In this case one of the matrix functions by which the matrix function G in the formulations of the indicated theorems is multiplied may be chosen to be the identity.

In summary, for the Φ-factorization problem in the space L_2 on $\mathbb{T}$ we have derived criteria of non-negativity, non-positivity, and equality to zero of partial indices. In view of its particular importance we now still want to formulate the criterion of stability.

THEOREM 7.15. The matrix function $G \in L_\infty$ given on $\mathbb{T}$ is Φ-factorable in L_2 with a stable tuple of partial indices if and only if one can find an integer k and matrix functions $X_+ \in H_\infty^{\pm}$ such that $X_{\pm}^{-1} \in M_\infty^{\pm}$ and $\|I-t^{-k}GX_-\| < 1$, $\|I-t^{-k-1}X_+G\| < 1$.

7.6. ON PARTIAL INDICES OF CONTINUOUS MATRIX FUNCTIONS

In Chapter 6 we have already used the fact that the additional assumption $G \in L_\infty^{\pm} + C$ excludes the dependence of the Φ-factorability property and the values of partial indices on the parameter value p. In this way, for $G \in L_\infty^{\pm} + C$, Theorems 7.14, 7.15 and Corollary 7.11 proved above for the factorization in L_2 pass into criteria of non-negativity, stability and equality to zero of partial indices related to factorization in arbitrary L_p , $1 < p < \infty$. In particular, this remark applies to continuous matrix functions G .

Supposing the requirement of factorability in C (which is stronger than the condition $G^{\pm 1} \in C$) to be fulfilled, it seems that we may go even further. Namely, one can claim that the conditions of non-negativity (non-positivity, equality to zero, stability) of partial indices mentioned in Section 6.5 will remain necessary even in case the additional demand of rationality is imposed upon the matrix functions $X_{\pm}$, $Y_{\pm}$ involved in them. It should be noted that in this case the proof of necessity is not based on the sophisticated Lemma 7.3. Now we are going to present the exact formulation and the proof for the situation when the partial indices are equal to zero.

THEOREM 7.16. Assume the matrix function G defined on $\mathbb{T}$ to be factorable in C and all of its partial indices to be equal to zero. Then there can be found polynomial matrix functions X_1 and X_2 whose zeros of the determinant lie outside the unit disk and such that

$$\|I - X_1 G\| < 1 \ , \ \|I - GX_2^*\| < 1 \ . \tag{7.26}$$

Proof. By assumption, the factorization of the matrix function G is of the form $G = AB^*$, where $A_-^{\pm 1}$, $B_-^{\pm 1} \in C^+$. Therefore, the matrix functions $Y_1 = \mu BA^{-1}$ and $Y_2 = \mu AB^{-1}$ also belong to C^+ and are non-degenerate in the unit disk for arbitrarily chosen $\mu \neq 0$. Since $I - Y_1 G = I - \mu BB^*$, $I - GY_2^* = I - \mu AA^*$, then choosing μ from the interval $(0, \min\{\|A\|^{-2}, \|B\|^{-2}\})$, we may ensure the validity of the inequalities $\|I - Y_1 G\| < 1$, $\|I - GY_2^*\| < 1$. The condition $Y_{1,2} \in C^+$ enables us to uniformly approximate the matrix functions $Y_{1,2}$ by matrix polynomials with arbitrary degree of accuracy. Choosing as $X_{1,2}$ matrix polynomials sufficiently close to $Y_{1,2}$ we may guarantee both the validity of inequality (7.26) and the non-degeneracy of $X_{1,2}$ in the unit disk, which proves Theorem 7.16. ≡

Finally, we intend to present a proposition which is obtained from Theorem 7.11 under the additional requirement of continuity of the matrix function G.

THEOREM 7.17. The partial indices of a continuous strictly non-degenerate matrix function are equal to each other.

Proof. With regard to Definition 6.3 the condition $0 \notin H(G(t))$ is fulfilled for all $t \in \mathbb{T}$. Owing to the convexity of the numerical domain, we may claim that there exists a straight line l_t separating $H(G(t))$ from zero. As the matrix function G is continuous, the straight line l_t will separate from zero also all the sets $H(G(\tau))$ with τ close enough to t. In this way, the conditions of Theorem 7.11 are satisfied. Due to this theorem, the partial indices of G (coinciding with its partial 2-indices) are equal to each other, which proves Theorem 7.17. ≡

<u>COROLLARY 7.12.</u> Suppose the matrix function G is continuous on $\mathbb{T}$ and for all $t \in \mathbb{T}$ G(t) is normal, and the convex hull of the spectrum of G(t) does not contain zero. Then the partial indices of G are equal to each other.

The assertion of the corollary is correct, because the numerical domain of a normal matrix coincides with the convex hull of the spectrum. In particular, if G is a unitary matrix function, then G(t) is, for all $t \in \mathbb{T}$, a normal matrix with a spectrum concentrated on the unit circle. Therefore the following statement is true.

<u>COROLLARY 7.13.</u> If U is a unitary matrix function continuous on $\mathbb{T}$ whose eigenvalues, for any $t \in \mathbb{T}$, are concentrated on an arc of the circle the end points of which are seen at an angle less than π, then all partial indices of U coincide.

<u>COROLLARY 7.14.</u> Assume G to be a continuous second-order matrix function given on $\mathbb{T}$, where, for all $t \in \mathbb{T}$, G(t) is a normal matrix with eigenvalues $\lambda_1(t)$ and $\lambda_2(t)$. For the coincidence of the partial indices of G, it is sufficient for the quotient $\lambda_1(t)/\lambda_2(t)$ to be non-negative for any $t \in \mathbb{T}$.

Indeed, the numerical domain of the matrix function G(t) is an interval with the end points $\lambda_1(t)$ and $\lambda_2(t)$. The condition imposed on $\lambda_1(t)/\lambda_2(t)$ just means that this interval does not contain the zero point.

Incidentally, the structure of the numerical domain for second-order matrices can be easily described, even if they fail to be normal (HALMOS [1]). Namely, if λ_1 and λ_2 are eigenvalues of the second-order matrix A and x_1 and x_2 are normed eigenvectors associated with them, then H(A) is an ellipse with focuses λ_1 and λ_2 and a large axis

$$\frac{|\lambda_1-\lambda_2|}{(1-|(x_1,x_2)|^2)^{1/2}},$$

if $\lambda_1 \neq \lambda_2$, and a disk of radius $\frac{1}{2}\|A-\lambda I\|$ and centre λ, if $\lambda_1 = \lambda_2 = \lambda$. From this we derive the next result.

COROLLARY 7.15. Let G be a continuous second-order matrix function. Furthermore, assume that $\lambda_1(t)$ and $\lambda_2(t)$ are the eigenvalues of the matrix $G(t)$ and $x_1(t)$ and $x_2(t)$ the normed eigenvectors associated with them. The following condition is sufficient for the coincidence of partial indices of G :

$$|\lambda_1(t)| + |\lambda_2(t)| > |\lambda_1(t)-\lambda_2(t)|(1-|x_1(t),x_2(t))|^2)^{-1/2}$$

must hold at those points $t \in \mathbb{T}$ at which $\lambda_1(t) \neq \lambda_2(t)$, and

$$2|\lambda(t)| > \|G(t) - \lambda(t)I\|$$

is valid at those points $t \in \mathbb{T}$ at which $\lambda_1(t) = \lambda_2(t)$ $(= \lambda(t))$.

In connection with Corollary 7.14 the following example is of some significance. Let

$$G(t) = \frac{1}{2}\begin{pmatrix} t^k+t^{-k} & -t^k+t^{-k} \\ t^k-t^{-k} & -t^k-t^{-k} \end{pmatrix},$$

where $k \geq 0$ is integer.

The matrix $G(t)$ is simultaneously Hermitian and unitary, its eigenvalues do not depend on t and are equal to $\lambda_1(t) = 1$ and $\lambda_2(t) = -1$. At the same time,

$$G(t) = \frac{1}{2}\begin{pmatrix} 1 & 1 \\ 1 & -1 \end{pmatrix}\begin{pmatrix} 0 & t^k \\ t^{-k} & 0 \end{pmatrix}\begin{pmatrix} 1 & 1 \\ 1 & -1 \end{pmatrix},$$

so that the partial indices of G are equal to k and $-k$. For $k = 0$, they coincide, although the assumption of Corollary 7.14 is not fulfilled; for $k > 0$, the partial indices of the matrix function G do not coincide. Thus, the sufficient condition for coincidence of partial indices established in Corollary 7.14 is essential but not necessary.

7.7. COMMENTS

The relationship between factorizations of the matrix functions G and G^* in case of Hölder matrix functions mentioned in Theorems 7.1 and 7.1' was established by SHMUL'YAN [2]. Relation (7.5) from Theorem 7.2 for the same case was also proved by him.

Theorem 7.3 and its Corollary 7.5 are given in SPITKOVSKIĬ [6]. Theorem 7.4 and Corollary 7.8 for the case of matrix functions with Hölder elements were proved in NIKOLAĬCHUK, SPITKOVSKIĬ [1,2]; in SPITKOVSKIĬ [7] they were extended to the general case. A special kind of factorization of Hermitian matrix functions with zero partial indices is presented in SHMUL'YAN [2]. Corollary 7.6 is also proved there. Theorem 7.4 may be used for the classification of shifts in a space with indefinite metric in case of a finite-dimensional isotropic subspace (concerning this matter, see the note of one of the authors in the review Referativnyĭ Zhurnal Matematika 1983, 3B, 1001 of the article BALL, HELTON [1], where the inverse way of reasoning was gone: Theorem 7.6 was deduced from results related to shift classification).

A Φ-factorability criterion in L_2 as well as a method for constructing a factorization and calculating partial indices of a Hermitian second-order matrix function with negative determinant and definite diagonal elements are described in LITVINCHUK, SPITKOVSKIĬ [1,2]. In particular, in these papers it is established that the general case of such a matrix function can be reduced to the study of a matrix function of the kind

$$\Omega = \begin{pmatrix} |\omega|^2-1 & \omega \\ \bar{\omega} & 1 \end{pmatrix} \qquad (\omega \in L_\infty) .$$

In this case the matrix function Ω is Φ-factorable if and only if 1 does not belong to the limit spectrum of the operator $H(\omega)H(\omega)^*$ ($H(\omega) = Q\omega P$ is a Hankel operator with the symbol ω) and its partial indices are $\pm\, l$, where l is the multiplicity of 1 as an s-number of the operator $H(\omega)$ (i.e. as an eigenvalue of $H(\omega)H(\omega)^*$).

The proof scheme of Theorem 7.4 given here was used by DIDENKO and CHERNETSKIĬ [1] in studying the factorization problem for orthogonal matrix functions. Namely, in this article it is shown that, for a Hölder orthogonal matrix function G, equations (7.5) are fulfilled and there always exists a factorization (2.1) subjected to the additional conditions $G_+^{\prime}G_+ = G_-G_-^{\prime} = T$, where T is the matrix defined by equation (7.3).

Lemma 7.1 is a result of SZEGŐ (see, e.g., HOFFMAN [1]) obtained by him as a generalization of the Fejer-Riesz lemma which asserts that any trigonometric polynomial non-negative on $\mathbb{T}$ coincides with the square of the modulus of some algebraic polynomial. Lemma 7.2 and Theorem 7.7 are reformulations of an important proposition from the theory of stochastic processes (see, for example, ROZANOV [1]). The extension of this statement to the sectorial case and the history of the problem can be found in KREĬN, SPITKOVSKIĬ [1,2]. In the article KREĬN, SPITKOVSKIĬ [3] the results of the papers just mentioned, in particular, the theorems on factorization of sectorial matrix functions were applied for obtaining generalizations of the Szegö limit theorem. In turn, these generalizations can be used for the discussion of some problems of statistical physics in a similar manner as the corresponding results for the scalar case were used in VLADIMIROV, VOLOVICH [1,2].
We would like to remark that methods and results of factorization theory have been used for extending the Szegö limit theorem before the paper of KREĬN, SPITKOVSKIĬ [3], too. Let us refer, for instance, to one result from WIDOM [3] due to which, for a matrix function F from the class $H_\infty + C$, the left and right partial indices are equal to zero,

$$\lim_{n \to \infty} \frac{\Delta_{n+1}}{\Delta_n} = \lim_{\varrho \to 1} \exp \frac{1}{2\pi} \int_0^{2\pi} \log \det G_\varrho(e^{i\theta})d\theta .$$

Here G_ϱ are the values of the harmonic continuation of G on the circle with radius ϱ (< 1) and Δ_n is the determinant of the block-Toeplitz matrix $(G_{i-j})_{i,j=0}^{\infty}$ constructed by the Fourier coefficients G_j of the matrix function G.

In case of a contracting positively definite matrix function G, the material of Ch. 5 of the book SZ.-NAGY, FOIAS [1] is also related to Theorem 7.7. The special kind (7.15) of factorization of a positively definite matrix function satisfying a Hölder condition was established by SHMUL'YAN [1]. Theorems 7.5 and 7.9 are explicitly formulated (as corollaries of more general propositions) in SPITKOVSKIĬ [2], however, as a matter of fact, they were known even earlier.

The boundedness of the factorization factors of a positively definite matrix function proved in Theorem 7.9 generalizes (for $\Gamma = \mathbb{T}$) the result of Lemma 6.5 from the scalar case. In Chapter 6 the proposition which stated that the multiplication by a positive function α invertible in L_∞ does not go beyond the class of Φ-factorable matrix functions was easily derived from this lemma. The latter result, however, cannot be transferred to the case of a positively definite matrix function G , even if $\Gamma = \mathbb{T}$: in the paper of KRUPNIK and ROZENBERG [1] it was proved that there exist piecewise continuous 2×2 matrix functions A and B such that A is Φ-factorable in L_p, B is uniformly positively definite, but the product AB fails to be Φ-factorable in L_p . An example of two uniformly positively definite piecewise continuous matrix functions of second order the product of which is not Φ-factorable in L_2 was constructed by one of the authors in SPITKOVSKIĬ [4].

Theorem 7.8 is due to SIMONENKO [4]. The equality to zero of the partial indices of a matrix function factorable in C and with uniformly positive real part was shown by GOHBERG and KREĬN [3]. The factorability in L_2 and the equality to zero of the partial indices of matrix functions of the type $I + F$ with $\|F\| < 1$ were established by WIENER and MASANI [1]. Notice that every matrix function with a uniformly positive real part may be transformed into the type just mentioned via multiplication by a positive constant.

In connection with Theorem 7.3 we also note that on every connected rectifiable closed contour different from the circle there exists a rational matrix function with uniformly positive real part and non-zero partial indices (VIROZUB, MATSAEV [1]). Such matrix functions exist even for $n = 2$ (MARKUS, MATSAEV [2]).

Theorem 7.10 has been proved by one of the authors (SPITKOVSKIĬ [10]). A slightly different formulation of this theorem is given in SPITKOVSKIĬ [5]. In case of unitary matrix functions Theorem 7.10 changes over into a result of KRUPNIK, NYAGA [1] (see also KRUPNIK [4]) coinciding with the reformulation of Corollary 6.4, where equations (7.19) are taken into account. This theorem also covers the factorability criterion of a matrix function G with zero partial indices which is discussed in VERBITSKIĬ, KRUPNIK [2]. Furthermore, notice that the questions of Fredholmness, index and one-sided invertibility of the operator

$$Tf(s) = sf(s) + \frac{B^*(s)}{\pi} \int_E \frac{B(t)f(t)}{s-t} dt$$

which was examined by another method in FAOUR NAZIH [1] (concerning this topic, see the note of one of the authors in the review Referativnyĭ Zhurnal, Matematika 1980, 10 B, 674 of the paper in question) may be studied with the aid of Theorem 7.10.

The factorization problem of locally sectorial (i.e. satisfying the condition $H(F(\tau)) \subseteq S_t$ $(\tau \in \gamma_t)$ of Theorem 7.10) but, generally speaking, unbounded matrix functions F was studied in SPITKOVSKIĬ [7]. In this paper the notion of canonical factorization was introduced. On the one hand, it generalizes the corresponding notion from KREĬN, SPITKOVSKIĬ [1,2] (especially, the representation of a positively definite matrix function as the product of an outer matrix function and its conjugate) and, on the other hand, the notion of factorization in L_2 with coinciding partial indices. Moreover, it is shown there that, for locally sectorial matrix functions, a canonical factorization is determined up to constant multipliers. In connection with this it should be mentioned that till now a definition of factorization on the circle which comprehends in a certain sense both factorization in L_p and representations of the form (7.15) and is unique in the sense that it could be reconstructed by the factor Λ with the same degree of arbitrariness of a factorization in L_p has not been found yet. From our point of view, the problem of finding such a definition is very important for the needs of a logically well-composed structure of factorization theory.

Theorem 7.11 in the scalar case was proved by DOUGLAS and WIDOM [1]. In this case the conditions of Theorem 7.11 may be formulated in a more elegant fashion. Namely, the function F satisfies the conditions of Theorem 7.11 (for $n = 1$) if and only if the convex hull of the set of its essential limits at every point $t \in \mathbb{T}$ does not contain zero. With this in mind, in the paper DOUGLAS, WIDOM [1] there was posed the following problem: Is the condition of non-degeneracy at every point $t \in \mathbb{T}$ of all matrices from the convex hull of the essential limits of a matrix function F $(\in L_\infty)$ given on $\mathbb{T}$ sufficient for the Φ-factorability of F in L_2 with zero partial indices? This question was positively answered by CLANCEY [1] under the additional supposition that, at every point $t \in \mathbb{T}$, the matrix function F has no more than two limits. In the general case the answer to this question is negative: In the article AZOFF, CLANCEY [1] one can find examples of matrix functions F satisfying the Douglas-Widom demands, but whose partial 2-indices are not equal to zero. Moreover, there are cited examples of matrix functions F satisfying these demands, but in general being not factorable in L_2 at all.

Lemma 7.3 for the scalar case was proved in ADAMYAN, AROV, KREĬN [1], DUKHOVNYĬ [1] and for the matrix case (and the case of an operator function, which we do not touch upon) in ADAMYAN, AROV, KREĬN [2], NEHARI [1]. The main ideas of the proof described here are borrowed from ADAMYAN, AROV, KREĬN [1], POUSSON [1]. In the present book we do not mention the following sophisticated question naturally arising in connection with Lemma 7.3: Under which conditions is the matrix function X_0 (Y_0, respectively) on which the minimum in (7.20) is attained unitary and to which degree are the properties in which the matrix function G is peculiar acquired by the matrix function $G - X_0$ ($G - Y_0$) ? It appears that the last question is closely related to the properties of the factorization factors of G ; concerning this subject, see the paper ADAMYAN, AROV, KREĬN [1] quoted above. In this connection we still refer to another paper (SILBERMANN [1]), where it is shown that the best approximation of a function G $(\in L_\infty)$ analytic at all but one points $t \in \mathbb{T}$ can be everywhere discontinuous. In this way, the local principle does not work here.

Theorem 7.12 in the scalar case was proved by LEE and SARASON [1]

Theorems 7.13 and 7.14 in the scalar case were established by WIDOM [1] and DEVINATZ [1], and in the matrix case but for zero partial indices by POUSSON [1] and RABINDRANATHAN [1] (in other words, in the latter two papers Corollaries 7.10 and 7.11 were shown). In a general form Theorems 7.13 - 7.15 were presented by one of the authors (SPITKOVSKIǏ [2,10]).

The device of transition to a unitary matrix function described in Lemma 7.4 was suggested by RABINDRANATHAN [1]. In the paper SPITKOVSKIǏ [6] a modification of the Rabindranathan method was proposed which consists in the multiplication of the studied matrix function G by A^{-1} on the left and by $(B^*)^{-1}$ on the right, where A and B are outer matrix functions from the representations $AA^* = (GG^*)^{1/2}$ and $BB^* = (G^*G)^{1/2}$. In particular, on such a multiplication Hermitian matrix functions change into matrix functions which are Hermitian and unitary simultaneously (applying a notion usual in matrix theory, such matrix functions are called $\mathfrak{J}$-matrix functions). There are two situations in which the factorization problem for $\mathfrak{J}$-matrix functions can be solved trivially. This is the scalar case, where we simply deal with a function having the values ± 1, and the definite case, in which an $\mathfrak{J}$-matrix function may be reduced to a constant one which equals I or $-I$. On the strength of this simple consideration in SPITKOVSKIǏ [6] a generalization of Theorem 7.6 to the case $p \neq 2$ is proved. Moreover, it is clarified that the requirement for the total index to be equal to zero can be omitted in Corollary 7.9. Incidentally, Theorem 7.6 and Corollary 7.9 themselves, as far as the authors know, have not been published previously.

We intend to note that for an arbitrary $\mathfrak{J}$-matrix function, certainly, there exists a criterion for the partial indices to be equal to zero formulated in terms of the behaviour (dependence on t) of the subspace of its invariant vectors, since the matrix function itself may be reconstructed uniquely by this subspace. One sufficient condition of this type is presented in the article SPITKOVSKIǏ [6]. Unfortunately, a criterion itself has not been obtained yet.

In connection with the theory of canonical differential equations the factorization of unitary matrix functions defined on the real line has been studied by KREǏN and MELIK-ADAMYAN [1,2]. Among other results they proved, in principle, that, for a given matrix function $X \in H_\infty^+$, one can find a matrix function $Y \in H_\infty^-$ such that $X + Y$ is unitary almost everywhere on $\mathbf{T}$ and has zero partial indices if and only if $\|PXQ\| < 1$. A procedure of finding the matrix function Y, which is uniquely defined by X, is also described there.

Concerning other work dedicated to the specific character of factorization of matrix functions having one or another additional algebraic property, we mention the article of FEINSTEIN, SHAMASH [1]. In this paper an algorithm for constructing a factorization of the form $G(s) = X(s)X'(-s)$ for a rational matrix function G considered on the real line with $G(s) = G'(-s)$, $G(is) \geq 0$ is presented.
Theorem 7.16 was proved in SPITKOVSKIǏ [10], cf. also SPITKOVSKIǏ [2,3]; Theorem 7.17 and its Corollaries 7.12 - 7.15 are borrowed from SPITKOVSKIǏ [1], wheras the example inserted after Corollary 7.15 is taken from SHMUL'YAN [1].

In terms of Toeplitz operators (i.e. operators of the form $T_p(G)$) the theory of the factorization problem in L_2 on the circle for the scalar case is explained in detail in Ch. 7 of the book DOUGLAS [2] [1]. In particular, in the book just mentioned one can find an interesting result on the connectivity of the spectrum of the operator $T_p(G)$ for arbitrary $G \in L_\infty$ obtained by WIDOM [2] as well as an analogue of this result for the case of an essential spectrum. When diagonal matrix functions were first dealt with, we already noticed that the property of the spectrum and the essential spectrum just mentioned disappears in passing over to the matrix case. In the examples known to the authors the number of connected components of the (essential) spectrum does not exceed the order of the matrix. It is of some interest to find out whether this law remains true for all matrix functions from L_∞.

---

1) See also the monographs HALMOS, SUNDER [1] and BÖTTCHER, SILBERMANN [1].

CHAPTER 8. CONDITIONS OF Φ-FACTORABILITY IN THE SPACE L_p. CRITERION OF Φ-FACTORABILITY IN L_2 OF BOUNDED MEASURABLE MATRIX FUNCTIONS

In this comparatively small chapter we shall be concerned with classes of matrix functions from L_∞ defined on a contour of class $\mathcal{R}$ and Φ-factorable in the spaces $L_p(\Gamma)$, where we pursue the aim to select such classes which are as wide as possible. For the construction of classes of matrix functions from the classes studies previously in Chapters 5, 6 and 7 which admit a Φ-factorization we shall use the ε-local principle (Theorem 3.22) and the properties of a matrix function $F \in L_\infty$ to preserve Φ-factorability on multiplication by a matrix function from the classes $L_\infty^{\pm} + C$ (Theorem 5.5). As a matter of fact, this general approach forced us from the very start to give up any attempts to obtain, simultaneously with conditions of Φ-factorability, any conclusions about the values of partial indices. The conditions of Φ-factorability in L_p derived below are sufficient. However, for $p = 2$ in case of a Lyapunov contour Γ, we are also able to substantiate their necessity. A criterion of Φ-factorability of a matrix function G from L_∞ in the spaces L_p with $p \neq 2$ fails to be known hitherto.

Now we intend to describe the contents of the present chapter in more detail. Section 8.1 is of auxiliary character. On the basis of the ε-local principle the operation of transition from a certain class A of matrix functions from L_∞ to a wider class $\mathfrak{A}$ preserving the property of Φ-factorability is introduced in it. In addition, in 8.1 properties and estimates for the radius $\delta'_{p,n}(\Gamma)$ of the largest neighbourhood of a unitary matrix function entirely consisting of matrix functions which are Φ-factorable in L_p will be established.

The preliminary results are used in Section 8.2 in order to formulate a sufficient condition of Φ-factorability in L_p.

This condition consists in the membership of the matrix function G to the class $B_{p,n}(\Gamma)$ which is constructed by some class of matrix functions F from L_∞ with the help of the method described in 8.1 and is determined by one of the conditions ensuring Φ-factorability of F in L_p. In case of a Lyapunov contour Γ the conditions determining the class $B_{p,n}(\Gamma)$ can be weakened. If $p = 2$ and Γ is a Lyapunov contour, then the condition $G \in B_{2,n}(\Gamma)$ proves to be an exact condition of Φ-factorability. This result is explained in Section 8.3. Comments on current literature are given in 8.4.

8.1. AUXILIARY RESULTS

DEFINITION 8.1. Let A be a certain class of matrix functions from L_∞. The class of all matrix functions G satisfying the following requirements will be denoted by $\widetilde{A}$: for every point $t \in \Gamma$, there exist matrix functions $F_t \in A$ and $G_{\pm,t} \in L_\infty$ such that

1) $G_{+,t}^{\pm 1} \in L_\infty^+ + C$, $G_{-,t}^{\pm 1} \in L_\infty^- + C$,

2) the matrix functions G and $G_{+,t}F_tG_{-,t}$ are ε-locally equivalent at the point t.

It is clear by the very definition that the class $\widetilde{A}$ contains A. The operation "$\sim$" of transition from A to $\widetilde{A}$ is idempotent: choosing the class $B = \widetilde{A}$ as the initial one and constructing by it the class $\widetilde{B}$, we see that it does not contain any new matrix functions (in comparison with $\widetilde{A}$), i.e. $\widetilde{\widetilde{A}} = \widetilde{A}$.

The operation "$\sim$" is of interest for us, since it does not violate the Φ-factorability of a matrix function. To be more exact, the following result holds.

THEOREM 8.1. Assume A to be an arbitrary subclass of the class L_∞ and U ($\subseteq (1,\infty)$) a set lying in a certain component of the Φ-factorability domain of every matrix function from A. Then U is a subset of some component of the Φ-factorability domain of all matrix functions from class $\widetilde{A}$.

In case of a one-point set U ($U = \{p\}$) Theorem 8.1 simply means that Φ-factorability in L_p of all matrix functions of the class A implies Φ-factorability in L_p of the matrix functions of the class $\widetilde{A}$.

Proof. Starting from the matrix function $G \in \mathfrak{A}$ and the point $t \in \Gamma$, we reconstruct the matrix functions F_t and $G_{\pm,t}$ involved in Definition 8.1.

Let p be any point of the set U. Then the matrix function F_t $(\in A)$ is Φ-factorable in L_p and, according to Theorem 5. , the matrix function $G_t = G_{+,t}F_tG_{-,t}$ is also Φ-factorable in L_p. Since, for all $t \in \Gamma$, the matrix functions G and G_t are ε-locally equivalent at the point t, Theorem 3.22 enables us to make a conclusion about Φ-factorability of the matrix function G in L_p.

In this way, we have verified that the set U lies in the domain of Φ-factorability of every matrix function G from the class $\tilde{A}$. Now we are still obliged to prove that this set belongs entirely to one component of the Φ-factorability domain, i.e., for any $p_1, p_2 \in U$ $(p_1 < p_2)$, the total p_1- and p_2-indices of G coincide. By assumption, such a coincidence holds for all matrix functions of the class A and, especially, for the matrix function F_t. Owing to the relation $G_{\pm,t} \in L_\infty^{\pm} + C$, the total index of the matrix function $G_{\pm,t}$ does not depend on p and, according to Theorem 5.5, the total p_1- $(p_2$-$)$ index of G_t is equal to the sum of the total p_1- $(p_2$-$)$ index of F_t and the total indices of $G_{\pm,t}$. Thus, the total p_1-index of the matrix function G_t coincides with its total p_2-index. But then, as follows from Corollary 2.2, the matrix function G_t admits one and the same factorization in L_{p_1} and L_{p_2}, where in view of Theorem 3.8 this factorization is a Φ-factorization (in L_{p_1} and L_{p_2}). From Theorem 3.16 we deduce that in this case it is possible to indicate a regularizer of the operator $P + G_tQ$ in the space $L_{p_1}^n$ such that its restriction on $L_{p_2}^n$ is a regularizer of $P + G_tQ$ in this space. Using the method of constructing a regularizer of a local type operator (in this case, the operator $P + GQ$) by its local regularizers (in this case, by the regularizers of the operators $P + G_tQ$, $t \in \Gamma$) described in Theorem 1.14, we find that for the operator $P + GQ$ there exists also a regularizer R in the space $L_{p_1}^n$ the restriction of which on the space $L_{p_2}^n$ is a regularizer for $P + GQ$ in this space.

Evidently, the index of an arbitrary bounded operator does not increase with the growth of p. Since the index of the product $(P + GQ)R$ is equal to zero in either of the spaces $L^n_{p_1}$ and $L^n_{p_2}$, from this and Theorem 1.6 we deduce that the index of the operator $P + GQ$ in $L^n_{p_1}$ and $L^n_{p_2}$ is one and the same.

In other words, the total p_1-index of the matrix function G coincides with its total p_2-index, which proves Theorem 8.1. ≡

For obtaining new concrete criteria of Φ-factorability with the aid of Theorem 8.1, it is necessary to choose as A one of the classes of Φ-factorable matrix functions which are already known.

In particular, we may assume the class A to agree with the class of matrix functions satisfying the conditions of one of the Theorems 6.6 - 6.11'. For the moment, however, only the Φ-factorability of matrix functions from the class A is essential for us, but not any other information about their partial indices, because the latter gets lost in any case in passing to the class $\mathfrak{X}$. Therefore, in describing the class A, without any loss we may replace the values $\delta_{p,n}(\Gamma)$ involved in Theorems 6.6 - 6.11 by, generally speaking, larger values $\delta'_{p,n}(\Gamma)$. The legality of such a substitution will be founded in Section 8.2. Here we state the definition of these values and discuss some of their properties.

<u>DEFINITION 8.2.</u> By $\delta'_{p,n}(\Gamma)$ we denote the radius of the largest spherical neighbourhood of the $n{\times}n$ matrix function I consisting entirely of matrix functions which are Φ-factorable in L_p.

Recall that we denote by Λ_p the interval of the real line connecting the point p with the point $q\ (= p/(p-1))$.

<u>LEMMA 8.1.</u> 1) For any contour Γ and all $p \in (1,\infty)$, the following relations hold:

$$\delta_{p,n}(\Gamma) \leq \delta'_{p,n}(\Gamma)\,, \tag{8.1}$$

$$\delta'_{p,n}(\Gamma) \leq \delta'_{p,1}(\Gamma) \leq \delta_{p,1}(\Gamma)\,, \tag{8.2}$$

$$\delta'_{q,n}(\Gamma) = \delta'_{p,n}(\Gamma)\,, \tag{8.3}$$

$$\delta'_{r,n}(\Gamma) \geq \delta'_{p,n}(\Gamma) \quad \text{if} \quad r \in A_p \,; \tag{8.4}$$

2) if the contour Γ is composed of closed disjoint curves Γ_j, then

$$\delta'_{p,n}(\Gamma) = \min_j \delta'_{p,n}(\Gamma_j) \,;$$

3) for all simple closed smooth contours Γ, the quantity $\delta'_{p,n}(\Gamma)$ takes one and the same value.

Proof. 1) By definition, the $\delta_{p,n}(\Gamma)$-neighbourhood of the matrix function I consists only of matrix functions which are Φ-factorable in L_p with zero partial indices. Hence, this neighbourhood lies in the $\delta'_{p,n}(\Gamma)$-neighbourhood of I, which implies the relation (8.1). The inequality $\delta'_{p,n}(\Gamma) \leq \delta'_{p,1}(\Gamma)$ results from Corollary 4.2, according to which the diagonal $n\times n$ matrix function fI fails to be Φ-factorable in L_p as soon as the scalar function f is not Φ-factorable in L_p.

Now, let us note that the total p-index of every matrix function from the $\delta'_{p,n}(\Gamma)$-neighbourhood of I is equal to zero. Indeed, owing to its stability and integralness, the total p-index is constant on connected open subsets of the set of matrix functions being Φ-factorable in L_p and, in particular, on the $\delta'_{p,n}(\Gamma)$-neighbourhood of I. In case $n = 1$, this fact simply means that the indices of all functions from the $\delta'_{p,1}(\Gamma)$-neighbourhood of the identity matrix are equal to zero, i.e., this neighbourhood belongs to its $\delta_{p,1}(\Gamma)$-neighbourhood. Thus $\delta'_{p,1}(\Gamma) \leq \delta_{p,1}(\Gamma)$, which together with inequality (8.1) completes the proof of relations (8.2) for $n = 1$.

Proceeding to the verification of equation (8.3), we consider the mapping $Y = (1-\varepsilon^2)(X')^{-1}$. In the proof of Lemma 6.2 it was already mentioned that, for every $\varepsilon \in (0,1)$, the ε-neighbourhood of the identity matrix function I remains invariant under this mapping. Furthermore, the Φ-factorability of the matrix function X in L_p is equivalent to the Φ-factorability of the matrix function Y in L_q. Thus we conclude that, for every $\varepsilon < 1$, the inequalities $\varepsilon < \delta'_{p,n}(\Gamma)$ and $\varepsilon < \delta'_{q,n}(\Gamma)$ are equivalent and, therefore, $\min\{1,\delta'_{p,n}(\Gamma)\} = \min\{1,\delta'_{q,n}(\Gamma)\}$.

But relations (8.2) and the inequality $\delta_{p,1}(\Gamma) \leq 1$ imply that the values $\delta'_{p,n}(\Gamma)$ and $\delta'_{q,n}(\Gamma)$ do not exceed one. Hence, relation (8.3) is true.

Finally, consider an arbitrary matrix function G from the $\delta'_{p,n}(\Gamma)$-neighbourhood of I. Due to equation (8.3), this matrix function is Φ-factorable not only in L_p but also in L_q. Besides, as it was shown above, its total p- (q-) index is equal to zero. In this way, the interpolation Theorem 3.9 can be applied, according to which the matrix function G is Φ-factorable in all spaces L_r, $r \in A_p$.

In summary, all matrix functions from the $\delta'_{p,n}(\Gamma)$-neighbourhood of I are Φ-factorable in L_r, $r \in A_p$. Hence $\delta'_{r,n}(\Gamma) \geq \delta'_{p,n}(\Gamma)$, which completes the proof of assertion 1).

2) Let G be a certain matrix function given on Γ, and assume (as in Theorem 3.21) G_j to be the restriction of this matrix function on Γ_j. The inequality $\|I-G\| < \varepsilon$ is fulfilled iff $\|I-G_j\| < \varepsilon$ for any j. Therefore, if $\varepsilon < \min_j \delta_{p,n}(\Gamma_j)$, then every matrix function G_j is left and right Φ-factorable on Γ_j in L_p (here we used equation (8.3) proved above and Theorem 3.7'). With regard to assertion 2) of Theorem 3.21, from this the Φ-factorability of the matrix function G in L_p results.

In this way, the condition $\|I-G\| < \varepsilon$ guarantees the Φ-factorability of G in L_p, i.e. $\varepsilon \leq \delta'_{p,n}(\Gamma)$. Thus we have proved that $\min_j \delta'_{p,n}(\Gamma_j) \leq \delta'_{p,n}(\Gamma)$. Now we choose a contour Γ_{j_0} on which $\min_j \delta'_{p,n}(\Gamma_j)$ is attained. Moreover, on this contour we take a matrix function G_{j_0} which is not Φ-factorable in L_p (on the left if $j_0=0$, and on the right if $j_0 > 0$) but lies at a distance of $\delta'_{p,n}(\Gamma_{j_0})$ from I.

Finally, set $G_j = I$ for $j \neq j_0$. Then we obtain a matrix function G which is not Φ-factorable in L_p (by Theorem 3.21) and for which $\|I-G\| = \delta'_{p,n}(\Gamma_{j_0})$. Therefore $\delta'_{p,n}(\Gamma) \leq \delta'_{p,n}(\Gamma_{j_0})$, which completes the proof of proposition 2).

Proposition 3) may be deduced from proposition 1) of Theorem 3.21 in an analogous manner. ≡

Owing to inequality (8.1), the lower bounds for $\delta_{p,n}(\Gamma)$ indicated in proposition 1) of Lemma 6.2 are simultaneously lower bounds for $\delta'_{p,n}(\Gamma)$. However, it turns out that more precise estimates are available, in which the norms of the operators S and Q are replaced by their factor norms $|S|_{L_p^n}$ and $|Q|_{L_p^n}$ [1].

In other words, the following statement is true.

LEMMA 8.2. Either of the values $|Q|^{-1}_{L_p^n}$ and $\dfrac{2|S|_{L_p^n}}{1+|S|^2_{L_p^n}}$ is a lower bound for $\delta'_{p,n}(\Gamma)$.

Proof. We intend to show, for instance, that $|Q|^{-1}_{L_p^n} \le \delta'_{p,n}(\Gamma)$.

Suppose that the condition $\|I-G\| < |Q|^{-1}_{L_p^n}$ is satisfied. By definition of the factor norm, there exists an operator T compact in the space L_p^n such that $\|I-G\| < \|Q+T\|^{-1}_{L_p^n}$.

Thanks to the contracting mapping principle, in this case the operator $V = I-(I-G)(Q+T) = P+GQ-(I-G)T$ is invertible. The operator $P + GQ$ differing from V by the compact summand $(I-G)T$ will be Fredholm in view of Theorem 1.5. In this way, the Φ-factorability in L_p of all matrix functions from the $|Q|^{-1}_{L_p^n}$-neighbourhood of I and, together with it, the desired estimate have been proved.

In connection with the second estimate of Lemma 8.2 we would like to note that the value $|S|_{L_p^n}$ does not change under smooth mappings β of the contour Γ. Indeed, for such mappings $\beta : L \to \Gamma$, in the proof of Theorem 3.21 the existence of an isometric invertible operator $W : L_p^n(\Gamma) \to L_p^n(L)$ was established for which the operator WSW^{-1} differs from the operator S_o of singular integration along L only by

[1] We remind the reader that the definition of the factor norm was given in Section 1.1.

a compact summand and, possibly, by sign. But then $|WSW^{-1}|_{L_p^n(L)} = |S_o|_{L_p^n(L)}$. At the same time, due to the fact that the operator W is isometric, we have $|WSW^{-1}|_{L_p^n(L)} = |S|_{L_p^n(\Gamma)}$, which proves the invariance of the factor norm of the operator S for sufficiently smooth mappings β.

For smooth contours Γ one may obtain a result of final nature concerning the values $\delta'_{p,n}(\Gamma)$ and $|S|_{L_p^n}$.

<u>LEMMA 8.3.</u> Let the contour Γ be smooth. Then

$$\delta'_{p,n}(\Gamma) = \sin(\pi/\max(p,q)) \tag{8.5}$$

and

$$|S|_{L_p^n} = \operatorname{ctg}(\pi/2\max(p,q)) .$$

<u>Proof.</u> Every simply-connected smooth contour Γ is the image of the circle $\mathbb{T}$ under a certain diffeomorphism $\beta : \mathbb{T} \to \Gamma$.

According to proposition 3) of Lemma 8.1, for an arbitrary contour of this type, the equation

$$\delta'_{p,n}(\Gamma) = \delta'_{p,n}(\mathbb{T}) \tag{8.6}$$

holds.

But then, owing to assertion 2) of Lemma 8.1, the equation (8.6) is also correct for a compound contour Γ the components of which are smooth curves.

Furthermore, as it was clarified in Chapter 7, equations (7.19) are valid for any natural n. Thus, owing to relations (8.1) and (8.2), the relation $\delta'_{p,n}(\Gamma_o) = \sin(\pi/\max(p,q))$ follows. Comparing this result with equation (8.6), we obtain the first of the relations to be proved.[1)]

From the estimate $\frac{2|S|}{1+|S|^2} \le \delta'_{p,n}(\Gamma)$ and equation (8.5) we deduce that $|S|_{L_p^n} \ge \operatorname{ctg}(\pi/2\max(p,q))$. Since the value $|S|_{L_p^n}$ as also $\delta'_{p,n}(\Gamma)$

---

1) Thus, for the case of a circle, the inequalities in relations (8.1) and (8.2) become equalities.

is one and the same for all smooth contours, it suffices to verify the opposite inequality for $\Gamma = \mathbb{T}$. But in this case the inequality $|S|_{L_p^n} \le \mathrm{ctg}(\pi/2\max(p,q))$ results from relation (7.18). Thus Lemma 8.3 is completely proved. ≡

Remark that, for any contour Γ of class $\tilde{\mathcal{R}}$, proposition 1) of Lemma 6.2 along with inequality (8.2) enable us to claim that $\delta'_{p,n}(\Gamma) \le \sin(\pi/\max(p,q))$. In this way, for smooth contours, the quantities $\delta'_{p,n}(\Gamma)$ attain the largest possible value for contours of class $\tilde{\mathcal{R}}$. Clearly, at the same time the value $|S|_{L_p^n}$ takes the smallest of all possible values.

8.2. SUFFICIENT CONDITIONS OF Φ-FACTORABILITY

DEFINITION 8.3. To the class $B_{p,n}(\Gamma)$ we assigne those nxn matrix functions G given on Γ for which, for every point $t \in \Gamma$, one can specify an arc γ_t containing it as well as matrix functions $G_{\pm,t} \in L_\infty^{\pm} + C$ such that $G_{\pm,t}^{-} \in L_\infty^{\pm} + C$ and, for $F_t = G_{+,t}GG_{-,t}$, at least one of the following relations is fulfilled:

1) $\operatorname*{ess\,sup}_{\tau\in\gamma_t} \|I-F_t(\tau)\| < \delta'_{p,n}(\Gamma)$,

2) $\operatorname*{ess\,inf}_{\tau\in\gamma_t} d(F_t(\tau)) > \sqrt{1-(\delta'_{p,n}(\Gamma))^2}\ \operatorname*{ess\,sup}_{\tau\in\gamma_t} \|F_t(\tau)\|$,

3) the set $\dfrac{1}{\operatorname{ess\,sup}\|F_t(\tau)\|} \bigcup_{\tau\in\gamma_t} H(F_t(\tau))$ is separated from zero by a straight line whose distance to zero is greater than $\sqrt{1-\delta'_{p,n}(\Gamma)^2}$,

4) there exists a disk Δ_t which is visible from the origin at an angle $\alpha_t < 2\arcsin \delta'_{p,n}(\Gamma)$ and such that almost everywhere on γ_t the matrix $F_t(\tau)$ is normal and their eigenvalues are located in Δ_t.

It turns out that all matrix functions from the class $B_{p,n}(\Gamma)$ are Φ-factorable in L_p. Moreover, the following result is true.

THEOREM 8.2. The interval A_p is completely contained in a certain component of the domain of Φ-factorability of any matrix function from the class $B_{p,n}(\Gamma)$.

Proof. Consider the class A of those matrix functions F_t $(= F)$ for which at least one of the requirements 1) - 4) of Definition 8.3 is fulfilled, and that on the curve γ_t coinciding with the whole of the contour Γ. Evidently, the class $\tilde{A}$ constructed by A in accordance with Definition 8.1 coincides with the class $B_{p,n}(\Gamma)$. With regard to Theorem 8.1 it is possible to conclude that Theorem 8.2 will be proved as soon as we establish the correctness of its proposition with respect to matrix functions from the class A.
However, the Φ-factorability with one and the same total index in all L_r $(r \in A_p)$ of an arbitrary matrix function F satisfying condition 1) of Definition 8.3 for $\gamma_t = \Gamma$ results directly from Definition 8.2 of the values $\delta'_{p,n}(\Gamma)$ and inequality (8.4). The case when F satisfies one of the conditions 2) - 4) of Definition 8.3 can be reduced to the previous one by methods used in the arguments of Lemma 6.4, Theorems 6.11 and 6.10, respectively. Thus Theorem 8.2 is proved. ≡

Still preserving the claim of Theorem 8.2, in case of a smooth contour Γ one can weaken the restrictions on the class $B_{p,n}(\Gamma)$ to a certain degree. Namely, conditions 1) - 4) from Definition 8.3 related to a Lyapunov contour Γ will be replaced by the following:

1') $\operatorname{ess\,sup}_{\tau\in\gamma_t} \|I-F_t(\tau)\| < \sin(\pi/\max(p,q))$,

2') $d(F_t(\tau)) \geq \|F_t(\tau)\|\cos(\pi/\max(p,q))+\varepsilon_t$, $\varepsilon_t > 0$,

3') the set $\bigcup_{\tau\in\gamma_t} \|F_t(\tau)\|^{-1}H(F_t(\tau))$ is separated from zero by some straight line whose distance to zero is greater than $\cos(\pi/\max(p,q))$

4') there exist a sector S_t with vertex at the origin of apex angle $\alpha_t < 2\pi/\max(p,q)$ and a number $\varepsilon_t > 0$ such that $H(F_t(\tau)) \subset S_t$ and $h(F_t(\tau)) \geq \varepsilon_t$ a.e. on γ_t.

In Chapters 6 and 7 it was already mentioned that the conditions of the type 1) - 4) and 1') - 4') are not independent. For instance, 2) can be reduced to 1), and 3) to 2) by multiplying them by a suitable constant. At the same time, 2) is a special case of 3). Conditions 1') - 3') are interrelated in a similar manner. Furthermore, condition 4') is a consequence of any of the conditions 1') - 3'). Making use of this remark, one could relieve the definition of the class $B_{p,n}(\Gamma)$ and in case of a smooth contour Γ leave over only condition 4') (from all the conditions 1') - 4')). However, we do not intend to do this, because in concrete problems the check of one of the conditions 1) - 4) and 1') - 4') may prove to be easier than that of another condition.

THEOREM 8.3. Let the contour Γ be smooth. Then for all matrix functions of the class $B_{p,n}(\Gamma)$ (in the definition of which the conditions 1) - 4) are replaced by conditions 1') - 4')), the interval A_p lies entirely inside a certain component of the Φ-factorability domain.

Proof. As also in Theorem 8.2, it suffices to pay attention to matrix functions of the class A, to which we assign those matrix functions from L_∞ which possess one of the properties 1') - 4'), however, with the change of γ_t by Γ. From what was mentioned above it is clear that the class A consists exactly of those matrix functions F $(=F_t)$ which satisfy condition 4') for $\gamma_t = \Gamma$.

In case when the contour Γ is a circle, the Φ-factorability of such matrix functions F in L_r $(r \in A_p)$ with zero partial (and, thus, also total) indices results from Theorem 7.10. Since condition 4') is exclusively formulated in terms of values of G, it is invariant with respect to mappings $\beta : L \to \Gamma$ of contours for which the matrix function G given on Γ is replaced by the matrix function $G_0 = G \circ \beta$ defined on L. Therefore, using statement 1) of Theorem 3.21, one can assert that matrix functions F given on an arbitrary simple smooth contour Γ are Φ-factorable in L_r $(r \in A_p)$ with zero total index as soon as they satisfy condition 4') for $\gamma_t = \Gamma$. The passage from a simple smooth contour to a composite one can be accomplished with the aid of statement 2) of the same Theorem 3.21. Thus Theorem 8.3 is completely proved. ☰

8.3. CRITERION OF Φ-FACTORABILITY IN L_2

With the aid of Theorems 8.3 and 7.14 the problem of Φ-factorability in L_2 of matrix functions from the class L_∞ given on a smooth contour Γ may be solved to the very end. Before formulating the corresponding result, we note that, for $p = 2$, $\sin(\pi/\max(p,q)) = 1$, $\cos(\pi/\max(p,q)) = 0$ and, therefore, condition 2) from the definition of the class $B_{2,n}(\Gamma)$ is equivalent to the requirement of uniformly positiveness of the real part of the matrix function F on γ_t, and conditions 1'), 3') and 4') change over into 2'), if F_t is multiplied by a certain constant.

<u>THEOREM 8.4.</u> For a matrix function $G \in L_\infty$ defined on the smooth contour Γ, the following statements are equivalent:

1) $2 \in \Phi(G)$,
2) $G = G_{(o)}B$, where $B^{\pm 1} \in M_\infty^-$ and $\|I-G_{(o)}\| < 1$,
3) $G = G_{(o)}B$, where $B^{\pm 1} \in M_\infty^-$ and the real part of the matrix function $G_{(o)}$ is uniformly positive on Γ,
4) $G \in B_{2,n}(\Gamma)$.

<u>Proof.</u> The equivalence of assertions 2) and 3) was already mentioned above. Evidently, 3) ==> 4). The implication 4) ==> 1 is a special case (for $p = 2$) of Theorem 8.3. It remains to prove that 1) implies 2).

Let the matrix function G be Φ-factorable in L_2 and $\varkappa_n$ be the smallest of its partial 2-indices. Then the matrix function $G_1(t) = t^{-\varkappa_n}G(t)$ is Φ-factorable in L_2 and all its partial 2-indices are non-negative. If the contour Γ is the unit circle, then Theorem 7.14 can be applied, according to which $G_1 = A_1G_{(o)}^{(1)} = G_{(o)}^{(2)}B$, where $A_1 \in H_\infty^+$, $A_1^{-1} \in M_\infty^+$, $B_1 \in M_\infty^-$, $B_1^{-1} \in H_\infty^-$ and $G_{(o)}^{(j)}$ $(j = 1,2)$ are matrix functions with uniformly positive real part. Setting $A(z) = z^{\varkappa_n}A_1(z)$, $B(z) = z^{\varkappa_n}B_1(z)$, we find

$$G = A\, G_{(o)}^{(1)} = G_{(o)}^{(2)}\, B, \tag{8.7}$$

where $A^{\pm 1} \in M_\infty^+$, $B^{\pm 1} \in M_\infty^-$. Thus, if $\Gamma = \mathbb{T}$, then the proposition to be proved is correct.

Now, let Γ be a simple closed smooth contour, and assume ω to be a conformal mapping of the unit disk onto the domain $\mathcal{D}^+$ bounded by Γ. According to proposition 1) of Theorem 3.21, the matrix function G given on Γ is Φ-factorable in L_2 only simultaneously with the matrix function $G \circ \omega$ given on $\mathbb{T}$. By what was proved above, Φ-factorability of $G \circ \omega$ in L_2 means that it is possible to represent it in the form $G \circ \omega = AG_{(o)}$, where $A^{\pm 1} \in M^+_\infty(\mathbb{T})$ and $G_{(o)}$ is a matrix function with a uniformly positive real part. From the last equation we obtain that $G = (A \circ \omega^{-1})(G_{(o)} \circ \omega^{-1})$. Since $(A \circ \omega^{-1})^{\pm 1} \in M^+_\infty(\Gamma)$ and the ranges of the matrix functions $G_{(o)}$ and $G_{(o)} \circ \omega^{-1}$ agree, then the existence of the first of the representations (8.7) for G has been proved. The existence of the second representation can be established by means of a conformal mapping of the exterior of the unit disk onto the domain $\mathcal{D}^-$.

Now we proceed to the general case, when Γ is a collection of m connected contours $\Gamma(j)$, $j=0,\dots,m-1$. Due to assertion 2) of Theorem 3.21 (and in its notations), the matrix function G is Φ-factorable in L_2 if and only if the matrix function G_0 is Φ-factorable in L_2 from the left and G_j, $j=1,\dots,m-1$ from the right. Consequently, Φ-factorability (from the left) of G in L_2 implies Φ-factorability in L_2 (from the left) of the matrix functions G_0 and G'_j ($j=1,\dots,m-1$). Owing to what was proved above, the relations

$$G_0 = F_0 B_0 , \quad G'_j = A'_j H'_j , \quad j=1,\dots,m-1 \tag{8.8}$$

are valid, where the matrix functions F_j ($j=0,\dots,m-1$) are given on $\Gamma(j)$ and have uniformly positive real parts, $B_0^{\pm 1} \in M^-_\infty(\Gamma(0))$, $A_j^{\pm 1} \in M^+_\infty(\Gamma(j))$. Equations (8.8) mean that $G = FB$, where $F|_{\Gamma_j} = F_j$ ($j=0,\dots,m-1$), $B|_{\Gamma(0)} = B_0$, $B|_{\Gamma(j)} = A_j$ ($j=1,\dots,m-1$). Moreover, $B^{\pm 1} \in M^-_\infty(\Gamma)$ and F is a matrix function with a uniformly positive real part. Thus, the proof of Theorem 8.4 is complete. ≡

From Theorem 8.4 we obtain a necessary condition of Φ-factorability making the result of Corollary 3.5 more precise for $p = 2$.

COROLLARY 8.1. For the Φ-factorability in L_2 of the matrix function $G \in L_\infty$ given on the smooth contour Γ, it is necessary for G^{-1} to belong to the closed subalgebra $L_\infty^-[G]$ of the algebra L_∞ generated by the algebra $L_\infty^- + C$ and the matrix function G.

Proof. According to Theorem 8.4, from the Φ-factorability of the matrix function G in L_2 we deduce that $G = G_{(o)}B$, where $\|G_{(o)}-I\| < 1$ and $B^{\pm 1} \in M_\infty^-$. But then we have

$$G^{-1} = B^{-1}G_{(o)}^{-1} = B^{-1} \sum_{k=o}^{\infty} (I-G_{(o)})^k = \sum_{k=o}^{\infty} B^{-1}(I-GB^{-1})^k .$$

Every summand of the series obtained is a polynomial of G and B^{-1} and, therefore, lies in the algebra $L_\infty^-[G]$. Taking into account that this series converges in the metric of L_∞, we observe that the inclusion $G^{-1} \in L_\infty^-[G]$ holds, too.

If $G \in L_\infty^- + C$, then obviously $L_\infty^-[G] = L_\infty^- + C$, and the necessary condition of Φ-factorability stated in Corollary 8.1 coincides with the necessary and sufficient condition described in Theorem 5.2. As to the general case, the relation $G^{-1} \in L_\infty^-[G]$ does not yet guarantee Φ-factorability of G in L_2. An appropriate example is provided by every matrix function G not belonging to $L_\infty^- + C$ for which $G^{-1} \in L_\infty^- + C$.

8.4. COMMENTS

The properties of the values $\delta'_{p,n}(\Gamma)$ proved in Lemma 8.1 are analogous to the well-known property of the factor norm of the operators S and Q (see, e.g., Ch. 7 of the book GOHBERG, KRUPNIK [4]). In connection with Lemma 8.3 it should be noted that in the paper KRUPNIK, POLONSKIĬ [1], for $n = 1$, the coincidence of the norm of the operator S on the circle with its factor norm was established. Furthermore, their common value was found using a result of PICHORIDES [1]. The independence of this value of n is proved in KRUPNIK [4] (see also VERBITSKIĬ, KRUPNIK [1,2]). The coincidence of the factor norm of S (and also of P and Q) for all Lyapunov curves was mentioned e.g. in GOHBERG, KRUPNIK [4]. In the article of NYAGA [1] it is shown that, if one permits the existence of corner points on Γ, then the factor norms of the operators P, Q and S do depend on Γ. The problem of exactness of the estimates derived in Lemma 8.2 in case of a nonsmooth contour Γ remains unsolved. Also, the problem of precisely describing the dependence of the quantities $\delta'_{p,n}(\Gamma)$ on n has not been solved yet for such a contour.

Theorems 8.1 - 8.3 are certain extensions of corresponding results of SIMONENKO [4,6], DANILYUK [4,5] (see also [6]), KRUPNIK and NYAGA [1] and one of the authors (SPITKOVSKIĬ [2,10]). Theorem 8.4 for $n = 1$ can be found in SIMONENKO [6] and, for $n > 1$, in SPITKOVSKIĬ [2]. From Theorem 8.3, applied to the scalar case, the following proposition obtained by SIMONENKO [4,6] results. Let Γ be a smooth contour (which, for the sake of simplicity, is assumed to be connected). To the class $S_p(\Gamma)$ we assign those functions f given on Γ which can be represented in the form $f(t) = \varphi(t)t^k h(t)$, where $\varphi^{\pm 1} \in L_\infty^+$, k is an integer, $h^{\pm 1} \in L_\infty$, $|\arg h(t)| \leq \alpha$ almost everywhere on Γ for a certain $\alpha < 2\pi/\max(p,q)$ and $q = p/(p-1)$. Then all the functions of the class $S_p(\Gamma)$ are Φ-factorable in L_p and L_q with the same index value (equal to k).

KRUPNIK [2] showed that the set of functions which are Φ-factorable in L_p and L_q with equal value of the index is exhausted by the functions of class $S_p(\Gamma)$. This implies, in particular, that the class $\tilde{S}_p(\Gamma)$ constructed by $S_p(\Gamma)$ in accordance with Definition 8.1 agrees with $S_p(\Gamma)$ and $B_{p,1}(\Gamma)$.

The question whether the mentioned result can be transferred to the matrix case, i.e., whether the sufficient conditions of Φ-factorability in L_p and L_q with the same value of the total index indicated in Theorem 8.3 are necessary, is of some significance. For $p = 2$, Theorems 8.4 yields a positive answer to this question.

Clearly, the class $S_p(\Gamma)$ does not comprehend all functions which are Φ-factorable in L_p, because such functions are not necessarily Φ-factorable in L_q (all the more, they may or may not have coinciding p- and q-indices). Especially, not all piecewise continuous functions which are Φ-factorable in L_p belong to the class $S_p(\Gamma)$. The investigation of the problem of Φ-factorability of products of a piecewise continuous function multiplied by a function of the class $S_p(\Gamma)$ was initiared by DANILYUK [3]. The corresponding results from DANILYUK [3] and their extension obtained by DANILYUK, SHELEPOV [2] and SHELEPOV [1] are explained in detail in Ch. 5 of the monograph DANILYUK [6]. In FROLOV [2] (see also Section 8.6 in GOHBERG, KRUPNIK [4]) it is proved that, if the contour Γ is Lyapunov and the jumps of the argument of the non-degenerate piecewise continuous factor are included between $\min\{0, \frac{2\pi}{p} - \frac{2\pi}{q}\}$ and $\max\{0, \frac{2\pi}{p} - \frac{2\pi}{q}\}$, then the products of the indicated kind form the class $M_p(\Gamma)$ consisting only of functions which are Φ-factorable in L_p.

KOKILASHVILI and PAATASHVILI [2] have extended this result of Frolov to the case of contours from some wider class T (which is, however, a subclass of $\mathfrak{R}$). It is not hard to see that the class $M_p(\Gamma)$ contains, apart from the class $S_p(\Gamma)$, also all piecewise continuous functions being Φ-factorable in L_p.

The nonvoid proper subset of the class $M_p(\Gamma)$ consists of those products for which the points of discontinuity of the piecewise continuous factor are points of continuity of the factor from $S_p(\Gamma)$. The Φ-factorability in L_p of such functions was proved in KOKILASHVILI, PAATASHVILI [1] for contours of the class T and, for contours of an even wider subclass $\mathfrak{T}^*$ of the class $\mathfrak{R}$, in KOKILASHVILI, PAATASHVILI [3,4]. Let us explain that a contour Γ belongs to class $\mathfrak{T}^*$ if it may be partitioned into a finite number of arcs for each of which there exists a simple smooth curve γ such that

$$\operatorname*{ess\,sup}_{0\leq\sigma\leq1} \int_0^1 \left|\frac{t'(s)}{t(s)-t(\sigma)} - \frac{\tau'(s)}{\tau(s)-\tau(\sigma)}\right| ds < \infty ,$$

where $\tau(s)$ and $t(s)$, $0 \leq s \leq 1$ are natural parametrizations of the curves γ and Γ, respectively, and if, in addition, (1.12) is satisfied.

The class T is distinguished from $\mathfrak{T}^*$ by the conditions

$\gamma = \{\zeta : |\zeta| = 1\}$ and $t([0,1]) = \Gamma$.

The result of Frolov has been recently extended to the matrix case by one of the authors. The corresponding result, which simultaneously generalizes Theorem 8.3 (case 4')), reads as follows: Let the matrix function G given on the smooth contour Γ have the property that, for every point $t \in \Gamma$, there exist a matrix A_t , a number $\theta_t \in \in [0, 2\pi(r-p)/p]$ and a sector S_t with vertex at zero and an apex angle less than $2\pi/\max(p,q)$ such that, for all essential limits F of the matrix function G at the point t from the left (from the right), the numerical domain of the matrices $A_t F$ lies in the sector $S_t(e^{i\theta_t} S_t)$. Then G is Φ-factorable in L_p .

In the scalar case the problem of Φ-factorability of functions with discontinuities of almost-periodic (GOHBERG, KRUPNIK [4], GOHBERG, SEMENTSUL [1], PILIDI [1], SEMENTSUL [1] and semi-almost periodic type (SAGINASHVILI [1-3], SARASON [3]) was studied, too. For $p = 2$, there are also investigations concerning multiplicatively periodic weakly oscillating functions (ABRAHAMSE [1]) and functions from certain algebras generated by them (POWER [1]). The problem of Φ-factorability in L_2 of functions from the algebra generated by piecewise continuous (PC) and quasi-continuous (QC) functions, i.e. functions belonging to $H_\infty + C$ along with their complex conjugates, was also examined (SARASON [4]). A corresponding result for $H_\infty + PC$ fails to be known. One of the difficulties arising in the study of the latter class consists in the fact that it, being a subspace, is not an algebra (BONSALL, GILLESPIE [1]). In the paper ROCHBERG [1] (see also SPITKOVSKIǏ [6,14]) a criterion of Φ-factorability of functions G with p-index $\varkappa$ which is formulated in terms of condition (3.21) was obtained for $\varrho = \exp(-p\tilde{w}/2)$, where $\tilde{w}$ is the harmonic conjugate to a branch w of the argument of the function $G(t)t^{-\varkappa}$ chosen in a suitable manner. Analogues of all these results for the case $n > 1$ fail to be known hitherto. Concerning this topic, up to now certain results were obtained only for matrix functions with discontinuities of semi-almost periodic type. In KARLOVICH,

SPITKOVSKIǏ [1] it is shown that, under certain conditions, the Φ-factorability problem for such matrix functions can be reduced to the problem of existence of a so-called P-factorization of an almost-periodic function F given on the real line, i.e., of a representation

$$F(t) = F_+(t)(\delta_{kj}e^{i\nu_j t})_{k,j=1}^n F_-(t) ,$$

where $F_+^{\pm 1}$ ($F_-^{\pm 1}$) are almost-periodic matrix functions with non-negative (non-positive) Fourier exponents and $\nu_j \in \mathbb{R}$.

Some classes of matrix functions admitting a P-factorization are selected in GRUDSKIǏ, KHEVELEV [1], KARLOVICH, SPITKOVSKIǏ [1], SPITKOVSKIǏ [15], KHLGATYAN [1]. However, the existence problem of a P-factorization is very complicated even for second-order triangular matrix functions with almost-periodic polynomials as elements.

It should be mentioned that P-factorization may be viewed as a factorization with, generally speaking, infinite partial indices. The study of such a type of factorization and of the corresponding Riemann problem is very complicated even in the scalar case (see the pioneer work of GOVOROV [1,2], but also ALEKHNO [1], GRUDSKIǏ [2], GRUDSKIǏ, DYBIN [1,2], DYBIN, DODOKHOVA [1,2]). On the other hand, in the matrix case research related to this subject is only beginning to evolve.

In connection with Corollary 8.1 we want to note that, if $G \notin L_\infty^-$, then the algebra $L_\infty^-[G]$ agrees with the smallest closed subalgebra of L_∞ containing L_∞^- and G . It is not hard to derive this result from Lemmas 5.2 and 5.3 and the fact proved in HOFFMAN, SINGER [1] that every closed subalgebra of L_∞ containing H_∞ and not coinciding with H_∞ contains C , too. For the scalar case on the circle Corollary 8.1 is, in fact, established in LEE [1] [1].

[1] LEE [1] has discussed the case $G \in H_\infty + C$, where the algebra $H_\infty[G]$ was defined as generated by H_∞ and G; it was claimed that the demand $G^{-1} \in H_\infty[G]$ is equivalent to the Φ-factorability of the function G. However, in the proof of the necessity the condition $G \in H_\infty + C$ was not used, but the sufficience is a simple consequence of Theorem 5.2 which does not need any additional arguments.

Finally, we intend to note that the class of smooth contours, apparently, does not seem to be the most general class for which Theorems 8.3, 8.4 and Corollary 8.1 remain valid. The problem of extending this class is of some significance.

The generalized Riemann boundary value problem (also known as the Markushevich problem or the general boundary value problem of linear conjugation) on the unit circle $\mathbb{T}$ consists in the determination of functions φ^+ ($\in H_p^+$) and φ^- ($\in H_p^-$) by the boundary condition on $\mathbb{T}$

$$\varphi^+(t) + a(t)\varphi^-(t) + b(t)\overline{\varphi^-(t)} = c(t) , \qquad (9.1)$$

where c ($\in L_p$) and a,b ($\in L_\infty$) are given functions.

In view of the presence of conjugation in the boundary condition (9.1), the generalized Riemann boundary value problem is linear only then, when L_p and $H_p^\pm$ are considered as spaces over the field of real numbers. Therefore, speaking about the number of linearly independent solutions of the homogeneous $(c(t) \equiv 0)$ problem (9.1) or about the number of solvability conditions of the inhomogeneous problem, we shall understand the linear independence as the linear independence over the field of real numbers.

The study of the boundary value problem (9.1) is based on its reduction to the Riemann boundary value problem (9.4) for a two-dimensional vector with a certain matrix coefficient G. In doing so, the images of problems (9.1) and (9.4) are closed only simultaneously; the codimensions of the images and the dimensions of the kernels of problem (9.1) and (9.4), respectively, coincide, which allows us to employ the results of the preceding chapters for the study of problem (9.1).

On the basis of the mentioned relationship between problems (9.1) and (9.4) in Section 9.1 a criterion of Fredholmness of the generalized Riemann boundary value problem in L_p will be established and formulae for its defect numbers will be derived. It turns out that a necessary and sufficient condition of Fredholmness of problem (9.1) consists in the membership of the function a^{-1} to the class L_∞ and the Φ-factorability of the matrix coefficient G of problem (9.4), where the defect numbers are expressed by the partial indices of the matrix function G. In 9.1 it will also be established that the perturbation of the coefficient b by a function of class $H_\infty + C$ does not influence on the Fredholmness of problem (9.1). Hence, for $b \in H_\infty + C$, the Fredholmness of problem (9.1) is completely determined by the function a. In Section 9.2 the boundary value problem (9.1) is considered in the space L_2 under the assumption that $a = a_1 a_0 \overline{a_2}$, where $a_1^{\pm 1}, a_2^{\pm 1} \in H_\infty$, $a_0 \in C$. A condition of Fredholmness of the boundary value problem (9.1) in L_2 will be stated and estimates for its defect numbers as well as a stability condition for problem (9.1) understood as stability of the partial indices of G will be established. Corresponding results for the so-called elliptic, parabolic and hyperbolic case of problem (9.1) will be derived as consequences.

Section 9.3 is dedicated to the boundary value problem (9.1) with continuous coefficients $a(t)$ and $b(t)$. In this case the results of 9.2 allow an essential strengthening and, at the same time, may be formulated much more simply and elegantly. In particular, if the matrix function G can be factored with continuous factors, then the sufficient condition of stability of problem (9.1) presented in Section 9.2 becomes also necessary.

Section 9.4 contains comments on published papers.

9.1. CRITERION OF FREDHOLMNESS OF THE GENERALIZED RIEMANN BOUNDARY VALUE PROBLEM IN THE SPACE L_p

For functions φ of class H_p^+ $(\overset{\circ}{H}{}_p^-)$, we shall denote by $\hat{\varphi}$ the function which is defined by the equation $\hat{\varphi}(z) = z^{-1}\overline{\varphi(z)}$, where obviously $\hat{\varphi} \in \overset{\circ}{H}{}_p^-$ (H_p^+).

Besides of problem (9.1) we shall consider the system

$$\begin{cases} \varphi_1^+(t) + tb(t)\varphi_2^+(t) + a(t)\varphi_1^-(t) = g_1(t) , \\ \overline{a(t)}t\varphi_2^+(t) + \overline{b(t)}\varphi_1^-(t) + t\varphi_2^-(t) = g_2(t) , \end{cases} \tag{9.2}$$

where $g_1, g_2 \in L_p$ are known and $\varphi_j^+ \in H_p^+$, $\varphi_j^- \in \overset{\circ}{H}{}_p^-$ $(j=1,2)$ are the desired functions. System (9.2) may be rewritten in the form

$$(AP + BQ)\tilde{\varphi} = g ,$$

where $g = \begin{pmatrix} g_1 \\ g_2 \end{pmatrix}$, $\tilde{\varphi} = \begin{pmatrix} \varphi_1 \\ \varphi_2 \end{pmatrix} \in L_p^2$ $(P\varphi_j = \varphi_j^+ , Q\varphi_j = \varphi_j^- , j = 1,2)$,

$$A = \begin{pmatrix} 1 & tb \\ 0 & t\overline{a} \end{pmatrix} , \quad B = \begin{pmatrix} a & 0 \\ \overline{b} & t \end{pmatrix} .$$

To the latter equation the theory developed in the preceding sections may be applied. At the same time, as we shall see now, system (9.2) is closely associated with the initial problem (9.1), a fact, which is crucial for the examination of this problem.

LEMMA 9.1. If $\{\varphi^+,\varphi^-\}$ is a solution of problem (9.1), then, setting $\varphi_1^{\pm} = \varphi^{\pm}$, $\varphi_2^{\pm} = \hat{\varphi}^{\pm}$, we obtain a solution of system (9.2) for $g_1 = c$, $g_2 = \overline{c}$. Vice versa, if $\left\{\begin{pmatrix} \varphi_1^+ \\ \varphi_2^+ \end{pmatrix} , \begin{pmatrix} \varphi_1^- \\ \varphi_2^- \end{pmatrix}\right\}$ is a solution of system (9.2), then $\left\{\begin{pmatrix} \hat{\varphi}_2^- \\ \hat{\varphi}_1^- \end{pmatrix} , \begin{pmatrix} \hat{\varphi}_2^+ \\ \hat{\varphi}_1^+ \end{pmatrix}\right\}$ is a solution of the same system but with the right-hand side $\begin{pmatrix} \overline{g_2} \\ \overline{g_1} \end{pmatrix}$ and $\varphi^+ = \frac{1}{2}(\varphi_1^+ + \hat{\varphi}_2^-)$, $\varphi^- = \frac{1}{2}(\varphi_1^- + \hat{\varphi}_2^+)$ is a solution of problem (9.1).

The proof of Lemma 9.1 is reduced to a simple calculation. ≡

A similar connection exists between the solutions of the problem

$$a(t)\psi^+(t) - \overline{b(t)t^2\psi^+(t)} + \psi^-(t) = d(t) , \tag{9.1'}$$

which is called the associate to problem (9.1), and the solutions of the system

$$\begin{aligned} a(t)\psi_1^+(t) + \psi_1^-(t) - \overline{tb(t)}\psi_2^-(t) &= h_1(t) , \\ -t^2b(t)\psi_1^+(t) + t\psi_2^+(t) + t\overline{a(t)}\psi_2^-(t) &= h_2(t) . \end{aligned} \tag{9.2'}$$

Lemma 9.1 shows that system (9.2) with the right side $\begin{pmatrix} g_1 \\ g_2 \end{pmatrix}$ is solvable if and only if the same system with the right-hand side $\begin{pmatrix} \overline{g_2} \\ \overline{g_1} \end{pmatrix}$ is solvable. The identity

$$\begin{pmatrix} g_1 \\ g_2 \end{pmatrix} = \frac{1}{2}\begin{pmatrix} g_1 + \overline{g_2} \\ \overline{g_1} + g_2 \end{pmatrix} + \frac{1}{2i}\begin{pmatrix} i(g_1 - \overline{g_2}) \\ i(g_2 - \overline{g_1}) \end{pmatrix}$$

permits us to represent the set $\mathfrak{L}$ of right-hand sides $\begin{pmatrix} g_1 \\ g_2 \end{pmatrix}$ for which system (9.2) is solvable in the form of a sum $\mathcal{L}_0 + i\,\mathcal{L}_0$, where $\mathcal{L}_0$ consists of elements from $\mathcal{L}$ of the type $\begin{pmatrix} g \\ \bar{g} \end{pmatrix}$.

Clearly, $\mathcal{L}$ is a linear space over the field of complex and $\mathcal{L}_0$ over the field of real numbers, both linear spaces being closed only simultaneously.

In addition, Lemma 9.1 shows that problem (9.1) with the right-hand side c is solvable if and only if $\begin{pmatrix} c \\ \bar{c} \end{pmatrix} \in \mathcal{L}_0$. Consequently, the closedness of the image of problem (9.1) is equivalent to the closedness of $\mathcal{L}_0$ and, thus, of $\mathcal{L}$. From this we conclude the validity of the next assertion.

<u>COROLLARY 9.1.</u> The image of problem (9.1) is closed only simultaneously with the image of the operator $AP + BQ$.

Lemma 9.1 enables us also to establish relationships between solutions of the homogeneous problems (9.1) and (9.2). Owing to this lemma, the pair $\left\{\begin{pmatrix} \hat{\varphi}_2^- \\ \hat{\varphi}_1^- \end{pmatrix}, \begin{pmatrix} \hat{\varphi}_2^+ \\ \hat{\varphi}_1^+ \end{pmatrix}\right\}$ is, together with a certain pair $\left\{\begin{pmatrix} \varphi_1^+ \\ \varphi_2^+ \end{pmatrix}, \begin{pmatrix} \varphi_1^- \\ \varphi_2^- \end{pmatrix}\right\}$, also a solution of the homogeneous problem (9.2), which allows for writing the lineal M of solutions of the homogeneous problem (9.2) in the form $M = M_0 + iM_0$, where $M_0 \subseteq M$ consists of pairs of vector functions of the type $\left\{\begin{pmatrix} \varphi^+ \\ \hat{\varphi}^- \end{pmatrix}, \begin{pmatrix} \varphi^- \\ \hat{\varphi}^+ \end{pmatrix}\right\}$ (compare with similar considerations concerning the image of problem (9.2)). Furthermore, $\{\varphi^+, \varphi^-\}$ is a solution of the homogeneous problem (9.1) iff $\left\{\begin{pmatrix} \varphi^+ \\ \hat{\varphi}^- \end{pmatrix}, \begin{pmatrix} \varphi^- \\ \hat{\varphi}^+ \end{pmatrix}\right\}$ is a solution of the homogeneous problem (9.2). Thus, an isomorphism between the solution space of the homogeneous problem (9.1) and M_0 is established (both of them are regarded over the field of real numbers). Since the dimension of the lineal M_0 (over the field of real numbers) coincides with the dimension of M (over the complex field), the following result is valid.

<u>COROLLARY 9.2.</u> The number l of linearly independent solutions (over the field of real numbers) of the homogeneous problem (9.1) is

equal to the number of linearly independent (over the field of complex numbers) solutions of the homogeneous problem (9.2).

The following result can be verified analogously.

COROLLARY 9.2'. The number l' of linearly independent solutions (over the field of real numbers) of the homogeneous problem (9.1') coincides with the number of linearly independent solutions (over the complex field) of the homogeneous problem (9.2'). For the space M' of solutions of the homogeneous problem (9.2) we have the representation $M' = M'_0 + iM'_0$, where M'_0 consists of all elements from M' of the form $\left\{\begin{pmatrix}\psi^+\\ \hat{\psi}^-\end{pmatrix}, \begin{pmatrix}\psi^-\\ \hat{\psi}^+\end{pmatrix}\right\}$. Moreover, $\left\{\begin{pmatrix}\psi^+\\ \hat{\psi}^-\end{pmatrix}, \begin{pmatrix}\psi^-\\ \hat{\psi}^+\end{pmatrix}\right\}$ belongs to M'_0 if and only if $\{\psi^+,\psi^-\}$ is a solution of the homogeneous problem (9.1').

Corollaries 9.1 and 9.2 illustrate that for the normal solvability and finite dimensionality of the kernel of problem (9.1), it is necessary and sufficient that $AP + BQ$ is a Φ_+-operator.
From this we deduce the following proposition.

THEOREM 9.1. For finite dimensionality of the kernel and normal solvability of problem (9.1), it is necessary that $a^{-1} \in L_\infty$, i.e., for some $\delta > 0$, the inequality

$$|a(t)| \geq \delta \tag{9.3}$$

holds a.e. on $\mathbb{T}$.

Proof. We employ Theorem 3.18, due to which for $AP + BQ$ to be a Φ_+-operator, it is necessary that the conditions $A^{-1}, B^{-1} \in L_\infty$ be fulfilled. In the case under consideration, $\det A = t\bar{a}$, $\det B = ta$, therefore, either of the requirements $A^{-1} \in L_\infty$, $B^{-1} \in L_\infty$ is equivalent to condition (9.3), which proves Theorem 9.1. ≡
Condition (9.3) is necessary, in particular, for the Fredholmness of problem (9.1). In the sequel, this condition is supposed to be fulfilled. Assuming that $a^{-1} \in L_\infty$, we can rewrite the system (9.2) in the form

$$(P + GQ)\tilde{\varphi} = \tilde{g}, \tag{9.4}$$

where

$$G = A^{-1}B = \bar{a}^{-1}\begin{pmatrix} |a|^2-|b|^2 & -tb \\ \overline{tb} & 1 \end{pmatrix}, \quad \tilde{g} = A^{-1}g = \begin{pmatrix} g_1 - b\bar{a}^{-1}g_2 \\ t^{-1}\bar{a}^{-1}g_2 \end{pmatrix}. \quad (9.5)$$

In turn, the system (9.2') may be rewritten in the form

$$(Q + G'P)\tilde{\Psi} = \tilde{h}\ , \qquad (9.4')$$

where G' is the matrix function transposed to G , and

$$\tilde{h} = \begin{pmatrix} h_1 - t^{-2}\bar{b}\ \bar{a}^{-1}\ h_2 \\ t^{-1}\ \bar{a}^{-1}\ h_2 \end{pmatrix}.$$

Above (Corollary 9.1) it was established that problem (9.1) is normally solvable if and only if the image of the operator $AP + BQ$ or, which is equivalent, the image of the operator $P + GQ$ is closed, where the matrix function G is defined by equation (9.5). Now we want to complete this statement by describing the connection between the codimensions of the images of problems (9.1) and (9.4).

LEMMA 9.2 The image of problem (9.1) is a lineal (over the field of real numbers) the closure of which is the subspace defined by the condition

$$\operatorname{Re} \int_{\mathbb{T}} c(t)\psi^+(t)dt = 0\ , \qquad (9.6)$$

where ψ^+ runs over the "+"-components of the solutions of the homogeneous problem (9.1').

Proof. According to Lemma 9.1, problem (9.1) with the right-hand side c is solvable simultaneously with problem (9.2) with the right-hand side $\begin{pmatrix} c \\ \bar{c} \end{pmatrix}$ or, in other words, with problem (9.4) in which the right-hand side is equal to $\tilde{g} = \begin{pmatrix} c - b\bar{c}\ \bar{a}^{-1} \\ t^{-1}\ \bar{a}^{-1}\ \bar{c} \end{pmatrix}$.

As mentioned in Theorem 3.1, a necessary condition for solvability of problem (9.4) consists in the orthogonality of its right-hand side to the "+"-components of all solutions of the homogeneous associate problem, i.e. of problem (9.4') with zero right-hand side. Evidently, the solutions of the homogeneous problems (9.4') and (9.2') coincide.

The orthogonality of the vector function $\tilde{g}$ to the "+"-components of all vector functions from M' is equivalent to its orthogonality to the "+"-components of all vector functions from M'_0, i.e. to vector functions of the type $\begin{pmatrix} \psi^+ \\ \hat{\psi}^- \end{pmatrix}$, where $\{\psi^+, \psi^-\}$ is a solution of the homogeneous problem (9.1').

But

$$\int_{\mathbb{T}} \tilde{g}' \begin{pmatrix} \psi^+ \\ \hat{\psi}^- \end{pmatrix} dt = \int_{\mathbb{T}} ((c - b\bar{c}\bar{a}^{-1})\psi^+ + t^{-1}\bar{a}^{-1}\bar{c}\ \overline{t\psi^-})dt =$$

$$\int_{\mathbb{T}} \bar{a}^{-1}t^{-2}(c\bar{a}t^2\psi^+ - \bar{c}bt^2\psi^+ + \overline{c\psi^-})dt .$$

Using the fact that $\overline{bt^2\psi^+ - \psi^-} = a\psi^+$, we may rewrite the right-hand side in the following manner:

$$\int_{\mathbb{T}} \bar{a}^{-1}t^{-2}(c\bar{a}t^2\psi^+ - \bar{c}\overline{a\psi^+})dt = \int_{\mathbb{T}} c\psi^+ dt - \int_{\mathbb{T}} \bar{c}\overline{\psi^+}t^{-2}dt .$$

Since the contour under consideration is the unit circle, we have $\overline{dt} = -t^{-2}dt$, so that we finally get:

$$\int_{\mathbb{T}} \tilde{g} \begin{pmatrix} \psi^+ \\ \hat{\psi}^- \end{pmatrix} dt = 2 \operatorname{Re} \int_{\mathbb{T}} c(t)\psi^+(t)dt .$$

Thus, condition (9.6) coincides precisely with the condition of orthogonality of $\tilde{g}$ to the "+"-components of the solutions of the homogeneous problem (9.4). Therefore, it is necessary for the solvability of problem (9.1).

Now, let the function c $(\in L_p)$ satisfy the condition (9.6). Then in every neighbourhood of the vector function $\tilde{g} = \begin{pmatrix} c - b\bar{c}\,\bar{a}^{-1} \\ t^{-1}\,\bar{a}^{-1}\,\bar{c} \end{pmatrix}$ there exists a vector function $\tilde{f}$ belonging to the image of problem (9.4). The vector function $f = A\tilde{f} = \begin{pmatrix} f_1 \\ f_2 \end{pmatrix}$ belongs to the image of problem (9.2). With regard to Lemma 9.1, the function $\frac{1}{2}(f_1+\bar{f}_2)$ lies in the image of problem (9.1). Due to the closeness of the vector functions $\tilde{g}$ and $\tilde{f}$ it is possible to make the vector functions $A\tilde{g} = \begin{pmatrix} c \\ \bar{c} \end{pmatrix}$ and $A\tilde{f} = f$ as close as desired and, consequently, also the functions c and $\frac{1}{2}(f_1+\bar{f}_2)$. Hence, the image of problem (9.1) is dense in the subspace generated by conditions (9.6), which proves Lemma 9.2. ≡

COROLLARY 9.3. The codimension l' of the closure of the image of problem (9.1) (over the field of real numbers) agrees with the codimension of the closure of the image of problem (9.4) (over the complex field).

Indeed, Lemma 9.2 demonstrates that the number l' coincides with the number of linearly independent (over the field of real numbers) solutions of the homogeneous problem (9.1'), which, according to Corollary 9.2, is equal to the dimension (over the complex field) of the kernel of problem (9.2'). It remains to use the coincidence of the kernels of problems (9.2') and (9.4').

Now we are going to formulate the main theorem of the present section.

THEOREM 9.2. The generalized Riemann boundary value problem (9.1) is Fredholm in L_p iff

1) condition (9.3) is fulfilled,
2) the matrix function G defined by equation (9.5) is Φ-factorable in L_p.

If the conditions 1) and 2) are satisfied, then the index of problem (9.1) coincides with the total index of G, the number l of linearly independent solutions of the homogeneous problem is equal to the sum of positive partial indices, whereas the number l' of solvability conditions for the inhomogeneous problem is opposite to the sum of negative partial indices.

Proof. The necessity of condition 1) for the Fredholmness of problem (9.1) has been stated by Theorem 9.1. If this condition is satisfied, then, owing to Corollaries 9.1 - 9.3, problem (9.1) is Fredholm only simultaneously with problem (9.4). Thanks to Theorem 3.16, the Fredholmness of problem (9.4) is equivalent to the Φ-factorability of the matrix function G.

According to Corollary 9.2, the number l coincides with the dimension of the kernel of problem (9.4), i.e. with the sum of positive partial indices of G (by Theorem 3.16). The formula for l' is established on the strength of Corollary 9.3. Now, from the formulae for l and l

it is not hard to obtain the formula for the index of problem (9.1). Hence, Theorem 9.2 is proved. ≡

We would like to mention that the formulae for l and l' can be written in the following manner: Let $\varkappa_1$ and $\varkappa_2$ be the partial indices of the matrix function G. Then

$$\begin{aligned} l &= \max\{0,\varkappa_1+\varkappa_2\}\,, \quad l' = \max\{0,-\varkappa_1-\varkappa_2\}\,, \text{ if } \varkappa_1\varkappa_2 \geq 0\,; \\ l &= \varkappa_1\,, \quad l' = -\varkappa_2\,, \quad \text{if } \varkappa_1\varkappa_2 < 0\,. \end{aligned} \tag{9.7}$$

DEFINITION 9.1. The problem (9.1) will be said to be stable, if the partial indices of the corresponding matrix function (9.5) are stable.

If $\varkappa_1\varkappa_2 \geq 0$, then, due to formulae (9.7), the numbers l and l' are defined uniquely by the total index of the matrix function (9.5). Therefore, they remain unchanged under small perturbations of the coefficients a and b. Thus, the condition $\varkappa_1\varkappa_2 \geq 0$ (all the more, the condition of stability of problem (9.1.)) is sufficient for the stability of the numbers l and l'.

The next statement, which often proves to be useful in the study of problem (9.1), results directly from Theorem 9.2.

THEOREM 9.3. The substitution of the coefficient b in problem (9.1) by $b-\varphi$ with $\varphi \in H_\infty + C$ does not influence neither on the Fredholmness of the problem not on the value of its index. If $t\varphi \in H_\infty$, then the numbers l and l' of problem (9.1) also remain unchanged.

Proof. We take advantage of the identity

$$\bar{a}^{-1}\begin{pmatrix} |a|^2-|b-\varphi|^2 & -t(b-\varphi) \\ \overline{t(b-\varphi)} & 1 \end{pmatrix} = \begin{pmatrix} 1 & t_\varphi \\ 0 & 1 \end{pmatrix}\bar{a}^{-1}\begin{pmatrix} |a|^2-|b|^2 & -tb \\ \overline{tb} & 1 \end{pmatrix}\begin{pmatrix} 1 & 0 \\ -\overline{t\varphi} & 1 \end{pmatrix}, \tag{9.8}$$

which is true for any choice of the function φ. If $\varphi \in H_\infty + C$, then the matrix function $\begin{pmatrix} 1 & t\varphi \\ 0 & 1 \end{pmatrix}$, together with its inverse, belongs to the class $H_\infty^+ + C$, whereas $\begin{pmatrix} 1 & 0 \\ -\overline{t\varphi} & 1 \end{pmatrix}$ belongs to $H_\infty^- + C$ together with its inverse.

Applying Theorem 5.5, we observe that the matrix functions

$$\bar{a}^{-1}\begin{pmatrix} |a|^2-|b-\varphi|^2 & -t(b-\varphi) \\ \overline{t(b-\varphi)} & 1 \end{pmatrix} \text{ and } \bar{a}^{-1}\begin{pmatrix} |a|^2-|b|^2 & -tb \\ \overline{tb} & 1 \end{pmatrix}$$

are Φ-factorable in L_p only simultaneously, where their total indices differ by the sum of total indices of the matrix functions $\begin{pmatrix} 1 & t\varphi \\ 0 & 1 \end{pmatrix}$ and $\begin{pmatrix} 1 & 0 \\ -\overline{t\varphi} & 1 \end{pmatrix}$. The latter two matrix functions are triangular and the indices of their diagonal elements are equal to zero. According to Theorem 4.6, their partial (and, thus, also total indices) are equal to zero. Hence, the total indices of the matrix functions

$$\bar{a}^{-1}\begin{pmatrix} |a|^2-|b-\varphi|^2 & -t(b-\varphi) \\ \overline{t(b-\varphi)} & 1 \end{pmatrix} \text{ and } \bar{a}^{-1}\begin{pmatrix} |a|^2-|b|^2 & -tb \\ \overline{tb} & 1 \end{pmatrix}$$

coincide. This proves the first statement of the theorem.

If $t\varphi \in H_\infty$, then identity (9.8) shows that not only the total but also the partial indices of the matrix functions

$$\bar{a}^{-1}\begin{pmatrix} |a|^2-|b-\varphi|^2 & -t(b-\varphi) \\ \overline{t(b-\varphi)} & 1 \end{pmatrix} \text{ and } \bar{a}^{-1}\begin{pmatrix} |a|^2-|b|^2 & -tb \\ \overline{tb} & 1 \end{pmatrix}$$

agree. Making use of formulae (9.6), we get the second statement of the theorem. ≡

<u>COROLLARY 9.4.</u> If $b \in H_\infty + C$, then problem (9.1) is Fredholm if and only if the function a is Φ-factorable in L_p. In the latter case the index of problem (9.1) coincides with the double p-index of the function a.

In fact, for $b \in H_\infty + C$, problem (9.1) is Fredholm only along with problem (9.1) with the same coefficient a and $b \equiv 0$, whereas the indices of these problems coincide. At the same time, for $b \equiv 0$, problem (9.1) changes into the ordinary Riemann problem $\varphi^+ + a\varphi^- = c$. In order to avoid possible misunderstandings, note that the index of problem (9.1), for $b \equiv 0$, is the double index of the corresponding Riemann problem (i.e., does not agree with it), because the problem (9.1) is considered over the field of real numbers, while the Riemann problem is regarded over the complex field.

Thus, the index of problem (9.1) with a coefficient b from the class $H_\infty + C$ (in particular, with a continuous coefficient b) is necessarily even.

9.2. SUFFICIENT CONDITIONS OF FREDHOLMNESS AND STABILITY. ESTIMATES FOR THE DEFECT NUMBERS OF THE GENERALIZED RIEMANN BOUNDARY VALUE PROBLEM IN THE SPACE L_2

In this section we shall be concerned with problem (9.1) in the class L_2, assuming that the coefficient a can be represented in the form $a = a_1 a_0 \overline{a}_2$, where a_1 and a_2 are invertible elements of H_∞ and a_0 is a continuous, non-vanishing function. Applying Theorem 3.10 and Lemma 6.3, we recognize that the matrix function (9.5) is Φ-factorable only simultaneously with the matrix function

$$G_0(t) = \begin{pmatrix} |a(t)|^2-|b(t)|^2 & -tb(t) \\ \overline{tb(t)} & 1 \end{pmatrix}, \tag{9.9}$$

and the partial indices of the matrix function (9.5) are obtained from the partial indices of the matrix function (9.9) by shift on the index $\varkappa$ of the function a (coinciding with the index of a_0). Furthermore, multiplying the matrix function G_0 by the constant matrix $\begin{pmatrix} -1 & 0 \\ 0 & 1 \end{pmatrix}$ from the left, it turns into the Hermitian matrix function

$$F(t) = \begin{pmatrix} |b(t)|^2-|a(t)|^2 & tb(t) \\ \overline{tb(t)} & 1 \end{pmatrix} \tag{9.10}$$

with negative determinant. In accordance with formula (7.5), the partial 2-indices of F (and, consequently, also of G_0) are equal to k (≥ 0) and $-k$.

Therefore, the partial indices of the matrix function G are equal to $\varkappa_1 = \varkappa + k$ and $\varkappa_2 = \varkappa - k$. Formulae (9.7) for the numbers l and l' may be rewritten in the following form:

$$\begin{aligned} l &= \max\{0,2\varkappa\}, \quad l' = \max\{0,-2\varkappa\}, \quad \text{if } k \leq |\varkappa|, \\ l &= k+\varkappa, \quad l' = k-\varkappa, \quad \text{if } k > |\varkappa|. \end{aligned} \tag{9.11}$$

Thus, on condition that $k \le |\varkappa|$, the numbers l and l' of problem (9.1) are stable, while the stability of problem (9.1) itself is equivalent to the requirement $k = 0$.

THEOREM 9.4. Suppose the functions $\varphi_1, \varphi_2 \in M_\infty^+$ to have no common poles in $\mathcal{D}^+$, to satisfy the inequalities

$$\operatorname*{ess\,sup}_{t\in\mathbb{T}} \left| \frac{tb(t)-\varphi_1(t)}{a(t)} \right| < 1 < \operatorname*{ess\,inf}_{t\in\mathbb{T}} \left| \frac{tb(t)-\varphi_2(t)}{a(t)} \right| \tag{9.12}$$

and moreover,

$$(\varphi_1 - \varphi_2)^{-1} \in M_\infty^+ . \tag{9.13}$$

Then problem (9.1) is Fredholm in L_2 and for the numbers l and l' the relations

$$\begin{aligned} &l = \max(0, 2\varkappa), \quad l' = \max(0, -2\varkappa), \quad \text{if } N \le |\varkappa|, \\ &\max(0, 2\varkappa) \le l \le \varkappa + N, \quad l' = l - 2\varkappa, \quad \text{if } N > |\varkappa| \end{aligned} \tag{9.11'}$$

hold. Here N is the number of zeros (taking into account their multiplicity) of the function $\varphi_1 - \varphi_2$ in $\mathcal{D}^+$.

Proof. We represent the matrix function (9.9) in the form

$$G_0 = |\varphi_1 - \varphi_2|^{-2} \begin{pmatrix} \psi_2 & -\psi_1 \\ -\chi_2 & \chi_1 \end{pmatrix} G_1 \begin{pmatrix} \overline{\psi_2} & \overline{\chi_2} \\ \overline{\psi_1} & \overline{\chi_1} \end{pmatrix}.$$

Here $\varphi_1 = \psi_1/\chi_1$, $\varphi_2 = \psi_2/\chi_2$ ($\psi_j \in H_\infty$, χ_j is a polynomial the zeros of which are located in $\mathcal{D}^+$ and do not coincide with the zeros of ψ_j, $j=1,2$) are representations existing thanks to the condition $\varphi_1, \varphi_2 \in M_\infty^+$, and

$$G_1 = \begin{pmatrix} |\chi_2|^{-2}(|a|^2 - |tb-\varphi_1|^2) & -\bar{\chi}_1^{-1}\chi_2^{-1}(|a|^2 - |b|^2 + \varphi_1\overline{tb} + \overline{\varphi}_2 tb - \varphi_1\overline{\varphi}_2) \\ \chi_1^{-1}\bar{\chi}_2^{-1}(|a|^2 - |b|^2 + \overline{\varphi}_1 tb + \varphi_2\overline{tb} - \overline{\varphi}_1\varphi_2) & |\chi_1|^{-2}(|tb-\varphi_2|^2 - |a|^2) \end{pmatrix}.$$

Since $\operatorname{Re} G_1 = \operatorname{diag}[|\chi_2|^{-2}(|a|^2 - |tb-\varphi_1|^2), |\chi_1|^{-2}(tb-\varphi_2|^2 - |a|^2)]$, the conditions (9.12) guarantee the uniform positiveness of $\operatorname{Re} G_1$ and, according to Theorem 7.8, the Φ-factorability of the matrix function G_1 in L_2 with zero partial indices. The factor $A_+ = \begin{pmatrix} \psi_2 & -\psi_1 \\ -\chi_2 & \chi_1 \end{pmatrix}$ belongs to H_∞, while its inverse, in virtue of condition (9.13), belongs to M_∞^+ and, therefore, has no influence on the Φ-factorability

(Theorem 3.10). The estimates for the partial indices given in Theorem 2.11 allow us to claim that the partial indices of the matrix function A_+G_1 are included between 0 and N. Analogously, it can be verified that the product $A_+G_1A_-$ with $A_- = \begin{pmatrix} \overline{\psi_2} & \overline{\chi_2} \\ \overline{\psi_1} & \overline{\chi_1} \end{pmatrix}$ is Φ-factorable in L_2 and the partial indices of this product do not exceed N taken absolutely. In view of condition (9.13), $|\varphi_1 - \varphi_2|^{-2}$ is a positive function belonging to the class L_∞ together with its inverse. Applying Lemma 6.5 to this function, we find that the matrix functions G_0 and $A_+G_1A_-$ are Φ-factorable only simultaneously and their partial indices coincide.

Summarizing, we have proved that the matrix function G_0 is Φ-factorable in L_2, so that problem (9.1) is Fredholm and, in addition, $k \leq N$. In order to complete the proof of the theorem, it remains only to use formulae (9.11). ≡

<u>COROLLARY 9.5.</u> Let the function $\varphi \in M_\infty^+$ satisfy the requirement

$$\operatorname*{ess\,sup}_{t \in \mathbb{T}} \left| \frac{tb(t) - \varphi(t)}{a(t)} \right| < 1 . \tag{9.14}$$

Then problem (9.1) is Fredholm and for the numbers l and l' the relations

$$l = \max\{0, 2\varkappa\}, \quad l' = \max\{0, -2\varkappa\}, \quad \text{if } \mathcal{P}(\varphi) \leq |\varkappa| ,$$

$$\max\{0, 2\varkappa\} \leq l \leq \varkappa + \mathcal{P}(\varphi), \quad \text{if } \mathcal{P}(\varphi) > |\varkappa|$$

are fulfilled.

Here $\mathcal{P}(\varphi)$ is the number of poles (counting their multiplicity) of the function φ in $\mathcal{D}^+$.

Corollary 9.5 follows immediately from Theorem 9.4 by setting $\varphi_1 = \varphi$ and taking as φ_2 a sufficiently large constant C. In fact, in this case the conditions (9.12) and (9.13) are satisfied and the number of zeros of the function $\varphi_1 - \varphi_2$ is the number of points $t \in \mathcal{D}^+$ with $\varphi(t) = C$ and, therefore (if C is large enough), coincides with the number of poles of φ. ≡

<u>COROLLARY 9.6.</u> Suppose that the functions $\varphi_1, \varphi_2 \in M_\infty^+$ have no common poles in $\mathcal{D}^+$, coincide (with reference to the multiplicity)

at no more than $|\varkappa|$ points and satisfy the conditions (9.12) and (9.13). Then problem (9.1) is Fredholm and the numbers l and l' of this problem are stable.

Let us emphasize a sufficient condition for stability of problem (9.1).

THEOREM 9.5. Assume that the functions $\varphi_1, \varphi_2 \in M_\infty^+$ have no common poles in $\mathcal{D}^+$ and satisfy the inequalities (9.5) and the requirement $(\varphi_1 - \varphi_2)^{-1} \in H_\infty$. Then problem (9.1) is Fredholm and stable in L_2.

Indeed, the requirements imposed on φ_1 and φ_2 in Theorem 9.5 coincide with the requirements involved in Theorem 9.4 completed by the condition $N = 0$. In Theorem 9.4 it was proved that $k \leq N$. Consequently, under the conditions of Theorem 9.5, $k = 0$. ≡

From Corollary 9.5 we may derive a sufficient condition of stability of problem (9.1) (which is, of course, a special case of Theorem 9.5).

COROLLARY 9.7. Let the function $\varphi \in H_\infty$ satisfy the condition (9.14). Then problem (9.1) is Fredholm and stable in L_2.

In particular, problem (9.1) will be Fredholm and stable in L_2 in the so-called elliptic case:[1] $\operatorname{ess\,sup}_{t\in\mathbb{T}} |b(t)/a(t)| < 1$ (it suffices to choose $\varphi \equiv 0$ in Corollary 9.7).

Now we proceed to the so-called parabolic case

$$|b(t)| = |a(t)| \quad \text{a.e. on } \mathbb{T}. \tag{9.15}$$

In this case the matrix function G_0 becomes triangular, is Φ-factorable only simultaneously with the matrix function

$$\begin{pmatrix} tb & 0 \\ 1 & \overline{tb} \end{pmatrix} \tag{9.16}$$

and has the same tuple of partial indices.

THEOREM 9.6. Let the condition (9.15) be satisfied. Then the following assertions are equivalent:

[1] The concept of elliptic case in this sense and the concepts of parabolic and hyperbolic cases as well were introduced in MIKHAILOV [3,4].

1) problem (9.1) is Fredholm in L_2 ,

2) $T_Q(tb)$ is a Φ_--operator ,

3) there exists a function $\varphi \in M_\infty^+$ for which

$$\operatorname*{ess\,sup}_{t\in\mathbb{T}} \left| \frac{tb(t) - \varphi(t)}{b(t)} \right| < 1 , \tag{9.14'}$$

4) there exists a function $\varphi \in H_\infty + C$ satisfying the condition (9.14').

If the statements just mentioned are satisfied, then the defect numbers l and l' of problem (9.1) can be calculated by formulae (9.11) in which the quantity k may be replaced either by the defect number $\beta(T_Q(tb))$ or by the smallest possible (with regard to the multiplicity) number ν of poles in the unit disk of the function $\varphi \in M_\infty^+$ satisfying the relation (9.14).

Proof. Problem (9.1) is Fredholm if and only if the matrix function (9.16) is Φ-factorable. Therefore, the equivalence of assertion 1) and 2) results from Theorem 4.4. According to just this theorem, the relation $k = \beta(T_Q(tb))$ is valid. Thus, it remains to prove the equivalence of assertions 2) - 4) and to verify the equation $\nu = \beta(T_Q(tb))$. Assume $T_Q(tb)$ to be a Φ_--operator. Then, owing to Theorem 3.13, $b^{-1} \in L_\infty$. Applying Lemma 7.4 (which is trivial in the considered scalar case), we write down the representation $tb = u\psi$, where $\psi^{\pm 1} \in H_\infty$ and the absolute value of the function u is equal to 1 a.e. on $\mathbb{T}$. Then $T_Q(tb) = T_Q(\psi)T_Q(u)$ and, since the operator $T_Q(\psi)$ is invertible, the property of $T_Q(tb)$ to be a Φ_--operator implies that $T_Q(u)$ is a Φ_--operator, too. Moreover, the defect numbers of these operators coincide.

Now we are going to consider separately the cases of zero and positive values of $\beta(T_Q(tb))$.

a) Suppose $\beta(T_Q(tb)) = 0$. Then $T_Q(tb)$ is not only a Φ_--operator but also invertible from the right. Together with it the operator $T_Q(u)$ is also invertible from the right and, by Theorem 7.12, there exists a function $\chi \in H_\infty$ such that $\|u-\chi\| < 1$. Setting $\varphi = \chi\psi$ and taking into account that $u = tb\psi^{-1}$ and $|\psi| = |b|$, we deduce inequality (9.14') with a function $\varphi \in H_\infty$. Thus, condition 3) is satisfied, where $\nu = 0$.

b) Let $\beta(T_Q(tb)) > 0$. Then, due to assertion 3) of Theorem 3.1, $\alpha(T_Q(tb)) = 0$ and the Φ_--operator $T_Q(tb)$ proves to be Fredholm. Thus, the operator $T_Q(u)$ is also Fredholm. In addition, its index (i.e, the 2-index of the function u) is opposite to the number $\beta(T_Q(tb))$. By virtue of the equivalence of assertions1) and 3) of Theorem 7.13 (the case of non-positive indices), we find that there exists a function χ of class M_∞^+ such that $\chi^{-1} \in H_\infty$ and $\|u-\chi\| < 1$. According to the same theorem, the number of poles of such a functions in the unit disk is opposite to the index of the function u, i.e., they coincides with $\beta(T_Q(tb))$. Setting $\varphi = \chi\psi$, we come, as also in case a), to inequality (9.14'), however, already with a function φ of class M_∞^+ and a number of poles in the unit disk which is equal to $\beta(T_Q(tb))$. In summary, we have proved the implication 2) ==> 3) as well as the inequality $\nu \leq \beta(T_Q(tb))$.

The implication 3) ==> 4) is obvious.

Now we want to assume that condition 4) is fulfilled. Then, of course, $b^{-1} \in L_\infty$. Therefore, there exists again a representation $tb = u\psi$. With the aid of this representation condition (9.14) may be rewritten as follows: $\|1-\bar{u}\chi\| < 1$, where $\chi = \varphi\psi^{-1} \in H_\infty + C$. In view of the contracting mapping principle, the last inequality guarantees the invertibility of the operator $T_Q(\bar{u}\chi)$. But this operator differs from the product $T_Q(\chi)T_Q(\bar{u})$ only by the compact summand $Q\chi P\bar{u}Q$. Due to Theorem 1.5, the product $T_Q(\chi)T_Q(\bar{u})$ is Fredholm. This fact as well as Theorem 1.9 imply that $T_Q(\bar{u})$ is a Φ_+-operator. Now, Corollary 1.2 allows us to conclude that $T_Q(u)$ is a Φ_--operator. Finally, together with this operator, the operator $T_Q(tb)$ obtained from $T_Q(u)$ by multiplying it by the invertible operator $T_Q(\psi)$ is also a Φ_--operator. Finally, it must be said that if the operator $T_Q(tb)$ turned out to be Fredholm, then the operator $T_Q(\chi)$ is also Fredholm and, moreover, the indices of these operators coincide. If, in addition, $\varphi \in M^+_\infty$, then $\chi \in M^+_\infty$ and, by Theorem 2.6, the number of poles of the function χ in the unit disk is an upper bound for the value $-\operatorname{ind} T_Q(\chi)$. Taking into consideration that the number of poles of the function χ and φ is one and the same and that, for $\beta(T_Q(tb)) > 0$, $\operatorname{ind} T_Q(\chi) = -\beta(T_Q(tb))$, we deduce that the quantity $\beta(T_Q(tb))$ is a lower bound for the number of poles in the unit disk for an arbitrary function $\varphi \in M^+_\infty$ satisfying condition (9.14').

Thus, the implication 4) ==> 1) and the inequality $\nu \geq \beta(T_Q(tb))$ have been proved and, together with them, the complete Theorem 9.6. ≡

<u>COROLLARY 9.8.</u> Let condition (9.15) be satisfied (i.e., the parabolic case holds) and the function b be Φ-factorable in L_2 with the index λ. Then problem (9.1) is Fredholm and its defect numbers are calculated by formulae (9.11) in which one has to set $k = \max\{0,-\lambda-1\}$.

In fact, the Φ-factorability of the function b is equivalent to the Fredholmness of the operator $T_Q(tb)$, i.e. to a property which is stronger than the property to be a Φ_--operator. The equation $k = \max\{0,-\lambda-1\}$ follows from the relation $k = \beta(T_Q(tb))$ already mentioned and the formulae for the defect numbers proved in Chapter 3. ≡

<u>COROLLARY 9.9.</u> Under the condition (9.15) (i.e., in the parabolic case) for the stability of problem (9.1) in L_2, it is necessary and sufficient that there exists a function $\varphi \in H_\infty$ satisfying inequality (9.14'). The Φ-factorability of the function b in L_2 with index $\lambda \geq -1$ is a sufficient condition for stability.

<u>Proof.</u> It suffices to remember that the stability of problem (9.1) in L_2 is equivalent to its Fredholmness under the additional condition $k = 0$. After that we have to use the equality $k = \nu$ in the general case and the relation $k = \max\{0,-\lambda-1\}$ in case of a Φ-factorable function b.

We would like to note that in the parabolic case, i.e., under the additional condition (9.15), inequality (9.14) is equivalent to inequality (9.14'). Thus, in the parabolic case the sufficient conditions of Fredholmness and stability indicated in Corollaries 9.5 and 9.7 are necessary and sufficient. Moreover, the bounds for the defect numbers stated in Corollary 9.5 are exact in the parabolic case.

For the so-called hyperbolic case

$$\operatorname*{ess\,inf}_{t\in\mathbb{T}} |b(t)/a(t)| > 1 \tag{9.17}$$

we do not have such a complete solution of the question of Fredholness of problem (9.1) and the values of l and l' as for the elliptic and parabolic case. Here we only want to present a criterion of stability of the problem based on the representation

$$|b(t)|^2 - |a(t)|^2 = |\psi(t)|^2 \tag{9.18}$$

$(\psi^{\pm 1} \in H_\infty)$, which is possible by Theorem 7.10 in virtue of condition (9.17).

THEOREM 9.7. Assume the condition (9.17) to be satisfied, and let the convex hull of the range of the function $tb\psi^{-1}$ have a distance from zero which is greater than 1. Then the problem (9.1) is Fredholm and stable in L_2.

Proof. We represent the matrix function (9.9) in the form

$$G_0 = \begin{pmatrix} -\psi & 0 \\ 0 & 1 \end{pmatrix} \begin{pmatrix} tb\psi^{-1} & 1 \\ 1 & \frac{}{tb\psi^{-1}} \end{pmatrix} \begin{pmatrix} 0 & 1 \\ \overline{\psi} & 0 \end{pmatrix}.$$

From this representation it is clear that the matrix function G_0 is Φ-factorable only simultaneously with the matrix function

$$G_1 = \begin{pmatrix} tb\psi^{-1} & 1 \\ 1 & \frac{}{tb\psi^{-1}} \end{pmatrix}$$

and has the same tuple of partial indices. Furthermore, it should be noticed that the function ψ from the representation (9.18) is defined up to a constant coefficient with absolute value 1. Due to the choice of this multiplier and the condition imposed on the range of the function $tb\psi^{-1}$, we can ensure that $\operatorname{Re}(tb(t)\psi(t)^{-1}) \geq 1+\delta$ for some $\delta > 0$ a.e. on $\mathbb{T}$. Since

$$\operatorname{Re} G_1 = \begin{pmatrix} \operatorname{Re}(tb\psi^{-1}) & 1 \\ 1 & \operatorname{Re}(tb\psi^{-1}) \end{pmatrix},$$

the condition $\operatorname{Re}(tb(t)\psi(t)^{-1}) \geq 1+\delta$ guarantees the uniform positiveness of the matrix function $\operatorname{Re} G_1$ and, hence, the Φ-factorability of G_1 (and, along with it, also of G_0) in L_2 with zero partial indices, which proves Theorem 9.7. ≡

9.3. THE GENERALIZED RIEMANN BOUNDARY VALUE PROBLEM WITH CONTINUOUS COEFFICIENTS. A STABILITY CRITERION

Let us consider problem (9.1) with continuous coefficients a and b. From Theorem 9.2 and Corollary 9.4 we deduce directly the following criterion of Fredholmness of problem (9.1).

<u>THEOREM 9.8.</u> Problem (9.1) with continuous coefficients a and b is Fredholm (independently of the value $p \in (1,\infty)$) iff $a(t) \neq 0$ for all $t \in \mathbb{T}$. If this condition is satisfied, then the defect numbers l and l' of problem (9.4) do not depend on the parameter p either, and the index of the problem is equal to the double index $\varkappa$ of the function a.

We would like to explain that the independence of the numbers l and l' of the parameter value p can be seen from formulae (9.7) and from the fact that the partial indices of a continuous non-singular matrix function do not depend on p.

Thus, the numbers l and l' of problem (9.1) are, for all values of p, the same as for $p = 2$. Therefore, they can be calculated by formulae (9.11).

The estimates for the numbers l and l' mentioned in Theorem 9.4, 9.5 and their corollaries may be written in a somewhat simpler form.

<u>THEOREM 9.4'.</u> Let the functions a and b be continuous on $\mathbb{T}$, and assume the functions φ_1 and φ_2 to be meromorphic in $\mathcal{D}^+$, continuous extendable onto $\mathbb{T}$, to have no common poles and to coincide at no more than N points (counting the multiplicities) of $\mathcal{D}^+$.

If, for all $t \in \mathbb{T}$,

$$|tb(t) - \varphi_1(t)| < |a(t)| < |tb(t) - \varphi_2(t)|, \tag{9.19}$$

then for the numbers l and l' the relations (9.11') are valid.

Proof. Condition (9.19) means, especially, that $a(t) \neq 0$ and $\varphi_1(t) \neq \varphi_2(t)$ for all $t \in \mathbb{T}$. This implies that problem (9.1) is Fredholm and the function $(\varphi_1-\varphi_2)^{-1}$ is meromorphic in $\mathcal{D}^+$ and continuously extendable onto $\mathbb{T}$. Thus, condition (9.13) is satisfied. In addition, in view of the continuity of the functions $a, b, \varphi_1, \varphi_2$ on $\mathbb{T}$, from (9.19) we deduce (9.12).
Consequently, Theorem 9.4 can be applied and, hence, formulae (9.11) are valid for the case under study. This completes the proof of Theorem 9.4'. ≡

COROLLARY 9.6. Let the functions φ_1 and φ_2 be meromorphic in $\mathcal{D}^+$, continuously extendable onto $\mathbb{T}$, not have any common poles in $\mathcal{D}^+$, coincide at no more than $|\varkappa|$ points of $\mathcal{D}^+$ (with regard to the multiplicities) and satisfy the requirements (9.19). Then the numbers l and l' of problem (9.1) are calculated by the formulae $l = \max\{0,2\varkappa\}$, $l' = \max\{0,-2\varkappa\}$ (and, hence, are stable).

From Theorem 9.4 we derive a sufficient condition of stability of problem (9.1) with continuous coefficients a and b.

THEOREM 9.5'. Let the functions φ_1 and φ_2 be meromorphic in $\mathcal{D}^+$, continuously extendable onto $\mathbb{T}$ and satisfy inequalities (9.19) and the requirement $\varphi_1(z) \neq \varphi_2(z)$ for all $z \in \mathcal{D}^+$. Then problem (9.1) is stable.

It appears that the sufficient condition established in Theorem 9.5 becomes also necessary, if we require that the factorization factors of the matrix function G_0 defined via formula (9.9) be continuous (in other words, that G_0 be factorable in C). This condition is satisfied [1], e.g., if the functions a and b satisfy a Hölder condition,

[1] as results from Theorem 5.8. Other theorems of Section 5.2 yield other sufficient factorability conditions of G_0 in C.

THEOREM 9.9. Let the coefficients a and b of problem (9.1) be such that the matrix function (9.9) is factorable in C. For the stability of problem (9.1), it is necessary and sufficient that there exist rational functions r_1 and r_2 satisfying the requirements

$$|tb(t)-r_1(t)| < |a(t)| < |tb(t)-r_2(t)| \quad \text{for} \quad t \in \mathbb{T}, \tag{9.19'}$$

$$r_1(z) \neq r_2(z) \quad \text{for} \quad z \in \mathfrak{D}^+ . \tag{9.20}$$

Proof. Sufficiency. The condition (9.19') shows, in particular, that the function r_1 does not have poles on $\mathbb{T}$. If the function r_2 has also no poles on $\mathbb{T}$, then, setting $\varphi_j = r_j$ $(j=1,2)$, from Theorem 9.5 we may conclude the stability of problem (9.1).

Now we assume that the function r_2 has poles on $\mathbb{T}$. Using the representations $r_j = p_j/q_j$, where p_j, q_j $(j=1,2)$ are polynomials, we rewrite the second of the inequalities (9.19') and the condition (9.20) in the form

$$|a(t)q_2(t)| < |tb(t)q_2(t)-p_2(t)| \quad \text{for} \quad t \in \mathbb{T}, \tag{9.21}$$

$$p_1(z)q_2(z) - p_2(z)q_1(z) \neq 0 \quad \text{for} \quad z \in \mathfrak{D}^+ . \tag{9.22}$$

Moreover, from (9.19') we deduce that $r_1(t) \neq r_2(t)$ for all $t \in \mathbb{T}$, so that inequality (9.22) continues to be valid for any $z \in \mathfrak{D}^+ \cup \mathbb{T}$. Now we introduce a polynomial $\tilde{q}_2$ that has no zeros on $\mathbb{T}$ but is arbitrarily close to q_2 in such a way that conditions (9.21) and (9.22) (the latter for any $z \in \mathfrak{D}^+ \cup \mathbb{T}$) remain true, if we replace q_2 by $\tilde{q}_2$.

Then the conditions of the theorem are preserved, if we replace r_2 by $\tilde{r}_2 = p_2/\tilde{q}_2$. The function $\tilde{r}_2$ does not have poles on $\mathbb{T}$. Hence, due to what was proved above, problem (9.1) is stable.

Necessity. Let the problem (9.1) be stable, i.e., the partial indices of the matrix function (9.9) are equal to zero. Then the partial indices of the Hermitian matrix function (9.10) with negative determinant are also equal to zero. According to Theorem 7.4, the matrix function (9.10) can be factored in the form

$$F = A_o \begin{pmatrix} 1 & 0 \\ 0 & -1 \end{pmatrix} A_o^* . \tag{9.23}$$

Since the matrix function G_o (and, together with it, the matrix function F) is factorable in C, then by Corollary 7.7 the matrix function

$$A_o = \begin{pmatrix} \alpha & \beta \\ \gamma & \delta \end{pmatrix} ,$$

which is analytic in $\mathfrak{D}^+$, is continuous and non-singular in $\mathfrak{D}^+ \cup \mathbb{T}$. Consequently

$$\alpha(z)\delta(z) - \beta(z)\gamma(z) \neq 0 \quad \text{for any} \quad z \in \mathfrak{D}^+ \cup \mathbb{T} . \tag{9.24}$$

Writing the factorization (9.23) elementwise, we find that

$$|b|^2-|a|^2 = |\alpha|^2-|\beta|^2 , \quad tb = \alpha\overline{\gamma} - \beta\overline{\delta} , \quad 1 = |\gamma|^2-|\delta|^2 . \tag{9.25}$$

After some transformations we obtain from this

$$|\alpha\delta-\beta\gamma| = |a| , \quad tb\gamma-\alpha = (\alpha\delta-\beta\gamma)\overline{\delta} , \quad tb\delta-\beta = (\alpha\delta-\beta\gamma)\overline{\gamma} ,$$

so that

$$|tb\gamma-\alpha| = |a\delta| , \quad |tb\delta-\beta| = |a\gamma|. \tag{9.26}$$

By virtue of (9.25), $|\gamma| > |\delta|$, therefore, from (9.26) it follows that

$$|tb\gamma-\alpha| < |a\gamma| , \quad |tb\delta-\beta| > |a\delta| . \tag{9.27}$$

The functions $\alpha, \beta, \gamma, \delta$, which are analytic in $\mathfrak{D}^+$ and continuous in $\mathfrak{D}^+ \cup \mathbb{T}$, can be uniformly approximated by polynomials with arbitrary degree of accuracy. We choose polynomials p_1, q_1, p_2, q_2 sufficiently close to $\alpha, \beta, \gamma, \delta$, respectively, in such a way that, replacing $\alpha, \beta, \gamma, \delta$ by p_1, q_1, p_2, q_2, inequalities (9.24) and (9.26) remain valid. Setting $r_j = p_j/q_j$ $(j=1,2)$, we can satisfy requirements (9.19) and (9.20), which proves Theorem 9.9. ≡

9.4. COMMENTS

Beginning with the paper of MARKUSHEVICH [1] the boundary value problem (9.1) (for $\mathbb{T}$ replacing by a general contour Γ) was considered by a number of authors under various assumptions for Γ and the coefficients a, b, c (BOJARSKI [1,2], LITVINCHUK [1], MIKHAǏLOV [1-4], NIKOLAǏCHUK [1], NIKOLAǏCHUK, SPITKOVSKIǏ [1,2], PRIMACHUK [1], SABITOV [1,2]).

A detailed historical explanation of this subject is contained in Ch. 5 of the monograph LITVINCHUK [3].

The method of reducing problem (9.1) on the unit circle to the Riemann problem for two pairs of functions was proposed by one of the authors (LITVINCHUK [1,2]).[1] Lemmas 9.1, 9.2 and the corollaries of them yield a detailed description of this method. We would like to note that the approaches used in the proof of Lemmas 9.1 and 9.2 go back to MANDZHAVIDZE's paper [1]. Theorems 9.1 - 9.3 in the form stated here are borrowed from the article SPITKOVSKIǏ [8]. In the special case $t\varphi \in H_\infty$ Theorem 9.3 generalizes a result of NIKOLAǏCHUK [1]. The definition of stability of problem (9.1) was introduced by LITVINCHUK [1].

Section 9.2 is essentially the paper SPITKOVSKIǏ [8], in which the case $p \neq 2$ was considered, too. Here we restricted ourselves to the theory of problem (9.1) in the space L_2, since for this case the results obtained are more complete and easy to formulate. Formulae for the numbers l and l' in the elliptic case of problem (9.1) were first obtained by BOJARSKI [2] for Hölder coefficients a and b and, for coefficients a, b from the class L_∞, by MIKHAǏLOV [3,4].

Corollary 9.9 on the solvability of problem (9.1) in the parabolic case under the factorability condition of the coefficient b generalizes results of MIKHAǏLOV [3,4] and LITVINCHUK [1,2].

The proof of the equivalence of statements 2) and 4) from Theorem 9.6, in principle, reproduces the proof of the criterion for $T_Q(G)$ to be a Φ_--operator, which was discussed in the Comments from Chapter 4. Theorem 9.7 associated with the hyperbolic case, generalizes the correspondent result from SPITKOVSKIǏ [1].
Let us remark that the assumption concerning the coefficient a stipulated in Section 9.2 can be replaced by the weaker requirement $a \in \mathfrak{M}$[2], as it was done in SPITKOVSKIǏ [8]. In the authors' papers LITVINCHUK, SPITKOVSKIǏ [1,2] there was obtained a strengthening of Theorem 9.4

[1] By the way, notice that the results obtained with the help of this method in the Fredholm theory of problem (9.1) may be transferred to the case of a smooth contour.

[2] The definition of the class $\mathfrak{M}$ can be found in the Comments to Chapter 6.

consisting in the claim that, actually, $l = \varkappa + \max\{\varkappa, -\varkappa, N\}$ as soon as there exists a function φ_1 satisfying conditions (9.12), while the number N is chosen to be the smallest possible. Also, there is given a complete classification of problem (9.1) (which generalizes that proposed by Mikhaĭlov and makes it more precise), a stability criterion for the defect numbers and a stability criterion for the problem itself generalizing from the parabolic case Corollary 9.9. In the papers LITVINCHUK, SPITKOVSKIǏ [1,2] the question of relationships between problem (9.1) and certain problems from theory of approximation by functions with partially fixed poles is discussed either. Here we have no possibility to deal with these questions in detail which require large volumes of additional information (mainly from ADAMYAN, AROV, KREĬN [1,2] and other papers of these authors). Thus, the reader is referred to the article LITVINCHUK, SPITKOVSKIǏ [2], in which all background information needed as well as a systematic explanation of the results themselves is contained.

Theorem 9.8 is due to BOJARSKI [1] (for Hölder coefficients) and MIKHAĬLOV [3,4] (in the general case). Another way of proving this theorem was proposed by VEKUA in [4], see also VEKUA, KVESELAVA [1].

Theorems 9.4, 9.5' and 9.9 extend corresponding results from NIKOLAĬCHUK, SPITKOVSKIǏ [1,2] to the case of continuous coefficients a and b. Several special cases of Theorem 9.4' were discussed by SABITOV [1,2] and PRIMACHUK [1].

Problem (9.1) with a piecewise continuous coefficient a (and $b \in L_\infty$) was considered for the first time in MIKHAĬLOV [4]. Employing Theorem 9.2 and the criterion of Φ-factorability of piecewise continuous matrix functions (Theorem 5.6), A.I. YATSKO and S.I. YATSKO [1,2] obtained a criterion of Fredholmness for problem (9.1) with piecewise continuous coefficients a and b in the classes L_p $(1 < p < \infty)$. In doing so, they discovered that unlike the situation described by Theorem 9.8, the Fredholmness of problem (9.1) depends on the coefficient b (and, naturally, on the parameter value p). These results have also been extended to more general coefficients a and b.

Problem (9.1) on a composite contour was studied in YATSKO [1] and in spaces with weight - in YATSKO [2]. The paper of KHVOSHCHINSKAYA [2] is devoted to the explicit solution of problem (9.1) with piecewise constant coefficients which have no more than three points of discontinuity. She made use of the reduction of (9.1) to the vector-valued Riemann boundary value problem (9.4) and applied those results from KHVOSHCHINSKAYA [1] which were mentioned in the Comments to Chapter 5.

Finally, we would like to remark that problem (9.1) with matrix coefficients a and b of dimension $n \times n$ can be reduced to a Riemann boundary value problem for $2n$ pairs of functions with the aid of the method described in the present chapter (see KAPANADZE [1,2], LITVINCHUK [1,2]). The method of reduction to a vector-valued Riemann boundary value problem proved to be effective for the study of other multi-term boundary value problems from the theory of analytic functions, too. Thus, recently the authors together with Yu.D. LATUSHKIN succeeded in obtaining new results concerning Fredholmness and bounds for the defect numbers of a generalized Carleman boundary value problem with the help of this method (the statement of this problem and related results known previously may be found in Ch. 5 of the book LITVINCHUK [3]; the latest results themselves have not been published yet).

REFERENCES

Abrahamse, M. B.

[1] The spectrum of a Toeplitz operator with a multiplicatively periodic symbol.- J. Funct. Anal., 1979, 31, N.2, p. 224-233.

Adamyan, V.M., Arov D.Z., Krein,M.G(Адамян В.М., Аров Д.З., Крейн М.Г.)

[1] О бесконечных ганкелевых матрицах и обобщенных задачах Каратеодори-фейера и Ф. Рисса. - Функц. анализ и его прил., 1968, 2, No. I, с. I-I9.

[2] Бесконечные блочно-ганкелевы матрицы и связанные с ними проблемы продолжения.- Изв. АН Арм.ССР, 1971, 6, No. 2-3, с. 87-112.

Alekhno, A. G.(Алехно А. Г.)

[1] О краевой задаче Римана с конечным числом точек завихрения - ДАН БССР, 1979, 23, No. I2, с. I069-I072.

Ambartsumyan, G. V.(Амбарцумян Г. В.)

[1] О методе редукции для одного класса теплицевых матриц.- Матем. исслед., 1973, 8, No. 2, с. I6I-I69.

[2] Об обращении некоторых теплицевых матриц.- Матем. исслед., 1973, 8, No. 3, с. I40-I44.

Antontsev, S.N. (Антонцев С. Н.)

[1] Обобщенная система Коши-Римана с почти регулярными коэффицентами. - В кн.: Матрич. вопр. теории функций и отображений. Вып. 7: Материалы 4-го Коллоквиума, Донецк, 1974 г. Киев: Наук. думка, 1975, с. 3-I7.

Azoff, E., Clancey, K. F.

[1] Toeplitz operators with sectorial matrix-valued symbols. - Indiana Univ. Math. J., 1977, 26, N.5, p. 933-938.

Babaev, A.A., Salaev, V. V. (Бабаев А. А., Салаев В. В.)

[1] Краевые задачи и сингулярные уравнения на спрямляемом контуре.- Матем. заметки, 1982, 3I, No. 4, с. 57I-580.

Babeshko, V.A. (Бабешко В. А.)

[1] Факторизация одного класса матриц-функций и её приложения. - ДАН СССР, 1975, 223, No. 5, с. I094-I097.

[2] К факторизации одного класса матриц-функций, встречающихся в теории упругости. - ДАН СССР, 1975, 223, No. 6, с. I333-I356.

[3] Эффективный способ приближенной факторизации матриц-функций. - ДАН СССР, 1979, 247, No. 5, с. I089-I093.

Ball, J., Helton, J.

[1] Factorization results related to shifts in an indefinite metric.- Integr. Equat. and Oper. Theory, 1982, 5, N 5, 632-658

Bart, H., Gohberg, I., Kaashoek, M. A.

[1] Minimal factorization of matrix and operator functions. - Operator Theory: Advances and Applications, Vol. 1. Basel - Boston - Stuttgart 1979: Birkhäuser-Verlag

[2] Wiener-Hopf factorization of analytic operator functions and realization. - Vrije Universiteit Amsterdam, Rapport nr. 231 1983

[3] Exponentially dichotomous operators and inverse Fourier transforms.- Report 8511/M (1985). Erasmus University Rotterdam.

Belarmino G.D. (Беларминo Г. Д.)

[1] Краевая задача Римана и сингулярные интегральные уравнений. - Науч. тр. Азерб. ун-та, Сер. физ.-мат.н., Но. 6, с. 76-85.

Belokopytova L.V., Ivanenko O.A., Fil'shtinskiĭ L.A.
(Белокопытова Л. В., Иваненко О.А., Фильшеинский Л.А.)

[1] Передача нагрузки от упругого ребра к полубесконечной пьезокерамической пластине. - Изв. АН Арм. ССР. Механика, I98I, Но. 5 с. 4I-5I.

Bonsall F.F., Gillespie T.A.

[1] Hankel operators with PC symbols and the space H_∞ + PC. - Proc. Royal Soc. Edinburg, 1981, 89 A, p. 17-24.

Bojarski B. (Боярский Б. В.)

[1] Об устойчивости задачи Гильберта для голоморфного вектора. - Сообщ. АН СССР, I958, 2I, Но. 4, с. 39I-398.

[2] Об обобщенной граничной задаче Гильберта. - Сообщ. АН Груз. ССР, I960, 25, Но. 4, с. 385-390.

[3] Анализ разрешимости граничных задач теории функций. - В кн.: Исслед. по совр. пробл. теории функций комплексного переменного. М.: Физматгиз, I96I, с. 57-59.

[4] On the index problem for systems of singular integral equations.- Bull. Acad. polon. Sci., 1963, XI No. 10; 653-655; 1965, XIII, No. 9, 627-631, 633-637.

Böttcher,A., Silbermann B.

[1] Invertibility and asymptotics of Toeplitz matrices, Berlin: Akademie-Verlag, 1983.

Bourbaki N. (Бурбаки Н.)

[1] Функции действительного переменного.- М.: Наука, I965 transl. from: Eléments de matématique.Paris: Herman.

Budyanu M.S. (Будяну М.С.)

[1] Одна теорема о факторизации оператор-функций. - Изв. АН Молд. ССР, I965, Но. 7, с. 22-3I

Budyanu M.S., Gohberg I. (Будяну М.С., Гохберг И.Ц.)

[1] О задаче факторизации в абстрактных банаховых алгебрах. I. Распадающиеся алгебры. - Матем. исслед., I967, 2, Но. 2, с. 25-5I.

[2] О задаче факторизации в абстрактных банаховых алгебрах. II. Нераспадающиеся алгебры. - Матем. исслед., I967, 2, Но. 3, с. 3-I9.

[3] Общие теоремы о факторизации матриц-функций. I. Основная теорема. - Матем. исслед., I968, 3, Но. 2, с. 87-I03. English transl.: Amer. Math. Soc. Transl. 1973, 102, 1-14

[4] Общие теоремы о факторизации матриц-функций. II. Некоторые признаки и их следствия. - Матем. исслед., I968, 3, Но. 3, с. 3-I8. English transl.: Amer. Math. Soc. Transl. 1973, 102, 15-26.

Calderon A.P.

[1] Cauchy integrals on Lipschitz curves and related operators.- Proc. Nat. Acad. Sci. USA, 1977, 74, No. 4, p. 1324-1327.

Chakrabarti A.

[1] Derivation of the solution of certain singular integral equations. - J: Indian Inst. Sci., 1980, 62, No. 10, p. 147-157.

[2] On a system of Wiener-Hopf equations associated with a mixed diffraction problem. - Z. angew. Math. und Mech., 1981, 61, No. 7, p. 339-341.

Chebotarev G.N. (Чеботарев Г. Н.)

[1] К решению в замкнутой форме краевой задачи Римана для системы n пар функций. - Уч. зап. Казанск. Ун-та, I956, II6, Но. 4, с. 3I-58.

[2] Частные индексы краевой задачи Римана с треугольной матрицей второго порядка. - Успехи матем. наук, I956, II, вып. 3, с. I92-202.

[3] Некоторые матричные уравнения и их применение к решению в замкнутой форме краевой задачи Римана. - Тр. Всесоюзного матем. Съезда, I956, I, с. III.

Chebotarev G.N., Gakhov F.D. (Чеботарев Н. Г., Гахов Ф. Д.)

[1] О краевой задаче Римана для системы n пар функций. - Уч. зап. Казанск. ун-та, I950, II0, Но.7,с.45-50.

Chebotaru I.S. (Чеботару И.С.)

[1] Сведение уравнений Винера-Хопфа к системам с нулевыми индексами. Изв. АН Молд. ССР, I967, Но. 8, с. 54-66.

Chelidze V.G., Dzhvarsheĭshvili G.G. (Челидзе В.Г., Джваршейшвили А.Г.)

[1] Интеграл типа Коши. - Изв. вузов. Математика, I978, Но. 6, с. II7-I28.

Cherepanov G.P. (Черепанов Г. П.)

[1] Решение одной линейной краевой задачи для двух функций и её приложение к некоторым смешанным задачам теории упругости. - ПММ, I962, 26, Но. 5, с. 907-9I2.

[2] Задача Римана-Гильберта для внешности разрезов вдоль прямой или вдоль окружности. - ДАН СССР, I964, I56, Но. 2, с. 275-277.

[3] Об одном интегрируемом случае краевой задачи Римана для нескольких функций. - ДАН СССР, I965, I6I, Но. 6, с. I285-I288.

Choriev Kh. (Чориев Х.)

[1] Устойчивость частичных индексов и численный метод решения задач Римана и Римана-Гильберта для матриц. - Научн. труны Ташк. ун-та, I974, 460,с. I63-I68.

[2] Регулярная устойчивость краевой задачи Римана и вычисление частичных индексов. - Сб. научн. трудов. Ташк. ун-та, I977, 548, с. I20-I23.

[3] Регулярная устойчивость краевой задачи Римана и вычисление частичных индексов. - В кн.: Вопр. метрич. теории отображений и её применение: Материалы 5-го коллоквиума, Донецк, I976, г. Киев: Наук. думка, I978, с. I46-I48.

Clancey K.F.

[1] A local result for systems of Riemann-Hilbert barrier problems.- Trans. Amer. Math. Soc., 1974, 200, p. 315-325.

Clancey K.F., Gohberg I.

[1] Local and global factorizations of matrix valued functions. - Trans. Amer. Math. Soc., 1977, 232, p. 155-167.

[2] Localization of singular integral operators. - Math. Zeitschr., 1979, 169, p. 105-117.

[3] Factorization of matrix functions and singular integral operators. Basel-Boston-Stuttgart: Birkhäuser-Verlag, 1981.

Clancey K.F., Gosselin J.A.

[1] On the local theory of Toeplitz operators. - Ill. J. Math., 1978, 22, N 3, p. 449-458.

Coburn L.A.

[1] Weyl's theorem for non-normal operators. - Michigan Math. J., 1966, 13, p. 285-286.

Cotlar M.A.

[1] A unified theory of Hilbert transforms and ergodic theorems. - Rev. Mat. Guyana, 1955, 1, N 2, p. 105-167.

Danilov E.A. (Данилов Е.А.)

[1] Зависимость числа решений однородной задачи Римана от контура и модуля коэффициента. - ДАН СССР, 1982 г., 264, Но. 6, с. 1305-1308.

Danilyuk I.I. (Данилюк И.И.)

[1] О задаче Гильберта с измеримыми коэффициентами. - Сибирск. матем. ж., 1960, I, Но. 2, с. 171-197.

[2] К теории одномерных сингулярных уравнений. - В кн.: Проблемы механики сплошной среды. М.: Изд-во АН СССР, 1961, с. 135-144.

[3] Лекции по краевым задачам для аналитических функций и сингулярным интегральным уравнениям. - Новосибирск: Новосиб. ун-т 1964.

[4] Про загальну линийну граничну задачу з вимирними коэффициентами для багатьок аналитичных функций в класси E_p. - ДАН УРСР, сер. А, 1971, 9, с. 774-777.

[5] Об общей линейной граничной задаче с измеримыми коэффициентами для многих аналитических функций в классе E_p. - В кн.: Мех. сплошн. среды и родств. пробл. анализа. М.: Наука, 1972, с. 175-179.

[6] Нерегулярные граничные задачи на плоскости. - М.: Наука, 1975.

Danilyuk I.I., Shelepov V.Yu. (Данилюк И.И., Шелепов В.Ю.)

[1] Об ограниченности в L_p сингулярного оператора с ядром Коши вдоль кривой ограниченного вращения. - ДАН СССР, 1974, Но. 3, с. 514-517.

[2] При обмежнисть у зважених просторах L_p сингулярных интегральних операторов вздовж линий з обмежним обертанням. - ДАН УРСР, сер. А., 1969, 3, с. 199.

Devinatz A.

[1] Toeplitz operators on H^2 spaces. - Trans. Amer. Math. Soc., 1964, 112, p. 304-307.

Devinatz A., Shinbrot M.

[1] General Wiener-Hopf operators. - Trans. Amer. Math. Soc., 1969, 145, p. 467-494.

Didenko V.D. (Диденко В.Д.)

[1] Сходимость коллокационного метода и метода механических квадратур для систем сингулярных интегральных уравнений. - Изв. вузов Математика, 1979, Но. 1, с. 76-79.

[2] Метод механических квадратур для систем сингулярных интегральных уравнений. - Изв. вузов. Математика, 1979, Но. 3, с. 73-76.

[3] Приближенное решение систем сингулярных интегральных уравнений в полупространствах непрерывных функций. - ДАН СССР, 1980, 254, Но. 6, с. 1314 - 1317.

Didenko V.D., Chernetskiĭ V.A. (Диденко В.Д., Чернецкий В.А.)

[1] Краевая задача Римана с комплексной ортогональной матрицей. - Матем. заметки, 1978, 23, вып. 3, с. 405-416.

Didenko V.D., Tikhonenko N.Ya. (Диденко В.Д., Тихоненко Н.Я.)

[1] О приближенном решении матричной задачи Римана. - Изв. вузов. Математика, 1980, Но. 1, с. 16-19.

[2] О приближенном решении матричной задачи Римана. - Дифференц. уравнения, 1981, 17, Но. 11, с. 2087-2089.

Douglas R.G.

[1] Toeplitz and Wiener-Hopf operators in $H^\infty + C$. - Bull. Amer. Math. Soc., 1968, 74, N 5, p. 895-899.

[2] Banach algebra techniques in operator theory. - New York & London: Academic Press, 1972.

Douglas R.G., Sarason D.E.

[1] Fredholm Toeplitz Operators. - Proc. Amer. Math. Soc., 1970, 26, p. 117-120.

Douglas R.G., Widom H.

[1] Toeplitz operators with locally sectorial symbols. - Indiana Univ. Math. J., 1970, 20, Nr. 4. p. 385-388.

Dukhovnyĭ A.M. (Духовный А.М.)

[1] Одномерное случайное блуждание, зависящее от параметра. - ДАН УССР. Сер. А., 1962, Но. 3, с. 9-12.

Duracz T., Zelazny R.

[1] Solutions to some Riemann-Hilbert problems in two-group neutron transport theory. - Trans. Theory and Statist. Phys., 1982, 11, Nr. 1, p. 5-28.

Duren P.L.

[1] Theory of H^p spaces. - New York & London: Academic Press, 1970.

Duren P.L., Shapiro H.S., Shields A.L.

[1] Singular measures and domains not of Smirnov type. - Duke Math. J., 1966, 13, Nr. 2, p. 247-254.

Dybin V.B., Dodokhova G.V. (Дыбин В. Б., Додохова Г.В.)

[1] Корректная постановка краевой задачи Римана на прямой с почти-периодическим разрывом коэффициента. - ВИНИТИ, Но. 1497-81 Деп., 1981.

[2] Корректная постановка краевой задачи Римана на замкнутом контуре в случае почти-периодических разрывов у её коэффициента. - ВИНИТИ, Но. 3579-82 Деп., 1982.

Dzhvarsheĭshvili A.G. (Джваршейшвили А.Г.)

[1] Замечание об одной граничной задаче. - Сообщ. АН Груз ССР, 1981, 102, Но. 2, с. 297-299.

Emets Yu.P. (Емец Ю.П.)

[1] О некоторых приложениях краевой задачи Римана в магнитной гидродинамике. - В кн.: Материали Всес. конференции по краев. задачам. Казань: Казанск. ун-та, 1970, с. 101-106.

Engibaryan N.B. (Енгибарян Н.Б.)

[1] Факторизация матриц-функций и нелинейные интегральные уравнения. - Изв. АН Арм. ССР. Математика, 1980, 15, Но. 3, с. 233-244.

Faour Nazih S.

[1] The Fredholm index of a class of vector-valued singular integral operators. - Indian J. Pure and Appl. Math., 1980, 11, Nr. 2, p. 135-146.

Feinstein J., Shamash Y.

[1] Spectral factorization of a rational matrix. - IEEE Trans. Inform. Theory, 1977, 23, Nr. 4, p. 534-538.

Frolov V.D. (Фролов В.Д.)

[1] К теории сингулярных интегральных уравнений с измеримыми коэффициентами. - ДАН СССР, 1968, 189, Но. 6, с. 1185-1188.

[2] О сингулярных интегральных уравнениях с измеримыми коэффициентами в пространствах L_p с весом. - Матем. исслед., 1970, 5, Но. 1, с. 141-151.

Gabdulkhaev B.G. (Габдулхаев Б.Г.)

[1] Некоторые вопросы теории приближенных методов. - Изв. вузов, Математика, 1971, Но. 6, с. 15-23.

Gakhov F.D. (Гахов Ф.Д.)

[1] О краевой задаче Римана для систем n пар. функций. - ДАН СССР, 1949, 67, Но. 4, с. 601-606.

[2] Один случай краевой задачи Римана для системы n пар функций. - Изв. АН СССР, сер. матем., 1950, 14, Но. 6, с. 549-568.

[3] Краевая задача Римана для систем n пар функций. - Успехи матем. наук, 1952, 7, Но. 4, с. 3-54.

[4] Краевые задачи. - М.: Наука, 1977.

Gakhov F.D., Cherskiĭ Yu.I. (Гахов Ф.Д., Черский Ю.И.)

[1] Уравнения типа свертки. - М.: Наука, 1978.

Ganin M.Ts. (Ганин М.Ц.)

[1] Об интегральном уравнении Фредгольма с ядром, зависящим от разности аргументов. - Изв. вузов. Математика, 1963, Но. 2, с. 31-43.

Gantmakher F.R. (Gantmacher F.R., Гантмахер Ф. Р.)

[1] Теория матриц. - М.: Наука, 1967.
English transl. of 1st ed.: New York, Chelsea, 1959;
German transl: Berlin, Deutscher Verlag der Wiss., 1970

Gavdzinskiĭ V.N., Spitkovskiĭ I.M. (Гавдзинский В.Н., Спитковский И.М.)

[1] Об одном способе эффективного построения факторизации. - Украинск. матем. ж., 1982, 34, Но. 1, с. 15-19.

Gerus O.F. (Герус О.Ф.)

[1] Об одном особом интегральном уравнении и краевой задаче Римана. - Украинск. матем. ж., 1981, 33, Но. 3, с. 282-285.

Glazman I.M., Lyubich Yu.I. (Глазман И.М., Любич Ю.И.)

[1] Конечномерный линейный анализ в задачах. - М.: Наука, 1969.

Glebov A.V., Deundyak V.M. (Глебов А.В., Деундяк В.М.)

[1] Гомотопическая классификация нетеровых систем сингулярных интегральных операторов с разрывными коэффициентами. - Функцион. анализ и его прил., 1978, 12, Но, 3, с. 76-77.

Gohberg I. (Гохберг И.Ц.)

[1] О числе решений однородного сингулярного интегрального уравнения с непрерывными коэффициентами. - ДАН СССР, 1958, 122, Но. 3, с. 327-330.

[2] О границах частных индексов матриц-функций. - Успехи матем. наук, 1959, 14, вып. 4, с. 159-164.

[3] Общая задача о факторизации матриц-функций в нормированных кольцах и её приложения. - ДАН СССР, 1962, 146, Но. 2, с. 284-287.

[4] Задача факторизации в нормированных кольцах, функции от изометрических и симметрических операторов и сингулярные интегральные уравнения. - Успехи матем. наук, 1964, 19, вып. 1, с, 71-124.

Gohberg I., Feldman I.A. (Гохберг И.Ц., Фельдман И.А.)

[1] Уравнения в свертках и проекционные методы их решения. - М.: Наука, 1971.
English transl.; Convolution equations and projection methods for their solution. Transl. Math. Mon., vol. 41, 1974, Providence, R.I.
German transl.: Faltungsgleichungen und Projektionsverfahren zu ihrer Lösung. Akademie-Verlag Berlin 1974.

[2] Одно замечание о стандартной факторизации матриц-функций. - Уч. зап. Бельцкого пedин-та, 1960, 5, с. 65-69.

[3] Об индексах кратных расширений матриц-функций. - Изв. АН Молд. ССР, 1967, 8, с. 76-80.

Gohberg, I., Kaashoek M.A., van Shagen F.

[1] Similarity of operator blocks and canonical forms. II. Infinite dimensional case and Wiener-Hopf factorization. - Top. Mod. Oper. Theory. 5 Int. Conf. Oper. Theory. Timisoara and Herculane. June 2-12 1980, - Basel e.a., 1981, p. 121-170.

Gohberg I., Krein M.G. (Гохберг И.Ц., Крейн М.Г.)

[1] Основные положения о дефектных числах, корневых векторах и индексах,линейных операторов. - Успехи матем. наук, I957, I2, вып. 2, с. 43-II8. (English transl. Amer. Math. Soc. transl., 1960, 13, p. 185-264).

[2] Об устойчивой системе частных индексов Гильберта для нескольких неизвестных функций. - ДАН СССР, I958, II9, Но. 5, с. 854-857.

[3] Системы интегральных уравнений на полупрямой с ядрами, зависящими от разности аргументов. - Успехи матем. наук, I958, I3, вып. 2, с. 3-72. (English trans.: Amer. Math. Soc. transl. 1960, 2, p. 217-287).

[4] Введение в теорию линейных несамосопряженных операторов. - М.: Наука, I965. (English transl.: Transl. Math. Monographs, vol. 18, 1969, Providence, R.I.)

[5] Теория вольтерровых операторов в гильбертовом пространстве и её приложения. - М.: Наука, I967. (English transl.: Transl. Math. Monographs, 1970, Providence, R.I.)

Gohberg I., Krupnik N.Ya. (Гохберг И.Ц., Крупник Н.Я.)

[1] Система сингулярных интегральных уравнений в пространстве L_p с весом. - ДАН СССР, I969, Но. 5, с. 998-I00I.

[2] Сингулярные интегральные операторы с кусочно-непрерывными коэффициентами и их символы. - Изв. АН СССР, сер. матем. I97I, 35, Но. 4, с. 940-964.

[3] Об одном локальном принципе и алгебрах, порожденных теплицевыми матрицами. - Annakle ştiintifice ale univ. "Al. I. Cuza", Iaşi, Sect. I.a) Matematica, 19, 1, 1973.

[4] Введение в теорию одномерных сингулярных интегральных операторов. - Кишинев: Штиинца, I973. German transl.: Einführung in die Theorie der eindimensionalen singulären Integraloperatoren - Basel - Boston - Stuttgart, Birkhäuser Verlag, 1979.

Gohberg I., Leiterer J. (Гохберг И.Ц., Лайтерер Ю.)

[1] Общие теоремы о канонической факторизации оператор-функций относительно контура. - Матем. исслед., I972, 25, Но. 3, с. 87-I34.

[2] Факторизация оператор-функций относительно контура. - I. Mathem. Nachr. 1972, N. 52, 259-282. - II. Mathem. Nachr. 1972, N 54, 41-74. - III. Mathem. Nachr. 1973, N 55, 33-61.

Gohberg I., Sementsul A.A. (Гохберг И.Ц., Семенцул А.А.)

[1] Теплицевы матрицы, составленные из коэффициентов Фурье функций с разрывами почти-периодического типа. - Матем. исслед., I970, 5, Но. 4, с. 63-83.

Goluzin G.M. (Голузин Г.М.)

[1] Геометрическая теория функций комплексного переменного. - М.: Наука, I966.

Gordadze E.G. (Гордадзе Э.Г.)

[1] О задаче Римана-Привалова в случае негладкой граничной линии. - Тр. Тбилисс. мат. ин-та ГрузССР, I967, 33, с. 25-3I.

[2] О сингулярном интегральном операторе с кусочно-непрерывным коэффициентом. - Сообщ. АН ГрузССР, I97I, 63, Но. 2, с. 277-280.

[3] О сингулярных интегралах с ядром Коши. - Тр. Тбилисс. мат. ин-та АН ГрузССР, I972, 42, с. 5-I7.

[4] О сингулярном интегральном операторе на негладких линиях. - Тр. Симпоз. по мех. сплошн. среды и родствен. проб. анализа, I97I. Тбилиси: Мецниереба, I974, 2. с. 74-85.

[5] О граничной задаче линейного сопряжения. - Сообщ. АН ГрузССР, I976, 8I, Но. 3, с. 545-548.

[6] О граничной задаче линейного сопряжения для линий Радона. - Сообщ. АН ГрузССР, I976, 84, Но. I, с. 29-32.

Gordadze E.G., Khvedelidze B.V. (Гордадзе Э.Г., Хведелидзе Б. В.)

[1] О сингулярных интегральных уравнениях и задаче регуляризации. - Тр. Тбилис. мат. ин-та АН ГрузССР, I976, 53, с. I5-I7.

Gordienko V.N. (Гордиенко В.Н.)

[1] Факторизация матриц-функций частного вида. - Украинск. матем. ж., I97I, 23, Но. I, с. 8I-88.

Gorodzha L.V., Emets Yu.P., Zhukova N.I., Zverovich E.I.
(Городжа Л.В., Емец Ю.П., Жукова Н.И., Зверович Э.И.)

[1] О применении обобщенной краевой задачи Римана к расчету электрических полей. - ДАН БССР, I979, 23, Но. 2, с. II8-I20.

Govorov N.V. (Говоров Н.В.)

[1] О краевой задаче Римана с бесконечным индексом. - ДАН СССР, I964, I54, Но. 6, с. I247-I249.

[2] Об ограниченных решениях однородной краевой задачи Римана с бесконечным индексом степенного порядка. - Теория функций, функц. анадиз и их прил., I969, II, с. 3-34.

Grudskiǐ S.M. (Грудский С.М.)

[1] О компактности одного интегрального оператора. - ВИНИТИ, Но. 4856-80 Деп., I980, I0 с.

[2] Краевая задача Римана с разрывами почти-периодического типа в классе $L_\infty(\Gamma)$. - Дифференц. и интеграль. уравнений и их прил. Элиста, I982, с. 30-4I.

Grudskii S.M., Dybin V.B. (Грудский С.М., Дыбин В.Д.)

[1] Краевая задача Римана с разрывами почти-периодического типа у её коэффициента. - ДАН СССР, I977, 237, Но. I, с. 2I-24.

[2] Краевая задача Римана в пространстве $L_p(\Gamma,\rho)$ с почти-периодическими разрывами у её коэффициента. - Матем. исслед., I980, 54, с. 36-49.

Grudskii S.M., Khevelev A.V. (Грудский С.М., Хевелев А.В.)

[1] Об обратимости в $L_2(R)$ сингулярных интегральных операторов с периодическими коэффициентами и сдвигом. - ДАН СССР, I983, 269, Но. 6, с. I303-I306.

Gusak D.V. (Гусак Д.В.)

[1] Метод факторизации в граничных задачах для одного класса процессов на цепи Маркова. I - Киев: Препринт ИМ АН УССР 78.6, 1978.

[2] Метод факторизации в граничных задачах для одного класса процессов на цепи Маркова. II - Киев: Препринт ИМ АН УССР 78.II, 1978.

Halmos P.

[1] A Hilbert space problem book. - Princeton, New Jersey: Van Nostrand Company, Inc., 1967.

Halmos P., Sunder V.S.

[1] Bounded operators on L^2 spaces. - Berlin: Springer, 1978.

Hartman P.

[1] On completely continuous Hankel matrices. - Proc. Amer. Math. Soc., 1958, 9, N 6, p. 862-866..

Hartman P., Wintner A.

[1] The spectra of Toeplitz's matrices. - Amer. Math. J., 1954, 76, p. 867-882.

Heinig G. (Хайниг Г.)

[1] Об обратимости сингулярных интегральных операторов. - Сообщ. АН ГрузССР, 1979, 96, No. I, с. 29-32.

[2] Struktur des Kernes und partielle Indizes bei allgemeinen linearen Operatoren.- Preprint P - 36/80. IMath. Berlin, 1980.

Heinig G., Rost K.

[1] Algebraic methods for Toeplitz-like matrices and operators. - Mathematical Research vol. 19, Berlin: Akademie Verlag, 1984. - Operator Theory: Advances and Appl., vol. 13, Basel-Boston-Stuttgart: Birkhäuser Verlag 1984.

Heinig G., Silbermann B.

[1] Factorization of matrix functions in algebras of bounded functions. - In: Spectral theory of linear operators and related topics. Operator Theory: Advances and Appl., vol. 14, p. 157-177; Basel: Birkhäuser Verlag, 1984.

Heins A.E.

[1] The Sommerfeld half-plane problem revisited, I. The solution of a pair of coupled Wiener-Hopf integral equations. - Math. Meth. Appl. Sci., 1982, 4, N.1, p. 74-90.

[2] The Sommerfeld half-plane problem revisited, II. The factoring of a matrix of analytic functions. - Math. Meth. Appl. Sci., 1983, 5, N.1, p. 14-21.

Hoffman K.

[1] Banach spaces of analytic functions. - Prentice-Hall, Englewood Cliffs, New Jersey, 1962.

Hoffman K., Singer I.M.

[1] Maximal algebras of continuous functions. - Acta Math., 1960, 103, p. 217-241.

Hunt R.A., Muckenhoupt B., Wheeden R.L.

[1] Weighted norm inequalities for the conjugate function and Hilbert transform. - Trans. Amer. Math. Soc., 1973, 176, p. 227-252.

Hurd R.A.

[1] A note on the solvability of simultaneous Wiener-Hopf equations. - Canad. J. Phys., 1979, 57, N 3, p. 402-403.

Idemen M.

[1] A new method to obtain exact solutions of vector Wiener-Hopf equations. - Z. angew. Math. Mech., 1979, 59, p. 656-658.

[2] On an integral transform with kernel and its applications to second order canonical problems of GTD. - SIAM J. Appl. Math., 1982, 42, N.3, p. 636-652.

Isakhanov R.S. (Исаханов Р.С.)

[1] Об одной задаче линейного сопряжения для кусочно-голоморфных векторов. - Сообщ. АН ГрузССР, 1969, 53, No. 3, с. 537-540.

Ishchenko E.V. (Ищенко Е.В.)

[1] Скалярная разрывная граничная задача линейного сопряжения в случае общей кусочно-гладкой кривой. - Сообщ. АН Груз. ССР, 1982, 108, No. 3, с. 489-492.

[2] О факторизации кусочно-непрерывных матриц-функций. - Сообщ. АН ГрузССР, 1982, 106, No. 2, с. 245-248.

[3] Векторная разрывная задача линейного сопряжения. - Сообщ. АН ГрузССР, 1983, 109, No. I, с. 37-40.

Iskenderov B.B. (Искендеров Б.Б.)

[1] Об одной нелинейной краевой задаче для кусочно-аналитических функций. - Науч. тр. Азерб. ун-та. Сер. физ.-мат. наук, 1979, 5, с. 30-38.

Its A.R. (Итс А.Р.)

[1] Асимптотика решений нелинейного уравнения Шредингера и изомонодромные деформации систем линейных дифференциальных уравнений. - ДАН СССР, 1981, 261, No. I, с. 14-18.

Ivanov V.V. (Иванов В.В.)

[1] Некоторые свойства особых интегралов типа Коши и их приложения. - ДАН СССР, 1958, 121, No. 5, с. 793-794.

Jonckheere E., Delsarte P.

[1] Inversion of Toeplitz operators, Levinson equations, and Gohberg-Krein factorization - A simple and unified approach for the rational case. - J. Math. Anal. and Appl., 1982, 87, N.1, p. 295-310.

Jonckheere E., Silverman L.

[1] Spectral theory of the linear-quadratic optimal control problem: analytic factorization of rational matrix-valued functions. - SIAM J. Control and optimization, 1981, 19, N 2, p. 262-281.

Kadushin V.P. (Кадушин В.П.)

[1] К прямым методам решения одного класса сингулярных интегральных уравнений. - Изв. вузов. Математика, I976, Но. II, с. I09-III.

Kapanadse G.A. (Капанадзе Г.А.)

[1] Обобщенная граничная задача Гильберта для нескольких неизвестных функций. - Сообщ. АН ГрузССР, I973, 72, Но. 3, с. 537-540.

[2] Об одной обобщенной граничной задаче Гильберта для нескольких неизвестных функций в случае круга единичного радиуса. - Сообщ. АН ГрузССР, I974, Но. I, с. 25-28.

Karapetyants N.K., Samko S.G. (Карапетянц Н.К., Самко С.Г.)

[1] Сингулярные интегральные операторы со сдвигом Карлемана в случае кусочно-непрерывных коэффициентов. I - Изв. вузов Математика, I975, Но. 2, с. 43-54.

Karlovich Ju.I., Spitkovskiĭ I.M. (Карлович Ю.И., Спитковский И.М.)

[1] О нетеровости некоторых сингулярных интегральных операторов с матричными коэффициентами класса SAP и связанных с ними систем уравнений свертки на конечном промежутке. - ДАН СССР, I983, 269, Но. 3,

Kato T.

[1] Perturbation theory for linear operators.-Berlin: Springer-Verlag, 1966.

Kats B.A. (Кац Б.А.)

[1] Краевая задача Римана с осциллирующим коэффициентом. - Труды семинара по краевым задачам. Казань, I977, вып. I4, с. II0-I20.

[2] О краевой задаче Римана с коэффициентом, допускающим разрывы колебательного типа. - ДАН СССР, I979, 244, Но. 3, с. 52I-525.

[3] Задача Римана на замкнутой жордановой кривой. - Изв. вузов. Математика, I983, Но. 4, с. 68-80.

Khavin V.P. (Хавин В.П.)

[1] Граничные свойства интегралов типа Коши и гармонически сопряженных функций в областях со спрямляемой границей. - Матем. сб., I965, 68, Но. 4, с. 499-5I7.

Khavinson S.Ya. (Хавинсон С.Я.)

[1] Экстремальные задачи для некоторых классов аналитических функций в конечно-связных областях. - Матем. сб., I955, 36, Но. 3, с. 445-478.

Khlgatyan R.G. (Хлгатян Р.Г.)

[1] Некоторые вопросы теории систем разностных уравнений Винера-Хопфа. - ВИНИТИ, Но. 227-80 Деп., I980.

Khrapkov A.A. (Храпков А.А.)

[1] Некоторые случаи упругого равновесия бесконечного клина с несимметричным надрезом в вершине под действием сосредоточенных сил. - Прикл. матем. и мех., I97I. 35, Но. 4, с. 677-689.

Khvedelidze B.V. (Хведелидзе Б.В.)

[1] Линейные разрывные граничные задачи функций, сингулярные интегральные уравнения и некоторые их приложения. - Тр. Тбилисс. мат. ин-та ГрузССР, 1956, 23, с. 3-158.

[2] Замечания к моей работе "Линейные разрывные граничные задачи теории функций, сингулярные интегральные уравнения и некоторые их приложения", - Сообщ. АН ГрузССР, 1958, 21 Но. 2, с. 129-130.

[3] Граничная задача Римана-Привалова с кусочно-непрерывным коэффициентом. - Тр. Груз. политех. ин-та, 1962, 81, Но. 1, с. 11-29.

[4] Метод интегралов типа Коши в разрывных граничных задачах теории голоморфных функций одной комплексной переменной. - В кн. Итоги науки и техники, Сер. "Современные проблемы математики". М., 1975, 7, с. 5-162.

[5] О задаче линейного сопряжения и характеристических сингулярных интегральных уравнениях. - В кн. Комплексный анализ и его приложения. М.: Наука, 1978, с. 577-585.

Khvedelidze B.V., Ishchenko E.V. (Хведелидзе Б.В., Ищенко Е.В.)

[1] О разрывной задаче линейного сопряжения с кусочно-непрерывным коэффициентом. - Сообщ. АН ГрузССР, 1980. 97, Но. 3, с. 529-532.

[2] Разрывная граничная задача линейного сопряжения с кусочно-непрерывным коэффициентом. - Тр. Тбилисс. мат. ин-та АН ГрузССР, 1982, 69, с. 108.

Khvoshchinskaya L.A. (Хвощинская Л.А.)

[1] Однородная краевая задача Римана для двух функций с кусочно-постоянной матрицей в случае двух или трех особых точек. - ВИНИТИ, Но. 5157-81 Деп., 1981, 48, с.

[2] Решение некоторых задач, сводящихся к краевой задаче Римана для двух пар функций с кусочно постоянной матрицей. - ВИНИТИ, Но. 6531-82, Деп., 1982.

Kirillov A.A., Gvishiani A.D. (Кириллов А.А., Гвишиани А.Д.)

[1] Теоремы и задачи функционального анализа. - М.: Наука, 1979.

Kokilashvili V.M. (Кокилашвили В.М.)

[1] О весовых неравенствах для сингулярных интегралов с ядром Коши на гладких контурах. - Сообщ. АН ГрузССР, 1978, 90, Но. 3, с. 537-540.

Kokilashvili V.M., Paatashvili V.A. (Кокилашвили В.М., Пааташвили В.А.)

[1] О краевой задаче линейного сопряжения с измеримыми коэффициентами. - ДАН СССР, 1975, 224, Но. 5, с. 1008-1011.

[2] Краевая задача линейного сопряжения с измеримыми коэффициентами. - Тр. Тбилисс. матем. ин-та АН ГрузССР, 1977, 55, с. 59-92.

[3] Задача линейного сопряжения с измеримыми коэффициентами для одного класса граничных кривых. - Сообщ. АН ГрузССР, 1978, 91, Но. 1, с. 25-27.

[4] О разрывной задаче линейного сопряжения и сингулярных интегральных уравнениях. - Дифференц. уравнения, I980, I6, Но. 9, с. I650-I659.

Kolmogorov A.N., Fomin S.V. (Колмогоров А.Н., Фомин С.В.)

[1] Элементы теории функций и функционального анализа. - М.: Наука, I972.

Komyak I. I. (Комяк И.И.)

[1] Об интегральном уравнении типа свертки с N ядрами. - ДАН СССР, I968, I79, Но. 2, с. 279-282.

[2] О решении в квадратурах интегрального уравнения Фредгольма с ядром, зависящим от разности аргументов. - Изв. АН БССР. Сер. физ-мат. н., I973, Но. 2, с. 37-42.

[3] Об одном случае разрешимости в квадратурах интегрального уравнения с ядром, зависящим от разности. - Вестник БГУ. Сер. I, I974, Но. I, с. 70-72.

[4] Формула обращения для уравнения Вольтерра с разностным ядром. ДАН БССР, I976, 20, Но. 2, с. I06-I09.

Koppelman W.

[1] Singular integral equations, boundary value problem and the Riemann-Roch theorem. - J. Math. Mech., 1961, 10, N2, p.247-277.

Krasnosel'skiĭ M.I., Zabreĭko P.P., Pustyl'nik E.I., Sobolevskiĭ P.E. (Красносельский М.И., Забрейко П.П., Пустыльник Е.И., Соболевский П.Е.)

[1] Интегральные операторы в пространствах суммируемых функций. - М.: Наука, I966. English version: Integral operators in spaces of summable functions. Leyden: Noordhoff Intern. Publish. 1976.

Kravchenko V.G., Nikolaĭchuk A.M. (Кравченко В.Г., Николайчук А.М.)

[1] Об эквивалентности одного типа краевой Римана для системы n пар функций полному сингулярному уравнению с ядром Коши. - Дифференц. уравнения, I973, 9, Но. 2, с. 343-376.

[2] О частных индексах задачи Римана для двух пар функций. - ДАН СССР, I974, 2I6, Но. I, с. 53-56.

Kreĭn M.G. (Крейн М.Г.)

[1] Интегральные уравнения на полупрямой с ядром, зависящим от разности аргументов. - Успехи матем. наук, I958, I3, вып. 5, с. 3-I20.

Kreĭn M.G., Krasnosel'skiĭ M.I., Mil'man D.P. (Крейн М.Г., Красносельский М.А., Мильман Д.П.)

[1] О дефектных числах линейных операторов в банаховом пространстве и о некоторых геометрических вопросах. - Сб. трудов ин-та матем. АН УССР, I948, II, с. 97-II2.

Kreĭn M.G., Melik-Adamyan F.E. (Крейн М.Г., Мелик-Адамян Ф.Э.)

[1] К теории S-матриц канонических дифференциальных уравнений с суммируемым потенциалом. - ДАН СССР, I968, 46, Но. 4, с. I50-I55.

[2] Некоторые приложения теоремы о факторизации унитарной матрицы. - Функцион. анализ и его прил., I970 4, с. 73-75.

Krein M.G., Spitkovskii I.M. (Крейн М.Г., Спитковский И.М.)

[1] О факторизации матриц-функций на единичной окружности. ДАН СССР, 1977, 234, Но. 2, с. 287-290.

[2] О факторизации α -секториальных матриц-функций на единичной окружности. - Матем. исслед., 1978, Но. 47, с. 41-63.

[3] О некоторых обобщениях первой предельной теоремы Сегё. - Anal. Math. 1983, 9, N. I, 23-41.

Krein S. G. (Крейн С.Г.)

[1] Линейные уравнения в Банаховом пространстве. - М.: Наука, 1971.

Krichever I.M. (Кричевер И.М.)

[1] Аналог формулы Даламбера для уравнений главного кирального поля и уравнения - ДАН СССР, 1980, 253, Но. 2, с. 288-292.

[2] Авнеомодельные решения уравнений типа Кортевега-де Фриза. - Функц. анализ и его прил., 1980, 14, Но 3, с. 83-84.

Kruglov V.E. (Круглов В.Е.)

[1] Решение задачи Римана на одной n-листной римановской поверхности. - Матем. исслед., 1974, 9, Но. 2, с. 230-236.

[2] Абелевы дифференциалы и уравнения поверхности, заданные циклической группой подстановок. - Сообщ. АН ГрузССР, 1978, 92, Но. 3, с. 537-540.

[3] Частные индексы, абелевы дифференциалы I рода и уравнение поверхности, заданные конечной абелевой группой подстановок.- Сибирск. матем. ж., 1981, 22, Но. 6, с. 87-101.

[4] Частные индексы и одно приложение факторизации некоторых матриц подстановочного типа не выше четвертого порядка, I. - ВИНИТИ, Но. 3278-82 Деп., 1982,

[5] Частные индексы и одно приложение факторизации некоторых матриц подстановочного типа не выше четвертого, II. - ВИНИТИ, Но 3279-82, Деп., 1982.

[6] Частные индексы и одно приложение факторизации некоторых матриц подстановочного типа не выше четвертого порядка, III.- ВИНИТИ, Но. 3280-82, Деп., 1982,

Krupnik N.Ya. (Крупник Н.Я.)

[1] О фактор-норме сингулярного оператора. - Матем. исслед., 1975, Но.2, 10, с. 255-263.

[2] Критерий нетеровости сингулярных интегральных операторов с измеримыми коэффициентами. - Сообщ. АН ГрузССР, 1975, 80, Но. 3, с. 533-536.

[3] Некоторые общие вопросы теории одномерных сингулярных интегральных уравнений с матричными коэффициентами. - Матем. иссл. 1976, Но. 42, с. 91-112.

[4] О сингулярных интегральных операторах с матричными коэффициентами. - Матем. иссл., 1977, Но. 45, с. 93-99.

[5] Некоторые следствия из теоремы Ханта, Макенхаупта и Видена. - Матем. иссл., 1978, Но. 47, с. 64-70.

[6] Банаховы алгебры с символом и сингулярные интегральные операторы. - Кишиниев: Штиинца, 1984.

Krupnik N.Ya., Nyaga V.I. (Крупник Н.Я., Няга В.И.)

[1] О сингулярных интегральных операторах в случае некладкого контура. - Матем. исслед., 1975, 10, Но. I, с. 144-164.

Krupnik N.Ya., Polonskii E.P. (Крупник Н.Я., Полонский Е.П.)

[1] О норме оператора сингулярного интегрирования. - Функцион. анализ и его прил., 1975, 9, Но. 4, с. 73-74.

Krupnik N.Ya., Rosenberg S.M. (Крупник Н.Я., Розенберг С.М.)

[1] Один контрпример в теории сингулярных интегральных операторов. В кн.: Исслед. по алгебре, мат. анализу и их прил. Мат. науки. Кишинев: Штиинца, 1977, с. 89-90.

Kuchment P.A. (Кучмент П.А.)

[1] О нетеровых операторах в паре Банаховых пространств. - Труды НИММ ВГУ, вып. 3, Воронеш, 1971, с. 61-77.

Kuliev V.D., Sadykhov A.E. (Кулиев В.Д., Садыхов А.Э.)

[1] Проблема Римана для двух пар функций и её применение в теории упругости. - Изв. АН АрмССР. Механика, 1979, 32, Но. 2, с. 26-37.

Kvitko A.N. (Квитко А.Н.)

[1] Векторно-матричная задача Римана для эллиптической системы дифференциальных уравнений первого порядка в случае сложного контура на римановой поверхности. - Мат. методы и физ.-мех. поля, 1980, Но. II, с. 12-15.

Lagvilava E.T. (Лагвилава Э.Т.)

[1] О факторизации матриц-функций. - Сообщ. АН ГрузССР, 1978, 89, Но. 2, с. 317-319.

Lappo-Danilevskii I.A. (Лаппо-Данилевский И.А.)

[1] Теория функции от матриц и системы линейных дифференциальных уравнений. - М.-Л.: ГИТЛ, 1934.

Lax P.D.

[1] On the factorization of matrix-valued functions. - Comm. pure and appl. math., 1976, 29, N.6, p. 683-688.

Lee M.

[1] On Toeplitz-operators. - J. Math. Soc. Jap., 1971, 23, N.2, p. 320-322.

Le-Din Zon (Ле-Динь Зон)

[1] Об одном случае решения в замкнутом виде задачи Гильберта для вектор-функции. - Математический анализ и его приложения. Ростов-на-Дону, 1974, 5, с. 189-193.

Lee M., Sarason D.

[1] The spectra of some Toeplitz operators. - J. Math. Anal. and Appl., 1971, 33, N.3, p. 529-543.

Leiterer J. (Лайтерер Ю.)

[1] О факторизации матриц- и оператор функций. - Сообщ. АН Груз ССР, 1977, 88, Но. 3, с. 541-544.

Lindenstrauss J., Tzafriri L.

[1] On the complemented subspace problem. - Israel J. Math., 1971, 9, p. 263-269.

Litvinchuk G.S. (Литвинчук Г.С.)

[1] Об устойчивости одной краевой задачи теории аналитических функций. - ДАН СССР, 1967, 174, No. 6, с. 1268-1270.

[2] Две теоремы об устойчивости частных индексов краевой задачи Римана и их приложения. - Изв. вузов Математика, 1967, No. 1, с. 47-54.

[3] Краевые задачи и сингулярные интегральные уравнения со сдвигом. - М.: Наука, 1977,

Litvinchuk G.S., Nikolaĭchuk A.M., Spitkovskiĭ I.M. (Литвинчук Г.С., Николайчук А.М., Спитковский И.М.)

[1] Некоторые теоремы об устойчивости и оценках частных индексов краевой задачи Римана и их приложения. - В кн.: Проблемы развития прикладных математических исследованиях: IУ Республиканская конференция математиков Белоруссии: Тезисы докладов. Минск, 1975, ч. 2, с. 105.

Litvinchuk G.S., Spitkovskiĭ I.M. (Литвинчук Г.С., Спитковский И.М.)

[1] Точные оценки дефектных чисел краевой задачи Римана - ДАН СССР, 1980, 255, No. 5, с. 1042-1046.

[2] Точные оценки дефектных чисел обобщенной краевой задачи Римана, факторизация эрмитовых матриц-функций и некоторые проблемы приближения мероморфными функциями. - Матем. сб., 1982, 117, No. 2, с. 196-215.

Lowengrub M., Walton J.

[1] Systems of generalized Abel equations. - SIAM J. Math. Anal., 1979, 10, N.4, p. 794-807.

Magnaradze L.G. (Магнарадзе Л.Г.)

[1] Об одной линейной граничной задаче теории функций комплексного переменного. - ДАН СССР, 1949, 88, No. 4, с. 657-660.

Maister A.V. (Майстер А.В.)

[1] О разрешимости систем интегральных уравнений с обобщенными степенными ядрами. - ВИНИТИ, No. 5781-82 Деп., 1982.

Mal'tsev A.A. (Мальцев А.А.)

[1] Основы линейной алгебры. - М.: Наука, 1970.

Malyshev V.A. (Малышев В.А.)

[1] Уравнения Винера-Хопфа и их применения в теории вероятностей. В кн.: Итоги наука и техники, Сер. "Теория вероятностей, математическая статистика, теоретическая кибернетика". М., 1976, 13, с. 5-35.

Mandzhavidze G.F. (Манджавидзе Г.Ф.)

[1] Об одном сингулярном интегральном уравнении с разрывными коэффициентами и его применении в теории упругости. - Прикл. матем. и мех., 1951, 15, вып. 3, с. 279-296.

[2] О приближенном решении граничных задач теории функций комплексного переменного. - Сообщ. АН ГрузССР, 1953, 14, Но. 10, с. 577-582.

[3] О приближенном решении граничных задач теории аналитических функций. - Тр. Третьего Всесоюзного матем. съезда, 1956, I, с. 88.

[4] Приближенное решение граничных задач теории аналитических функций. - В кн.: Исслед. по совр. пробл. теории функций комплексного переменного. М.: Физматгиз, 1960, с. 365-370.

[5] О поведении решений граничной задачи линейного поярження. - Тр. Тбилис. мат. ин-та ГрузССР, 1969, 35, с. 173-182.

[6] Граничная задача линейного сопряжения с кусонно-непрерывным матричным коэффициентом. - В кн.: Механика сплошной среды и родств. пробл. анализа, М.: Наука, 1972, с. 297-304.

[7] О применении теории обобщенных аналитических функций к граничной задаче сопряжения со смещением. - ДАН СССР, 237, 1977 Но. 6, с. 1285-1288.

[8] Об одном семействе граничных задач линейного сопряжения. - Сообщ. АН ГрузССР, 1979, 95, Но. 2, с. 289-292.

[9] Применение теории обобщенных аналитических функций к изучению граничных задач сопряжения со смещением. - Диффер. и интегральн. уравнения и краев. задачи - Тбилиси 1979, с. 165-186.

Mandzhavidze G.F., Khvedelidze B.V. (Манджавидзе Г.Ф., Хведелидзе Б. В.)

[1] О задаче Римана-Привалова с непрерывными коэффициентами. - ДАН СССР, 1958, 123, Но. 5, с. 791-794.

[2] О задаче линейного сопряжения сингулярных интегральных уравнениях с ядром Коши с непрерывными коэффициентами. - Тр. Тбилис. мат. ин-та ГрузССР, 1962, 28, с. 85-105.

Markus A.S., Matsaev V.I. (Маркус А.С., Мацаев В.И.)

[1] О спектральных свойствах голоморфных оператор-функций в гильбертовом пространстве. - Матем. исслед., 1974, 9, Но. 4, с. 79-91.

[2] Два замечания о факторизации матриц-функций. - Матем. исслед. 1976, Но. 42, с. 216-223.

Marcus M., Minc H.

[1] A survey of matrix theory and matrix inequalities. - Boston: Allyn and Bacon, Inc., 1964.

Markushevich A.I. (Маркушевич А.И.)

[1] Об одной граничной задаче теории аналитических функций. - Уч. зап. Моск. ун-та, 146, 100, с. 20-30.

Maskudov F.G., Veliev S.G. (Маскудов Ф. Г., Велиев С.Г.)

[1] Факторизация матрицы рассеяния для системы уравнений Дирака на всей оси.- Изв. АН АзССР. Серия физ.-техн. и мат. наук, 1975, Но. 2, с. 70-75.

van der Mee C.V.M.

[1] Spectral analysis of the transport equation. I. Nondegenerate and multigroup case. - Integr. Equat. and Oper. Theory, 1980, 3, p. 529-573.

[2] Semigroup and factorization methods in transport theory. - Amsterdam: Math. Centre Tract., 1981, p. 146-169.

Meister E.

[1] Das Riemannsche Randwertproblem. - Neuere Ergebnisse und Anwendungsgebiete, Sitzungsber. - Berlin Math. Ges., 1969 - 1971, s.l.s.a., p. 36-37.

Meunargiya O.V. (Меунаргия О.В.)

[1] Об одной системе граничных задач линейного сопряжения. - Сообщ. АН ГрузССР, 1976, 82, Но. I, с. 17-20.

[2] О построении эффективного решения задачи линейного сопряжения для нескольких неизвестных функций. - Теорет. и мат. физика, 1978, 37, Но. 3, с. 423-426.

[3] Многокомпонентная граничная задача линейного сопряжения. - Теорет. и мат. физика, 1981, 47, Но. 3, с. 419-424.

Miamee A.G., Salehi H.

[1] On the factorization of a nonnegative operator valued function. - Lect. Notes Math., 1978, 656, p. 129-137.

Mikhailov L.G. (Михайлов Л.Г.)

[1] Общая краевая задача о бесконечно малых изгибаниях склеенных поверхностей. - Изв. вузов. Математика, 1960, Но. 5, с.99-109.

[2] Об одной граничной задаче линейного сопряжения. - ДАН СССР, 1961, 139, Но. 2, с. 294-297.

[3] Общая задача сопряжения аналитических функций и её применения.- Изв. АН СССР, Сер. Матем. 1963, 27, Но. 5, с. 969-992.

[4] Новый класс особых интегральных уравнений и его применение к дифференциальным уравнениям с сингулярными коэффициентами. - Душанбе: Изд-во АН ТаджССР, 1963.

Mikhlin S.G. (Михлин С.Г.)

[1] Сингулярные интегральные уравнения с непрерывными коэффициентами. ДАН СССР, 1948, 59, Но. 3, с. 435-438.

Michlin S., Prößdorf S.

[1] Singuläre Integraloperatoren. - Berlin: Akademie Verlag, 1980

Mishchishin I.I. (Мищишин И.И.)

[1] Об одной задаче линейного сопряжения с кусочно постоянными коэффициентами. - Исслед. по соврем. пробл. суммир. и приближ. функций и их прил., 6. Днепропетровск, 1975, с. 188-194.

[2] Метод нахождения частных решений однородной задачи линейного сопряжения. - В кн.: Актуальн. пробл. ЭВМ и программир. Днепропетровск, 1981, с. 96-100.

Morozov V.V. (Морозов В.В.)

[1] О коммутативных матрицах.- Уч. зап. Казанск. ун-та, I952, II2, Но. 9, с. I7-20.

Mossakovskiĭ V.I., Mishchishin I.I. (Моссаковский В.И., Мищишин И.И.)

[1] Об одной задаче линейного сопряжения. - Гидроаэромеханика и теория упругости. 8, Харьков, I968.

Mückenhoupt S.

[1] Weighted norm inequalities for the Hardy maximal function. - Trans. Amer. Math. Soc., 1972, 165, p. 207-226.

Muskhelishvili N.I. (Мусхелишвили Н.И.)

[1] Сингулярные интегральные уравнения. - М.: Наука, I968. English transl. (of 1st ed.), Groningen:Noordhoff, 1953. German transl. Berlin: Akademie-Verlag, 1965.

Muskhelishvili N.I., Vekua N.P. (Мусхелишвили Н.И., Векуа Н.П.)

[1] Краевая задача Римана для нескольких неизвестных функций и её приложение к системам сингулярных интегральных уравнений.- Тр. Тбилис. мат. ин-та АН ГрузССР, I943, I2, с. I-46.

Sz.-Nagy B., Foiaş C.

[1] Analyse harmonique des opérateurs de l'espace de Hilbert. - Masson et Cie, Académia Kíadó, 1967.

Nakazi Takahiko

[1] A note on the factorization of operator valued functions.- Proc. Amer. Math. Soc., 1981, 81, N.4, p. 591-594.

Nehari Z.

[1] On bounded bilinear forms. - Ann. Math., 1957, 65, N.1, p. 153-162.

Nikolaĭchuk A.M. (Николайчук А.М.)

[1] Некоторые оценки для частных индексов краевой задачи Римана.- Украинск. матем. ж., I97I, 23, Но. 6, с. 793-798.

[2] Об устойчивости краевой задачи Маркушевича. - Украинск. матем. ж., I974, 26, Но. 4, с. 558-559.

Nikolaĭchuk A.M., Spitkovskiĭ I.M. (Николайчук А.М., Спитковский И.М.)

[1] О краевой задаче Римана с эрмитовой матрицей. - ДАН СССР, I975, 22I, Но. 6, с. I280-I283. English Transl. Sov. Math. Dokl. 1975, N 6, p. 533-536

[2] Факторизация эрмитовых матриц-функций и её приложения к граничным задачам. - Украинск. Матем. ж., I975, 27, Но. 6, с. 767-779.

Nikolenko P.V. (Николенко П.В.)

[1] Об устойчивости системы частных индексов семейства матриц-функций. - ВИНИТИ, Но. 5525-8I Деп., I98I, I7 с.

[2] Об отсутствии стандартной факторизации матриц-функций. - ВИНИТИ, Но. 3666-82, Деп., I982, 6 с.

Novikov S.P. (ed.)

[1] Теория солитонов: Метод обратной задачи/Под ред. С.П. Новикова. М.: Наука, 1980.

Novokshenov V.Yu. (Новокшенов В.Ю.)

[1] Уравнения в свертках на конечном отрезке и факторизация эллиптических матриц. - Матем. заметки, 1980, 27, Но. 6, с. 935-946.

[2] Асимптотика при $t \to \infty$ решения задачи Коши для нелинейного уравнения Шредингера. - ДАН СССР, 1980, 251, Но. 4, с. 799-802.

[3] Асимптотика решений при $t \to \infty$ двумерного обобщения цепочки Тоды: ДАН СССР, 1982, 265, Но. 6, с. 1320-1324.

Nyaga V.I. (Няга В.И.)

[1] О символе сингулярных интегральных операторов в случае кусочно-ляпуновского контура. - Матем. исслед., 1974, 9, Но. 2, с. 109-125.

[2] О сингулярных интегральных операторах в случае неограниченного контура. - В кн.: Исслед. по алгебре, матем. анализу и их прил. Кишинев: Штиинца, 1977, с. 91-95.

[3] О сингулярных интегральных уравнениях в пространствах с весом.- Изв. вузов Математика. - 1979, Но. 2, с. 73-75.

Paatashvili V.A. (Пааташвили В.А.)

[1] О сингулярных интегралах Коши. - Сообщ. АН ГрузССР, 1969, 53, Но.3, с. 529-532.

Paatashvili V.A., Khuskivadze G.A. (Пааташвили В.А., Хускивадзе Г.А.)

[1] Об ограниченности сингулярного оператора Коши в пространствах Лебега в случае негладких контуров. - Тр. Тбилис. мат. ин-та, АН ГрузССР, 1982, 69, с. 93-107.

Page B.L.

[1] Bounded and compact vectorial Hankel operators. - Trans. Amer. Math. Soc., 1970, 150, N 2, p. 529-539.

Palais R.

[1] Seminar on the Atiyah-Singer index theorem. - Princeton: Princeton Univ. Press, 1965.

Pal'tsev B.V. (Пальцев Б.В.)

[1] Об одном признаке непрерывности канонической матрицы решения задачи Гильберта. - ДАН СССР, 1976, 226, Но. 6, с. 1271-1274.

[2] О задаче Дирихле для одного дифференциального оператора, встречающегося в теории случайных процессов. - Изв. АН СССР. Сер. матем., 1977, 41, Но. 6, с. 1348-1387.

[3] Об одном классе уравнений свертки на конечном интервале. - ДАН СССР, 1979, 247, Но. 1, с. 41-44.

[4] Уравнения свертки на конечном интервале для одного класса символов, имеющих степенную асимптотику на бесконечности. - Изв. АН СССР, Сер. матем., 1980, 44, Но. 2, с. 322-394.

[5] Обобщение метода Винера-Хопфа для уравнений свертки на конечном интервале с символами, имеющими степенную асимптотику на бесконечности. - Матем. сб., 1980, 113, Но. 3, с. 355-399.

[6] Об одном методе построения канонической матрицы решений задачи Гильберта, возникающей при решении уравнений свертки на конечном интервале. - Изв. АН СССР. Сер. матем., 1981, 45, No. 6, с. 1382-1390.

Panchenko I.F. (Панченко И.Ф.)

[1] Задача Римана для n пар функций на римановой поверхности в случае сложного контура в пространстве $L_p^n(\Gamma)$. - Исслед. по функц. анализу и дифференц. уравнениям, Кишинев, 1978, с.68-75.

Peller V.V.

[1] Vectorial Hankel operators, commutators and related operators of the Schatten- von Neumann class.-Integr. Equat. and Oper. Theory, 1982, 5, N.2, p. 244-272.

Petrov N.N. (Петров Н.Н.)

[1] О разрешимости линейных уравнений в произведении банаховых пространств. - В кн.: Топологические пространства и их отображения. Рига, 1979, с. 102-106.

Pichorides S.K.

[1] On the best values of the constants in the theorems of M. Riesz, Zygmund and Kolmogorov. - Studia Math., 1972, 19, N.2, p. 165-179.

Pilidi Z.S. (Пилиди З.С.)

[1] Априорные оценки для некоторого класса одномерных сингулярных интегральных операторов с разрывными коэффициентами. - Матем. заметки, 1979, 26, No. 2, с. 227-234.

Plemelj J.

[1] Riemannsche Funktionenscharen mit gegebener Monodromiegruppe. - Monatsh. für Math. und Phys., 1908, 19, p. 211-245.

Popov Yu.A. (Попов Ю.А.)

[1] Задача дифракции плоской электромагнитной волны на трех полубесконечных плоскостях. - В кн.: Материалы 5-й конф. молод. ученных, 1980,: МФТИ, ВИНИТИ, No. 2849 - 80 Деп., 1980, с.88-91.

Pousson H.R.

[1] Systems of Toeplitz operators on H^2. - Proc. Amer. Math. Soc., 1968, 19, N.3, p. 603-608.

[2] Systems of Toeplitz operators on H^2. II.-Trans. Amer. Math. Soc., 1968, 133, N.2, p. 527-536.

Power S.C.

[1] Fredholm Toeplitz operators and slow oscillation. - Can. J. Math., 1980, 32, N 5, p. 1058-1071.

Primachuk L.P. (Примачук Л.П.)

[1] О краевой задаче с сопряжением. - Изв. АН БССР, сер. физ.-мат. наук, 1967, No. 4, с. 59-62.

[2] О частных индексах задачи Римана с треугольной матрицей. - ДАН БССР, 1970, 14, No. 1, с. 5-7.

[3] Задача Римана для внешности разрезов вдоль прямой с подстановочными матрицами. - ДАН БССР, 1978, 22, No. 2, с. 115-118.

[4] Об одном интегрируемом случае задачи Римана с подстановочной матрицей. - ДАН БССР, 1978, 22, Но. 4, с. 310-313.

Privalov I.I. (Привалов И.И.)

[1] Об одной граничной задаче в теории аналитических функций. - Матем. сб., 1934, 41, Но. 4, с. 519-526.

[2] Граничные свойства аналитических функций. - М.-Л.: ГИТЛ, 1950.

Prößdorf S.

[1] Einige Klassen singulärer Gleichungen. - Berlin: Akademie-Verlag, 1974.

Prößdorf S., Schmidt G.

[1] Necessary and sufficient conditions for the collocation method for singular integral equations.- Math.Nachr. 1979, 89, p.203-215.

Prößdorf S., Silbermann B.

[1] Projektionsverfahren und die näherungsweise Lösung singulärer Gleichungen.-Leipzig: Teubner-Text, 1977.

Rabindranathan M.

[1] On the inversion of Toeplitz operators. - J. Math. and Mech., 1969, 19, N 3, p. 195-206.

Radon I. (Радон И.)

[1] О краевых задачах для логарифмического потенциала. - Успехи матем. наук, 1946, 1, вып. 3-4, с. 96-124.

Rajamaki M.

[1] The fundamental matrix of the Hilbert problem in transport theory.- Transp. Theory and Statist. Phys., 1973, 3, N.4, p. 175-197.

Rawlins A.D., Williams W.E.

[1] Matrix Wiener-Hopf factorization. - Quart. J. Mech. and Appl. Math., 1981, 34, N.1, p. 1-8.

Reyman A.G., Semenov-Tian-Shansky M.A.

[1] Reduction of Hamiltonian systems, Affine Lie algebras and Lax equations. - Inventiones Math., 1979, 54, p. 81-100.

[2] Reduction of Hamiltonian systems, Affine Lie algebras and Lax equations. II.- Inventiones Math., 1981, 63, p. 423-432.

Rochberg R.

[1] Toeplitz operators on weighted H^p spaces. - Indiana Univ. Math. J., 1977, 26, N.2, p. 291-298.

Rodin Yu. L. (Родин Ю.Л.)

[1] Структура общего решения краевой задачи Римана для голоморфного вектора на компактной римановой поверхности. - ДАН СССР, 1977, 232, Но. 5, с. 1019-1022.

[2] Структура общего решения краевой задачи Римана для голоморфного вектор-функции на компактной римановой поверхности. - В кн.: Вопр. матрич. теории отображения и её применение: Материалы 5-го Коллоквиума, Донецк, 1976, г. Киев: Наук. Думка, 1978, с. 103-120.

Rodin Yu.L., Turakulov A. (Родин Ю.Л., Туракулов А.)

[1] Краевая задача Римана для обобщенных аналитических функций с сингулярными коэффициентами на компактной римановой поверхности.- Сообщ. АН ГрузССР, 1979, 96, No. I, с. 21-24.

Röhrl H.

[1] On holomorphic families of fiber bundles over the Riemannian sphere. - Mem. Coll. Sci. Univ. Kyoto, 1961,33,N.3, p. 435-477.

[2] Über das Riemann-Privalovsche Randwertproblem. - Math. Ann., 1963, 151, p. 365-423.

Rozanov Yu.A. (Розанов Ю.А.)

[1] Стационарные случайные процессы. - М.: Наука, 1963.

Sabitov I.Kh. (Сабитов И.Х.)

[1] Об общей краевой задаче линейного сопряжения на окружности. - Сибирск. матем. ж., 1964, 5, No. I, с. 124-129.

[2] Об одной граничной задачей линейного сопряжения.- Матем. сб., 1964, No. 2, с. 262-274.

Saginashvili A.I. (Сагинашвили А.И.)

[1] Сингулярные интегральные операторы с коэффициентами, имеющими разрывы полу-почти-периодического типа. - Сообщ. АН ГрузССР, 1979, 94, No. 2, с. 289-291.

[2] Сингулярные интегральные операторы с полу-почти-периодическими разрывами у коэффициентов. - Сообщ. АН ГрузССР, 1979, 95, No.3, 541-543.

[3] Сингулярные интегральные уравнения с коэффициентами, имеющими разрывы полу-почти-периодического типа. - Тр. Тбилисс. мат. ин-та АН ГрузССР, 1980, 66, с. 84-95.

Sarason D.E.

[1] Generalized interpolation on H^{∞}. - Trans. Amer. Math. Soc., 1967, 127, p. 179-203.

[2] Algebras of functions on the unit circle. - Bull. Amer. Math. Soc., 1972, 79, N.2, p. 286-299.

[3] Toeplitz operators with semi-almost-periodic symbols. - Duke Math. J., 1977, 44, N.2, p. 357-364.

[4] Toeplitz operators with piecewise quasicontinuous symbols. - Indiana Univ.Math. J., 1977, 26, N.5, p. 817-838.

Seifullaev R.K. (Сейфуллаев Р.К.)

[1] Краевая задача Римана на негладкой разомкнутой кривой. - Матем. сб., 1980,112, No. 2, с. 147-161.

Seleznev V.A. (Селезнев В.А.)

[1] Системы сингулярных уравнений на ГQ -контурах. - Динамика сплошной среды, 1974, вып. 18, с. 243-248.

[2] Линейные сингулярные уравнения на квазиконформых контурах и задача линейного сопряжения для голоморфного вектора на замкнутых римановых поверхностях. - В кн.: Вопр. матрич. теории отображения и её применение. Материалы 5-го Коллоквиума, Донецк, 1976, г. Киев: Наук. думка, 1978, с. 125-135.

[3] Краевая задача Римана в классах жордановых границ. - В кн.: Метрич. вопросы теории функций. Киев: Наук. думка, 1980, с. 125-132

Sementsul A.A. (Семенцул А.А.)

[1] О сингулярных интегральных уравнениях с коэффициентами, имеющими разрывы почти-периодического типа. - Матем. исслед. 1971, 6, Но. 3, с. 92-114.

Sergeev A.G. (Сергеев А.Г.)

[1] Факторизация оператор-функций, непрерывных по Гельдеру. - УМН, 1972, 27, Но. 6, с. 253.

[2] Локальный L_p-принцип в задаче факторизации. - УМН, 1974, 29, Но. 6, с. 175-176.

Shamir E. (Шамир Е.)

[1] Решение систем Римана-Гильберта с кусочно-непрерывными коэффициентами в L_p.- ДАН СССР, 1966, 167, Но. 5, с. 1000-1003.

Shelepov V.Yu. (Шелепов В.Ю.)

[1] О задаче Римана в областях, граница которых имеет ограниченное вращение. - ДАН СССР, 1968, 181, Но. 3, с. 565-568.

Sherman D.I. (Шерман Д.И.)

[1] О приемах решения некоторых сингулярных интегральных уравнений. - ПММ, 1948, 12, Но. 4, с. 423-452.

Shestopalov V.P. (Шестопалов В.П.)

[1] Метод задачи Римана-Гильберта в теории дифракций. - Харьков: ХГУ, 1971.

Shmul'yan Yu.L. (Шмульян Ю.Л.)

[1] Задачи Римана с положительно определенной матрицей. - Успехи матем. наук, 1953, 8, вып. 2, с. 143-145.

[2] Задача Римана с эрмитовой матрицей. - Успехи матем. наук, 1954, 9, вып. 4, стр. 243-248.

Shneiberg I.Ya. (Шнейберг И.Я.)

[1] О разрешимости линейных уравнений в интерполяционных семействах банаховых пространств. - ДАН СССР, 1973, 212, Но. 1, с. 57-59.

[2] Спектральные свойства линейных операторов в интерполяционных семействах банаховых пространств. - Матем. исслед., 1974, 9, Но. 2, 214-229.

Shubin M.A. (Шубин М.А.)

[1] Факторизация зависящих от параметра матриц-функций в нормированных кольцах и связанные с ней вопросы теории нетеровых операторов. - Матем. сб., 1967, 73, Но. 4, с. 610-629.

[2] О локальном принципе в задаче факторизации. - Матем. исслед., 1971, 6, Но. 1, с. 174-180.

[3] Псевдодифференциальные операторы и спектральная теория. - М., Наука, 1978.

Siewert C.E., Kelley S.T.

[1] An analytical solution to a matrix Riemann-Hilbert problem. - Z. angew. Math. und Phys., 1980, 31, N 3, p. 344-351.

Siewert C.E., Kelley C.T., Garcia R.D.M.

[1] An analytical expression for the H matrix relevant to Rayleigh scattering. - J. Math. Anal. and Appl., 1981, 84, N 2, p. 509-518.

Silbermann B.

[1] Lokale Theorie des Reduktionsverfahrens für Toeplitzoperatoren. Math. Nachr., 1981, 104, p. 137-146.

Simonenko I.B. (Симоненко И.Б.)

[1] Краевая задача Римана с непрерывным коэффициентом. - ДАН СССР, 1959, 124, Но. 2, с. 278-281.

[2] Краевая задача Римана для n пар функций с непрерывными коэффициентами. - Изв. вузов. Математика, 1961, Но. 1, с. 140-145.

[3] Краевая задача Римана для n пар функций с измеримыми коэффициентами и её применение к исследованию сингулярных интегралов в пространствах L_p с весами. - ДАН СССР, 1961, 141, Но. 1, с. 36-39.

[4] Краевая задача Римана для n пар функций с измеримыми коэффициентами и её применение к исследованию сингулярных интегралов в пространствах L_p с весами. - Изв. АН СССР, сер. мат. 1964, 28, Но. 2, с. 277-306.

[5] Новый общий метод исследования линейных операторных интегральных уравнений. - I.- Изв. АН СССР, сер. мат., 1965, 29, Но. 3, с. 567-586.

[6] Некоторые общие вопросы теории краевой задачи Римана. - Изв. АН СССР, сер. мат., 1968, 32, Но. 5, с. 1138-1146.

[7] Эквивалентность локальной факторизуемости измеримой функции и локальный нетеровости порожденного ею сингулярного оператора. - ВИНИТИ, Но.2194-80, Деп., 1980, 21 с.

[8] Эквивалентность факторизуемости и локальной факторизуемости измеримых функций, определенных на контурах типа. - ВИНИТИ, Но. 2193-80, Деп., 1980, 51 с.

[9] О факторизуемости и локальной факторизуемости измеримых функций. - ДАН СССР, 1980, 250, Но. 5, с. 1063-1066.

[10] О связи локальной факторизуемости и локальной нетеревости. Сообщ. АН ГрузССР, 1980, 98, Но. 2, с. 281-283.

[11] О глобальной и локальной факторизуемости измеримой матрицы-функции и нетеровости порожденного ею сингулярного оператора. - Изв. вузов. Математика, 1983, Но. 4, с. 81-87.

Soldatov A.P. (Солдатов А.П.)

[1] К теории сингулярных интегральных операторов классического типа. - Дифференц. уравнения, 1979, 15, Но. 3, с. 529-544.

[2] Краевая задача линейного сопряжения теории функций. - Изв. АН СССР, сер. мат., 1979, 43, Но. 1, с. 184-202.

Speck, F.-O.

[1] General Wiener-Hopf factorization methods. - Boston - London - Melbourne: Pitman; Research Notes in Mathematics, vol. 19, 1985.

Spitkovskiĭ, I.M. (Спитковский И.М.)

[1] Устойчивость частных индексов краевой задачи Римана со строго невырожденной матрицей. - ДАН СССР, 1974, 218, Но. 1, с. 46-49.

[2] Задача факторизации измеримых матриц-функций. - ДАН СССР, 1976, 227, Но. 3, с. 576-579.

[3] О частных индексах непрерывных матриц-функций. - ДАН СССР, 1976, 229, Но. 5, с. 1059-1062.

[4] О множителях, не влияющих на факторизуемость. - ДАН СССР, 1976, 231, Но. 6, с. 1300-1303.

[5] О факторизации матриц-функций, хаусдорфово множество которых расположено внутри угла. - Сообщ. АН ГрузССР, 1977, 86, Но.3 с. 561-564.

[6] К вопросу о факторизуемости измеримых матриц-функций. - ДАН СССР, 1978, 240, Но. 3, с. 541-544.

[7] Факторизация измеримых матриц-функций и её приложения к краевым задачам для аналитических функций. - Канд. дисс., Одесса, 1978.

[8] К теории обобщенной краевой задачи Римана в классах L_p. - Украинск. матем. ж., 1979, 31, Но. 1, с. 63-73.

[9] О множителях, не влияющих на факторизуемость. - Матем. заметки, 1980, 27, Но. 2, с. 291-299.

[10] Некоторые оценки для частных индексов измеримых матриц-функций. - Матем. сб., 1980, 111, Но. 2, с. 227-248.

[11] О блочных операторах и связанных с ними вопросах теории факторизации матриц-функций. - ДАН СССР, 1980, 254, Но. 4, с. 816-820.

[12] Критерий нетеровости блочно-треугольных операторов и связанные с ними вопросы теории факторизации матриц-функций. - ВИНИТИ, Но. 2543-81, Деп., 1981.

[13] Факторизация измеримых матриц-функций, связанные с ней теории систем сингулярных интегральных уравнений и векторной краевой задачи Римана, I.- Дифференц. уравнения, 1981, 17, Но. 4, с. 697-709.

[14] Факторизация измеримых матриц-функций, связанные с ней вопросы вопросы теории систем сингулярных интегральных уравнений и векторной краевой задачи Римана, II. - Дифференц. уравнения, 1982, 18, Но. 3.

[15] Факторизация некоторых классов полу-почти-периодических матриц-функций и её приложения к системам уравнений типа свертки. - Изв. вузов. Математика, 1983, Но. 4, с. 88-94.

[16] О факторизации матриц-функций из классов $\tilde{A}_n(p)$ и TL. - Украинск. матем. ж., 1983, 33, Но. 4.

Storozh O. G. (Сторож О.Г.)

[1] К вопросу об обратимости треугольных операторных матриц второго порядка. - Мат. методы и физ.-мех. поля. Киев, 1980, с. 85-87.

Stray A., Фума К.О.

[1] On interpolating functions with minimal norm. - Proc. Amer. Math. Soc., 1978, 68, N.1, p. 75-78

Suciu I.

[1] Factorization theorems for operator valued functions on multiply connected domains. - Rev. Roum. Math. pures et appl., 1979, 24, N 8, p. 1251-1269.

Tolokonnikov L.A., Pen'kov V.B. (Толоконников Л.А., Пеньков В.Б.)

[1] Приложение краевой задачи Римана с разрывным матричным коэффициентом к механике. - Изв. вузов Математика, 1980, Но. 12, с. 55-59.

Troitskiĭ V.E. (Троицкий В.Е.)

[1] Об одном способе нахождения матрицы Иоста. - Теорет. и мат. физика, 1978, 37, Но. 2, с. 243-245.

Tsitskishvili A.R. (Цицкишвили А.Р.)

[1] Эффективное решение задач сопряжения для нескольких неизвестных функций в случае кусочно-постоянной матрицы. - Тр. Тбилис. мат. ин-та АН ГрузССР, 1969, 35, с. 67-103.

[2] Об эффективном решении задачи сопряжения. - Сообщ. АН ГрузССР, 1970, 58, с. 17-20.

[3] О фильтрации в земляных плотинах. - Тр. Тбилисск. ун-та, Математика, механика, астрономия, 1980, 210, с. 12-40.

[4] О фильтрации через треугольное ядро земляной плотины. - Тр. Тбилисск. ун-та. Математика, механика, астрономия, 1980, 210, с. 42-51.

Tumarkin G.Ts., Khavinson S.Ya. (Тумаркин Г.Ц., Хавинсон С.Я.)

[1] К определению аналитических функций класса E_p в многосвязных областях. - Успехи матем. наук, 1958, 13, вып. 1, с. 201-206

[2] О теореме разложения для аналитических функций класса E_p в многосвязных областях. - Успехи матем. наук, 1958, 13, вып. 2, с. 223-228.

[3] Классы аналитических функций в многосвязных областях. - В кн.: Исслед. по совр. пробл. теории функций комплексного переменного. М.: Физматгиз, 1960, с. 45-77.

Vasil'ev I.L. (Васильев И.Л.)

[1] О единственности решения системы уравнений Абеля с постоянными коэффициентами. - ДАН БССР, 1981, 25, Но. 2, с.105-107.

[2] Системы интегральных уравнений с ядром Абеля на отрезке вещественной оси. - Изв. АН БССР. Сер. физ.-мат. наук, 1982, Но. 2, с. 47-53.

Vekua I.N. (Векуа И.Н.)

[1] Обобщенные аналитические функции. - М.: Физматгиз, 1959.

Vekua N. P. (Векуа Н. П.)

[1] Краевая задача Гильберта с рациональными коэффициентами для нескольких неизвестных функций. - Сообщ. АН ГрузССР, 1946, 7, Но. 9-10, с. 595-600.

[2] Об одной задаче теории функций комплексного переменного. - ДАН СССР, 1952, 86, Но. 3, с. 457-460.

[3] Об одной задаче Гильберта для нескольких неизвестных функций. Тр. Тбилис. мат. ин-та АН ГрузССР, 1968, 34, с. 5-12.

[4] Системы сингулярных интегральных уравнений. - М.: Наука, 1970.

Vekua N.P., Kveselava D.A. (Векуа Н. П., Квеселава Д. А.)

[1] Об одной краевой задаче теории функций комплексного переменного. - Сообщ. АН ГрузССР, 1941, II, Но. 3, 223-240.

[2] Об одной краевой задаче теории функций комплексного переменного и её применении к решению системы сингулярных интегральных уравнений. - Тр. Тбилис. мат. ин-та АН ГрузССР, 1941, 9, с. 38-48.

Verbitskiĭ I.E. (Вербицкий И. Э.)

[1] О мультипликаторах в пространствах l_p с весом. - Матем. исслед., 1977, 45, с. 3-16.

Verbitskiĭ I.E., Krupnik N.Ya. (Вербицкий И.Э., Крупник Н.Я.)

[1] Точные константы в теоремах Бабенко К.И., Хведелидзе Б.В. об ограниченности сингулярного оператора. - Сообщ. АН ГрузССР, 1977, 85, Но. 1, с. 21-24.

[2] Точные константы в теоремах об ограниченности сингулярных операторов в пространствах L_p с весом и их приложения. - Матем. исслед., 1980, 54, с. 21-35.

Virozub A.I., Matsaev V.I. (Вирозуб А.И., Мацаев В.И.)

[1] Одна теорема о канонической факторизации оператор-функций. - Матем. исслед., 1973, 8, Но. 3, с. 145-150.

Vladimirov V.S., Volovich I.V. (Владимиров В.С., Волович И.В.)

[1] Уравнение Винера-Хопфа, задача Римана-Гильберта и ортогональные многочлены. - ДАН СССР, 1982, 266, Но. 4, с. 788-791.

[2] Об одной модели статистической физики. - Теорет. и мат. физика., 1983, 54, Но. 1, с. 8-22.

Vorob'ev V.L. (Воробьев В.Л.)

[1] Изгиб полубесконечной пластинки, лежащей на линейно-деформируемом основании с учетом сил сцепления: Дис. Канд. физ-мат. наук. - Одесса, 1973.

Vorovich I.I., Aleksandrov V.M., Babeshko V.A.
(Ворович И.И., Александров В.М., Бабешко В.А.)

[1] Неклассические смешанные задачи теории упругости. - М.: Наука, 1974.

Walsh J.L. (Уалш Дж.Л.)

[1] Интерполяция и аппроксимация рациональными функциями в комплексной области.-М.: Изд-во иностр. лит., I96I.

Walton J.R.

[1] Systems of generalized Abel integral equations with applications to simultaneous dual relations. - SIAM J. Math. Anal., 1979, 10, N.4, p. 808-822.

Widom H.

[1] Inversion of Toeplitz matrices. II. - Illinois J. Math., 1960, 4, p. 88-99.

[2] On the spectrum of Toeplitz matrices. - Pacif. J. Math., 1964, 14, p. 365-375.

[3] Perturbing Fredholm operators to obtain invertible operators.- J. Funct. Anal., 1975, 20, N.1, p. 26-31.

[4] Asymptotic behavior of block Toeplitz matrices and determinants. II. - Advanc. Math., 1976, 21, N.1, p. 1-29.

Wiener N., Masani P.

[1] The prediction theory of multivariate stochastic processes. II. - Acta Math., 1958, 99, p. 93-137.

Yandarov O.V. (Яндаров О.В.)

[1] Об одном классе В - пространств и его применении к теории сингулярных интегральных операторов. - Дифференц. уравнения, I982, I8, Но. 2, с. 356-359.

Yatsko A.I. (Яцко А.И.)

[1] Критерий нетеровости обобщенной краевой задачи Римана для сложного контура. - Изв. вузов. Математика, I98I, Но. II, 86-87.

[2] Обобщенная краевая задача Римана в пространствах L_p с весом.- Украинск. матем. ж., I98I, 33, с. 283-286.

Yatsko A.I., Yatsko S.I. (Яцко А.И., Яцко С.И.)

[1] К теории обобщенной краевой задачи Римана с кусочно-непрерывными коэффициентами. - В кн.: Теоретические и прикладные вопросы дифференциальных уравнений и алгебры. Киев: Наук. думка, I978, с. 250-253.

[2] Обобщенная краевая задача Римана с кусочно-непрерывными коэффициентами. - Украинск. матем. ж., I978, 30, Но. 5, с. 646-653.

Zakharov V.E., Shabat A.B. (Захаров В.Е., Шабат А.Б.)

[1] Интегрирование нелинейных уравнений математической физики методом обратной задачи рассеяния. II-Функц. анализ и его прил. I979, I3, вып. 3, с. I3-22.

Zalcman L.

[1] Bounded analytic functions on domains of infinite connectivity. Trans. Amer. Math. Soc., 1969, 144, p. 241-269.

Zapuskalova T.A., Kats B.A. (Запускалова Т.А., Кац Б.А.)

[1] Краевая задача Римана на спиралеобразном контуре. - В кн.: Тр. семинара по краев. задачам. Казань: Казанск. ун-т, I978, с. 53-6I.

Zolotarevskiĭ V.A. (Золотаревский В.А.)

[1] Сходимость коллокационного метода и метода механических квадратур для систем сингулярных уравнений. - Изв. вузов Математика, 1976, Но. 6, с. 105-108.

Zolotarevskiĭ V.A., Chebotaru I.S. (Золотаревский В.А., Чеботару И.С.)

[1] О приближенном решении систем уравнений Винера-Хопфа с ненулевыми частными индексами. - Изв. вузов. Математика, 1978, Но. 7, с. 102-105.

Zverovich È.I. (Зверович Э.И.)

[1] Краевые задачи теории аналитических функций в гельдеровских классах на римановых поверхностях. - Успехи матем. наук, 1971, 26, вып. 1, с. 113-179.

Zverovich L.F. (Зверович Л.Ф.)

[1] Задача Римана для нескольких неизвестных функций в случае сложного контура. - В кн.: Теория функций комплексного переменного и краевые задачи. - Чебоксары.: Чувашский ун-т 1974, вып. 2, с. 21-38.

[2] Задача Римана для n пар функций на римановой поверхности в случае сложного контура. - Сибирск. матем. ж., 1975, 16, Но. 3, - с. 510-519.

Zverovich È.I., Panchenko V.F. (Зверович Э.И., Панченко В.Ф.)

[1] О краевой задаче Римана для n пар функций на римановой поверхности в пространстве $L_n(\rho(t))$. - Вестн. Белорус. ун-та. сер. 1. Математика, физика, механика, 1978, Но. 3, с.71-72.

Zverovich È.J., Pomerantseva L.I. (Зверович Э.И., Померанцева Л.И.)

[1] Задача Римана для n пар функций с матрицами подстановочного типа. - ДАН СССР, 1974, 217, Но. 1, с. 20-23.

SUBJECT INDEX

NOTATION INDEX